# PHYSICIANS' GUIDE TO RARE DISEASES

SECOND EDITION

# Physicians' Guide to Rare Diseases

## Second Edition

*Jess G. Thoene, M.D., Editor*

*Nancy P. Coker, Managing Editor*

### EDITORIAL BOARD

*William F. Balistreri, M.D.*
*Laurence A. Boxer, M.D.*
*Russell W. Chesney, M.D.*
*Angelo M. DiGeorge, M.D.*
*Nancy Burton Esterly, M.D.*
*Robert Fekety, M.D.*
*David N. Finegold, M.D.*
*Raymond H. Flores, M.D.*
*Thomas P. Foley, Jr., M.D.*
*Robert H. Gray, Ph.D.*
*Marc C. Hochberg, M.D., M.P.H.*
*Richard Alan Lewis, M.D., M.S.*
*Steven C. Martin, M.D.*
*Amnon Rosenthal, M.D.*
*Melvin H. Van Woert, M.D.*

DOWDEN PUBLISHING COMPANY INC.
MONTVALE, N.J.

Prepared in association with
the National Organization for Rare Disorders

Dowden Publishing Company
110 Summit Avenue
Montvale, NJ 07645
Telephone (201) 391-9100    Fax (201) 391-2778


Library of Congress Catalog Card Number 95-68451
ISBN 0-9628716-1-3

# CONTENTS

**EDITOR**

# JESS G. THOENE, M.D.
Professor of Pediatrics
Associate Professor of Biological Chemistry
Chief, Pediatric Biochemical Genetics and Metabolism
The University of Michigan Medical Center
Ann Arbor, Michigan

Chairman of the Board of Directors
National Organization for Rare Disorders

Chair
National Commission on Orphan Diseases


**MANAGING EDITOR**
NANCY P. COKER

**EDITORIAL DIRECTOR**
LEWIS A. MILLER

# ACKNOWLEDGMENTS

The National Organization for Rare Disorders (NORD) is grateful to the corporations, trade groups, foundations, and other philanthropic benefactors without whom NORD's Rare Disease Database and this book would not have been possible. NORD is particularly indebted to the Catt Family Foundation and the Robert Leet & Clara Guthrie Patterson Trust.

The editors express their gratitude to Katherine S. Balch and Doris C. Smith, professional medical editors and writers, for their unflagging effort and indispensable collaboration in this project, and to Nafi Coker, president of Troy Technologies, for his expert computer advice and support. Gratitude is also extended to Abbey S. Meyers, president of NORD, and her staff, especially Joy E. Yacolucci, director of information services, and Debra L. Madden, senior writer, for their diligent work and extensive updating of material for this second edition. Many people at Dowden Publishing Company have provided invaluable support, most notably Carroll V. Dowden, president; Robert J. Osborn, Jr., vice president and group publisher; and Jean Di Pietro, manager of special projects. Thanks are also due to Katherine S. Balch, who updated and assembled the Master Resources List; to Barbara F. Wood of Intermedica, Inc., who researched and compiled the Directory of Orphan Drugs; and to Philip Denlinger, who designed this book. Lastly, the members of the Editorial Board are thanked for their close and active role in the revision and expansion of this book.

—*Nancy P. Coker*
*Managing Editor*

# EDITOR'S PREFACE TO THE SECOND EDITION

The first edition of this volume received good critical reviews and in many ways accomplished the goal of the Editorial Board and the National Organization for Rare Disorders: to assist physicians in primary care by enabling them to focus quickly on the correct diagnosis in persons presenting with symptoms of rare disorders. Further, it was hoped that the book would provide a valuable index of support groups and of centers for specialized testing and referral. Numerous letters have confirmed the usefulness of the book in these areas. The second edition represents an expansion of the first work, with approximately 250 additional rare disease entries. We also have lengthened the introductory material of each chapter and have introduced a chapter on alternative medicine by Dr. Steven C. Martin of Albert Einstein College of Medicine. Persons with rare diseases are always at risk for unproved and fruitless remedies as a result of the frequent failure of orthodox medicine to offer meaningful therapeutic intervention. This does not, however, mean that such persons should be the prey of unscrupulous practitioners, whatever their medical frame of reference, seeking to profit from the misfortune of these patients. In a very thoughtful manner, Dr. Martin undertakes to explore these ramifications and to provide help to physicians in primary care in answering the legitimate questions about alternative therapy that persons with rare disorders frequently ask of their practitioners.

We note with deep regret the passing of Dr. Martin Carter. A professor and senior physician at Rockefeller University, Dr. Carter was a highly respected colleague. His wit and clinical expertise, as well as solid understanding of the problems of persons with rare disorders, will be sorely missed.

We are pleased to welcome newcomers to the Editorial Board. In addition to Dr. Steven Martin, they include Dr. Thomas P. Foley, Jr., and Dr. David N. Finegold, who coedited the chapter on Endocrine Disorders in this edition. Also new to the Editorial Board are Dr. Nancy Burton Esterly, who replaced Dr. Carter as editor of the chapter on Dermatologic Disorders, and Dr. Raymond H. Flores, who, together with Dr. Marc C. Hochberg, coedited the chapter on Arthritis and Connective Tissue Diseases. We are also pleased to welcome Nancy P. Coker as managing editor.

We live in rapidly changing times. In the next five years, the face of medicine will in many ways not be a happy one from either the physician's or patient's perspective. The impact of managed health care on current referral practices threatens to disrupt established patterns that have been very painstakingly developed to enable persons with rare disorders to reach the one or two best specialists in the nation for medical treatment. Persons enrolled in HMOs may not receive optimal care in a timely manner. NORD's mission, and the purpose of this book, is to facilitate, insofar as is possible, the timely referral of persons with rare disorders to those physicians best able to meet the patients' needs.

*—Jess G. Thoene, M.D.*
*Editor*

# EDITOR'S PREFACE TO THE FIRST EDITION

The physician caring for a person with a rare disease (one affecting fewer than 200,000 Americans) often is hard pressed to find accurate and timely information about the condition. In a busy practice, an encounter with such a patient can be burdensome. Not in the common stream of daily events, the person's symptoms may be perplexing and the diagnostic tests required may not be readily available. A survey by the National Commission on Orphan Diseases of the rare disease experiences of 247 physicians demonstrated that between 20 percent and 40 percent of physicians could neither find information on the availability or location of appropriate treatment or on the existence of support groups, nor access printed information for patients regarding rare diseases.

The National Commission on Orphan Diseases studied the problems of persons with these rare conditions for two years. Their findings demonstrated that about one-third of these patients do not receive correct diagnoses for over five years. Fifteen percent of these persons went without a diagnosis for over six years. Furthermore, persons with rare diseases desperately want and need information on research projects for patient participation, knowledge of new treatments and research advances, easy-to-understand written information about their rare conditions, and details of the location of treatment centers. None of these is readily available, although the National Organization for Rare Disorders has attempted to meet this need with the introduction of the Rare Disease Database on CompuServe, providing comprehensible information in lay terms on over 800 rare diseases. Additionally, through its networking function, NORD assists patients with rare diseases in finding other persons with the same conditions and maintains a registry of treatment centers.

To address the problem of providing more and better information to physicians, NORD and Dowden Publishing Company have collaborated to produce this first edition of PHYSICIANS' GUIDE TO RARE DISEASES. This work is an adaptation of the rare disease database entries for close to 700 rare diseases and has been revised to address the concerns of physicians in primary care specialties. The intent of the volume is not to provide specialists in rare diseases with comprehensive data about these conditions, but rather to assist someone who encounters rare diseases infrequently by providing ready access to signs and symptoms for help in differential diagnosis, to availability of therapy, and to the location of support groups for these patients.

Each major section of the Guide opens with an overview article by a specialist on the Editorial Board. This introduction is intended as a helpful guide to the diseases covered in that section. Because of its synoptic nature, this book is necessarily inadequate with regard to the details of pathophysiology, diagnosis, and treatment. However, by identifying the rare condition and its major presenting symptomatology, it should shorten the time needed to achieve a correct diagnosis, as well as provide ready access to further information and the location of support groups. This last feature is unique to this book, and we hope it will be most helpful to the practicing physician.

Also featured in this first edition is a full-color atlas of visual diagnostic signs, a directory of "orphan" drugs organized by use and providing the name of a key contact person at each research center, and a detailed index of symptoms and key words.

The reader's comments will be most welcome so that we can make the next edition of PHYSI-CIANS' GUIDE TO RARE DISEASES even more valuable. Please address these to me in care of the publisher, Dowden Publishing Company, 110 Summit Avenue, Montvale, New Jersey 07645.

I am grateful to the Editorial Board, who undertook to review each article for medical accuracy, and for the outstanding support of Doris Smith, managing editor, and Carroll Dowden, president of Dowden Publishing Company, who pushed the project along most rapidly. Finally, Abbey Meyers, executive director of NORD, has been the driving force on behalf of rare disease patients in this country for many years, and without her none of this project would have been realized.

*—Jess G. Thoene, M.D.*
*Editor*

# ALTERNATIVE MEDICINE AND RARE DISEASES
*By Steven C. Martin, M.D.*

Alternative healing practices are used by a wide variety of patients and enjoy a level of social acceptance today that is unprecedented for the twentieth century. Physicians who treat patients with rare diseases should expect to be confronted by the issues surrounding alternative medicine. Surveys indicate that roughly one-third of Americans utilize alternative medical practices. Many studies of populations with life-threatening illnesses, such as cancer or acquired immune deficiency syndrome **(AIDS),** reveal a 50 to 60 percent use of unorthodox practices, with some studies reporting rates of 80 percent.

Physicians tend to underestimate the use of alternative medicine by their patients. Traditionally, doctors have viewed unorthodox medicine with skepticism, assuming that those who use alternative healers are either weird, ignorant, desperate, or all three. However, research over the past two decades has repeatedly demonstrated that the use of alternative medicine cuts across all socioeconomic lines. Educated, white, upper-middle-class patients are slightly more likely to employ alternative healing practices. Another misconception common among physicians is that those individuals who seek out alternative healers will shun orthodox medical care. The reality is that the vast majority of patients, roughly 95 percent, see practitioners of orthodox and unorthodox medicine simultaneously for their problem.

Not only has the use of alternative medicine increased, but its level of social respectability has improved. Forty years ago patients engaged in unorthodox practices were likely to keep it hidden from their physicians, friends, and family. Today many people consider using alternative practices a mark of independent thinking and courage.

Popular culture mirrors this attitude. Mainstream media frequently present materials approving of alternative medicine. The popular movie *Lorenzo's Oil* favorably depicts a family that, in the face of orthodox medical opposition, develops an unorthodox dietary treatment for adrenoleukodystrophy. Instead of depicting alternative medicine as a cruel hoax, as would likely have been done thirty years earlier, the movie portrays this unorthodox approach in a heroic light, implying that the embattled parents have saved their child from a disastrous fate. Although further research has demonstrated that Lorenzo's oil does not cure adrenoleukodystrophy, the popular image of orthodox medicine as intransigent and alternative medicine as heroic remains.

Even within orthodox medicine, alternative practices are being seriously considered. Prestigious medical publications like the *New England Journal of Medicine,* the *Annals of Internal*

*Medicine*, and the *British Medical Journal* no longer simply publish denunciations of alternative practices, but report randomized clinical trials, epidemiologic studies, and meta-analyses, and review articles. Many medical schools now offer course work in alternative medicine.

In 1992 the National Institutes of Health, arguably the preeminent symbol of modern scientific medicine, opened an Office of Alternative Medicine **(OAM).** Although formed by congressional command rather than at the request of the scientific community, the establishment of the OAM epitomizes the new attitude toward alternative medicine as an area worthy of scientific examination rather than scorn, and reflects the growing acceptance of its broad appeal to Americans.

Unfortunately, recognizing the growing respectability and popularity of alternative medicine does not provide guidance to physicians on how they should respond to this reality. The excesses of patent medicine vendors, charlatans, and frauds of all types remain deeply embedded in medicine's collective professional conscience. The battle against quackery has been central to medical ethics for centuries. How should physicians now respond to those who make claims the medical community finds difficult to accept? What should doctors reply to patients who question them about the appropriateness of alternative medicine? Has the time come when physicians should refer patients to alternative practitioners? Is it appropriate to enter into professional collaborations with alternative practitioners? Are there any limits to these relationships?

## Alternative Medicine in Historical Perspective: The Nineteenth Century

The answers to these questions must be shaped by an understanding of the historical relationship between alternative and orthodox medicine. It would be naive for physicians to believe that the current fascination with alternative medicine is simply related to discovering and evaluating new therapeutic approaches to illness. Alternative medicine has historically represented a sweeping critique of medicine, challenging its intellectual, social, clinical, and therapeutic assumptions, and this remains true today.

In America, this challenge peaked between 1825 and 1875. During most of the nineteenth century, physicians were held in low regard. There was deep skepticism about medicine's efficacy, a skepticism that was well founded, given that the most popular treatments included emetics, cathartics, and vigorous bleeding. Furthermore, medicine lacked strong institutions. Early in the century, medical education was by apprenticeship. Later, proprietary medical schools were founded, but many were merely diploma mills designed to earn their founders substantial income. Medical journals were rare, and professional societies weak. Although the medical elite were highly regarded, rank-and-file physicians were often men of little distinction, considered unfit for more prestigious occupations. These conditions combined with the radical egalitarianism of the Jacksonian era to nearly eliminate medical licensure.

Unorthodox healers rejected medicine's claim to superiority and argued that each patient ought to be allowed to determine what medical treatment he or she desired. The state, in their view, had no right imposing its belief on its citizens. Unorthodox practitioners argued that medicine simply represented one theory among many possible theories for understanding health and disease. Many alternative practitioners claimed their interventions were milder, more effective, and cheaper than orthodox medical care. Physicians were portrayed as autocratic elitists who sought to suppress their competition primarily to advance their economic position.

These criticisms of medicine resonated with the American populace. The absence of obvious differences in efficacy, the unimpressive quality of medical training, an unwillingness to cede authority to the government, and stubborn individualism all helped a series of medical sectarian movements to flourish.

Physicians opposed sectarians on several grounds. First, they argued that the claims of sectarians and quacks were not believable in light of the accumulated experience of the profession. It seemed patently absurd to physicians that homeopaths, using medications that by the laws of chemistry could no longer contain any active ingredient, could be effectively treating disease. The obvious corollary to this was that alternative medicine was dangerous, in some cases because of the noxious quality of the treatment provided, but in all cases because it deprived the patient of proper medical treatment.

The next series of reasons were class based. Physicians argued that the education of sectarians was inferior and that their social behavior was not gentlemanly. Association with these sectarian healers harmed the medical profession by falsely legitimizing the irregulars and concomitantly lowering the status of the regular profession. Interestingly, these complaints remain at the core of medical opposition to alternative medicine.

Medicine's efforts to suppress sectarians met with limited success until the late nineteenth century. The engine that transformed the relationship between alternative and orthodox medicine was the growing emphasis by physicians on laboratory science. The emergence of experimental physiology, germ theory, and bacteriology fundamentally reorganized medical thought.

In part, the new intellectual climate allowed physicians to begin to argue more persuasively that their interventions were more effective than those of the sectarians. Although in hindsight there were relatively few effective therapies introduced circa 1900, the development of diphtheria antitoxin, rabies vaccine, and aseptic surgery provided dramatic examples that received widespread publicity.

More importantly, physicians could now argue that the competition between orthodox and alternative medicine was more than a difference of therapeutic opinion. Instead, medicine argued that science was a neutral arbiter that could objectively judge all comers. One physician declared that "there can be in medicine no heresy, because there is no orthodoxy." Abraham Flexner, writing in his enormously influential 1910 report to the Carnegie Foundation, *Medical Education in the United States and Canada*, argued that "modern medicine has . . . as little sympathy for allopathy as for homeopathy. It simply denies outright the relevancy or value of either doctrine. It wants not dogma but facts. . . . No man is asked in whose name he comes—whether that of Hahnemann, Rush, or of some more recent prophet. But all are required to undergo rigorous cross-examination." And science was the cross-examiner.

Concomitant with this intellectual shift were important social and political changes. Americans gradually accepted state-licensed professions as critical to the functioning of an increasingly specialized and industrialized society. The emphasis on unfettered, individualistic capitalism was checked by the excesses of the robber barons.

The reorganization of the American Medical Association (**AMA**) in 1900 epitomized these trends. The AMA became a powerful advocate for the new scientific medicine. Using savvy political skills and an effective organizational structure, the AMA introduced stringent licensing reform. These medical practice laws made it illegal to practice medicine without a license.

The AMA used not only licensure but science as a powerful lever to suppress alternative practitioners. Patent medicines proved a perfect foil. Using a tool of science—the chemistry lab—the AMA demonstrated that most patent medicines (the most popular being alcohol and opium) contained few active ingredients. Nostrum vendors were vulnerable to attacks on their honesty, integrity, and the commercial nature of their product, and provided a perfect example for physicians of how unscientific practices and unethical behavior went hand in hand. A major public relations campaign of the AMA helped lead to the passing of the Pure Food and Drug Act of 1906.

In its certainty that science was the answer to alternative medicine, orthodox medicine did little to distinguish among the wide array of alternative practices. Physicians defined what was scientific and what was not, so anything labeled unscientific by the AMA was ethically suspect. The result was that the AMA tarred all alternative practitioners with the same brush, which was often, but not always, deserved.

## Alternative Medicine in Historical Perspective: The Twentieth Century

There were limits to how much authority Americans were willing to cede medicine, and orthodox medicine achieved only a partial victory over alternative medicine. Despite active medical opposition, chiropractic became licensed in the majority of states during the 1920s. A 1929 survey revealed that 4 percent of health care expenditures were devoted to alternative medicine.

The growth of alternative medicine was fueled by persistent skepticism about medicine and science. Even with medicine's ascendancy, there remained deep within American culture images of the scientist as reclusive, weird, dangerous, amoral, or blatantly immoral. This subtext in American culture, which has been revived in recent times, was kept alive in part by alternative healers. Physicians were labeled atheistic materialists. Vivisection was decried as an affront to morality. Iatrogenic deaths were labeled murders.

Despite these reservations, medicine enjoyed broad social support during the first two-thirds of the century. After World War II, dramatic advances, such as the introduction of effective antibiotics and chemotherapy, and the development of a polio vaccine, created a golden age for medicine. Government support for research dramatically increased, and the National Institutes of Health expanded dramatically.

In this context, medicine continued its opposition to alternative medicine. In 1963, at the peak of medicine's power and authority, the AMA established a Committee on Quackery. However, over the course of the next two decades, the AMA's policies against quackery were sharply criticized. During this time, the AMA was engaged in a lengthy legal battle with the chiropractic community, a dispute from which chiropractors emerged victorious, with the courts ruling that the AMA's policies against chiropractic violated antitrust laws.

One key shift was the erosion of faith in the cornerstone of modern medicine—science. Science as an unalloyed good was being challenged. There was a growing recognition of the vast destructive power of science, demonstrated by atomic weaponry and by insecticides, as documented in Rachel Carson's groundbreaking 1962 classic *Silent Spring*.

Within medicine, the naive optimism that science could cure all disease met the hard reality of chronic diseases. Slowly and seemingly inexorably, medicine had developed a series of halfway technologies. The way patients died was troubling, hospitalized under the ministration of physicians who viewed death as the enemy. What physicians failed to appreciate was that their victories began to become Pyrrhic. Adding an extra few weeks or months of life by keeping patients in hospitals with tubes attached to every natural orifice (and, if that wasn't sufficient, creating some new orifices) proved unsatisfactory to patient and physician alike. As the title of one book succinctly described the situation, we were "doing better, feeling worse."

Not only was there a growing recognition of the unexpected, untoward effects of modern science, but the ethical purity of science itself was being challenged. The horrors of Nazi Germany revealed cruelty inflicted by scientists in the name of a greater scientific good. Although this was dismissed as the aberration of an evil society, a seed of doubt was planted. This seed was nourished in part by the cultural memory of the centrality of German expertise to the rise of modern science in general and medical science in particular.

In 1966, Americans were stunned by an article published in the *New England Journal of Medicine*. Henry Beecher, professor and chairman of Harvard Medical School's Department of Anesthesiology, revealed a series of ethically questionable practices, including injecting cancer cells into patients without their permission and inducing hepatitis in mentally retarded children. In the early 1970s, an even more nefarious medical experiment, carried out under the auspices of the United States Public Health Service, was exposed. Government researchers and academics had collected a cohort of black men infected with syphilis in the 1930s and had assiduously prevented them from receiving therapy. The study had been continued over four decades, surviving multiple reviews, including one in 1969. The suspicion developed that unethical human experimentation was not simply an aberration committed by unscrupulous researchers but was deeply embedded in the research culture. The phrase "Trust me, I'm a doctor" grew increasingly hollow. Another powerful influence on medicine was the dramatic social upheaval of the late 1960s and early 1970s. Suddenly the word *authoritative* was transformed into *authoritarian*. In an echo of Jacksonian America, the commoner was assumed to be able to control his or her own destiny without relying entirely on the expert. The new egalitarian impulse challenged the assumption that somehow physicians and experts are preeminent and therefore entitled to be paternalistic. Patients were increasingly viewed as consumers, who ought to be in the position of informed, rather than ignorant, buyers. Instead of a professional model of relations, a business model was established. One wouldn't buy a car or appliance on the say-so of a salesperson. Neither should a patient passively accept the judgment of a physician without a careful explanation. The cornerstone of the ethical relationship between physician and patient changed. Rather than beneficence, as determined by physicians, being the central principle, autonomy came to dominate medical ethics. In an exchange between equals, informed consent was essential.

Autonomy, consumerism, and egalitarianism had a powerful effect on the relationship between orthodox and alternative medicine. The growing willingness to define medicine in business terms eroded many distinctions traditionally drawn by physicians. Perhaps the most prominent example is advertising, which professional ethics had always prohibited and which alternative practitioners had embraced. When the courts ruled that prohibitions against advertising were anticompetitive and therefore illegal, one of the standard distinctions between medicine and quackery crumbled. Similarly, medicine's opposition to alternative practitioners was now framed in business terms. Attempts to suppress alternative medicine were no longer perceived to be the altruistic efforts of a profession devoted to the public good, but instead a push by physicians to suppress economic competition.

The loss of faith in science and the emphasis on a business ethic diminished the gap between orthodox medicine and alternative medicine by lowering medicine's status, rather than by raising alternative medicine's status. However, as a result of dramatic reports from China about the efficacy of acupuncture, the status of alternative medicine began to rise. Respected journalists, including James Reston of *The New York Times*, witnessed surgery under acupuncture anesthesia. It was difficult to believe this was a hoax. Suddenly, the notion that alternative medicine had something tangible to offer that orthodox medicine did not gained respectability.

The rising stature of alternative medicine rested on more than the possibility that it could be effective. The discontent with medicine that had been growing since the 1960s included the argument that medicine had become too technocratic, materialistic, and reductionist. Critics argued that medicine had ceased to be humane.

It was a short step from arguing that medicine was coldhearted, to focusing on the growing interest in the relationship between spirituality and medicine. Many alternative practices rested on assumptions about the interconnectedness of mind, body, and spirit. These alternative practices argued that they addressed the quality of life better than orthodox medicine. These arguments dovetailed with a growing shift in the definition of health from the traditional formulation that equated health with the absence of disease, to a new formulation of health as an optimal state of being, in all spheres of life.

The decline of medicine's status and authority, along with the rise of alternative medicine's stature in terms of its presumed efficacy, morality, and eagerness to address issues neglected by medicine, has resulted in the resurgence of interest in alternative medicine. Arguably, alternative medicine is now as popular as it was during its heyday in the mid-nineteenth century. However, the social environment of the late twentieth century contrasts sharply to that of the mid-nineteenth century. In a marked departure from its previously dogged opposition to alternative medicine, the AMA, in 1980, adopted a revised version of its Principles of Medical Ethics, stating that physicians were "free to choose whom to serve, with whom to associate, and the environment in which to provide medical services."

## Alternative and Orthodox Medicine Today

Although physicians are free to associate with whom they wish, they are still left with the problem of whether they *wish* to associate with alternative practitioners. What criteria should shape medicine's response to alternative medicine?

Part of the answer lies in taking the critique of medicine embodied in alternative medicine seriously. Perhaps the most important of these criticisms is that medicine fails to adequately address the emotional and spiritual needs of patients. This complaint has several roots. In part, it represents a paucity of communication skills among physicians. Flaws in communication range from the mundane, when physicians fail to spend sufficient time with patients, to more subtle shortcomings, such as failing to ask open-ended questions, interpret body language, and assume a nonjudgmental and supportive role. This can be especially problematic when physicians lack ready answers and are required to provide supportive and palliative care, rather than the curative interventions that both patient and physician find so satisfying.

At a deeper level, the critique of medicine finds fault with a stubbornly reductionist conception of health and disease. Many people are convinced that there are fundamentally important relationships between emotional, spiritual, mental, and physical health and fear that medicine actively rejects this assumption. Ironically, clinicians have always recognized these relationships, even if a clear scientific basis was lacking. Recently, such relationships have become the focus of increased study, spawning the discipline of psycho-neuro-immunology.

One fundamental response to alternative medicine by physicians ought to be an acknowledgment of concerns about the interrelationship of mind, body, and spirit, and a recognition that these interrelationships have important clinical manifestations. Minimally, this approach takes into consideration the emotional well-being of their patients; maximally, it has the potential for extending both the quality and quantity of life.

At the same time that it actively addresses the criticisms implicit in alternative medicine, orthodox medicine needs to remain skeptical. Science remains an essential tool in evaluating alternative practices. In recent years, we have developed an increasingly sophisticated ability to evaluate clinical interventions. Randomized clinical trials, quasi-experimental designs, and case control studies—in short, the entire panoply of clinical epidemiology—can be called into service to determine the efficacy of alternative medicine. The great advantage of such research is that it does not require assumptions about the underlying mechanisms of therapeutic interventions. Increasingly, investigators have used such scientific techniques to investigate alternative practices. For example, laetrile was debunked as an anticancer agent, while spinal manipulation has been confirmed as a useful treatment for lower back pain. Both had been vigorously opposed by physicians; clinical science helped to distinguish useless from useful.

Clinical trials, however, are not accepted by some supporters of alternative medicine. Clinical trials assume that one can evaluate patients grouped by diagnosis and intervention. Some alternative practitioners reject the assumption that one can make any judgments from group averages, arguing that each patient can be understood only as a unique individual whose disease and response to therapy cannot play a role in predicting the response of others. Given this assumption, the very idea of clinical trials makes little sense.

Some alternative practitioners accept the idea of clinical trials, but reject orthodox diagnostic categories. If physicians seek to study what they perceive as a single clinical entity, and if others argue that this group of patients does not actually suffer from a single disease but rather from a series of disparate diseases, such as different spinal subluxations or interference with different energy points, it becomes impossible for a clinical trial to answer questions to the satisfaction of both orthodox and alternative practitioners. Clinical trials can still be performed using the assumptions of a given healing system, but translating results between orthodox and alternative medicine may be difficult.

The unwillingness of some alternative healers to accept the basic assumptions of orthodox science highlights what I believe is an underappreciated aspect of the rise of alternative medicine. Many alternative systems reject the fundamental assumptions of medical epistemology. Orthodox science may establish the efficacy of acupuncture or chiropractic for particular conditions to our satisfaction, but this does not mean that alternative healers embrace orthodox medicine. Many continue to postulate that the world does not operate on the physical principles that orthodox science takes for granted. There is much emphasis on energy forces and other intangibles in the alternative literature.

At its core, such an approach is an assault on modern biomedical science and represents a dangerous phenomenon. Just as creation science has attracted significant support but represents a threat to modern biology, elements of alternative medicine clearly threaten orthodox science. At a time when alternative medicine has achieved growing respectability, physicians need to be vigilant and actively oppose those aspects of alternative medicine that undermine rational, scientific inquiry.

The recent history of AIDS clinical trials provides a cautionary tale. In an effort to streamline a cumbersome evaluation process, a wide array of new types of clinical trials were promoted. With the passage of time, reassessment of some of these trials suggests that an absence of methodological rigor and sophistication has made the results difficult or impossible to interpret.

The response to alternative medicine by physicians who treat patients with rare diseases needs to be multifaceted. When caring for individual patients, physicians need to assess nonjudgmentally what course of action the patient wishes to pursue and what the patient hopes to gain from pursuing such a course. Acquiring this information can allow physicians to frame a rough risk/benefit analysis of each patient's case. This analysis must take into consideration the efficacy and side effects of conventional medical practices and of alternative practices (if such information is available), the possible interactions between the two courses of action, the sense of control and independence that is important to each patient, the roles both conventional and alternative practices play in the emotional and psychological health of the patient, and the fine line between hope and false hope. Patients should not make the mistake of rejecting the possibility that alternative practices have tangible physical benefits, but instead should take a skeptical yet open-minded approach in evaluating all new therapies, conventional or alternative.

At a broader level, physicians should actively analyze the arguments of alternative medicine. Historically, these have included valid criticisms that have helped medicine improve itself. For example, the growth of homeopathy spurred the decline of heroic bleeding and purging. Alternative practices hold the possibility of adding to medicine's therapeutic armamentarium. Even if these practices are demonstrated to be ineffective, medicine's willingness to evaluate them demonstrates an open-mindedness that is demanded by intellectual honesty, an honesty and open-mindedness that all too many patients are convinced medicine lacks.

By addressing our patients' concerns, both explicit and implicit, about alternative medicine, we as physicians will be responding to our patients' needs in the broadest sense. Utilizing the best of our scientific approaches, remaining simultaneously receptive but skeptical, we can evolve an ethical response to alternative medicine that avoids the excesses of adamant rejection and open-armed acceptance. Alternative medicine includes both quacks and colleagues, and we need to be vigilant to distinguish between the two.

### References

Alternative Medicine: Expanding Medical Horizons: A report to the National Institutes of Health on alternative medical systems and practices in the United States, prepared under the auspices of the Workshop on Alternative Medicine, Chantilly, VA, September 14–16, 1992; Washington, D.C., Government Printing Office, 1994.

Unconventional Medicine in the United States: D.M. Eisenberg, et al.; N. Engl. J. Med., 1993, vol. 328, pp. 246–252.

Other Healers: Unorthodox Medicine in America: N. Gevitz, ed.; The Johns Hopkins University Press, 1988.

### Resources for Physicians

Office of Alternative Medicine, National Institutes of Health, Rockville, MD 20892. Tel.: (301) 402-2467. Recently founded and still working toward defining its role. Takes alternative medicine seriously. Is principally devoted to funding research and is not well organized to handle consumer or physician inquiries. May be aware of clinical trials involving alternative medicine.

National Council Against Health Fraud, P.O. Box 1276, Loma Linda, CA 92354. Tel.: (909) 824-4690. An organization that hearkens back to traditional medical efforts to expose and combat health fraud and quackery. An excellent resource in that it maintains files on nearly all current forms of alternative practices. Demands high levels of proof before accepting alternative practices as reputable.

American Cancer Society, 1599 Clifton Rd., N.E., Atlanta, GA 30329-4251. Tel.: (404) 320-3333. Has up-to-date information specifically related to alternative cancer therapies. Because many alternative practices are promoted for a wide array of diseases, the information supplied by the American Cancer Society may be more broadly applicable.

# PHYSICIANS' GUIDE TO RARE DISEASES

SECOND EDITION

# 1 GENETIC DISEASES AND DYSMORPHIC SYNDROMES
*By Angelo M. DiGeorge, M.D.*

In this section are included a few disorders readily recognizable by physicians and lay persons alike, such as Down syndrome, and other disorders so rare and esoteric that thus far only a few affected patients have been described. Even physicians with a special interest in rare disorders cannot be expected to instantly recognize or be knowledgeable about every one of them. After 45 years of clinical practice in a busy children's hospital, I have personally seen only about 50 percent of the disorders in this chapter. Considering that about half of these disorders have been described during the past three decades, I have missed my share of diagnoses. Gorlin's encyclopedic monograph describes about 700 syndromes that involve the head and neck,[1] and new entities are being reported in the medical journals every year.

How can the practicing pediatrician or family physician be expected to diagnose such a growing hodgepodge of abstruse conditions? For the serious student of dysmorphology, I recommend Dr. Jon M. Aase's book on the systematic approach to the diagnosis of the dysmorphology syndromes.[2]

The most important requirement of physicians who seek to enhance their diagnostic acumen is an abiding curiosity about unusual clinical findings or odd associations of common manifestations. One cannot repeat too often the importance of a detailed history and complete physical examination. Dr. John A. Kolmer, one of my professors in medical school, was fond of admonishing us over and over again, "More mistakes are made in medicine by not looking than by not knowing." Even after assembling the abnormal historical and physical findings, the physician should not be surprised that in many instances these do not immediately conjure up a diagnosis. The next step, as I tell my students, is to "look it up."

Where does one start? Begin with the index of symptoms and key words in this compendium. But do not begin by looking up minor or prevalent abnormalities such as micrognathia, low-set ears, cleft lip, scoliosis, or clinodactyly. These manifestations are common to many disorders and are likely to lead you to a jumble of a differential diagnosis. Always begin by looking up the most uncommon, unusual, strange, or exotic finding. For example, a low-pitched growling cry will lead you to Cornelia de Lange syndrome; a kittenlike mewing cry will lead to cri du chat syndrome (deletion of the short arm of chromosome 5). Likewise, freckles on the lips will lead to Peutz-Jeghers syndrome, and freckling of the axilla to neurofibromatosis type I. Unusual abnormalities of the eyes are particularly helpful in zeroing in on a diagnosis. Aniridia (Wilms tumor association), heterochromia of the irides (Waardenburg syndrome), dislocated lens (Marfan syndrome and homocystinuria), and optic nerve hypoplasia (septo-optic dysplasia) are examples of this bull's-eye approach to diagnosis. Similarly, clear-to-yellow or brown nodules on the surface of the iris (Lisch nodules) are diagnostic of neurofibromatosis type I; and retinal angiomatosis is often the only manifestation in children with von Hippel–Lindau disease. This is, of course, an oversimplified approach that only works for about 25 percent of these disorders, but I have seen children whose diagnoses were unduly delayed for lack of physician curiosity, and failure of even the most cursory inquiry.

Only 30 of the more common chromosomal disorders are included here. The phenotypes of Down, trisomy 13, trisomy 18, or cri du chat syndromes can be recognized in the neonatal period and the diagnosis readily confirmed cytogenetically. Many girls with Turner syndrome can also be detected in the newborn period if lymphedema is present; if not, short stature with or without other associated abnormalities should suggest the diagnosis in childhood. On the other hand, males with Klinefelter syndrome are often not recognized until they present as adults with small testes, gynecomastia, and/or infertility.

The physician who uses this compendium should be aware that another 60 or more chromosomal syndromes have been delineated but are not included here. Although each is very rare, their large number obliges chromosomal analysis in all patients with an undiagnosed constellation of congenital anomalies, dysmorphism, and/or mental retardation. Moreover, small chromosomal deletions or duplications are cytogenetically visible in only a proportion of patients with certain syndromes described in this section; examples include the Prader-Willi (del 15q11.2–q12), Angelman (del 15q11.2–q12), DiGeorge (del 22q11), Shprintzen (del 22q11), trichorhinophalangeal type I (del 8q24.12) and type II (del 8q24.11–24.13), WAGR (del 11p13), Williams (del 7q11.23), and Beckwith-Wiedemann (dup 11p15.5) syndromes. Fluorescent in situ hybridization (**FISH**) technology is becoming increasingly available to detect patients with these disorders who do not have a visible deletion.

Imaging is another important diagnostic tool for this group of patients. Radiographs are required for patients with disproportionate short stature and skeletal anomalies and for assessment of osseous maturation. Computerized tomography and magnetic resonance are essential for imaging of the central nervous system and other organs. These technologies are particularly important for the detection of tumors in patients having syndromes with a known predisposition to malignancy, such as neurofibromatosis types I and II, and von Hippel–Lindau, Peutz-Jeghers, Beckwith-Wiedemann, and Sotos syndromes.

Genetic counseling is obligatory for most of these conditions. The most comprehensive single source of information for the physician is McKusick's *Mendelian Inheritance in Man*.[3] However, unraveling some of these arcane entities presents a challenge even for the expert geneticist because of the heterogeneity of many similar-appearing syndromes. Two examples of heterogeneity are chondrodysplasia punctata, which occurs in X-linked dominant, X-linked recessive, and autosomal recessive forms, with each having markedly different prognoses; and the oral-facial-digital syndrome, which has been subdivided into seven different phenotypes.

Other persuasive reasons to seek expert genetic counseling are the quickening rate at which it is becoming possible to establish diagnoses at the DNA level for some of these conditions and, more importantly, the revision of cherished genetic dogma, emanating from meticulous study of certain selected syndromes.

The discovery that an identical gene may behave quite differently depending on whether it was inherited from the mother or the father has shaken the long-held precept that the parental source of a given gene has no bearing on phenotype. The clearest evidence of this is provided by the Prader-Willi and Angelman syndromes; a percentage of each has an identical cytogenetic deletion of chromosome 15 but, surprisingly, markedly different phenotypes. It has been established that in Prader-Willi syndrome, the deletion occurs on the paternally derived chromosome 15, whereas in

Angelman syndrome the deletion occurs on the maternally derived chromosome 15. These findings implicate genetic imprinting, a phenomenon in which the expression of genes is influenced by their parental origin.

With the accelerating delineation of disease-causing mutations, there is great interest in relating phenotype to genotype. For many disorders, the variability is readily explained by allelic variants of the same gene where mutations in different parts of the gene can produce different phenotypes. It is now clear that mutations in the COL 2A1 gene may result in Stickler syndrome, late-onset spondyloepiphyseal dysplasia, Kniest dysplasia, spondyloepiphyseal dysplasia congenita, hypochondroplasia, spondylometaepiphyseal dysplasia, and achondrogenesis type II. Even more recently it has been revealed that a mutation of fibroblast growth factor receptor 2 (**FGFR2**) can result in Apert, Crouzon, Jackson-Weiss, and Pfeiffer syndromes.[4]

Even with identical mutations within a family, there may be considerable phenotypic diversity as occurs with neurofibromatosis type I and many other genetic disorders. The terms *incomplete penetrance* and *variable expressivity* have a long history to describe this inexplicable phenomenon, but the concept that the *genetic background* (modifier genes) in which the mutant finds itself plays an important role in phenotype seems to have a brighter future.[5]

Treatment is the short suit of dysmorphology. For most of these conditions, there are as yet no known specific treatment modalities. However, through the application of corrective surgical procedures and supportive, medical, and paramedical technology, a large proportion of affected patients can lead normal and productive lives. Another important way the physician can help these individuals and their families is by remembering to make them aware of the many voluntary organizations dedicated to specific diseases; this manual is one of the most complete sources of such information. These groups consist of caring, compassionate individuals skilled in teaching patients about their conditions and possessing firsthand knowledge of coping mechanisms and available resources. In addition, they promote physicians' and public education programs; they raise funds for research; and they lobby government agencies for increased research funding, and pharmaceutical companies for development of orphan drugs.

Finally, a word of caution to the young physician. In your lifetime the number of rare diseases will almost surely double. The function of only a small percentage of all the genes is known. Every patient with a rare disease cannot be pigeonholed into one of the known entities. Always be alert to the possibility of a "new" rare disease.

### References
1. Syndromes of the Head and Neck, 3rd ed.: R.J. Gorlin, M.M. Cohen, Jr., L.S. Levin; Oxford University Press, 1990.
2. Diagnostic Dysmorphology: J.M. Aase; Plenum Publishing Corporation, 1990.
3. Mendelian Inheritance in Man, 11th ed.: V.A. McKusick; The Johns Hopkins University Press, 1994.
4. Craniofacial Syndromes: No Such Thing As a Single Gene Disease: J.J. Mulvihill; Nat. Genet., 1995, vol. 9, pp. 101–103.
5. Phenotypic Diversity, Allelic Series and Modifier Genes: G. Romeo and V.A. McKusick; Nat. Genet., 1994, vol. 7, pp. 451–453.

# GENETIC DISEASES AND DYSMORPHIC SYNDROMES
*Listings in This Section*

# AARSKOG SYNDROME

**Description** The characteristic features of Aarskog syndrome include short stature and abnormalities of the face, hands, and genitals.

**Synonyms**

Aarskog-Scott Syndrome

Facial-Digital-Genital Syndrome

Faciogenital Dysplasia

**Signs and Symptoms** Facial abnormalities include ocular hypertelorism; ptosis; a short, broad nose; broad philtrum; widow's peak; and low-set, floppy ears. Dental deformities and pectus excavatum may be present. Hands are short and broad, joints are highly extendable, and feet are short, broad, and flat. Characteristic genital abnormalities include cryptorchidism, encircling scrotal folds, and inguinal hernia. Intelligence is usually normal.

Growth deficiency may or may not be apparent at birth but is usually evident by ages 1 to 3 years. A mild mental deficiency may be present.

**Etiology** Inheritance is X-linked dominant; females are less severely affected. The genetic defect is located on chromosome Xp11.21. A putative gene has been isolated that seems to involve a guanine nucleotide exchange factor.

**Epidemiology** Males are affected more often and more severely than females.

**Related Disorders** See *Oral-Facial-Digital Syndrome; Nager Syndrome.*

**Juberg-Hayward syndrome (orocraniodigital syndrome)** is characterized by short stature resulting from growth hormone deficiency. Affected individuals have microcephaly, cleft lip and palate, and deformities of the thumbs and toes.

**Treatment—Standard** Surgical correction of some abnormalities may be required, as may orthodontic treatment. Genetic counseling is advised.

**Treatment—Investigational** Families with this disorder having 2 generations of affected individuals should contact Richard A. Lewis, M.D., Departments of Ophthalmology, Medicine, Pediatrics, and the Institute for Molecular Genetics, Baylor College of Medicine, Houston, Texas. The following physicians are conducting research on Aarskog syndrome: Dagfinn Aarskog, M.D., Haukeland Hospital, Newline, Norway, and Jerome Gorski, M.D., University of Michigan Medical Center.

Please contact the agencies listed under Resources, below, for the most current information. Addresses and telephone numbers of these agencies, as well as of individual experts and research centers, may be found in the Master Resources List.

**Resources**

**For more information on Aarskog syndrome:** National Organization for Rare Disorders (NORD); NIH/National Institute of Child Health and Human Development; Aarskog Syndrome Support Group; The Arc (a national organization on mental retardation).

**For genetic information and genetic counseling referrals:** March of Dimes Birth Defects Foundation; Alliance of Genetic Support Groups.

**References**

Isolation and Characterization of the Faciogenital Dysplasia (Aarskog-Scott) Gene: A Putative Rho/Rac Guanine Nucleotide Exchange Factor: N.G. Pasteris; Cell, 1994, vol. 79, pp. 669–678.

Mendelian Inheritance in Man, 11th ed.: V.A. McKusick; The Johns Hopkins University Press, 1994, pp. 2353–2354.

Aarskog Syndrome: Syndrome of the Month: M.S.M. Porteous and D.R. Goudie; J. Med. Genet., 1991, vol. 28, pp. 44–47.

Smith's Recognizable Patterns of Human Malformation, 4th ed.: K.L. Jones; W.B. Saunders Company, 1988, pp. 110–111.

# AASE-SMITH SYNDROME

**Description** Aase-Smith syndrome is characterized by congenital hypoplastic anemia accompanied by triphalangeal thumb and other abnormalities.

**Synonyms**

Anemia–Congenital Triphalangeal Thumb Syndrome

Triphalangeal Thumb Syndrome

**Signs and Symptoms** Features of the syndrome are present at birth. Skin pallor is accompanied by anemia and variable leukocytopenia. There is a mild growth deficiency. Associated abnormalities include triphalangeal thumbs, hypoplastic radii, narrow shoulders, and late closure of fontanelles. Possible cardiac anomalies include ventricular septal defect. Hepato- and splenomegaly may be present. The anemia often diminishes as the child grows.

**Etiology** The cause is unknown. An autosomal recessive inheritance has been suggested.

**Epidemiology** Both males and females appear to be affected.

**Treatment—Standard** Hypoplastic anemia is treated by bone marrow transplantation from HLA-compatible siblings. Blood transfusions and, in some cases, corticosteroid therapy may also be appropriate.

**Treatment—Investigational** Please contact the agencies listed under Resources, below, for the most current information. Addresses and telephone numbers of these agencies, as well as of individual experts and research centers, may be found in the Master Resources List.

**Resources**

**For more information on Aase-Smith syndrome:** National Organization for Rare Disorders (NORD); NIH/National Heart, Lung and Blood Institute; Human Growth Foundation; NIH/National Institute of Child Health and Human Development.

**For genetic information and genetic counseling referrals:** March of Dimes Birth Defects Foundation; Alliance of Genetic Support Groups.

**References**

Mendelian Inheritance in Man, 11th ed.: V.A. McKusick; The Johns Hopkins University Press, 1994, p. 1625.

Aase Syndrome: A.V. Hing; Am. J. Med. Genet., February 1993, vol. 15(45 pt. 4), pp. 413–415.

Birth Defects Encyclopedia: M.L. Buyse, ed.-in-chief; Blackwell Scientific Publications, 1990, pp. 134–135.

Smith's Recognizable Patterns of Human Malformation, 4th ed.: K.L. Jones; W.B. Saunders Company, 1988, p. 277.

# ACHONDROGENESIS

**Description** The disorder has been categorized into 3 forms. Major features include extreme short-limbed small stature and lack of development of the ribs and other major bone formations. The head may be either soft or enlarged depending on the type of achondrogenesis involved. Types I and II are usually fatal either in utero or shortly after birth; the Grebe type is quite different.

**Synonyms**

> Achondrogenesis Type I
>> Achondrogenesis Type IA
>> Parenti-Fraccaro Type Achondrogenesis
>
> Achondrogenesis Type II
>> Achondrogenesis-Hypochondrogenesis Type II
>> Achondrogenesis Type IB
>> Chondrogenesis Imperfecta
>> Langer-Saldino Achondrogenesis
>
> Achondrogenesis, Grebe Type
>> Achondrogenesis Type II
>> Brazilian Achondrogenesis
>> Grebe Chondrodysplasia
>> Grebe Dysplasia

**Signs and Symptoms Achondrogenesis type I** is characterized by premature birth, fetal hydrops, either a soft or abnormally large head due to edema of the soft tissues, and a short neck and trunk. The limbs are extremely short and the ribs, vertebra, and other skeletal bones improperly developed. The abdomen is prominent. Other anomalies include cleft palate, corneal clouding, ear deformities, and underdeveloped testicles and rectum. There is deficient ossification of lumbar vertebrae and absent ossification of sacral, pubic, and ischial bones. The ribs are thin and often show multiple fractures.

**Achondrogenesis type II** is also characterized by severe micromelia, a soft but normal-sized head, premature birth, and edema throughout the body. There is virtual absence of ossification of the vertebral column, sternum, and pubic bones. The ribs are also very short, but they do not show fractures as do the ribs of the infants with achondrogenesis type I. Stillbirths are fewer and survival may be longer.

**Achondrogenesis, Grebe type,** is characterized by very short limbs, but the head and trunk are normal. There may be absent or extra fingers or toes, or these digits may be very small. The hands and feet are extremely short and stubby. This form of achondrogenesis does not result in death and bears little resemblance to achondrogenesis types I and II.

**Etiology** Achondrogenesis is inherited as an autosomal recessive trait in all forms except for type II, which may be autosomal dominant as well as recessive. One patient with type II showed a defect in the metabolism of sulfate; another showed a mutation in the COL 2A1 gene.

**Epidemiology** The Grebe form is usually found in a highly inbred Brazilian population and in Miao Chinese. There is also a form that affects certain persons of German heritage. Males and females are affected in equal numbers.

**Related Disorders** See *Camptomelic Syndrome; Kniest Dysplasia.*

**Treatment—Standard** Ultrasound of the mother in the 3rd trimester can often warn of the condition of the fetus. Treatment of the condition is to maintain the mother's health. Genetic counseling may be helpful. Other treatment is symptomatic and supportive.

**Treatment—Investigational** Please contact the agencies listed under Resources, below, for the most current information. Addresses and telephone numbers of these agencies, as well as of individual experts and research centers, may be found in the Master Resources List.

**Resources**

**For more information on achondrogenesis:** National Organization for Rare Disorders (NORD); NIH/National Institute of Child Health and Human Development; International Center for Skeletal Dysplasia; Magic Foundation for Children's Growth; Human Growth Foundation; Parents of Dwarfed Children; Little People of America; Short Stature Foundation.

**For genetic information and genetic counseling referrals:** March of Dimes Birth Defects Foundation; Alliance of Genetic Support Groups.

**References**

A Defect in the Metabolic Activation of Sulfate in a Patient with Achondrogenesis Type IB: A. Superti-Fuga; Am. J. Hum. Genet., 1994, vol. 55, pp. 1137–1145.

Mendelian Inheritance in Man, 11th ed.: V.A. McKusick; The Johns Hopkins University Press, 1994, pp. 1573–1575.

Birth Defects Encyclopedia: M.L. Buyse, ed.-in-chief; Blackwell Scientific Publications, 1990, pp. 8, 9, 10, 13.

Achondrogenesis Type II (Langer-Saldino) in Association with Jugular Lymphatic Obstruction Sequence: K.D. Wenstrom, et al.; Prenat. Diagn., July 1989, vol. 9(7), pp. 527–532.

Achondrogenesis Type I: Delineation of Further Heterogeneity and Identification of Two Distinct Subgroups: Z. Borochowitz, et al.; J. Pediatr., January 1988, vol. 112(1), pp. 23–31.

Smith's Recognizable Patterns of Human Malformation, 4th ed.: K.L. Jones; W.B. Saunders Company, 1988, pp. 280–281, 312.

Type II Achondrogenesis-Hypochondrogenesis: Morphologic and Immunohistologic Studies: M.Godfrey, et al.; Am. J. Hum. Genet., December 1988, vol. 43(6), pp. 894–904.

# ACHONDROPLASIA

**Description** Achondroplasia is a hereditary, congenital disorder that results in short stature because of an impairment of endochondral bone formation. Craniofacial abnormalities are among the associated conditions.

**Signs and Symptoms** The vault of the skull is usually large in order to accommodate the enlarged brain, making the forehead broad. Hydrocephalus may be present. Brain stem compression due to abnormalities of the craniocervical junction may occur and result in death in young children.

A low nasal bridge is characteristic. The limbs are short; the trunk appears longer than the extremities. The hands are short and broad, with a trident appearance. A dorsal kyphosis is usually present, and the legs may be bowed. Most adult males are under 4½ feet tall, and females are about 3 inches shorter.

Achondroplasia does not cause any mental deficiencies, and life expectancy in infants who survive their first 4 years is normal.

**Etiology** Achondroplasia is inherited as an autosomal dominant trait, but about 80 to 90 percent of cases are caused by new mutations. Children of fathers of advanced age are more likely to be born with a fresh achondroplasia mutation.

When both parents have achondroplasia, there is a 25 percent chance that an offspring will have a double dose of the mutant gene. Such children have a much more severe form of the disorder and die within the first year of life.

Achondroplasia is caused by a mutation in the fibroblast growth factor receptor 3; the gene is on the short arm of chromosome 4 (4p16.3). Virtually all affected patients have identical mutations. Prenatal diagnosis is possible.

**Epidemiology** Onset occurs during gestation. Achondroplasia is one of the most common forms of congenital bone disturbances present from birth and occurs between 1:15,000 and 1:40,000 live births.

**Related Disorders** A distinct mutation of the same gene causing achondroplasia, **FGFR3,** results in **thanatophoric dysplasia,** a lethal neonatal skeletal dysplasia.

**Treatment—Standard** Ultrasonography of the brain in infancy is done to determine the presence of hydrocephalus. Orthopedic surgery may be beneficial. Genetic counseling is useful. Little People of America is an organization providing social contact for persons with achondroplasia. The organization also acts as an advocate on their behalf.

**Treatment—Investigational** The Titanium Rib Project oversees the implantation of expandable ribs in children with disorders involving missing, underdeveloped, or malformed rib cages or chest walls. Contact Robert Campbell, M.D., at Santa Rosa Children's Hospital, San Antonio, Texas, for more information.

Please contact the agencies listed under Resources, below, for the most current information. Addresses and tele-

phone numbers of these agencies, as well as of individual experts and research centers, may be found in the Master Resources List.

### Resources

**For more information on achondroplasia:** National Organization for Rare Disorders (NORD); NIH/National Arthritis and Musculoskeletal and Skin Diseases Information Clearinghouse; International Center for Skeletal Dysplasia; Little People of America; Human Growth Foundation; Short Stature Foundation; Magic Foundation for Children's Growth; Parents of Dwarfed Children; Association for Research into Restricted Growth.

**For genetic information and genetic counseling referrals:** March of Dimes Birth Defects Foundation; Alliance of Genetic Support Groups.

### References

Achondroplasia Is Defined by Recurrent G-380R Mutations of FGFR3: G.A. Bellus, et al.; Am. J. Med. Genet., 1995, vol. 56, pp. 368–373.

Health Supervision for Children with Achondroplasia: Committee on Genetics; Pediatrics, 1995, vol. 95, pp. 443–451.

Prospective Assessment of Risks for Cervico-Medullary Junction Compression in Infants with Achondroplasia: R.M. Paul, et al.; Am. J. Med. Genet., 1995, vol. 56, pp. 732–744.

Mendelian Inheritance in Man, 11th ed.: V.A. McKusick; The Johns Hopkins University Press, 1994, pp. 12–15.

Cecil Textbook of Medicine, 19th ed.: J.B. Wyngaarden, et al., eds.; W.B. Saunders Company, 1992, pp. 1435–1436.

Nelson Textbook of Pediatrics, 14th ed.: R.E. Behrman, ed.-in-chief; W.B. Saunders Company, 1992, pp. 1733–1734.

Birth Defects Encyclopedia: M.L. Buyse, ed.-in-chief; Blackwell Scientific Publications, 1990, pp. 11–12.

Smith's Recognizable Patterns of Human Malformation, 4th ed.: K.L. Jones; W.B. Saunders Company, 1988, pp. 298–303.

# ACROCALLOSAL SYNDROME, SCHINZEL TYPE

**Description** Acrocallosal syndrome, Schinzel type, is an inherited disorder characterized by craniofacial, digital, muscular, and mental abnormalities.

**Synonyms**

Hallux Duplication, Postaxial Polydactyly, and Absence of Corpus Callosum

Schinzel Acrocallosal Syndrome

**Signs and Symptoms** Agenesis of the corpus callosum, polydactyly, mental retardation, hypotonia, and craniofacial abnormalities are primary characteristics.

Facial features include macrocephaly; a bulging forehead; a short, broad nose; hypertelorism; strabismus; and down-slanting eyes.

Abnormalities of the fingers and toes may include an additional or partial duplication of the large toe; additional fingers and/or toes; bifid terminal; and syndactyly.

Postnatal hypoxia as well as feeding difficulties and frequent respiratory infections are common. Other abnormalities include seizures, hydrocephaly, cleft lip and cleft palate, cerebellar hypoplasia, cryptorchidism, bone malformations, and abnormal kidney development

**Etiology** Schinzel acrocallosal syndrome is thought to be inherited as an autosomal recessive trait.

**Epidemiology** Males and females are affected in equal numbers. Approximately 15 cases have been reported.

**Related Disorders** See *Greig Cephalopolysyndactyly; Oral-Facial-Digital Syndrome.*

**Treatment—Standard** Surgery may be performed to separate and remove additional fingers and/or toes.

Hydrocephalus is treated by inserting a shunt to drain the cerebrospinal fluid. In growing children the shunt may have to be lengthened periodically.

Treatment of clefting requires a team of specialists: pediatricians, dental specialists, surgeons, speech pathologists, and others. Cleft palate may be repaired by surgery or covered with a prosthesis. Cleft lip can be corrected by surgery in a series of operations, beginning in the patient's infancy. Braces are usually effective to treat dental complications; sometimes dental prosthetics are needed to replace missing teeth.

Anticonvulsant drugs are used to help control seizures.

Genetic counseling may benefit patients and their families. Other treatment is symptomatic and supportive.

**Treatment—Investigational** Researchers are studying a Teflon-glycerine paste that is applied to the rear of the pharynx in a minor surgical procedure to bring the pharynx and palate into proper relationship. For further information, contact William N. Williams, D.D.S., at the University of Florida.

Please contact the agencies listed under Resources, below, for the most current information. Addresses and telephone numbers of these agencies, as well as of individual experts and research centers, may be found in the Master Resources List.

### Resources

**For more information on acrocallosal syndrome, Schinzel type:** National Organization for Rare Disorders (NORD); NIH/National Institute of Child Health and Human Development; The Arc (a national organization on mental retardation); American Cleft Palate Cranial Facial Association; Hydrocephalus Parent Support Group;

National Hydrocephalus Foundation; Hydrocephalus Association; Epilepsy Foundation of America.

**For genetic information and genetic counseling referrals:** March of Dimes Birth Defects Foundation; Alliance of Genetic Support Groups.

### References

Mendelian Inheritance in Man, 11th ed.: V.A. McKusick; The Johns Hopkins University Press, 1994, pp. 1576–1577.

Acrocallosal Syndrome: H.J. Hendriks, et al.; Am. J. Med. Genet., March 1990, vol. 35(3), pp. 443–446.

Birth Defects Encyclopedia: M.L. Buyse, ed.-in-chief; Blackwell Scientific Publications, 1990, p. 34.

Acrocallosal Syndrome: Additional Manifestations: A.C. Casamassima, et al.; Am. J. Med. Genet., March 1989, vol. 32(3), pp. 311–317.

Acrocallosal Syndrome: New Findings: J.B. Moeschler, et al.; Am. J. Med. Genet., March 1989, vol. 32(3), pp. 306–310.

The Acrocallosal Syndrome: M.M. Nelson, et al.; Am. J. Med. Genet., June 1982, vol. 12(2), pp. 195–199.

## ACRODYSOSTOSIS

**Description** Acrodysostosis is a very rare genetic disorder primarily characterized by short stature, mental retardation, and bony deformities of the face and extremities.

**Synonyms**

    Peripheral Dysostosis

**Signs and Symptoms** Short stature is apparent at birth, and growth retardation continues over the years. The head is brachycephalic, and facial characteristics include hypertelorism, a short and flattened nose, underdeveloped maxilla, prognathism, and malaligned teeth. The hands and feet are short and stubby, with broad, short nails. Bones in the arms, legs, and elbows are deformed, and early fusion of these bones occurs. Mental deficiency is present in most cases.

**Etiology** The cause is not known; an autosomal dominant inheritance is suggested. It has been found that paternal age is usually more advanced than usual.

**Related Disorders** Reported cases of acrodysostosis may represent other disorders, such as pseudohypoparathyroidism.

**Treatment—Standard** Plastic surgery may be required in severe cases of acrodysostosis. Genetic counseling may be beneficial.

**Treatment—Investigational** Please contact the agencies listed under Resources, below, for the most current information. Addresses and telephone numbers of these agencies, as well as of individual experts and research centers, may be found in the Master Resources List.

**Resources**

**For more information on acrodysostosis:** National Organization for Rare Disorders (NORD); International Center for Skeletal Dysplasia; NIH/National Institute of Child Health and Human Development; Human Growth Foundation; Parents of Dwarfed Children.

**For genetic information and genetic counseling referrals:** March of Dimes Birth Defects Foundation; Alliance of Genetic Support Groups.

**References**

Mendelian Inheritance in Man, 11th ed.: V.A. McKusick; The Johns Hopkins University Press, 1994, p. 22.

Smith's Recognizable Patterns of Human Malformation, 4th ed.: K.L. Jones; W.B. Saunders Company, 1988, pp. 392–393.

## ADAMS-OLIVER SYNDROME

**Description** Adams-Oliver syndrome is a very rare genetic disorder in which congenital scalp and skull defects occur, along with peripheral skeletal abnormalities.

**Synonyms**

    Absence Defect of Limbs, Scalp, and Skull

    Hemimelia and Scalp-Skull Defects

    Scalp-Skull and Limbs, Absence Defect of

**Signs and Symptoms** Bald, ulcerated areas on the vertex of the scalp, usually with underlying bony defects of the skull, are present at birth. These skull and scalp abnormalities usually heal spontaneously during the first few months of life, but in a few cases plastic surgery may be necessary.

Severity of the limb abnormalities varies. Digits may be short or absent, and metacarpals may be missing. In the most severe cases, lower extremities below mid-calf may also be absent. A wide variety of other anomalies have been reported in different patients.

**Etiology** Adams-Oliver syndrome is transmitted through autosomal dominant inheritance.

**Epidemiology** The syndrome is present at birth and is extremely rare. Males and females are affected equally.

**Related Disorders** See *Holt-Oram Syndrome; Split-Hand Deformity; Aplasia Cutis Congenita.*

**Treatment—Standard** Healing of skin defects generally occurs spontaneously; surgical repair of ulcerated areas may, however, be necessary. Other treatment is symptomatic and supportive. Genetic counseling is advised.

**Treatment—Investigational** Please contact the agencies listed under Resources, below, for the most current information. Addresses and telephone numbers of these agencies, as well as of individual experts and research centers, may be found in the Master Resources List.

**Resources**

**For more information on Adams-Oliver syndrome:** National Organization for Rare Disorders (NORD); NIH/National Arthritis and Musculoskeletal and Skin Diseases Information Clearinghouse.

**For genetic information and genetic counseling referrals:** March of Dimes Birth Defects Foundation; Alliance of Genetic Support Groups.

**References**

Adams-Oliver Syndrome: A Family with Extreme Variability in Clinical Expression: J.S. Bamfort, et al.; Am. J. Clin. Genet., 1994, vol. 49, pp. 393–396.

Mendelian Inheritance in Man, 11th ed.: V.A. McKusick; The Johns Hopkins University Press, 1994, pp. 4–5.

Congenital Scalp Defects with Distal Limb Reduction Anomalies: J.P. Fryns; J. Med. Genet., August 1987, vol. 24(8), pp. 493–496.

# AMELOGENESIS IMPERFECTA

**Description** Amelogenesis imperfecta is a rare genetic disorder in which formation of dental enamel is defective. Fourteen different subclassifications have been described; hypocalcified (hypomineralized), hypomaturation (snow-capped teeth), and hypoplastic (hypoplastic-explastic) are some of these.

**Synonyms**

Brown Enamel, Hereditary

**Signs and Symptoms** The disorder is characterized by defective or missing tooth enamel. Secondary effects include early tooth loss, heightened susceptibility to periodontal and alveolar disease, and increased sensitivity to hot and cold. The dental pulp (pulpa) in the root canal is exposed in some cases, and an open bite may occur because the upper and lower jaws do not align properly. Psychological problems can arise because of the unsightly teeth.

**Hypocalcified type:** Suspected autosomal recessive cases of this form of amelogenesis imperfecta are more severe than those resulting from autosomal dominant inheritance. Unerupted and newly erupted teeth are covered by a light yellow-brown enamel. After eruption, the enamel turns brown or black from food stains. The enamel crumbles easily and wears off rapidly, so that by the ages of 10 to 12 years only the cores of the teeth, consisting of dentin, remain. Enamel of the cervical portion of the teeth may be better calcified. Incomplete closing of the upper and lower jaws produces an anterior open bite. The teeth are overly sensitive to temperature changes. On x-ray the enamel appears less dense than the dentin of the core. The crown of the affected tooth appears to have small irregular holes, with a dense line of calcified enamel at the neck of the tooth. The hypocalcified type of amelogenesis imperfecta is the most frequently occurring variant of the disorder.

**Hypomaturation type (snow-capped teeth):** In this sex-linked recessive form of amelogenesis imperfecta, the enamel of the primary teeth in males looks white and has the appearance of ground glass. The enamel of the permanent teeth is mottled and yellow. The soft enamel can be penetrated by a sharp dental instrument under pressure. In females, the enamel of the primary teeth shows vertical bands of abnormal white enamel that looks like ground glass randomly alternating with bands of translucent normal enamel. The enamel of the permanent teeth shows vertical bands of either opaque white or opaque yellow enamel randomly alternating with bands of translucent normal enamel.

**Pigmented autosomal recessive hypomaturation type:** Both primary and secondary teeth are involved. The enamel is clear-to-cloudy light brown and of normal thickness. It is, however, softer than normal, can be penetrated by a sharp dental instrument, and tends to break off from the dentin core. X-rays show a lack of contrast between enamel and dentin.

**Hypoplastic types:** In the **pitted autosomal dominant hypoplastic type,** the enamel is thin with random pits from pinpoint to pinhead size primarily on the surfaces of permanent teeth facing the lips or cheeks (labial or buccal). In both primary and permanent dentition, some teeth may be normal. X-rays show a normal contrast between the enamel and the dentin core of the teeth. In the **rough autosomal dominant hypoplastic type,** the enamel is thin, brown, and very hard, with a granular vitreous surface. There is lack of contact between adjacent teeth. On x-ray the teeth appear outlined by a thin layer of enamel. A high contrast between enamel and dentin is seen. In the **rough autosomal recessive hypoplastic type,** the tooth surface is rough, grainy, and light yellow-brown in color. Lack of contact between adjacent teeth occurs. X-rays show the lack of enamel. Many teeth are unerupted and partially resorbed into the jaws. Microscopically, the only evidence of enamel is the laminated agatelike glassy calcification on the surface of the tooth core.

In the **smooth autosomal dominant hypoplastic type** of amelogenesis imperfecta, the enamel is thin, brown, smooth, and glossy, except where it is hypocalcified at contact points. Lack of contact occurs between adjacent teeth. X-rays show many unerupted teeth with resorption of the crowns in the jaw bones. Small calcified spots may be seen adjacent to unerupted teeth. In the **smooth sex-linked dominant hypoplastic form,** both males and females are affected. In males, the enamel is thin, brown or yellow-brown, smooth, and shiny. In females, alternating vertical bands of normal and abnormal enamel (Lyon effect) occur. These bands are visible on x-ray. In the **local autosomal dominant hypoplastic** variant, only the baby teeth are affected. Pits and grooves of hypoplastic enamel occur horizontally across the middle third of a tooth. Defective enamel may be present in all or only some of the teeth. The most frequently affected teeth are the incisors, or the baby molars.

Diagnosis of amelogenesis imperfecta is usually made by x-ray examination at the time the teeth erupt. By 1 to 2 years of age, the diagnosis can be made by visual examination.

**Etiology** As noted above, amelogenesis imperfecta is inherited through autosomal dominant, autosomal recessive, and X-linked transmission. Two amelogenin genes have been identified. A mutation of one of these genes, mapped to Xp21.1–22.3, has been reported and molecular defects characterized.

**Epidemiology** Amelogenesis imperfecta affects between 1:14,000 to 1:16,000 children in the United States. Some 40 percent of them have the hypocalcified dominant type. The autosomal dominant and recessive forms of the disorder affect males and females in equal numbers. The sex-linked dominant type of the disorder affects twice as many males as females. The sex-linked recessive type affects only males.

**Related Disorders** See *Trichodentoosseous Syndrome.*

The genetic disorder **taurodontism,** which may be a form of trichodentoosseous syndrome, is characterized by large cavities in the jaw bones in which the tooth pulp rests. Molars are usually the most severely affected. The disorder is most often found in Eskimos who use their teeth for cutting hides.

**Treatment—Standard** The condition may be corrected with orthodontics and restorative procedures. Desensitizing toothpaste can prevent painful sensitivity to heat and cold. Good oral hygiene is important. Genetic counseling is recommended for families of affected children.

**Treatment—Investigational** Please contact the agencies listed under Resources, below, for the most current information. Addresses and telephone numbers of these agencies, as well as of individual experts and research centers, may be found in the Master Resources List.

**Resources**

**For more information on amelogenesis imperfecta:** National Organization for Rare Disorders (NORD); National Foundation for Ectodermal Dysplasias; NIH/National Institute of Dental Research.

**For genetic information and genetic counseling referrals:** March of Dimes Birth Defects Foundation; Alliance of Genetic Support Groups.

**References**

Characterization of Molecular Defects in X-Linked Amelogenesis Imperfecta (A1H1: H.J. Lench and G.B. Winter; Hum. Mutat., 1995, vol. 5, pp. 251–259.

Mendelian Inheritance in Man, 11th ed.: V.A. McKusick; The Johns Hopkins University Press, 1994, pp. 81, 1622, 2301–2308.

A New Classification of Heritable Human Enamel Defects and a Discussion of Dentin Defects: E.D. Shields; Birth Defects, 1983, vol. 19(1), pp. 107–127.

A Clinical, Genetic, and Ultrastructural Study of Snow-Capped Teeth: Amelogenesis Imperfecta, Hypomaturation Type: V.H. Escobar, et al.; Oral Surg., December 1981, vol. 52(6), pp. 607–614.

# AMNIOTIC BANDS

**Description** When the fetus is constrained in its fetal habitat, a variety of extrinsic deformations may be produced in an otherwise normal fetus. Important causes of fetal constraint are serious deficiency of amniotic fluid and pregnancy in a bicornuate uterus. When constrictive amniotic bands occur late in pregnancy, they may result in defective development of limbs or parts of limbs, whereas when they occur early in pregnancy, they often cause deformities of the spine, chest, and face, and even may result in fetal death.

**Synonyms**

Early Constraint Defects

Oligohydramnios Sequence

**Signs and Symptoms** Compression of the chest in utero can result in underdevelopment of the lungs, making the infant incapable of independent breathing. Vascular constriction may cause reduction in the size of limbs. Compression of legs or arms may result in joint stiffness and dislocations. Scoliosis and clubfeet are common deformations. Craniofacial deformities include flattening of the nose and ears.

Premature rupture of the amniotic sac may cause problems during delivery, since the neonate cannot maneuver properly.

Decreased amniotic fluid may be detected early in the 2nd trimester by α-fetoprotein screening.

**Etiology** Early rupture of the amniotic sac can occur idiopathically; rarely, it is the result of amniocentesis. Oligohydramnios can also result from a fetal kidney disorder, since in the later stages of pregnancy fetal urine comprises a large portion of the amniotic fluid. Bilateral renal agenesis is the most common cause of oligohydramnios. When oligohydramnios is the result of insufficient fetal urine output, first-degree family members should be checked for hereditary kidney disease.

**Epidemiology** Both males and females are affected. Infants with amniotic bands are more commonly born to young women with preeclampsia.

**Related Disorders** See *Pierre Robin Syndrome; Clubfoot; Renal Agenesis, Bilateral.*

**Potter syndrome (oligohydramnios tetrad)** is characterized by facial anomalies, pulmonary hypoplasia, limb deformities, and hypoplastic or absent kidneys. The disorder results from inadequate urinary output from the fetus, or from chronic leakage of amniotic fluid.

**Treatment—Standard** Treatment is symptomatic and supportive. Genetic counseling may benefit families of infants with certain forms of inherited kidney disease that can cause amniotic bands.

**Treatment—Investigational** Artificial instillation of amniotic fluid is being investigated for treatment of women with severe oligohydramnios, when conservative measures have proved ineffective.

Please contact the agencies listed under Resources, below, for the most current information. Addresses and telephone numbers of these agencies, as well as of individual experts and research centers, may be found in the Master Resources List.

**Resources**

**For more information on amniotic bands:** National Organization for Rare Disorders (NORD); NIH/National Institute of Child Health and Human Development.

**For genetic information and genetic counseling referrals:** March of Dimes Birth Defects Foundation; Alliance of Genetic Support Groups.

**References**

Artificial Instillation of Amniotic Fluid As a New Technique for the Diagnostic Evaluation of Cases of Oligohydramnios; U. Gembruch, et al.; Prenat. Diagn., January 1988, vol. 8(1), pp. 33–45.

Smith's Recognizable Patterns of Human Malformation, 4th ed.: K.L. Jones; W.B. Saunders Company, 1988, pp. 572–573.

Acute Development of Oligohydramnios in a Pregnancy Complicated by Chronic Hypertension and Superimposed Pre-Eclampsia: P.J. Weinbaum, et al.; Am. J. Perinatol., January 1986, vol. 3(1), pp. 47–49.

Elevated Maternal Serum Alpha-Fetoprotein, Second-Trimester Oligohydramnios, and Pregnancy Outcome: W.L. Koontz, et al.; Obstet. Gynecol., September 1983, vol. 62(3), pp. 301–304.

Oligohydramnios; Clinical Associations and Predictive Value for Intrauterine Growth Retardation: E.H. Philipson, et al.; Am. J. Obstet. Gynecol., June 1, 1983, vol. 146(3), pp. 271–278.

# ANENCEPHALY

**Description** Anencephaly is a developmental brain disorder characterized by the absence of the cranial vault. The cerebral hemispheres are missing or grossly defective. Spina bifida and anencephaly are generally considered one entity.

**Signs and Symptoms** Because of the absence of brain tissue, infants cannot perform basic functions, such as movement, and do not survive more than a few days or weeks. Amniocentesis and ultrasound examination can detect anencephaly.

**Etiology** Anencephaly is the result of defective closure of the anterior portion of the neural tube. Both autosomal dominant and recessive inheritances have been reported.

**Epidemiology** Both males and females are affected.

**Related Disorders** See *Spina Bifida.*

**Treatment—Standard** Counseling concerning medical intervention is beneficial.

**Treatment—Investigational** Please contact the agencies listed under Resources, below, for the most current information. Addresses and telephone numbers of these agencies, as well as of individual experts and research centers, may be found in the Master Resources List.

**Resources**

**For more information on anencephaly:** National Organization for Rare Disorders (NORD); Fighters for Encephaly Support Group; NIH/National Institute of Neurological Disorders and Stroke.

**For genetic information and genetic counseling referrals:** March of Dimes Birth Defects Foundation; Alliance of Genetic Support Groups.

**References**
Mendelian Inheritance in Man, 11th ed.: V.A. McKusick; The Johns Hopkins University Press, 1994, pp. 1377–1378, 1627–1628.
Smith's Recognizable Patterns of Human Malformation, 4th ed.: K.L. Jones; W.B. Saunders Company, 1988, pp. 548–549, 659–660.
Neural Tube Defect-Specific Acetylcholinesterase: Its Properties and Quantitation in the Detection of Anencephaly and Spina Bifida: J.R. Bonham, et al.; Clin. Chim. Acta, November 1987, 170(1), pp. 69–77.
When Is Termination of Pregnancy During the Third Trimester Morally Justifiable?: F.A. Chervenak, et al.; N. Engl. J. Med., February 1984, 310(8), pp. 501–504.
Diagnostic Effectiveness of Ultrasound in Detection of Neural Tube Defect: The South Wales Experience of 2509 Scans (1977–1982) in High-Risk Mothers: C.J. Roberts, et al.; Lancet, November 1983, pp. 1068–1069.

# ANGELMAN SYNDROME

**Description** Angelman syndrome is characterized by severe congenital mental retardation, and unusual facies and muscular abnormalities that were first unfortunately described as the happy puppet syndrome.

**Signs and Symptoms** Characteristic features are microcephaly with an occipital groove, a protruding mandible, and an open mouth with a visible tongue. Patients seem to smile continually and they laugh inappropriately, features that do not seem to occur because of happiness but may be a result of a brain stem defect. Mental retardation is severe, and speech is absent. Motor development is slowed and muscle tone decreased, and jerky limb movements and hand flapping are characteristic. Patients also have poor balance. Epilepsy usually develops between 18 and 24 months of life.

**Etiology** In 50 to 80 percent of patients, depending on whether cytogenetic or molecular analysis is used, there is a cytogenetic deletion of chromosome 15q11.2–q12. The deletion occurs on the maternally derived chromosome 15.

In a few patients with normal chromosomes, both chromosomes 15 have been paternal in origin (paternal uniparental disomy).

Although the identical cytogenetic deletion occurs in Prader-Willi syndrome, it is the paternally derived chromosome that is involved.

**Epidemiology** Males and females are affected equally.

**Treatment—Standard** Multidisciplinary evaluations should include geneticists, neurologists, orthopedists, physical therapists, nutritionists, social workers, educators, ophthalmologists, psychologists or psychiatrists, and dentists. Family and individual psychiatric counseling, as well as genetic counseling, may be beneficial. Other treatment is symptomatic and supportive.

**Treatment—Investigational** Please contact the agencies listed under Resources, below, for the most current information. Addresses and telephone numbers of these agencies, as well as of individual experts and research centers, may be found in the Master Resources List.

**Resources**

**For more information on Angelman syndrome:** National Organization for Rare Disorders (NORD); Angelman Syndrome Support Group; NIH/National Institute of Child Health and Human Development.

**For genetic information and genetic counseling referrals:** March of Dimes Birth Defects Foundation; Alliance of Genetic Support Groups.

**References**
Angelman Syndrome Due to Paternal Uniparental Disomy of Chromosome 15: A Milder Phenotype: A. Bottani, et al.; Am. J. Med. Genet., 1994, vol. 51, pp. 35–40.
Mendelian Inheritance in Man, 11th ed.: V.A. McKusick; The Johns Hopkins University Press, 1994, pp. 98–101.
Angelman Syndrome: B.B. Schneider, et al.; J. Am. Optom. Assoc., July 1993, vol. 65(7), pp. 502–506.
Molecular Mechanisms in Angelman Syndrome: A Survey of 24 Patients: C-T. J. Chan, et al.; J. Med. Genet., 1993, vol. 30, pp. 895–902.
Nondisjunction of Chromosome 15: Origin and Recombination: W.P. Robinson, et al.; Am. J. Hum. Genet., September 1993, vol. 53(3), pp. 740–751.
Uniparental Disomy Revisited: The First Twelve Years: E. Engel; J. Med. Genet., March 1993, vol. 46, pp. 670–674.
Chromosome 15 Uniparental Disomy Is Not Frequent in Angelman Syndrome: J. H. Knoll, et al.; Am. J. Hum. Genet., January 1991, vol. 48(1), pp. 16–21.
Birth Defects Encyclopedia: M.L. Buyse, ed.-in-chief; Blackwell Scientific Publications, 1990, pp. 140–141.
Dictionary of Medical Syndromes, 3rd ed.: S.I. Magalini, et al., eds.: J.B. Lippincott Company, 1990, p. 389.
Syndromes of the Head and Neck, 3rd ed.: R.J. Gorlin, et al.; Oxford University Press, 1990, pp. 616–617.
Smith's Recognizable Patterns of Human Malformation, 4th ed.: K.L. Jones; W.B. Saunders Company, 1988, pp. 168–169.
The Angelman ("Happy Puppet") Syndrome: C.A. Williams, et al.; Am. J. Genet., April 1982, vol. 11(4), pp. 453–460.

# ANODONTIA

**Description** Anodontia is a genetic condition in which all or most of the primary and secondary teeth are missing. It is usually associated with a group of nonprogressive syndromes called ectodermal dysplasias, in which the skin, skin appendages, and mucous membranes are affected.

**Synonyms**

> Anodontia Vera
> Complete Anodontia
> Partial Anodontia (Hypodontia)

**Signs and Symptoms** Anodontia may be either complete or partial. Patients are known who have normal primary dentition but do not develop secondary teeth. This is inherited in an autosomal recessive form. In partial anodontia, only some teeth are missing.

**Etiology** When the disorder is associated with ectodermal dysplasia, it is inherited as either an X-linked recessive or autosomal recessive trait.

**Epidemiology** Anodontia is congenital. In the X-linked disorder, about 60 to 75 percent of female carriers are minimally affected and can be ascertained by careful clinical evaluation.

**Related Disorders Ectodermal dysplasia** syndromes are hereditary and nonprogressive. They affect the skin and other organs that develop from the ectodermal germ layer during gestation. Respiratory infection is a common serious complication that develops because those affected tend to exhibit a weakened immune system and impaired respiratory mucus glands.

**Treatment—Standard** Complete anodontia is treated by fitting the patient with dentures. Partial anodontia that results in missing front teeth can be treated with a bridge that consists of an acrylic tooth that is attached to 3 orthodontic wires, which form a support for the device.

**Treatment—Investigational** Please contact the agencies listed under Resources, below, for the most current information. Addresses and telephone numbers of these agencies, as well as of individual experts and research centers, may be found in the Master Resources List.

**Resources**

For more information on anodontia: National Organization for Rare Disorders (NORD); National Foundation for Ectodermal Dysplasias; NIH/National Institute of Dental Research.

For genetic information and genetic counseling referrals: March of Dimes Birth Defects Foundation; Alliance of Genetic Support Groups.

**References**

Prevalence of Tooth Agenesis Correlated with Jaw Relationship and Dental Crowding: L.R. Dermaut, et al.; Am. J. Orthod. Dentofacial Orthop., September 1986, vol. 90(3), pp. 204–210.

A Review of Tooth Formation in Children with Cleft Lip/Palate: R. Ranta; Am. J. Orthod. Dentofacial Orthop., July 1986, vol. 90(1), pp. 11–18.

New Technique for Semipermanent Replacement of Missing Incisors: J. Artun, et al.; Am. J. Orthod. Dentofacial Orthop., May 1984, vol. 85(5), pp. 367–375.

# ANTLEY-BIXLER SYNDROME

**Description** The very rare Antley-Bixler syndrome is characterized by multiple skeletal fusions, especially of the skull, the hip bones, and part of the arm bones.

**Synonyms**

> Craniosynostosis, Choanal Atresia, Radiohumeral Synostosis
> Multisynostotic Osteodysgenesis
> Trapezoidocephaly–Multiple Synostosis Syndrome

**Signs and Symptoms** Craniofacial abnormalities include craniosynostosis, frontal bossing, and midface hypoplasia, with a depressed nasal bridge, proptosis, and choanal atresia. Ear development is abnormal. Other characteristics include radiohumeral synostosis, and femoral bowing and fractures. Intelligence is normal.

Prenatal diagnosis can be made with ultrasound.

**Etiology** The cause is not known; an autosomal recessive inheritance is suspected.

**Epidemiology** Males and females are both affected.

**Related Disorders** See *Camptomelic Syndrome.*

Features of **acrocephalosyndactyly syndromes** include abnormalities related to craniosynostosis, and syndactyly.

**Treatment—Standard** Treatment for Antley-Bixler syndrome is symptomatic and supportive.

**Treatment—Investigational** Please contact the agencies listed under Resources, below, for the most current information. Addresses and telephone numbers of these agencies, as well as of individual experts and research centers, may be found in the Master Resources List.

**Resources**

    **For more information on Antley-Bixler syndrome:** National Organization for Rare Disorders (NORD); FACES—National Association for the Craniofacially Handicapped; Society for the Rehabilitation of the Facially Disfigured; National Craniofacial Foundation; NIH/National Institute of Dental Research; International Center for Skeletal Dysplasia; NIH/National Institute of Child Health and Human Development.

    **For genetic information and genetic counseling referrals:** March of Dimes Birth Defects Foundation; Alliance of Genetic Support Groups.

**References**

Mendelian Inheritance in Man, 11th ed.: V.A. McKusick; The Johns Hopkins University Press, 1994, p. 1630.

Radiohumeral Synostisis, Femoral Bowing, Other Skeletal Anomalies, and Anal Atresia: A Variant Example of Antley-Bixler Syndrome?: J. Antich, et al.; Genet. Couns., 1993, vol. 4(3), pp. 207–211.

Antley-Bixler Syndrome: Description of Two Patients: E. Bianchi, et al.; Skeletal Radiol., 1991, vol. 20(5), pp. 339–343.

Harrison's Principles of Internal Medicine, 12th ed.: J.D. Wilson, et al.; McGraw-Hill, 1991, pp. 2058–2059.

Birth Defects Encyclopedia: M.L. Buyse, ed.-in-chief; Blackwell Scientific Publications, 1990, p. 154.

Dictionary of Medical Syndromes, 3rd ed.: S.I. Magalini, et al., eds.: J.B. Lippincott Company, 1990, p. 57.

Smith's Recognizable Patterns of Human Malformation, 4th ed.: K.L. Jones; W.B. Saunders Company, 1988, pp. 378–379.

# APERT SYNDROME

**Description** Apert syndrome is an inherited disorder in which characteristic malformations of the head, fingers, and toes occur, along with mental deficiency.

**Synonyms**

    Acrocephalosyndactyly, Type I

    Syndactylic Oxycephaly

    Vogt Cephalodactyly

**Signs and Symptoms** Acrocephaly (resulting from craniostenosis) and syndactyly are the key identifying features of the syndrome. Other symptoms may include hypertelorism, exophthalmos, cataracts, and a high, pointed palate. Vertebral deformities and radioulnar synostosis may occur. Most patient have normal intelligence; of those, the IQ is above 70.

**Etiology** The disorder is autosomal dominant; however, a large number of cases are considered to be fresh mutations. Above-average parental age has been associated with sporadic cases. Very recently mutations have been reported involving fibroblast growth factor receptor 2 **(FGFR2).**

**Epidemiology** Both males and females may be affected by Apert syndrome. Birth prevalence is 1:65,000.

**Related Disorders** See *Crouzon Disease; Pfeiffer Syndrome.*

    Jackson-Weiss syndrome has recently been shown to also involve FGFR2 in most affected patients. See also *Jackson-Weiss Syndrome.*

**Treatment—Standard** Syndactyly and vertebral deformities may be corrected surgically. Reconstructive surgery is performed for facial and cranial deformities. Special education classes are necessary.

**Treatment—Investigational** Please contact the agencies listed under Resources, below, for the most current information. Addresses and telephone numbers of these agencies, as well as of individual experts and research centers, may be found in the Master Resources List.

**Resources**

    **For more information on Apert syndrome:** National Organization for Rare Disorders (NORD); NIH/National Institute of Child Health and Human Development; Apert Syndrome Support Group.

    **For information about congenital heart defects:** American Heart Association; Congenital Heart Anomalies Support, Education, and Resources.

    **For information about craniofacial research and treatments:** Forward Face; FACES—National Association for the Craniofacially Handicapped; National Foundation for Facial Reconstruction; Craniofacial Family Association; Craniofacial Support Group; The Arc (a national organization on mental retardation).

    **For genetic information and genetic counseling referrals:** March of Dimes Birth Defects Foundation; Alliance of Genetic Support Groups.

**References**

Apert Syndrome Results from Localized Mutation of FGFR2 and Is Allelic with Cruzon Syndrome: O.M.W. Andrew, et al.; Nat. Genet., 1995, vol. 9, pp. 165–171.

Apert Syndrome: Quantitative Assessment by CT Scan of Presenting Deformity and Surgical Results After First-Stage Reconstruction: J.C. Posnick, et al.; Plast. Reconstr. Surg., March 1994, vol. 93(3), pp. 489–497.

Mendelian Inheritance in Man, 11th ed.: V.A. McKusick; The Johns Hopkins University Press, 1994, pp. 19–20.

Growth Pattern in the Apert Syndrome: M.M. Cohen, et al.; Am. J. Med. Genet., October 1993, vol. 47(5), pp. 617–623.

Skeletal Abnormalities in the Apert Syndrome: M.M. Cohen, et al.; Am. J. Med. Genet., October 1993, vol. 47(5), pp. 624–632.

An Updated Pediatric Perspective on the Apert Syndrome: M.M. Cohen, et al.; Am. J. Dis. Child., September 1993, vol. 147(9), pp. 989–993.

Birth Prevalence Study of the Apert Syndrome: M.M. Cohen, et al.; Am. J. Med. Genet., March 1992, vol. 42(5), pp. 655–659.

Cecil Textbook of Medicine, 19th ed.: J.B. Wyngaarden, et al., eds.; W.B. Saunders Company, 1992, p. 1146.

Nelson Textbook of Pediatrics, 14th ed.: R.E. Behrman, ed.-in-chief; W.B. Saunders Company, 1992, p. 1491.

Harrison's Principles of Internal Medicine, 12th ed.: J.D. Wilson, et al.; McGraw-Hill, 1991, p. 924.

Birth Defects Encyclopedia: M.L. Buyse, ed.-in-chief; Blackwell Scientific Publications, 1990, pp. 39–40.

The Central Nervous System in Apert Syndrome: M.M. Cohen, et al.; January 1990, vol. 35 (1), pp. 36–45.

Smith's Recognizable Patterns of Human Malformation, 4th ed.: K.L. Jones; W.B. Saunders Company, 1988, pp. 372–373.

# ARTHROGRYPOSIS MULTIPLEX CONGENITA (AMC)

**Description** AMC is characterized by hypomobility of multiple joints due to fibrous ankylosis. This is a heterogeneous group of disorders that includes neurogenic AMC, myopathic AMC, Guerin-Stern syndrome, amyoplasia congenita, and dozens of other congenital disorders that have multiple contractures as a feature.

**Synonym**
Congenital Multiple Arthrogryposis
Fibrous Ankylosis of Multiple Joints

**Signs and Symptoms** The deformities are present at birth. The primary feature of typical AMC is limited or fixed flexion contracture of joints. Soft tissue webbing may have developed over the flexed joints, and the muscles may be hypoplastic. The long bones of the skeleton are exceptionally slender, but skeletal x-rays are otherwise normal. Cleft palate and cryptorchidism may be present. Intelligence usually is normal.

**Etiology** The cause is unknown. Most types of AMC are not hereditary. Autosomal recessive inheritance has been reported in one large inbred Arabic kindred in Israel. A gene for an autosomal dominant form of arthrogryposis (**distal arthrogryposis type I**) has been localized to the pericentric region of chromosome 9.

There is evidence of nervous system involvement, and electromyographic studies show muscle fiber changes, suggesting a myopathic origin.

**Epidemiology** Males and females are affected equally.

**Related Disorders** See *Pterygium Syndrome, Multiple.*

**Popliteal pterygium syndrome** is an autosomal dominant disorder characterized by popliteal webbing, pits in the lower lip, cleft lip and palate, and genital and digital anomalies.

In **amyoplasia congenita,** a generalized lack of muscular development is accompanied by multiple joint contractures.

**Treatment—Standard** Physiotherapy in the newborn period and early infancy is beneficial. Splints can be made to augment the stretching exercises to increase range of motion. Removable splints for the knees and feet that permit regular muscle exercise are recommended. Surgery may be required on ankles, knees, hips, elbows, or wrists to achieve better position or greater range of motion. In some cases, tendon transfers have been performed.

**Treatment—Investigational** Please contact the agencies listed under Resources, below, for the most current information. Addresses and telephone numbers of these agencies, as well as of individual experts and research centers, may be found in the Master Resources List.

**Resources**

**For more information on arthrogryposis multiplex congenita:** National Organization for Rare Disorders (NORD); AVENUES, A National Support Group for Arthrogryposis Multiplex Congenita; Arthrogryposis Support Group; NIH/National Arthritis and Musculoskeletal and Skin Diseases Information Clearinghouse; Human Growth Foundation; Short Stature Foundation.

**For genetic information and genetic counseling referrals:** March of Dimes Birth Defects Foundation; Alliance of Genetic Support Groups.

**References**

A Gene for Distal Arthrogryposis Type I Maps to the Pericentric Region of Chromosome 9: M. Bamshad, et al.; Am. J. Med. Genet., 1994, vol. 55, pp. 1153–1158.

Mendelian Inheritance in Man, 11th ed.: V.A. McKusick; The Johns Hopkins University Press, 1994, pp. 165–166, 1639–1642, 2316.

Smith's Recognizable Patterns of Human Malformation, 4th ed.: K.L. Jones; W.B. Saunders Company, 1988, pp. 140–141.

# ASPHYXIATING THORACIC DYSTROPHY (ATD)

**Description** ATD is a genetic disorder of the thoracic bone structure. Major features include a small thoracic cage, shortened bones of the arms and legs, and renal dysfunction.

**Synonyms**
> Asphyxiating Thoracic Dysplasia
> Jeune Syndrome
> Thoracic-Pelvic-Phalangeal Dystrophy

**Signs and Symptoms** The characteristic bell-shaped chest cavity in the newborn leaves the infant unable to breathe properly and susceptible to pulmonary infections. Other findings include hypertension, pancreatic cysts, and polydactyly. These patients have insufficient growth of the pelvic bones, and shortened long bones of the arms and legs. Problems in respiration, and chronic nephritis leading to renal failure are the most serious complications.

Prenatal diagnosis of ATD can be made using ultrasound imaging.

**Etiology** ATD is caused by hardening of the endochondral bone in the fetal thorax. It is inherited as an autosomal recessive trait.

**Epidemiology** About 1:120,000 live births are affected. Males and females are affected in equal numbers.

**Related Disorders Chondroectodermal dysplasia** is characterized by shortened extremities and short stature. Polydactyly, fused wrists, and dystrophy of the fingernails are seen, along with lip abnormalities and heart defects.

**Metatrophic short stature,** noticed in infancy, is characterized by a long narrow thorax, flattening of the vertebral bones, and relatively short limbs. Progressive deformity of the bones of the thorax and spine causes kyphoscoliosis and a marked shortening of the trunk, resulting in short-spine short stature and severe skeletal dysplasia.

**Treatment—Standard** To facilitate breathing, the chest may be surgically expanded by removal of cartilage in the sternum or by implantation of an acrylic device to expand the rib cage. Renal dysfunction is managed with dialysis or transplantation. Genetic counseling may benefit families affected by this disorder. Other treatment is symptomatic and supportive.

**Treatment—Investigational** The Titanium Rib Project oversees the implantation of expandable ribs in children with disorders involving missing, underdeveloped, or malformed rib cages or chest walls. Contact Robert Campbell, M.D., at Santa Rosa Children's Hospital, San Antonio, Texas, for more information.

Please contact the agencies listed under Resources, below, for the most current information. Addresses and telephone numbers of these agencies, as well as of individual experts and research centers, may be found in the Master Resources List.

**Resources**

**For more information on asphyxiating thoracic dystrophy:** National Organization for Rare Disorders (NORD); NIH/National Arthritis and Musculoskeletal and Skin Diseases Information Clearinghouse; International Center for Skeletal Dysplasia; Human Growth Foundation.

**For genetic information and genetic counseling referrals:** March of Dimes Birth Defects Foundation; Alliance of Genetic Support Groups.

**References**

Mendelian Inheritance in Man, 11th ed.: V.A. McKusick; The Johns Hopkins University Press, 1994, pp. 1645–1646.

Smith's Recognizable Patterns of Human Malformation, 4th ed.: K.L. Jones; W.B. Saunders Company, 1988, pp. 292–295.

A Thoracic Expansion Technique for Jeune's Asphyxiating Thoracic Dystrophy: D.W. Todd, et al.; J. Pediatr. Surg., February 1986, vol. 21(2), pp. 161–163.

Asphyxiating Thoracic Dysplasia. Clinical, Radiological, and Pathological Information on Ten Patients: R. Oberklaid, et al.; Arch. Dis. Child, October 1977, vol. 52(10), pp. 758–765.

# BALLER-GEROLD SYNDROME

**Description** Major features of this disorder are craniosynostosis; a short, curved ulnar; and a missing or underdeveloped radius.

**Synonyms**
> Craniosynostosis–Radial Aplasia Syndrome

**Signs and Symptoms** Premature closure of cranial sutures, causing a cone-shaped head, is apparent at birth. The ulnar is short and curved, and the radius is underdeveloped or missing. Most patients are very short and have a high nasal bridge and a prominent lower jaw. Hearing loss; absent or underdeveloped thumbs and bones of the hand; abnormalities of the pelvis and spine; epicanthal folds; close-set eyes; small, abnormally developed ears; skin that sheds; and mental or motor delay may also be present. Deformities of the hands and arms may cause difficulty with fine motor skills.

**Etiology** Baller-Gerold syndrome is thought to be inherited as an autosomal recessive trait.

**Epidemiology** Males and females are affected in equal numbers. Approximately 12 cases have been reported in the medical literature.

**Related Disorders** See *Apert Syndrome; Carpenter Syndrome; Crouzon Disease.*

**Treatment—Standard** Craniosynostosis requires surgical separation of the bony sections and the lining of the seams to prevent fusion. The younger the patient, the better the results. Surgery to correct other skeletal deformities may be indicated, and physical as well as occupational therapy may improve fine motor skills.

Genetic counseling may benefit patients and their families. Other treatment is symptomatic and supportive.

**Treatment—Investigational** Please contact the agencies listed under Resources, below, for the most current information. Addresses and telephone numbers of these agencies, as well as of individual experts and research centers, may be found in the Master Resources List.

**Resources**

**For more information on Baller-Gerold syndrome:** National Organization for Rare Disorders (NORD); National Craniofacial Foundation; Forward Face; FACES—National Association for the Craniofacially Handicapped; Children's Craniofacial Association; AboutFace; Craniofacial Family Association; NIH/National Institute of Child Health and Human Development.

**For genetic information and genetic counseling referrals:** March of Dimes Birth Defects Foundation; Alliance of Genetic Support Groups.

**References**

Mendelian Inheritance in Man, 11th ed.: V.A. McKusick; The Johns Hopkins University Press, 1994, p. 1725.

Baller-Gerold Syndrome: An 11th Case of Craniosynostosis and Radial Aplasia: J.M. Boudreaux, et al.; Am. J. Med., December 1990, vol. 37(4), pp. 447–450.

Birth Defects Encyclopedia: M.L. Buyse, ed.-in-chief; Blackwell Scientific Publications, 1990, p. 2791.

Smith's Recognizable Patterns of Human Malformation, 4th ed.: K.L. Jones; W.B. Saunders Company, 1988, pp. 380–381.

# BARDET-BIEDL SYNDROME (BBS)

**Description** BBS is a recessively inherited disorder characterized by polydactyly, mental retardation, retinitis pigmentosa, obesity, and hypogonadism. Most investigators believe that this disorder actually consists of 2 distinct syndromes: Laurence-Moon (less common) and Bardet-Biedl (more common).

**Synonyms**

Adipogenital–Retinitis Pigmentosa–Polydactyly Syndrome
Bardet-Biedl Syndrome
Laurence-Moon-Bardet-Biedl Syndrome
Laurence-Moon Syndrome

**Signs and Symptoms** Polydactyly of one or more extremities is present on the lateral (small digit) side at birth. This may range from a tiny skin tag to a complete bony digit. Obesity occurs after age 1 year. Onset of retinitis pigmentosa typically begins in the 2nd half of the first decade of life. Hypogonadism, more evident in males, is accompanied by delayed onset of puberty and development of secondary sex characteristics. Boys may be sterile and develop breastlike tissue; girls may be amenorrheic and fail to develop breasts. Mental retardation is another distinguishing feature of the disorder. The presence of a progressive retinal dystrophy and at least 3 of the cardinal features confirms the diagnosis.

Other abnormalities may also occur. Kidney disease is common, including structural and functional abnormalities (microcystic and macrocystic renal disease and malfunction, horseshoe kidneys, etc.). Diabetes may also occur in adolescence. Congenital heart defects are rare.

**Etiology** BBS is inherited as an autosomal recessive trait. In 17 of 31 North American families, the gene has been assigned to chromosome 11q13. In 1 of 2 large Bedouin tribes, the gene locus is chromosome 16q. These studies suggest nonallelic genetic heterogeneity for BBS.

**Epidemiology** More than 600 cases have been reported. The incidence is greatest among Bedouin Arabs.

**Related Disorders** See *Alstrom syndrome; Prader-Willi Syndrome.*

**Weiss syndrome** is characterized by deafness, obesity, hypogonadism, and mental retardation.

**Biemond II syndrome** resembles BBS except that eye abnormalities affect the iris, not the retina.

**Treatment—Standard** Surgery may be indicated to correct polydactyly. Visual aids may help those who have retained some useful vision. A strictly controlled diet may help manage appetite and control weight. Endocrine therapy may be required in hypogonadal individuals.

**Treatment—Investigational** Research is being conducted at the Cullen Eye Institute of the Baylor College of Medicine in Houston, Texas, on the subject of inherited retinal diseases, including Bardet-Biedl syndrome. Families with at least one living affected member and both parents living are needed to participate in the program.

Please contact the agencies listed under Resources, below, for the most current information. Addresses and telephone numbers of these agencies, as well as of individual experts and research centers, may be found in the Master Resources List.

### Resources

**For more information on Bardet-Biedl syndrome:** National Organization for Rare Disorders (NORD); Laurence-Moon-Bardet-Biedl Syndrome; NIH/National Institute of Child Health and Human Development; Foundation Fighting Blindness.

**For services to persons visually impaired:** American Council of the Blind; American Foundation for the Blind; American Printing House for the Blind; National Association for Parents of the Visually Impaired; National Library Service for the Blind and Physically Handicapped; National Society to Prevent Blindness; Vision Foundation; National Association for the Visually Handicapped; Council of Families with Visual Impairment.

**For genetic information and genetic counseling referrals:** March of Dimes Birth Defects Foundation; Alliance of Genetic Support Groups.

### References

Bardet-Biedl Syndrome Is Linked to DNA Markers on Chromosome 11q and Is Genetically Heterogeneous: M. Leppert, et al.; Nat. Genet., 1994, vol. 7, 108–111.

Mendelian Inheritance in Man, 11th ed.: V.A. McKusick; The Johns Hopkins University Press, 1994, pp. 1659–1660.

Birth Defects Encyclopedia: M.L. Buyse, ed.-in-chief; Blackwell Scientific Publications, 1990, pp. 1038.

Focal Sclerosing Glomerulonephritis in a Child with Laurence-Moon-Biedl Syndrome: A.J. Barakat; Child Nephrol. Urol., 1990, vol. 10(2), pp. 109–111.

The Spectrum of Renal Disease in Laurence-Moon-Biedl Syndrome: J.D. Harnett, et al.; N. Engl. J. Med., September 8, 1988, vol. 319(10), pp. 615–618.

Retinal and Neurologic Findings in the Laurence-Moon-Bardet-Biedl Phenotype: E.L. Berson, et al.; Ophthalmology, 1986, vol. 93, pp. 1452–1456.

Renal Disease: A Sixth Cardinal Feature of the Laurence-Moon-Bardet-Biedl Syndrome: D.N. Churchill, et al.; Clin. Nephrol., 1981, vol. 16, pp. 151–154.

# BECKWITH-WIEDEMANN SYNDROME

**Description** Beckwith-Wiedemann syndrome is a rare congenital disorder characterized by macroglossia, omphalocele, macrosomia, and ear creases.

### Synonyms

Exomphalos-Macroglossia-Gigantism Syndrome.

**Signs and Symptoms** Almost all patients have macroglossia, which may cause feeding and breathing problems; it is often mistaken for congenital hypothyroidism. The majority of patients have pre- or postnatal gigantism (height greater than 90th percentile) and abdominal wall defects ranging from omphalocele to diastasis recti. Renal abnormalities, facial flame nevus, and neonatal hypoglycemia are also common findings. Ear creases or ear pits of the helix is a distinctive finding that occurs in about 75 percent of patients. A few patients may have cardiac abnormalities or mental retardation. Mild asymmetry or hemihypertrophy occurs in about 25 percent of patients. Inguinal hernia and cryptorchidism are common in males.

Both malignant and benign tumors may develop. Malignant tumors occur in 5 to 10 percent of patients. The most common types are Wilms tumor, adrenocortical carcinoma, hepatoblastoma, rhabdomyosarcoma, gonadoblastoma, and neuroblastoma. Benign tumors include adenoma of the adrenal cortex, cardiac hamartoma, umbilical myxoma, and ganglioneuroma.

As children with Beckwith-Wiedemann syndrome grow older, the characteristics of the disorder are less noticeable. Excess growth rate often slows after the first few years of life.

**Etiology** An autosomal dominant inheritance with incomplete penetrance appears to be the cause in familial cases. In some patients there is a cytogenetic abnormality of chromosome 11p15. In some patients there is a paternally derived duplication of chromosome 11p15. The genetics of this disorder is complex and the subject of continuing investigation.

**Epidemiology** Males and females are affected equally. Over 300 cases of the disorder have been reported in the medical literature since 1963.

**Related Disorders** See *Simpson-Golabi-Behmel Syndrome.*

**Treatment—Standard** Treatment may include surgery to repair omphalocele and hypospadias. If malignant or benign tumors develop, they must be treated and/or removed through surgery. Neonatal hypoglycemia, if present, is usually transient and is treated by intravenous glucose. If left untreated, hypoglycemia can be life-threatening and can cause mental retardation.

Beckwith-Wiedemann patients should be screened at 6-month intervals by abdominal ultrasound examination to monitor the growth of internal organs and tumors; and α-fetoprotein measurements should be monitored until patients are 7 years old.

Genetic counseling may benefit patients and their families. Other treatment is symptomatic and supportive.

**Treatment—Investigational** Please contact the agencies listed under Resources, below, for the most current information. Addresses and telephone numbers of these agencies, as well as of individual experts and research centers, may be found in the Master Resources List.

**Resources**

**For more information on Beckwith-Wiedemann syndrome:** National Organization for Rare Disorders (NORD); Beckwith-Wiedemann Support Network; NIH/National Institute of Child Health and Human Development; The Arc (a national organization on mental retardation).

**For genetic information and genetic counseling referrals:** March of Dimes Birth Defects Foundation; Alliance of Genetic Support Groups; Barbara Biesecker, M.D., National Center for Human Genome Research.

**References**

Beckwith-Wiedemann Syndrome: M. Elliott and E.R. Maher; J. Med. Genet., 1994, vol. 31, pp. 560–564.

Genetic Events in the Development of Wilms' Tumor: M. Copped, et al.; N. Engl. J. Med., September 1994, vol. 9(331), pp. 586–590.

Mendelian Inheritance in Man, 11th ed.: V.A. McKusick; The Johns Hopkins University Press, 1994, pp. 464–467.

Beckwith-Wiedemann Syndrome: A Demonstration of the Mechanisms Responsible for the Excess of Transmitting Females: C. Mantou, et al.; J. Med. Genet., April 1992, vol. 29(4), pp. 217–220.

Birth Defects Encyclopedia: M.L. Buyse, ed.-in-chief; Blackwell Scientific Publications, 1990, pp. 218–219.

Smith's Recognizable Patterns of Human Malformation, 4th ed.: K.L. Jones; W.B. Saunders Company, 1988, pp. 136–139.

# BLOOM SYNDROME

**Description** Bloom syndrome is an inherited disorder characterized by short stature, facial telangiectasia, photosensitivity, susceptibility to infections, and, later in life, to malignancies. Except for the susceptibility to infections and cancer, affected persons generally have good health, particularly in infancy and childhood.

**Synonyms**

Short Stature, Telangiectatic Erythema of the Face

**Signs and Symptoms** Affected infants are small at birth. Normal size is not achieved, but body proportions are normal. The face is often small and narrow, and is characteristically covered with telangiectasia during the first year. Areas of abnormal pigmentation may occur on the rest of the body. The skin is highly photosensitive, especially on the affected areas on the face. Typically there are immunologic abnormalities that lead to vulnerability to infection. In addition, almost 50 percent of patients eventually develop a wide variety of malignancies, especially leukemia and squamous cell carcinoma. Occasionally, abnormalities of the eyes, ears, hands, and feet may be present.

**Etiology** Bloom syndrome is inherited as an autosomal recessive trait. Cytogenetic characteristics include chromosomal breakage and sister chromatid exchanges.

**Epidemiology** The syndrome most often affects persons of Ashkenazic Jewish ancestry. A slight male predominance is unexplained. The recent finding of a patient with both Bloom syndrome and Prader-Willi syndrome permitted localization of the gene for Bloom syndrome on the long arm of chromosome 15. (See *Prader-Willi Syndrome.*)

**Treatment—Standard** Sunscreen should be used. Treatment is symptomatic, with antibiotics and cancer therapy as necessary.

**Treatment—Investigational** Please contact the agencies listed under Resources, below, for the most current information. Addresses and telephone numbers of these agencies, as well as of individual experts and research centers, may be found in the Master Resources List.

**Resources**

**For more information on Bloom syndrome:** National Organization for Rare Disorders (NORD); NIH/National Institute of Child Health and Human Development; Bloom's Syndrome Registry; Human Growth Foundation; National Foundation for Jewish Genetic Diseases.

**For genetic information and genetic counseling referrals:** March of Dimes Birth Defects Foundation; Alliance of Genetic Support Groups.

**References**

Bloom Syndrome and Maternal Uniparental Disomy for Chromosome 15: T. Woodage, et al.; Am. J. Hum. Genet., 1994, vol. 55, pp. 74–80.

Mendelian Inheritance in Man, 11th ed.: V.A. McKusick; The Johns Hopkins University Press, 1994, pp. 1667–1670.

Bloom Syndrome: A Mendelian Prototype of Somatic Mutational Disease: J. German; Medicine, November 1993, vol. 72(6), pp. 393–406.

Human Genetic Instability Syndromes: Single Gene Defects with Increased Risk for Cancer: M. Digweed; Toxicol. Lett., April 1993, vol. 67(1–3), pp. 259–281.

Cecil Textbook of Medicine, 19th ed.: J.B. Wyngaarden, et al., eds.; W.B. Saunders Company, 1992, pp. 944, 1049.

Long-Term Study of the Immunodeficiency of Bloom's Syndrome: N. Kundo, et al.; Acta Paediatr., January 1992, vol. 81(1), pp. 86–90.

Nelson Textbook of Pediatrics, 14th ed.: R.E. Behrman, ed.-in-chief; W.B. Saunders Company, 1992, pp. 291, 1651.

Birth Defects Encyclopedia: M.L. Buyse, ed.-in-chief; Blackwell Scientific Publications, 1990, pp. 230–231.

Clinical Dermatology, 2nd ed.: T.P. Habif, ed.; C.V. Mosby Company, 1990, p. 640.

Smith's Recognizable Patterns of Human Malformation, 4th ed.: K.L. Jones; W.B. Saunders Company, 1988, pp. 94–95.

# BLUE RUBBER BLEB NEVUS

**Description** Blue rubber bleb nevus is a very rare congenital vascular disorder that affects the skin and internal organs. The primary feature is multiple distinctive hemangiomas, which are rubbery and blisterlike. The tumors vary in color, size, shape, number, and site. They may be tender and are usually benign.

**Synonyms**

Bean Syndrome

**Signs and Symptoms** Blue rubber bleb nevus is characterized by soft, tender, elevated blue, blue-black, or purplish-red hemangiomas, some of which are present at birth. They are blood-filled and compressible, refilling immediately after compression. Hyperhidrosis may occur in the surrounding areas, and nocturnal pain is common. External hemangiomas are usually located on the upper arms or trunk. Internal hemangiomas may be found in the liver, lungs, spleen, gallbladder, kidney, and skeletal muscles. Nevi in the gastrointestinal tract may produce bleeding and chronic anemia; in the brain, they may result in hemorrhage and increased cranial pressure.

**Etiology** Blue rubber bleb nevus is inherited as an autosomal dominant trait.

**Epidemiology** Males and females are affected in equal numbers.

**Related Disorders** See *Maffucci Syndrome; von Hippel–Lindau Syndrome.*

**Treatment—Standard** Carbon dioxide laser surgery is recommended for removal of external hemangiomas. For internal hemangiomas, conventional surgery usually is necessary. Surgical resection may be required to treat growths in the gastrointestinal tract. Genetic counseling may benefit patients and their families. Other treatment is symptomatic and supportive.

**Treatment—Investigational** Please contact the agencies listed under Resources, below, for the most current information. Addresses and telephone numbers of these agencies, as well as of individual experts and research centers, may be found in the Master Resources List.

**Resources**

**For more information on blue rubber bleb nevus:** National Organization for Rare Disorders (NORD); NIH/National Institute of Arthritis, Musculoskeletal and Skin Diseases Information Clearinghouse.

**For genetic information and genetic counseling referrals:** March of Dimes Birth Defects Foundation; Alliance of Genetic Support Groups.

**References**

Mendelian Inheritance in Man, 11th ed.: V.A. McKusick; The Johns Hopkins University Press, 1994, pp. 212–213.

Blue Rubber Bleb Nevus Syndrome Presenting with Recurrence: K.S. Sandhu, et al.; Dig. Dis. Sci., February 1987, vol. 32(2), pp. 214–219.

Central Nervous System Involvement in Blue Rubber Bleb Nevus Syndrome: S. Satya-Murti, et al.; Arch. Neurol., November 1986, vol. 43(11), pp. 1184–1186.

# BORJESON SYNDROME

**Description** Major characteristics include unusual facies, mental retardation, seizures, short stature, delayed sexual development, hypotonia, and obesity. The syndrome is seen primarily in males; females typically have symptoms and signs that are less severe and more variable.

**Synonyms**

Borjeson-Forssman-Lehmann Syndrome

**Signs and Symptoms** Craniofacial features include microcephaly, prominent supraorbital ridges, ptosis, and deepset eyes, giving the face a coarse appearance. A short neck is also often present.

The majority of affected males have severe mental deficiency; in some it is mild to moderate. In affected females the range is mild to moderate. Some female carriers of the gene have normal to above average intelligence.

Delayed growth and sexual development, including micropenis and cryptorchidism, is present in all affected males, and hypogonadism is found in most. Some females experience a delay in sexual development also.

Less frequently occurring features include eye and skeletal abnormalities, tapering fingers, widely spaced toes, and hyperkyphosis.

**Etiology** Inheritance is X-linked dominant, with reduced penetrance in females. The defective gene is located in the region of Xq26–q27. A mutation in the SOX 3 may be the cause of this disorder.

**Epidemiology** The disorder is rare. Males and females are affected in equal numbers. Six family groups with the disorder have been reported in the medical literature.

**Related Disorders** See *Bardet-Biedl Syndrome; Coffin-Lowry Syndrome; Noonan Syndrome; Prader-Willi Syndrome.*

**Treatment—Standard** Treatment is symptomatic and supportive. Some affected individuals may benefit from special education and related services. Those with severe mental and physical deficiencies may need a sheltered environment. Genetic counseling will be helpful for patients and their families.

**Treatment—Investigational** Please contact the agencies listed under Resources, below, for the most current information. Addresses and telephone numbers of these agencies, as well as of individual experts and research centers, may be found in the Master Resources List.

**Resources**

For more information on Borjeson syndrome: National Organization for Rare Disorders (NORD); The Arc (a national organization on mental retardation); NIH/National Institute of Child Health and Human Development.

For genetic information and genetic counseling referrals: March of Dimes Birth Defects Foundation; Alliance of Genetic Support Groups.

**References**

Mendelian Inheritance in Man, 11th ed.: V.A. McKusick; The Johns Hopkins University Press, 1994, pp. 2317–2318.

Birth Defects Encyclopedia: M.L. Buyse, ed.-in-chief; Blackwell Scientific Publications, 1990, pp. 232–233.

Syndromes of the Head and Neck, 3rd ed.: R.J. Gorlin, et al.; Oxford University Press, 1990, pp. 351–352.

Linkage Location of Borjeson-Forssman-Lehmann Syndrome: K.D. Mathews, et al.; Am. J. Med.Gen., December 1989, vol. 34(4), pp. 470–474.

Smith's Recognizable Patterns of Human Malformation, 4th ed.: K.L. Jones, ed.; W. B. Saunders Company, 1988, p. 524.

The Borjeson-Forrsmann-Lehmann Syndrome: A.M. Dereymaeker, et al.; Clin. Gen., April 1986, vol. 29(4), pp. 317–320.

Borjeson-Forssman-Lehmann Syndrome: Further Delineation in Five Cases: H.H. Ardinger, et al.; Am. J. Med. Gen., December 1984, vol. 19(4), pp. 653–654.

The Borjeson-Forssman-Lehmann Syndrome: L.K. Robinson, et al.; Am. J. Med. Gen., July 1983, vol. 15(3), pp. 457–468.

# BOWEN HUTTERITE SYNDROME

**Description** Bowen Hutterite syndrome is a genetic disorder characterized by anomalies of the head, joints, and feet.

**Synonyms**

Bowen-Conradi Hutterite Syndrome

Bowen-Conradi Syndrome

Hutterite Syndrome, Bowen-Conradi Type

**Signs and Symptoms** Typically the affected infant presents with microcephaly, micrognathia, a prominent nose, low birth weight, unusual facial features, rocker-bottom feet, joint limitations (especially of the hip), and failure to thrive. Poor sucking and recurrent pneumonia are common. Other symptoms include cryptorchidism, inguinal hernia, camptodactyly, clouding of the cornea, anomalies of the central nervous and renal systems, and underdeveloped nails of the fingers and toes.

**Etiology** Bowen Hutterite syndrome is inherited as an autosomal recessive trait. All reported cases of this disorder have been the result of inbreeding.

**Epidemiology** Males and females are affected in equal numbers. Of the approximately 20 reported cases, most have come from the Hutterite community.

**Related Disorders** See *Cerebro-Oculo-Facio-Skeletal Syndrome.*

**Chromosome 18, Trisomy 18** is caused by the presence of an extra chromosome 18. Symptoms include slowed growth, failure to thrive, cryptorchidism, poor sucking ability, rocker-bottom feet, an unusual face with a small head, and clenched fists with overlapping fingers. Abnormalities of the kidneys and heart may also occur.

**Treatment—Standard** Treatment of Bowen Hutterite syndrome is symptomatic and supportive. Gastrostomy may be required in some cases. Genetic counseling may benefit families of patients with this disorder.

**Treatment—Investigational** Please contact the agencies listed under Resources, below, for the most current information. Addresses and telephone numbers of these agencies, as well as of individual experts and research centers, may be found in the Master Resources List.

**Resources**

**For more information on Bowen Hutterite syndrome:** National Organization for Rare Disorders (NORD); NIH/National Institute of Child Health and Human Development.

**For genetic information and genetic counseling referrals:** March of Dimes Birth Defects Foundation; Alliance of Genetic Support Groups.

**References**

Mendelian Inheritance in Man, 11th ed.: V.A. McKusick; The Johns Hopkins University Press, 1994, p. 1671.

Birth Defects Encyclopedia: M.L. Buyse, ed.-in-chief; Blackwell Scientific Publications, 1990, pp. 883–884.

The Bowen-Conradi Syndrome: An Autosomal Recessive Syndrome of Microcephaly, Micrognathia, Low Birth Weight, and Joint Deformities: A.G. Hunter et al.; Am. J. Med. Genet., 1979 vol. 3(3), pp. 201–204.

# BRANCHIO-OCULO-FACIAL SYNDROME

**Description** The hallmarks of the syndrome are gill-like hemangiomatous clefts behind and below the ears; a protruding, narrow, ridged philtrum; and cleft lip/cleft palate.

**Synonyms**

Hemangiomatous Branchial Clefts–Lip Pseudocleft Syndrome

Lip Pseudocleft–Hemangiomatous Branchial Cyst Syndrome

**Signs and Symptoms** Besides the hallmark features, other characteristics include some ear malformation and possible hearing loss, nasal duct obstruction, a broad nasal bridge, and hypertelorism. Ocular deficits range from anophthalmos to cataracts, strabismus, and retinal and optic nerve abnormalities. The infant's birth weight may be low, and the child's hair may start graying before the teen years.

**Etiology** The syndrome is transmitted through autosomal dominant genes. In most cases at least one parent has a deformity of the lip or mouth, and premature graying of the hair.

**Epidemiology** The syndrome is very rare. Males and females are affected in equal numbers.

**Related Disorders** See *Cerebro-Costo-Mandibular Syndrome; Cerebro-Oculo-Facio-Skeletal Syndrome; Oral-Facial-Digital Syndrome.*

**Treatment—Standard** Reconstructive surgery will repair facial deformities and obstructed nasal ducts, and correct strabismus. Genetic counseling is recommended for patients and their families. Other treatment is symptomatic and supportive.

**Treatment—Investigational** Please contact the agencies listed under Resources, below, for the most current information. Addresses and telephone numbers of these agencies, as well as of individual experts and research centers, may be found in the Master Resources List.

**Resources**

**For more information on branchio-oculo-facial syndrome:** National Organization for Rare Disorders (NORD); FACES—National Association for the Craniofacially Handicapped; National Craniofacial Foundation; Let's Face It; National Foundation for Facial Reconstruction.

**For genetic information and genetic counseling referrals:** Alliance of Genetic Support Groups; March of Dimes Birth Defects Foundation;

**References**

Mendelian Inheritance in Man, 11th ed.: V.A. McKusick; The Johns Hopkins University Press, 1994, pp. 221–222.

Syndromes of the Head and Neck, 3rd ed.: R.J. Gorlin, et al.; Oxford University Press, 1990, pp. 728–729.

# BRANCHIO-OTO-RENAL SYNDROME

**Description** The disorder is characterized by preauricular pits or tags, branchial fistulas and cysts, hearing loss, and renal dysplasia.

**Synonyms**

Melnick-Fraser Syndrome

**Signs and Symptoms** The majority of patients with branchio-oto-renal syndrome have some type of hearing loss, either sensorineural or conductive, or both. The degree of loss varies from mild to severe. Preauricular pits and tags are common, as are anomalies of the outer, middle, and inner ear. A branchial fistula and an opening, cyst, or mass in the tonsil area are often present.

Kidney abnormalities, ranging from mild to severe, are found in approximately 66 percent of patients. These abnormalities may include an unusually shaped kidney, duplication of the collecting system, or renal agenesis.

Other, less common, features include cleft palate and mental retardation.

**Etiology** The syndrome is inherited as an autosomal dominant trait.

**Epidemiology** Symptoms and signs can first appear from early childhood to the young adult years. About 1:40,000 persons are afflicted. Occurrence in the profoundly deaf is about 2 percent. Males and females are affected in equal numbers.

**Related Disorders** See *Branchio-Oculo-Facial Syndrome.*

**Treatment—Standard** When structural defects of the ear are present, surgery may be indicated. Patients may require hearing aids. Severe kidney problems may warrant surgery or kidney transplantation. Genetic counseling will benefit patients and their families. Other treatment is symptomatic and supportive.

**Treatment—Investigational** W.J. Kimberling, Ph.D., and Shrawan Kumar, Ph.D., of Boys Town National Research Hospital are conducting research to identify and describe the branchio-oto-renal syndrome gene located on chromosome 8. Volunteers are needed and will be asked to provide a family history, medical records, and a small blood sample. Selected individuals may be asked to have certain routine medical tests performed to provide needed data. The researchers will pay for or reimburse any expenses resulting from these requests. Please contact Tom Fowler.

Please contact the agencies listed under Resources, below, for the most current information. Addresses and telephone numbers of these agencies, as well as of individual experts and research centers, may be found in the Master Resources List.

**Resources**

**For more information on branchio-oto-renal syndrome:** National Organization for Rare Disorders (NORD); American Society for Deaf Children; National Kidney Foundation; American Kidney Fund; NIH/National Institute of Diabetes, Digestive and Kidney Diseases.

**For genetic information and genetic counseling referrals:** March of Dimes Birth Defects Foundation; Alliance of Genetic Support Groups.

**References**

Mendelian Inheritance in Man, 11th ed.: V.A. McKusick; The Johns Hopkins University Press, 1994, pp. 222–223.

Birth Defects Encyclopedia: M.L. Buyse, ed.-in-chief; Blackwell Scientific Publications, 1990, pp. 243–244.

The Branchio-Oto-Renal Syndrome: Report of Two Family Groups: M. Raspino, et al.; J. Laryngol. Otol., February 1988, vol. 102(2), pp. 138–141.

Smith's Recognizable Patterns of Human Malformation, 4th ed.: K.L. Jones; W.B. Saunders Company, 1988, p. 206.

The Branchio-Oto-Renal (BOR) Syndrome: Report of Bilateral Renal Agenesis in Three Sibs: R. Carmi, et al.; Am. J. Med. Genet., April 1983, vol. 14(4), pp. 625–627.

# C SYNDROME

**Description** C syndrome is characterized by craniofacial abnormalities, joints that are bent or in a fixed position, and loose skin. All recorded patients except one have had mental retardation.

**Synonyms**

Opitz Trigonocephaly Syndrome

Trigonocephaly C Syndrome

**Signs and Symptoms** Trigonocephaly is the distinguishing feature of C syndrome. Other characteristics include a broad nasal bridge with a short nose, epicanthus, a deeply furrowed palate, abnormalities of the outer ear, strabismus, fixed or dislocated joints, and loose skin. Secondary characteristics include abnormalities of the sternum, lower jaw, heart, and renal and pulmonary systems; hypotonia; facial palsy; webbed fingers and toes; short limbs; cryptorchidism; and/or seizures.

**Etiology** C syndrome is thought to be inherited as an autosomal recessive trait.

**Epidemiology** Males and females are affected in equal numbers. Approximately 25 cases have been reported.

**Related Disorders** Symptoms of the following disorders can be similar to those of C syndrome. Comparisons may be useful for a differential diagnosis.

**Trigonocephaly autosomal dominant type** is caused by premature closure of the bones, which can result in compression of the brain. A small head and skin tags on the ears have been found in several cases. Mental development is normal in all cases. This disorder affects males 5 times more often than females.

**Trigonocephaly autosomal recessive type** causes malformations in the olfactory nerves. Multiple affected siblings have been reported.

**Trigonocephaly X-linked type** causes short stature and developmental delay. In addition, related patients have had a closed space between the bones at the back of the skull, a narrow forehead, ocular hypertelorism, a small head circumference, low weight, and slow mental and physical development.

Typically the borders or joints of the skull close between the ages of 28 and 32 years. Patients with trigonocephaly with short stature and developmental delay have closure between the ages of 2 and 3 years. The 5 related patients described in the medical literature were all males.

**Treatment—Standard** Severe trigonocephaly requires surgery to relieve the pressure on the brain and to cosmetically improve facial appearance. Other treatment is symptomatic and supportive. Genetic counseling may benefit patients and their families.

**Treatment—Investigational** Please contact the agencies listed under Resources, below, for the most current information. Addresses and telephone numbers of these agencies, as well as of individual experts and research centers, may be found in the Master Resources List.

**Resources**

For more information on C syndrome: National Organization for Rare Disorders (NORD); National Craniofacial Foundation; FACES—National Association for the Craniofacially Handicapped; NIH/National Institute of Child Health and Human Development.

For genetic information and genetic counseling referrals: March of Dimes Birth Defects Foundation; Alliance of Genetic Support Groups.

**References**

Mendelian Inheritance in Man, 11th ed.: V.A. McKusick; The Johns Hopkins University Press, 1994, pp. 1674–1675.

Birth Defects Encyclopedia: M.L. Buyse, ed.-in-chief; Blackwell Scientific Publications, 1990, pp. 251–252.

"C" Trigonocephaly Syndrome: Clinical Variability and Possibility of Surgical Treatment: F. Lalatta, et al.; Am. J. Med. Genet., December 1990, vol. 37(4), pp. 451–456.

Modification in the Surgical Correction of Trigonocephaly: A.M. Sadove, et al.; Plast. Reconstr. Surg., June 1990, vol. 85(6). pp. 853–858.

# CAMPTOMELIC SYNDROME

**Description** Camptomelic syndrome is a congenital skeletal disorder characterized by angulation and bowing of long bones as well as by other skeletal anomalies.

**Synonyms**

Camptomelic Dwarfism

**Signs and Symptoms** The osteochondrodysplasia is characterized by bowed tibia and angular-shaped long bones of the legs. Eleven sets of ribs instead of the usual 12 may be present. Underdeveloped pelvis and scapula, flat facies with ocular hypertelorism, and micrognathia are also common. Respiratory distress due to insufficient space for lung growth in the underdeveloped rib cage is the most serious symptom; the condition is frequently fatal.

The bowed bones of the legs are short and unusually wide. Premature closure of the fontanelle causes the formation of 3 cranial lobes and a cloverleaf appearance to the head. Hydrocephalus, talipes equinovarus, underdeveloped lungs, and cardiac and renal abnormalities may also occur.

Complete sex-reversal is common; of the 50 reported chromosomal male patients, more than two-thirds are phenotypically female.

**Etiology** Camptomelic syndrome is inherited as an autosomal dominant disorder. It has been recently established that the sex-reversal and other abnormalities are caused by a mutation in the SRY-related gene (SOX 9).

**Epidemiology** Approximately 100 cases of this disorder have been reported.

**Related Disorders** See *Achondroplasia; Hypophosphatasia; Osteogenesis Imperfecta.*

**Treatment—Standard** Treatment of respiratory problems consists of mechanical or physical breathing assistance. Orthopedic medical care including surgery may help correct some of the more serious bone deformities.

Genetic counseling may benefit patients and their families. Other treatment is symptomatic and supportive.

**Treatment—Investigational** The Titanium Rib Project oversees the implantation of expandable ribs in children with disorders involving missing, underdeveloped, or malformed rib cages or chest walls. Contact Robert Campbell, M.D., at Santa Rosa Children's Hospital, San Antonio, Texas, for more information.

Please contact the agencies listed under Resources, below, for the most current information. Addresses and telephone numbers of these agencies, as well as of individual experts and research centers, may be found in the Master Resources List.

**Resources**

For more information on camptomelic syndrome: National Organization for Rare Disorders (NORD); International Center for Skeletal Dysplasia; NIH/National Arthritis and Musculoskeletal and Skin Diseases Information Clearinghouse; Short Stature Foundation; Human Growth Foundation.

For genetic information and genetic counseling referrals: March of Dimes Birth Defects Foundation; Alliance of Genetic Support Groups.

**References**

Autosomal Sex Reversal and Camptomelic Dysplasia Are Caused by Mutations in and Around the SRY-Related Gene SOX9: T. Wagner, et al.; Cell, 1994, vol. 79, pp. 1111–1120.

Mendelian Inheritance in Man, 11th ed.: V.A. McKusick; The Johns Hopkins University Press, 1994, pp. 1677–1678.

Birth Defects Encyclopedia: M.L. Buyse, M.D., ed.-in-chief; Blackwell Scientific Publications, 1990, pp. 252–253.

Camptomelic Dysplasia: R.I. Macpherson, et al.; Pediatr. Radiol., 1989, vol. 20(1–2), pp. 90–93.

Dental Abnormalities Associated with Camptomelic Syndrome: Case Report: G.L. Roberts, et al.; Pediatr. Dent., March 1989, vol. 11(1), pp. 43–46.

Smith's Recognizable Patterns of Human Malformation, 4th ed.: K.L. Jones; W.B. Saunders Company, 1988, p. 296.

Bronchoscopic Evaluation of Airway Obstruction in Camptomelic Dysplasia: R. Grad, et al.; Pediatr. Pulmonol., September–October 1987, vol. 3(5), pp. 364–367.

# CARDIO-FACIO-CUTANEOUS SYNDROME

**Description** The syndrome is characterized by mental retardation and multiple congenital anomalies, which include ectodermal abnormalities, cardiac defects, and characteristic facial features.

**Synonyms**

Facio-Cardio-Cutaneous Syndrome

**Signs and Symptoms** Craniofacial characteristics include an unusually high forehead, downward slanting palpebral fissures, hypoplasia of the supraorbital ridges, depressed bridge of the nose, and angled-back ears with prominent cartilage on the outer ear.

Skin abnormalities vary from hyperkeratosis to ichthyosis. The most common heart defects are pulmonary valve stenosis and atrial septal defect. In some cases the following are present: growth failure; mental retardation; sparse, curly hair; hydrocephaly; and hemangiomatosis.

**Etiology** All of the reported cases of cardio-facio-cutaneous syndrome have been sporadic. None of the parents have been affected, and consanguinity has not been a factor.

**Epidemiology** Approximately 16 cases, in the United States, Australia, and Europe, have been reported in the medical literature. Males and females are affected in equal numbers.

**Related Disorders** See *Hydrocephalus; Ichthyosis.*

**Treatment—Standard** Therapy is symptomatic and supportive, and appropriate for the specific associated conditions.

**Treatment—Investigational** Please contact the agencies listed under Resources, below, for the most current information. Addresses and telephone numbers of these agencies, as well as of individual experts and research centers, may be found in the Master Resources List.

**Resources**

**For more information on cardio-facio-cutaneous syndrome:** National Organization for Rare Disorders (NORD); Forward Face; Cardio-Facial-Cutaneous Syndrome Support Network; Foundation for Ichthyosis and Related Skin Types; American Heart Association; Magic Foundation for Children's Growth; Human Growth Foundation; The Arc (a national organization on mental retardation); NIH/National Institute of Child Health and Human Development.

**For genetic information and genetic counseling referrals:** March of Dimes Birth Defects Foundation; Alliance of Genetic Support Groups.

**References**

Mendelian Inheritance in Man, 11th ed.: V.A. McKusick; The Johns Hopkins University Press, 1994, pp. 253–254.

Birth Defects Encyclopedia: M.L. Buyse, ed.-in-chief; Blackwell Scientific Publications, 1990, p. 282.

# CARPENTER SYNDROME

**Description** Carpenter syndrome is a rare genetic disorder in which characteristic anomalies of the head, hands, and genitalia occur. Mental retardation is also present in affected individuals.

**Synonyms**

Acrocephalopolysyndactyly II

**Signs and Symptoms** Carpenter syndrome is a form of craniosynostosis. In addition to skull deformities, brachydactyly with webbing, duplication of the big toe, and cryptorchidism are present. Down-slanting eyes, a flattened nose, low-set ears, and mandibular hypoplasia are characteristic features, along with obesity and cardiac anomalies. Mental retardation is common, but intelligence is normal in some patients.

**Etiology** Carpenter syndrome is inherited as an autosomal recessive trait.

**Epidemiology** Males and females are affected in equal numbers.

**Related Disorders** See *Oral-Facial-Digital Syndrome; Apert Syndrome; Nager Syndrome; Goodman Syndrome.*

**Treatment—Standard** Early craniofacial surgery may relieve intracranial pressure and limit the severity of mental retardation, as well as correct the characteristic facial anomalies. Additional surgical intervention is indicated for the correction of cardiac and digital abnormalities. Genetic counseling is advised.

**Treatment—Investigational** Please contact the agencies listed under Resources, below, for the most current information. Addresses and telephone numbers of these agencies, as well as of individual experts and research centers, may be found in the Master Resources List.

**Resources**

For more information on Carpenter syndrome: National Organization for Rare Disorders (NORD); NIH/National Institute of Child Health and Human Development; FACES—National Association for the Craniofacially Handicapped; National Craniofacial Foundation; Institute of Reconstructive Plastic Surgery.

For genetic information and genetic counseling referrals: March of Dimes Birth Defects Foundation; Alliance of Genetic Support Groups.

**References**

Mendelian Inheritance in Man, 11th ed.: V.A. McKusick; The Johns Hopkins University Press, 1994, p. 1577.

Acrocephalopolysyndactyly Type II Carpenter Syndrome: Clinical Spectrum and Attempt at Unification with Goodman and Summit Syndromes: D.M. Cohen; Am. J. Med. Genet., October 1987, vol. 28(2), pp. 311–324.

Carpenter Syndrome: Natural History and Clinical Spectrum: L.K. Robinson; Am. J. Med. Genet., March 1985, vol. 20(3), pp. 461–469.

# CARTILAGE-HAIR HYPOPLASIA

**Description** Cartilage-hair hypoplasia is a progressive genetic disorder characterized by short-limbed short stature caused by abnormal development of long-bone cartilage.

**Synonyms**

Metaphyseal Chondrodysplasia, McKusick Type

**Signs and Symptoms** Cartilage-hair hypoplasia primarily affects the peripheral bones, resulting in short-limbed small stature. Adult height is about 120 cm. The range of symptoms is wide and includes abnormalities of the spine; hypermobile fingers; and fine, thin hair on the head, eyebrows, and eyelashes. Decreased cell-mediated immunity and increase rate of malignancy have been described. Hirschsprung disease has also occurred in some patients (see *Hirschsprung Disease*).

**Etiology** The disorder is inherited through an autosomal recessive gene, which has been assigned to 9p21–p13.

**Epidemiology** Cartilage-hair hypoplasia is rare. It is most often diagnosed in Finland, although it was first described in the Amish communities of the United States. Males and females are affected equally.

**Related Disorders** See *Hypochondroplasia; Metaphyseal Chondrodysplasia, Schmid Type.*

Metaphyseal chondrodysplasia, Jansen type (chondrodysplasia, Murk-Jansen type) is another type of short-limbed small stature, which is inherited through an autosomal dominant pattern. Distortion of the spine, pelvis, and lower legs is present. The skull bones, including those of the inner ear, are sclerosed, causing deafness. Patients also exhibit a receding chin and abnormally short fingers. This disorder is often associated with asymptomatic hypercalcemia and hypophosphatemia. The etiology is a constitutively active mutant PTH-PTHrP receptor.

**Treatment—Standard** Some patients may benefit from physiotherapy and orthopedic treatment. Genetic counseling may be helpful for patients and their families.

**Treatment—Investigational** Please contact the agencies listed under Resources, below, for the most current information. Addresses and telephone numbers of these agencies, as well as of individual experts and research centers, may be found in the Master Resources List.

**Resources**

For more information on cartilage-hair hypoplasia: National Organization for Rare Disorders (NORD); Human Growth Foundation; Little People of America; Parents of Dwarfed Children; Short Stature Foundation.

For genetic information and genetic counseling referrals: March of Dimes Birth Defects Foundation; Alliance of Genetic Support Groups.

**References**

Cartilage-Hair Hypoplasia: O. Makitie, et al.; J. Med. Genet., 1995, vol. 32, pp. 39–43.

A Constitutively Active Mutant PTH-PTHrP Receptor in Jansen-Type Metaphyseal Chondrodysplasia: E. Schipani, et al.; Science, 1995, vol. 268, pp. 98–100.

Mendelian Inheritance in Man, 11th ed.: V.A. McKusick; The Johns Hopkins University Press, 1994, pp. 1993–1994.

Metaphyseal Chondrodysplasia, Schmid Type: Clinical and Radiographic Delineation with a Review of the Literature: R.S. Lachman, et al.; Pediatr. Radiol., 1988, vol. 18(2), pp. 93–102.

The Jansen Type of Metaphyseal Chondrodysplasia: Confirmation of Dominant Inheritance and Review of Radiographic Manifestations in the Newborn and Adult: J. Charrow, et al.; Am. J. Med. Genet., June 1984, vol. 18(2), pp. 321–327.

# CAUDAL REGRESSION SYNDROME

**Description** The syndrome is characterized by abnormal development of the fetal caudal region, resulting in a wide range of abnormalities. Neurologic impairment may occur in severe cases.

**Synonyms**

> Caudal Dysplasia Sequence
> Sacral Agenesis, Congenital

**Signs and Symptoms** Abnormalities associated with this disorder include agenesis or hypoplasia of the lower vertebrae, pelvis, and coccyx; paralysis or numbness of the legs; urinary and fecal incontinence; dislocation of the hip; permanently fixed joints; underdeveloped muscles; clubfoot; intestinal volvulus; multiple cysts or partial fusion of the kidneys; displacement of the external genitalia; and hypospadias.

Abnormalities found less commonly include hydrocephaly; partial or complete absence of the pituitary; cleft palate or lip; micrognathia; cardiac defects; imperforate anus; extra digits.

Ultrasound will detect the syndrome during the 2nd trimester of pregnancy.

**Etiology** The cause is not known in most cases. Autosomal dominant inheritance has been suggested in some instances. Nearly 16 percent of affected persons have had diabetic mothers.

**Epidemiology** Males and females are affected in equal numbers. It is estimated that approximately 3:100,000 newborns will have the syndrome.

**Related Disorders** See *Sirenomelia Sequence.*

**Treatment—Standard** Surgery can correct or improve such conditions as imperforate anus, hydrocephaly, cleft palate or lip, and extra digits. Orthopedic devices may be used to help problems of the hip, back, and legs. Other treatment is symptomatic and supportive.

**Treatment—Investigational** Please contact the agencies listed under Resources, below, for the most current information. Addresses and telephone numbers of these agencies, as well as of individual experts and research centers, may be found in the Master Resources List.

**Resources**

**For more information on caudal regression syndrome:** National Organization for Rare Disorders (NORD); NIH/National Institute of Child Health and Human Development.

**For genetic information and genetic counseling referrals:** March of Dimes Birth Defects Foundation; Alliance of Genetic Support Groups.

**References**

Mendelian Inheritance in Man, 11th ed.: V.A. McKusick; The Johns Hopkins University Press, 1994, pp. 1377–1378.

Birth Defects Encyclopedia: M.L. Buyse, ed.-in-chief; Blackwell Scientific Publications, 1990, pp. 296–297.

Partial Transposition of the Penis and Scrotum with Anterior Urethral Diverticulum in a Child Born with the Caudal Regression Syndrome: A.M. Shanberg, et al.; J. Urol., October 1989, vol. 424, pp. 1060–1062.

Smith's Recognizable Patterns of Human Malformation, 4th ed.: K.L. Jones; W.B. Saunders Company, 1988, p. 575.

# CEREBRO-COSTO-MANDIBULAR SYNDROME

**Description** Cerebro-costo-mandibular syndrome is a rare genetic disorder in which severe micrognathia and palatal defects are present, along with multiple rib abnormalities. Mental retardation may also occur.

**Synonyms**

> Rib Gap Defects with Micrognathia

**Signs and Symptoms** The syndrome is characterized by severe micrognathia, glossoptosis, abnormalities of the palate, and multiple rib defects, particularly between the 3rd and 7th pairs. The thorax is small and bell-shaped with gaps between the posterior ossified and anterior cartilaginous ribs. Rarely, hearing loss may result from a defect of the middle ear, and speech development may be delayed. Moderate-to-severe mental retardation occurs in about one-third of patients. Rib fractures and pseudarthrosis of the ribs usually improve with age.

The infant's difficulty with nipple feeding may lead to failure to thrive. Respiratory distress may be a significant problem, and increased susceptibility to respiratory infections may be life-threatening. Pneumonia and otitis media often recur. Almost half of the children die in the first year.

**Etiology** The inheritance pattern is not established. The syndrome appears to have been transmitted through autosomal recessive inheritance in one family, and as an autosomal dominant trait in others.

**Epidemiology** Males and females tend to be affected in equal numbers.

**Related Disorders** See *Pierre Robin Syndrome.*

**Treatment—Standard** Intensive medical intervention may be necessary for respiratory distress, feeding difficulty, and respiratory infections. Surgical correction of the palate may be required. Genetic counseling is advisable.

**Treatment—Investigational** Please contact the agencies listed under Resources, below, for the most current information. Addresses and telephone numbers of these agencies, as well as of individual experts and research centers, may be found in the Master Resources List.

**Resources**

**For more information on cerebro-costo-mandibular syndrome:** National Organization for Rare Disorders (NORD); National Craniofacial Foundation; FACES—National Association for the Craniofacially Handicapped; Craniofacial Family Association; NIH/National Institute of Child Health and Human Development.

**For genetic information and genetic counseling referrals:** March of Dimes Birth Defects Foundation; Alliance of Genetic Support Groups.

**References**

Mendelian Inheritance in Man, 11th ed.: V.A. McKusick; The Johns Hopkins University Press, 1994, p. 279.

Smith's Recognizable Patterns of Human Malformation, 4th ed.: K.L. Jones; W.B. Saunders Company, 1988, pp. 534–535.

Cerebrocostomandibular Syndrome: Case Report and Literature Review: K.G. Smith, et al.; Clin. Pediatr. (Phila.), April 1985, vol. 24(4), pp. 223–225.

# CHARGE ASSOCIATION

**Description** CHARGE is the acronym for a very rare disorder that results from several defects in early fetal development. A minimum of 4 of the following characteristics are necessary for the diagnosis: (**C**)oloboma of the eye; (**H**)eart defects; (**A**)tresia of the choanae; (**R**)etardation of growth and development, and central nervous system abnormalities; (**G**)enital hypoplasia in males; and (**E**)ar abnormalities and loss of hearing.

**Signs and Symptoms** Coloboma is present in over three-fourths of CHARGE patients. About 80 percent of affected individuals have cardiac abnormalities. These include ventricular and atrial septal defects, patent ductus arteriosus, and tetralogy of Fallot. Choanal atresia occurs in over half of patients, and retarded growth and development as well as mental deficiency and/or central nervous system abnormalities are present in about 90 percent. Approximately three-fourths of males with CHARGE association have microphallus and testicular hypoplasia. Close to 90 percent of patients have ear abnormalities: the ears may be short, wide, and cup-shaped, and may differ in shape. There may be mild-to-severe hearing loss.

In addition to those anomalies included in the CHARGE acronym, affected infants may also have feeding difficulties, microcephaly, micrognathia, cleft lip and palate, and tracheoesophageal fistulas. There may also be rib and renal anomalies. Some patients have features of DiGeorge syndrome; of 18 patients with CHARGE association, one was reported to have a 22q11.2 deletion characteristic of DiGeorge syndrome (see ***DiGeorge Syndrome).***

**Etiology** Most instances are sporadic. The etiology is heterogeneous. In some cases the disorder is transmitted as an autosomal recessive trait. Recurrences of certain abnormalities have been observed within families.

**Epidemiology** CHARGE association is very rare, affecting only approximately 200 persons in the United States. Females are affected twice as often as males.

**Treatment—Standard** A full heart evaluation is recommended for all children with coloboma or choanal atresia in whom CHARGE association is a possible diagnosis. All patients with conotruncal or aortic arch defects and abnormalities in other parts of the body should be evaluated for CHARGE association and DiGeorge syndrome.

Surgery to correct cardiac and other anomalies may be appropriate.

**Treatment—Investigational** Please contact the agencies listed under Resources, below, for the most current information. Addresses and telephone numbers of these agencies, as well as of individual experts and research centers, may be found in the Master Resources List.

**Resources**

**For more information on CHARGE association:** National Organization for Rare Disorders (NORD); NIH/National Institute of Child Health and Human Development.

**For genetic information and genetic counseling referrals:** March of Dimes Birth Defects Foundation; Alliance of Genetic Support Groups.

**References**

Mendelian Inheritance in Man, 11th ed.: V.A. McKusick; The Johns Hopkins University Press, 1994, pp. 1700–1701.

Smith's Recognizable Patterns of Human Malformation, 4th ed.: K.L. Jones; W.B. Saunders Company, 1988, pp. 606–608.

Familial Charge Syndrome: Clinical Report with Autopsy Findings: L.A. Metlay, et al.; Am. J. Med. Genet., March 1987, vol. 26(3), pp. 577–581.

The Pattern of Cardiovascular Malformation in Charge Association: A.E. Lin, et al.; Am. J. Dis. Child., September 1987, vol. 141(9), pp. 1010–1013.

The CHARGE Association: How Well Can They Do?: E. Goldson, et al.; Am. J. Dis. Child., September 1986, vol. 140(9), pp. 918–921.

# CHROMOSOME 3, MONOSOMY 3P2

**Description** Chromosome 3, monosomy 3p2 is a very rare chromosomal disorder in which the distal portion of the short arm of chromosome 3 is missing. Major symptoms include failure of the fetus to grow during pregnancy and severely delayed growth of the child after birth. Mental retardation may also occur.

**Synonyms**

> Chromosome 3, Distal 3p Monosomy
> Chromosome 3, Deletion of Distal 3p
> Monosomy 3p2

**Signs and Symptoms** Major symptoms include failure of the fetus to grow during pregnancy and/or severely delayed growth of the child after birth. Other symptoms include mental retardation, severe to profound developmental delays, and craniofacial dysmorphism. The facial abnormalities most frequently seen in individuals with chromosome 3, monosomy 3p2 include microcephaly, hypertrichosis, and eyebrows that grow together (synophrys).

Other symptoms include a triangular face, an abnormally long head (dolichocephaly), slightly raised areas on the frontal bones above the eyes (frontal bossing), and micrognathia. Ptosis, hypertelorism, and epicanthal folds may also be present. Symptoms of this disorder may also include low-set and malformed ears; a broad, flat nose; down-turned mouth; finger abnormalities; pectus excavatum; and scoliosis. Hypogenitalia has been reported in males with chromosome 3, monosomy 3p2.

The following congenital malformations have been present in 1 or 2 cases of chromosome 3, monosomy 3p2: cardiac defects, hiatal hernia, optic atrophy, fetal lobulation of the kidneys, renal dysplasia, and hypoplastic clavicles.

Prenatal diagnosis of chromosome 3, monosomy 3p2 is possible by chorionic villus sampling or amniocentesis.

**Etiology** The exact cause of the chromosomal deletion is not known. The majority of documented cases may be the result of a complex rearrangement of the chromosomes of a parent. This rearrangement occurs when a portion of chromosome 3 breaks off from one arm of the chromosome, then attaches to the other arm of the same chromosome. The result is that one arm of the chromosome has more than the normal amount of genetic material (duplication), while the other arm of the chromosome is missing genetic material (deficiency). This rearrangement is usually harmless to the carrier but is associated with a high risk of unbalanced chromosomes in the carrier's offspring and abnormal development.

In some cases, chromosome 3, monosomy 3p2 may be the result of de novo deletion. In these cases it is unlikely that subsequent offspring would have the same chromosomal abnormality.

**Epidemiology** Chromosome 3, monosomy 3p2 affects males and females in equal numbers. There have been approximately 12 cases reported in the medical literature.

**Treatment—Standard** Treatment is symptomatic and supportive. Special education, physical therapy, and other medical, social, or vocational services may benefit the patient, and are often necessary for the child to reach his or her full potential. Genetic counseling may benefit affected individuals and their families.

**Treatment—Investigational** Please contact the agencies listed under Resources, below, for the most current information. Addresses and telephone numbers of these agencies, as well as of individual experts and research centers, may be found in the Master Resources List.

**Resources**

**For more information on chromosome 3, monosomy 3p2:** National Organization for Rare Disorders (NORD); Chromosome Deletion Outreach; The Arc (a national organization on mental retardation); NIH/National Institute of Child Health and Human Development.

**For genetic information and genetic counseling referrals:** March of Dimes Birth Defects Foundation; Alliance of Genetic Support Groups.

**References**

Birth Defects Encyclopedia: M.L Buyse, ed.-in-chief; Blackwell Scientific Publications, 1990, p. 332.

Loss of the 3p25.3 Band Is Critical in the Manifestation of Del(3p) Syndrome: Karyotype-Phenotype Correlation in Cases with Deficiency of the Distal Portion of the Short Arm of Chromosome 3: J. Narahara, et. al.; Am. J. Med. Genet., February 1990, vol. 35(2), pp. 269–273.

# CHROMOSOME 4 RING

**Description** Chromosome 4 ring is a rare chromosomal disorder in which the patient has a breakage of chromosome 4 at both ends, and the ends of the chromosome join together to form a ring. The amount of genetic material lost at the 2 ends of the chromosome can vary. As a result, a patient with very little absent genetic material may have fewer symptoms than an individual with a significant part of the chromosomal ends missing.

Chromosome 4 ring is usually detected at birth or during prenatal testing.

**Synonyms**

Ring Chromosome 4

**Signs and Symptoms** The symptoms seen most often in individuals with chromosome 4 ring are low birth weight, growth and developmental retardation, and microcephaly. Micrognathia, a broad nose, and cleft plate may also be present. Clinodactyly, ptosis, mental retardation, hypospadias, and abnormal ears have also been found in some affected individuals. Speech is often delayed along with other developmental skills.

**Etiology** The cause is unknown. Most chromosomal deletions occur de novo. The parents of the affected child typically have normal chromosomes and a very low probability of having another child with a chromosomal abnormality. The majority of cases of this disorder have been a deletion of the sections of the 4th chromosome identified as 4p16 and 4q35, or 4q36.

**Epidemiology** Chromosome 4 ring affects males and females in equal numbers.

**Treatment—Standard** Special education as well as speech therapy will benefit children with chromosome 4 ring. Genetic counseling may benefit patients and their families. Other treatment is symptomatic and supportive.

**Treatment—Investigational** Please contact the agencies listed under Resources, below, for the most current information. Addresses and telephone numbers of these agencies, as well as of individual experts and research centers, may be found in the Master Resources List.

**Resources**

**For more information on chromosome 4 ring:** National Organization for Rare Disorders (NORD); Chromosome Deletion Outreach; NIH/National Institute of Child Health and Human Development; The Arc (a national organization on mental retardation).

**For genetic information and genetic counseling referrals:** March of Dimes Birth Defects Foundation; Alliance of Genetic Support Groups.

**References**

Birth Defects Encyclopedia: M.L Buyse, ed.-in-chief; Blackwell Scientific Publications, 1990, pp. 336–337.

Ring Chromosome 4 in a Child with Duodenal Atresia: F. Halal, et al.; Am. J. Med. Genet., September 1990, vol. 37(1), pp. 79–82.

# CHROMOSOME 6 RING

**Description** Chromosome 6 ring causes mental and psychomotor retardation, growth delays, and craniofacial anomalies.

**Synonyms**

Ring Chromosome 6

**Signs and Symptoms** Cytogenetic studies are an essential way to distinguish among the many chromosomal disorders associated with mental retardation. Severity depends on the amount of genetic material lost on the small and long arms of the chromosome before it formed a ring. Primary features of chromosome 6 ring include a small head circumference, micrognathia, low-set ears, a flat nasal bridge and/or abnormalities of the eyes, mild to severe mental retardation, and psychomotor retardation. Other manifestations include ocular hypertelorism, epicanthal folds, a high-arched palate, clubfoot, hydrocephalus, syndactyly, a short neck, downward slanting eyes, and/or widely spaced nipples. Some cases are asymptomatic.

**Etiology** Chromosome 6 ring occurs as an isolated event in the early stages of embryonic development. The parents of the affected child typically have normal chromosomes and a very low probability of having another child with a chromosomal abnormality.

**Epidemiology** Males are slightly more affected than females. There have been approximately 17 cases reported.

**Treatment—Standard** Patients with chromosome 6 ring and poor muscle tone may benefit from physical therapy. Special education and related services are of benefit to children with this disorder.

Genetic counseling may benefit patients and their families. Other treatment is symptomatic and supportive.

**Treatment—Investigational** Please contact the agencies listed under Resources, below, for the most current information. Addresses and telephone numbers of these agencies, as well as of individual experts and research centers, may be found in the Master Resources List.

**Resources**

**For more information on chromosome ring 6:** National Organization for Rare Disorders (NORD); Chromosome Deletion Outreach; Spotlight 6 (Chromosome 6 Disorders); The Arc (a national organization on mental retardation); NIH/National Institute of Child Health and Human Development.

**For genetic information and genetic counseling referrals:** March of Dimes Birth Defects Foundation; Alliance of Genetic Support Groups.

**References**

Birth Defects Encyclopedia: M.L. Buyse, ed.-in-chief; Blackwell Scientific Publications, 1990, p. 343.

Ring Chromosome 6: Clinical and Cytogenetic Behavior: C. Paz-y-Mino, et al.; Am. J. Med. Genet., April 1990, vol. 35(4), pp. 481–483.
Ring Chromosome 6: Report of a Patient and Literature Review: D. Chitayat, et al.; Am. J. Med. Genet., January 1987, vol. 35(4), pp. 145–151.

# CHROMOSOME 9 RING

**Description** Chromosome 9 ring causes craniofacial and mental abnormalities.

**Synonyms**

Ring Chromosome 9

**Signs and Symptoms** Cytogenetic studies are indicated to distinguish among the many chromosomal disorders associated with mental retardation. Severity depends on the amount of genetic material lost on the small and long arms of the 9th chromosome before it formed a ring. Craniofacial abnormalities include microcephaly, trigono-cephaly, down-slanting eyes that protrude outward, an exaggerated arch to the eyebrows, a small chin, and/or a short neck. Mental retardation is common. Some individuals become agitated easily, while others are very shy. Cardiac and skeletal anomalies, including cleft palate, are less common. A few affected males have abnormal external genitalia and/or hypospadias.

**Etiology** Chromosome 9 ring occurs as an isolated event, probably in the early stages of embryonic development. A parent with chromosome 9 ring and few apparent symptoms may transmit the disorder to a child and has a 50 percent chance of having another child with this disorder.

**Epidemiology** Males and females are affected equally. Twelve cases have been reported, though several hundred may go unreported.

**Treatment—Standard** Special education and related services are beneficial to children with chromosome 9 ring. Cleft palate requires a team of surgeons, psychologists, speech pathologists, and dental specialists. Cleft lip can be corrected by surgery, beginning in the patient's infancy. Cleft palate may also be treated surgically or by a prosthesis.

Genetic counseling may benefit families of patients. Other treatment is symptomatic and supportive.

**Treatment—Investigational** Researchers are studying a Teflon-glycerine paste that is applied to the rear of the pharynx in a minor surgical procedure to bring the pharynx and palate into proper relationship. For further information, contact William N. Williams, D.D.S., University of Florida.

Please contact the agencies listed under Resources, below, for the most current information. Addresses and telephone numbers of these agencies, as well as of individual experts and research centers, may be found in the Master Resources List.

**Resources**

**For more information on chromosome 9 ring:** National Organization for Rare Disorders (NORD); Chromosome Deletion Outreach; The Arc (a national organization on mental retardation); American Cleft Palate Cranial Facial Association.

**For genetic information and genetic counseling referrals:** March of Dimes Birth Defects Foundation; Alliance of Genetic Support Groups.

**References**

Birth Defects Encyclopedia: M.L. Buyse, ed.-in-chief; Blackwell Scientific Publications, 1990, p. 354.
Ring Chromosome 9: Case Report and Review of the Literature: S. Manouvrier-Hanu et al.; Ann. Genet., 1988, vol. 31(4), pp. 250–253.
Apparent Prader-Willi Phenotype in a Woman with Ring Chromosome 9: R.O. Hess, et al.; Am. J. Med. Genet., 1987, vol. 3(suppl.), pp. 133–138.

# CHROMOSOME 14 RING

**Description** Chromosome 14 ring causes distinct facial features, growth delays, mental retardation, seizures, and microcephaly.

**Synonyms**

Ring Chromosome 14

**Signs and Symptoms** Cytogenetic studies are necessary to distinguish among the many chromosomal disorders associated with mental retardation. Severity depends on the amount of genetic material lost before the 2 ends of the chromosome formed a ring. Primary symptoms include an elongated face, microcephaly with a high forehead, ocular hypertelorism, epicanthal folds, a broad nasal bridge, a down-turned mouth, micrognathia, a high-arched palate, and a thin upper lip. Growth delays, mental retardation, and psychomotor difficulties are apparent. Low-set ears, a short neck, a palmar simian crease, vitiligo, and café au lait spots are less common.

Epileptic seizures typically start at an early age, although a few patients have no seizures. In addition, hyperactivity, athetosis of the extremities, intention tremors, ataxia, narrowing of the aorta and the pulmonary artery, and joint contractures may occur.

**Etiology** Chromosome 14 ring occurs as an isolated event in the early stages of embryonic development. The parents of the affected child typically have normal chromosomes and very little chance of having another child with a chromosomal abnormality. If one parent has chromosome 14 ring, the chances are much greater of having another child with this disorder.

**Epidemiology** Males are affected slightly more often than females. Over 30 cases have been reported.

**Treatment—Standard** Physical therapy may help prevent contractures. Special education and related services will benefit children. Anticonvulsant drugs can prevent and control seizures associated with epilepsy.

Genetic counseling may benefit patients and their families. Other treatment is symptomatic and supportive.

**Treatment—Investigational** Please contact the agencies listed under Resources, below, for the most current information. Addresses and telephone numbers of these agencies, as well as of individual experts and research centers, may be found in the Master Resources List.

**Resources**

**For more information on chromosome 14 ring:** National Organization for Rare Disorders (NORD); Epilepsy Foundation of America; The Arc (a national organization on mental retardation); NIH/National Institute of Child Health and Human Development.

**For genetic information and genetic counseling referrals:** March of Dimes Birth Defects Foundation; Alliance of Genetic Support Groups.

**References**

Ring Chromosome 14 Syndrome: Report of Two Cases, Including Extended Evaluation of a Previously Reported Patient and Review: L. Zelante, et al.; Ann. Genet. Italy, 1991, vol. 34(2), pp. 93–97.

Birth Defects Encyclopedia: M.L. Buyse, ed.-in-chief; Blackwell Scientific Publications, 1990, pp. 372–373.

# CHROMOSOME 15 RING

**Description** Chromosome 15 ring causes delayed growth, microcephaly, a triangular-shaped face, hypotonia, and mental retardation.

**Synonyms**

Ring Chromosome 15

**Signs and Symptoms** This disorder is usually detected at birth or during prenatal testing. Severity depends on the amount of genetic material lost on the chromosome before it formed a ring. Craniofacial abnormalities include microcephaly, mental retardation, growth delays, hypotonia, micrognathia, ocular hypertelorism, and hypogonadism. Other symptoms include congenital heart defects, short bones of the hands and feet, syndactyly, scoliosis, seizures, renal abnormalities, and café au lait pigmentation.

**Etiology** Chromosome 15 ring occurs as an isolated event, probably in the early stages of embryonic development. The parents of the affected child typically have normal chromosomes and a very low probability of having another child with a chromosomal abnormality. However, in several cases, an asymptomatic parent with chromosome 15 ring has had a child with the disorder. Some cases have resulted from a parent with a balanced translocation.

**Epidemiology** Females are affected more often than males.

**Treatment—Standard** Patients with chromosome 15 ring and hypotonia may benefit from physical therapy. Special education and related services will benefit patients with this disorder.

Genetic counseling may benefit families of patients with this disorder.

**Treatment—Investigational** Please contact the agencies listed under Resources, below, for the most current information. Addresses and telephone numbers of these agencies, as well as of individual experts and research centers, may be found in the Master Resources List.

**Resources**

**For more information on chromosome 15 ring:** National Organization for Rare Disorders (NORD); Chromosome Deletion Outreach; The Arc (a national organization on mental retardation); NIH/National Institute of Child Health and Human Development.

**For genetic information and genetic counseling referrals:** March of Dimes Birth Defects Foundation; Alliance of Genetic Support Groups.

**References**

Birth Defects Encyclopedia: M.L. Buyse, ed.-in-chief; Blackwell Scientific Publications, 1990, pp. 375–376.

Two Patients with Ring Chromosome 15 Syndrome: M.G. Butler, et al.; Am. J. Med. Genet., January 1988, vol. 29(1), pp. 149–154.

Phenotypic Delineation of Ring Chromosome 15 and Russell-Silver Syndromes: G.N. Wilson, et al.; J. Med. Genet., June 1985, vol. 22(3), pp. 233–236.

# CHROMOSOME 18 RING

**Description** Chromosome 18 ring causes mental retardation, unusual facial features, microcephaly, and hypotonia.

**Synonyms**

Ring Chromosome 18

**Signs and Symptoms** This disorder is usually detected at birth or during prenatal testing. Cytogenetic studies distinguish among the many chromosomal disorders associated with mental retardation. Severity depends on the amount of genetic material lost on the chromosome before it formed a ring. Craniofacial abnormalities include microcephaly, mental retardation, growth retardation, hypotonia, and recurrent infections during infancy. More than half of patients have such ocular abnormalities as hypertelorism, ptosis, an abnormally small eyeball or one that is displaced in a downward position or crossed, an absent or defective iris, and nystagmus. Unusually developed external ears, narrow eustachian tubes, ears set very low on the head, and deafness are common.

Other symptoms include a high-arched palate, small tongue, small or protruding mandible, down-turned mouth, vertebrae and genital anomalies, small arms and legs, fingers that curve inward, overlying toes, and/or a decrease in the antibody IgA.

Some patients present with symptoms uncommon to any other patient with chromosome 18 ring.

**Etiology** Chromosome 18 ring occurs as an isolated event, probably in the early stages of embryonic development. The parents of the affected child typically have normal chromosomes and a very low possibility of having another child with a chromosomal abnormality. However, in several cases, a parent with chromosome 18 ring has had a child with the disorder. Some cases have resulted from a parent with a balanced translocation.

**Epidemiology** Females are affected slightly more often than males. Approximately 70 cases have been reported.

**Treatment—Standard** Patients with chromosome 18 ring and poor muscle tone may benefit from physical therapy. Special education and related services will benefit children with this disorder. When hearing is impaired, speech may be delayed, and the patient may benefit from speech therapy as well as from a hearing aid.

Genetic counseling may benefit patients and their families. Other treatment is symptomatic and supportive.

**Treatment—Investigational** Please contact the agencies listed under Resources, below, for the most current information. Addresses and telephone numbers of these agencies, as well as of individual experts and research centers, may be found in the Master Resources List.

**Resources**

**For more information on chromosome 18 ring:** National Organization for Rare Disorders (NORD); Chromosome 18 Registry and Research Society; The Arc (a national organization on mental retardation); NIH/National Institute of Child Health and Human Development.

**For genetic information and genetic counseling referrals:** March of Dimes Birth Defects Foundation; Alliance of Genetic Support Groups.

**References**

Birth Defects Encyclopedia: M.L. Buyse, ed.-in-chief; Blackwell Scientific Publications, 1990, p. 384.

Chronic Arthritis in Two Children with Partial Deletion of Chromosome 18: R.E. Petty, et al.; J. Rheumatol., June 1987, vol. 14(3), pp. 586–587.

Ring Chromosome 18 in a Mother and Child: M.A. Donlan, et al.; Am. J. Med. Genet., May 1986, vol. 24(1), pp. 171–174.

# CHROMOSOME 21 RING

**Description** Chromosome 21 ring is a rare chromosomal disorder in which the affected individual has a breakage of chromosome 21 at both ends, and the ends of the chromosome join together to form a ring. The amount of genetic material lost at the 2 ends of the chromosome can vary. As a result, a patient with very little absent genetic material may have no or few apparent symptoms, while a patient with a significant part of the chromosomal ends missing may have severe symptoms.

**Synonyms**

Ring Chromosome 21

**Signs and Symptoms** Individuals with a significant amount of missing genetic material may have microcephaly, down-slanting eyes, down-turned mouth, underdeveloped jaws, dislocated joints, seizures, mental retardation, eye abnormalities, and skeletal abnormalities. Some individuals have abnormalities of the internal organs, dysgenesis of the anterior segment of the eye, and hemifacial microsomia.

Infertility and/or miscarriages have occurred in asymptomatic patients who were later found to have chromosome 21 ring.

Chromosome 21 ring is usually detected at birth or during prenatal testing.

**Etiology** The cause is unknown. The parents of an affected child typically have normal chromosomes and a very low probability of having another child with the chromosomal abnormality. However, there have been a few cases of chromosome 21 ring in which an asymptomatic parent has transmitted the disorder to the child. When this is the case, the parent has a 50 percent chance of having another child with chromosome 21 ring.

**Epidemiology** Chromosome 21 ring affects males and females in equal numbers.

**Treatment—Standard** Special education and related services will benefit children with chromosome 21 ring. Genetic counseling may benefit patients and their families. Other treatment is symptomatic and supportive.

**Treatment—Investigational** Please contact the agencies listed under Resources, below, for the most current information. Addresses and telephone numbers of these agencies, as well as of individual experts and research centers, may be found in the Master Resources List.

**Resources**

**For more information on chromosome 21 ring:** National Organization for Rare Disorders (NORD); Chromosome Deletion Outreach; The Arc (a national organization on mental retardation); NIH/National Institute of Child Health and Human Development.

**For genetic information and genetic counseling referrals:** March of Dimes Birth Defects Foundation; Alliance of Genetic Support Groups.

**References**

Birth Defects Encyclopedia: M.L Buyse, ed.-in-chief; Blackwell Scientific Publications, 1990, p. 391.

Acute Lymphoblastic Leukemia in a Child with Constitutional Ring Chromosome 21: A.M. Falchi, et al.; Cancer Genet. Cytogenet., August 1987, vol. 27(2), pp. 219–224.

Familial Transmission of a Ring Chromosome 21: J.M. Hertz, et al.; Clin. Genet., July 1987, vol. 32(1), pp. 35–39.

Ring 21 Chromosome: The Mild End of the Phenotypic Spectrum: R.J. Gardner, et al.; Clin. Genet., December 1986, vol. 30(6), pp. 466–470.

Ring Chromosome 21: Characterization of DNA Sequences at Sites of Breakage and Reunion: H.H. Kazazian, Jr., et al.; Ann. N. Y. Acad. Sci., 1985, vol. 450, pp. 33–42.

Ring Chromosome 21 in a Phenotypically Normal but Infertile Man: J.L. Huret, et al.; Clin. Genet., December 1985, vol. 28(6), pp. 541–545.

# CHROMOSOME 22 RING

**Description** Chromosome 22 ring causes mental retardation, psychomotor difficulties, and hypotonia.

**Synonyms**

Ring Chromosome 22

**Signs and Symptoms** Cytogenetic studies are a critical way to distinguish among the many chromosomal disorders associated with mental retardation. Severity depends on the amount of genetic material lost on the small and long arms of the chromosome before it formed a ring. Chromosome 22 ring is usually detected at birth or prenatally. In addition to the primary signs of hypotonia and mental and psychomotor retardation, patients may also present with such craniofacial anomalies as a smaller-than-normal nose or a large, rounded nose; large ears; a high-arched palate; ocular hypertelorism; epicanthal folds; and/or ptosis. A few patients have underdeveloped toenails, syndactyly, small eyes, long eyelashes, and heart defects. Some cases are asymptomatic.

**Etiology** Chromosome 22 ring occurs as an isolated event in the early stages of embryonic development. The parents of the affected child typically have normal chromosomes and very little chance of having another child with a chromosomal abnormality. A very small number of cases have been reported as familial.

**Epidemiology** Males are affected more often than females. More than 40 cases have been reported.

**Treatment—Standard** Patients with hypotonia may benefit from physical therapy. Special education and related services are of benefit to children with this disorder.

Genetic counseling may benefit patients and their families. Other treatment is symptomatic and supportive.

**Treatment—Investigational** Please contact the agencies listed under Resources, below, for the most current information. Addresses and telephone numbers of these agencies, as well as of individual experts and research centers, may be found in the Master Resources List.

**Resources**

**For more information on chromosome 22 ring:** National Organization for Rare Disorders (NORD); Chromosome Deletion Outreach; The Arc (a national organization on mental retardation); NIH/National Institute of Child Health and Human Development.

**For genetic information and genetic counseling referrals:** March of Dimes Birth Defects Foundation; Alliance of Genetic Support Groups.

**References**

Ring Chromosome 22: A Case Report: C. Severien, et al.; Klin. Padiatr., November–December 1991, vol. 203(6), pp. 467–469.

Birth Defects Encyclopedia: M.L. Buyse, ed.-in-chief; Blackwell Scientific Publications, 1990, p. 394.
Deleted Ring Chromosome 22 in a Mentally Retarded Boy: K.H. Gustavson, et al.; Clin. Genet., April 1986, vol. 29(4), pp. 337–341.

# CHROMOSOME 4Q- SYNDROME

**Description** The syndrome is caused by a partial deletion of the long arm of chromosome 4. Severity and type of abnormalities depend on the size and location of the missing chromosomal piece.

**Signs and Symptoms** The head may be microcephalic and the nose short, with a depressed bridge and anteverted nostrils. The ears are usually low-set, the eyes wide-set and slanted upward, and cleft palate and micrognathia are often present. In some cases there may be agenesis of the corpus callosum.

The hands and feet are usually small, and a clinodactylic, pointed 5th finger is characteristic. Cardiac and genitourinary defects, hypotonia, and poor or delayed growth all may be present. Mental retardation when it occurs is moderate to severe. In some cases, delayed growth and mental retardation may be present without obvious physical abnormalities, making diagnosis difficult.

**Etiology** The syndrome is caused by a partial deletion of the long arm of chromosome 4. Whether the deletion is interstitial or terminal usually determines the symptoms and severity of the disorder.

**Epidemiology** Over 30 cases have been described. Males and females are affected in equal numbers.

**Related Disorders** See *Chromosome 11q- Syndrome; Down Syndrome; Greig Cephalopolysyndactyly Syndrome; Trisomy; Wolf-Hirschhorn Syndrome.*

**Treatment—Standard** Special education, physical therapy, and vocational services may be of benefit, as may genetic counseling. Other treatment is symptomatic and supportive.

**Treatment—Investigational** Please contact the agencies listed under Resources, below, for the most current information. Addresses and telephone numbers of these agencies, as well as of individual experts and research centers, may be found in the Master Resources List.

**Resources**

**For more information on chromosome 4q- syndrome:** National Organization for Rare Disorders (NORD); Retarded Infant Services; Federation of Families for Children's Mental Health; The Arc (a national organization on mental retardation); NIH/National Institute of Child Health and Human Development.

**For genetic information and genetic counseling referrals:** March of Dimes Birth Defects Foundation; Alliance of Genetic Support Groups.

**References**

Syndromes of the Head and Neck, 3rd ed.: R.J. Gorlin, et al.; Oxford University Press, 1990, pp. 728–729.
Interstitial Deletion, Del (4)(q33q35.1), in a Mother and Two Children: M.A. Curtis, et al.; J. Med. Genet., October 1989, vol. 26(10), pp. 652–654.
A New Interstitial Deletion of 4q (q21.1::q22.1): K. Fagan and A. Gill; J. Med. Genet., October 1989, vol. 26(10), pp. 644–647.
Interstitial and Terminal Deletions of the Long Arm of Chromosome 4: Further Delineation of Phenotypes: A.E. Lin, et al.; Am. J. Med. Genet., November 1988, vol. 31(3), pp. 533–548.
A Patient with an Interstitial Deletion of the Proximal Portion of the Long Arm of Chromosome 4: M.H. Beall, et al.; Am. J. Med. Genet., November 1988, vol. 31(3), pp. 553–557.

# CHROMOSOME 11Q- SYNDROME

**Description** Chromosome 11q- syndrome is a genetic disorder affecting the long arm of chromosome 11. Characteristics include a narrow, prominent forehead; abnormally shaped nose and mouth; ocular disorders; and mental retardation. Related chromosome 11 disorders are deletion on the short arm of chromosome 11 and partial trisomy of 11q.

**Synonyms**

Deletion on Long Arm of Chromosome 11

**Signs and Symptoms** Hypertelorism, strabismus, and ptosis are the ocular manifestations of chromosome 11q-syndrome. Other facial abnormalities include a narrow, protruding forehead; broad nasal root; short upturned tip of the nose; fishlike mouth; and receding chin. The ears may be misshapen, and there may be simian creases in the hands. Mental retardation is also present. Various congenital heart defects are common.

**Etiology** Chromosome 11q- syndrome results from a deletion on the long arm (q) of chromosome 11. The cause of the chromosome break is unknown; its size and location determine the severity of the disorder and the forms of abnormality.

**Epidemiology** Chromosome 11q- syndrome is present at birth, and over 80 percent of affected individuals are female. About 25 percent die before the age of 2 years.

**Related Disorders** See *Trisomy 13 Syndrome; Trisomy 18 Syndrome; Down Syndrome.*

An interstitial deletion on the short arm of chromosome 11 (11p13) is associated with aniridia and, in 50 percent of patients, with Wilms tumor, the most common form of renal cancer in children. (See *Aniridia; Wilms Tumor.)*

**Partial trisomy 11q** characteristics may include severe psychomotor retardation, microcephaly, cleft palate, large beaked nose, micrognathia, short hands, and displaced thumbs.

**Treatment—Standard** Symptomatic treatment with special education, physical therapy, and vocational services is appropriate. Genetic counseling is advised.

**Treatment—Investigational** Please contact the agencies listed under Resources, below, for the most current information. Addresses and telephone numbers of these agencies, as well as of individual experts and research centers, may be found in the Master Resources List.

**Resources**

**For more information on chromosome 11q- syndrome:** National Organization for Rare Disorders (NORD); Support Organization for Trisomy 18, 13 and Related Disorders; The Arc (a national organization on mental retardation); NIH/National Institute of Child Health and Human Development.

**For genetic information and genetic counseling referrals:** March of Dimes Birth Defects Foundation; Alliance of Genetic Support Groups.

**References**

Syndromes of the Head and Neck, 3rd ed.: R.J. Gorlin, et al.; Oxford University Press, 1990, p. 85.

# CHROMOSOME 13Q- SYNDROME

**Description** Chromosome 13q- syndrome, a chromosomal disorder caused by a partial deletion of the long arm of chromosome 13, is characterized primarily by mental and growth deficiencies; other abnormalities include microcephaly and retinoblastoma. Syndromes that involve other deviations of chromosome 13 are chromosome 13q- mosaicism, monosomy 13, intrachromosomal insertion (inversion) of chromosome 13, chromosome 13 ring, translocation 13, and trisomy 13.

**Synonyms**

13q- Chromosomal Syndrome

**Signs and Symptoms** Abnormalities of infants born with chromosome 13q- syndrome include microcephaly, trigonocephaly, holoprosencephaly, large low-set ears, a prominent nasal bridge, hypertelorism, ptosis, coloboma, retinoblastoma, microphthalmia, a prominent maxilla, micrognathia, and a short webbed neck. Digital abnormalities, including small or absent thumbs, clinodactyly, and short big toes, may occur. The soles of the feet may be permanently flexed, so that patients walk on their toes. Genitourinary anomalies in males include cryptorchidism and hypospadias. In females, the urethra may open into the vagina. There may be cardiac, pelvic, and renal defects.

**Etiology** In partial deletion of the long arm (q) of chromosome 13, the severity and type of abnormalities depend on the size and location of the missing genetic information.

**Epidemiology** This rare congenital disorder affects males and females in equal numbers.

**Related Disorders** See *Trisomy 13 Syndrome; Wolf-Hirschhorn Syndrome.*

**Chromosome 13q- mosaicism** is a disorder in which some cells of the body have a partial deletion in the long arm of chromosome 13 while other cells are normal. Chromosome 13q- mosaicism has features similar to those of chromosome 13q- syndrome but with a greater variability in type and severity because of the presence of normal cells.

**Monosomy 13** may refer to any deletion of chromosome 13, or to the absence of one of the pair of chromosomes. Features may be similar to those of chromosome 13q- syndrome.

**Intrachromosomal insertion of chromosome 13** involves the breaking off of a section of chromosome 13 and its subsequent reattachment in a different way, e.g., inversion. Mental deficiency, personality defects, psychosis, and other symptoms and signs may occur.

In **chromosome 13 ring,** chromosome 13 has a ringlike shape. When parts of the chromosome are missing, abnormalities can be similar to those of chromosome 13q- syndrome.

**Translocation 13** is identified by the exchange of parts between chromosome 13 and another chromosome. Some characteristics are similar to those of chromosome 13q- syndrome, including retinoblastoma and developmental delay.

**Treatment—Standard** Special education classes and physical therapy may benefit these patients. Genetic counseling is advised.

**Treatment—Investigational** Please contact the agencies listed under Resources, below, for the most current information. Addresses and telephone numbers of these agencies, as well as of individual experts and research centers, may be found in the Master Resources List.

**Resources**

**For more information on chromosome 13q- syndrome:** National Organization for Rare Disorders (NORD); Support Organization for Trisomy 18, 13 and Related Disorders; NIH/National Institute for Child Health and Human Development.

**For genetic information and genetic counseling referrals:** March of Dimes Birth Defects Foundation; Alliance of Genetic Support Groups.

**References**

Smith's Recognizable Patterns of Human Malformation, 4th ed.: K.L. Jones; W.B. Saunders Company, 1988, pp. 54–55, 38–41, 56–59.

Interstitial Del (13)(q21.3q31) Associated with Psychomotor Retardation, Eczema, and Absent Suck and Swallowing Reflex: P.J. Peet, et al.; J. Med. Genet., December 1987, vol. 24(12), pp. 786–788.

Intrachromosomal Insertion of Chromosome 13 in a Family with Psychosis and Mental Subnormality: S.H. Roberts, et al.; J. Ment. Defic. Res., September 1986, vol. 30(pt. 3), pp. 227–232.

# CHROMOSOME 18P- SYNDROME

**Description** Among the primary features of chromosome 18p- syndrome (deletion of the short arm of chromosome 18) are unusual facial characteristics and mild-to-severe mental retardation.

**Synonyms**

Short Arm 18 Deletion Syndrome

**Signs and Symptoms** Physical characteristics include hypertelorism, ptosis, epicanthal folds, low nasal bridge, downturned mouth, a rounded face, micrognathia, and large protruding ears. Microcephaly and mental retardation, a tendency toward hypotonia, and mild-to-moderate growth deficiency are also usually present. The patient often has an IQ averaging between 45 and 50, although some patients have no mental deficiency at all. The ability to speak simple sentences may be delayed until 7 years of age or older. Poor concentration, emotional lability, and restlessness may be characteristic. Other features that may be present include relatively small hands and feet, pectus excavatum, and a high occurrence of dental caries.

**Etiology** Chromosome 18p- syndrome is caused by the deletion of the short arm (p) of chromosome 18.

**Epidemiology** Symptoms are apparent at birth. Females are affected at least twice as often as males. Older parental age may be related to the occurrence of chromosome 18p- syndrome in offspring.

**Related Disorders** See *Down Syndrome; Trisomy 13 Syndrome; Trisomy 18 Syndrome.*

**Partial trisomy 14** results in mental, motor, and growth retardation. Ptosis, malformed ears, and cardiac and genital anomalies may also be present. Seizures may occur.

**Treatment—Standard** Affected children may benefit from early intervention programs in special education and language development, along with physical therapy. Genetic counseling is recommended.

**Treatment—Investigational** Please contact the agencies listed under Resources, below, for the most current information. Addresses and telephone numbers of these agencies, as well as of individual experts and research centers, may be found in the Master Resources List.

**Resources**

**For more information on chromosome 18p- syndrome:** National Organization for Rare Disorders (NORD); Chromosome 18 Registry and Research Society; Support Organization for Trisomy 18, 13 and Related Disorders; NIH/National Institute of Child Health and Human Development; The Arc (a national organization on mental retardation).

**For genetic information and genetic counseling referrals:** March of Dimes Birth Defects Foundation; Alliance of Genetic Support Groups.

**References**

Duplication 18p- with Mild Influence on the Phenotype: B. Johansson, et al.; Am. J. Med. Genet., April 29, 1988, vol. 4, pp. 871–874.

Smith's Recognizable Patterns of Human Malformation, 4th ed.: K.L. Jones; W.B. Saunders Company, 1988, pp. 56–57.

# CHROMOSOME 18Q- SYNDROME

**Description** Chromosome 18q- syndrome is a congenital disorder characterized by mental retardation, short stature, and craniofacial anomalies.

**Synonyms**

Chromosome 18 Long Arm Deletion Syndrome

Chromosome 18, Monosomy 18q

Monosomy 18q Syndrome

**Signs and Symptoms** This disorder is usually detected at birth or during prenatal testing. Severity depends on the amount of genetic material deleted from the long arm of chromosome 18. Primary symptoms include mental retardation, short stature, a flat midface, hypotonia, and microcephaly.

In addition, down-turned mouth, a cleft or high palate, a broad nasal bridge, epicanthal folds, hypertelorism, and an outward curl of the ear may occur. Malformation of the optic nerve; nystagmus; strabismus; long, tapering fingers and toes; low-set thumbs; palmar simian crease; fleshy tips of the fingers; abnormal placement of the second toe; and genu varum may also occur. Abnormalities of the genitals, such as a small penis, cryptorchidism, and a small or absent labia minor have been found in many patients.

An increased number of whorl patterns on the fingertips, congenital heart disease, impaired hearing, deficient IgA, closed or narrow eustachian tubes, widely spaced nipples, and seizures are less common. Delayed speech and behavior problems have also been reported.

**Etiology** Chromosome 18q- syndrome occurs as an isolated event, probably in the early stages of embryonic development. The parents of the affected child typically have normal chromosomes and a very low probability of having another child with a chromosomal abnormality. However, in several cases, a parent with chromosome 18q- syndrome has had a child with the disorder. Nineteen cases have resulted from an asymptomatic parent with a balanced translocation. These parents have a high probability of having a child with a chromosome 18 deletion .

**Epidemiology** Females are affected more often than males. More than 50 cases have been reported.

**Treatment—Standard** Patients with chromosome 18q- syndrome and hypotonia may benefit from physical therapy. Cleft palate may be treated surgically or by a prosthesis. Special education and related services will benefit children with this disorder.

Genetic counseling may benefit patients and their families. Other treatment is symptomatic and supportive.

**Treatment—Investigational** Researchers are studying a paste that is applied to the rear of the pharynx in a minor surgical procedure to bring the pharynx and palate into proper relationship. For further information, contact William N. Williams, D.D.S., University of Florida.

Please contact the agencies listed under Resources, below, for the most current information. Addresses and telephone numbers of these agencies, as well as of individual experts and research centers, may be found in the Master Resources List.

**Resources**

**For more information on chromosome 18q- syndrome:** National Organization for Rare Disorders (NORD); Chromosome 18 Registry and Research Society; Chromosome Deletion Outreach; The Arc (a national organization on mental retardation); NIH/National Institute of Child Health and Human Development.

**For genetic information and genetic counseling referrals:** March of Dimes Birth Defects Foundation; Alliance of Genetic Support Groups.

**References**

The 18q- Syndrome: Analysis of Chromosomes by Bivariate Flow Karyotyping and the PCR Reveals a Successive Set of Deletion Breakpoints Within 18q21.2–q22.2: G.A. Silverman, et al.; Am. J. Hum. Genet, 1995, vol. 56, pp. 926–937.

Interstitial Deletion of Chromosome 18 [Del (18) (q11.2q12.2 or q12.2q21.1]: L.C. Surh, et al.; Am. J. Med. Genet., October 1991, vol. 41(1), pp. 15–17.

Birth Defects Encyclopedia: M.L. Buyse, ed.-in-chief; Blackwell Scientific Publications, 1990, pp. 382–383.

The Brain in the 18q- Syndrome: H. Vogel, et al.; Dev. Med. Child Neurol., August 1990, vol. 32(8), pp. 732–737.

Chronic Arthritis in Two Children with Partial Deletion of Chromosome 18: R.E. Petty, et al.; J. Rheumatol., June 1987, vol. 14(3), pp. 586–587.

# CHROMOSOME 5, TRISOMY 5P

**Description** Chromosome 5, trisomy 5p is a very rare genetic disorder caused by a duplication of all or part of the short arm of chromosome 5.

**Synonyms**

Trisomy 5p

**Signs and Symptoms** Symptoms are usually apparent at birth and include mental retardation, microcephaly, facial dysmorphism, hypotonia, and psychomotor retardation. Although birth weight is normal, postnatal growth failure and seizures may occur. Other symptoms include a weak cry, a downward slant to the eyes, extra epicanathal folds, hypertelorism, and low-set and malformed ears. A depressed nasal bridge, macroglossia, thick cheeks, arachnodactyly, bilateral cryptorchidism, and congenital heart disease may also be present. In a very few rare cases, eye abnormalities, macrocephaly, micrognathia, and clubfoot has been reported in children with chromosome 5, trisomy 5p. Recurrent respiratory infections and feeding problems may also afflict affected children.

The severity of symptoms appears to depend on the length of the duplicated portion of chromosome 5. More severe symptoms may appear in individuals with **complete trisomy 5p** (5p11–pter) than in individuals with **par-**

tial trisomy 5p (5p13–ter or 14–pter). In some cases of partial trisomy 5p, the physical symptoms may be nearly absent.

Chromosomal testing is necessary for a definite diagnosis.

**Etiology** The exact cause of the chromosomal duplication is not known.

**Complete trisomy 5p** may be the result of a spontaneous unbalanced translocation. An unbalanced translocation occurs very early in embryonic development when, for unknown reasons, a piece of one chromosome breaks off and connects to another chromosome. A spontaneous unbalanced translocation is not related to the chromosomes of the parents.

**Partial trisomy 5p** may be the result of an error during the development of the gametes if one parent has a balanced translocation. A translocation is balanced if pieces of 2 or more chromosomes break off and trade places, creating an altered but balanced set of chromosomes. Balanced translocations are usually harmless to the carrier but are associated with a high risk of abnormal chromosomal development in the carrier's offspring.

**Epidemiology** Chromosome 5, trisomy 5p affects twice as many females as males. Three cases of complete trisomy 5p and 21 cases of partial trisomy 5p have been reported.

**Treatment—Standard** Treatment of chromosome 5, trisomy 5p is symptomatic and supportive. Special education, physical therapy, and other medical, social, or vocational services are of benefit to the affected individual and are often necessary for the child to reach his or her full potential. Genetic counseling may benefit affected individuals and their families.

**Treatment—Investigational** Please contact the agencies listed under Resources, below, for the most current information. Addresses and telephone numbers of these agencies, as well as of individual experts and research centers, may be found in the Master Resources List.

**Resources**

**For more information on chromosome 5, trisomy 5p:** National Organization for Rare Disorders (NORD); Support Organization for Trisomy 18, 13 and Related Disorders; Support Organization for Trisomy Canada; The Arc (a national organization on mental retardation); NIH/National Institute of Child Health and Human Development.

**For genetic information and genetic counseling referrals:** March of Dimes Birth Defects Foundation; Alliance of Genetic Support Groups.

**References**

Birth Defects Encyclopedia: M.L. Buyse, ed.-in-chief; Blackwell Scientific Publications, 1990, pp. 340–341.

Trisomy 5p: A Report of 2 Cases: J. Alvarez-Coca, et. al.; An. Esp. Pediatr., March 1985, vol. 22(4), pp. 288–292.

A New Case of Trisomy 5p: V.G. Antonenko, et al.; Genetika, December 1985, vol. 21(12), pp. 2066–2070.

"Complete 5p" Trisomy: 1 Case and 19 Translocation Carriers in 6 Generations: F.S. Brimblecombe, et al.; J. Med. Genet., August 1977, vol. 14(4), pp. 271–274.

Duplication (5p Leads to Pter): Prenatal Diagnosis and Review of the Literature: G.S. Khodr, et al.; Am. J. Med. Genet., May 1982, vol. 12(1), pp. 43–49.

# CHROMOSOME 14, TRISOMY MOSAIC

**Description** Chromosome 14, trisomy mosaic is a very rare chromosomal disorder in which an extra chromosome 14 is present in some, but not all, of the cells of the affected individual. This disorder is usually apparent at birth, and may be diagnosed pre- or postnatally by genetic testing. Chromosomal analysis is necessary for a definitive diagnosis.

**Synonyms**

Mosaic Trisomy 14 Syndrome

Trisomy 14 Mosaicism

**Signs and Symptoms** The severity of symptoms may depend on the percentage of cells having the extra chromosome.

Characteristic features of chromosome 14, trisomy mosaic include delayed growth of the fetus during pregnancy and of the child after birth, developmental delays, and mental retardation. Heart disease is present at birth in most individuals with this disorder.

Other symptoms include a prominent forehead, hypertelorism, a wide nasal bridge, and small, low-set ears. Micrognathia, a highly arched or cleft palate, a short neck, cryptorchidism, and an abnormally small penis frequently occur.

Unusual patterns of skin coloration, ptosis, microphthalmia, a large mouth, and a narrowed opening between the eyelids may also appear in this disorder. Symptoms that are less common include a translucent film over the eyes and uneven, asymmetrical development of the body, with one side developing more quickly than the other.

**Etiology** The cause is unknown.

**Epidemiology** Chromosome 14, trisomy mosaic is reported in females more often than males. Approximately 15 cases have been documented in the medical literature.

**Related Disorders** See *Tetralogy of Fallot.*

**Treatment—Standard** Treatment is symptomatic and supportive. Special education, physical therapy, and other medical, social, or vocational services may benefit the affected individual and are often necessary for the child to reach his or her full potential. Genetic counseling may benefit affected individuals and their families.

Treatment may also include surgery to help correct congenital heart defects. If surgical correction is not possible, a shunt may be inserted to facilitate blood flow through the heart. Medication may be needed to treat arrhythmia. Individuals with tetralogy of Fallot are susceptible to bacterial endocarditis and should be given prophylactic antibiotics prior to surgery or dental procedures. Respiratory infections should also be treated vigorously and early.

**Treatment—Investigational** Please contact the agencies listed under Resources, below, for the most current information. Addresses and telephone numbers of these agencies, as well as of individual experts and research centers, may be found in the Master Resources List.

**Resources**

**For more information on chromosome 14, trisomy mosaic:** National Organization for Rare Disorders (NORD); Support Organization for Trisomy 18, 13 and Related Disorders; Support Organization for Trisomy Canada; The Arc (a national organization on mental retardation); NIH/National Institute of Child Health and Human Development.

**For genetic information and genetic counseling referrals:** March of Dimes Birth Defects Foundation; Alliance of Genetic Support Groups.

**References**

Natural History of Mosaic Trisomy 14 Syndrome: A. Fujimoto, et al.; Am. J. Med. Genet., September 1992, vol. 44(2), pp. 189–196.

Birth Defects Encyclopedia: M.L Buyse, ed.-in-chief; Blackwell Scientific Publications, 1990, pp. 373–374.

Trisomy 14 Mosaicism Syndrome: M.H. Lipson; Am. J. Med. Genet., March 1987; vol. 26(3), pp. 541–544.

# CHROMOSOME 22, TRISOMY MOSAIC

**Description** Chromosome 22, trisomy mosaic is a rare chromosomal disorder in which an extra chromosome 22 is present in some, but not all, of the cells of the affected individual. This disorder is usually apparent at birth, and may be diagnosed pre- or postnatally) through specialized genetic testing. Chromosomal analysis is necessary for a definitive diagnosis.

**Synonyms**

Mosaic Trisomy 14 Syndrome

Trisomy 22 Mosaicism

**Signs and Symptoms** The severity of symptoms may depend on the percentage of cells having the extra chromosome.

Major symptoms of chromosome 22, trisomy mosaic include hemidystrophy, which may be accompanied by unilateral hearing loss; hypoplastic fingers and/or toes; flexion creases on the palms of the hands; abnormal or missing nails on the fingers and toes; areas of unusual skin coloration (linear pigmentations); and/or a shortened limb. Ptosis, a webbed neck, and a low posterior hairline may also be present. Intelligence may be mildly impaired.

Individuals affected by this disorder may have malformations of the major coronary blood vessels (e.g., the aortic arch), renal defects, malformation of the elbow (cubitus valgus), and multiple pigmented skin nevi. Delayed sexual development, undeveloped ovaries or testes (streak gonads), and absent ovaries and fallopian tubes may also occur.

**Etiology** The cause is unknown.

**Epidemiology** Chromosome 22, trisomy mosaic appears to affect females more frequently than males.

**Related Disorders** See *Turner Syndrome; Noonan Syndrome.*

**Treatment—Standard** Treatment is symptomatic and supportive. Special education, physical therapy, and other medical, social, or vocational services may benefit the affected individual and are often necessary for the child to reach his or her full potential. Genetic counseling may benefit affected individuals and their families.

**Treatment—Investigational** Please contact the agencies listed under Resources, below, for the most current information. Addresses and telephone numbers of these agencies, as well as of individual experts and research centers, may be found in the Master Resources List.

**Resources**

**For more information on chromosome 22, trisomy mosaic:** National Organization for Rare Disorders (NORD); Support Organization for Trisomy 18, 13 and Related Disorders; Support Organization for Trisomy Canada; The

Arc (a national organization on mental retardation); NIH/National Institute of Child Health and Human Development.

**For genetic information and genetic counseling referrals:** March of Dimes Birth Defects Foundation; Alliance of Genetic Support Groups.

### References

Birth Defects Encyclopedia: M.L Buyse, ed.-in-chief; Blackwell Scientific Publications, 1990, p. 395.

Trisomy 22 Mosaicism Limited to Skin Fibroblasts in a Mentally Retarded, Dysmorphic Girl: H.T. Lund, et al.; Acta Paediatr. Scand., June–July 1990, vol. 79(6–7), pp. 714–718.

Trisomy 22 Mosaicism with Normal Blood Chromosomes: Case Report with Literature Review: M.L. Lessick, et al.; Clin. Pediatr., September 1988, vol. 27(9), pp. 451–454.

Trisomy 22 Mosaicism Syndrome and Ullrich-Turner Stigmata: W. Wertelecki, et al.; Am. J. Med. Genet., March 1986, vol. 23(3), pp. 739–749.

Incomplete Trisomy 22: III. Mosaic Trisomy 22 and the Problem of Full Trisomy 22: A. Schinzel, et al.; Hum. Genet., 1981, vol. 56(3), pp. 269–273.

Unilateral Radial Aplasia and Trisomy 22 Mosaicism: F. Dulitzky, et al.; J. Med. Genet., December 1981, vol. 18(6), pp. 473–476.

# CLEIDOCRANIAL DYSPLASIA

**Description** Cleidocranial dysplasia is a hereditary skeletal disorder that also involves dentition.

**Synonyms**

       Cleidocranial Dysostosis

       Dysplasia, Osteodental

       Marie-Sainton Disease

**Signs and Symptoms** Primary characteristics are premature closure of the coronale, causing the forehead to bulge outward; a wide face; delayed fontanelle closure, causing a bulge in the skull cap; complete or partial absence of the clavicles; and narrow, drooping shoulders. There may also be abnormalities of the muscles in the clavicular area, allowing for a wide range of shoulder movement; moderately short stature; and fingers that are abnormal in length.

Other bone abnormalities include a wide pelvic joint, delayed growth of the pubic bone, coxa vara, coxa valga, genu valgum, failure of the lower jaw bones to unite, scoliosis, and a small scapula.

Dental abnormalities include a delay in tooth eruption, incomplete development or absence of teeth, underdeveloped enamel, and extra teeth. Cysts may form around the unerupted or displaced teeth in some cases.

A high-arched or a cleft palate may be present as well as other minor abnormalities.

**Etiology** Cleidocranial dysplasia is usually inherited as an autosomal dominant trait with complete penetrance and marked expressivity. Approximately one-third of cases are due to a mutation. Linkage to chromosome 6p has been demonstrated in 2 families.

**Epidemiology** Males and females are affected in equal numbers. Over 500 cases have been reported. The incidence of the disorder is believed to be approximately 1:1,000,000.

**Related Disorders Mandibuloacral dysplasia** is inherited as an autosomal recessive trait and is characterized by limited joint movement, delayed growth of the jaw, atrophic skin, underdeveloped fingers, a wide fontanelle, limited joint movement, absent or underdeveloped clavicle, and coxa valga. Males and females are affected equally.

**Pyknodysostosis** is a very rare disorder that affects males and females equally and is inherited as an autosomal recessive trait. A delay in closure of the skull bones, short stature, an increase in bone density, an underdeveloped jaw, and abnormalities of the fingers are characteristic. A small receding chin, dental abnormalities, and short arms and legs may also be present.

**Treatment—Standard** Protective head gear may be worn until the skull bones close. Appropriate dental care should be provided. Surgery may be performed to correct the cleft palate. Speech and language may need to be assessed by a speech pathologist.

Genetic counseling may benefit patients and their families. Other treatment is symptomatic and supportive.

**Treatment—Investigational** Researchers are studying a paste that is applied to the rear of the pharynx in a minor surgical procedure to bring the pharynx and palate into proper relationship. For further information, contact William N. Williams, D.D.S., University of Florida.

Please contact the agencies listed under Resources, below, for the most current information. Addresses and telephone numbers of these agencies, as well as of individual experts and research centers, may be found in the Master Resources List.

**Resources**

**For more information on cleidocranial dysplasia:** National Organization for Rare Disorders (NORD); National Craniofacial Foundation; FACES—National Association for the Craniofacially Handicapped; American Cleft

Palate Cranial Facial Association; NIH/National Institute of Arthritis Musculoskeletal and Skin Diseases.

**For genetic information and genetic counseling referrals:** March of Dimes Birth Defects Foundation; Alliance of Genetic Support Groups.

### References

Genetic Mapping of Cleidocranial Dysplasia and Incidence of a Microdeletion in One Family: S. Mundlos, et al.; Hum. Mol. Genet., 1995, vol. 4, pp. 71–75.

Mendelian Inheritance in Man, 11th ed.: V.A. McKusick; The Johns Hopkins University Press, 1994, pp. 309–310.

Intrafamilial Variability in Cleidocranial Dysplasia: A Three-Generation Family: D. Chitayat, et al.; Am. J. Med. Genet., February 1992, vol. 42(3), pp. 298–303.

Birth Defects Encyclopedia: M.L. Buyse, ed.-in-chief; Blackwell Scientific Publications, 1990, pp. 417.

Cleidocranial Dysplasia: H.D. Kerr; J. Rheumatol., February 1988, vol. 15(2), pp. 359–361.

# CLUBFOOT

**Description** The term *clubfoot* is a word used to describe several kinds of congenital ankle and foot deformities. The defect can be mild or severe, unilateral or bilateral.

**Synonyms**

> Calcaneal Valgus
> Calcaneovalgus
> Metatarsus Varus
> Talipes Calcaneus
> Talipes Equinovarus
> Talipes Equinus
> Talipes Valgus
> Talipes Varus
> Valgus Calcaneus

**Signs and Symptoms** The several types of clubfoot are shown in the synonyms, above. In the most common form, **calcaneal valgus,** the heel turns outward from the midline and the anterior part of the foot is elevated. In **equino-varus,** the heel turns inward from the midline of the leg; the foot is plantar flexed, and the Achilles tendon is very tight. In **metatarsus adductus,** the forefoot deviates toward the midline. In **metatarsus varus,** the inner border of the foot does not reach the ground, so that the patient must walk on the outer border of the foot. Clubfoot is not painful and causes no difficulties until the infant begins to stand and walk. At that point, the defect forces the child to walk as if on a peg leg. If both feet are affected, the child usually walks on the balls of the feet. In severe cases, the child may walk on the sides or even the dorsum of the feet. Without the protection of the thick skin of the sole of the foot, the sides and dorsum may become ulcerated. Growth of the entire extremity may be affected.

**Etiology** The cause is unclear. The most likely explanation is a combination of hereditary factors and environmental influences, such as infection, drugs, and disease, which may affect prenatal growth.

It has been suggested that 2 etiologic types of clubfoot may occur. One is characterized by an even sex ratio, normal maternal age curve, recurrence risk of about 10 percent, and probable dominant inheritance with about 40 percent penetrance. The other group is described as born to younger mothers; affected persons are predominantly male and show no clear pattern of inheritance.

Uterine constraint may be associated with clubfoot (see *Amniotic Bands).* Children with spina bifida (see *Spina Bifida)* sometimes develop a form of clubfoot. In such cases, muscle imbalance or spasticity may cause twisting of a normal foot.

**Epidemiology** Clubfoot is usually present at birth. In the United States, it affects approximately 9,000 infants (about 1:400 live births). Boys are affected twice as often as girls.

**Treatment—Standard** Treatment of clubfoot is begun soon after birth. Serial casting for 3 to 6 months is usually required, with frequent follow-up by an orthopedist. In milder cases, splinting and night bracing may be sufficient. Surgical correction is required in more severe cases, especially when heel cord lengthening is needed.

When initiated early, conservative treatment is successful in more than half of cases. With expert early treatment, most patients are able to wear regular shoes, participate in sports, and lead active lives. Left untreated, however, the deformity becomes fixed, and growth of the entire extremity may be affected. Surgery after infancy may successfully treat the foot, but the rest of the leg may be permanently deformed.

**Treatment—Investigational** Please contact the agencies listed under Resources, below, for the most current information. Addresses and telephone numbers of these agencies, as well as of individual experts and research centers, may be found in the Master Resources List.

**Resources**

**For more information on clubfoot:** National Organization for Rare Disorders (NORD); NIH/National Institute of Child Health and Human Development.

**For genetic information and genetic counseling referrals:** March of Dimes Birth Defects Foundation; Alliance of Genetic Support Groups.

**References**

Mendelian Inheritance in Man, 11th ed.: V.A. McKusick; The Johns Hopkins University Press, 1994, p. 310.

Clubfoot: Public Health Education Information Sheet, Health Education Information Sheet, March of Dimes, 1983.

# COCKAYNE SYNDROME

**Description** Cockayne syndrome is a progressive disorder with characteristics that include growth retardation, photosensitivity, and a prematurely aged appearance.

**Synonyms**

Progeroid Nanism

**Signs and Symptoms** Infants affected by Cockayne syndrome generally appear normal at birth, with features of the disorder manifesting during the 2nd year of life. A few cases of prenatal onset have been reported.

Craniofacial abnormalities include microcephaly, a thin nose, sunken eyes, lack of subcutaneous facial fat, and prognathism. Dental caries may occur. The individual will be short of stature but have disproportionately long arms and legs, and large hands and feet. Joints may be large and habitually flexed, and there may be kyphosis. The extremities may feel cold and have a bluish color, and the patient may experience tremor and unsteady gait. Affected individuals are highly photosensitive and may be mentally deficient and partially deaf. Ocular involvement includes optic atrophy with retinal pigmentation, and cataracts. Hepatomegaly may occur. Older patients may be sexually underdeveloped. There appears to be no predisposition to malignancy.

**Etiology** Cockayne syndrome has autosomal recessive inheritance. Failure of RNA synthesis to recover to normal levels after UV irradiation occurs in about 60 percent of affected patients.

**Epidemiology** Fewer than 200 cases of all forms of the disorder have been reported.

**Related Disorders** See *Hutchinson-Gilford Syndrome,* some aspects of which are similar to Cockayne syndrome.

**Treatment—Standard** Treatment is symptomatic and supportive.

**Treatment—Investigational** Please contact the agencies listed under Resources, below, for the most current information. Addresses and telephone numbers of these agencies, as well as of individual experts and research centers, may be found in the Master Resources List.

**Resources**

**For more information on Cockayne syndrome:** National Organization for Rare Disorders (NORD); NIH/National Institute of Child Health and Human Development; Human Growth Foundation; Research Trust for Metabolic Diseases in Children; Share and Care Cockayne Syndrome Network; Magic Foundation for Children's Growth.

**For genetic information and genetic counseling referrals:** March of Dimes Birth Defects Foundation; Alliance of Genetic Support Groups.

**References**

Cockayne's Syndrome: Correlation of Clinical Features with Cellular Sensitivity of RNA Synthesis to UV Irradiation: A.R. Lehman, et al.; J. Med. Genet., August 1993, vol. 30(8), pp. 679–682.

Deficient Repair of the Transcribed Strand of Active Genes in Cockayne's Syndrome Cells: A. Van Hoffen, et al.; Nucleic Acids Res., December 1993, vol. 21(25), pp. 5890–5895.

DNA Repair: D.E. Barnes, et al.; Curr. Opin. Cell. Biol., June 1993, vol. 5(3), pp. 424–433.

Xeroderma Pigmentosum–Cockayne Syndrome Complex in Two Patients: Absence of Skin Tumors Despite Severe Deficiency of DNA Excision Repair: R.J. Scott, et al.; J. Am. Acad. Dermatol., November 1993, vol. 29(5 pt. 2) pp. 883–889.

Xeroderma Pigmentosum Complementation Group G Associated with Cockayne Syndrome: W. Vermeulen, et al.; Am. J. Hum. Genet., July 1993, vol. 53(1), pp. 185–192.

Cockayne Syndrome: Review of 140 Cases: M.A. Nance, et al.; Am. J. Med. Genet., January 1992, vol. 42(1), pp. 68–84.

Cranial CT and MRI in Diseases with DNA Repair Defects: P. Demaerel, et al.; Neuroradiology, 1992, vol. 34(2), pp. 117–121.

Demyelinating Peripheral Neuropathy in Cockayne Syndrome: A Histopathologic and Norphometric Study: J. Sasaki, et al.; Brain Dev., March 1992, vol. 14(2), pp. 114–117.

Mendelian Inheritance in Man, 10th ed.: V.A. McKusick; The Johns Hopkins University Press, 1992, pp. 1290–1291.

Nelson Textbook of Pediatrics, 14th ed.: R.E. Behrman, ed.-in-chief; W.B. Saunders Company, 1992, p. 1650.

Ocular Findings in Cockayne Syndrome: E.I. Traboulsi, et al.; Am. J. Ophthalmol., November 1992, vol. 114(5), pp. 579–583.

Apparent Late-Onset Cockayne Syndrome and Interstitial Deletion of the Long Arm of Chromosome 10 (del [10][q11.23q21.3]): J.P. Fryns, et al.; Am. J. Med. Genet., September 1991, vol. 40(3), pp. 343–344.

Cockayne's Syndrome: Literature Review and Case Report: R.A. Boraz; Pediatr. Dent., July –August 1991, vol. 13(4), pp. 227–230.

Comparison of Cellular Sensitivity to UV Killing with Neuropsychological Impairment in Cockayne Syndrome Patients: K. Sugita, et al.; Brain Dev., May 1991, vol. 13(3), pp. 163–166.

Birth Defects Encyclopedia: M.L. Buyse, ed.-in-chief; Blackwell Scientific Publications, 1990, pp. 420–422.

Dictionary of Medical Syndromes, 3rd ed.: S.I. Magalini, et al., eds.: J.B. Lippincott Company, 1990, pp. 191–192.

Syndromes of the Head and Neck, 3rd ed.: R.J. Gorlin, et al.; Oxford University Press, 1990, pp. 492–494.

The Metabolic Basis of Inherited Disease, 6th ed.: C.R. Scriver, et al., eds.; McGraw-Hill, 1989, pp. 2962–2964.

Smith's Recognizable Patterns of Human Malformation, 4th ed.: K.L. Jones; W.B. Saunders Company, 1988, pp. 122–123.

# COFFIN-LOWRY SYNDROME

**Description** Coffin-Lowry syndrome is characterized by short stature, mental retardation, hypotonia, and various facial and skeletal abnormalities.

**Synonyms**

> Coffin Syndrome
>
> Mental Retardation with Osteocartilaginous Anomalies

**Signs and Symptoms** Affected individuals have a prominent square forehead, narrow temples, prominent chin and ears, hypertelorism, downward slanting palpebral fissures, a broad nose with thick alar cartilage, thick lips, and an open mouth. There may be feeding and respiratory problems.

Patients are short in stature. Hands are large and soft, with thick, tapering fingers and prominent hypothenar. Pectus carinatum or pectus excavatum may be present. An awkward gait is characteristic in both males and females. In males, the skin is loose and easily stretched. Affected males are severely mentally retarded. Only 20 percent of females are severely mentally deficient, and 20 percent are normal.

**Etiology** Coffin-Lowry syndrome has X-linked inheritance; the gene is on the short arm of the X chromosome (Xp22.2). Female heterozygotes are usually less severely affected.

**Epidemiology** Males and females seem to be affected in equal numbers, but symptoms may be more severe in males and usually progress with age.

**Treatment—Standard** Treatment for Coffin-Lowry disease is symptomatic and supportive. Genetic counseling will be helpful for patients and their families.

**Treatment—Investigational** Please contact the agencies listed under Resources, below, for the most current information. Addresses and telephone numbers of these agencies, as well as of individual experts and research centers, may be found in the Master Resources List.

**Resources**

**For more information on Coffin-Lowry syndrome:** National Organization for Rare Disorders (NORD); NIH/National Institute of Neurological Disorders and Stroke; NIH/National Arthritis and Musculoskeletal and Skin Diseases Information Clearinghouse.

**For genetic information and genetic counseling referrals:** March of Dimes Birth Defects Foundation; Alliance of Genetic Support Groups.

**References**

Mendelian Inheritance in Man, 11th ed.: V.A. McKusick; The Johns Hopkins University Press, 1994, pp. 2330–2331.

Syndromes of the Head and Neck, 3rd ed.: R.J. Gorlin, et al.; Oxford University Press, 1990, pp. 827–829.

Smith's Recognizable Patterns of Human Malformation, 4th ed.: K.L. Jones; W.B. Saunders Company, 1988, pp. 236–237.

Early Clinical Signs in Coffin-Lowry Syndrome: J.S. Vles, et al.; Clin. Genet., November 1984, vol. 26(5), pp. 448–452.

Forearm Fullness in Coffin-Lowry Syndrome: A Misleading Yet Possible Early Diagnostic Clue: J.H. Hersh, et al.; Am. J. Med. Genet., June 1984, vol. 18(2), pp. 195–199.

Brief Clinical Report: Early Recognition of the Coffin-Lowry Syndrome: W.G. Wilson, et al.; Am. J. Med. Genet., 1981, vol. 8(2), pp. 215–220.

# COFFIN-SIRIS SYNDROME

**Description** Coffin-Siris syndrome is a congenital disorder in which mental retardation, short stature, and malformations of the 5th digit are present from birth in affected individuals. Feeding problems and frequent respiratory infections are typical.

**Synonyms**

> Fifth Digit Syndrome
>
> Mental Retardation with Hypoplastic 5th Fingernails and Toenails
>
> Short Stature–Onychodysplasia

**Signs and Symptoms** Characteristic facies includes a wide nose and/or mouth, low nasal bridge, and thick lips. Scalp hair may be sparse or excessive. Nails on the 5th finger and toe may be hypoplastic or absent. Short stature and mental deficiency are typical, and there may be joint laxity (dislocated elbows are common) and mild-to-severe hypotonia. Dental and motor development may be retarded. Feeding problems, vomiting, and recurrent respiratory infections are early manifestations. Occasionally, patients have variable skin, skeletal, genital, and cardiac defects, as well as Dandy-Walker syndrome.

**Etiology** The cause is unknown; an autosomal recessive inheritance may be involved.

**Epidemiology** Females are affected 4 times as frequently as males; lethality in males is suspected.

**Related Disorders** See *Dandy-Walker Syndrome.*

**Treatment—Standard** Treatment is symptomatic and supportive.

**Treatment—Investigational** Please contact the agencies listed under Resources, below, for the most current information. Addresses and telephone numbers of these agencies, as well as of individual experts and research centers, may be found in the Master Resources List.

**Resources**

For more information on **Coffin-Siris syndrome:** National Organization for Rare Disorders (NORD); NIH/National Institute of Child Health and Human Development; Short Stature Foundation; Human Growth Foundation.

For **genetic information and genetic counseling referrals:** March of Dimes Birth Defects Foundation; Alliance of Genetic Support Groups.

**References**

Mendelian Inheritance in Man, 11th ed.: V.A. McKusick; The Johns Hopkins University Press, 1994, p. 531.

Syndrome of Developmental Retardation, Facial and Skeletal Anomalies, and Hyperphosphatasia in Two Sisters: Nosology and Genetics of the Coffin-Siris Syndrome: P. Rabe, et al.; Am. J. Med. Genet., December 1991, vol. 41(3), pp. 350–354.

Birth Defects Encyclopedia: M.L. Buyse, ed.-in-chief; Blackwell Scientific Publications, 1990, pp. 422–423.

The Coffin-Siris Syndrome: Q.H. Qazi, et al.; J. Med. Genet., May 1990, vol. 27(5), pp. 333–336.

Dictionary of Medical Syndromes, 3rd ed.: S.I. Magalini, et al., eds.: J.B. Lippincott Company, 1990, pp. 193–194.

Smith's Recognizable Patterns of Human Malformation, 4th ed., K.L. Jones; W.B. Saunders Company, 1988, pp. 522–523.

# COHEN SYNDROME

**Description** The syndrome is characterized primarily by hypotonia, truncal obesity, prominent incisors, and mental retardation.

**Synonyms**

Pepper Syndrome

**Signs and Symptoms** The infant will have low birth weight and delayed growth, and be hypotonic. The head may be microcephalic. Facial characteristics include a high nasal bridge, mild downward slanting of palpebral fissures, short philtrum, and an open mouth. As the child grows, prominent upper central incisors are seen, and the jaw may develop abnormally. By mid-childhood, truncal obesity occurs. The hands and toes are long and slender, and there may be syndactyly of the fingers and deformities of the knees, elbows, and spine, including mild scoliosis.

Ocular deficits include hemeralopia and decreased clarity of vision; a narrowing of the visual field; and retinitis pigmentosa. Cryptorchidism and delayed puberty may be present. Leukopenia, seizures, and mitral valve prolapse are among the features seen infrequently.

**Etiology** Cohen syndrome is inherited as an autosomal recessive trait.

**Epidemiology** The disorder is rare and occurs more frequently in persons of eastern European Jewish descent and in Finns. Mottled retina appears to occur predominantly in Finnish patients.

**Related Disorders** See *Marfan Syndrome; Prader-Willi Syndrome; Retinitis Pigmentosa; Sotos Syndrome.*

**Treatment—Standard** Treatment may include surgery to correct the facial deformities, visual problems, syndactyly, and cryptorchidism. Genetic counseling may benefit patients and their families. Other treatment is symptomatic and supportive.

**Treatment—Investigational** Please contact the agencies listed under Resources, below, for the most current information. Addresses and telephone numbers of these agencies, as well as of individual experts and research centers, may be found in the Master Resources List.

**Resources**

For more information on **Cohen syndrome:** National Organization for Rare Disorders (NORD); NIH/National Institute of Child Health and Human Development.

For **genetic information and genetic counseling referrals:** March of Dimes Birth Defects Foundation; Alliance of Genetic Support Groups.

**References**

Mendelian Inheritance in Man, 11th ed.: V.A. McKusick; The Johns Hopkins University Press, 1994, pp. 1711–1712.
Syndromes of the Head and Neck, 3rd ed.: R.J. Gorlin, et al.; Oxford University Press, 1990, pp. 349–359.
Cohen Syndrome: A Connective Tissue Disorder?: K. Mehes, et al.; Am. Med. Genet., September 1988, vol. 31(1), pp. 131–133.
Smith's Recognizable Patterns of Human Malformation, 4th ed.: K.L. Jones; W.B. Saunders Company, 1988, p. 174.
Cohen Ureteral Reimplantation: Sonographic Appearance: P. Mezzacappa, et al.; Radiology, December 1987, vol. 165(3), pp. 851–852.
Intrafamilial Variation in Cohen Syndrome: I. Young, et al.; J. Med. Genet., August 1987, vol. 24(8), pp. 488–492.
Cohen Syndrome in Israel: J. Sack, et al.; Isr. J. Med. Sci., November 1986, vol. 22(11), pp. 766–770.
Cohen Syndrome with Bull's Eye Macular Lesion: K. Resnick, et al.; Ophthalmic Paediatr. Genet., March 1986, vol. 7(1), pp. 1–8.

# CONRADI-HÜNERMANN SYNDROME

**Description** Conradi-Hünermann syndrome, a form of chondrodysplasia punctata, affects infants and young children and is characterized by facial abnormalities, mild-to-moderate growth deficiencies, large skin pores, and sparse but coarse hair. The term *chondrodysplasia punctata* refers to a group of skeletal dysplasias characterized by abnormal calcium deposition in regions of endochondral bone formation.

**Synonyms**

       Chondrodysplasia Punctata
       Chondrodystrophia Calcificans Congenita
       Conradi Disease
       Dysplasia Epiphysialis Punctata

**Signs and Symptoms** Affected children have a short neck and a broad, flat nose. Large pores in the skin, resembling orange peel, may occur on the body, and scalp hair tends to be coarse and sparse. Ichthyotic skin lesions may be present (see ***Ichthyosis).*** Epiphyseal calcification slows growth in the extremities, and scoliosis may occur even in infancy. Buildup of fibrous tissue around joints may limit mobility. Cataracts may develop, and a small percentage of patients may be mentally retarded.

**Etiology** Conradi-Hünermann syndrome is the X-linked dominant form of chondrodysplasia punctata. Chondrodysplasia punctata is heterogeneous both at the genetic and clinical levels. The X-linked form of this condition is caused by a mutation in a sulfatase gene on Xp22.3.

**Epidemiology** This extremely rare syndrome is present at birth and seems to affect only females, since the gene defect is lethal for hemizygous males.

**Related Disorders Chondrodysplasia (rhizomelic type)** is a form of chondrodysplasia punctata inherited as an autosomal recessive trait. Affected individuals may have facial anomalies, cardiac and vision disorders, and a predisposition to recurrent infections. Spasticity and mental retardation are also present. Calcifications of hip and shoulder joints inhibit growth in the extremities. The condition is usually lethal in the first year of life.

**Fetal warfarin syndrome** has features similar to those of Conradi-Hünermann syndrome, including growth deficiency, unusual facies, and recurrent infection, along with mental retardation. The condition results from maternal use of warfarin during pregnancy. It appears that warfarin embryopathy is caused by drug-induced inhibition of the sulfatase gene.

**Treatment—Standard** Orthopedic surgery may be useful in the correction of problems associated with bone growth abnormalities, and problems with vision may be treated surgically or with corrective lenses. Dermatologic conditions should be treated symptomatically. Genetic counseling is advised.

**Treatment—Investigational** Please contact the agencies listed under Resources, below, for the most current information. Addresses and telephone numbers of these agencies, as well as of individual experts and research centers, may be found in the Master Resources List.

**Resources**

   **For more information on Conradi-Hünermann syndrome:** National Organization for Rare Disorders (NORD); NIH/National Arthritis and Musculoskeletal and Skin Diseases Information Clearinghouse; NIH/National Eye Institute; International Center for Skeletal Dysplasia; Human Growth Foundation; Parents of Dwarfed Children; Little People of America; Short Stature Foundation.

   **For more information on scoliosis:** National Scoliosis Foundation.

   **For genetic information and genetic counseling referrals:** March of Dimes Birth Defects Foundation; Alliance of Genetic Support Groups.

**References**

A Cluster of Sulfatase Genes on Xp22.3: Mutations in Chondrodysplasia Punctata (CDPX) and Implications for Warfarin Embryopathy: B. Franco; Cell, 1995, vol. 85, pp. 15–25.
Mendelian Inheritance in Man, 11th ed.: V.A. McKusick; The Johns Hopkins University Press, 1994, p. 297.

Syndromes of the Head and Neck, 3rd ed.: R.J. Gorlin, et al.; Oxford University Press, 1990, pp. 188–190.
Smith's Recognizable Patterns of Human Malformation, 4th ed.: K.L. Jones; W.B. Saunders Company, 1988, pp. 338–339.

# CORNELIA DE LANGE SYNDROME

**Description** Individuals with Cornelia de Lange syndrome greatly resemble each other. Major characteristics include skeletal and facial anomalies, excessive hairiness, and severe mental retardation.

**Synonyms**
>Amsterdam Dwarf Syndrome of de Lange
>Brachmann–de Lange Syndrome

**Signs and Symptoms** Neonates have low birth weight (under 5 lb) and feeding difficulties. Typical craniofacial features include microcephaly; a small, broad nose; thin, down-turned lips; thick, bushy eyebrows; and long eyelashes. Cleft palate may occur. Hands and feet are small, and limb abnormalities include phocomelia and oligodactyly. Other characteristics include hirsutism, hearing loss, seizures, and cardiac and gastrointestinal abnormalities. Stature is small. Mental retardation is severe and speech may be impaired.

**Etiology** The syndrome is suspected to be genetic in origin, but the mode of transmission is unknown. A gene on the long arm of chromosome 3 may be responsible. Most cases are sporadic.

**Epidemiology** Males and females appear to be affected in equal numbers. There is a 2 to 4 percent recurrence rate within families. The syndrome is estimated to occur in less than 1:100,000 births.

**Treatment—Standard** Physical and occupational therapy, special education, hearing aids, and prosthetic limbs may all be beneficial. Genetic counseling is recommended.

**Treatment—Investigational** Please contact the agencies listed under Resources, below, for the most current information. Addresses and telephone numbers of these agencies, as well as of individual experts and research centers, may be found in the Master Resources List.

**Resources**
**For more information on Cornelia de Lange syndrome:** National Organization for Rare Disorders (NORD); Cornelia de Lange Syndrome Foundation; NIH/National Institute of Child Health and Human Development.

**For genetic information and genetic counseling referrals:** March of Dimes Birth Defects Foundation; Alliance of Genetic Support Groups.

**References**
Mendelian Inheritance in Man, 11th ed.: V.A. McKusick; The Johns Hopkins University Press, 1994, pp. 367–369.
Smith's Recognizable Patterns of Human Malformation, 4th ed.: K.L. Jones; W.B. Saunders Company, 1988, pp. 80–83.
Normal Language Skills and Normal Intelligence in a Child with De Lange Syndrome: T.H. Cameron, et al.; J. Speech Hear. Discord., May 1988, vol. 53(2), pp. 219–222.
Mild Brachmann–de Lange Syndrome: Changes of Phenotype with Age: F. Greenberg, et al.; Am. J. Med. Genet., January 1989, vol. 32(1), pp. 90–92.

# CRANIOMETAPHYSEAL DYSPLASIA

**Description** Craniometaphyseal dysplasia is a rare genetic disorder in which characteristic craniofacial and skeletal anomalies occur, accompanied by hearing loss.

**Synonyms**
>Osteochondroplasia

**Signs and Symptoms** The disorder is usually evident at birth, and is characterized by hyperostosis of the bones of the cranial vault, face, and mandible. The thickening is especially evident at the nasal bridge, and the nasal passages are abnormally small as a result of bony encroachment. Hypertelorism and proptosis occur, and there may be mandibular malocclusion. If cranial pressure is not relieved, facial paralysis, deafness, and loss of vision may occur. The limbs may be affected by sclerosis or metaphyseal splaying. Intelligence is usually normal.

**Etiology** The cause is not known. Both autosomal dominant and recessive forms have been described. The recessive form is more severe than the dominant form.

**Epidemiology** Males and females are equally affected.

**Related Disorders** See *Osteopetrosis.*

**Pyle disease (metaphyseal dysplasia),** often confused with craniometaphyseal dysplasia, is a rare genetic disorder with few clinical findings, and the skull is only mildly affected. It is characterized by marked splaying of the long bones, which is more severe than that seen in craniometaphyseal dysplasia.

**Frontometaphyseal dysplasia** is a rare genetic disorder characterized by a wide nasal bridge, incomplete development of the sinuses, hypertelorism, supraorbital bossing, micromandible, and multiple deformities of the teeth and bones. Mental retardation may also occur.

**Treatment—Standard** Early surgical treatment to relieve cranial pressure and correct the facial deformities may also help eliminate vision and hearing complications. Genetic counseling may be beneficial.

**Treatment—Investigational** Please contact the agencies listed under Resources, below, for the most current information. Addresses and telephone numbers of these agencies, as well as of individual experts and research centers, may be found in the Master Resources List.

**Resources**

**For more information on craniometaphyseal dysplasia:** National Organization for Rare Disorders (NORD); NIH/National Institute of Child Health and Human Development; National Craniofacial Foundation; National Foundation for Facial Reconstruction; FACES—National Association for the Craniofacially Handicapped.

**For genetic information and genetic counseling referrals:** March of Dimes Birth Defects Foundation; Alliance of Genetic Support Groups.

**References**

Mendelian Inheritance in Man, 11th ed.: V.A. McKusick; The Johns Hopkins University Press, 1994, pp. 373, 1724.

Smith's Recognizable Patterns of Human Malformation, 4th ed.: K.L. Jones; W.B. Saunders Company, 1988, p. 349.

Autosomal Dominant Craniometaphyseal Dysplasia: Clinical Variability: A. Carnevale, et al.; Clin. Genet., January 1983, vol. 23(1), pp. 17–22.

Optic Atrophy and Visual Loss in Craniometaphyseal Dysplasia: C. Puliafito, et al.; Am. J. Ophthalmol., November 1981, vol. 92(5), pp. 696–701.

# CRANIOSYNOSTOSIS, PRIMARY

**Description** Primary craniosynostosis is a congenital disorder in which premature closure of the sutures results in an abnormally shaped head. The severity of symptoms and shape of the skull depend on which bones are affected.

**Synonyms**

Craniostenosis
Kleeblattschadel Deformity
Plagiocephaly
Scaphocephaly
Trigonocephaly
Turricephaly

**Signs and Symptoms** Primary craniosynostosis comprises several types of premature cranial closures:

**Kleeblattschadel deformity** is craniosynostosis of multiple or all sutures. The head assumes a cloverleaf shape. Hydrocephaly may cause the head to appear larger.

**Plagiocephaly** is the closure of one side of the coronal joint, causing the head to look twisted or lopsided. The forehead and orbit of the eye are flat on one side. Bulging of the forehead may be apparent. Females are affected more often than males.

In **scaphocephaly,** the most common form of craniosynostosis, the sagittal joint is closed prematurely, resulting in a long, narrow head.

**Trigonocephaly** causes premature closure of the metopic suture, a keel-shaped forehead, and hypotelorism. Abnormal development of the forebrain may occur.

**Turricephaly** is characterized by premature closure of both the coronal and sagittal joints, resulting in a long, narrow head with a pointed top.

**Etiology** Primary craniosynostosis is inherited as an autosomal recessive or autosomal dominant trait. A mutation in the MSX2 gene on chromosome 5q34–q35 is the cause of Boston-type craniosynostosis but not of other forms of craniosynostosis.

**Epidemiology** Males are affected slightly more often than females. The genetically recessive cases of this disorder in the United States have been associated with the Amish in Ohio.

**Related Disorders** See *Apert Syndrome; Carpenter Syndrome; Crouzon Disease; Pfeiffer Syndrome; Saethre-Chotzen Syndrome.*

**Treatment—Standard** Surgery is indicated for multiple premature closures of the skull to prevent intracranial pressure and possible brain damage. Surgery may also be performed for cosmetic reasons.

Genetic counseling may benefit patients and their families. Other treatment is symptomatic and supportive.

**Treatment—Investigational** Please contact the agencies listed under Resources, below, for the most current information. Addresses and telephone numbers of these agencies, as well as of individual experts and research centers, may be found in the Master Resources List.

**Resources**

**For more information on primary craniosynostosis:** National Organization for Rare Disorders (NORD); FACES—National Association for the Craniofacially Handicapped; National Craniofacial Foundation; Forward Face; Children's Craniofacial Association; Craniofacial Family Association; AboutFace; NIH/National Institute of Child Health and Human Development.

**For genetic information and genetic counseling referrals:** March of Dimes Birth Defects Foundation; Alliance of Genetic Support Groups.

**References**

Mendelian Inheritance in Man, 11th ed.: V.A. McKusick; The Johns Hopkins University Press, 1994, pp. 373–375.

Craniosynostosis: A.D. Hockley; Lancet, July 1993, vol. 342(8865), pp. 189–190.

Nelson Textbook of Pediatrics, 14th ed.: R.E. Behrman, ed.-in-chief; W.B. Saunders Company, 1992, pp. 1490–1491.

Birth Defects Encyclopedia: M.L. Buyse, ed.-in-chief; Blackwell Scientific Publications, 1990, p. 464.

A Population-Based Study of Craniosynostosis: L.R. French, et al.; J. Clin. Epidemiol. 1990, vol. 43(1), pp. 69–73.

Craniosynostosis: An Analysis of the Timing, Treatment, and Complications in 164 Consecutive Patients: L.A. Whitaker, et al.; Plast. Reconstr. Surg., August 1987, vol. 80(2), pp. 195–212.

# CRI DU CHAT SYNDROME

**Description** Cri du chat syndrome is characterized in infants by a high, shrill, mewing, kittenlike cry that fades in later infancy. Other abnormalities are present.

**Synonyms**

Cat's Cry Syndrome

Chromosome 5p- Syndrome

Le Jeune Syndrome

**Signs and Symptoms** The characteristic plaintive cry similar to the mewing of a cat is present during the first weeks of life. Birth weight usually is low, and growth is slow. Almost all patients are microcephalic and mentally deficient. The typical infant has a round face with hypertelorism, epicanthal folds, strabismus, low-set and/or malformed ears, a small chin, prominent nose, and facial asymmetry. Palmar simian creases are common. More than three-quarters of infants are hypotonic; as infants grow older this is replaced with hyperreflexia.

Abnormalities that occur less frequently include myopia, cleft lip and cleft palate, bifid uvula, clinodactyly, hemivertebra, inguinal hernia, cryptorchidism, absent kidney and spleen, clubfoot, and flat feet. Seven of 13 adults in one study had scoliosis, and 11 patients had short metacarpals and metatarsals. A great deal of phenotypic heterogeneity occurs in this syndrome.

**Etiology** A partial deletion of the short arm of chromosome 5 causes cri du chat syndrome. The larger the deletion, the more severe the effect on intelligence, height, and weight. The majority of deletions are de novo; parental translocations account for 10 percent of cases.

**Epidemiology** Cri du chat syndrome was first described in 1963; since then over 100 cases have been reported. It has been estimated that the syndrome occurs in about 1:50,000 births and accounts for approximately 1 percent of institutionalized mentally retarded patients.

**Treatment—Standard** Treatment for cri du chat syndrome is symptomatic and supportive.

**Treatment—Investigational** Please contact the agencies listed under Resources, below, for the most current information. Addresses and telephone numbers of these agencies, as well as of individual experts and research centers, may be found in the Master Resources List.

**Resources**

**For more information on cri du chat syndrome:** National Organization for Rare Disorders (NORD); Cri-du-Chat Society; 5p- Society; NIH/National Institute of Child Health and Human Development; Chromosome Deletion Outreach.

**For genetic information and genetic counseling referrals:** March of Dimes Birth Defects Foundation; Alliance of Genetic Support Groups.

**References**

Molecular Definition of Deletions of Different Segments of Distal 5p That Result in Distinct p Phenotypic Features: D.M. Church, et al.; Am. J. Hum. Genet., 1995, vol. 56, pp. 1162–1172.

Syndromes of the Head and Neck, 3rd ed.: R.J. Gorlin, et al.; Oxford University Press, 1990, pp. 48–49.

Smith's Recognizable Patterns of Human Malformation, 4th ed.: K.L. Jones; W.B. Saunders Company, 1988, pp. 40–41.

Psychomotor Development in 65 Home-Reared Children with Cri-du-Chat Syndrome: L.E. Wilkins, et al.; J. Pediatr., 1980, vol. 97, p. 401.

# CROUZON DISEASE

**Description** Crouzon disease is a form of craniosynostosis in which characteristic facial anomalies occur, accompanied by mental retardation and disturbances in vision and hearing.

**Synonyms**
>Acrocephalosyndactyly II
>Craniofacial Dysostosis
>Crouzon Craniofacial Dysostosis

**Signs and Symptoms** Acrocephaly, hypertelorism, exophthalmos, strabismus, a parrot-beaked nose with deviated septum, hypoplastic maxilla, and mandibular prognathism are present in affected individuals. In more than 50 percent of cases, progressive vision loss and conductive hearing loss occur. Mental retardation is evident, and spinal anomalies are present in about one-third of patients. Abnormal cranial growth begins in the first year of life and is completed by age 3 years. Life expectancy is normal.

**Etiology** The disease is inherited as an autosomal dominant trait. Mutations in the fibroblast growth factor receptor 2 (**FGFR2**) gene is the cause of Crouzon disease.

**Epidemiology** Males and females are affected in equal numbers.

**Related Disorders** Most patients with Apert syndrome and Jackson-Weiss syndrome and many with Pfeiffer syndrome also have mutations at FGFR2. See *Apert Syndrome; Jackson-Weiss Syndrome; Pfeiffer Syndrome.*

**Treatment—Standard** Surgery is indicated to relieve intracranial pressure and to correct craniofacial anomalies. Vision loss may be treated with corrective lenses or with ophthalmic surgical procedures. Genetic counseling is recommended.

**Treatment—Investigational** Drs. Amy Feldman Lewanda and Ethylin Wang Jabs at Johns Hopkins Hospital in Baltimore are investigating the genes responsible for craniofacial disorders.

Please contact the agencies listed under Resources, below, for the most current information. Addresses and telephone numbers of these agencies, as well as of individual experts and research centers, may be found in the Master Resources List.

**Resources**

**For more information on Crouzon disease:** National Organization for Rare Disorders (NORD); National Craniofacial Foundation; FACES—National Association for the Craniofacially Handicapped; Society for the Rehabilitation of the Facially Disfigured; AboutFace.

**For genetic information and genetic counseling referrals:** March of Dimes Birth Defects Foundation; Alliance of Genetic Support Groups.

**References**
Mutations in the Fibroblast Growth Factor Receptor 2 Gene Cause Cruzon Syndrome: W. Reardon, et al.; Nat. Genet., 1994, vol. 8, pp. 98–103.

The Encyclopedia of Genetic Disorders and Birth Defects: J. Wynbrandt and M.D. Ludman, eds.; Facts on File, 1991, pp. 88–89.

Developmental Abnormalities: A.B. Baker and R.J. Joynt; *in* Clinical Neurology, revised edition, Harper and Row, 1986, pp. 71–74.

Three-Dimensional Cat Scan Reconstruction–Pediatric Patients: K.E. Salyer, et al.; Clin. Plast. Surg., July 1986, vol. 13(3), pp. 463–474.

Premature Closure of the Cranial Sutures: L.P. Roland and C. Kennedy; *in* Merritt's Textbook of Neurology, 7th ed., Lea and Febiger, 1984, pp. 376–379.

# CYSTIC HYGROMA

**Description** Cystic hygroma, a cystic lymphangioma, usually occurs at the nape of the neck.

**Synonyms**
>Cystic Lymphangioma
>Fetal Cystic Hygroma
>Hygroma Colli

**Signs and Symptoms** Cystic hygroma may be present at birth or can begin during early childhood. The sac, filled with lymphatic fluid and cells, is thin-walled and compressible, and it grows rapidly upward toward the ear, or down toward the axilla. Rarely it may originate in the axilla, groin, retroperitoneal cavity, chest wall, hip, or the coccygeal region. Surgical or drug treatment usually prevents the cyst from greatly enlarging; however, it may become progressive, causing hydrops.

Cystic hygroma can be detected during pregnancy through ultrasonography and through testing for an elevated level of $\alpha$-1-fetoprotein in the amniotic fluid.

**Etiology** Cystic hygroma is probably inherited through autosomal recessive genes. The hygroma is thought to be caused by a failure of the lymphatic system to properly connect with the cervical blood vessels.

**Epidemiology** Males and females are affected in equal numbers.

**Related Disorders** Cystic hygroma may be seen in persons with ***Turner Syndrome.*** See also ***Lymphangioma, Cavernous.***

**Treatment—Standard** Prenatal testing through ultrasonography may reveal a greatly elevated level of α-1-feto-protein. Treatment may include surgery as well as use of bleomycin in a microsphere-in-oil emulsion. Recurrence of the hygroma is possible after treatment.

**Treatment—Investigational** Please contact the agencies listed under Resources, below, for the most current information. Addresses and telephone numbers of these agencies, as well as of individual experts and research centers, may be found in the Master Resources List.

**Resources**

**For more information on cystic hygroma:** National Organization for Rare Disorders (NORD); National Lymphatic and Venous Diseases Foundation; American Cancer Society; NIH/National Cancer Institute Physician Data Query Phoneline.

**For genetic information and genetic counseling referrals:** March of Dimes Birth Defects Foundation; Alliance of Genetic Support Groups.

**References**

Mendelian Inheritance in Man, 11th ed.: V.A. McKusick; The Johns Hopkins University Press, 1994, p. 2082.

Nelson Textbook of Pediatrics, 14th ed.: R.E. Behrman, ed.-in-chief; W.B. Saunders Company, 1992, p. 481.

Treatment of Cystic Hygroma and Lymphangioma with the Use of Bleomycin Fat Emulsion: N. Tanigawa, et al.; Cancer, August 1987, vol. 60(4), pp. 741–749.

Fetal Cystic Hygroma Colli: Antenatal Diagnosis, Significance, and Management: A.S. Garden, et al.; Am. J. Obstet. Gynecol., February 1986, vol. 154(2), pp. 221–225.

Fetal Cystic Hygroma and Turner's Syndrome: R.F. Carr, et al.; Am. J. Dis. Child., June 1986, vol. 140(6), pp. 580–583.

# DENTIN DYSPLASIA, CORONAL

**Description** Coronal dentin dysplasia is a genetic disorder characterized by opalescent deciduous teeth and normal-appearing, but abnormal, secondary dentition.

**Synonyms**

Anomalous Dysplasia of Dentin
Dentin Dysplasia, Type II
Pulp Stones
Pulpal Dysplasia

**Signs and Symptoms** The deciduous teeth have a brownish-blue opalescent look. On x-ray, they show obliterated pulp chambers and reduced root canals. The permanent teeth are normal in color but contain flame-shaped pulp chambers, often with an extension reaching into the root, and numerous pulp stones. Root formation in the permanent teeth is usually normal.

**Etiology** Coronal dentin dysplasia is inherited as an autosomal dominant trait.

**Epidemiology** Males and females are affected in equal numbers.

**Related Disorders** See ***Dentin Dysplasia, Radicular; Dentinogenesis Imperfecta, Type III.***

**Treatment—Standard** Coronal dentin dysplasia may be treated by curettage around the tips of the roots and retrograde amalgam seal, or by more conventional root canal therapy. However, preventive dental care provides the best available means of maintaining the teeth.

Genetic counseling is recommended for families of children with coronal dentin dysplasia.

**Treatment—Investigational** Please contact the agencies listed under Resources, below, for the most current information. Addresses and telephone numbers of these agencies, as well as of individual experts and research centers, may be found in the Master Resources List.

**Resources**

**For more information on coronal dentin dysplasia:** National Organization for Rare Disorders (NORD); National Foundation for Ectodermal Dysplasias; NIH/National Institute of Dental Research.

**For genetic information and genetic counseling referrals:** March of Dimes Birth Defects Foundation; Alliance of Genetic Support Groups.

**References**

Mendelian Inheritance in Man, 11th ed.: V.A. McKusick; The Johns Hopkins University Press, 1994, p. 412.

Dentinal Dysplasia: A Clinicopathological Study of Eight Cases and Review of the Literature: N.E. Steidler, et al.; Br. J. Maxillofac. Surg., August 1984, vol. 22(4), pp. 274–286.

A Scanning Electron Microscopic Study of Dentin Dysplasia Type II in Primary Dentition: J.R. Jasmin, et al.; Oral Surg., July 1984, vol. 58(1), pp. 57–63.

# DENTIN DYSPLASIA, RADICULAR

**Description** Radicular dentin dysplasia is a genetic disorder characterized by atypical formation of the dentin, resulting in abnormal roots and pulp chambers.

**Synonyms**
>Dentin Dysplasia, Type I
>Rootless Teeth

**Signs and Symptoms** The teeth generally are of normal shape and color, although in some cases there is an opalescent shine. X-rays reveal half-moon–shaped or obliterated pulp chambers in the roots. Areas around the abnormally short roots may appear radiolucent.

Both the deciduous and permanent teeth are affected. The teeth are often poorly aligned and can be chipped easily. Without treatment, persons with radicular dentin dysplasia may lose their teeth by age 30 to 40 years.

**Etiology** Radicular dentin dysplasia is inherited as an autosomal dominant disorder.

**Epidemiology** Radicular dentin dysplasia affects about 1:100,000 persons. Males and females are affected in equal numbers.

**Related Disorders** See *Dentin Dysplasia, Coronal; Dentinogenesis Imperfecta, Type III.*

**Treatment—Standard** Filling the tips of the root canals permits the teeth to remain in their natural positions. Sometimes the affected teeth must be extracted and replaced with dentures.

Genetic counseling is recommended for families of children with radicular dentin dysplasia.

**Treatment—Investigational** Please contact the agencies listed under Resources, below, for the most current information. Addresses and telephone numbers of these agencies, as well as of individual experts and research centers, may be found in the Master Resources List.

**Resources**

**For more information on radicular dentin dysplasia:** National Organization for Rare Disorders (NORD); National Foundation for Ectodermal Dysplasias; NIH/National Institute of Dental Research.

**For genetic information and genetic counseling referrals:** March of Dimes Birth Defects Foundation; Alliance of Genetic Support Groups.

**References**

Mendelian Inheritance in Man, 11th ed.: V.A. McKusick; The Johns Hopkins University Press, 1994, pp. 411–412.

Dentin Dysplasia Type I: A Clinical Report: J.A. Petrone, et al.; J. Am. Dent. Assoc., December 1981, vol. 103(6), pp. 891–893.

Dentin Dysplasia Type I: A Scanning Electron Microscopic Analysis of the Primary Dentition: M. Melnick, et al.; Oral Surg., October 1980, vol. 50(4), pp. 335–340.


# DENTINOGENESIS IMPERFECTA, TYPE III

**Description** Dentinogenesis imperfecta, type III, is an inherited dental disorder in which the primary and secondary teeth erode early and the pulp is revealed. Other genetic anomalies often occur concomitantly with this dental disorder.

**Synonyms**
>Brandywine Type Dentinogenesis Imperfecta
>Dentinogenesis Imperfecta, Shields Type III

**Signs and Symptoms** The crowns of both primary and secondary teeth decay, sometimes exposing the pulp. The pulp is smooth and amber-colored and reflects an iridescent light. Secondary teeth may be characterized by absent or partially absent pulp chambers and root canals, whereas those of the primary teeth may be larger than normal. Secondary teeth may also be pitted.

The teeth of carriers may appear normal, but the pulp chamber may be larger than normal, and the enamel may be quite thin. This condition is referred to as shell teeth.

**Etiology** Dentinogenesis imperfecta, type III, is inherited as an autosomal dominant trait.

**Epidemiology** First diagnosed in the Brandywine, Maryland, community, dentinogenesis imperfecta, type III, is also found in the Ashkenazic Jewish population.

**Related Disorders** See *Dentin Dysplasia, Radicular; Dentin Dysplasia, Coronal.*

**Dentinogenesis imperfecta, type I (DGI 1; opalescent dentin; opalescent teeth without osteogenesis imperfecta; dentinogenesis imperfecta, Shields type II; capdepont teeth; hereditary brown teeth)** is a genetic condition in which the teeth are bluish-gray or amber-colored and reflect an iridescent light, without concomitant brittle bones. The teeth have bulbous crowns. Roots, root canals, and pulp chambers are absent or too small. Bringing the teeth together, as occurs when chewing, causes the enamel to separate from the ivory.

**Treatment—Standard** Children are fitted with dental crowns as early as possible for cosmetic benefit; adults may undergo tooth extraction and replacement with dentures.

Families of affected children may benefit from genetic counseling.

**Treatment—Investigational** Please contact the agencies listed under Resources, below, for the most current information. Addresses and telephone numbers of these agencies, as well as of individual experts and research centers, may be found in the Master Resources List.

**Resources**

**For more information on dentinogenesis imperfecta, type III:** National Organization for Rare Disorders (NORD); National Foundation for Ectodermal Dysplasias; NIH/National Institute of Dental Research.

**For genetic information and genetic counseling referrals:** March of Dimes Birth Defects Foundation; Alliance of Genetic Support Groups.

**References**

An Autosomal-Dominant Form of Juvenile Periodontitis: Its Localization to Chromosome 4 and Linkage to Dentinogenesis Imperfecta and Gc; J. Craniofac. Genet. Dev. Biol., 1986, vol. 6(4), pp. 341–350.

An Unusual Presentation of Opalescent Dentin and Brandywine Isolate Hereditary Opalescent Dentin in an Ashkenazic Jewish Family: A. Heimler, et al.; Oral Surg. Oral Med. Oral Pathol., June 1985, vol. 59(6), pp. 608–615.

Dentinogenesis Imperfecta in the Brandywine Isolate (DI Type III): Clinical, Radiologic, and Scanning Electron Microscopic Studies of the Dentition: L.S. Levin, et al.; Oral Surg., September 1983, vol. 56(3), pp. 267–274.

# DIASTROPHIC DYSPLASIA

**Description** Diastrophic dysplasia is a hereditary growth disorder characterized by short limbs, abnormally curved bones, joint and hand deformities, and clubfeet. Intelligence is usually normal.

**Synonyms**

Chondrodystrophy with Clubfeet

**Signs and Symptoms** Onset is prenatal. Infants are short in stature. Abnormalities of the spine generally include scoliosis, kyphosis, and cervical spina bifida. Pelvic bones, the femoral head, and the coccyx may be malformed. On weight-bearing, the hip and knee joints tend to dislocate. The thumb is extended in a characteristic hitchhiker position, and synostosis of proximal interphalangeal joints is present. Severe bilateral clubfeet may occur.

Craniofacial abnormalities include cleft palate (about 25 percent of patients) and occasionally a beak-shaped nose and facial hemangioma. In early infancy the pinna of the ear may have cystlike swellings; later these may develop into cauliflower-like shapes with or without ossification.

**Etiology** The genetic defect, transmitted by autosomal recessive genes, affects the manner in which cartilage is converted to bone. Mutations involving a novel sulfate transporter (**DTDST**) have been recently reported as a cause for the condition.

**Epidemiology** Males and females are affected in equal numbers. The disorder is particularly prevalent in Finland.

**Related Disorders** See ***Achondroplasia; Arthrogryposis Multiplex Congenita.***

**Treatment—Standard** Treatment consists of orthopedic management, including surgery, braces, casts, and manipulations. Dental treatment and surgical closure of the cleft palate are used when necessary. Corticosteroids are injected into the ear to treat the cartilage deformity. Genetic counseling is recommended.

**Treatment—Investigational** Please contact the agencies listed under Resources, below, for the most current information. Addresses and telephone numbers of these agencies, as well as of individual experts and research centers, may be found in the Master Resources List.

**Resources**

**For more information on diastrophic dysplasia:** National Organization for Rare Disorders (NORD); NIH/National Arthritis and Musculoskeletal and Skin Diseases Information Clearinghouse; Little People of America; Human Growth Foundation; Short Stature Foundation; International Center for Skeletal Dysplasia.

**For genetic information and genetic counseling referrals:** March of Dimes Birth Defects Foundation; Alliance of Genetic Support Groups.

**References**

The Diastrophic Dysplasia Gene Encodes a Novel Sulfate Transporter: Positional Cloning by Fine-Structure Linkage Disequilibrium Mapping: J. Hastbacka; Cell, 1994, vol. 78, pp. 1073–1087.

Mendelian Inheritance in Man, 11th ed.: V.A. McKusick; The Johns Hopkins University Press, 1994, pp. 1766–1767.

Smith's Recognizable Patterns of Human Malformation, 4th ed.: K.L. Jones; W.B. Saunders Company, 1988, pp. 326–327.

Disorders of the Spine in Diastrophic Dwarfism: D. Bethem, et al.; J. Bone Joint Surg. Am., 1980, vol. 62(4), pp. 529–536.

# DiGeorge Syndrome

**Description** DiGeorge syndrome results from developmental defects of the 3rd and 4th pharyngeal pouches and the 4th branchial arch. The disorder consists of abnormalities of the heart, thymus, and parathyroid glands.

**Synonyms**

Third and Fourth Pharyngeal Pouch Syndrome

**Signs and Symptoms** Since the original description by DiGeorge, the spectrum of the disorder has been considerably expanded. The majority of children have a congenital heart defect, mainly conotruncal defects such as interrupted aortic arch, truncus, or tetralogy of Fallot. Other defects, as well as multiple cardiac defects, may occur.

Neonatal hypocalcemia is common. It may be severe and unremitting owing to aplasia of the parathyroids, whereas in patients with hypoplasia of the parathyroids the hypocalcemia remits or may not have its onset until childhood.

Aplasia of the thymus and severe immunodeficiency are rare. More often, some thymic tissue that failed to descend into the chest is present in the neck. Absence of a thymic shadow radiographically or even during cardiac surgery does not usually mean the thymus is aplastic. Patients with ectopia of the thymus have mild degrees of immunodeficiency and are usually clinically asymptomatic.

Facial, pharyngeal, and palatal abnormalities are common. Urogenital and skeletal anomalies and developmental retardation occur in some patients.

**Etiology** Most often the condition occurs sporadically. In 20 percent of cases, a cytogenetic deletion of the long arm of chromosome 22 (22q11) is found. However, DNA probes have revealed that 90 percent of patients have the 22q11 deletion. In about 10 percent of cases, the disorder is inherited from a parent with only minor stigmata who carries the 22q11 deletion. Prenatal diagnosis is possible.

Patients with Shprintzen syndrome (velo-cardio-facial syndrome) have many of the same phenotype findings as well as the same 22q11 deletion as patients with DiGeorge syndrome (see **Shprintzen Syndrome**). The DiGeorge phenotype may also occur in infants of diabetic mothers, in retinoic acid embryopathy, and in the CHARGE association (see **CHARGE Association**). Faulty development of the cephalic neural crest is believed to be the common pathogenetic mechanism involved in all of these conditions.

**Epidemiology** Males and females seem to be affected in equal numbers.

**Related Disorders** See *Nezelof Syndrome; Severe Combined Immunodeficiency; Wiskott-Aldrich Syndrome.*

**Treatment—Standard** To control infantile seizures, blood calcium levels must be increased. Orally administered calcium and vitamin D are indicated. Mild immunodeficiency usually improves spontaneously after the first few years of life unless the thymus is completely absent. Transplantation of fetal thymus tissue, bone marrow transplantation, and administration of various thymic hormones have been used to treat severe cases. Optimal treatment is still evolving.

Patients with severe immunodeficiency must be protected as much as possible from infectious agents. They should not be immunized with live viral vaccines. Corticosteroids and immunosuppressant drugs must be avoided. Should blood transfusions be necessary, the blood must be irradiated to remove all viable lymphocytes that might cause graft-versus-host disease. Cardiac surgery is often necessary for life-threatening heart defects.

Genetic counseling may benefit patients and their families. Parents of affected patients should be tested for the 22q11 deletion.

**Treatment—Investigational** Transplantation of fetal thymus tissue, bone marrow transplantation, and administration of various thymic hormones have been used experimentally to treat severe cases of DiGeorge syndrome. More research is needed to determine the safety and efficacy of such procedures.

Please contact the agencies listed under Resources, below, for the most current information. Addresses and telephone numbers of these agencies, as well as of individual experts and research centers, may be found in the Master Resources List.

**Resources**

**For more information on DiGeorge syndrome:** National Organization for Rare Disorders (NORD); NIH/National Institute of Child Health and Human Development; Immune Deficiency Foundation; Angelo M. DiGeorge, M.D., St. Christopher's Hospital for Children, Philadelphia; Frank Greenberg, M.D., Baylor College of Medicine, Houston; Craig B. Langman, M.D., and Samuel S. Gidding, M.D., Children's Memorial Hospital, Chicago, Illinois.

**For genetic information and genetic counseling referrals:** March of Dimes Birth Defects Foundation; Alliance of Genetic Support Groups.

**References**

Mendelian Inheritance in Man, 11th ed.: V.A. McKusick; The Johns Hopkins University Press, 1994, pp. 1439–1441.

DiGeorge Syndrome: Part of CATCH 22: D.I. Wilson, et al.; J. Med. Genet., 1993, vol. 30, pp. 852–856.

A Genetic Etiology for DiGeorge Syndrome: Consistent Deletions and Microdeletions of 22q11: D.A. Driscoll; Am. J. Hum. Genet., May 1992, vol. 50(5), pp. 924–933.

Nelson Textbook of Pediatrics, 14th ed.: R.E. Behrman, ed.-in-chief; W.B. Saunders Company, 1992, pp. 553–554.

The DiGeorge Anomaly: R. Hong; Immunodefic. Rev., 1991, vol. 3(1), pp. 1–14.

Recognizable Patterns of Human Malformation, 4th ed.: K.L. Jones; W.B. Saunders Company, 1988, pp. 556–557.

Immunodeficiency: R.H. Buckley; J. Allergy Clin. Immunol., December 1983, vol. 6(72), pp. 627–641.

# Down Syndrome

**Description** Down syndrome is the most common and readily identifiable genetic condition associated with mental retardation. Facial, skeletal, and frequently cardiac anomalies are among the more than 50 clinical signs seen in the syndrome, although it is rare to find all or even most of them in one person.

**Synonyms**

> Mongolism
>
> Trisomy 21 Syndrome

**Signs and Symptoms** Some common characteristics include microcephaly, small mouth, flat nasal bridge, Brushfield spots in the iris, epicanthal folds, small ears sometimes folded over at the tops, short neck, a simian crease on the palm, and poor muscle tone.

All children with Down syndrome have some degree of mental retardation, usually in the mild-to-moderate range, but sometimes profound.

Approximately 50 percent of affected children have congenital heart disease. They are prone to respiratory, eye, and ear problems. They are 20 times more likely to develop leukemia than the general population, but it is believed that leukemia itself is not inherited but results from an increased genetic susceptibility to leukemia-causing environmental factors. Life expectancy is close to normal.

**Etiology** In Down syndrome, the mental and physical abnormalities are caused by the presence of an extra chromosome contributed by either the egg or sperm cell, i.e., a total of 47 chromosomes instead of the normal 46. Trisomy 21, with 3 copies of chromosome 21, is the most common form of Down syndrome.

**Epidemiology** Approximately 1:800 live births, or 7,000 children annually, are born in the United States with Down syndrome. The incidence is higher for children born to women and men over 35. The most common forms of the syndrome do not usually occur more than once in a family. All races and societal economic levels are affected equally.

**Treatment—Standard** The basic neurologic disorder cannot be altered, but early intervention can benefit affected children (see Resources, below, for organizations that can recommend helpful programs). Education of both parent and child can begin in the postnatal period. Learning, language, mobility, self care, and socialization skills can be developed early, followed up by toddler and preschool programs. Many of the children can be educated in the public schools, learn basic academic and prevocational skills with special training, and perform many daily living activities independently.

Surgery during infancy or childhood may be indicated for cardiac defects.

**Treatment—Investigational** Please contact the agencies listed under Resources, below, for the most current information. Addresses and telephone numbers of these agencies, as well as of individual experts and research centers, may be found in the Master Resources List.

**Resources**

**For more information on Down syndrome:** National Organization for Rare Disorders (NORD); Association for Children with Down Syndrome; National Down Syndrome Congress; National Down Syndrome Society; National Center for Down's Syndrome; NIH/National Institute of Child Health and Human Development; Children's Brain Diseases Foundation for Research; The Arc (a national organization on mental retardation); National Institute of Mental Retardation (Canadian Association for the Mentally Retarded).

**For genetic information and genetic counseling referrals:** March of Dimes Birth Defects Foundation; Alliance of Genetic Support Groups.

**References**

Nelson Textbook of Pediatrics, 14th ed.: R.E. Behrman, ed.-in-chief; W.B. Saunders Company, 1992, pp. 282–284.

Birth Defects Encyclopedia: M.L. Buyse, ed.-in-chief; Blackwell Scientific Publications, 1990, pp. 391–392.

Clinical Aspects of Down Syndrome from Infancy to Adulthood: S.M. Pueschel; Am. J. Med. Genet., 1990, vol. 7 (suppl.), pp. 52–56.

Smith's Recognizable Patterns of Human Malformation, 4th ed.: K.L. Jones; W.B. Saunders Company, 1988, pp. 10–15, 659–661.

# DUBOWITZ SYNDROME

**Description** Dubowitz syndrome, a very rare developmental disorder, is characterized by short stature and an unusual facies.

**Synonyms**

Intrauterine Short Stature

**Signs and Symptoms** Onset is intrauterine or immediately postnatal. Affected children have low birth weight, usually about 5 lb at full term. Short stature is a prominent feature. Facial abnormalities include a relatively high nasal bridge, hypoplasia of supraorbital ridges, ocular hypertelorism, ptosis, blepharophimosis, prominent ears, delayed eruption of teeth as well as dental decay, abnormalities of the jaw area (zygoma, malar eminence, mandible), and, occasionally, cleft palate. The voice is often high-pitched, the hair is sparse, and eczema may be present on the face, knees, and elbows. Intelligence is usually normal, with some memory deficits or learning disabilities, although some patients are mildly retarded and speech usually is impaired. These children may be hyperactive.

**Etiology** The condition is considered to be autosomal recessive. The genetic defect causes intrauterine or postnatal growth retardation.

**Epidemiology** Males and females are equally affected.

**Related Disorders** See *Bloom Syndrome.*

**Treatment—Standard** Treatment is symptomatic and supportive.

**Treatment—Investigational** Please contact the agencies listed under Resources, below, for the most current information. Addresses and telephone numbers of these agencies, as well as of individual experts and research centers, may be found in the Master Resources List.

**Resources**

**For more information on Dubowitz syndrome:** National Organization for Rare Disorders (NORD); NIH/National Institute of Child Health and Human Development; Human Growth Foundation; Short Stature Foundation; Dubowitz Syndrome Parent Support Network.

**For genetic information and genetic counseling referrals:** March of Dimes Birth Defects Foundation; Alliance of Genetic Support Groups.

**References**

Mendelian Inheritance in Man, 11th ed.: V.A. McKusick; The Johns Hopkins University Press, 1994, p. 1776.

Blepharophimosis, Eczema, and Growth and Developmental Delay in a Young Adult: Late Features of Dubowitz Syndrome?: S. Lyonnet, et al.; J. Med. Genet., January 1992, vol. 29(1), pp. 68–69.

Cecil Textbook of Medicine, 19th ed.: J.B. Wyngaarden, et al., eds.; W.B. Saunders Company, 1992, p. 1494.

Nelson Textbook of Pediatrics, 14th ed.: R.E. Behrman, ed.-in-chief; W.B. Saunders Company, 1992, p. 1731.

Birth Defects Encyclopedia: M.L. Buyse, ed.-in-chief; Blackwell Scientific Publications, 1990, pp. 547–548.

Dictionary of Medical Syndromes, 3rd ed.: S.I. Magalini, et al., eds.: J.B. Lippincott Company, 1990, pp. 263–264.

Smith's Recognizable Patterns of Human Malformation, 4th ed.: K.L. Jones; W.B. Saunders Company, 1988, pp. 92–93.

# DUODENAL ATRESIA OR STENOSIS

**Description** Absence or complete closure of a portion of the lumen within the duodenum, or partial obstruction due to narrowing of the duodenum, is present. The defect may be located in the area where the pancreatic and bile ducts join as they open into the duodenum (ampulla of Vater), or in the portion of the duodenum furthest from the opening of the ampulla of Vater. There may be an absence of the channel at the top of the small intestine, a ring or web in the duodenum, an abnormally small channel at the top of the small intestines, or the duodenum may end with just a short cord going to the bowel. These obstructions in the digestive tract prevent proper absorption of food. Other associated abnormalities may be found in over half of those affected with duodenal atresia or duodenal stenosis.

**Signs and Symptoms** Symptoms usually become apparent during infancy. Symptoms of complete blockage of the duodenum may include bilious vomiting (a yellow-green secretion arising from the liver or in some cases a clear or light-brown granular matter) typically beginning a few hours after birth, distention or swelling of the upper abdomen, constipation resistant to treatment, and jaundice. Polyhydramnios may be detected before birth through ultrasound.

Symptoms of partial duodenal blockage vary, depending on the severity. They may wax and wane, not appearing for weeks, months, or years. Prolonged vomiting along with dehydration may also occur.

Other problems associated with this disorder may include intestines that are shorter than normal, low birth weight, premature birth, and an imbalance of electrolytes. Twenty to 30 percent of affected individuals have Down syndrome, and 22 percent have heart disease. An abnormal rotation of the colon, annulas pancreas, tracheoesophageal fistula, and kidney malformations can also be associated with duodenal atresia or stenosis.

Duodenal atresia may be recognized through ultrasound by the presence of a "double bubble" that can be seen in the abdominal area.

**Etiology** The majority of cases of duodenal atresia or stenosis are of unknown origin. There are 2 theories as to why the abnormalities may occur. Blood vessel defects in the embryo may cause the absence or closure of the duodenum by decreasing the blood supply in the affected area, or there may be an overgrowth of cells in the duodenum, obstructing the lumen during the 6th or 7th week of fetal development.

A few cases of duodenal atresia have been inherited as an autosomal recessive genetic trait.

**Epidemiology** Duodenal atresia or stenosis occurs in approximately 1:17,000 births. Males and females are affected in equal numbers, and there is no racial prevalence.

**Related Disorders** See *Jejunal Atresia.*

**Multiple intestinal atresia** is a rare disorder in which there are multiple areas of the intestines with an absence of a normal opening or space, resulting in intestinal blockage. The atresias typically involve the duodenum, the jejunum, the ileum, and the rectum. Infants born with this condition may have persistent vomiting and swelling just below the sternum, an empty anal canal, and scaphoid abdomen.

**Pyloric stenosis** is a digestive disorder that may be apparent soon after birth or during the first few months of life. It may also occur in adults. The development of projectile vomiting immediately after eating is one of the first symptoms. Because too little food reaches the intestines, constipation is a frequent complication, as is failure of the infant to gain weight. The signs and symptoms of adult pyloric stenosis are similar to those in the infant.

**Treatment—Standard** The earlier the disorder is recognized and surgery is performed, the better the outcome. The surgery most often performed is a duodenojejunostomy. When the atresia is located in the first part of the duodenum, a gastrojejunostomy may be the treatment of choice. A duodenoduodenostomy is another surgical procedure sometimes used to connect the 2 portions of the divided duodenum.

Parenteral nutrition may be needed for a period of time. Genetic counseling may benefit patients and their families with the hereditary form of the disorders.

**Treatment—Investigational** Please contact the agencies listed under Resources, below, for the most current information. Addresses and telephone numbers of these agencies, as well as of individual experts and research centers, may be found in the Master Resources List.

**Resources**

**For more information on duodenal atresia or stenosis:** National Organization for Rare Disorders (NORD); American Society of Parenteral and Enteral Nutrition; NIH/National Digestive Diseases Information Clearinghouse.

**For genetic information and genetic counseling referrals:** March of Dimes Birth Defects Foundation; Alliance of Genetic Support Groups.

**References**

Mendelian Inheritance in Man, 11th ed.: V.A. McKusick; The Johns Hopkins University Press, 1994, p. 1766.

Nelson Textbook of Pediatrics, 14th ed.: R.E. Behrman, ed.-in-chief; W.B. Saunders Company, 1992, pp. 950–952.

Birth Defects Encyclopedia: M.L Buyse, ed.-in-chief; Blackwell Scientific Publications, 1990, pp. 549–550.

Prenatal Diagnosis of Duodenal Atresia: Does It Make Any Difference?: R. Romero, et al.; Obstet. Gynecol., May 1988, vol. 71(5), pp. 739–741.

Newborn Duodenal Atresia: An Improving Outlook: D. Mooney, et al.; Am. J. Surg., April 1987, vol. 153(4), pp. 347–349.

Duodenal Atresia: A Comparison of Techniques of Repair: T.R. Weber, et al.; J. Pediatr. Surg., December 1986, vol. 21(12), pp. 1133–1136.

Value of Serial Sonography in the In Utero Detection of Duodenal Atresia: L.H. Nelson, et al.; Obstet. Gynecol., May 1982, vol. 59(5), pp. 657–660.

# DYGGVE-MELCHIOR-CLAUSEN (DMC) SYNDROME

**Description** DMC syndrome is characterized by abnormal growth and development of the skeleton, and by mental retardation. A form of the disorder, **Smith-McCort dwarfism,** has all the features of DMC syndrome except mental retardation.

**Signs and Symptoms** Patients with DMC syndrome typically have short-trunk small stature, a bulging sternum, barrel chest, restricted movement of the joints, and a waddling gait, as well as mental retardation.

Scoliosis, kyphosis, lordosis, flattening of the vertebrae and iliac crest, and genu valgum and varum may be present. The metacarpals and phalanges are shorter than normal.

Differential diagnosis with the mucopolysaccharidoses (see under Related Disorders, below) is aided by the fact that DMC patients have normal excretion of mucopolysaccharides.

**Etiology** The syndrome is inherited through an autosomal recessive trait.

**Epidemiology** Males and females are affected in equal numbers. Cases have been reported in Greenland, Lebanon, and Norway.

**Related Disorders** See *Hurler Syndrome; Morquio Syndrome; Spondyloepiphyseal Dysplasia Congenita; Spondyloepiphyseal Dysplasia Tarda.*

**Treatment—Standard** Treatment is symptomatic and supportive. When partial dislocation of the cervical vertebrae is present, the joint between the 2 vertebrae can be fused. This procedure should be done in order to prevent damage to the cervical portion of the spinal cord.

Children may benefit from early intervention programs and special education. Genetic counseling is helpful for patients and their families.

**Treatment—Investigational** Please contact the agencies listed under Resources, below, for the most current information. Addresses and telephone numbers of these agencies, as well as of individual experts and research centers, may be found in the Master Resources List.

**Resources**

**For more information on Dyggve-Melchior-Clausen syndrome:** National Organization for Rare Disorders (NORD); Magic Foundation for Children's Growth; Human Growth Foundation; The Arc (a national organization on mental retardation); NIH/National Institute of Child Health and Human Development; Parents of Dwarfed Children.

**For genetic information and genetic counseling referrals:** March of Dimes Birth Defects Foundation; Alliance of Genetic Support Groups.

**References**

Mendelian Inheritance in Man, 11th ed.: V.A. McKusick; The Johns Hopkins University Press, 1994, pp. 1777–1778.

Birth Defects Encyclopedia: M.L. Buyse, ed.-in-chief; Blackwell Scientific Publications, 1990, pp. 563–564.

Smith's Recognizable Patterns of Human Malformation, 4th ed.: K.L. Jones; W.B. Saunders Company, 1988, p. 315.

Dyggve-Melchior-Clausen Syndrome: A Histochemical Study of the Growth Plate: W.A. Horton, et al.; J. Bone Joint Surg., March 1982, vol. 64(3), pp. 408–415.

Dyggve-Melchior-Clausen Syndrome: Genetic Studies and Report of Affected Sibs: S.P. Toledo, et al.; Am. J. Med. Genet., 1979, vol. 4(3), pp. 255–261.

# DYSCHONDROSTEOSIS

**Description** Major features of this disorder are Madelung deformity of the wrist and mesomelic short stature.

**Synonyms**

Leri-Weill Syndrome

Mesomelic Dwarfism–Madelung Deformity

**Signs and Symptoms** The forearm and wrist of persons with dyschondrosteosis are bowed as a result of Madelung deformity's curvature of the lower radius. Partial dislocation of the radius and ulna can result.

Abnormally short forearms and lower legs (mesomelic short stature) are also present in dyschondrosteosis.

When one or more family members have both Madelung deformity and mesomelic short stature, a relative who has the wrist deformity without the short stature is also considered to have dyschondrosteosis.

Other characteristics of dyschondrosteosis include deformity of the humerus; exostoses of the tibia; short, thick metacarpals and phalanges; cubitus valgus; coxa valga; and osteoarthritis.

**Etiology** The disorder is inherited through an autosomal dominant trait. Male-to-male transmission has also been recorded in the medical literature.

**Epidemiology** Both males and females are affected; the female-to-male ratio is 4:1.

**Related Disorders** See *Acrodysostosis; Ellis–van Creveld Syndrome; Robinow Syndrome.*

**Madelung deformity due to trauma or infection** can also occur, causing dislocation of the bones of the forearm. Short stature is not involved.

Forms of mesomelic dysplasia such as **Langer, Nievergelt, Reinhardt-Pfeiffer,** and **Werner** also display some of the same symptoms as dyschondrosteosis.

**Treatment—Standard** Orthopedic surgery will relieve the pain and increase mobility in persons with severe Madelung deformity.

Bone growth in patients with dyschondrosteosis should be monitored regularly during the growth period. In severe cases surgery may be performed to equalize the length of the 2 legs.

Genetic counseling will benefit patients and their families.

**Treatment—Investigational** Please contact the agencies listed under Resources, below, for the most current information. Addresses and telephone numbers of these agencies, as well as of individual experts and research centers, may be found in the Master Resources List.

**Resources**

**For more information on dyschondrosteosis:** National Organization for Rare Disorders (NORD); International Center for Skeletal Dysplasia; Magic Foundation for Children's Growth; Human Growth Foundation; Little People of America; Parents of Dwarfed Children; Short Stature Foundation; NIH/National Institute of Child Health and Human Development.

**For genetic information and genetic counseling referrals:** March of Dimes Birth Defects Foundation; Alliance of Genetic Support Groups.

### References

Mendelian Inheritance in Man, 11th ed.: V.A. McKusick; The Johns Hopkins University Press, 1994, pp. 439–440.
Birth Defects Encyclopedia: M.L. Buyse, ed.-in-chief; Blackwell Scientific Publications, 1990, pp. 565–566.
Smith's Recognizable Patterns of Human Malformation, 4th ed.: K.L. Jones; W.B. Saunders Company, 1988, p. 388.
Madelung's Deformity and Dyschondrosteosis: R.H. Gelberman, et al.; J. Hand Surg., July 1980, vol. 5(4), pp. 338–340.
Sex-Influenced Expression of Madelung's Deformity in a Family of Dyschondrosteosis: J.R. Lichtenstein, et al.; J. Med. Genet., February 1980, vol. 17(1), pp. 41–43.

# DYSPLASIA EPIPHYSEALIS HEMIMELICA

**Description** Dysplasia epiphysealis hemimelica is characterized by overgrowth of the epiphyseal cartilage of one or more of the carpal or tarsal bones. Less often, the cartilage on other bones, e.g., the ankle, knee, or hip joint, can be affected.

### Synonyms
Chondrodystrophy, Epiphyseal
Epiphyseal Osteochondroma, Benign
Tarsoepiphyseal Aclasis
Tarsomegaly
Trevor Disease

**Signs and Symptoms** Onset of symptoms usually is between 2 and 4 years of age. Pain and discomfort occur because of the excessive cartilage growth. Usually only one limb is involved, and the limbs may be unequal in length.

**Etiology** The cause is unknown. No familial cases have been reported.

**Epidemiology** The disorder affects males 3 times more often than females.

**Related Disorders Chondrodysplasia punctata** consists of a group of disorders characterized by a pug nose, scaly skin lesions, and abnormalities in epiphyseal cartilage. See **Conradi-Hünermann Syndrome,** an X-linked dominant form of chondrodysplasia punctata that affects infants and young children.

**Treatment—Standard** Treatment consists of surgical removal of cartilage overgrowth in joints where it causes pain and discomfort. Other treatment is symptomatic and supportive.

**Treatment—Investigational** Please contact the agencies listed under Resources, below, for the most current information. Addresses and telephone numbers of these agencies, as well as of individual experts and research centers, may be found in the Master Resources List.

### Resources

**For more information on dysplasia epiphysealis hemimelica:** National Organization for Rare Disorders (NORD); NIH/National Arthritis and Musculoskeletal and Skin Diseases Information Clearinghouse.

### References

Mendelian Inheritance in Man, 11th ed.: V.A. McKusick; The Johns Hopkins University Press, 1994, pp. 441–442.
The Variable Manifestations of Dysplasia Epiphysealis Hemimelica: E.M. Azouz, et al.; Pediatr. Radiol., 1985, vol. 15(1), pp. 44–49.
Dysplasia Epiphysealis Hemimelica: R. Cruz-Conde, et al.; J. Pediatr. Orthop., September 1984, vol. 4(5), pp. 625–629.
Dysplasia Epiphysealis Hemimelica: A Clinical and Genetic Study: J.M. Horan, et al.; J. Bone Joint Surg. Br., May 1983, vol. 65(3), pp. 350–354.

# ECTRODACTYLY–ECTODERMAL DYSPLASIA–CLEFT LIP/PALATE (EEC) SYNDROME

**Description** EEC syndrome is a genetic disorder characterized by multiple physical deformities of the face, digits, and urinary tract.

**Signs and Symptoms** The primary symptoms of this multisystem disorder are ectrodactyly, with abnormalities of the 3rd digit, and syndactyly.

Eye disorders include the absence of a lacrimal gland or a meibomian gland orifice, an abnormally narrow nasolacrimal duct, infections, scarring, and vision difficulties.

Cleft palate or cleft lip may be present, accompanied by hypertelorism and/or slanted eyes. In the absence of clefting, micrognathia, a short groove in the center of the upper lip, and a broad nasal tip may occur.

Renal disorders include an obstructed ureter and resultant hydronephrosis; pyelonephritis; and the absence or duplication of a kidney

Ectodermal dysplasia is a typical finding: hair that is dry, light colored, fine, and sparse; the absence of eyebrows and eyelashes; dry skin; and teeth that are missing, abnormally small, or lacking enamel.

Macules, slowed voluntary movement, an abnormally small brain, and the lack of long bones of the extremities have been associated with EEC syndrome.

**Etiology** An autosomal dominant genetic inheritance is suspected.

**Epidemiology** Males and females are affected in equal numbers. A high proportion of patients live in Denmark.

**Related Disorders Rapp-Hodgkins syndrome** is a rare form of ectodermal dysplasia inherited as an autosomal dominant trait. An inability to sweat, cleft lip and palate, dental abnormalities, and lack of hair are common.

**Treatment—Standard** Surgery may be performed on fingers and toes to correct syndactyly and malformations. Dermatologic treatment is often beneficial. Clefting requires a team of specialists: pediatricians, surgeons, psychologists, speech pathologists, and dental specialists. Cleft palate may be repaired by surgery or covered with a prosthesis.

Special education and related services are of benefit to children with learning delays.

Hydronephrosis is treated by temporary drainage of the urine. Surgery may be indicated if there is pain or infection or if renal function is compromised.

Genetic counseling may benefit patients and their families. Other treatment is symptomatic and supportive.

**Treatment—Investigational** Researchers are studying a Teflon-glycerine paste that is applied to the rear of the pharynx in a minor surgical procedure to bring the pharynx and palate into proper relationship. For further information contact William N. Williams, D.D.S., University of Florida.

Please contact the agencies listed under Resources, below, for the most current information. Addresses and telephone numbers of these agencies, as well as of individual experts and research centers, may be found in the Master Resources List.

**Resources**

**For more information on ectrodactyly–ectodermal dysplasia–cleft lip/palate syndrome:** National Organization for Rare Disorders (NORD); National Foundation for Ectodermal Dysplasias; NIH/National Arthritis and Musculoskeletal and Skin Disease Information Clearinghouse; American Cleft Palate Cranial Facial Association.

**For genetic information and genetic counseling referrals:** March of Dimes Birth Defects Foundation; Alliance of Genetic Support Groups.

**References**

Mendelian Inheritance in Man, 11th ed.: V.A. McKusick; The Johns Hopkins University Press, 1994, p. 451.

Nelson Textbook of Pediatrics, 14th ed.: R.E. Behrman, ed.-in-chief; W.B. Saunders Company, 1992, p. 1629.

Birth Defects Encyclopedia: M.L. Buyse, ed.-in-chief; Blackwell Scientific Publications, 1990, pp. 607–608.

EEC Syndrome: Report on 20 New Patients, Clinical and Genetic Considerations: E.S. Rodini, et al.; Am. J. Genet., September 1990, vol. 37(1), pp. 42–53.

Genitourinary Anomalies Are a Component Manifestation in the Ectodermal Dysplasia, Ectrodactyly, Cleft Lip/Palate (EEC) Syndrome: B.R. Rollnick, et al.; Am. J. Med. Genet., January 1988, vol. 29(1), pp. 131–136.

Smith's Recognizable Patterns of Human Malformation, 4th ed.: K.L. Jones; W.B. Saunders Company, 1988, p. 252.

Growth Hormone Deficiency Associated with the Ectrodactyly–Ectodermal Dysplasia–Clefting Syndrome: J. Knudtzon, et al.; Pediatrics, March 1987, vol. 79(3), pp. 410–412.

# ELLIS–VAN CREVELD SYNDROME

**Description** Ellis–van Creveld syndrome is an achondroplastic disorder associated with polydactyly, abnormal development of fingernails, and cardiac defects.

**Synonyms**

Chondroectodermal Dysplasia

Mesoectodermal Dysplasia

**Signs and Symptoms** Short-limbed small stature and polydactyly are evident in all cases. Underdeveloped fingernails, a partial cleft lip, teeth at birth that erupt and shed very early, genu valgum, and wrist bone abnormalities are common. More than half of patients present with congenital cardiac anomalies, with atrial septal defect as the most common. A few patients present with one heart chamber missing.

Dandy-Walker malformation, epispadias, cryptorchidism, talipes equinovarus, mental retardation, scant or fine hair, and renal agenesis occur in a minority of cases of Ellis–van Creveld syndrome.

**Etiology** Ellis–van Creveld syndrome is inherited as an autosomal recessive trait.

**Epidemiology** Ellis–van Creveld syndrome affects males and females in equal numbers. More than 100 cases have been found among the Amish in Lancaster County, Pennsylvania. Other ethnic groups are affected only rarely.

**Treatment—Standard** Treatment is symptomatic. Surgery may be used to correct the genu valgum, partial cleft palate, and polydactyly; to repair the atrial septal defect; and to drain accumulated cerebrospinal fluid. Patients with mental retardation may benefit from special education.

Genetic counseling may benefit patients and their families.

**Treatment—Investigational** Please contact the agencies listed under Resources, below, for the most current information. Addresses and telephone numbers of these agencies, as well as of individual experts and research centers, may be found in the Master Resources List.

**Resources**

**For more information on Ellis–van Creveld syndrome:** National Organization for Rare Disorders (NORD); Magic Foundation for Children's Growth; Human Growth Foundation; NIH/National Institute of Child Health and Human Development; Parents of Dwarfed Children.

**For genetic information and genetic counseling referrals:** March of Dimes Birth Defects Foundation; Alliance of Genetic Support Groups.

**References**

Mendelian Inheritance in Man, 11th ed.: V.A. McKusick; The Johns Hopkins University Press, 1994, pp. 1788–1789.

Birth Defects Encyclopedia: M.L. Buyse, ed.-in-chief; Blackwell Scientific Publications, 1990, pp. 322–323.

Dandy-Walker Malformation in Ellis–van Creveld Syndrome: K.M. Zangwill, et al.; Am. J. Med. Genet., September 1988, vol. 31(1), pp. 123–129.

Smith's Recognizable Patterns of Human Malformation, 4th ed.: K.L. Jones; W.B. Saunders Company, 1988, p. 324.

Brief Clinical Report: Condroectodermal Dysplasia (Ellis–van Creveld) with Anomalies of CNS and Urinary Tract: S. Rosemberg, et al.; Am. J. Med. Genet., June 1983, vol. 15(2), pp. 291–295.

Ellis–van Creveld Syndrome: Report of 15 Cases in an Inbred Kindred: E.O. da Silva, et al.; J. Med. Genet., October 1980, vol. 17(5), pp. 349–356.

# ENGELMANN DISEASE

**Description** The major features of Engelmann disease, a rare genetic bone disorder, include diaphyseal dysplasia, muscle weakness, bone pain, an unusual gait, extreme fatigue, and anorexia, leading to a malnourished appearance.

**Synonyms**

Camurati-Engelmann Disease

Osteopathia Hyperostotica Multiplex Infantilis

Progressive Diaphyseal Dysplasia

**Signs and Symptoms** Onset is usually in childhood. Normal muscle development is lacking, and weakness in the leg muscles results in an unusual waddling walk. Bone pain is severe, especially in the femur. The bones at the base of the skull, the bones of the hands and feet, and rarely the jaw bone may be affected. Overgrowth of the bones near the eye sockets may occur and can result in loss of vision. Fatigue, headache, and poor appetite may be present.

**Etiology** Engelmann disease is inherited as an autosomal dominant trait.

**Epidemiology** Males and females are affected in equal numbers.

**Related Disorders** See *Muscular Dystrophy, Becker; Muscular Dystrophy, Duchenne; Muscular Dystrophy, Emery-Dreifuss; Myotonic Dystrophy; Paget Disease of Bone.*

**Treatment—Standard** Treatment usually involves corticosteroids, such as cortisone or prednisone, for relief of symptoms. Eye surgery to decompress the optic nerves is most often ineffective and usually not recommended. Genetic counseling may benefit patients and their families. Other treatment is symptomatic and supportive.

**Treatment—Investigational** Please contact the agencies listed under Resources, below, for the most current information. Addresses and telephone numbers of these agencies, as well as of individual experts and research centers, may be found in the Master Resources List.

**Resources**

**For more information on Engelmann disease:** National Organization for Rare Disorders (NORD); NIH/National Arthritis and Musculoskeletal and Skin Diseases Information Clearinghouse.

**For genetic information and genetic counseling referrals:** March of Dimes Birth Defects Foundation; Alliance of Genetic Support Groups.

**References**

Mendelian Inheritance in Man, 11th ed.: V.A. McKusick; The Johns Hopkins University Press, 1994, p. 475.

Smith's Recognizable Patterns of Human Malformation, 4th ed.: K.L. Jones; W.B. Saunders Company, 1988, pp. 428–429.

Progressive Diaphyseal Dysplasia (Camurati-Engelmann): Radiographic Follow-up and CT Findings: J.K. Kaftori, et al.; Radiology, September 1987, vol. 164(3), pp. 777–782.

Clinical and Scintigraphic Evaluation of Corticosteroid Treatment in a Case of Progressive Diaphyseal Dysplasia: L.A. Verbruggen, et al.; J. Rheumatol., August 1985, vol. 12(4), pp. 809–813.

Progressive Diaphyseal Dysplasia: Evaluation of Corticosteroid Therapy: Y. Naveh, et al.; Pediatrics, February 1985, vol. 75(2), pp. 321–323.

# ESOPHAGEAL ATRESIA AND/OR TRACHEOESOPHAGEAL FISTULA

**Description** Esophageal atresia and tracheoesophageal fistula is usually sporadic, but there may be genetic factors.

**Synonyms**

Atresia of Esophagus with or Without Tracheoesophageal Atresia

Tracheoesophageal Fistula with or Without Esophageal Atresia

**Signs and Symptoms** Abnormalities of the esophagus and tracheoesophageal fistula typically occur together, but one may appear without the other. Symptoms include excessive salivation, choking, and regurgitation. When tracheoesophageal fistula is present, the abdomen may be swollen as a result of air passing from the fistula to the stomach. Pneumonitis and atelectasis may occur.

Infection, dehydration, and electrolyte imbalance, in addition to abnormalities of the skeleton, kidney, heart, anus, and gastrointestinal tract, have been found in some patients.

**Etiology** Esophageal atresia and tracheoesophageal fistula may occur with no known cause. Familial cases are probably multifactorial.

**Epidemiology** Males and females are affected in equal numbers. Approximately 1:5,000 live births are affected with some form of these disorders.

**Related Disorders** See ***VACTERL Association.***

**Treatment—Standard** The disorder is detected when a catheter is unable to pass into the stomach or if air is found in the abdomen. Prior to surgical repair, oral feedings may be withheld and a tube inserted into the upper esophagus to prevent aspiration pneumonia. When the infant is more than 5.5 lb and free of other serious abnormalities, a gastrostomy is performed, followed by a repair to the esophageal atresia and/or fistula.

Genetic counseling may benefit patients and their families. Other treatment is symptomatic and supportive.

**Treatment—Investigational** Please contact the agencies listed under Resources, below, for the most current information. Addresses and telephone numbers of these agencies, as well as of individual experts and research centers, may be found in the Master Resources List.

**Resources**

**For more information on esophageal atresia and/or tracheoesophageal fistula:** National Organization for Rare Disorders (NORD); NIH/National Institute of Diabetes, Digestive and Kidney Diseases.

**For genetic information and genetic counseling referrals:** March of Dimes Birth Defects Foundation; Alliance of Genetic Support Groups.

**References**

Mendelian Inheritance in Man, 11th ed.: V.A. McKusick; The Johns Hopkins University Press, 1994, p. 1454.

Nelson Textbook of Pediatrics, 14th ed.: R.E. Behrman, ed.-in-chief; W.B. Saunders Company, 1992, pp. 474, 940–941.

Birth Defects Encyclopedia: M.L. Buyse, ed.-in-chief; Blackwell Scientific Publications, 1990, pp. 642–643.

Growth and Feeding Problems After Repair of Esophageal Atresia: J.W. Puntis, et al.; Arch. Dis. Child., January 1990, vol. 65(1), pp. 84–88.

Primary Repair Without Routine Gastrostomy Is the Treatment of Choice for Neonates with Esophageal Atresia and Tracheoesophageal Fistula: D.W. Shaul, et al.; Arch. Surg., October 1989, vol. 124(10), pp. 188–190.

Care of Infants with Esophageal Atresia, Tracheoesophageal Fistula, and Associated Anomalies: T.M. Holder, et al.; J. Thorac. Cardiovasc. Surg., December 1987, vol. 94(6), pp. 828–835.

# EXOSTOSES, MULTIPLE

**Description** An exostosis is a cartilaginous protrusion near the ends of long bones; these undergo calcification.

**Synonyms**

Diaphyseal Aclasis

External Chondromatosis Syndrome

Multiple Cartilaginous Exostoses

Osteochondromatosis

**Signs and Symptoms** Benign cartilaginous protuberances appear at tendon and muscle junctures, causing deformities of the forearms, knees, ankles, spine, and pelvis. Short stature may occur as a result of shortened legs. If the vertebrae are affected, spinal chord compression can cause numbness or paralysis. Urinary obstruction has been observed as a result of exostoses of the pelvic area. Growth of exostoses continues until shortly after puberty. Malignant transformation occurs in 0.9 to 2.8 percent of patients, usually in young adult life.

**Etiology** Multiple exostoses can be inherited as an autosomal dominant trait. Linkage studies have identified genes at 8q24.1, the pericentric region of 11, and 19p.

**Epidemiology** Males and females are affected in equal numbers. A high incidence of this disorder has been reported in the Chamorros of Guam. One general hospital in the United States reported 1:90,000 patient visits as having multiple exostoses.

**Related Disorders** See *Dysplasia, Epiphysealis Hemimelica; Maffucci Syndrome.*

**Enchondromatosis,** which affects males and females equally, is characterized by slow-growing tumors near the ends of the long bones. The tumors may cause the bone to bulge, bow, or be shorter than normal. Typically these growths stop at the end of adolescence. A single limb or multiple bones may be involved. Enchondromatosis occurs sporadically.

**Metachondromatosis** is a very rare disorder in which the patient has both enchondromatosis and multiple exostoses. It is thought to be inherited as an autosomal dominant trait.

**Treatment—Standard** Surgery is indicated for tumors that cause pain, compress nerves or tendons, or hinder movement. Genetic counseling may benefit patients and their families. Other treatment is symptomatic and supportive.

**Treatment—Investigational** Please contact the agencies listed under Resources, below, for the most current information. Addresses and telephone numbers of these agencies, as well as of individual experts and research centers, may be found in the Master Resources List.

**Resources**

**For more information on multiple exostoses:** National Organization for Rare Disorders (NORD); NIH/National Arthritis and Musculoskeletal and Skin Diseases Information Clearinghouse.

**For genetic information and genetic counseling referrals:** March of Dimes Birth Defects Foundation; Alliance of Genetic Support Groups.

**References**

Hereditary Multiple Exostoses and Chondrosarcoma: Linkage to Chromosome 11 and Loss of Heterozygosity for EXT-Linked Markers on Chromosomes 11 and 8: J.T. Hecht, et al.; Am. J. Hum. Genet., 1995, vol. 56, pp. 1125–1131.

Mendelian Inheritance in Man, 11th ed.: V.A. McKusick; The Johns Hopkins University Press, 1994, pp. 501–502.

Birth Defects Encyclopedia: M.L. Buyse, ed.-in-chief; Blackwell Scientific Publications, 1990, pp. 646–47.

Hand Involvement in Multiple Hereditary Exostoses: V.E. Molitor, et al.; Hand Clin., November 1990, vol. 6(4), pp. 685–692.

Multiple Hereditary Osteochondromata: H.A. Peterson; Clin. Orthop., February 1989, vol. (239), pp. 222–230.

Osteochondromatosis (Diaphyseal Aclasis): A Case Report and Literature Report: M.D. Perlman, et al.; J. Foot Surg., March–April 1989, vol. 28(2), pp. 162–165.

Cartilaginous Exostoses Arising from the Ventral Surface of the Scapula: A Case Report: O. Nercessiana, et al.; Clin. Orthop., November 1988, vol. (236), pp. 145–147.

Smith's Recognizable Patterns of Human Malformation, 4th ed.: K.L. Jones; W.B. Saunders Company, 1988, p. 384.

# FAIRBANK DISEASE

**Description** Fairbank disease is sometimes characterized by small, irregular, mottled epiphyses. Although the patient may not experience symptoms during early childhood, subsequent developmental hip abnormalities may cause pain in the hips, knees, or ankles, and restrict movement. This is a genetically heterogeneous group of disorders.

**Synonyms**

Multiple Epiphyseal Dysplasia

**Signs and Symptoms** The disease manifests between 2 and 5 years of age, when patients begin to waddle or walk awkwardly. Patients 5 to 14 years of age may experience pain in the hips, knees, or ankles because of continuing alterations in bone structure.

The most prominent symptom involves the hips and may be confused with bilateral Legg-Calvé-Perthe syndrome (see *Legg-Calvé-Perthe Syndrome).* Less commonly involved are the bones of the shoulders, feet, or hands. Vertebrae are usually normal but may be affected slightly. The femur, including the cartilage, can change shape and density and then recover. Although bone tissue reforms, the bones may be slightly shorter, and mild short stature results.

**Etiology** Fairbank disease is an inherited dominant trait. The gene for one form of Fairbank disease has been mapped to chromosome 19, and for another form, to the short arm of chromosome 1 in a region that encodes the gene for collagen 9A2.

**Epidemiology** Males and females are affected in equal numbers.

**Related Disorders** See *Conradi-Hünermann Syndrome.*

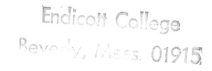

**Treatment—Standard** Hip surgery may alleviate restricted movement, and physical therapy and genetic counseling may be beneficial. Other treatment is symptomatic and supportive.

**Treatment—Investigational** Please contact the agencies listed under Resources, below, for the most current information. Addresses and telephone numbers of these agencies, as well as of individual experts and research centers, may be found in the Master Resources List.

**Resources**

**For more information on Fairbank disease:** National Organization for Rare Disorders (NORD); International Center for Skeletal Dysplasia; Human Growth Foundation; Little People of America; Parents of Dwarfed Children; Short Stature Foundation; NIH/National Institute of Child Health and Human Development.

**For genetic information and genetic counseling referrals:** March of Dimes Birth Defects Foundation; Alliance of Genetic Support Groups.

**References**

Genetic Heterogeneity in Multiple Epiphyseal Dysplasia: M. Deere, et al.; Am. J. Hum. Genet., 1995, vol. 56, pp. 698–704.

Genetic Mapping of a Locus for Multiple Epiphyseal Dysplasia (EDM2) to a Region of Chromosome 1 Containing Type IX Collagen Gene: M.D. Briggs, et al.; Am. J. Med. Genet., 1994, vol. 55, pp. 678–684.

Mendelian Inheritance in Man, 11th ed.: V.A. McKusick; The Johns Hopkins University Press, 1994, pp. 484–485.

Multiple Epiphyseal Dysplasia: A Family Study: T. Gibson, et al.; Rheumatol. Rehabil., November 1979, 18(4), pp. 239–242.

The Epiphyseal Dysplasias: J. Spranger; Clin. Orthop., January–February 1976, 114, pp. 46–59.

# FEMORAL-FACIAL SYNDROME

**Description** Major characteristics of femoral-facial syndrome are underdeveloped femurs and distinctive facies.

**Synonyms**

Femoral Dysgenesis, Bilateral–Robin Anomaly

Femoral Hypoplasia–Unusual Faces Syndrome

**Signs and Symptoms** Skeletal abnormalities include short stature due to femur deformity, restricted mobility at the elbow, Sprengel deformity, and deformities of the foot and ankle.

Craniofacial features include upslanting eyes, a short nose with a broad tip, a thin upper lip, and micrognathia. Cleft palate, small or abnormally shaped ears, webbing or fusion of the toes, and abnormalities of the vertebrae, ribs, and pelvis may also be present.

The following may be found in association with femoral-facial syndrome: astigmatism, esotropia, hypogonadism, cryptorchidism, polycystic kidneys, renal agenesis, and urinary complications.

**Etiology** The cause of femoral-facial syndrome is not known. Most cases of this disorder occur as isolated events. Two reported cases of affected relatives are thought to have been the result of an autosomal dominant inheritance.

**Epidemiology** Females are affected more often than males.

**Related Disorders** See *Camptomelic Syndrome; Caudal Regression Syndrome.*

**Treatment—Standard** Orthopedic care, including surgery, may correct the serious bone deformities associated with femoral-facial syndrome. Treatment of cleft palate requires a team of specialists: pediatricians, dental specialists, surgeons, speech pathologists, and others. Cleft palate may be repaired by surgery or covered with a prosthesis.

Genetic counseling may benefit patients and their families. Other treatment is symptomatic and supportive.

**Treatment—Investigational** Researchers are studying a Teflon-glycerine paste that is applied to the rear of the pharynx in a minor surgical procedure. For further information contact William N. Williams, D.D.S., University of Florida.

Please contact the agencies listed under Resources, below, for the most current information. Addresses and telephone numbers of these agencies, as well as of individual experts and research centers, may be found in the Master Resources List.

**Resources**

**For more information on femoral-facial syndrome:** National Organization for Rare Disorders (NORD); International Center for Skeletal Dysplasia; American Cleft Palate Cranial Facial Association; NIH/National Arthritis and Musculoskeletal and Skin Diseases Information Clearinghouse.

**For genetic information and genetic counseling referrals:** March of Dimes Birth Defects Foundation; Alliance of Genetic Support Groups.

**References**

Mendelian Inheritance in Man, 11th ed.: V.A. McKusick; The Johns Hopkins University Press, 1994, pp. 514–515.

Birth Defects Encyclopedia: M.L. Buyse, ed.-in-chief; Blackwell Scientific Publications, 1990, pp. 681–682.

Smith's Recognizable Patterns of Human Malformation, 4th ed.: K.L. Jones; W.B. Saunders Company, 1988, p. 268.

# FETAL ALCOHOL SYNDROME (FAS)

**Description** FAS refers to a wide range of mental and physical birth defects that affect the offspring of mothers who consume alcohol while pregnant.

**Synonyms**
>Alcoholic Embryopathy
>Alcohol-Related Birth Defects

**Signs and Symptoms** Characteristics of FAS infants include smaller-than-normal length, low birth weight, and microcephaly. Failure to thrive and physical and mental retardation are common.

The infants have a characteristic facies, including protruding forehead, short palpebral fissures, epicanthal folds, short upturned nose with a flattened bridge, retracted upper lip, micrognathia, cleft palate, and abnormally shaped ears. Some minor joint and limb abnormalities may occur, including a palmar simian crease. Cardiac complications consist mainly of septal defects.

Alcohol withdrawal occurs within the first 24 hours of life. Symptoms associated with withdrawal include irritability, tremors and convulsions, increased muscle tone, opisthotonos, rapid breathing, abdominal distention, and vomiting.

Infants may exhibit all or only some of these symptoms. There is a direct relationship between the severity of symptoms and the level of alcohol consumption.

**Etiology** It is not certain whether alcohol itself or a breakdown product causes the syndrome.

**Epidemiology** The incidence of FAS in the United States is 1:1,000 to 2:1,000 live births. Although the majority of Americans know about the risk of consuming alcohol during pregnancy, the incidence of FAS is not declining significantly.

**Related Disorders** FAS may be associated with upper respiratory abnormalities that contribute to the development of apnea, lung hypertension, and sudden infant death syndrome.

**Treatment—Standard** The syndrome can be prevented by total abstinence from alcohol by a woman during her pregnancy.

Treatment is generally symptomatic and supportive. Agencies that treat alcohol addiction, special education services, and agencies that provide services to mentally retarded individuals and their families may be beneficial.

**Treatment—Investigational** Research is under way to study the effects of alcohol on fetuses, to find a treatment and prevention for alcoholism, and to determine the stages of pregnancy during which alcohol-related birth defects are most likely to occur. Other studies are seeking ways to prevent FAS and other alcohol-related birth defects.

Please contact the agencies listed under Resources, below, for the most current information. Addresses and telephone numbers of these agencies, as well as of individual experts and research centers, may be found in the Master Resources List.

**Resources**

**For more information on fetal alcohol syndrome:** National Organization for Rare Disorders (NORD); Fetal Alcohol Education Program; U.S. Dept. of Health and Human Services Public Health Service; NIH/National Clearinghouse for Alcohol Information; Alcoholics Anonymous; NIH/National Institute of Mental Health.

**References**

Upper Airway Obstruction in Infants with Fetal Alcohol Syndrome: A.G. Usowicz, et al.; Am. J. Dis. Child., October 1986, vol. 140(10), pp. 1039–1041.

Alcohol Research: Meeting the Challenge: NIAAA, National Clearinghouse for Alcohol Information (NCALI). For sale by the Superintendent of Documents, U.S. Government Printing Office, Washington, D.C., p. 11.

# FETAL HYDANTOIN SYNDROME

**Description** Fetal hydantoin syndrome is caused by fetal exposure to phenytoin and is characterized by craniofacial abnormalities, growth deficiencies, underdeveloped nails of the fingers and toes, and developmental delays.

**Synonyms**
>Fetal Dilantin Syndrome

**Signs and Symptoms** The most consistent facial features in the newborn are a flat bridge of the nose and eyes that are down-slanted, widely spaced, and crossed. An underdeveloped philtrum, cleft lip and/or palate, ptosis, and mild webbing of the neck have also been reported. Growth deficiencies may include underdeveloped fingers and toes, malformed nails, and fingerlike thumbs. Microencephaly and associated mild-to-moderate mental retardation affect approximately 30 percent of patients.

**Etiology** Fetal hydantoin syndrome is caused by exposure of the fetus to the anticonvulsant phenytoin (Dilantin). Enzyme differences may be a factor in determining which sibling is affected.

**Epidemiology** Males and females are affected in equal numbers. Approximately 11 percent of infants exposed to hydantoin in utero are affected.

**Related Disorders** See *Aarskog Syndrome; Noonan Syndrome.*

**Treatment—Standard** A mother receiving phenytoin (Dilantin) whose infant is affected with fetal hydantoin syndrome should be given a different anticonvulsant drug during future pregnancies. However, the effects of other seizure medications on a fetus are not always well understood.

Cleft lip can be corrected by surgery, beginning in the patient's infancy. Cleft palate may also be treated surgically or by a prosthesis. Special education and related services will benefit children with learning delays. Other treatment is symptomatic and supportive.

**Treatment—Investigational** Researchers are studying a Teflon-glycerine paste that is applied to the rear of the pharynx in a minor surgical procedure to bring the pharynx and palate into proper relationship. For further information, contact William N. Williams, D.D.S., University of Florida.

Please contact the agencies listed under Resources, below, for the most current information. Addresses and telephone numbers of these agencies, as well as of individual experts and research centers, may be found in the Master Resources List.

**Resources**

**For more information on fetal hydantoin syndrome:** National Organization for Rare Disorders (NORD); The Arc (a national organization on mental retardation); NIH/National Institute of Child Health and Human Development.

**For more information on cleft palate:** For information on local cleft teams, contact the American Cleft Palate Cranial Facial Association.

**For genetic information and genetic counseling referrals:** March of Dimes Birth Defects Foundation; Alliance of Genetic Support Groups.

**References**

Birth Defects Encyclopedia: M.L. Buyse, ed.-in-chief; Blackwell Scientific Publications, 1990, pp. 714–715.

Prenatal Prediction of Risk of the Fetal Hydantoin Syndrome: B.A. Buehler, et al.; N. Engl. J. Med., May 1990, vol. 322(22), pp. 1567–1572.

Smith's Recognizable Patterns of Human Malformation, 4th ed.: K.L. Jones; W.B. Saunders Company, 1988, p. 495.

Fetal Hydantoin Syndrome in Triplets: A Unique Experiment of Nature: S.A. Bustamante, et al.; Am. J. Dis. Child., October 1978, vol. 132(10), pp. 978–9.

Risks to the Offspring of Women Treated with Hydantoin Anticonvulsants, with Emphasis on the Fetal Hydantoin Syndrome: J.W. Hanson, et al.; J. Pediatr., October 1976, vol. 89(4), pp. 662–668.

# FETAL VALPROATE SYNDROME

**Description** Fetal valproate syndrome is a rare congenital disorder caused by exposure of the fetus to valproic acid (Dalpro, Depakene, Depakote, Depakote Sprinkle, Divalproex, Epival, myproic acid) during the first 3 months of pregnancy. Symptoms of this disorder may include spina bifida, distinctive facial features, and other musculoskeletal abnormalities.

**Synonyms**

> Dalpro, Fetal Effects from
> Depakene, Fetal Effects from
> Depakote, Fetal Effects from
> Depakote Sprinkle, Fetal Effects from
> Divalproex, Fetal Effects from
> Epival, Fetal Effects from
> Myproic Acid, Fetal Effects from
> Valproic Acid, Fetal Effects from

**Signs and Symptoms** Infants with fetal valproate syndrome may be born with spina bifida. Affected infants may also have epicanthal folds; a small, upturned nose with a flat bridge; microstomia; a long, thin upper lip; a downturned mouth; and minor abnormalities of the ears.

Other abnormalities sometimes found include underdeveloped nails of the fingers and toes, dislocation of the hip, arachnodactyly, overlapping fingers and toes, diastasis recti, absence of the first rib, hypospadias, abnormalities of the heart, tracheomalacia, and clubfoot.

Growth deficiency and microcephaly may also occur when valproic acid is taken in combination with other anticonvulsant drugs during pregnancy.

**Etiology** Valproic acid, the causative agent, is an anticonvulsant drug used to control certain types of seizures in the treatment of epilepsy. It is believed that valproic acid crosses the placenta and acts as a teratogen. The severity of defects caused by valproic acid may be dose related.

**Epidemiology** Fetal valproate syndrome affects males and females in equal numbers. Spina bifida is found in approximately 1 to 5 percent of infants exposed to valproic acid as fetuses. Facial abnormalities have been found in almost half of the children exposed to valproic acid in utero. There were approximately 175 cases of fetal valproate syndrome reported internationally between 1974 and 1988.

**Related Disorders** Fetal abnormalities caused by other anticonvulsant drugs may be similar to those of fetal valproate syndrome. The determining factor is the identification of the drugs the mother was taking during the first 3 months of pregnancy.

**Treatment—Standard** See *Spina Bifida* (Treatment—Standard; Treatment—Investigational).

Surgery may be necessary to correct heart defects as well as other major malformations that may be present. Other treatment is symptomatic and supportive.

**Treatment—Investigational** Please contact the agencies listed under Resources, below, for the most current information. Addresses and telephone numbers of these agencies, as well as of individual experts and research centers, may be found in the Master Resources List.

**Resources**

**For more information on fetal valproate syndrome:** National Organization for Rare Disorders (NORD); Epilepsy Foundation of America; Spina Bifida Association of America; NIH/National Institute of Child Health and Human Development; Spina Bifida Association of Canada; International Federation for Hydrocephalus and Spina Bifida.

**For genetic information and genetic counseling referrals:** March of Dimes Birth Defects Foundation.

**References**

Birth Defects Encyclopedia: M.L Buyse, ed.-in-chief; Blackwell Scientific Publications, 1990, p. 730.

Verification of the Fetal Valproate Syndrome Phenotype: H.H. Ardinger, et al.; Am. J. Med. Genet., January 1988, vol. 29(1), pp. 171–185.

Fetal Valproate Syndrome: Is There a Recognizable Phenotype?: R.M. Winter, et al.; J. Med. Genet., November 1987, vol. 24(11), pp. 692–695.

The Fetal Valproate Syndrome: J.H. DiLiberti, et al.; Am. J. Med. Genet., November 1984, vol. 19(3), pp. 473–481.

# FG SYNDROME

**Description** FG syndrome is an uncommon hereditary disorder that affects males. Characteristics vary, but a large head, mental retardation, imperforate anus, absence of the corpus callosum, and congenital hypotonia are present in a large percentage of cases. The syndrome gets its name from the classification system employed by John M. Opitz, M.D., in which he used the initials of patients' surnames.

**Synonyms**

Opitz-Kaveggia Syndrome

**Signs and Symptoms** The presence and severity of symptoms vary from patient to patient. Affected individuals seem to have a specific personality type and are often friendly, outgoing, and hyperactive, with a short attention span. They may be easily frustrated and prone to temper tantrums. Some female carriers may have certain physical characteristics related to FG syndrome.

Features include postnatal megalencephaly, mental retardation, severe perinatal hypotonia, seizures, delayed motor development, multiple joint contractures, syndactyly, vertebral defects of the spine, a sacral dimple, or cryptorchidism. Thumbs and big toes are usually broad. The anus may be imperforate, abnormally placed, or stenotic. Constipation is a factor in three-quarters of patients. Hypospadias may be present. Stature is variable.

Craniofacial abnormalities also include a prominent forehead, short palpebral fissures that most often slant downward, a frontal upswept cowlick, hypertelorism, epicanthal folds, long philtrum, prominent lower lip, and small ears. The palate may be narrow or have a cleft. Facial skin is sometimes wrinkled.

Occasionally, other skull abnormalities occur, such as craniosynostosis, hydrocephalus, or absence of the corpus callosum. Rarely, intestinal abnormalities, heart defects, or dilation of the urinary tract are present. Sensorineural deafness occurs in some patients and may be severe.

To date, mothers of males with FG syndrome have shown normal intelligence. Some may have a broad forehead, cowlick, epicanthal folds, hypertelorism, or abnormal placement of the anus.

**Etiology** The syndrome is inherited as an X-linked recessive trait.

**Epidemiology** The disorder is very rare; over 30 cases have been noted. Only males are affected; some female carriers show a few of the syndrome's characteristics.

**Related Disorders** See *Townes-Brocks Syndrome; VACTERL Association.*

**Treatment—Standard** Surgery can correct some malformations. Special education services and genetic counseling are helpful. Other treatment is symptomatic and supportive.

**Treatment—Investigational** Please contact the agencies listed under Resources, below, for the most current information. Addresses and telephone numbers of these agencies, as well as of individual experts and research centers, may be found in the Master Resources List.

**Resources**

**For more information on FG syndrome:** National Organization for Rare Disorders (NORD); FG Syndrome Support Group; The Arc (a national organization on mental retardation); NIH/National Institute of Child Health and Human Development; John M. Opitz, M.D., Shodar Children's Hospital, Helena, Montana.

**For genetic information and genetic counseling referrals:** March of Dimes Birth Defects Foundation; Alliance of Genetic Support Groups.

**References**

Mendelian Inheritance in Man, 11th ed.: V.A. McKusick; The Johns Hopkins University Press, 1994, p. 2355.

Syndromes of the Head and Neck, 3rd ed.: R.J. Gorlin, et al.; Oxford University Press, 1990, pp. 882–883.

FG Syndrome Update 1988: Note of 5 New Patients and Bibliography: J. M. Opitz, et al.; Am. J. Med. Genet., May–June 1988, vol. 30(1–2), pp. 309–328.

Smith's Recognizable Patterns of Human Malformation, 4th ed.: K.L. Jones; W.B. Saunders Company, 1988, pp. 240–241.

The FG Syndrome: 7 New Cases: E.M. Thompson, et al.; Clin. Genet., June 1985, vol. 27(6), pp. 582–594.

Sensorineural Deafness in the FG Syndrome: Report on Four New Cases: G. Neri, et al.; Am. J. Med. Genet., October 1984, vol. 19(2), pp. 369–377.

# FIBROMATOSIS, CONGENITAL GENERALIZED

**Description** Congenital generalized fibromatosis is a rare disorder characterized by multiple noncancerous tumors. It is an invasive and recurring disorder that can involve the bones, internal organs, skin, and muscles. These tumors are usually present at, or may occur within a few months of, birth.

**Synonyms**

Myofibromatosis, Juvenile

**Signs and Symptoms** The tumors can range from 3 to 18 cm in size, and very often do not cause symptoms. Soft tissue and bony tumors will sometimes resolve without treatment. If the abdominal cavity or chest is involved, the tumors may cause an obstruction of the intestinal tract, constipation, diarrhea; or respiratory difficulties.

**Etiology** The cause is unknown. The disorder may be inherited as an autosomal recessive trait.

**Epidemiology** Newborn males and females are affected in equal numbers.

**Related Disorders** See *Gardner Syndrome; Neurofibromatosis.*

**Congenital fibrosarcoma** is a rare, highly malignant bone tumor formed from fibroblasts. It usually occurs between the ages of 10 and 20 years, but can occur at any age.

**Treatment—Standard** Treatment generally consists of surgical removal of the tumor. Chemotherapeutic drugs such as vincristine, actinomycin D, and cyclophosphamide may be prescribed alone or in conjunction with radiation therapy and surgery. Some tumors disappear without treatment but should be closely followed by a physician. Genetic counseling may benefit patients and their families. Other treatment is symptomatic and supportive.

**Treatment—Investigational** The drug tamoxifen is being studied for its effectiveness in treating certain types of fibromatosis.

A new orphan drug, toremifene (Estrinex) has been designated for use in treating congenital generalized fibromatosis. The long-term safety and effectiveness of this drug require further investigation. For more information on toremifene, contact Adria Laboratories.

Please contact the agencies listed under Resources, below, for the most current information. Addresses and telephone numbers of these agencies, as well as of individual experts and research centers, may be found in the Master Resources List.

**Resources**

**For more information on congenital generalized fibromatosis:** National Organization for Rare Disorders (NORD); Laura S. Nye Research Fund for Desmoid Tumors; American Cancer Society; NIH/National Cancer Institute Physician Data Query Phoneline.

**For genetic information and genetic counseling referrals:** March of Dimes Birth Defects Foundation; Alliance of Genetic Support Groups.

**References**

Mendelian Inheritance in Man, 11th ed.: Victor A. McKusick; The Johns Hopkins University Press, 1994, pp. 1813–1814

Congenital Multiple Fibromatosis (Infantile Myofibromatosis): L. Burgess, et al.; Arch. Otolaryngol. Head Neck Surg., February 1988, vol. 114(2), pp. 207–209.

Challenges in the Treatment of Childhood Fibromatosis: B. Rao, et al.; Arch. Surg., November 1987, vol. 122(11), pp. 1296–1298.

Infantile (Desmoid Type) Fibromatosis with Extensive Ossification: F. Fromowitz, et al.; Am. J. Surg. Pathol., January 1987, vol. 11(1), pp. 66–75.

Nonsurgical Management of Children with Recurrent or Unresectable Fibromatosis: B. Raney, et al.; Pediatrics, March 1987, vol. 79(3), pp. 394–398.

Remission of Rapidly Growing Desmoid Tumors After Tamoxifen Therapy: B. Ritter, et al.; Cancer, December 15, 1983, vol. 52(12), pp. 2201–2204.

# FIBROUS DYSPLASIA

**Description** Fibrous dysplasia is a medullary bone disease in which benign cysts occur as a result of irregular bone development. A single bone may be involved (monostotic fibrous dysplasia or Jaffe-Lichtenstein disease), or multiple bones may be affected (polyostotic fibrous dysplasia).

**Synonyms**

> Jaffe-Lichenstein Disease
> Monostotic Fibrous Dysplasia
> Polyostotic Fibrous Dysplasia

**Signs and Symptoms Monostotic fibrous dysplasia** first appears during childhood, and the cysts usually stop developing at puberty. The lesions can be painful, deforming, and widespread. An affected individual may have cysts of a craniofacial bone, vertebra, or long bone. The loss of density where the bone is being replaced by fibrous tissue is usually detected by x-ray. The cortical walls may atrophy, and the medullary cavity may expand.

The bone lesions of **polyostotic fibrous dysplasia** are usually present during childhood and may involve a large percentage of the skeleton. A skeletal x-ray is used to detect this disorder often as a result of complaints by the patient of bone and joint pain or repeated fractures. There may be femur deformity and a discrepancy in leg length ("shepherd's-crook") as well as facial disfigurement. Affected individuals may also have McCune-Albright syndrome (see *McCune-Albright Syndrome*), in which precocious puberty and skin pigmentation (café au lait spots) also occur.

**Etiology** The cause is not known. Most cases seem to occur sporadically.

**Epidemiology** Males and females seem to be affected equally. About 50 percent of females with polyostotic fibrous dysplasia have McCune-Albright syndrome with early sexual development.

**Treatment—Standard** Orthopedic procedures are used in treatment. Packing with bone chips and curettage has been found to be most successful in patients over 18 years of age. Internal fixation may be used on lesions in the lower extremities of patients under 18 years of age.

**Treatment—Investigational** See *McCune-Albright Syndrome*, if the patient has this disorder in association with fibrous dysplasia.

Please contact the agencies listed under Resources, below, for the most current information. Addresses and telephone numbers of these agencies, as well as of individual experts and research centers, may be found in the Master Resources List.

**Resources**

**For more information on fibrous dysplasia:** National Organization for Rare Disorders (NORD); International Center for Skeletal Dysplasia; NIH/National Arthritis and Musculoskeletal and Skin Diseases Information Clearinghouse.

**References**

Birth Defects Encyclopedia: M.L. Buyse, ed.-in-chief; Blackwell Scientific Publications, 1990, pp. 738–739.

Fibrous Dysplasia of Bone: B.E. Stompro, et al.; Am. Fam. Physicians, March 1989, vol. 39(3), pp. 179–184.

Cecil Textbook of Medicine, 18th ed.: J.B. Wyngaarden and L.H. Smith, Jr., eds.; W.B. Saunders Company, 1988, pp. 1519–1520.

Fibrous Dysplasia: An Analysis of Options for Treatment: R.B. Stephenson, et al.; J. Bone Joint Surg. Am., March 1987, vol. 69(3), pp. 400–409.

Internal Medicine, 2nd ed.: J.H. Stein, ed.-in-chief; Little, Brown and Company, 1987, pp. 2117–2118.

# FILIPPI SYNDROME

**Description** Filippi syndrome is a very rare disorder characterized by syndactyly, clinodactyly, microcephaly, mild-to-severe mental and physical retardation, and an unusual facial appearance.

**Synonyms**

Syndactyly Type I with Microcephaly and Mental Retardation

**Signs and Symptoms** Individuals with Filippi syndrome have microcephaly and unusual facies, with a characteristic broad-based nose. Syndactyly of fingers 3 and 4 and of toes 2, 3, and 4 is also present. In addition, there is clinodactyly of the 5th finger as well as a simian crease across the palms of the hands. In males, sexual organs do not develop fully, and there is cryptorchidism. Growth retardation as well as mild to severe mental retardation is also present.

**Etiology** Filippi syndrome is thought to be inherited as an autosomal recessive trait.

**Epidemiology** Filippi syndrome is a very rare disorder. Three affected families have been recorded in the medical literature.

**Related Disorders KBG syndrome** is a very rare disorder that can be inherited as an autosomal dominant trait or can occur sporadically. Symptoms of this disorder include mental retardation, short stature, an unusual face, bow-shaped lips, and skeletal abnormalities. KBG syndrome affects males and females equally.

**Scott craniodigital syndrome with mental retardation** is a rare disorder thought to be inherited as an X-linked recessive trait. Characteristics of this disorder include mental and growth retardation, syndactyly, and unusual facial features.

**Treatment—Standard** Language and oral speech therapy as well as special education may benefit individuals with Filippi syndrome. Surgery may be performed to improve the function of the hand. Genetic counseling may benefit patients and their families. Other treatment is symptomatic and supportive.

**Treatment—Investigational** Please contact the agencies listed under Resources, below, for the most current information. Addresses and telephone numbers of these agencies, as well as of individual experts and research centers, may be found in the Master Resources List.

**Resources**

**For more information on Filippi syndrome:** National Organization for Rare Disorders (NORD); The Arc (a national organization on mental retardation); NIH/National Institute of Child Health and Human Development.

**For genetic information and genetic counseling referrals:** March of Dimes Birth Defects Foundation; Alliance of Genetic Support Groups.

**References**

Mendelian Inheritance in Man, 11th ed.: V.A. McKusick; The Johns Hopkins University Press, 1994, p. 2210.

Nelson Textbook of Pediatrics, 14th ed.: R.E. Behrman, ed.-in-chief; W.B. Saunders Company, 1992, p. 1720.

Birth Defects Encyclopedia: M.L. Buyse, ed.-in-chief; Blackwell Scientific Publications, 1990, p. 1619.

Unusual Facial Appearance, Microcephaly, Growth and Mental Retardation, and Syndactyly: A New Syndrome: G. Filippi, Am. J. Med. Genet., December 1985, vol. 22(4), pp. 821–824.

# FLOATING-HARBOR SYNDROME

**Description** Floating-Harbor syndrome is characterized by short stature, delayed language skills, and a triangular-shaped face. The disorder was named for the first 2 patients who were seen at Boston Floating Hospital and Harbor General Hospital in California.

**Signs and Symptoms** During infancy, growth delays typically become apparent. A delay in bone age causes the head to appear relatively large, while the limbs and trunk are in proportion. At the age 3 or 4, distinctive facial features become apparent: a broad nose and nasal bridge; a wide mouth with thin lips; deep-set eyes; abnormally long eyelashes; and a small, triangular-shaped face. Dental abnormalities are common. Delayed expressive language is found in all patients, and some may also have delayed learning ability. Most children appear to be slightly behind in school, but retardation has not been recorded.

Clinodactyly of the 5th finger, clubbing of the fingers, and hirsutism have been found in some. Celiac sprue, pulmonary stenosis, constipation, and an additional thumb are less common.

**Etiology** The exact cause is not known. There have been no reported recurrences within a family. It is thought that Floating-Harbor syndrome may be a new dominant mutation.

**Epidemiology** Males and females are affected in equal numbers. Approximately 20 cases have been reported, but it is thought that many cases go unrecognized.

**Related Disorders** See ***Dubowitz Syndrome; Russell-Silver Syndrome.***

**Three M syndrome** is a characterized by low birth weight; short stature; narrow face; clinodactyly; thin, slender long bones; a prominent mouth; and a short neck. The head appears large and the face triangular. The syndrome is inherited as an autosomal recessive trait.

**Treatment—Standard** Treatment includes special educational programs and speech therapy. Genetic counseling may benefit patients and their families. Other treatment is symptomatic and supportive.

**Treatment—Investigational** Please contact the agencies listed under Resources, below, for the most current information. Addresses and telephone numbers of these agencies, as well as of individual experts and research centers, may be found in the Master Resources List.

**Resources**

**For more information on Floating-Harbor syndrome:** National Organization for Rare Disorders (NORD); Floating-Harbor Syndrome Support Group; NIH/National Arthritis and Musculoskeletal and Skin Diseases Information Clearinghouse; Human Growth Foundation; Short Stature Foundation; Association for Research into Restricted Growth (U.K.).

**For genetic information and genetic counseling referrals:** March of Dimes Birth Defects Foundation; Alliance of Genetic Support Groups.

**References**

Mendelian Inheritance in Man, 11th ed.: V.A. McKusick; The Johns Hopkins University Press, 1994, p. 534.

Floating-Harbor Syndrome: M.A. Patton, et al.; J. Med. Genet., 1991, vol. 28, pp. 201–204.

Floating-Harbor Syndrome and Celiac Disease: A.E. Chudley, et al.; Am. J. Med. Genet., March 1991, vol. 38(4), pp. 562–564.

# FRAGILE X SYNDROME

**Description** Fragile X syndrome is an X chromosome defect that causes mental retardation and a wide range of associated signs and symptoms.

**Synonyms**

FRAXA

Marker X Syndrome

Martin-Bell Syndrome

X-Linked Mental Retardation and Macro-orchidism

**Signs and Symptoms** The face is typically long and narrow. A high-arched palate, large ears, otitis media, strabismus, and dental problems are present. Other common characteristics include hyperextensible joints, hypotonia, and heart problems, including mitral valve prolapse. In males abnormally large testes are a distinctive feature.

In young children, delayed motor development, hyperactivity, behavioral problems, toe walking, and occasional seizures can occur. Autism is suggested by poor eye contact, hand flapping, hand biting, and self-stimulating behaviors (see **Autism).**

Poor sensory skills and mathematical ability are sometimes found in conjunction with good reading skills. Speech and language problems can include echolalia, perseveration, poor language content, and cluttering (dropping of letters or syllables when speaking). Affected girls tend to be shy and socially withdrawn, and to have particular difficulty with mathematics.

**Etiology** The condition results from a defect on the X chromosome near the end of the long arm (Xq27.3). In karyotyping, the tip of the X chromosome is susceptible to breakage under certain conditions (fragile site). A special cell culture must be used in cytogenetic studies when searching for this defect.

**Epidemiology** Fragile X syndrome occurs with more frequency and greater severity among males than females (4:1). It is estimated that 1:1,000 males and 1:700 females have the fragile X chromosome. About 20 percent of males who inherit the mutation have no clinical manifestations of the disorder. About one-third of carrier females have some evidence of mental retardation. About 1:350 persons carries the fra(X) mutation. Affected individuals do not reproduce. The explanation for these puzzling findings is now known to be related to the size of CCG trinucleotide repeat of the gene. A large increase in the number of trinucleotide repeats results in the disorder. A small increase in trinucleotide repeats (premutation) results in normal transmitting males and unaffected carrier females. When premutation is passed through female meiosis, the trinucleotide repeats may greatly expand in number, resulting in the full-blown syndrome.

**Related Disorders Renpenning syndrome** is a form of inherited X-linked mental retardation caused by the presence of the genetic defect at a different site than that of fragile X (marXq28). This disorder occurs more frequently in males, although some females may also be affected.

**Treatment—Standard** Treatment includes special education; speech, occupational, and sensory integration training; and behavior modification programs. Surgical correction of heart defects is sometimes necessary. Genetic counseling will benefit families of affected persons. Other treatment is symptomatic and supportive.

**Treatment—Investigational** Folic acid has been found to improve hyperactivity and attention deficits in some preadolescent males with fragile X syndrome. However, further study of this treatment is warranted to determine long-term benefits and possible side effects.

Families with children who have the fragile X chromosome and who wish to participate in clinical research may contact Valerie Simon, Michael Reiss, M.D., and Lisa Freund, Ph.D., at the Kennedy Institute, Baltimore, Maryland.

Please contact the agencies listed under Resources, below, for the most current information. Addresses and telephone numbers of these agencies, as well as of individual experts and research centers, may be found in the Master Resources List.

### Resources

**For more information on fragile X syndrome:** National Organization for Rare Disorders (NORD); Fragile X Foundation; Fragile X Association of Michigan; Institute for Basic Research in Developmental Disabilities; NIH/National Institute of Child Health and Human Development.

**For genetic information and genetic counseling referrals:** March of Dimes Birth Defects Foundation; Alliance of Genetic Support Groups.

### References

Frequency and Stability of the Fragile X Premutation: A.L. Reiss, et al.; Hum. Mol. Genet., 1994, vol. 3, pp. 393–398.

Mendelian Inheritance in Man, 11th ed.: V.A. McKusick; The Johns Hopkins University Press, 1994, pp. 2452–2461.

Diagnosing Fragile X Syndrome: I.D. Young; Lancet, October 1993, vol. 342(8878), pp. 1004–1005.

Molecular Advances in Fragile X Syndrome: J.C. Tarleton and R.A. Sarl; J. Pediatr., 1993, vol. 122, pp. 169–185.

Folic Acid As an Adjunct in the Treatment of Children with the Autism Fragile-X Syndrome (AFRAX): C. Gillberg, et al.; Dev. Med. Child Neurol., October 1986, vol. 28(5), pp. 624–627.

Genetics and Expression of the Fragile X Syndrome: W.T. Brown, et al.; Ups. J. Med. Sci. Suppl., 1986, vol. 44, pp. 137–154.

# FRASER SYNDROME

**Description** Fraser syndrome is a rare genetic disorder characterized by multiple physical abnormalities that include craniofacial anomalies, renal malformation or agenesis, and incomplete development of the sexual organs.

### Synonyms

Cryptophthalmos-Syndactyly Syndrome

**Signs and Symptoms** Craniofacial abnormalities include cryptophthalmos, malformation of the lacrimal ducts, a broad nose with a flattened bridge, a high or cleft palate, a malformed or absent larynx, and deformities of the middle and outer ear. Hair growth may extend from the forehead to the eyebrows. Other characteristics may include syndactyly, malformed or absent kidneys, a displaced navel, widely spaced nipples, and malformation of the pubic bones. In males, there may be hypospadias or cryptorchidism; in females, clitoromegaly, fused labia, bicornuate uterus, or malformed fallopian tubes.

Mental deficiency may be present.

**Etiology** Fraser syndrome is an autosomal recessive genetic disorder.

**Epidemiology** Males and females are affected in equal numbers.

**Related Disorders** See *Renal Agenesis, Bilateral; Branchio-Oto-Renal Syndrome.*

**Cat's-eye syndrome** is characterized by coloboma of the iris and anal atresia. Other abnormalities may include renal agenesis, severe psychomotor retardation, and congenital heart disease.

**Treatment—Standard** Treatment may include surgical correction of some malformations. Other treatment is symptomatic and supportive. Genetic counseling may benefit families of affected children.

**Treatment—Investigational** Please contact the agencies listed under Resources, below, for the most current information. Addresses and telephone numbers of these agencies, as well as of individual experts and research centers, may be found in the Master Resources List.

### Resources

**For more information on Fraser syndrome:** National Organization for Rare Disorders (NORD); NIH/National Institute of Child Health and Human Development; National Kidney Foundation; American Kidney Fund; National Craniofacial Foundation; FACES—National Association for the Craniofacially Handicapped; National Foundation for Facial Reconstruction.

**For genetic information and genetic counseling referrals:** March of Dimes Birth Defects Foundation; Alliance of Genetic Support Groups.

### References

Mendelian Inheritance in Man, 11th ed.: V.A. McKusick; The Johns Hopkins University Press, 1994, pp. 1727–1728.

ENT Abnormalities Associated with Fraser Syndrome: Case Report and Literature Review: M. Mina, et al.; J. Otolaryngol., August 1988, vol. 17(5), pp. 233–236.

Fraser Syndrome (Cryptophthalmos-Syndactyly Syndrome): A Review of Eleven Cases with Postmortem Findings: P. Boyd, et al.; Am. J. Med. Genet., September 1988, vol. 31(1), pp. 159–168.

Smith's Recognizable Patterns of Human Malformation, 4th ed.: K.L. Jones; W.B. Saunders Company, 1988, pp. 204–205.

The Clinical Spectrum of the Fraser Syndrome: Report of Three New Cases and Review: J. Gattuso, et al.; J. Med. Genet., September 1987, vol. 24(9), pp. 549–555.

# FREEMAN-SHELDON SYNDROME

**Description** Freeman-Sheldon syndrome, a very rare genetic disorder that is present at birth, is characterized by abnormal muscle and skeletal development. The face, eyes, hands, and feet are most often affected. Patients usually have normal intelligence, although mental deficiency can occur.

**Synonyms**

> Craniocarpotarsal Dystrophy
> Whistling Face Syndrome
> Whistling Face–Windmill Vane Hand Syndrome

**Signs and Symptoms** Patients have stiffened muscles. Abnormalities in the interior bone structure of the skull are often present. Other characteristics include a round forehead (sometimes with ridges across the lower portion); a flat, expressionless face with full cheeks and a small mouth, giving a typical whistling appearance; and a small nose with flared nostrils and a broadened bridge. The tongue is small, the roof of the mouth is high, and speech has a nasal quality. The patient may have deep-set eyes and strabismus, a long philtrum, and an H-shaped dimple on the chin. Infants may fail to thrive because of dysphagia and vomiting.

The 2nd through 5th fingers are permanently flexed toward contracted thumbs, and the skin is thickened over the first finger. Clubfeet with contracted toes may occur, and occasionally spina bifida. (See *Clubfoot; Spina Bifida.*) In males, an inguinal hernia or cryptorchidism may be present. Low birth weight, small stature, scoliosis, or dislocation of the hip may be present in some children.

**Etiology** Freeman-Sheldon syndrome is usually inherited as an autosomal dominant trait, but autosomal recessive inheritance has been reported in a few families.

**Epidemiology** Males and females are affected in equal numbers. Over 65 cases of Freeman-Sheldon syndrome have been identified worldwide since the disorder was first recognized in 1938.

**Related Disorders** See *Arthrogryposis Multiplex Congenita.*

**Treatment—Standard** Treatment usually involves multiple surgical procedures (which can be difficult because of muscle stiffness and thickened tissues) or the use of splints or casts to improve bent fingers or feet. Correction of the thumb deformity may be the first surgery in the long-term treatment of many cases. Cosmetic facial or hand and foot restructuring surgery can improve appearance. Genetic counseling will benefit patients and their families. Other treatment is symptomatic and supportive.

**Treatment—Investigational** It has been suggested that agents other than halothane and succinyicholine be given to Freeman-Sheldon syndrome patients with a family history of malignant hyperthermia in order to avoid jaw spasms.

The Department of Plastic Surgery at the University of Virginia, Charlottesville, is reviewing surgical procedures for Freeman-Sheldon syndrome.

The Division of Pediatric Genetics at the University of Utah has undertaken a gene mapping study of Freeman-Sheldon syndrome.

Please contact the agencies listed under Resources, below, for the most current information. Addresses and telephone numbers of these agencies, as well as of individual experts and research centers, may be found in the Master Resources List.

**Resources**

**For more information on Freeman-Sheldon syndrome:** National Organization for Rare Disorders (NORD); Freeman-Sheldon Parent Support Group; NIH/National Arthritis and Musculoskeletal and Skin Diseases Information Clearinghouse.

**For genetic information and genetic counseling referrals:** March of Dimes Birth Defects Foundation; Alliance of Genetic Support Groups.

**References**

Mendelian Inheritance in Man, 11th ed.: V.A. McKusick; The Johns Hopkins University Press, 1994, pp. 1546–1547.

Muscle Rigidity Following Halothane Anesthesia in Two Patients with Freeman-Sheldon Syndrome: R. Jones, M.D., et al.; Anesthesiology, September 1992, vol. 77(3), pp. 599–600.

Smith's Recognizable Patterns of Human Malformation, 4th ed.: K.L. Jones; W.B. Saunders Company, 1988, pp. 182–183.

Freeman-Sheldon Syndrome: A Disorder of Congenital Myopathic Origin?: J. Vanek, et al.; J. Med. Genet., June 1986, vol. 23(3), pp. 231–236.

New Evidence for Genetic Heterogeneity of the Freeman-Sheldon (FS) Syndrome: M. Sanchez, et al.; Am. J. Med. Genet., November 1986, vol. 25(3), pp. 507–511.

Ocular Abnormalities in the Freeman-Sheldon Syndrome: M. O'Keefe, et al.; Am. J. Ophthalmol., September 1986, vol. 102(3), pp. 346–348.

# FRONTO-FACIO-NASAL DYSPLASIA

**Description** Fronto-facio-nasal dysplasia is a congenital disorder of the skull and face.

**Synonyms**

> Facio-Fronto-Nasal Dysplasia
> Fronto-Facio-Nasal Dysostosis
> Nasal-Fronto-Facial Dysplasia

**Signs and Symptoms** Cleft palate and cleft lip are the 2 major features of this disorder. Premature coronal suture in an infant causes side-to-side growth. Other signs include blepharophimosis, ptosis, an S-shaped opening between the upper and lower eyelids, dermoid of the eye, coloboma, missing or sparse eyelashes, lagophthalmos, adhesions between the upper and lower eyelids, and hypertelorism. Cranium bifidum occultum, encephalocele, as well as lipomata on the frontal lobe of the brain may also be present.

**Etiology** Fronto-facio-nasal dysplasia is inherited as an autosomal recessive trait.

**Epidemiology** Of the 4 cases of fronto-facio-nasal dysplasia reported in the medical literature, 2 (a brother and sister) were from the same family.

**Related Disorders Cranio-fronto-nasal dysplasia** is thought to be inherited as an autosomal dominant trait with a wide variance in expression. Ocular hypertelorism, a missing or grooved tip of the nose, and a broad nasal bridge are typically present. Other abnormalities include syndactyly; split nails; a broad index finger; a wide mouth; a malformed clavicle; and a high, broad forehead.

**Median cleft-face syndrome** occurs sporadically. This disorder affects males and females equally and is characterized by a widely spaced central portion of the face. The nasal groove varies greatly in severity from a missing nasal tip to separation of the nose into 2 parts. Ocular hypertelorism may occur, and some patients have a split anterior skull as well as a widow's peak.

**Treatment—Standard** Treatment of cleft lip and palate requires a team of specialists: pediatricians, dental specialists, surgeons, speech pathologists, and others. Cleft palate may be repaired by surgery or covered with a prosthesis.

Routine hearing tests are recommended for preschool children with cleft palate. Myringotomy may be required to drain the eustachian tubes.

Surgery is indicated for encephalocele or cranium bifidum occultum.

Genetic counseling may benefit patients and their families. Other treatment is symptomatic and supportive.

**Treatment—Investigational** Researchers are studying a Teflon-glycerine paste that is applied to the rear of the pharynx in a minor surgical procedure to bring the pharynx and palate into proper relationship. For further information contact William N. Williams, D.D.S., University of Florida.

Drs. Amy Feldman Lewanda and Ethylin Wang Jabs at Johns Hopkins Hospital in Baltimore are trying to identify the genes responsible for craniofacial disorders.

Please contact the agencies listed under Resources, below, for the most current information. Addresses and telephone numbers of these agencies, as well as of individual experts and research centers, may be found in the Master Resources List.

**Resources**

**For more information on fronto-facio-nasal dysplasia:** National Organization for Rare Disorders (NORD); National Craniofacial Foundation; FACES—National Association for the Craniofacially Handicapped; Society for the Rehabilitation of the Facially Disfigured; Forward Face; Children's Craniofacial Association; Craniofacial Family Association; AboutFace; NIH/National Institute of Child Health and Human Development.

**For genetic information and genetic counseling referrals:** March of Dimes Birth Defects Foundation; Alliance of Genetic Support Groups.

**References**

Mendelian Inheritance in Man, 11th ed.: V.A. McKusick; The Johns Hopkins University Press, 1994, p. 1821.

Birth Defects Encyclopedia: M.L. Buyse, ed.-in-chief; Blackwell Scientific Publications, 1990, p. 749.

Frontofacionasal Dysplasia: Evidence for Autosomal Recessive Inheritance: T.R. Gollop, et al.; Am. J. Med. Genet., October 1984, vol. 19(2), pp. 301–305.

# FRYNS SYNDROME

**Description** Fryns syndrome is a multisystem disorder of the face, hands, feet, lungs, and urogenital areas.

**Signs and Symptoms** Unusual facial features are usually present at birth and include a broad nasal bridge, micrognathia, cleft palate and lip, and a coarse appearance. Corneal opacities, a short neck, deformed finger and toe nails, and anomalies of the hands and feet may also be present.

Cysts, hydrocephalus, and missing areas or unusual development of the brain may occur. Diaphragmatic hernia, poor lung development, and the misplacement of abdominal organs into the rib cage may affect the pulmonary and cardiac functions of the infant.

When all of the above characteristics are present, chances of survival are poor. However, if diaphragmatic hernia and poor lung development are absent, the prognosis is better. The affected child is often mentally retarded.

**Etiology** Fryns syndrome is usually caused by autosomal recessive inheritance. Some cases occur as isolated events for which a genetic cause cannot be found.

**Epidemiology** Fryns syndrome has occurred both sporadically and in the offspring of blood-related couples. Males and females are affected in equal numbers. Approximately 35 cases have been reported. Estimated occurrence is 1:10,000 births.

**Related Disorders** See *Pentalogy of Cantrell; Dandy-Walker Syndrome; Oral-Facial-Digital Syndrome.*

**Treatment—Standard** Fryns syndrome can be detected prenatally by ultrasound; such testing is recommended if a sibling has been diagnosed with the disorder. Fryns syndrome can be treated with surgical correction of internal malformations in those infants who survive. Cleft lip can be corrected by surgery, beginning in the patient's infancy. Cleft palate may also be treated surgically or by a prosthesis.

Genetic counseling will benefit the families of Fryns syndrome infants. Other treatment is symptomatic and supportive.

**Treatment—Investigational** Researchers are studying a Teflon-glycerine paste that is applied to the rear of the pharynx in a minor surgical procedure to bring the pharynx and palate into proper relationship. For further information, contact William N. Williams, D.D.S., University of Florida.

Please contact the agencies listed under Resources, below, for the most current information. Addresses and telephone numbers of these agencies, as well as of individual experts and research centers, may be found in the Master Resources List.

**Resources**

**For more information on Fryns syndrome:** National Organization for Rare Disorders (NORD); NIH/National Institute of Child Health and Human Development.

**For genetic information and genetic counseling referrals:** March of Dimes Birth Defects Foundation; Alliance of Genetic Support Groups.

**References**

Mendelian Inheritance in Man, 11th ed.: V.A. McKusick; The Johns Hopkins University Press, 1994, pp. 1824–1825.

Birth Defects Encyclopedia: M.L. Buyse, ed.-in-chief; Blackwell Scientific Publications, 1990, pp. 752–753.

Fryns Syndrome: A Predictable, Lethal Pattern of Multiple Congenital Anomalies: A. Samueloff, et al.; Am. J. Obstet. Gynecol., January 1987, vol. 156(1), pp. 86–88.

A Case Of Fryns Syndrome: I.D. Young, et al.; J. Med. Genet., February 1986, vol. 23(1), pp. 82–84.

Fryns Syndrome: An Autosomal Recessive Disorder Associated with Craniofacial Anomalies, Diaphragmatic Hernia, and Distal Digital Hypoplasia: C. Cunniff, et al.; Pediatrics, April 1990, vol. 85(4), pp. 499–504.

The Fryns Syndrome: Diaphragmatic Defects, Craniofacial Dysmorphism, and Distal Digital Hypoplasia: Further Evidence for Autosomal Recessive Inheritance: P. Meinecks, et al.; Clin. Genet., December 1985, vol. 28(6), pp. 516–520.

# GASTROSCHISIS

**Description** Gastroschisis is characterized by a small abdominal cavity with herniated intestines usually on the right of the umbilical cord.

**Synonyms**

Aparoschisis

**Signs and Symptoms** Gastroschisis is apparent at birth and can be detected prenatally with ultrasound. Through the defect on the right side of the umbilical chord can be seen herniated intestines, which appear swollen and shortened due to exposure to amniotic fluid. The abdominal cavity is smaller than normal, and there is no membranous sac covering the intestines. Other symptoms include low birth weight, infection, dehydration, hypothermia, volvulus and resultant obstruction, midgut infarction, and metabolic acidosis.

**Etiology** The exact cause of gastroschisis is not known. Rupture of an omphalocele in utero has been suggested. The sac may be reabsorbed prenatally in the case of gastroschisis. Another theory is a dysfunction in the omphalomesenteric artery. Several cases of gastroschisis have occurred in siblings, which suggests an autosomal recessive inheritance.

**Epidemiology** This disorder affects approximately 1:6,000 live births. Males are more frequently affected than females; the male-to-female ratio is 5:1.

**Related Disorders** See *Beckwith-Wiedemann Syndrome.*

**Prune belly syndrome** is a congenital disorder characterized by underdevelopment of the abdominal muscles associated with intestinal and urogenital abnormalities. The abdomen appears large and lax, the abdominal wall is thin, and the intestinal loops can be seen through the thin abdominal wall.

**Treatment—Standard** Diagnosis is by ultrasound prenatally. Closure of the defective wall is done as soon as possible postnatally. If the abdominal cavity is too small to hold the intestines, a covering of a soft pliable plastic in the shape of a chimney is placed over the protrusion until the cavity can accommodate the intestines.

Genetic counseling may benefit patients and their families. Other treatment is symptomatic and supportive.

**Treatment—Investigational** Please contact the agencies listed under Resources, below, for the most current information. Addresses and telephone numbers of these agencies, as well as of individual experts and research centers, may be found in the Master Resources List.

**Resources**

**For more information on gastroschisis:** National Organization for Rare Disorders (NORD); NIH/National Digestive Diseases Information Clearinghouse.

**For genetic information and genetic counseling referrals:** March of Dimes Birth Defects Foundation; Alliance of Genetic Support Groups.

**References**

Mendelian Inheritance in Man, 11th ed.: V.A. McKusick; The Johns Hopkins University Press, 1994, p. 1838.

Is Primary Repair of Gastroschisis and Omphalocele Always the Best Operation?: E.R. Sauter, et al.; Am. Surg., March 1991, vol. 57(3), pp. 142–144.

Birth Defects Encyclopedia: M.L. Buyse, ed.-in-chief; Blackwell Scientific Publications, 1990, pp. 768–769.

Ultrasonographic Assessment of Intestinal Damage in Fetuses with Gastroschisis: Is It of Clinical Value?: R.R. Lenke, et al.; Am. J. Obstet. Gynecol., September 1990, vol. 163(3), pp. 995–998.

The Effect of Initial Operative Repair on the Recovery of Intestinal Function in Gastroschisis: M.S. Bryant, et al.; Am. Surg., April 1989, vol. 55(4), pp. 209–211.

# GOLDENHAR SYNDROME

**Description** Goldenhar syndrome encompasses a wide spectrum of ear, eye, facial, vertebral, and other congenital malformations. The disorder is almost always more severe on one side.

**Synonyms**

>Auriculo-Oculo-Vertebral Syndrome
>Facio-Auriculo-Vertebral Anomaly
>First and Second Branchial Arch Syndrome
>Goldenhar-Gorlin Syndrome
>Mandibulofacial Dysostosis with Epibulbar Dermoids
>Oculo-Auriculo-Vertebral Spectrum

**Signs and Symptoms** The syndrome is commonly associated with varying combinations of the following abnormalities, many of which are often asymmetric and unilateral: macrostomia; malar, maxillary, and mandibular hypoplasia; absent or closed nares; frontal bossing; microtia; middle ear anomalies; deafness; anomalies of the tongue and soft palate; and hemivertebra.

Less common abnormalities associated with Goldenhar syndrome include epibulbar dermoid, strabismus, microphthalmia, inner ear anomalies, cleft lip, and cleft palate. Neurologic, cardiac, pulmonary, renal, and gastrointestinal anomalies occur.

**Hemifacial microsomia (HFM),** now thought to be part of the spectrum of Goldenhar syndrome, is characterized by facial abnormalities that may be bilateral but are always quite asymmetrical, and by the fairly frequent finding of facial nerve paralysis. The wide variety of features in HFM includes mandibular hypoplasia with tilting of the jaw to one side, macrostomia, unilateral microtia, and variable hypoplasia of the cheek and eye on the affected side.

**Etiology** The cause of Goldenhar syndrome is not known. Most cases are sporadic; some are autosomal dominant. Expression within a family may be variable.

**Epidemiology** Goldenhar syndrome occurs in about 1:45,000 newborn infants.

**Related Disorders** See *Spina Bifida; Treacher Collins Syndrome.*

**Treatment—Standard** Spinal and/or facial deformities may be managed surgically. Speech and language therapy and special education may be beneficial. The child may also benefit from supportive counseling.

**Treatment—Investigational** Advances in tissue and bone grafts currently under investigation may be useful in treating Goldenhar syndrome.

Drs. Amy Feldman Lewanda and Ethylin Wang Jabs at Johns Hopkins Hospital in Baltimore are investigating the genes responsible for craniofacial disorders.

Please contact the agencies listed under Resources, below, for the most current information. Addresses and telephone numbers of these agencies, as well as of individual experts and research centers, may be found in the Master Resources List.

**Resources**

**For more information on Goldenhar syndrome:** National Organization for Rare Disorders (NORD); Goldenhar Syndrome Research and Information Fund; International Center for Skeletal Dysplasia; Society for the Rehabilitation of the Facially Disfigured; FACES—National Association for the Craniofacially Handicapped; National Craniofacial Foundation; Orofacial Guild; AboutFace; NIH/National Institute of Child Health and Human Development.

**For genetic information and genetic counseling referrals:** March of Dimes Birth Defects Foundation; Alliance of Genetic Support Groups.

**References**

Mendelian Inheritance in Man, 11th ed.: V.A. McKusick; The Johns Hopkins University Press, 1994, pp. 1039–1040.

Syndromes of the Head and Neck, 3rd ed.: R.J. Gorlin, et al.; Oxford University Press, 1990, pp. 641–649.

Smith's Recognizable Patterns of Human Malformation, 4th ed.: K.L. Jones; W.B. Saunders Company, 1988, pp. 584–587.

Congenital Absence of the Portal Vein in Oculoauriculovertebral Dysplasia (Goldenhar Syndrome): J.H. Seashore, et al., Pediatr. Radiol., 1986, vol. 16(5), pp. 437–439.

Goldenhar's Syndrome: A Case Study: L. Belenchia; J. Commun. Disord., October 1985, vol. 18(5), pp. 383–392.

The Use of Microvascular Free Flaps for Soft Tissue Augmentation of the Face in Children with Hemifacial Microsomia: La Rossa; Cleft Palate J., April 1980, vol. 17(2), pp. 138–143.

# GOODMAN SYNDROME

**Description** Goodman syndrome (acrocephalopolysyndactyly type IV) is an extremely rare genetic disorder characterized by marked malformations of the head and face, abnormalities of the hands and feet, and congenital heart disease. Goodman syndrome may be a variant of Carpenter syndrome (acrocephalopolysyndactyly type II). There are 4 types of acrocephalopolysyndactyly: Noack syndrome (type I), Carpenter syndrome (type II), Sakati syndrome (type III), and Goodman syndrome (type IV). All of these types are characterized by acrocephaly, polydactyly, and syndactyly.

**Synonyms**

Acrocephalopolysyndactyly Type IV

**Signs and Symptoms** Craniosynostosis occurs, causing the head to grow upward. As a result, the head appears elongated, narrow, and pointed at the top (acrocephaly). Characteristic facial abnormalities include a prominent nose; large, protruding ears; high-arched eyebrows; slightly slanted palpebral fissures; and epicanthal folds that may cover the eyes' inner corners.

Goodman syndrome is also characterized by several abnormalities of the hands and feet, including syndactyly, postaxial polydactyly, and 5th fingers that are abnormally bent (clinodactyly) and permanently flexed (camptodactyly). Other features include a deviation of the ulna, knees that may be abnormally close together and ankles that are abnormally far apart (genu valgum), and congenital heart disease. All affected individuals described in the medical literature have exhibited normal intelligence.

**Etiology** Goodman syndrome is inherited as an autosomal recessive trait.

**Epidemiology** Goodman syndrome affects males and females in equal numbers. Three cases within one family of closely related parents have been reported.

**Related Disorders** Goodman syndrome may be a variant of Carpenter syndrome. The presence of camptodactyly and clinodactyly combined with deviation of the ulna is mainly what distinguishes Goodman syndrome from Carpenter syndrome. See *Carpenter Syndrome.*

See also *Pfeiffer Syndrome; Nager Syndrome; Oral-Facial-Digital Syndrome; Antley-Bixler Syndrome; Summitt Syndrome.*

**Treatment—Standard** Early craniofacial surgery may be performed to correct craniosynostosis and to improve appearance. Additional craniofacial surgery may be done later in life as well as surgery to correct deformities of the hands and feet. Infants with Goodman syndrome who have congenital heart defects may also be treated surgically. Other treatment is symptomatic and supportive. Genetic counseling may benefit patients and their families.

**Treatment—Investigational** Please contact the agencies listed under Resources, below, for the most current information. Addresses and telephone numbers of these agencies, as well as of individual experts and research centers, may be found in the Master Resources List.

**Resources**

For more information on Goodman syndrome: National Organization for Rare Disorders (NORD); NIH/National Institute of Child Health and Human Development.

For information about heart defects: NIH/National Heart, Lung and Blood Institute Information Center; American Heart Association; Congenital Heart Anomalies Support, Education, and Resources.

For information about craniofacial research and treatments: Forward Face; FACES—National Association for the Craniofacially Handicapped; Let's Face It; National Craniofacial Foundation; National Foundation for Facial Reconstruction; AboutFace; Craniofacial Family Association; Craniofacial Support Group.

For genetic information and genetic counseling referrals: March of Dimes Birth Defects Foundation; Alliance of Genetic Support Groups.

**References**

Mendelian Inheritance in Man, 11th ed.: V.A. McKusick; The Johns Hopkins University Press, 1994, p. 1577.

Online Mendelian Inheritance in Man (OMIM): V.A. McKusick; last edit date 3/30/94, entry number 201000; last edit date 3/12/94, entry number 272350; last edit date 3/11/94, entry number 101120.

Carpenter's Syndrome (Acrocephalopolysyndactyly Type II) with Normal Intelligence: M.N. Jamil, et al.; Br. J. Neurosurg., 1992, vol. 6(3), pp. 243–247.

Birth Defects Encyclopedia: M.L Buyse, ed.-in-chief; Blackwell Scientific Publications, 1990, pp. 36–37.

Acrocephalopolysyndactyly Type II—Carpenter Syndrome: Clinical Spectrum and an Attempt at Unification with Goodman and Summitt Syndromes: D.M. Cohen, et al.; Am. J. Med. Genet., October 1987, vol. 28(2), pp. 311–324.

Carpenter Syndrome: Marked Variability of Expression to Include the Summitt and Goodman Syndromes: R. Gershoni-Baruch; Am. J. Med. Genet., February 1990, vol. 35(2), pp. 236–240.

# GORDON SYNDROME

**Description** Gordon syndrome, one of a group of genetic musculoskeletal disorders called the distal arthrogryposes, is characterized by camptodactyly, a cleft palate, and clubfoot. Other developmental abnormalities may also occur.

**Synonyms**

Arthrogryposis Multiplex Congenita, Distal, Type IIA

Camptodactyly–Cleft Palate–Clubfoot

Distal Arthrogryposis, Type IIA

**Signs and Symptoms** Major features are 1 or 2 permanently flexed fingers, a cleft palate, and clubfoot. An affected fetus usually has limited movement in utero. An omphalocele is sometimes present at birth, and there may be cutaneous syndactyly and abnormalities in the fingerprints. Fertility of adults with Gordon syndrome may be lessened or absent.

**Etiology** The syndrome has autosomal dominant inheritance.

**Epidemiology** Onset is in utero. Females and males are affected in equal numbers.

**Related Disorders** See *Arthrogryposis Multiplex Congenita.*

**Treatment—Standard** Gordon syndrome can be diagnosed in utero. Abnormalities associated with this disorder can often be corrected through surgery and physical therapy.

**Treatment—Investigational** Please contact the agencies listed under Resources, below, for the most current information. Addresses and telephone numbers of these agencies, as well as of individual experts and research centers, may be found in the Master Resources List.

**Resources**

For more information on Gordon syndrome: National Organization for Rare Disorders (NORD); AVENUES, a National Support Group for Arthrogryposis Multiplex Congenita; NIH/National Arthritis and Musculoskeletal and Skin Diseases Information Clearinghouse.

**References**

Mendelian Inheritance in Man, 11th ed.: V.A. McKusick; The Johns Hopkins University Press, 1994, p. 241.

Three Distinct Types of X-Linked Arthrogryposis Seen in 6 Families: J.G. Hall, et al.; Clin. Genet., February 1982, vol. 21(2), pp. 81–97.

The Gordon Syndrome: Autosomal Dominant Cleft Palate, Camptodactyly, and Club Feet: M. Robinow, et al.; Amer. J. Med. Genet., 1981, vol. 9(2), pp. 139–146.

# GOTTRON SYNDROME

**Description** Gottron syndrome is a mild inherited form of **progeria** that appears to be limited to the extremities. The prognosis for a normal life is good.

**Synonyms**

      Acrogeria, Familial

**Signs and Symptoms** From infancy on, patients seem older than their age as a result of thin, parchment-like skin on their hands and feet, which remain small into adulthood. Veins on the chest are prominent because of the small amount of subcutaneous fat. Physical and mental development are normal.

**Etiology** Gottron syndrome is inherited as an autosomal recessive trait.

**Epidemiology** Males and females are affected equally.

**Related Disorders** See *Hutchinson-Gilford Syndrome,* a more severe form of progeria that affects children; and *Werner Syndrome,* another form of progeria that affects adults.

**Treatment—Standard** Treatment is symptomatic and supportive. Genetic counseling may benefit patients and their families.

**Treatment—Investigational** Please contact the agencies listed under Resources, below, for the most current information. Addresses and telephone numbers of these agencies, as well as of individual experts and research centers, may be found in the Master Resources List.

**Resources**

    **For more information on Gottron syndrome:** National Organization for Rare Disorders (NORD); Institute for Basic Research in Developmental Disabilities; Progeria International Registry; NIH/National Institute of Child Health and Human Development; Sunshine Foundation. (The Sunshine Foundation raises funds to bring all children with progeria together each year so that their progress can be studied while the children socialize in a vacation atmosphere.)

    **For genetic information and genetic counseling referrals:** March of Dimes Birth Defects Foundation; Alliance of Genetic Support Groups.

**References**

Mendelian Inheritance in Man, 11th ed.: V.A. McKusick; The Johns Hopkins University Press, 1994, p. 1579.

Cecil Textbook of Medicine, 19th ed.: J.B. Wyngaarden, et al., eds.; W.B. Saunders Company, 1992, p. 1145.

Nelson Textbook of Pediatrics, 14th ed.: R.E. Behrman, ed.-in-chief; W.B. Saunders Company, 1992, p. 1765.

Birth Defects Encyclopedia: M.L. Buyse, ed.-in-chief; Blackwell Scientific Publications, 1990, pp. 1411–1413.

Dictionary of Medical Syndromes, 3rd ed.: S.I. Magalini, et al., eds.; J.B. Lippincott Company, 1990, p. 363.

Smith's Recognizable Patterns of Human Deformation, 2nd ed.: J.M. Graham, Jr.; W.B. Saunders Company, 1988, pp. 118–119.

# GREIG CEPHALOPOLYSYNDACTYLY SYNDROME (GCPS)

**Description** GCPS is characterized by macrocephaly, an unusual facies, and multiple physical deformities of the hands and feet.

**Synonyms**

      Greig Syndrome

      Greig Polysyndactyly Craniofacial Dysmorphism Syndrome

**Signs and Symptoms** Craniofacial characteristics include macrocephaly; a high, prominent forehead; a broad nose; and ocular hypertelorism. Polysyndactyly, syndactyly, and enlarged thumbs and great toes are usually present. Occasionally there is camptodactyly as well as hydrocephalus and mild mental retardation.

**Etiology** GCPS is believed to be inherited as an autosomal dominant trait. The defective gene has been localized to the short arm of chromosome 7 (7p13). Evidence suggests that mutations in the GL13 gene are the cause of this disorder.

**Epidemiology** The syndrome is very rare. Males and females are affected in equal numbers.

**Related Disorders** See *Apert Syndrome.*

**Treatment—Standard** Corrective surgery may be performed for the syndactyly. Genetic counseling may benefit patients and their families. Other treatment is symptomatic and supportive.

**Treatment—Investigational** Please contact the agencies listed under Resources, below, for the most current information. Addresses and telephone numbers of these agencies, as well as of individual experts and research centers, may be found in the Master Resources List.

**Resources**

**For more information on Greig cephalopolysyndactyly syndrome:** National Organization for Rare Disorders (NORD); National Craniofacial Foundation; Society for the Rehabilitation of the Facially Disfigured; FACES—National Association for the Craniofacially Handicapped; NIH/National Institute of Child Health and Human Development.

**For genetic information and genetic counseling referrals:** March of Dimes Birth Defects Foundation; Alliance of Genetic Support Groups.

**References**

Mendelian Inheritance in Man, 11th ed.: V.A. McKusick; The Johns Hopkins University Press, 1994, pp. 1194–1195.

Chromosomal Localisation of a Developmental Gene in Man: Direct DNA Analysis Demonstrates That Greig Cephalopolysyndactyly Maps to 7p13 L: Brueton, et al.; Am. J. Med. Genet., December 1988, vol. 31(4), pp. 799–804.

Smith's Recognizable Patterns of Human Malformation, 4th ed.: K.L. Jones; W.B. Saunders Company, 1988, pp. 376–377.

Evaluation of a Uniform Operative Technique to Treat Syndactyly: D. Keret, et al.; J. Hand Surg., September 1987, vol. 12(5 pt. 1), pp. 727–729.

The Greig Cephalopolysyndactyly Syndrome: Report of a Family and Review of the Literature: T. Gallop, et al.; Am. J. Med. Genet., September 1985, vol. 22(1), pp. 59–68.

Greig Cephalopolysyndactyly: Report of 13 Affected Individuals in Three Families: M. Baraiter, et al.; Clin. Genet., October 1983, vol. 24(4), pp. 257–265.

# HALLERMANN-STREIFF SYNDROME

**Description** The syndrome is characterized by proportionate short stature and bony abnormalities of the calvaria, face, and jaw.

**Synonyms**

> François Dyscephalic Syndrome
> Hallermann-Streiff-François Syndrome
> Mandibulo-Oculo-Facial Dyscephaly
> Oculomandibulodyscephaly
> Oculomandibulofacial Syndrome

**Signs and Symptoms** Children are born with a birdlike face: a receding jaw; a narrow, beaked nose; and thinned or absent hair overlying the skull sutures. Eyebrows may be absent or underdeveloped. The eyeballs and corneas are abnormally small, and cataract or glaucoma, or both, may be present. Dental abnormalities include the presence of teeth at birth or at a few weeks of age, and the eruption of teeth that are not well anchored in the jaw and often fall out. Permanent teeth, which normally erupt during childhood, are usually absent except for the first permanent molars. Abnormalities of the skull and face may predispose some patients to respiratory disorders. Additionally, motor and mental retardation (15 percent), progeroid appearance, and atrophy of the elastic tissue of the skin may occur. There is proportionate short stature.

**Etiology** The cause is uncertain. In practically all instances chromosomal studies have been normal. Almost all cases have been sporadic. A few familial cases suggest autosomal recessive inheritance, but these are not accepted by all dysmorphologists.

**Epidemiology** Males and females are affected in equal numbers. Since the disorder was first identified in 1948, about 150 cases have been reported.

**Related Disorders** See *Treacher Collins Syndrome; Seckel Syndrome.*

**Treatment—Standard** Treatment is symptomatic and supportive. Vision problems can be successfully treated. Infections should be guarded against. A tracheostomy may be necessary for severe respiratory distress. Services that assist physically and mentally retarded individuals are helpful. Genetic counseling will benefit patients and their families.

**Treatment—Investigational** Please contact the agencies listed under Resources, below, for the most current information. Addresses and telephone numbers of these agencies, as well as of individual experts and research centers, may be found in the Master Resources List.

**Resources**

**For more information on Hallermann-Streiff syndrome:** National Organization for Rare Disorders (NORD); Hallermann-Streiff Parent Association; International Center for Skeletal Dysplasia; FACES—National Association for the Craniofacially Handicapped; Society for the Rehabilitation of the Facially Disfigured; National Craniofacial Foundation; AboutFace; NIH/National Institute of Child Health and Human Development.

**For genetic information and genetic counseling referrals:** March of Dimes Birth Defects Foundation; Alliance of Genetic Support Groups.

**References**

Mendelian Inheritance in Man, 11th ed.: V.A. McKusick; The Johns Hopkins University Press, 1994, p. 1878.

Smith's Recognizable Patterns of Human Malformation, 4th ed.: K.L. Jones; W.B. Saunders Company, 1988, pp. 102–103.

Hallermann-Streiff Syndrome: Report of a Case: A.J. Malerman, et al.; ASDC J. Dent. Child., July–August 1986, vol. 53(4), pp. 287–292.

Airway Management in Hallermann-Streiff Syndrome: R.T. Sataloff, et al.; Am. J. Otolaryngol., January–February 1984, vol. 5(1), pp. 64–67.

Dento-Alveolar Abnormalities in Oculomandibulodyscephaly (Hallermann-Streiff Syndrome): P.J. Slootweg, et al.; J. Oral Pathol., April 1984, vol. 13(2), pp. 147–154.

# HOLT-ORAM SYNDROME

**Description** Holt-Oram syndrome is a genetic disorder consisting primarily of congenital heart disease and upper limb abnormalities, typically of the forearm, fingers, and wrist.

**Synonyms**

> Atriodigital Dysplasia
> Heart-Hand Syndrome
> Upper Limb–Cardiovascular Syndrome

**Signs and Symptoms** The most common congenital cardiac findings are atrial and ventricular septal defects, although other anomalies may be present, including various disturbances of cardiac rhythm.

Upper limb involvement is a consistent feature of the syndrome, while the association of congenital heart disease is variable. The skeletal defects often occur bilaterally but may be unilateral. Most patients have abnormalities or absence of the thumbs and foreshortened arms; phocomelia may occur.

There is a range of severity in Holt-Oram syndrome, and bony abnormalities may also be quite mild.

Pregnant women at risk of having an affected child may undergo ultrasound imaging procedures prenatally to evaluate fetal development as early as 14 weeks into pregnancy.

**Etiology** The syndrome is inherited as an autosomal dominant trait. In 15 of 17 patients studied thus far, the gene has been mapped to chromosome 12q. The disorder may be heterogeneous.

**Epidemiology** The disorder occurs in about 1:100,000 live births. All ethnic groups and races can be affected. Males and females are affected in equal numbers.

**Related Disorders** See *Thrombocytopenia–Absent Radius Syndrome.*

**Treatment—Standard** Treatment is by surgical correction where necessary, both of the heart and skeletal problems. Services that benefit the physically handicapped may be helpful in some cases. Other treatment is symptomatic and supportive. Genetic counseling is recommended for patients and their families.

**Treatment—Investigational** Please contact the agencies listed under Resources, below, for the most current information. Addresses and telephone numbers of these agencies, as well as of individual experts and research centers, may be found in the Master Resources List.

**Resources**

**For more information on Holt-Oram syndrome:** National Organization for Rare Disorders (NORD); American Heart Association.

**For cardiac symptoms information:** NIH/National Heart, Lung and Blood Institute.

**For bone symptoms information:** NIH/National Arthritis and Musculoskeletal and Skin Diseases Information Clearinghouse; International Center for Skeletal Dysplasia.

**For genetic information and genetic counseling referrals:** March of Dimes Birth Defects Foundation; Alliance of Genetic Support Groups.

**References**

The Clinical and Genetic Spectrum of Holt-Oram Syndrome: C.T. Basson, et al.; N. Engl. J. Med., March 1994, vol. 330(13), pp. 885–891.

A Gene for Holt-Oram Syndrome Maps to the Distal Long Arm of Chromosome 12: D. Bonnet, et al.; Nat. Genet., 1994, vol. 6, pp. 405–408.

Holt-Oram Syndrome Is a Genetically Heterogeneous Disease with One Locus Mapping to Human Chromosome 12: J.A. Terrett, et al.; Nat. Genet., 1994, vol. 6, pp. 401–404.

Mendelian Inheritance in Man, 11th ed.: V.A. McKusick; The Johns Hopkins University Press, 1994, pp. 717–718.

Smith's Recognizable Patterns of Human Malformation, 4th ed.: K.L. Jones; W.B. Saunders Company, 1988, p. 272.

Cross-Sectional Echocardiographic Imaging of Supracardiac Total Anomalous Pulmonary Venous Drainage to a Vertical Vein in a Patient with Holt-Oram Syndrome: K.Z. Zhang, et al.; Chest, January 1981, vol. 79(1), pp. 113–115.

# HUTCHINSON-GILFORD SYNDROME

**Description** In this progeria syndrome, children age rapidly, are very short of stature, and have characteristic facies. Intelligence is normal.

**Synonyms**

Gilford Syndrome
Premature Senility Syndrome
Progeria (Childhood)
Souques-Charcot Syndrome

**Signs and Symptoms** Birth weight is normal, and the growth rate does not decelerate until about 1 year of age. At 10 years, most affected children have the height of the average 3-year-old. Lifetime height rarely exceeds that of a normal 5-year-old.

Craniofacial characteristics include a relatively large head but a small face, with a sharp, beaklike nose and receding chin. Because of the small size of the jaw, the teeth are often crowded and irregular. The eyes protrude and may have bluish sclerae and cloudy corneas. Patients may have no eyebrows and eyelashes and no hair on the scalp, revealing prominent veins; alternatively, the hair may turn gray.

The skin is dry, thin, and wrinkled, and often is a brownish color. Scarcity of subcutaneous fat leads to the wrinkling and appearance of age. The long bones are decalcified and thin, and the chest is narrow. The abdomen protrudes. There may be splenomegaly and umbilical or inguinal hernias. The sex organs remain undeveloped.

In adolescence, the patient becomes susceptible to strokes, atherosclerosis, occlusion of the coronary artery, and angina. These and assorted other complications are associated with high levels of blood lipoprotein. Very rarely, amino acids are lost in the urine. Life-threatening heart disease or stroke may occur.

**Etiology** The cause is unclear. There seems to be no familial pattern. High paternal age has been implicated in some studies, but this finding has not been conclusive.

**Epidemiology** The syndrome is very rare. Boys and girls are affected equally, and usually survive into their teens.

**Related Disorders** See *Werner Syndrome,* an adult form of progeria.

In *Gottron Syndrome* (acrogeria), only the hands and feet are involved; these remain unusually small and age much more rapidly than the rest of the body.

**Treatment—Standard** Treatment is supportive. Symptomatic therapy of heart conditions, stroke, etc., may be necessary.

**Treatment—Investigational** Please contact the agencies listed under Resources, below, for the most current information. Addresses and telephone numbers of these agencies, as well as of individual experts and research centers, may be found in the Master Resources List.

**Resources**

**For more information on Hutchinson-Gilford syndrome:** National Organization for Rare Disorders (NORD); Institute for Basic Research in Developmental Disabilities; Progeria International Registry; NIH/National Institute of Child Health and Human Development; Sunshine Foundation. (The Sunshine Foundation raises funds to bring all children with progeria together once each year so that their medical progress can be studied while the children socialize in a vacation atmosphere.)

**References**

Mendelian Inheritance in Man, 11th ed.: V.A. McKusick; The Johns Hopkins University Press, 1994, pp. 1235–1236.

Acrometageria: A Spectrum of "Premature Aging" Syndromes: J.M. Karnes, et al.; Am J. Med. Genet., October 1992, vol. 44(3), pp. 334–339.

Cecil Textbook of Medicine, 19th ed.: J.B. Wyngaarden, et al., eds.; W.B. Saunders Company, 1992, p. 1145.

Hyaluronic Acid in Progeria and the Aged Phenotype?: K.J. Sweeney, et al.; Gerontology, 1992, vol. 38(3), pp. 139–152.

Nelson Textbook of Pediatrics, 14th ed.: R.E. Behrman, ed.-in-chief; W.B. Saunders Company, 1992, p. 1765.

Progeria: A Human-Disease Model of Accelerated Aging: W.T. Brown; Am. J. Clin. Nutr., June 1992, vol. 55(6 suppl.), pp. 1222S–1224S.

Progeria: Report of a Case and Review of the Literature: Q.X. Yu, et al.; J. Oral. Pathol. Med., February 1991, vol. 20(2), pp. 86–88.

Progressive Early Dermatologic Changes in Hutchinson-Gilford Progeria Syndrome: P.J. Gillar, et al.; Pediatr. Dermatol., September 1991, vol. 8(3), pp. 199–206.

Birth Defects Encyclopedia: M.L. Buyse, ed.-in-chief; Blackwell Scientific Publications, 1990, pp. 1411–1414.

Dictionary of Medical Syndromes, 3rd ed.: S.I. Magalini, et al., eds.: J.B. Lippincott Company, 1990, p. 429.

Syndromes of the Head and Neck, 3rd ed.: R.J. Gorlin, et al.; Oxford University Press, 1990, pp. 482–485.

Smith's Recognizable Patterns of Human Malformation, 4th ed.: K.L. Jones; W.B. Saunders Company, 1988, pp. 118–119.

# HYPOCHONDROPLASIA

**Description** Hypochondroplasia is a type of chondrodystrophy characterized by short stature. It becomes evident during mid-childhood.

**Synonyms**

>Achondroplasia Tarda
>
>Atypical Achondroplasia

**Signs and Symptoms** At birth, those affected appear normal. Arms and legs do not develop properly, however, and the body becomes thick and shorter than normal. The patient has a normal-sized head, but arms, legs, hands, and feet, although shaped normally, are disproportionately small. Elbow flexibility is limited. Arms and legs are not usually bowed. Motor abilities may develop slowly, but intelligence is usually normal.

Hypochondroplasia can be distinguished from other forms of short-limbed small stature by clinical and radiologic examination of the skull and long bones of the arms and legs. The clinical and radiologic features tend to be milder than those of achondroplasia.

**Etiology** The disorder is inherited as an autosomal dominant trait. The gene responsible has been mapped to chromosome 4 (4p16.3). Thus far no mutation of the fibroblast growth factor receptor gene has been found, despite the marked similarity of this condition to achondroplasia.

**Epidemiology** Females appear to be affected more often than males.

**Related Disorders** See *Achondroplasia.*

**Kozlowski spondylometaphyseal dysplasia** is usually diagnosed by the time the patient is 2 years old, although onset generally occurs during the first year. The bones are affected, especially the spine and pelvis, by a reduction of calcification. The neck and trunk are short, the legs are bowed, and there is a waddling gait. Patients experience pain and a limited range of motion. Males and females are affected equally.

**Treatment—Standard** Treatment of hypochondroplasia may consist of orthopedic correction and physical therapy. Pregnant patients may require cesarean section. Genetic counseling may benefit patients and their families. Other treatment is symptomatic and supportive.

**Treatment—Investigational** Please contact the agencies listed under Resources, below, for the most current information. Addresses and telephone numbers of these agencies, as well as of individual experts and research centers, may be found in the Master Resources List.

**Resources**

**For more information on hypochondroplasia:** National Organization for Rare Disorders (NORD); International Center for Skeletal Dysplasia; NIH/National Arthritis and Musculoskeletal and Skin Diseases Information Clearinghouse; Human Growth Foundation; Parents of Dwarfed Children; Little People of America; Short Stature Foundation.

**For genetic information and genetic counseling referrals:** March of Dimes Birth Defects Foundation; Alliance of Genetic Support Groups.

**References**

Human Genetics Disorders; J. NIH Res., August 1994, vol. 6(8), pp. 115–134.

Mendelian Inheritance in Man, 11th ed.: V.A. McKusick; The Johns Hopkins University Press, 1994, pp. 769–770.

Achondroplasia and Hypochondroplasia: Clinical Variation and Spinal Stenosis: R. Wynne-Davies, et al., J. Bone Joint Surg. Br., 1981, vol. 63B(4), pp. 508–515.

# IMPERFORATE ANUS

**Description** Imperforate anus is a congenital disorder in which the anus is missing or abnormally located. An associated anomaly is the presence of a fistula that connects the vagina or bladder to the rectum or colon.

**Synonyms**

>Anal Atresia
>
>Anal Stenosis
>
>Anorectal Malformations

**Signs and Symptoms** Imperforate anus is congenital and is identified by an abnormal or absent anus. The rectum may open into the vagina in females or near the scrotum in males.

**Etiology** The disorder may be inherited either through autosomal recessive or through X-linked genes or may be multifactorial..

**Epidemiology** The incidence of imperforate anus in the United States is approximately 1:5,000 births. Six males are affected for every 4 females.

**Related Disorders** Since imperforate anus occurs as one manifestation in a number of multiple malformation syndromes, affected neonates must be carefully examined for other abnormalities. See **_VACTERL Association._**

**Treatment—Standard** Imperforate anus is surgically corrected by dilating, enlarging, or repositioning the external opening to allow for elimination of feces. Genetic counseling may benefit patients and their families.

**Treatment—Investigational** Please contact the agencies listed under Resources, below, for the most current information. Addresses and telephone numbers of these agencies, as well as of individual experts and research centers, may be found in the Master Resources List.

**Resources**

**For more information on imperforate anus:** National Organization for Rare Disorders (NORD); NIH/National Digestive Diseases Information Clearinghouse; United Ostomy Association.

**For genetic information and genetic counseling referrals:** March of Dimes Birth Defects Foundation; Alliance of Genetic Support Groups.

**References**

Imperforate Anus with Long but Apparent Low Fistula in Females: F.G. Cigerroa, et al.; J. Pediatr. Surg., January 1988, vol. 23(1 pt. 2), pp. 42–44.

The Genitourinary System in Patients with Imperforate Anus: G.A. McLorie, et al.; J. Pediatr. Surg., December 1987, vol. 22(12), pp. 1100–1104.

The Genital Tract in Female Children with Imperforate Anus: R. Hall, et al.; Am. J. Obstet. Gynecol., January 1985, vol. 151(2), pp. 169–171.

# IVEMARK SYNDROME

**Description** Ivemark syndrome is a rare progressive disorder characterized primarily by congenital asplenia or, sometimes, splenic hypoplasia or polysplenia, as well as malformations of the cardiovascular system and situs inversus.

**Synonyms**

Asplenia with Cardiovascular Anomalies

Bilateral Right-Sidedness Sequence

**Signs and Symptoms** Cardiovascular abnormalities may result in cyanosis and heart failure. Pulmonary involvement is characterized by isomerism, with both lungs resembling a normal right lung in asplenia; in polysplenia, left-sidedness predominates. The stomach may be displaced to the right or left side of the body, and the bowel may be rotated improperly and may have a volvulus. Renal anomalies may be present, and physical and mental development may be retarded. The patient is vulnerable to increased infection, especially of the skin and respiratory system.

Diagnosis of asplenia is confirmed by the presence of Heinz or Howell-Jolly bodies in erythrocytes. Prenatal diagnosis can be made by ultrasound examination.

**Etiology** Autosomal recessive inheritance is suggested.

**Epidemiology** Ivemark syndrome is a rare disorder that affects males 3 times more often than females.

**Treatment—Standard** Infections are treated with antibiotics. Surgery may be indicated to relieve some of the associated signs or abnormalities.

Genetic counseling may benefit patients and their families. Other treatment is symptomatic and supportive.

**Treatment—Investigational** Please contact the agencies listed under Resources, below, for the most current information. Addresses and telephone numbers of these agencies, as well as of individual experts and research centers, may be found in the Master Resources List.

**Resources**

**For more information on Ivemark syndrome:** National Organization for Rare Disorders (NORD); NIH/National Institute of Child Health and Human Development.

**For genetic information and genetic counseling referrals:** March of Dimes Birth Defects Foundation; Alliance of Genetic Support Groups.

**References**

Mendelian Inheritance in Man, 11th ed.: V.A. McKusick; The Johns Hopkins University Press, 1994, pp. 1646–1647.

Prenatal Diagnosis of Asplenia/Polysplenia Syndrome: D. Chitayat, et al.; Am. J. Obstet. Gynecol., May 1988, vol. 158(5), pp. 1085–1087.

Smith's Recognizable Patterns of Human Malformation, 4th ed.: K.L. Jones; W.B. Saunders Company, 1988, p. 543.

Prolonged and Functional Survival with the Asplenia Syndrome: M. Wolfe, et al.; Am. J. Med., December 1986, vol. 81(6), pp. 1089–1091.

# JACKSON-WEISS SYNDROME

**Description** Jackson-Weiss syndrome is a hereditary disorder characterized by craniosynostosis and abnormalities of the face and feet.

**Synonyms**

    Craniosynostosis, Midfacial Hypoplasia, and Foot Abnormalities

    Jackson-Weiss Craniosynostosis

**Signs and Symptoms** Symptoms vary from mild to severe. The craniosynostosis may cause headaches, vision disturbances, and intracranial pressure. Other common symptoms include micrognathia, hypertelorism, down-slanting eyes, ptosis, strabismus, abnormalities of the outer ear, a flat bridge of the nose, a beaked nose, a cleft or a high-arched palate, and hydrocephaly. Some patients have syndactyly, abnormalities of the digital bones, limited joint movement, mental retardation, and genu valgum.

**Etiology** Jackson-Weiss syndrome is inherited as an autosomal dominant trait with incomplete penetrance. It is now known that this syndrome is allelic with Crouzon disease and is caused by mutations in fibroblast growth factor receptor 2.

**Epidemiology** Males and females are affected in equal numbers. Over 130 cases have been reported.

**Related Disorders** See *Apert Syndrome; Carpenter Syndrome; Crouzon Disease; Pfeiffer Syndrome; Saethre-Chotzen Syndrome.*

**Treatment—Standard** Surgical correction of craniosynostosis, cleft palate, and abnormalities of the hands and feet is often indicated. Speech therapy is beneficial for cleft palate.

    Genetic counseling may benefit patients and their families. Other treatment is symptomatic and supportive.

**Treatment—Investigational** Researchers are studying a Teflon-glycerine paste that is applied to the rear of the pharynx in a minor surgical procedure to bring the pharynx and palate into proper relationship. For further information contact William N. Williams, D.D.S., University of Florida.

    Please contact the agencies listed under Resources, below, for the most current information. Addresses and telephone numbers of these agencies, as well as of individual experts and research centers, may be found in the Master Resources List.

**Resources**

    **For more information on Jackson-Weiss syndrome:** National Organization for Rare Disorders (NORD); National Craniofacial Foundation; FACES—National Association for the Craniofacially Handicapped; Forward Face; Children's Craniofacial Association; Craniofacial Family Association; AboutFace; American Cleft Palate Cranial Facial Association; The Arc (a national organization on mental retardation); NIH/National Institute of Child Health and Human Development;

    **For genetic information and genetic counseling referrals:** March of Dimes Birth Defects Foundation; Alliance of Genetic Support Groups.

**References**

Jackson-Weiss and Crouzon Syndromes Are Allelic with Mutations in Fibroblast Growth Factor Receptor 2: M.E. Jabs, et al.; Nat. Genet., 1994, vol. 8, pp. 275–279.

Mendelian Inheritance in Man, 11th ed.: V.A. McKusick; The Johns Hopkins University Press, 1994, p. 375.

Birth Defects Encyclopedia: M.L. Buyse, ed.-in-chief; Blackwell Scientific Publications, 1990, pp. 467–468.

Craniosynostosis, Midfacial Hypoplasia and Foot Abnormalities: An Autosomal Dominant Phenotype in a Large Amish Kindred: C.E. Jackson, et al.; J. Pediatr., June 1976, vol. 88(6), pp. 963–968.

# JARCHO-LEVIN SYNDROME

**Description** Multiple deformities, including those of the face and head, hands, thorax, and spine, characterize Jarcho-Levin syndrome.

**Synonyms**

    Spondylocostal Dysplasia

    Spondylothoracic Dysplasia

**Signs and Symptoms** Craniofacial anomalies include a large occiput, wide nasal bridge, anteverted nares, and upwardly slanted eyelids. Syndactyly and camptodactyly with long digits are also characteristic. The thorax is small, causing respiratory problems that are often fatal. Spinal abnormalities include neural defects and hemivertebrae. The neck and trunk are characteristically short. Genitourinary tract anomalies may be present. Occasionally, distention of the stomach and pelvis may occur as a result of bladder obstruction.

**Etiology** The inheritance is autosomal recessive. Autosomal dominant inheritance has also been reported.

**Epidemiology** Jarcho-Levin syndrome affects males and females equally. Most cases have occurred in Puerto Rican children.

**Related Disorders** Features of **thanatophoric dysplasia** include vertebral abnormalities, a narrow thorax and short pelvis, short limbs with short digits, hypotonia, a large cranium, a low nasal bridge, small facies, and early lethality.

**Treatment—Standard** Treatment is symptomatic and supportive. Genetic counseling may be beneficial.

**Treatment—Investigational** The Titanium Rib Project oversees the implantation of expandable ribs in children with disorders involving missing, underdeveloped, or malformed rib cages or chest walls. Contact Robert Campbell, M.D., at Santa Rosa Children's Hospital, San Antonio, Texas, for more information.

Please contact the agencies listed under Resources, below, for the most current information. Addresses and telephone numbers of these agencies, as well as of individual experts and research centers, may be found in the Master Resources List.

**Resources**

**For more information on Jarcho-Levin syndrome:** National Organization for Rare Disorders (NORD); NIH/National Institute of Child Health and Human Development.

**For genetic information and genetic counseling referrals:** March of Dimes Birth Defects Foundation; Alliance of Genetic Support Groups.

**References**

Mendelian Inheritance in Man, 11th ed.: V.A. McKusick; The Johns Hopkins University Press, 1994, pp. 2256–2257.

Neural Defects in Jarcho-Levin Syndrome: M.G. Reyes, et al.; J. Child Neurol., January 1989, 4(1), p. 51.

Prenatal Findings in a Case of Spondylocostal Dysplasia I (Jarcho-Levin) Syndrome: R. Romero, et al.; Obstet. Gynecol., June 1988, 6(2), p. 988.

Smith's Recognizable Patterns of Human Malformation, 4th ed.: K.L. Jones; W.B. Saunders Company, 1988, p. 536.

# JEJUNAL ATRESIA

**Description** Synonyms for this syndrome reflect the look of jejunal twisting around the marginal artery, resulting in blockage and its symptoms.

**Synonyms**

Apple Peel Syndrome

Christmas Tree Syndrome

**Signs and Symptoms** Characteristics include vomiting of bile; epigastric distention; and an absence of stools after birth.

Jejunal atresia can be determined prenatally by amniocentesis. This procedure is suggested if an earlier pregnancy resulted in the birth of a child with the disorder.

**Etiology** Jejunal atresia may be inherited as an autosomal recessive trait, or it may occur sporadically. The mechanism is agenesis of the mesentery, which causes the jejunal twisting.

**Epidemiology** Approximately 57 cases have been reported in the medical literature. Males and females are affected in equal numbers.

**Related Disorders** See *Duodenal Atresia or Stenosis.*

**Multiple intestinal atresia** is caused by blockages in the duodenum, jejunum, ileum, and rectum. Symptoms and signs include continual vomiting, epigastric swelling, scaphoid abdomen, and an empty anal canal. In some cases the disorder is inherited as an autosomal recessive trait.

**Treatment—Standard** Surgery is performed immediately to repair the intestinal obstruction. Parenteral nutrition is given for a period of time. Genetic counseling may benefit patients and their families. Other treatment is symptomatic and supportive.

**Treatment—Investigational** Please contact the agencies listed under Resources, below, for the most current information. Addresses and telephone numbers of these agencies, as well as of individual experts and research centers, may be found in the Master Resources List.

**Resources**

**For more information on jejunal atresia:** National Organization for Rare Disorders (NORD); Parent Education Network; NIH/National Digestive Diseases Information Clearinghouse.

**For genetic information and genetic counseling referrals:** March of Dimes Birth Defects Foundation; Alliance of Genetic Support Groups.

**References**

Mendelian Inheritance in Man, 11th ed.: V.A. McKusick; The Johns Hopkins University Press, 1994, pp. 1941–1942.

Birth Defects Encyclopedia: M.L. Buyse, ed.-in-chief; Blackwell Scientific Publications, 1990, pp. 993–994.

Apple Peel Jejunal Atresia: L.S. Ahlgren; J. Pediatr. Surg., May 1987, vol. 22(5), pp. 451–453.

Familial Apple Peel Jejunal Atresia: Surgical, Genetic, and Radiographic Aspects: J.H. Collins, et al.; Pediatrics, October 1987, vol. 80(4), pp. 540–544.

Identical Twins with Malrotation and Type IV Jejunal Atresia: L.M. Olson, et al.; J. Pediatr. Surg., November 1987, vol. 22(11), pp. 1015–1016.

# KABUKI MAKEUP SYNDROME

**Description** Kabuki makeup syndrome is characterized by mental retardation, short stature, unusual facial features, skeletal abnormalities, and unusual skin ridge patterns on the fingers, toes, palms of the hands, and soles of the feet.

**Synonyms**

Niikawakuroki Syndrome

**Signs and Symptoms** The primary characteristic of the syndrome is the facial expression, which closely resembles that of a Japanese Kabuki actor. The opening between the upper and lower eyelids is abnormally long, and one-third of the lower eyelid is turned outward. The tip of the nose may be broad and depressed, and the ears large and malformed. The eyebrows may be high and arched. A cleft or high-arched palate; malocclusion; scoliosis; a short 5th finger that curves inward; abnormalities of the vertebrae, hands, and hip joint; short stature; and abnormal skin ridge patterns on the fingers, toes, palms of the hands, and soles of the feet are common. Early breast development in females and cardiac defects are less common.

All patients with Kabuki makeup syndrome have mental retardation ranging from mild to severe.

**Etiology** The majority of cases appear to be isolated events. Three patients had abnormalities on the Y chromosome, leading researchers to suspect an autosomal dominant inheritance.

**Epidemiology** Males and females are affected in equal numbers. Most cases have occurred in people of Japanese ancestry, although the disorder has been reported in Canada, Italy, Germany, Libya, Latin America, and the United States.

**Related Disorders** See *Aarskog Syndrome; Coffin-Lowry Syndrome; Trichorhinophalangeal Syndrome, Type II.*

**KBG syndrome** is inherited as an autosomal dominant trait. Symptoms include mental retardation, short stature, skeletal abnormalities, and an unusual face with bow-shaped lips. Males and females are affected equally.

**Treatment—Standard** Physical therapy may help prevent scoliosis. Cosmetic surgery may also be beneficial. Treatment of cleft palate requires a team of specialists: pediatricians, dental specialists, surgeons, speech pathologists, and others. Cleft palate may be repaired by surgery or covered with a prosthesis.

Genetic counseling may benefit patients and their families. Other treatment is symptomatic and supportive.

**Treatment—Investigational** Researchers are studying a Teflon-glycerine paste that is applied to the rear of the pharynx in a minor surgical procedure to bring the pharynx and palate into proper relationship. For further information contact William N. Williams, D.D.S., University of Florida.

Please contact the agencies listed under Resources, below, for the most current information. Addresses and telephone numbers of these agencies, as well as of individual experts and research centers, may be found in the Master Resources List.

**Resources**

**For more information on Kabuki makeup syndrome:** National Organization for Rare Disorders (NORD); The Arc (a national organization on mental retardation); NIH/National Institute of Child Health and Human Development.

**For genetic information and genetic counseling referrals:** March of Dimes Birth Defects Foundation; Alliance of Genetic Support Groups.

**References**

Mendelian Inheritance in Man, 11th ed.: V.A. McKusick; The Johns Hopkins University Press, 1994, pp. 835–836.

Birth Defects Encyclopedia: M.L. Buyse, ed.-in-chief; Blackwell Scientific Publications, 1990, pp. 998–999.

# KARTAGENER SYNDROME

**Description** Kartagener syndrome is a genetic disorder characterized by sinusitis, bronchiectasis, and situs inversus.

**Synonyms**

Chronic Sinobronchial Disease and Dextrocardia

Dextrocardia, Bronchiectasis, and Sinusitis

Immotile Cilia Syndrome
Kartagener Triad
Primary Ciliary Dyskinesia
Situs Inversus, Bronchiectasis, and Sinusitis

**Signs and Symptoms** Kartagener syndrome is a congenital disease that usually manifests during infancy. The major symptoms–sinusitis, bronchiectasis, and situs inversus—persist into adulthood. Mucus accumulation in the sinuses leads to sinusitis; mucus accumulation in the lungs results in coughing, bronchitis, and bronchiectasis. Chronic ear infections and possible abnormalities of the inner ear may lead to hearing loss. Situs inversus is diagnosed by x-ray; if it is complete, cardiac complications may occur.

Reproductive complications can also be associated with Kartagener syndrome. Reduced sperm motility produces sterility in males. Women with the syndrome are fertile.

**Etiology** Kartagener syndrome is inherited as an autosomal recessive trait with incomplete penetrance.

**Epidemiology** Kartagener syndrome affects approximately 1:30,000 to 1:60,000 individuals.

**Related Disorders** See *Alveolitis, Fibrosing.*

**Bronchiectasis** is characterized by enlarged bronchial tubes. Congenital bronchiectasis is the result of abnormal fetal development. Acquired bronchiectasis may be caused by a variety of disorders, such as measles, sinusitis, chronic bronchitis, pneumonia, cystic fibrosis, emphysema, lung abscess, silicosis, lung cancer, or the presence of foreign substances in the lungs.

Patients may exhibit either a dry or mucus-producing cough from the accumulation of mucus in the bronchioles. The sputum is thick and has a foul odor. Infection and inflammation is usually partial; only rarely does it involve an entire lung. Antibiotic drugs are indicated to prevent deterioration of bronchial tubes and spread of infection.

**Polynesian bronchiectasis (immotile cilia syndrome)** is a type of ciliary dyskinesia that results in bronchial tube complications and reduced motility of cilia. The syndrome is primarily confined to Samoans and to the Maoris of New Zealand. It is differentiated from Kartagener syndrome through laboratory evaluation of the cilia.

**Treatment—Standard** Patients usually require daily postural drainage. Fever and systemic symptoms are treated with antibiotic therapy. Surgery may be indicated to correct abnormalities in circulation.

Other treatment is symptomatic and supportive. Genetic counseling is recommended for patients and their families.

**Treatment—Investigational** Please contact the agencies listed under Resources, below, for the most current information. Addresses and telephone numbers of these agencies, as well as of individual experts and research centers, may be found in the Master Resources List.

**Resources**

**For more information on Kartagener syndrome:** National Organization for Rare Disorders (NORD); American Lung Association; NIH/National Heart, Lung and Blood Institute.

**For genetic information and genetic counseling referrals:** March of Dimes Birth Defects Foundation; Alliance of Genetic Support Groups.

**References**

Mendelian Inheritance in Man, 11th ed.: V.A. McKusick; The Johns Hopkins University Press, 1994, pp. 1944–1946.

Internal Medicine, 2nd ed.: J.H. Stein, ed.; Little, Brown and Company, 1987, p. 691.

Kartagener's Syndrome with Motile Cilia and Immotile Spermatozoa: Axonemal Ultrastructure and Function: L.J. Wilton, et al.; Am. Rev. Respir. Dis., December 1986, vol. 40(4), pp. 1233–1236.

# KLINEFELTER SYNDROME (47,XXY)

**Description** The classic form of Klinefelter syndrome is the most common cause of primary hypogonadism in males. It is characterized by the presence of an extra X chromosome. It is usually not diagnosed until after puberty.

**Signs and Symptoms** Abnormally small testes have sclerosed tubules and are azoospermic. Gynecomastia often occurs. Secondary sexual characteristics may be attenuated, resulting in a high-pitched voice and diminished facial and body hair. Muscles are underdeveloped. Mental retardation generally is not present, although affected persons may not achieve higher-education levels. Personality disorder may occur.

Variants, such as 46,XY/47,XXY (mosaic), may be associated with fewer symptoms in adults. Other variants, such as 48,XXXY and 48,XXYY, occur.

**Etiology** Klinefelter syndrome results from the presence of an extra X chromosome, which is paternal in origin in 33 percent of patients and maternal in origin in 67 percent of patients.

**Epidemiology** Klinefelter syndrome occurs in 1:1,000 newborn males.

**Treatment—Standard** Androgens, such as testosterone enanthate or cypionate, are given to promote virilization. Affected patients are infertile. Patients may achieve cosmetic benefit from mastectomy. Genetic counseling may be beneficial to families of children with the disorder.

**Treatment—Investigational** Please contact the agencies listed under Resources, below, for the most current information. Addresses and telephone numbers of these agencies, as well as of individual experts and research centers, may be found in the Master Resources List.

**Resources**

**For more information on Klinefelter syndrome:** National Organization for Rare Disorders (NORD); Klinefelter's Syndrome Association of America; Klinefelter's Syndrome Support Group of Canada; NIH/National Institute of Child Health and Human Development.

**For genetic information and genetic counseling referrals:** March of Dimes Birth Defects Foundation; Alliance of Genetic Support Groups.

**References**

Cecil Textbook of Medicine, 19th ed.: J.B. Wyngaarden, et al., eds.: W.B. Saunders Company, 1992, pp. 1342–1344.

Growth During Puberty in the XYY Boy: S.G. Ratcliffe; Ann. Hum. Biol., November–December 1992, vol. 19(6), pp. 579–587.

Nelson Textbook of Pediatrics, 14th ed.: R.E. Behrman, ed.-in-chief; W.B. Saunders Company, 1992, pp. 1456–1457.

Textbook of Endocrinology, 8th ed.: J.D. Wilson and D.W. Foster, eds.; W.B. Saunders Company, 1992, pp. 879–884.

The Klinefelter Syndrome of Testicular Dysgenesis: I.D. Schwartz; Endocrinol. Metab. Clin. North Am., March 1991, vol. 20(1), pp. 153–163.

Klinefelter Syndrome: The Need for Early Identification and Treatment: M.W. Mandoki; Clin. Pediatr., March 1991, vol. 30(3), pp. 161–164.

Birth Defects Encyclopedia: M.L. Buyse, ed.-in-chief; Blackwell Scientific Publications, 1990, pp. 1014–1015.

Smith's Recognizable Patterns of Human Deformation, 2nd ed.: J.M. Graham, Jr.; W.B. Saunders Company, 1988, pp. 66–67.

# KLIPPEL-FEIL SYNDROME

**Description** Klippel-Feil syndrome is a congenital disorder that affects the spine. Associated complications include hearing loss and neurologic, cardiac, renal, and respiratory problems. The syndrome is categorized into types I, II, and III.

**Synonyms**

Congenital Cervical Synostosis

**Signs and Symptoms** The 3 types of Klippel-Feil syndrome are all characterized by scoliosis, fusion of neck vertebrae, and low hairline at the nape.

In **type I,** the neck and upper back vertebrae are fused into bony blocks. In **type II,** fusion occurs at only 1 or 2 disks. Patients with **type III** disease exhibit fusion in the neck and back or lower back. The presence of craniocervical fusion increases the risk of injury to the head and neck. Neurologic, cardiac, and respiratory complications result from compressed vertebrae. In some families, the disorder may be associated with sensorineural hearing loss. In 4 isolated cases, the disorder was associated with absent vagina and conductive deafness.

**Etiology** The syndrome is inherited as an autosomal dominant or autosomal recessive trait; it also occurs sporadically.

**Epidemiology** The syndrome is rare. Males and females are affected in equal numbers.

**Related Disorders** See *Wildervanck Syndrome.*

**Treatment—Standard** Treatment is supportive and symptomatic. Genetic counseling may benefit patients and their families.

**Treatment—Investigational** Please contact the agencies listed under Resources, below, for the most current information. Addresses and telephone numbers of these agencies, as well as of individual experts and research centers, may be found in the Master Resources List.

**Resources**

**For more information on Klippel-Feil syndrome:** National Organization for Rare Disorders (NORD); NIH/National Arthritis and Musculoskeletal and Skin Diseases Information Clearinghouse.

**For genetic information and genetic counseling referrals:** March of Dimes Birth Defects Foundation; Alliance of Genetic Support Groups.

**References**

Mendelian Inheritance in Man, 11th ed.: V.A. McKusick; The Johns Hopkins University Press, 1994, pp. 847–848, 1697.

Aural Abnormalities in Klippel-Feil Syndrome: I. Ohtani, et al.; Am. J. Otolaryngol., November 1985, vol. 6(6), pp. 468–471.

# KLIPPEL-TRENAUNAY SYNDROME

**Description** Klippel-Trenaunay syndrome is a triad characterized by cutaneous hemangiomata, varicosities, and limb overgrowth. Severity of disease and associated complications may vary widely in patients.

**Synonyms**

>Angio-Osteohypertrophy Syndrome
>Congenital Dysplastic Angiectasia
>Klippel-Trenaunay-Weber Syndrome

**Signs and Symptoms** The most common sign is a congenital nevus flammeus, which is apparent at birth, may extend over a large area, and usually deepens in color over time.

Vascular lesions consisting of masses of veins, lymph vessels, and capillaries can be detected in utero by ultrasonography. These obstructive lesions lead to development of varicose veins during infancy and early childhood. All or part of the limbs and digits, as well as the trunk, may be affected and may enlarge. Edema may develop rarely in response to compression or malformations of lymph vessels. Atrophy may occur in an affected limb.

Other associated features are adactyly, polydactyly, dilated pulmonary veins, partial overgrowth of the face without nevus flammeus, absence of an ear canal opening, thrombocytopenia, hypofibrinogenemia, spina bifida, congenital dislocation of the hips, larger-than-normal feet, and bilateral cryptorchidism. Skin ulcerations associated with constrictive blood flow can occur, as can eczema, flesh-colored warts, cellulitis, scoliosis, and hyperhidrosis. Thrombophlebitis may be present but is usually stationary.

Hemorrhage may occur because abnormal blood vessels do not contain sufficient clotting factor. Dilation of abdominal veins may lead to bleeding in the rectum, vagina, or vulva. In some cases, hypertrophy in the bladder or colon may cause bleeding, and compressing growths near the spinal cord may result in partial paralysis.

**Parkes-Weber syndrome,** a subdivision of Klippel-Trenaunay syndrome, is characterized by arteriovenous shunts.

**Etiology** The cause is unknown.

**Epidemiology** Klippel-Trenaunay syndrome is a rare disorder that affects males and females in equal numbers.

**Related Disorders** See *Sturge-Weber Syndrome.*

**Treatment—Standard** Treatment is symptomatic. Argon, yellow light, or carbon dioxide laser surgery may lighten or remove the nevus flammeus. Blood vessel abnormalities in the colon may require intestinal resection. Lesions in the bladder may be removed with a high-frequency electrical current, using a cystoscope. Pain from varicose veins may be relieved by wearing elastic support stockings.

Surgery to correct leg length discrepancy is usually not indicated in children if the difference is less than 1 cm. Instead, scoliosis may be prevented with the use of a compensating shoe lift. Leg length discrepancy should be monitored through x-ray every 6 months and surgically corrected if it becomes significant. Surgery is not indicated in children to treat varicose veins because of the risk of complications and recurrence.

Patients with cellulitis, thrombophlebitis, recurrent bleeding, or anemia may be treated with diuretics, antibiotics, or iron supplements. Ulcerations or eczema may require topical medication.

**Treatment—Investigational** The flashlamp-pulsed tunable dye laser is showing promising results for treating nevus flammeus in children under 18.

Please contact the agencies listed under Resources, below, for the most current information. Addresses and telephone numbers of these agencies, as well as of individual experts and research centers, may be found in the Master Resources List.

**Resources**

**For more information on Klippel-Trenaunay syndrome:** National Organization for Rare Disorders (NORD); Klippel-Trenaunay Syndrome Support Group; NIH/National Institute of Neurological Disorders and Stroke; Sturge-Weber Support Group.

**For genetic information and genetic counseling referrals:** March of Dimes Birth Defects Foundation; Alliance of Genetic Support Groups.

**References**

CT Findings in Splenic Hemangiomas in the Klippel-Trenaunay-Weber Syndrome: R.L. Pakter, et al.; J. Comput. Assist. Tomogr., January–February 1987, vol. 11(1), pp. 88–91.

A Retromedullary Arteriovenous Fistula Associated with the Klippel Syndrome: A Clinicopathologic Study: N. Benhaiem-Sigaux, et al.; Acta Neuropathol. (Berl.), 1985, vol. 66(4), pp. 318–324.

Surgical Implications of Klippel-Trenaunay Syndrome: Peter P. Gloriezk, et al.; Ann. Surg., March 1983, vol. 197, p. 353.

Correction of Leg Inequality in the Klippel-Trenaunay-Weber Syndrome: M. Peixinho, et al.; Int. Orthop., 1982, vol. 6(1), pp. 45–47.

# KNIEST DYSPLASIA

**Description** The disorder is primarily characterized by flat facies, disproportionately short stature with thick joints, and platyspondylisis. Intellect is usually normal.

**Synonyms**
> Metatropic Dysplasia II
> Swiss Cheese Cartilage Syndrome

**Signs and Symptoms** The newborn has abnormally short legs and a characteristic flat face. The eyes protrude, and there is a low nasal bridge. Cleft palate and chronic otitis media may be present. Eye involvement includes myopia and eventual retinal detachment and cataracts. As the patient matures, the joints may become enlarged, causing limited movement and pain. Limbs are short and often bowed, and contracted hips may cause walking difficulties. Vertebral flattening and kyphoscoliosis often result in truncal shortening.

Cartilage recovered on biopsy is soft to the touch and has the appearance of Swiss cheese. In some cases excessive excretion of keratan sulfate is found in the urine.

**Etiology** The disorder is inherited as an autosomal dominant trait. It appears to be caused by a mutation in COL 2A1, the gene for collagen type II.

**Epidemiology** Males and females are affected in equal numbers.

**Related Disorders** Other COL 2A1 mutations include achondrogenesis, hypochondrogenesis, spondyloepiphyseal dysplasia congenita, spondyloepimetaphyseal dysplasia, and Stickler syndrome. These diseases span a variety of phenotypes, from very mild to severe.

**Treatment—Standard** Treatment usually consists of stabilization of lax joints, surgery to prevent contractures, and repair of retinal detachments and cleft palate. Genetic counseling may benefit patients and their families. Other treatment is symptomatic and supportive.

**Treatment—Investigational** Please contact the agencies listed under Resources, below, for the most current information. Addresses and telephone numbers of these agencies, as well as of individual experts and research centers, may be found in the Master Resources List.

**Resources**

**For more information on Kniest dysplasia:** National Organization for Rare Disorders (NORD); Magic Foundation for Children's Growth; Human Growth Foundation; NIH/National Institute of Child Health and Human Development; Parents of Dwarfed Children; Little People of America; Short Stature Foundation.

**For genetic information and genetic counseling referrals:** March of Dimes Birth Defects Foundation; Alliance of Genetic Support Groups.

**References**

Mendelian Inheritance in Man, 11th ed.: V.A. McKusick; The Johns Hopkins University Press, 1994, pp. 938–939.

Kniest Dysplasia Is Characterized by an Apparent Abnormal Processing of the C-Propeptide of Type II Cartilage Collagen Resulting in Imperfect Assembly: A. Poole, et al.; J. Clin. Invest., February 1988, vol. 81(2), pp. 579–589.

Smith's Recognizable Patterns of Human Malformation, 4th ed.: K.L. Jones; W.B. Saunders Company, 1988, pp. 312, 313–314.

The Ocular Findings in Kniest Dysplasia: I. Maumenee, et al.; Am. J. Opthalmol., July 15, 1985, vol. 100(1), pp. 155–160.

Ocular Manifestations in Kniest Syndrome, Smith-Lemli-Opitz Syndrome, Hallerman-Streiff-Francois Syndrome, Rubenstein-Taybi Syndrome and Median Cleft Syndrome: A. Bardelli, et al.; Ophthalmic Paediatr. Genet., August 1985, vol. 6(1–2), pp. 343–347.

# LADD SYNDROME

**Description** LADD syndrome is characterized primarily by malformations of the upper limbs, the lacrimal network, the teeth, and the ears.

**Synonyms**
> Lacrimo-Auriculo-Dento-Digital Syndrome
> Levy-Hollister Syndrome
> Limb Malformations–Dento–Digital Syndrome

**Signs and Symptoms** Malformations of the upper limbs are a consistent finding in LADD syndrome. Forearm defects (shortening and also synostosis of the radius and ulna) are seen in all affected persons. Other upper limb anomalies include absent or hypoplastic thumb or 2nd finger; 3 bones in the thumb instead of 2; 5th finger clinodactyly; and syndactyly of the 2nd and 3rd fingers.

Lacrimal malformations have been found in three-quarters of LADD patients; these include nasolacrimal duct obstruction and aplasia or hypoplasia of the lacrimal puncta.

The ears are often small and cupped, and both sensorineural and conductive hearing loss may occur. Anomalies of the teeth include enamel dysplasia and thinning, hypodontia, peg-shaped incisors, and darkening of the teeth. There may be salivary gland aplasia or hypoplasia.

Less common features include genitourinary malformations, hypospadias, and renal agenesis.

**Etiology** LADD syndrome is inherited as an autosomal dominant trait. There has been one reported case of sporadic occurrence.

**Epidemiology** Approximately 12 cases have been described in the medical literature. The majority of reported cases have been in the white-American and Mexican-American population. Males and females are affected in equal numbers.

**Related Disorders** See *Split-Hand Deformity.*

**Treatment—Standard** Treatment is symptomatic, supportive, and appropriate to the associated conditions. Genetic counseling will benefit patients and their families.

**Treatment—Investigational** Please contact the agencies listed under Resources, below, for the most current information. Addresses and telephone numbers of these agencies, as well as of individual experts and research centers, may be found in the Master Resources List.

**Resources**

**For more information on LADD syndrome:** National Organization for Rare Disorders (NORD); International Center for Skeletal Dysplasia; NIH/National Arthritis and Musculoskeletal and Skin Diseases Information Clearinghouse.

**For genetic information and genetic counseling referrals:** March of Dimes Birth Defects Foundation; Alliance of Genetic Support Groups.

**References**

Mendelian Inheritance in Man, 11th ed.: V.A. McKusick; The Johns Hopkins University Press, 1994, p. 850.

Birth Defects Encyclopedia: M.L. Buyse, ed.-in-chief; Blackwell Scientific Publications, 1990, p. 1024.

Lacrimo-Auriculo-Dento-Digital (LADD) Syndrome with Renal and Foot Anomalies: A.M. Roodhooft, et al.; Clin. Genet., September 1990, vol. 38(3), pp. 228–232.

Smith's Recognizable Patterns of Human Malformation, 4th ed.: K.L. Jones; W.B. Saunders Company, 1988, p. 273.

# LARSEN SYNDROME

**Description** Larsen syndrome is a congenital genetic disorder that affects many systems of the body. Characteristics include dislocations and abnormalities of the bones, an abnormally high foot arch, unusual facies, and cylindrical fingers.

**Synonyms**

Sinding-Larsen-Johansson Disease

**Signs and Symptoms** Features of the syndrome include a prominent forehead, upturned nose with a flattened bridge, hypertelorism, and low-set ears. Dislocations of bones in the knees, hips, and elbow are common. Patients may have mild scoliosis or osteoporosis. The fingers are usually cylindrical in shape and may be syndactylic. Pes cavus and clubbing are common abnormalities of the feet.

Congenital heart or respiratory complications may occur. Some males may have cryptorchidism.

**Etiology** Larsen syndrome is inherited both as an autosomal dominant and as an autosomal recessive trait. Sporadic cases are also known. Symptoms are thought to result from a gestational embryonic disorder of the mesenchyma.

**Epidemiology** Larsen syndrome affects males and females equally.

**Related Disorders** See *Arthrogryposis Multiplex Congenita; Ehlers-Danlos Syndrome.*

**Treatment—Standard** Infants should be managed by manipulation of joints, and with casts or traction. Older children may benefit from orthopedic surgery to correct bone deformities or dislocations. Reconstructive surgery may be appropriate to repair heart valve and spinal abnormalities, or cleft palate or cleft lip. Speech therapy and services for physically or mentally impaired patients and their families may be helpful.

Genetic counseling may benefit patients and their families. Other treatment is symptomatic and supportive.

**Treatment—Investigational** Please contact the agencies listed under Resources, below, for the most current information. Addresses and telephone numbers of these agencies, as well as of individual experts and research centers, may be found in the Master Resources List.

**Resources**

**For more information on Larsen syndrome:** National Organization for Rare Disorders (NORD); NIH/National Institute of Child Health and Human Development; NIH/National Arthritis and Musculoskeletal and Skin Diseases Information Clearinghouse.

**For genetic information and genetic counseling referrals:** March of Dimes Birth Defects Foundation; Alliance of Genetic Support Groups.

**References**

Mendelian Inheritance in Man, 11th ed.: V.A. McKusick; The Johns Hopkins University Press, 1994, pp. 857–858, 1954–1955.

Spinal Deformities in Larsen's Syndrome: J.R. Bowen, et al.; Clin Orthop., July–August 1985, vol. 197, pp. 159–163.

Cardiovascular Manifestations in the Larsen Syndrome: E.A. Kiel, et al.; Pediatrics, June 1983, vol. 20(6), pp. 422–424.

Severe Cardiac Anomalies in Sibs with Larsen Syndrome: P. Strisciuglio, et al.; J. Med. Genet., December 1983, vol. 20(6), pp. 422–424.

Sinding-Larsen-Johansson Disease: Its Etiology and Natural History: R.C. Medlar, et al.; J. Bone Joint Surg. Am., December 1978, vol. 60(8), pp. 1113–1116.

# LEPRECHAUNISM

**Description** Leprechaunism is a rare hereditary endocrine disorder characterized by severe growth failure, decreased subcutaneous tissue, a pixie face, and insulin resistance.

**Synonyms**

Donohue Syndrome

**Signs and Symptoms** Growth retardation begins in utero. Subcutaneous fatty tissue usually disappears with advancing age. Affected children have an elfin face, with sunken cheeks, a pointed chin, a flat, broad nose, low-set ears, and ocular hypertelorism. Other features include hirsutism and dark pigmentation in skin creases. In girls, the nipples and clitoris may be enlarged, and ovaries may be enlarged and cystic. In boys, the penis may be larger than normal.

Patients with leprechaunism have hyperglycemia and hyperinsulinemia after fasting. They are also more susceptible to infections, and early death is common.

**Etiology** It has been established that the disorder is inherited as an autosomal recessive trait, and that parents of affected children are often consanguineous. The disorder is caused by a mutation in the gene coding for the insulin receptor. Surprisingly, homozygous deletion of the receptor gene has been found to be compatible with life.

**Epidemiology** Leprechaunism has been reported in about 50 patients, with twice as many females as males.

**Related Disorders** See *Williams Syndrome.*

**Patterson-David syndrome** is a very rare disorder that has been confused with leprechaunism. Affected children may have a normal birth weight, hyperpigmentation, loose skin on the hands and feet, unusual facies, severe mental retardation, bony deformities, and skeletal dysplasia.

**Treatment—Standard** Treatment is symptomatic and supportive. Genetic counseling may benefit families of affected children. Infections should be guarded against and aggressively treated.

**Treatment—Investigational** Please contact the agencies listed under Resources, below, for the most current information. Addresses and telephone numbers of these agencies, as well as of individual experts and research centers, may be found in the Master Resources List.

**Resources**

**For more information on leprechaunism:** National Organization for Rare Disorders (NORD); NIH/National Institute of Diabetes, Digestive and Kidney Diseases; Research Trust for Metabolic Disorders in Children.

**For genetic information and genetic counseling referrals:** March of Dimes Birth Defects Foundation; Alliance of Genetic Support Groups.

**References**

Mendelian Inheritance in Man, 11th ed.: V.A. McKusick; The Johns Hopkins University Press, 1994, pp. 819–823, 1958–1959.

Homozygous Deletion of the Human Insulin Receptor Gene Results in Leprechaunism: E. Wertheimer, et al.; Nat. Genet., 1993, vol. 5, pp. 72–73.

Smith's Recognizable Patterns of Human Malformation, 4th ed.: K.L. Jones; W.B. Saunders Company, 1988, p. 537.

Insulin Resistance in an Infant with Leprechaunism: H. Kashiwa, et al.; Acta Paediatr. Scand., September 1984, vol. 73(5), pp. 701–704.

The Patterson Syndrome, Leprechaunism, and Pseudoleprechaunism: T.J. David, et al.; J. Med. Genet., August 1981, vol. 18(4), pp. 294–298.

# MACROGLOSSIA

**Description** Macroglossia is a disorder in which the tongue is too large for the mouth, sometimes causing it to protrude. Macroglossia may be either congenital or acquired.

**Synonyms**

Enlarged Tongue

Giant Tongue

**Signs and Symptoms** In infants, macroglossia can complicate feeding. As the child matures, speech may be affected, and the jaw and teeth may not develop properly, resulting in dental abnormalities. The tip of the tongue may become ulcerative or necrotic.

**Etiology** Macroglossia may be associated with a wide variety of congenital and acquired syndromes and diseases, including the following: mandibulofacial dysostosis, Apert syndrome, hypothyroidism, Greig hypertelorism, amyloidosis, type 2 glycogen storage disease, Sturge-Weber syndrome, acromegaly, neurofibromatosis, Down syndrome, craniofacial dysostosis, Hurler syndrome, Beckwith-Wiedemann syndrome, and lymphangiomas.

**Epidemiology** Males and females are affected equally.

**Related Disorders** The tongue may become enlarged in persons who have lost their teeth and have not replaced them with dentures.

**Treatment—Standard** Congenital macroglossia may resolve as the child matures so that the tongue is relative in size to other oral structures.

Macroglossia in edentulous persons may resolve if the patient is fitted with dentures.

The tongue may be reduced in size by orthodontic procedures or by surgery with remodeling of the mouth.

**Treatment—Investigational** Please contact the agencies listed under Resources, below, for the most current information. Addresses and telephone numbers of these agencies, as well as of individual experts and research centers, may be found in the Master Resources List.

**Resources**

**For more information on macroglossia:** National Organization for Rare Disorders (NORD); Association for Glycogen Storage Diseases; NIH/National Institute of Dental Research; Smell and Taste Research Center, University of Pennsylvania Hospital; Chemosensory Clinical Research Center of Connecticut, University of Connecticut Health Center.

**References**

Macroglossia: Etiologic Considerations and Management Techniques: F.M. Rizer, et al.; Int. J. Pediatr. Otorhinolaryngol., July 1985, vol. 9(5), pp. 189–194.

Spontaneous Regression of Anterior Open Bite Following Treatment of Macroglossia: Maisels; Br. J. Plast. Surg., October 1979, vol. 32(4), pp. 309–314.

# MAFFUCCI SYNDROME

**Description** Maffucci syndrome is a congenital disorder characterized by hemangioma and enchondromatosis that may be present at birth or appear later in infancy or childhood.

**Synonyms**

> Dyschondrodysplasia with Hemangiomas
> Enchondromatosis with Multiple Cavernous Hemangiomas
> Hemangiomatosis Chondrodystrophica
> Kast Syndrome
> Multiple Angiomas and Enchondromas

**Signs and Symptoms** The skin lesions (cavernous or capillary hemangiomas) are unilateral in almost half of patients; when bilateral, they differ in size. Lesions may occur in some viscera, and in the mucous membranes, commonly the mouth but also the esophagus, ileum, and anus. The skin lesions do not necessarily overlie the bone lesions.

Endochondral involvement results in dyschondroplasia of the long bones. During early childhood, enchondromas may also develop in the small bones of the hands and feet.

Patients are usually short, and scoliosis may develop where there is severe unilateral enchondromatosis. Bone fractures are common.

Many patients develop malignancies, especially chondrosarcomas. Other connective tissue neoplasms include gliomas, fibrosarcomas, angiosarcomas, lymphangiosarcomas, granulosa cell ovarian tumors, and pancreatic adenocarcinomas.

**Etiology** The syndrome is inherited as an autosomal dominant trait.

**Epidemiology** Maffucci syndrome affects males and females in equal numbers. First identified in 1881, the syndrome is very rare. Fewer than 105 cases have been documented in the United States.

**Related Disorders** See ***Blue Rubber Bleb Nevus; Klippel-Trenaunay Syndrome; Ollier Disease.***

**Treatment—Standard** Because there are so many different symptoms and signs, an individual approach to treatment is necessary. Orthopedic treatment or surgery may be appropriate to correct differences in leg length, scoliosis, and bone deformities. There is some question as to the effectiveness of reconstructive surgery for the hemangiomas and enchondromas. Malignant neoplasms may respond to radiation therapy, chemotherapy, surgery, or a combination of these.

**Treatment—Investigational** Please contact the agencies listed under Resources, below, for the most current information. Addresses and telephone numbers of these agencies, as well as of individual experts and research centers, may be found in the Master Resources List.

**Resources**

**For more information on Maffucci syndrome:** National Organization for Rare Disorders (NORD); NIH/National Arthritis and Musculoskeletal and Skin Diseases Information Clearinghouse; NIH/National Heart, Lung and Blood Institute; American Cancer Society; NIH/National Cancer Institute Physician Data Query Phoneline.

**For genetic information and genetic counseling referrals:** March of Dimes Birth Defects Foundation; Alliance of Genetic Support Groups.

**References**

Chondrosarcoma in Maffucci's Syndrome: T.C. Sun, et al.; J. Bone Joint Surg. Am., October 1985, vol. 67(8), pp. 1214–1219.

Angiosarcoma Arising in a Patient with Maffucci Syndrome: T.I. Davidson, et al.; Eur. J. Surg. Oncol., December 1985, vol. 11(4), pp. 381–384.

# MALIGNANT HYPERTHERMIA

**Description** Malignant hyperthermia is a pharmacogenetic disorder in which the patient rapidly develops a high fever after anesthesia administration or some muscle relaxants. Offending drugs include halothane, cyclopropane, or succinylcholine.

**Synonyms**

Fulminating Hyperpyrexia
Hyperthermia of Anesthesia
Malignant Fever
Malignant Hyperpyrexia

**Signs and Symptoms** Patients may have been previously unaffected by anesthesia or injection of muscle relaxants, although a few may have reported previous episodes of muscle cramps or weakness. After anesthetic drugs or muscle relaxants are administered, the patient quickly develops a high fever, sometimes as high as 110° F. Muscles are characterized by twitching and rigidity. Headache, nausea, vomiting, hypotension, tachycardia, and cardiac arrhythmias may be present. Major complications include skeletal muscle degeneration (rhabdomyolysis), renal failure, pulmonary edema, and disruption of blood clotting mechanisms. Levels of muscle enzymes are markedly elevated. Some patients with central core disease, a rare myopathy, also develop malignant hyperthermia.

**Etiology** Persons inherit a predisposition to malignant hyperthermia through an autosomal dominant pattern. Only about 50 percent of affected patients have been found to have mutations of the ryanodine receptor (**RYR**) located on 19q13.1. Central core disease is also caused by mutations of RYR. Malignant hyperthermia is genetically heterogeneous, and other suspected genes have been mapped to 17q and 3q13.1.

**Epidemiology** Malignant hyperthermia occurs in 1:50,000 anesthetized patients. Males and females are affected equally.

**Related Disorders** Boys affected with **King syndrome** (characteristics include slanted eyes, low-set ears, receding chins, webbed necks, cryptorchidism, spinal abnormalities, and short stature), and perhaps *Noonan Syndrome,* may also experience malignant hyperthermia.

**Treatment—Standard** Immediate rapid treatment is indicated, with cooling of the body, support of respiration, and bicarbonate for metabolic acidosis. Dantrolene sodium, an antispasmodic, is effective. Procaine and verapamil may be useful.

Prevention includes elucidation of a history of abnormal response to involved drugs. Biopsy of the thigh muscle can aid diagnosis. Dantrolene sodium given the day before anesthesia has prevented malignant hyperthermia. Regional or local anesthesia may be indicated for at-risk individuals.

**Treatment—Investigational** Research is ongoing to develop a less invasive diagnostic test and more effective therapies.

Drs. Ron Gregg and Kirk Hogan at the University of Wisconsin, Madison, are developing a test to identify those at risk for malignant hyperthermia. Members of families in which 2 or more persons have developed the disorder are needed for the study.

Please contact the agencies listed under Resources, below, for the most current information. Addresses and telephone numbers of these agencies, as well as of individual experts and research centers, may be found in the Master Resources List.

**Resources**

**For more information on malignant hyperthermia:** National Organization of Rare Disorders (NORD); Malignant Hyperthermia Association of the United States; North American MH Registry.

**For names of on-call physicians available 24 hours/day to treat MH emergencies:** Medic Alert Foundation International.

**For malignant hypothermia clinics:** Mayo Clinic, Dept. of Anesthesiology, Rochester, MN; University of Texas, Medical Branch at Galveston, Dept. of Anesthesiology, Galveston, TX; Hahnemann University Medical School, Dept. of Anesthesiology, Philadelphia; Massachusetts General Hospital, Dept. of Anesthesiology, Boston; University of Toronto, MH Investigatory Unit, Toronto.

**For genetic information and genetic counseling referrals:** March of Dimes Birth Defects Foundation; Alliance of Genetic Support Groups.

**References**

Mendelian Inheritance in Man, 11th ed.: V.A. McKusick; The Johns Hopkins University Press, 1994, pp. 763–766, 910–911.

Mutations in the Ryanodine Receptor Gene in Central Core Disease and Malignant Hyperthermia: K.A. Quane; Nat. Genet., 1993, vol. 5, pp. 51–55.

Malignant Hyperthermia: J.L. Moore, et al.; Am. Fam. Physician, May 1992, vol. 45(5), pp. 2245–2251.

Internal Medicine, 3rd ed.: J.H. Stein, ed.-in-chief; Little, Brown and Company, 1990, p. 2416.

# MARFAN SYNDROME

**Description** Marfan syndrome is an inherited disorder that affects the connective tissues of the cardiovascular and musculoskeletal systems, and the eyes.

**Synonyms**

Arachnodactyly

**Signs and Symptoms** Affected persons are tall and thin. Both the face and limbs are abnormally long. Other features include excessive joint mobility, flat feet, hypotonia, a protruding or indented sternum, and scoliosis. Teeth may be crowded because of an abnormally high palate. Striae may appear on the skin.

Significant cardiovascular problems may be present. The most common is mitral valve prolapse, which is often asymptomatic. Enlargement and degeneration of the aorta, aortic aneurysm, and aortic regurgitation are also common and account for most deaths. Dissection of the ascending aorta is the leading cause of premature death.

The major ocular findings are severe myopia, ectopia lentis (about 50 percent of patients), increased axial globe length, corneal flatness, and occasionally retinal detachment.

Emphysema develops in almost all patients with Marfan syndrome. Pneumothorax occurs in about 5 percent of patients, either spontaneously or traumatically, and requires prompt treatment.

**Etiology** Marfan syndrome is transmitted through a single mutant autosomal dominant gene on chromosome 15. Penetrance is complete, but expression of clinical manifestations may be variable. The fibrillin gene (**FBN1**) is the site of mutations, and the mutation is unique in each family. This precludes rapid genetic diagnosis of this condition. A compound heterozygote for the gene resulted in a lethal phenotype.

**Epidemiology** The syndrome affects males and females in equal numbers. In the United States, about 25,000 to 30,000 persons are affected, many of whom have not been diagnosed. In about 25 percent of cases, there is no family history.

**Related Disorders** See *Acromegaly; Ehlers-Danlos Syndrome; Homocystinuria.*

**Treatment—Standard** Treatment is symptomatic. β-Adrenergic blocking agents (e.g., propranolol and atenolol) are used to treat cardiovascular symptoms. Because early mortality is usually the result of aortic dissection, patients should have annual evaluation for this. Malfunctioning valves may be treated medically, but surgical replacement of the aorta may eventually become necessary. Patients should minimize stress on the aorta by avoiding activities such as heavy lifting and sports.

Scoliosis and chest deformity are the most serious complications of the skeletal system. An orthopedic surgeon should be consulted if curvature of more than 10 degrees develops. Some children, especially girls, have been treated with estrogens in order to reduce the length of time of susceptibility to curvature. This therapy produces minimal physical side effects and may actually reduce final height, but may produce psychological problems as the child copes with early sexual maturation. Deformities of the sternum can be corrected surgically but should be postponed until mid-adolescence if the problem is solely cosmetic.

Failure to detect any of the ocular abnormalities may result in permanent visual disability. Increased risk of retinal detachment warrants special care, and patients should be counseled to avoid activities that may result in a blow to the eye.

Genetic counseling is essential to patients and their families.

**Treatment—Investigational** Other β-adrenergic blocking drugs are being investigated as possible therapies to treat cardiovascular symptoms.

Basic research continues on the etiology of Marfan syndrome, including studies of the biochemistry of connective tissue and of the location and nature of the genetic defect.

Bruce S. Alpert, M.D., at the University of Tennessee, Memphis, is conducting clinical trials on patients 25 years old or younger with a diagnosis of Marfan syndrome.

Please contact the agencies listed under Resources, below, for the most current information. Addresses and telephone numbers of these agencies, as well as of individual experts and research centers, may be found in the Master Resources List.

**Resources**

**For more information on Marfan syndrome:** National Organization for Rare Disorders (NORD); National Marfan Foundation; NIH/National Arthritis and Musculoskeletal and Skin Diseases Information Clearinghouse.

**For genetic information and genetic counseling referrals:** March of Dimes Birth Defects Foundation; Alliance of Genetic Support Groups.

**References**

Mendelian Inheritance in Man, 11th ed.: V.A. McKusick; The Johns Hopkins University Press, 1994, pp. 916–919.

A Molecular Approach to the Stratification of Cardiovascular Risk in Families with Marfan Syndrome: L. Pereira, et al.; N. Engl. J. Med., July 1994, vol. 331(3), pp. 148–153.

Cecil Textbook of Medicine, 19th ed.: J.B. Wyngaarden, et al., eds.; W.B. Saunders Company, 1992, pp. 1122–1123.

Birth Defects Encyclopedia: M.L. Buyse, ed.-in-chief; Blackwell Scientific Publications, 1990, pp. 1104–1105.

Internal Medicine, 3rd ed.: J.H. Stein, ed.-in-chief; Little, Brown and Company, 1990, pp. 226–227.

# MARINESCO-SJÖGREN SYNDROME

**Description** Marinesco-Sjögren syndrome is a neuromuscular disorder that results in cerebellar ataxia. Muscle spasticity, cataract, and mental deficiency are other major characteristics. Most patients are able to walk during childhood but will need a wheelchair as an adult.

**Synonyms**

       Marinesco-Sjögren-Garland Syndrome

       Moravcsik-Marinesco-Sjögren Syndrome

       Myopathy-Marinesco-Sjögren Syndrome

**Signs and Symptoms** Other common features of the syndrome include dysarthria, nystagmus, and strabismus. Some patients may have microcephaly, joint contractures, short stature, and skeletal deformities such as a bulging sternum, scoliosis, short metatarsals and metacarpals, cubitus valgus, and coxa valga. Hypergonadotropic hypogonadism, and delayed puberty are common.

**Etiology** The syndrome is inherited as an autosomal recessive trait.

**Epidemiology** Approximately 100 cases have been documented in the medical literature. The syndrome occurs more frequently in Italy, Scandinavia, and sections of Alabama in the United States. Males and females are affected in equal numbers.

**Related Disorders** See *Ataxia, Friedreich; Ataxia, Telangiectasia; Lowe Syndrome; Peripheral Neuropathy.*

**Treatment—Standard** Treatment is symptomatic and supportive. Genetic counseling may benefit patients and their families.

**Treatment—Investigational** After removal of the affected lens in children with congenital cataracts, an intraocular lens (**IOL**) has been implanted. If technically feasible, the IOL is implanted in the lens capsule. More research is needed before this implantation can be used more generally to preserve sight and reduce double vision.

Please contact the agencies listed under Resources, below, for the most current information. Addresses and telephone numbers of these agencies, as well as of individual experts and research centers, may be found in the Master Resources List.

**Resources**

**For more information on Marinesco-Sjögren syndrome:** National Organization for Rare Disorders (NORD); National Ataxia Foundation; The Arc (a national organization on mental retardation); National Scoliosis Foundation; NIH/National Institute of Neurological Disorders and Stroke; NIH/National Arthritis and Musculoskeletal and Skin Diseases Information Clearinghouse.

**For genetic information and genetic counseling referrals:** March of Dimes Birth Defects Foundation; Alliance of Genetic Support Groups.

**References**

Mendelian Inheritance in Man, 11th ed.: V.A. McKusick; The Johns Hopkins University Press, 1994, p. 1979.

Birth Defects Encyclopedia: M.L. Buyse, ed.-in-chief; Blackwell Scientific Publications, 1990, pp. 1105–1106.

The Marinesco-Sjögren Syndrome Examined by Computed Tomography, Magnetic Resonance, and 18F-2-Deoxy-D-Glucose and Positron Emission Tomography: M.B. Bromberg, et al.; Arch. Neurol., November 1990, vol. 47(11), pp. 1239–1242.

# MARSHALL SYNDROME

**Description** Major symptoms include a distinctive face characterized by a flattened nasal bridge, anteverted nares, and hypertelorism; myopia; cataracts; and hearing loss.

**Synonyms**

> Deafness–Myopia–Cataract–Saddle Nose, Marshall Type

**Signs and Symptoms** Craniofacial characteristics include a distinctive flat and sunken midface with saddle nose, anteverted nares, and hypertelorism. The calvaria is thicker than normal, and calcium deposits can be found in the cranium. Eye defects include myopia and cataract. Sensorineural hearing loss may be slight or severe.

Less common features include esotropia, hypertropia, retinal detachment, glaucoma, and protruding upper incisors.

**Etiology** The syndrome is inherited as an autosomal dominant trait.

**Epidemiology** Approximately 21 cases have been reported in the medical literature. Males and females are affected in equal numbers.

**Related Disorders** See *Spondyloepiphyseal Dysplasia Congenita; Stickler Syndrome; Syphilis, Congenital.*

**Wagner syndrome** is a rare disorder inherited as an autosomal dominant trait. Expression can be mild, moderate, or severe. Characteristics include facial abnormalities, an underdeveloped jaw, saddle nose, cleft palate, and vision abnormalities. Joint hyperextensibility in the fingers, elbows, and knees, and hip deformities may also occur. Patients with Wagner syndrome do not have retinal detachment as do those with Marshall and Stickler syndromes.

**Treatment—Standard** Treatment is symptomatic and supportive. Genetic counseling may benefit patients and their families.

**Treatment—Investigational** Please contact the agencies listed under Resources, below, for the most current information. Addresses and telephone numbers of these agencies, as well as of individual experts and research centers, may be found in the Master Resources List.

**Resources**

**For more information on Marshall syndrome:** National Organization for Rare Disorders (NORD); National Association for Craniofacially Handicapped; Let's Face It; National Foundation for Facial Reconstruction; American Society for Deaf Children; NIH/National Institute of Child Health and Human Development; NIH/National Eye Institute.

**For genetic information and genetic counseling referrals:** March of Dimes Birth Defects Foundation; Alliance of Genetic Support Groups.

**References**

Mendelian Inheritance in Man, 11th ed.: V.A. McKusick; Johns Hopkins University Press, 1994, pp. 919–920.

Birth Defects Encyclopedia: M.L. Buyse, ed.-in-chief; Blackwell Scientific Publications, 1990, pp. 504–505.

Smith's Recognizable Patterns of Human Malformation, 4th ed.: K.L. Jones; W.B. Saunders Company, 1988, p. 212.

# MARSHALL-SMITH SYNDROME

**Description** Bony maturation and linear growth are accelerated and are accompanied by severe respiratory problems, mental retardation, and other characteristic physical abnormalities.

**Signs and Symptoms** The infant is underweight in relation to height and fails to thrive. Respiratory complications are common and often fatal in the first year. Stridor and tongue obstruction of the air passage occur. Hypotonia, muscle weakness, and psychomotor retardation are often present.

Craniofacial abnormalities include prominent forehead and eyes, upturned nose with a low nasal bridge, and blue sclerae. Maldevelopment of the epiglottis and laryngomalacia may be present. Hypertrichosis is often a feature.

Some patients may have a short sternum, choanal atresia or stenosis, and omphalocele, as well as brain abnormalities, which can include cerebral atrophy, macrogyria, and an absent corpus callosum. Defects in the immune system are sometimes present.

**Etiology** The cause is unknown. There is no evidence of genetic inheritance.

**Epidemiology** The disorder is very rare; about 20 cases have been reported. Males and females are affected in equal numbers.

**Related Disorders** See *McCune-Albright Syndrome; Sotos Syndrome; Weaver Syndrome.*

**Treatment—Standard** Aggressive treatment of respiratory difficulties is necessary; otherwise, treatment is symptomatic and supportive. Special education and related services will be necessary during school years.

**Treatment—Investigational** Please contact the agencies listed under Resources, below, for the most current information. Addresses and telephone numbers of these agencies, as well as of individual experts and research centers, may be found in the Master Resources List.

**Resources**

For more information on **Marshall-Smith syndrome:** National Organization for Rare Disorders (NORD); Magic Foundation for Children's Growth; Human Growth Foundation; The Arc (a national organization on mental retardation); NIH/National Institute of Child Health and Human Development.

**References**

Syndromes of the Head and Neck, 3rd ed.: R.J. Gorlin, et al.; Oxford University Press, 1990, pp. 340–342.

Marshall-Smith Syndrome: New Aspects: A.M. Roodhooft, et al.; Neuropediatrics, November 1988, vol. 19(4), pp. 179–182.

Smith's Recognizable Patterns of Human Malformation, 4th ed.: K.L. Jones; W.B. Saunders Company, 1988, pp. 134–135.

Marshall-Smith Syndrome: Two Case Reports and a Review of Pulmonary Manifestations: J.P. Johnson, et al.; Pediatrics, February 1983, vol. 71(2), pp. 219–223.


# MAXILLOFACIAL DYSOSTOSIS

**Description** Maxillofacial dysostosis is characterized by anomalies of the upper jaw and eyelids and by malformations of the external ear.

**Synonyms**

Hypoplasia of the Maxilla, Primary Familial

**Signs and Symptoms** The primary symptoms include an underdeveloped maxilla, down-slanting eyelids, malformations of the external ear, and delayed speech with poor articulation. Other symptoms include nystagmus, strabismus, pectus excavatum, incomplete or underdeveloped nipples, a flat posterior skull, and a beaked nose with a flat nasal bridge. Language difficulties are not indicative of a patient's intelligence, which is usually normal. Educators should be informed, and the patient's progress should be monitored.

**Etiology** Maxillofacial dysostosis is inherited as an autosomal dominant trait.

**Epidemiology** Males and females are affected in equal numbers. Only 12 cases have been reported.

**Related Disorders** See *Acrodysostosis; Nager Syndrome; Treacher Collins Syndrome.*

**Treatment—Standard** Facial features improve with age and often appear normal by adulthood. Plastic surgery and orthodontic repair can be beneficial for severe malformations of the face.

Genetic counseling may benefit patients and their families. Other treatment is symptomatic and supportive.

**Treatment—Investigational** Please contact the agencies listed under Resources, below, for the most current information. Addresses and telephone numbers of these agencies, as well as of individual experts and research centers, may be found in the Master Resources List.

**Resources**

For more information on **maxillofacial dysostosis:** National Organization for Rare Disorders (NORD); NIH/National Institute of Child Health and Human Development; Forward Face; FACES—National Association for the Craniofacially Handicapped; National Craniofacial Foundation; Children's Craniofacial Association; Craniofacial Family Association; AboutFace.

For **genetic information and genetic counseling referrals:** March of Dimes Birth Defects Foundation; Alliance of Genetic Support Groups.

**References**

Mendelian Inheritance in Man, 11th ed.: V.A. McKusick; The Johns Hopkins University Press, 1994, p. 921.

Birth Defects Encyclopedia: M.L. Buyse, ed.-in-chief; Blackwell Scientific Publications, 1990, p. 1109.


# MAXILLONASAL DYSPLASIA, BINDER TYPE

**Description** Binder-type maxillonasal dysplasia is a disorder characterized by distinct facial features as well as abnormalities of the cervical spine.

**Synonyms**

Binder Syndrome

Maxillonasal Dysplasia
Nasomaxillary Hypoplasia

**Signs and Symptoms** A small, flat, low-set nose with a short underdeveloped nasal septum; "half-moon" nasal apertures; an absent or underdeveloped nasal spine; an elevated and rounded upper lip; and a protruding chin are characteristic. Other features include convergent strabismus, a cleft lip, a labiomaxillopalatine cleft, abnormalities of the cervical spine, protrusion of the lower jaw, and malocclusion.

Binder-type maxillonasal dysplasia may be a mild form of **chondrodysplasia punctata.** Misdiagnosis is usually the result of patients' seeking help at an older age when the x-ray features of chondrodysplasia punctata have disappeared. (See Related Disorders.)

**Etiology** Binder-type maxillonasal dysplasia may appear as an isolated event or be inherited as an autosomal dominant or autosomal recessive trait.

**Epidemiology** Males and females are affected in equal numbers. Although detectable at birth, the disorder may not be diagnosed until years later. Over 100 cases have been reported.

**Related Disorders** See *Conradi-Hünermann Syndrome.*

**Rhizomelic-type chondrodysplasia punctata** is a rare disorder inherited as an autosomal recessive trait. A flattened face, vision problems, and calcification in the hip and shoulder joints may also be present. Spasticity and mental retardation may also occur.

**Fetal warfarin syndrome** is a disorder of altered fetal development caused by the anticoagulant warfarin. Affected infants may have facial features similar to Binder-type maxillonasal dysplasia. The most consistent feature of this disorder is depression of the nasal bridge, resulting in an upturned, flattened appearance and a deep groove between the nostrils. Growth deficits, recurrent infections, and mental retardation may also occur.

**Treatment—Standard** Treatment consists of surgery to correct the abnormalities of the nose and jaw when the child is older. Cleft lip can be corrected by surgery, beginning in the patient's infancy. Cleft palate may also be treated surgically or by a prosthesis. A team of orthodontists as well as oral and plastic surgeons may be used.

Genetic counseling may benefit patients and their families. Other treatment is symptomatic and supportive.

**Treatment—Investigational** Researchers are studying a paste that is applied to the rear of the pharynx in a minor surgical procedure to bring the pharynx and palate into proper relationship. For further information, contact William N. Williams, D.D.S., University of Florida.

Please contact the agencies listed under Resources, below, for the most current information. Addresses and telephone numbers of these agencies, as well as of individual experts and research centers, may be found in the Master Resources List.

**Resources**

**For more information on Binder-type maxillonasal dysplasia:** National Organization for Rare Disorders (NORD); FACES—National Association for the Craniofacially Handicapped; Craniofacial Family Association; National Craniofacial Foundation; National Foundation for Facial Reconstruction; NIH/National Arthritis and Musculoskeletal and Skin Diseases Information Clearinghouse.

**For genetic information and genetic counseling referrals:** March of Dimes Birth Defects Foundation; Alliance of Genetic Support Groups.

**References**

Mendelian Inheritance in Man, 11th ed.: V.A. McKusick; The Johns Hopkins University Press, 1994, p. 921.

Birth Defects Encyclopedia: M.L. Buyse, ed.-in-chief; Blackwell Scientific Publications, 1990, pp. 1110–1111.

The Craniofacial Morphology in Persons with Maxillonasal Dysplasia (Binder Syndrome): A Longitudinal Cephalometric Study of Orthodontically Treated Children: M. Olow-Nordenram, et al.; Am. J. Orthod. Dentofacial Orthop., February 1989, vol. 95(2), pp. 148–158.

Maxillonasal Dysplasia (Binder's Syndrome): A Critical Review and Case Study: B.B. Horswell, et al.; J. Oral Maxillofac. Surg., February 1987, vol. 45(2), pp. 114–122.

Familial Variant of Maxillonasal Dysplasia: E. Gross-Kieselstein, et al.; J. Craniofac. Genet. Dev. Biol., 1986, vol. 6(3), pp. 331–334.

Surgical Correction of the Nose and Midface in Maxillonasal Dysplasia (Binder's Syndrome): H. Holmstrom; Plast. Reconstr. Surg., November 1986, vol. 78(5), pp. 568–580.

Clinical and Radiologic Aspects of Maxillonasal Dysostosis (Binder Syndrome): J. Delaire, et al.; Head Neck Surg., November–December, 1980, vol. 3(2), pp. 105–122.

Maxillonasal Dysplasia (Binder's Syndrome): I.R. Munro, et al.; Plast. Reconstr. Surg., May 1979, vol. 63(5), pp. 657–663.

# MECKEL SYNDROME

**Description** Meckel syndrome is a rare inherited disorder with a wide variety of manifestations, the most common of which are sloping forehead, posterior encephalocele, polydactyly, and polycystic kidney. Liver abnormalities are also common. Infants rarely live more than a few days or weeks.

**Synonyms**

Dysencephalia Splanchnocystica

Gruber Syndrome
Meckel-Gruber Syndrome

**Signs and Symptoms** Characteristic features are posterior encephalocele and other brain abnormalities, renal cysts, and abnormalities of the bile ducts of the liver. Polydactyly and shortening or bowing of the long bones of the arms and legs are common. In males the testicles may contain abnormal cysts and may fail to descend or grow properly.

**Etiology** Meckel syndrome is inherited as an autosomal recessive trait.

**Epidemiology** Males and females are affected in equal numbers. Estimates of the incidence of this syndrome vary in different populations from 1:9,000 to 1:140,000 births. The incidence appears to be higher in India, Finland, and among the Tatars in the Soviet Union.

**Related Disorders** See *Smith-Lemli-Opitz Syndrome.*

**Potter syndrome** is a rare hereditary disorder marked by congenital cysts of the kidneys and liver. Patients also suffer from cerebral hemorrhage, aortic aneurysm, and hypertension.

**Ullrich-Feichtiger syndrome** exhibits the same symptoms as Meckel syndrome, with the addition of some facial deformities that include micrognathia and cleft palate.

**Treatment—Standard** Meckel syndrome can be identified in pregnant women during the 5th month of pregnancy either through ultrasound testing or amniocentesis. Treatment is symptomatic and supportive. Genetic counseling is recommended for families affected by this disorder.

**Treatment—Investigational** Please contact the agencies listed under Resources, below, for the most current information. Addresses and telephone numbers of these agencies, as well as of individual experts and research centers, may be found in the Master Resources List.

**Resources**

**For more information on Meckel syndrome:** National Organization for Rare Disorders (NORD); NIH/National Institute of Child Health and Human Development.

**For genetic information and genetic counseling referrals:** March of Dimes Birth Defects Foundation; Alliance of Genetic Support Groups.

**References**

Mendelian Inheritance in Man, 11th ed.: V.A. McKusick; The Johns Hopkins University Press, 1994, pp. 1980–1981.

Smith's Recognizable Patterns of Human Malformation, 4th ed.: K.L. Jones; W.B. Saunders Company, 1988, pp. 152–153.

A New Syndrome with Features of the Smith-Lemli-Opitz and Meckel-Gruber Syndromes in a Sibship with Cerebellar Defects: A.C. Casamassima, et al.; Am. J. Med. Genet., February 1987, vol. 26(2), pp. 321–336.

Studies on the Elevated Amniotic Fluid sp 1 in Meckels' Syndrome; Modified Glycosylation of sp 1; M. Heikinheimo, et al.; Placenta, July–August 1987, vol. 8(4), pp. 427–432.

The Meckel Syndrome: Clinicopathological Findings in 67 Patients; R. Salonen, et al.; Am. J. Med. Genet., August 1984, vol. 18(4), pp. 671–689.

Are Bowing of Long Tubular Bones and Preaxial Polydactyly Signs of the Meckel Syndrome?: F. Majewski, et al.; Hum. Genet., 1983, vol. 65(2), pp. 125–133.

# MELNICK-NEEDLES SYNDROME

**Description** Melnick-Needles syndrome is a disorder in which bones develop abnormally. Characteristic features include hypertelorism, bowed arm and leg bones, and micrognathia.

**Synonyms**

Melnick-Needles Osteodysplasty
Osteodysplasty of Melnick and Needles

**Signs and Symptoms** Patients with this syndrome exhibit unique facial characteristics, including hypertelorism, micrognathia, small facial bones, a slow-developing skull, and an abnormal bite. The syndrome also affects the limbs. The humerus, phalanges, radius, fibula, and tibia may be shorter than normal, bowed, and flared.

Although patients usually achieve a normal height, their gait may be unusual, a result of the presence of coxa valga.

The upper trunk may also be affected. The thoracic cage may be smaller than normal, the ribs irregular, and the shoulders narrowed. Other symptoms include pectus excavatum, longer-than-normal vertebrae, and flared ilium. These deformities make the patients more susceptible to respiratory infections.

The pelvis may also be involved, and the hip may become dislocated. Osteoarthritis may affect the hip and spine. Complications relating to childbirth and kidney malfunction may also occur.

**Etiology** Melnick-Needles syndrome is a genetically transmitted disorder. The exact genetic mechanism is not known, but X-linked dominance with lethality in males appears most likely.

**Epidemiology** Melnick-Needles syndrome occurs at birth and affects females more often than males.

**Related Disorders Multiple epiphyseal dysplasia** is an inherited disorder that affects the bones. It is usually diagnosed when the patient is between 2 and 5 years and begins to exhibit an unusual gait. Osteoarthritis may develop in the joints. Patients reach normal height but exhibit smaller-than-normal hands and feet. Males and females are affected equally.

**Treatment—Standard** Treatment is symptomatic and supportive. Genetic counseling may benefit patients and their families.

**Treatment—Investigational** Please contact the agencies listed under Resources, below, for the most current information. Addresses and telephone numbers of these agencies, as well as of individual experts and research centers, may be found in the Master Resources List.

**Resources**

For more information on **Melnick-Needles syndrome:** National Organization for Rare Disorders (NORD); International Center for Skeletal Dysplasia; NIH/National Institute of Child Health and Human Development.

For **genetic information and genetic counseling referrals:** March of Dimes Birth Defects Foundation; Alliance of Genetic Support Groups.

**References**

Mendelian Inheritance in Man, 11th ed.: V.A. McKusick; The Johns Hopkins University Press, 1994, pp. 2446–2447.
Smith's Recognizable Patterns of Human Malformation, 4th ed.: K.L. Jones; W.B. Saunders Company, 1988, pp. 528–529.
Melnick-Needles Syndrome in Males: M. Krajewska-Walasek, et al.; Am. J. Med. Genet., May 1987, vol. 27(1), pp. 153–158.

# METAPHYSEAL CHONDRODYSPLASIA, SCHMID TYPE

**Description** Schmid-type metaphyseal chondrodysplasia is a progressive, inherited bone disorder that is the most common of a heterogeneous group of disorders characterized by abnormalities of the metaphyses.

**Synonyms**

Schmid Metaphyseal Chondrodysplasia
Schmid Metaphyseal Dysostosis

**Signs and Symptoms** X-rays show that the metaphyses are fragmented, cupped, and irregular and that the new bones have ossified. This results in moderately short stature, bowed legs, and a waddling gait, noticeable when the infant begins to walk. Coxa vara and genu varum are common. The shoulders, hips, wrists, knees, and ankles are affected. The front ends of the ribs may be cupped, and the lower rib cage is often flared. Bone density is normal. Noninflammatory arthralgia and stiffness may also be present.

**Etiology** Schmid-type metaphyseal chondrodysplasia is inherited as an autosomal dominant trait. A type X collagen mutation, COL 10A1, has been found in a large Mormon kindred and in a number of sporadic cases.

**Epidemiology** Males and females are affected in equal numbers. Several large kindred have been documented in the medical literature.

**Related Disorders** See *Rickets, Hypophosphatemic; Cartilage-Hair Hypoplasia.*

**Jansen-type metaphyseal chondrodysplasia** is a rare autosomal dominant disorder characterized by progressive, short-limbed small stature. This is the most severe of the metaphyseal dysplasias. Extreme genu varum, enlarged joints, and an underdeveloped jaw are typical. The spine and pelvis are distorted. Sclerosis of the cranial bones, including those of the inner ear, leads to deafness.

**Spahr-type metaphyseal chondrodysplasia** is a progressive bone disorder inherited as an autosomal recessive trait and is similar to the Schmid type except in the mode of inheritance. Genu varum is the most apparent feature.

**Treatment—Standard** Patients with Schmid-type metaphyseal chondrodysplasia may benefit from physical therapy as well as orthopedic care. Genetic counseling may benefit patients and their families. Other treatment is symptomatic and supportive.

**Treatment—Investigational** Please contact the agencies listed under Resources, below, for the most current information. Addresses and telephone numbers of these agencies, as well as of individual experts and research centers, may be found in the Master Resources List.

**Resources**

For more information on **Schmid-type metaphyseal chondrodysplasia:** National Organization for Rare Disorders (NORD); NIH/National Institute of Child Health and Human Development.

For **genetic information and genetic counseling referrals:** March of Dimes Birth Defects Foundation; Alliance of Genetic Support Groups.

**References**

Concentrations of Mutations Causing Schmid Metaphyseal Chondrodysplasia in the C-Terminal Noncollagenous Domain of Type X Collagen: I. McIntosh; Hum. Mutat., 1995, vol. 5, pp. 121–125.

Mendelian Inheritance in Man, 11th ed.: V.A. McKusick; The Johns Hopkins University Press, 1994, pp. 312–313.

Nelson Textbook of Pediatrics, 14th ed.: R.E. Behrman, ed.-in-chief; W.B. Saunders Company, 1992, p. 1739.

Birth Defects Encyclopedia: M.L. Buyse, ed.-in-chief; Blackwell Scientific Publications, 1990, p. 1133.

Metaphyseal Chondrodysplasia, Schmid Type: Clinical and Radiographic Delineation with a Review of the Literature: R.S. Lachman, et al.; Pediatr. Radiol., 1988, vol. 18(2), pp. 93–102.

Smith's Recognizable Patterns of Human Malformation, 4th ed.: K.L. Jones; W.B. Saunders Company, 1988, p. 332.

# MILLER SYNDROME

**Description** Major characteristics include upper and lower limb shortening, lower eyelid and ear abnormalities, and malar hypoplasia.

**Synonyms**

Genee-Wiedemann Syndrome

Postaxial Acrofacial Dysostosis

**Signs and Symptoms** Craniofacial abnormalities include micrognathia, malar hypoplasia, coloboma of the lower eyelid, downward slanting palpebral fissures, and cupped ears. The nose may be very broad at the base.

The fingers and toes may be missing, webbed, or incompletely formed, and the long bones in the arms and legs may be hypoplastic. Deformities of the palate or jaw may cause breathing and swallowing difficulties in the newborn, making insertion of breathing and feeding tubes necessary.

Occasionally other problems are present, such as cardiac defects, stomach or kidney reflux, hearing loss, and extra nipples.

**Etiology** The syndrome is thought to be caused by autosomal recessive inheritance. However, the mode of transmission is still under investigation.

**Epidemiology** In the cases reported thus far, males have been affected slightly more often than females.

**Related Disorders** See *Nager Syndrome; Oral-Facial-Digital Syndrome; Treacher Collins Syndrome.*

**Goldenhar-Gorlin syndrome** is a rare congenital disorder that involves unusual facial characteristics, such as asymmetry of the skull, sharply prominent forehead, partial absence of the upper eyelid, absent or closed nares, and cleft palate.

**Juberg-Hayward syndrome (orocraniodigital syndrome)** is a rare hereditary disorder characterized by cleft lip and palate, microcephaly, deformities of the thumbs and toes, and growth hormone deficiency resulting in short stature.

**Treatment—Standard** Insertion of breathing and feeding tubes may be necessary in some infants. Tubes may also need to be inserted into the ears. Multiple plastic surgeries may be necessary to correct eye and jaw defects. Physical therapy will improve walking and use of hands. Surgery and speech therapy are often necessary when cleft palate or lip is present. Genetic counseling may benefit patients and their families. Other treatment is symptomatic and supportive.

**Treatment—Investigational** To participate in the Human Genome Project, aimed at mapping every gene in the human body, families with individuals with Miller syndrome should contact Eric A. Wulfsberg, M.D., or Karen Supovitz, M.S., Division of Human Genetics, University of Maryland School of Medicine.

Please contact the agencies listed under Resources, below, for the most current information. Addresses and telephone numbers of these agencies, as well as of individual experts and research centers, may be found in the Master Resources List.

**Resources**

**For more information on Miller syndrome:** National Organization for Rare Disorders (NORD); Foundation for Nager and Miller Syndromes; NIH/National Institute of Child Health and Human Development; American Cleft Palate Cranial Facial Association; FACES—National Association for the Craniofacially Handicapped; National Craniofacial Foundation; American Society for Deaf Children.

**For genetic information and genetic counseling referrals:** March of Dimes Birth Defects Foundation; Alliance of Genetic Support Groups.

**References**

Mendelian Inheritance in Man, 11th ed.: V.A. McKusick; The Johns Hopkins University Press, 1994, p. 2144.

An Adaptation of the Miller Patient Classification System for the Postanesthesia Care Unit at Children's Hospital of Eastern Ontario: J. Kay, et al,; J. Postanesth. Nurs., August 1990, vol. 5(4), pp. 239–246.

Birth Defects Encyclopedia: M.L. Buyse, ed.-in-chief; Blackwell Scientific Publications, 1990, pp. 45–46.

Pathogenesis of Cleft Palate in Treacher Collins, Nager, and Miller Syndromes: K.K. Sulik, et al; Cleft Palate J., July 1989, vol. 26(3), pp. 209–216.

Smith's Recognizable Patterns of Human Malformation, 4th ed.: K.L. Jones; W.B. Saunders Company, 1988, pp. 214–215.

Miller's Syndrome: Anaesthetic Management of Postaxial Acrofacial Dysostosis: M. Richards; Anaesthesia, August 1987, vol. 42(8), pp. 871–874.

# MOEBIUS SYNDROME

**Description** Moebius syndrome is an inherited type of facial paralysis caused by absent or decreased 6th and 7th nerve development. Abnormalities of the facial muscles and jaw develop. Central nervous system abnormalities may also occur. Mental retardation is present in about 10 percent of cases.

**Synonyms**

> Congenital Facial Diplegia Syndrome
> Congenital Oculofacial Paralysis
> Sixth and Seventh Nerve Palsy

**Signs and Symptoms** From birth, patients exhibit a masklike expression, especially when crying or laughing. Nerve and muscle abnormalities cause the mouth and eyes to remain open during sleep, resulting in ocular ulcerations. Feeding during infancy is difficult. Speech problems may develop. Fluid secretions of the mouth may be breathed into the lungs, resulting in bronchopneumonia. Epicanthal folds, microphthalmos, and malformations of the jaw and tongue may also occur.

Many abnormalities of the hands and feet may be present, including polydactyly, oligodactyly, and clubfeet. Congenital dislocation of the hip may also occur.

**Etiology** Moebius syndrome is thought to be inherited as an autosomal dominant trait, but most often occurs sporadically.

**Epidemiology** The syndrome is very rare. Males and females are affected in equal numbers.

**Related Disorders** See *Muscular Dystrophy, Landouzy-Dejerine.*

**Treatment—Standard** Medical therapy may be indicated for dry or ulcerated eyes. Parenteral tube feeding may be necessary during infancy, and later, patients may require a special diet to avoid aspirating food into the lungs. Speech may improve with therapy and vocal cord surgery. Other surgery involving muscle transfer may be necessary to correct abnormalities of the eye, face, hands, or feet.

Other treatment is symptomatic and supportive. Genetic counseling will benefit patients and their families.

**Treatment—Investigational** Please contact the agencies listed under Resources, below, for the most current information. Addresses and telephone numbers of these agencies, as well as of individual experts and research centers, may be found in the Master Resources List.

**Resources**

**For more information on Moebius syndrome:** National Organization for Rare Disorders (NORD); NIH/National Institute of Neurological Disorders and Stroke; FACES—National Association for the Craniofacially Handicapped; Society for the Rehabilitation of the Facially Disfigured; AboutFace.

**For genetic information and genetic counseling referrals:** March of Dimes Birth Defects Foundation; Alliance of Genetic Support Groups.

**References**

Mendelian Inheritance in Man, 11th ed.: V.A. McKusick; The Johns Hopkins University Press, 1994, pp. 948–949.

Extraocular Muscle Aplasia in Moebius Syndrome: E.I. Traboulsi, et al.; J. Pediatr. Ophthalmol. Strabismus, May–June 1986, vol. 23(3), pp. 120–122.

Abnormal B.A.E.P. in a Family with Moebius Syndrome: Evidence for Supranuclear Lesion: M. Stabile, et al.; Clin. Genet., May 1984, vol. 25(5), pp. 459–463.

Moebius Syndrome: Case Report of a 30-Year Follow-Up: D.C. Morello, et al.; Plast. Reconstr. Surg., September 1977, vol. 60(3), pp. 451–453.

# NAGER SYNDROME

**Description** The syndrome is characterized primarily by malar hypoplasia, micrognathia, radial limb and thumb anomalies, and ear abnormalities.

**Synonyms**

> Acrofacial Dysostosis, Nager Type
> Mandibulofacial Dysostosis
> Split Hand Deformity–Mandibulofacial Dysostosis

**Signs and Symptoms** Besides the small jaw and underdeveloped cheekbones, craniofacial abnormalities include downward slanting eyes, internal and external ear deformities, absence of eyelashes, and clefting of the soft and hard palate. Facial hair may grow in an elongated sideburn effect.

The forearms are short and the thumbs hypoplastic. Missing, overlapping or webbing of the toes may occur. Clubfeet, hip dislocation, and underdeveloped ribs may occasionally be present, as may tetralogy of Fallot.

The syndrome is closely related to Miller syndrome, and in some cases has been misdiagnosed as Treacher Collins syndrome.

**Etiology** The cause is not known. Autosomoal recessive inheritance is suggested in some instances, and autosomal dominant in others.

**Epidemiology** The syndrome is apparent at birth. Males and females are affected in equal numbers.

**Related Disorders** See *Miller Syndrome; Oral-Facial-Digital Syndrome; Treacher Collins Syndrome.*

**Juberg-Hayward syndrome (orocraniodigital syndrome)** is a rare hereditary disorder characterized by cleft lip and palate, microcephaly, deformities of the thumbs and toes, and growth hormone deficiency resulting in short stature.

**Treatment—Standard** Insertion of breathing and feeding tubes may be necessary in some infants. Tubes may also need to be inserted into the ears. Multiple plastic surgeries may be necessary to correct eye and jaw defects. Physical therapy will improve walking and use of hands. Orthopedic surgery may be necessary to correct deformities of the arms, hands, feet, or toes. Speech therapy may be needed to aid in hearing and language development.

**Treatment—Investigational** Please contact the agencies listed under Resources, below, for the most current information. Addresses and telephone numbers of these agencies, as well as of individual experts and research centers, may be found in the Master Resources List.

**Resources**

**For more information on Nager syndrome:** National Organization for Rare Disorders (NORD); Foundation for Nager and Miller Syndromes; NIH/National Institute of Child Health and Human Development; American Cleft Palate Cranial Facial Association; Forward Face; FACES—National Association for the Craniofacially Handicapped); Let's Face It; National Craniofacial Foundation; American Society for Deaf Children.

**For genetic information and genetic counseling referrals:** March of Dimes Birth Defects Foundation; Alliance of Genetic Support Groups.

**References**

Mendelian Inheritance in Man, 11th ed.: V.A. McKusick; The Johns Hopkins University Press, 1994, pp. 912–913.

Birth Defects Encyclopedia: M.L. Buyse, ed.-in-chief; Blackwell Scientific Publications, 1990, pp. 44–45.

A Significant Feature of Nager's Syndrome: Palatal Agenesis: I.T. Jackson, et al.; Plast. Reconstr. Surg., August 1989, vol. 84(2), pp. 219–226.

Nager Acrofacial Dysostosis: Evidence for Apparent Heterogeneity: D.J. Goldstein, et al.; Am. J. Med. Genet., July 1988, vol. 30(3), pp. 741–746.

Smith's Recognizable Patterns of Human Malformation, 4th ed.: K.L. Jones; W.B. Saunders Company, 1988, pp. 216–217.

The Nager Acrofacial Dysostosis Syndrome with the Tetralogy of Fallot: E. Thompson, et al.; J. Med. Genet., October 1985, vol. 22(5), pp. 408–410.

# NAIL-PATELLA SYNDROME

**Description** Nail-patella syndrome is a rare genetic disorder characterized primarily by nail dysplasia, bone deformities, and, in some cases, renal abnormalities.

**Synonyms**

Fong Syndrome

Onycho-osteodysplasia, Hereditary

Turner-Kieser Syndrome

**Signs and Symptoms** The nails, especially the thumbs, are hypoplastic with splitting, ridges, discoloration, and abnormal moons. The patellae are hypoplastic or absent, and there often are abnormalities of the elbows affecting range of movement, abnormalities of the ilia (iliac spurs, seen in almost three-quarters of patients), and abnormalities of the scapulae. About half of patients have a cloverleaf pigmentation of the iris, and one-third of patients have renal signs (proteinuria, abnormal urinary sediment). The renal disease is usually benign, although it occasionally leads to early death. Other, less frequent, abnormalities are skeletal, ocular, muscular, and neurologic.

**Etiology** The syndrome is inherited as an autosomal dominant trait linked to the ABO blood group locus. The gene has been localized to 9q34.

**Related Disorders** See *Alport Syndrome.*

**Nail-patella-like renal disease** involves the kidneys without apparent bone and nail abnormalities. However, electron microscopy reveals histopathologic changes similar to nail-patella syndrome.

**Treatment—Standard** Renal dialysis and possibly kidney transplantation may be indicated in the treatment of kidney complications. Genetic counseling may benefit patients and their families. Other treatment is symptomatic and supportive.

**Treatment—Investigational** Please contact the agencies listed under Resources, below, for the most current information. Addresses and telephone numbers of these agencies, as well as of individual experts and research centers, may be found in the Master Resources List.

**Resources**

**For more information on nail-patella syndrome:** National Organization for Rare Disorders (NORD); National Kidney Foundation; NIH/National Kidney and Urologic Diseases Information Clearinghouse.

**For genetic information and genetic counseling referrals:** March of Dimes Birth Defects Foundation; Alliance of Genetic Support Groups.

**References**

Mendelian Inheritance in Man, 11th ed.: V.A. McKusick; The Johns Hopkins University Press, 1994, pp. 996–997.

Smith's Recognizable Patterns of Human Malformation, 4th ed.: K.L. Jones; W.B. Saunders Company, 1988, pp. 386–387.

An Autosomal Recessive Disorder, with Glomerular Basement Membrane Abnormalities Similar to Those Seen in the Nail Patella Syndrome: Report of a Kindred: J.R. Salcedo; Am. J. Med. Genet., 1984, vol. 19, pp. 579–584.

# NEUROFIBROMATOSIS (NF)

**Description** The term *neurofibromatosis* is used to describe what are now known to be 2 distinctly different disorders: the more common neurofibromatosis type I **(NF 1),** and the less common type II **(NF 2).** Both disorders are transmitted in an autosomal dominant fashion, but the genes involved are on separate chromosomes. Both conditions are characterized by the occurrence of multiple neurofibromas. In the recent past, great lay interest in neurofibromatosis has been sparked by the Broadway show and the movie based on the book by Sir Frederick Treves, *The Elephant Man and Other Reminiscences.* Lamentably, this led to the vogue of referring to NF 1 as Elephant Man disease; not only is this odious but it now appears that Treves' patient had Proteus syndrome rather than NF 1 (see ***Proteus Syndrome).***

**Synonyms**

Bilateral Acoustic Neurofibromatosis (NF 2)

Central Neurofibromatosis (NF 2)

Neurofibroma, Multiple

Recklinghausen Disease (NF 1)

von Recklinghausen Disease (NF 1)

**Signs and Symptoms** NF 1 usually has its onset during childhood. The disease is progressive and tends to become more active at puberty and during pregnancy. Although the course and symptoms of NF vary and are unpredictable, brown (café au lait) spots are usually the first sign. These spots measure approximately 0.5 cm in diameter in children and grow to 1.5 cm in diameter in adults. Six or more 0.5 café au lait macules and 2 or more neurofibromas are diagnostic in a child. Axillary or inguinal freckling or 2 or more Lisch nodules in the iris are other important diagnostic criteria.

The most common tumors, neurofibromas, occur in NF 1 and can form under the skin or in deeper areas in the body. Pain may or may not occur. Tumors can produce disfigurement and orthopedic problems, including scoliosis and pseudoarthrosis. Sexual development may be delayed or precocious, and learning disabilities may develop. Optic glioma, hamartomas, and other CNS lesions are common.

NF 2 develops later than NF 1, usually in the teens and 20s. Fewer café au lait spots and cutaneous neurofibromas develop. It is characterized by bilateral acoustic neuromas and may be associated with brain and spinal cord tumors. Buzzing or ringing in the ears and loss of hearing are the clinical manifestations of these neuromas.

**Etiology** NF 1 and 2 have autosomal dominant inheritance; however, about half of all cases are due to new mutations. The gene for NF 1 is on chromosome 17 (17q11.2). The gene for NF 2 is on chromosome 22 (22q). The NF 1 gene is a very large gene; only about 10 percent of mutations have been reported in more than 500 patients.

A localized (unilateral and not crossing the midline) form of neurofibromatosis appears to be caused by a somatic mutation, with little risk of recurrence.

**Epidemiology** NF 1 affects 1:4,000 individuals; NF 2 affects 1:50,000.

**Treatment—Standard** Once diagnosis is established, a systematic follow-up program is indicated. Quantitation of specific signs, such as café au lait macules, neurofibromas, and Lisch nodules is indicated. Tests, such as computed tomography, magnetic resonance imaging, and electroencephalography, are dictated by clinical findings. About 50 percent of patients require surgery to remove troublesome neurofibromas. Surgical indications for optic gliomas, acoustic neuromas, and other tumors must be individualized. Since management options are evolving, physicians must be aware of current consensus regarding treatment.

**Treatment—Investigational** Neurofibromatosis research is ongoing and includes recombinant DNA and nerve growth factor. Recent identification of chromosome markers for both types of NF may lead to genetic testing.

Families with one or more members who have central neurofibromatosis (NF 2) with bilateral acoustic neuromas are being sought for a clinical research study at the National Institute of Neurological Disorders and Stroke in Bethesda, MD. The study's goal is to establish methods for early detection and diagnosis. Clinicians who wish to refer potential candidates or obtain additional information should contact Donald Wright, M.D., at the Surgical Neurology Branch of NINDS.

Researchers are also investigating learning disabilities and neurologic changes in NF children from birth to 18 years of age. A controlled study is under way of NF children and siblings who do not have the disorder. Testing is being performed in conjunction with Children's Hospital, Washington, DC.

Ongoing research is directed toward understanding the genetic changes in tumor formation in neurofibromatosis. Known or suspected malignancy tissue is requested. Samples of neurofibromas from female patients are also requested. Please contact Gary R. Skuse, M.D., or Peter T. Rowley, M.D., Division of Genetics, University of Rochester Medical Center.

Brain tumors associated with NF 1 are being studied at the Georgetown University Medical Center, Washington, DC.

Brain and tissue banks that collect samples from patients with NF 1 are supported by the National Institute of Child Health and Human Development. For more information, contact the University of Maryland or the University of Miami School of Medicine.

Studies are ongoing at the National Institutes of Health on possible treatments for people with NF 2. Please contact Dilys Parry, Ph.D., NIH/National Cancer Institute, Medical Genetics/Epidemiology.

For information on other genetic studies of NF 2, including research on a test for its detection, please contact Mia McCollin, M.D., Molecular Neurogenetica Laboratory, Massachusetts General Hospital, or Guy Rouleau, Ph.D., McGill University, Montreal.

Please contact the agencies listed under Resources, below, for the most current information. Addresses and telephone numbers of these agencies, as well as of individual experts and research centers, may be found in the Master Resources List.

### Resources

**For more information on neurofibromatosis:** National Organization for Rare Disorders (NORD); Neurofibromatosis; National Neurofibromatosis Foundation; NF-2 Sharing Network; NIH/National Institute of Neurological Disorders and Stroke; National Association of the Deaf; NIH/National Institute on Deafness and Other Communication Disorders Information Clearinghouse..

**Clinical facilities:** Massachusetts General Hospital Neurofibromatosis Clinic, Department of Neurosurgery, Boston; Georgetown University Medical Center, Department of Neurosurgery, Washington, D.C.; Children's Hospital Neurofibromatosis Clinic, Washington, D.C.; Children's Hospital Neurofibromatosis Clinic, Philadelphia; Neurofibromatosis Program, University of Chicago; Cedars-Sinai Birth Defects Center, Los Angeles; Mount Sinai School of Medicine Neurofibromatosis Clinic, New York, NY.

**For genetic information and genetic counseling referrals:** March of Dimes Birth Defects Foundation; Alliance of Genetic Support Groups.

### References

Mendelian Inheritance in Man, 11th ed.: V.A. McKusick; The Johns Hopkins University Press, 1994, pp. 1005–1015.

Molecular Basis of Neurofibromatosis Type 1 (NF 1): Mutation Analysis and Polymorphisms in the NF 1 Gene: M. Upadhyaya, et al.; Hum. Mutat., 1994, vol. 4, pp. 83–101.

A Novel Moesin-, Ezrin-, Radixin-Like Gene Is a Candidate for the Neurofibromatosis 2 Tumor Suppressor: J.A. Trofatter, et al.; Cell, March 12, 1993, vol. 72, pp. 791–800.

Principles of Neurology, 5th ed.; R.D. Adams and M. Victor, eds; McGraw-Hill, 1993, pp. 1030–1033.

Cecil Textbook of Medicine, 19th ed.: J.B. Wyngaarden, et al., eds.; W.B. Saunders Company, 1992, pp. 2143–2144.

Nelson Textbook of Pediatrics, 14th ed.: R.E. Behrman, ed.-in-chief; W.B. Saunders Company, 1992, pp. 1509–1510.

Diseases of the Nose, Throat, Ear, Head and Neck, 14th ed.: J.J. Ballenger; Lea and Febiger, 1991, pp. 1205–1206.

Harrison's Principles of Internal Medicine, 12th ed.: J.D. Wilson, et al., eds.; McGraw-Hill, 1991, p. 2055.

Identification of the Type I Neurofibromatosis Gene (Interview): Neuroscience Forum, Summer 1991, vol. 1(2), pp. 1, 5, 11, 15.

1991 National Institutes of Health Consensus Development Conference Statement on Acoustic Neuroma.

Birth Defects Encyclopedia: M.L. Buyse, M.D., ed.-in-chief; Blackwell Scientific Publications, 1990, pp. 30–31, 1233–1234.

Current Therapy In Neurologic Diseases: R.T. Johnson, ed,; B.C. Becker, 1990, pp. 101–108.

Dictionary of Medical Syndromes, 3rd ed.: Sergio I. Magalini, et al., eds.: J.B. Lippincott Company, 1990, pp. 216–217, 914–915.

Neurofibromatosis 1 (Recklinghouse Disease) and Neurofibromatosis 2 (Bilateral Acoustic Neurofibromatosis): An Update: J.J. Mulvihill, et al.; Ann. Int. Med., 1990, vol. 113(1), pp. 39–52.

Smith's Recognizable Patterns of Human Malformation, 4th ed.: K.L. Jones; W.B. Saunders Company, 1988, pp. 452–453.

# NOONAN SYNDROME

**Description** Noonan syndrome is characterized by congenital heart defects, short stature, broad or webbed neck, and droopy eyelids.

**Synonyms**
>Turner-like Syndrome

**Signs and Symptoms** The most common cardiac defects are pulmonary valvular stenosis or atrial septal defect, occurring in two-thirds of patients. Average adult height of males is 64 inches, and that of females, 60 inches. A characteristic facies includes hypertelorism, epicanthus, an antimongoloid palpebral slant, ptosis, micrognathia, and ear abnormalities. Other findings include webbing of the neck, pectus carinatum or pectus excavatum, cubitum valgum, and, in males, undescended testes. Puberty usually occurs normally but is delayed 2 years on average. A bleeding diathesis and various hematologic disorders have been reported in some patients.

**Etiology** Noonan syndrome is inherited primarily through an autosomal dominant pattern, with highly variable expression. Many cases appear to be sporadic.

**Epidemiology** The syndrome is thought to occur in approximately 1:1,000 to 1:2,500 persons. The wide variety of symptoms may contribute to significant underdiagnosis and misdiagnosis.

**Related Disorders** See *Turner Syndrome.*

**Treatment—Standard** Cryptorchidism should be treated by 2 to 3 years of age. Severe ptosis can be surgically corrected. Severe pulmonary stenosis may require surgery or balloon dilation.

Genetic counseling is useful for families of children with Noonan syndrome.

**Treatment—Investigational** Human growth hormone treatment for the short stature of Noonan syndrome is at the investigational stage.

Please contact the agencies listed under Resources, below, for the most current information. Addresses and telephone numbers of these agencies, as well as of individual experts and research centers, may be found in the Master Resources List.

**Resources**

**For more information on Noonan syndrome:** National Organization for Rare Disorders (NORD); Noonan Syndrome Support Group; NIH/National Institute of Child Health and Human Development; Human Growth Foundation.

**For genetic information and genetic counseling referrals:** March of Dimes Birth Defects Foundation; Alliance of Genetic Support Groups.

**References**

Mapping a Gene for Noonan Syndrome to the Long Arm of Chromosome 12: C.R. Jamieson, et al.; Nat. Genet., 1994, vol. 8, pp. 357–360.

Mendelian Inheritance in Man, 11th ed.: V.A. McKusick; The Johns Hopkins University Press, 1994, pp. 1029–1030.

Noonan Syndrome: The Changing Phenotype: J.E. Allanson, et al.; Am. J. Med. Gen., July 1985, vol. 21(3), pp. 507–514.

Percutaneous Balloon Vulvoplasty for Pulmonary Valve Stenosis in Infants and Children: I.D. Sullivan, et al.; Br. Heart J., October 1985, vol. 54(4), pp. 435–441.

# OCULO-CEREBRO-CUTANEOUS SYNDROME

**Description** Oculo-cerebro-cutaneous syndrome is a congenital disorder of the brain, skin, and central nervous system.

**Synonyms**
>Delleman Syndrome
>Delleman-Oorthuys Syndrome
>Orbital Cyst with Cerebral and Focal Dermal Malformations

**Signs and Symptoms** Primary symptoms include cysts in the orbit of at least one eye; skin tags in front of the outer ear and in the orbit of the eyes; underdeveloped, "punched-out," or streaked skin lesions on the trunk and head; and seizures.

Colobomas; microphthalmos; the presence of the hyaloid artery; porencephalic cysts; agenesis of the corpus callosum; and abnormalities of the bones, genitalia, and hands and feet have also been found.

**Etiology** Most cases occur as isolated events. An autosomal dominant inheritance with varying severity is suspected.

**Epidemiology** Approximately 8 cases have been reported, 4 of them Dutch.

**Related Disorders** See *Agenesis of Corpus Callosum; Focal Dermal Hypoplasia.*

**Andermann syndrome** is an autosomal recessive trait characterized by a combination of agenesis of corpus callosum, mental retardation, and neuropathy. A long, triangular-shaped face with an underdeveloped jaw and low hairline are common. Scoliosis may cause heart and lung complications. Most reported cases have been traced to Quebec, Canada.

**Treatment—Standard** Surgical excision of cysts is usually indicated, followed by cosmetic surgery. Anticonvulsant drugs are used to prevent and control seizures.

Genetic counseling may benefit patients and their families. Other treatment is symptomatic and supportive.

**Treatment—Investigational** Experiments are being conducted on the anticonvulsant drugs nimodipine, praziquantel, clomiphene, and lorazapam. The orphan drug fosphentoin (manufactured by Warner-Lambert) is being tested as treatment for grand mal epileptic seizures.

Upsher-Smith Laboratories is sponsoring the testing of rectal administration of a diazepam viscous solution to control acute repetitive seizures. More research is required to determine the long-term safety and effectiveness of these drugs.

Please contact the agencies listed under Resources, below, for the most current information. Addresses and telephone numbers of these agencies, as well as of individual experts and research centers, may be found in the Master Resources List.

**Resources**

**For more information on oculo-cerebro-cutaneous syndrome:** National Organization for Rare Disorders (NORD); Agenesis of Corpus Callosum Network; Epilepsy Foundation of America; NIH/National Institute of Neurological Disorders and Stroke.

**For genetic information and genetic counseling referrals:** March of Dimes Birth Defects Foundation; Alliance of Genetic Support Groups.

**References**

Mendelian Inheritance in Man, 11th ed.: V.A. McKusick; The Johns Hopkins University Press, 1994, p. 1038.

Oculocerebrocutaneous Syndrome: J.J. Hoo, et al.; Am. J. Med. Genet., September 1991, vol. 40(3), pp. 290–293.

Birth Defects Encyclopedia: M.L. Buyse, ed.-in-chief; Blackwell Scientific Publications, 1990, p. 1274.

Oculocerebrocutaneous Syndrome: R.D. Wilson, et al.; Am. J. Ophthalmol., February 1985, vol. 99(2). pp. 142–148.

# OCULO-DENTO-DIGITAL DYSPLASIA

**Description** Oculo-dento-digital dysplasia is characterized by microcornea, defective teeth enamel, and syndactyly.

**Synonyms**

> Dento-Oculo-Osseous Dysplasia
> Oculo-Dento-Osseous Dysplasia
> Osseous-Oculo-Dento Dysplasia

**Signs and Symptoms** Primary symptoms include microcornea; defective teeth enamel; syndactyly of the 4th and 5th fingers; a slender nose with narrow nostrils; underdeveloped alae; and slow-growing, dry hair. Also in evidence may be a prominent lower jaw; abnormally small head or teeth; strabismus; glaucoma; a short, narrow opening between the upper and lower eyelids; a vertical fold over the inner corner of the eye; ocular atrophy; cleft lip and/or palate; clinodactyly of the 4th and 5th fingers; syndactyly and/or clinodactyly of the 2nd, 3rd, and 4th toes; and abnormalities in the bones of the toes and 5th finger.

A severe form of oculo-dento-digital dysplasia in which the ocular and skeletal changes are more pronounced may be inherited as an autosomal recessive trait. The eyes are smaller than normal, slanted, and set wide apart; blindness may occur. Skeletal abnormalities include overgrowth of the lower jaw; excessive thickening of cranial tissue; an abnormally wide clavicle; calcium deposits in the ear lobes; a long, narrow nose with underdeveloped outer flaring walls of the nostrils; irregular teeth with abnormal enamel; and syndactyly of the 4th and 5th fingers.

**Etiology** Oculo-dento-digital dysplasia may be inherited as an autosomal dominant trait or as a new mutation. An autosomal recessive form of the disorder has been documented, but there is insufficient evidence to support it.

**Epidemiology** Males and females are affected in equal numbers. Eighty-five cases have been reported.

**Related Disorders** See *Amelogenesis Imperfecta; Saethre-Chotzen Syndrome.*

**Oro-cranio-digital syndrome** is a very rare disorder that is thought to have an autosomal recessive inheritance. Symptoms include an abnormally small head, abnormalities of the thumbs and toes, growth retardation, and cleft lip and/or palate. This disorder affects females slightly more often than males.

**Treatment—Standard** Surgical repair of the webbed fingers and bone malformations may be of benefit. Full crown restorations can correct defective teeth enamel. Strabismus may be corrected at a young age by wearing a patch over the strong eye in order to strengthen the weak eye. Surgery may be indicated in some cases. Patients too old for this correction can be treated with the orphan drug oculinum, which is injected around the eye muscles every few months.

Genetic counseling may benefit patients and their families. Other treatment is symptomatic and supportive.

**Treatment—Investigational** Please contact the agencies listed under Resources, below, for the most current information. Addresses and telephone numbers of these agencies, as well as of individual experts and research centers, may be found in the Master Resources List.

**Resources**

**For more information on oculo-dento-digital dysplasia:** National Organization for Rare Disorders (NORD); National Foundation for Ectodermal Dysplasias; NIH/National Arthritis and Musculoskeletal and Skin Diseases Information Clearinghouse; NIH/National Institute of Dental Research.

**For genetic information and genetic counseling referrals:** March of Dimes Birth Defects Foundation; Alliance of Genetic Support Groups.

**References**

Mendelian Inheritance in Man, 11th ed.: V.A. McKusick; The Johns Hopkins University Press, 1994, pp. 1038–1039, 2083.
Birth Defects Encyclopedia: M.L. Buyse, ed.-in-chief; Blackwell Scientific Publications, 1990, pp. 1276-1277.

# OPITZ SYNDROME

**Description** Opitz syndrome was initially thought to represent 2 different hereditary disorders: Opitz G and Opitz BBB. The subtype names are the initials of the surnames of patients first seen with the disorder. Some research indicates that the 2 syndromes are really just a single condition with symptoms that vary both in type and severity from patient to patient.

**Synonyms**

> BBB Syndrome
> BBBG Syndrome
> G Syndrome
> Opitz BBBG Compound Syndrome
> Opitz-Frias Syndrome
> Opitz Hypertelorism-Hypospadias Syndrome
> Opitz Oculogenitolaryngeal Syndrome

**Signs and Symptoms**

**Features common to both subtypes:** hypertelorism; posterior angulation of the auricle of the ear; widow's peak; mild mental retardation; and hernia. Hypospadias, bifid scrotum, and cryptorchidism often occur in males. Females usually have normal genitalia. Occasional features that may be present in both forms include imperforate anus; cleft lip, palate, or uvula; an unusually short frenulum of the tongue; strabismus; downward slanting palpebral fissures; cranial asymmetry; and cardiac anomalies. Infrequently present are diastasis recti; agenesis of the gallbladder; renal defects; and duodenal stricture. Midline brain anomalies are common.

Twins, especially identical twins, may occur more often in families having this disorder (increased monozygotic twinning).

**Features common to Opitz G syndrome:** a weak, hoarse cry in infants; difficulty in swallowing or breathing, leading to recurrent aspiration and possibly caused by such malformations as malformed larynx, laryngotracheal cleft, and tracheoesophageal fistula; pulmonary hypoplasia; subglottic stenosis; and achalasia of the esophagus.

The bridge of the nose is usually broad and flat. Anteverted nares, micrognathia, and a high-arched palate may be present.

**Features common to Opitz BBB syndrome:** lack of respiratory and swallowing difficulties, and a hoarse voice; different facial characteristics, e.g., the bridge of the nose is often high, though also broad. Congenital heart disease, e.g., coarctation of the aorta and atrial septal defect; upper urinary tract anomalies; intestinal volvulus, and micropenis may also occur.

**Etiology** Both forms have autosomal dominant inheritance.

**Epidemiology** Both G and BBB forms are rare genetic disorders present at birth. Males are affected more often and more severely than females.

**Related Disorders** See *Imperforate Anus; VACTERL Association.*

**Treatment—Standard** Prenatal ultrasound testing may indicate the presence of Opitz syndrome. Fetal edema can be treated in utero.

Treatment often includes corrective surgery for malformations. Special education and related services may be helpful for children with this disorder. Genetic counseling will benefit patients and their families. Other treatment is symptomatic and supportive.

**Treatment—Investigational** Please contact the agencies listed under Resources, below, for the most current information. Addresses and telephone numbers of these agencies, as well as of individual experts and research centers, may be found in the Master Resources List.

## Resources

**For more information on Opitz syndrome:** National Organization for Rare Disorders (NORD); NIH/National Institute of Child Health and Human Development; John M. Opitz, M.D., Shodar Children's Hospital, Helena, Montana.

**For genetic information and genetic counseling referrals:** March of Dimes Birth Defects Foundation; Alliance of Genetic Support Groups.

## References

Mendelian Inheritance in Man, 11th ed.: V.A. McKusick; The Johns Hopkins University Press, 1994, pp. 759–761.

Brain Magnetic Resonance Imaging Findings in the Opitz G/BBB Syndrome: Extension of the Spectrum of Midline Brain Anomalies: M.R. MacDonald, et al.; Am. J. Med. Genet., 1993, vol. 46, pp. 706–711.

Syndromes of the Head and Neck, 3rd ed.: R.J. Gorlin, et al.; Oxford University Press, 1990, pp. 792–796.

BBBG Syndrome or Opitz Syndrome: New Family: A. Verloes, et al.; Am. J. Med. Genet., November 1989, vol. 34(3), pp. 313–316.

Prenatal Diagnosis of Opitz (BBB) Syndrome in the Second Trimester by Ultrasound Detection of Hypospadias and Hypertelorism: C. Hogdall, et al.; Prenat. Diagn., November 1989, vol. 9(11), pp. 783–793.

Smith's Recognizable Patterns of Human Malformation, 4th ed.: K.L. Jones; W.B. Saunders Company, 1988, pp. 114–117.

Congenital Anal Anomalies in Two Families with the Opitz G Syndrome: J.L. Tolmie, et al.; J. Med. Genet., November 1987, vol. 24(11), pp. 688–691.

The Opitz Hypertelorism-Hypospadias Syndrome: Further Delineation of the Spectrum of Clinical Findings: A.M. Dereymaeker, et al.; J. Genet. Hum., August 1987, 35(4), pp. 259–265.

The Opitz Syndrome: A New Designation for the Clinically Indistinguishable BBB and G Syndromes: M. Cappa, et al.; Am. J. Med. Genet., October 1987, vol. 28(2), pp. 303–309.

# ORAL-FACIAL-DIGITAL (OFD) SYNDROME

**Description** OFD syndrome is characterized by neuromuscular disturbances, mental disturbances, cleft palate and other facial malformations, shortened limbs, and deformities of the hands and feet. It is categorized into types I–IV.

**Synonyms**

Mohr Syndrome (Type II OFD)

Orofaciodigital Syndrome

**Signs and Symptoms** Symptoms common to all 4 types of the syndrome include neuromuscular disturbances; clefts of the tongue, jaw, and lip; overgrowth of the frenulum of the tongue; epicanthal folds; broad-based nose; syndactyly, brachydactyly, and clinodactyly; and extra divisions between skull sections.

**Type I** patients have coarse, thin hair, skin lesions, and unilateral polysyndactyly.

**Type II** is similar to type I, but polysyndactyly of the toes is bilateral.

**Type III** is characterized by the presence of extra teeth and jaw-winking.

**Type IV** patients have shortened limbs. Also present may be psychomotor retardation, clefts and other abnormalities of the jaw and tongue, and tooth malformations. Ocular manifestations include see-saw winking and exotropia.

**Etiology** OFD syndrome is believed to be inherited in types II, III, and IV as an autosomal recessive trait. Type I is X-linked dominant, and lethal in males.

**Epidemiology** The syndrome is very rare. Except for Type I, males and females are affected in equal numbers.

**Related Disorders** See *Joubert Syndrome; Nager Syndrome.*

**Juberg-Hayward syndrome (orocraniodigital syndrome)** is a rare hereditary disorder characterized by cleft lip and palate, microcephaly, thumb and toe abnormalities, and short stature due to growth hormone deficiency.

**Treatment—Standard** Reconstructive surgery for facial clefts may be necessary. Other treatment is symptomatic and supportive. Genetic counseling is recommended for patients and their families.

**Treatment—Investigational** Please contact the agencies listed under Resources, below, for the most current information. Addresses and telephone numbers of these agencies, as well as of individual experts and research centers, may be found in the Master Resources List.

## Resources

**For more information on oral-facial-digital syndrome:** National Organization for Rare Disorders (NORD); NIH/National Institute of Dental Research; FACES—National Association for the Craniofacially Handicapped; AboutFace; National Foundation for Facial Reconstruction.

**For more information on cleft palate:** American Cleft Palate Cranial Facial Association; Let's Face It.

**For genetic information and genetic counseling referrals:** March of Dimes Birth Defects Foundation; Alliance of Genetic Support Groups.

## References

Mendelian Inheritance in Man, 9th ed.: V.A. McKusick; The Johns Hopkins University Press, 1990, p. 1697.

Syndromes of the Head and Neck, 3rd ed.: R.J. Gorlin, et al.; Oxford University Press, 1990, pp. 676–686.

Prenatal Diagnosis of Mohr Syndrome by Ultrasonography: M. Iaccarino, et al.; Prenat. Diagn., November–December 1985, vol. 5(6), pp. 415–418.

The Spectrum of the Oro-Facial-Digital Syndrome: O.M. Fenton, et al.; Br. J. Plast. Surg., October l985, vol. 38(4), pp. 532–539.

Mohr Syndrome in Two Siblings: A. Gencik, et al.; J. Genet. Hum., December l983, vol. 31(4), pp. 307–315.

Syndrome of Acrofacial Dysostosis, Cleft Lip/Palate, and Triphalangeal Thumb in a Brazilian Family: A. Richieri-Costa, et al.; Am. J. Med. Genet., 1983, vol. 14, pp. 225–229.

Orocraniodigital (Juberg-Hayward) Syndrome with Growth Hormone Deficiency: H.M. Kingston, et al.; Arch. Dis. Child, October 1982, vol. 57(10), pp. 790–792.

A Case of The Orocraniodigital (Juberg-Hayward) Syndrome: N.C. Nevin, et al.; J. Med. Genet., December 1981, vol. 18(6), pp. 478–481.

# OSTEOGENESIS IMPERFECTA (OI)

**Description** Osteogenesis imperfecta is characterized by unusually fragile bones that fracture easily. There are generally considered to be 4 types, some with subtypes. The congenital form, type II, is the most severe; affected infants are either stillborn or die soon after birth of respiratory insufficiency.

**Synonyms**
>  Brittle Bone Disease
>  Lobstein Disease (Type I)
>  Vrolik Disease (Type II)

**Signs and Symptoms** Fractures, especially of the long bones of the legs, are common after even minimal trauma.

**Type I** is characterized by blue sclera, little or no deformity, normal stature, and hearing loss in about 50 percent of patients.

**Type II** is lethal in the newborn period. Infants are born with multiple fractures, marked long bone deformities, and compressed fractures.

Patients with **type III** have short stature and only a variable scleral hue. Hearing loss and dentinogenesis are common. Deformation of bones tends to be progressive.

Patients with **type IV** have normal sclera, mild bone deformity, and variable short stature. Dentinogenesis is common, but hearing loss is rare.

**Etiology** The most common form of inheritance is autosomal dominant, but a recessive pattern has been identified in a few patients. More than 50 mutations in the genes that encode the chains of type I collagen have been delineated. The nature of the mutation determines the phenotype.

**Epidemiology** Osteogenesis imperfecta occurs in 1:20,000 to 1:50,000 births in the United States.

**Treatment—Standard** Treatment is generally symptomatic. Physical therapy and hydrotherapy help strengthen muscles, increase weight-bearing capacity, and reduce the tendency to fracture.

Metal rods surgically placed in the long bones (rodding) can help prevent fracture. Plastic braces are preferable to plaster casts as protective devices because they permit greater mobility and are water-resistant. Inflatable suits can provide protection, especially to young children.

**Treatment—Investigational** Please contact the agencies listed under Resources, below, for the most current information. Addresses and telephone numbers of these agencies, as well as of individual experts and research centers, may be found in the Master Resources List.

**Resources**

**For more information on osteogenesis imperfecta:** National Organization for Rare Disorders (NORD); Osteogenesis Imperfecta Foundation; Michael P. Whyte, M.D., Shriners' Hospital for Crippled Children, St. Louis, Missouri; NIH/National Arthritis and Musculoskeletal and Skin Diseases Information Clearinghouse.

**For genetic information and genetic counseling referrals:** March of Dimes Birth Defects Foundation; Alliance of Genetic Support Groups.

**References**
Mendelian Inheritance in Man, 11th ed.: V.A. McKusick; The Johns Hopkins University Press, 1994, pp. 319–330, 2093–2095.

McKusick's Heritable Disorders of Connective Tissue, 5th ed.: P. Beighton, ed.; C.V. Mosby Company, 1993.

Cecil Textbook of Medicine, 19th ed.: J.B. Wyngaarden, et al., eds.; W.B. Saunders Company, 1992, pp. 1124–1125.

Osteogenesis Imperfecta: P.H. Byers, et al.; Ann. Rev. Med., 1992, vol. 43, pp. 269–282.

Brittle Bones–Fragile Molecules: Disorders of Collagen Gene Structure and Expression: P.H. Byers; Trends in Genetics, 1990, vol. 6, pp. 293–300.

Osteogenisis Imperfecta: J.M. Gertner and L. Root; Orthop. Clin. North Am., January 1990, vol. 21(1), pp. 151–162.

Smith's Recognizable Patterns of Human Malformation, 4th ed.: K.L. Jones; W.B. Saunders Company, 1988, pp. 432–437.

# OSTEOPETROSIS

**Description** Osteopetrosis is characterized by increased bone density and brittle bones, resulting in frequent fractures. Skeletal and other abnormalities may also be present. There is a severe, lethal form seen at birth and a milder form (Albers-Schönberg syndrome) with delayed manifestations.

**Synonyms**

> Albers-Schönberg Syndrome
> Generalized Congenital Osteosclerosis
> Ivory Bones
> Marble Bones

**Signs and Symptoms** The severe, lethal form of the disease is evident at birth and is diagnosed by skeletal x-rays. There is an increased density in bone and decreased density in marrow. Craniofacial abnormalities include macrocephaly, a deformity of the base of the skull, and delayed fontanelle closure. Dental defects, cataracts, deafness, chest deformity, growth retardation, pancytopenia, and brain damage may occur. Death usually occurs in infancy or childhood. A subtype of this form of osteopetrosis is associated with renal tubular acidosis and carbonic anhydrase II deficiency.

The delayed form (**Albers-Schönberg syndrome**) is milder and may not be diagnosed until adolescence or adulthood, when spinal pain or multiple bone fractures arouse suspicion. Vision problems, facial paralysis, and anemia may be present.

**Etiology** Lethal osteopetrosis is inherited as an autosomal recessive trait. The delayed form is generally considered to be autosomal dominant, but an autosomal recessive form has been described. The basic defect is unknown except in those patients with carbonic anhydrase II deficiency; mutations in the gene have been reported.

**Epidemiology** Males and females are equally affected in both forms of osteopetrosis.

**Related Disorders** See *Osteogenesis Imperfecta.*

**Melorheostosis** is a rare form of osteosclerosis or hyperostosis caused by a lack of calcium density in the bone. A genetic inheritance has not been established. The disorder results in shortening or deformity of at least one limb, with accompanying pain and restricted movement. Prognosis is guardedly favorable.

**Osteopoikilosis ("spotted bones")** is a rare autosomal dominant disorder that may occur concomitantly with melorheostosis, usually between the ages of 15 and 60. Although the disorder is often asymptomatic, joint pain and skin lesions may be present. Osteopoikilosis can be diagnosed by the presence of spotty shadows on x-rays of most bones.

**Treatment—Standard** For the severe form, bone marrow transplantation is curative for the bone disorder; but the outcome is largely dependent on the availability of a genotypically HLA-identical bone marrow. For patients with a mild course, bone marrow transplantation can be postponed until an HLA-identical unrelated donor is found.

**Treatment—Investigational** Please contact the agencies listed under Resources, below, for the most current information. Addresses and telephone numbers of these agencies, as well as of individual experts and research centers, may be found in the Master Resources List.

**Resources**

**For more information on osteopetrosis:** National Organization for Rare Disorders (NORD); NIH/National Arthritis and Musculoskeletal and Skin Diseases Information Clearinghouse; Research Trust for Metabolic Diseases in Children.

**For genetic information and genetic counseling referrals:** March of Dimes Birth Defects Foundation; Alliance of Genetic Support Groups.

**References**

Bone Marrow Transplantation for Autosomal Recessive Osteopetrosis: J.A. Gerritson, et al.; J. Pediatr., 1994, vol. 125, pp. 896–902.

Mendelian Inheritance in Man, 11th ed.: V.A. McKusick; The Johns Hopkins University Press, 1994, pp. 1081, 2097–2099.

Smith's Recognizable Patterns of Human Malformation, 4th ed.: K.L. Jones; W.B. Saunders Company, 1988, pp. 353–355.

Bone Marrow Transplantation: Research Report; U.S. Dept. of Health and Human Services, National Cancer Institute, September 1986, NIH publication No. 86-1178.

Juvenile Osteopetrosis: Effects on Blood and Bone of Prednisone and a Low Calcium, High Phosphate Diet: L.M. Dorantes, et al.; Arch. Dis. Child, July 1986, vol. 61(7), pp. 666–670.

# OTO-PALATO-DIGITAL SYNDROME

**Description** The syndrome is expressed in 2 forms, **OPD-I (Taybi syndrome)** and **OPD-II (Andre syndrome),** categorized in part by mode of inheritance. Major characteristics of both forms include cleft palate, hearing loss, and short, broad distal phalanges of thumbs and toes. OPD-I typically is milder, with fewer symptoms. Complete expression shows up only in males; females are mildly affected with some symptoms.

**Synonyms**

> Andre Syndrome (OPD-II)
> Digito-Oto-Palatal Syndrome
> Palatao-Oto-Digital Syndrome
> Taybi Syndrome (OPD-I)

**Signs and Symptoms** Male patients with **OPD-I** typically have frontal bone prominence, cleft palate, downward slanting palpebral fissures, conductive hearing loss, abnormal shortness of fingers and toes, and mild mental retardation and short stature. Also seen are hypoplastic facial bones; a broad bridge of the nose; short, broad thumbs and great toes; wide spaces between the toes; syndactyly; short fingernails; dislocation of the head of the radius; and slow speech development secondary to hearing loss and mental retardation.

Females carriers of OPD-I may have hypertelorism, frontal bone prominence, a depressed nasal bridge, and a flat midface.

Major characteristics in males with **OPD-II** include microcephaly, hypertelorism, broad forehead, downward slanting palpebral fissures, flat bridge of the nose, small mouth, cleft palate, micrognathia, flexed and overlapping short fingers, short toes, and bowing of the long bones of the forearms and legs. Mental retardation occasionally is present.

Female carriers for OPD-II have milder symptoms and signs, such as arched palate, broad face, downward slanting palpebral fissures, low-set ears, split uvula, and short stature.

**Etiology** OPD-I is inherited as an X-linked recessive trait with variable expression in females. OPD-II is inherited as an X-linked semi-dominant trait. Females with OPD-II may be mildly affected.

**Epidemiology** OPD-I and OPD-II affect males only. Carrier females are more mildly symptomatic; no cases of full expression in a female have been reported. Approximately 30 cases of OPD-I and 9 cases of OPD-II have been seen.

**Related Disorders** See *Craniometaphyseal Dysplasia; Larsen Syndrome; Oral-Facial-Digital Syndrome; Osteopetrosis.*

**Frontometaphyseal dysplasia** is characterized by coarse facial features that include a wide nasal bridge, hypertelorism, micrognathia, and sinus hypoplasia. Multiple deformities of the teeth and bones may also be present. Occasionally mental retardation may occur.

**Treatment—Standard** Therapy is symptomatic and supportive, and geared to specific individual conditions. Genetic counseling may be helpful.

**Treatment—Investigational** Please contact the agencies listed under Resources, below, for the most current information. Addresses and telephone numbers of these agencies, as well as of individual experts and research centers, may be found in the Master Resources List.

**Resources**

**For more information on oto-palato-digital syndrome:** National Organization for Rare Disorders (NORD); NIH/National Institute of Child Health and Human Development; National Craniofacial Foundation; Let's Face It; FACES—National Association for the Craniofacially Handicapped; National Foundation for Facial Reconstruction..

**For genetic information and genetic counseling referrals:** March of Dimes Birth Defects Foundation; Alliance of Genetic Support Groups.

**References**

Mendelian Inheritance in Man, 11th ed.: V.A. McKusick; The Johns Hopkins University Press, 1994, pp. 2504–2505.

Birth Defects Encyclopedia: M.L. Buyse, ed.-in-chief; Blackwell Scientific Publications, 1990, pp. 1340–1342.

Syndromes of the Head and Neck, 3rd ed.: R.J. Gorlin, et al.; Oxford University Press, 1990, pp.

Smith's Recognizable Patterns of Human Malformation, 4th ed.: K.L. Jones; W.B. Saunders Company, 1988, pp. 232–234.

Temporal Bone Findings in a Case of Otopalatodigital Syndrome: S.R. Shi; Arch. Otolaryngol., February 1985, vol. 111(2), pp. 119–121.

# PALLISTER-HALL SYNDROME

**Description** Pallister-Hall syndrome is a very rare developmental disorder characterized by hypothalamic hamartomablastoma, postaxial polydactyly, imperforate anus, and hypopituitarism. Unusual facial features, mental retardation, hydrocephalus, and cranial pressure may also occur. Symptoms are apparent at birth, and newborns must be monitored closely for signs of hypopituitarism that can lead to life-threatening complications if left untreated.

**Synonyms**

> Hall-Pallister Syndrome
>
> Hypothalamic Hamartoblastoma, Hypopituitarism, Imperforate Anus, and Postaxial Polydactyly

**Signs and Symptoms** The most significant feature of Pallister-Hall syndrome is a benign tumor in the hypothalamus. The tumor replaces the hypothalamus, and the anterior lobe of the pituitary gland may be missing. Hypopituitarism, imperforate anus, and postaxial polysyndactyly with underdeveloped or absent nails are other characteristic features of Pallister-Hall syndrome.

Symptoms of hypopituitarism may be present at birth and may include hypoglycemia, abnormal electrolyte levels, and metabolic acidosis. Lethargy and jaundice may also occur. Hypothalamic hamartoblastoma may block the circulation of cerebrospinal fluid, causing hydrocephalus. Increased cranial pressure may occur as a result of tumor enlargement.

Children with Pallister-Hall syndrome may also have ears that are unusually small and rotated toward the back of the head; a short, flat-bridged nose; and a longer-than-usual philtrum. Microglossia may be associated with malformations of the larynx and epiglottis. Affected children may show signs of puberty earlier than usual.

Some infants with Pallister-Hall syndrome may have natal teeth, buccal frenula, pes cavus, syndactyly, and palmar creases. Other symptoms may include a short neck, short limbs, dislocated hips, and spinal defects. Pulmonary hypoplasia with abnormal lung formation, malformed and/or displaced kidneys, and heart defects may also occur. Microphallus and cryptorchidism are common in affected males. As more affected patients are being detected, the spectrum of the disorder is expanding and more mildly affected patients are being reported.

**Etiology** Most diagnosed cases of Pallister-Hall syndrome have been isolated events, apparently due to an unexplained mutation in genetic material. Rarely, Pallister-Hall syndrome may be familial. Although the gene for Pallister-Hall syndrome has not been identified, some scientists suggest that Pallister-Hall syndrome may be inherited as an autosomal dominant trait in some individuals.

**Epidemiology** Pallister-Hall syndrome affects males twice as often as females. More than 2 dozen cases of this disorder have been documented in the medical literature.

**Related Disorders** There are 3 disorders known as midline malformation complexes: Pallister-Hall syndrome, oral-facial-digital syndrome, and hydrolethalus syndrome. These disorders appear to originate in the early stages of fetal development, resulting in abnormal formation of bones and tissue along the midline of the body. Although the syndromes are characterized by different features, overlapping symptoms can make it difficult to differentiate among them. See **Oral-Facial-Digital Syndrome.**

**Hydrolethalus syndrome** is a very rare developmental disorder characterized by severe central nervous system malformations and extra fingers and/or toes. Two great toes on each foot, underdeveloped eyes, a small lower jaw, and a poorly formed nose are common. Macrocephaly is present, with prominent frontal and occiptal regions. Lung and heart abnormalities may also occur.

See also **Smith-Lemli-Opitz Syndrome.**

**Treatment—Standard** Infants with Pallister-Hall syndrome who have hypopituitarism must be treated immediately with hormonal replacement therapy. Treatment of hypopituitarism usually resolves the associated symptoms (hypoglycemia, abnormal electrolyte levels, and/or metabolic acidosis). Close monitoring and prompt treatment is imperative to prevent severe life-threatening complications.

Periodic examinations with specialized equipment to monitor the brain tumor associated with this disorder are essential. Magnetic resonance imaging is often required since CT scan may not always detect hypothalamic hamartoblastomas. Surgical removal of a hamartoblastoma may be necessary if cranial pressure increases, hydrocephalus occurs, and other symptoms arise as a result of pressure on the brain.

**Treatment—Investigational** Researchers at the University of California at Los Angeles and the National Institutes of Health are conducting a research program for people affected by Pallister-Hall syndrome. The study hopes to identify the gene that is responsible for this disorder. Researchers also want to study and document the full range of symptoms that are associated with this disorder. Individuals who wish to be included in this study should meet at least 2 of the 4 criteria for the study. These criteria are: hypothalamic hamartoma or hamartoblastoma; polydactyly of one or more limbs; imperforate anus; and a family member affected with Pallister-Hall syndrome. For more information on this research program, please contact Leslie Biesecker, M.D., National Center for Human Genome Research, or John Graham, Jr., M.D., Cedars-Sinai Medical Center, Los Angeles.

Please contact the agencies listed under Resources, below, for the most current information. Addresses and telephone numbers of these agencies, as well as of individual experts and research centers, may be found in the Master Resources List.

**Resources**

**For more information on Pallister-Hall syndrome:** National Organization for Rare Disorders (NORD); The Arc (a national organization on mental retardation); NIH/National Institute of Child Health and Human Development; American Brain Tumor Association.

**For genetic information and genetic counseling referrals:** March of Dimes Birth Defects Foundation; Alliance of Genetic Support Groups.

**References**

Mendelian Inheritance in Man, 11th ed.: V.A. McKusick; The Johns Hopkins University Press, 1994, pp. 774–775.

Online Mendelian Inheritance in Man (OMIM): V.A. McKusick; last edit date 3/29/94, entry number 146510.

Recurrence of Pallister-Hall Syndrome in Two Sibs: H.M. Thomas, et al.; J. Med. Genet., 1994, vol. 31, pp. 145–147.

Autosomal Dominant Transmission of the Pallister-Hall Syndrome: K.F. Topf, et al.; December 1993, vol. 123(6), pp. 943–946.

Twin Fetuses with Abnormalities That Overlap with Three Midline Malformation Complexes: S.R. Hingorani, et al.; Am. J. Med. Genet., November 1, 1991, vol. 41(2), pp. 230–235.

Birth Defects Encyclopedia: M.L Buyse, ed.-in-chief; Blackwell Scientific Publications, 1990, pp. 932–934.

A Cluster of Pallister-Hall Syndrome Cases (Congenital Hypothalamic Hamartoblastoma Syndrome): J.M. Graham, et al.; Am. J. Med. Genet. Suppl., 1986, vol. 2, pp. 53–63.

# PALLISTER-KILLIAN SYNDROME

**Description** Features of Pallister-Killian syndrome include severe retardation, seizures, hypotonia, and distinctive facies.

**Synonyms**

>Isochromosome 12p- Mosaicism
>Killian Syndrome
>Mosaic Tetrasomy 12p-
>Pallister Mosaic Aneuploidy
>Pallister Mosaic Syndrome
>Teschler-Nicola/Killian Syndrome
>Teschler-Nicola Syndrome
>Tetrasomy 12p- Mosaicism

**Signs and Symptoms** Congenital manifestations are hypertelorism and distinctive facies. Growth deficiency, balding, and hypotonia develop during infancy and early childhood. Later in childhood, contractures, seizures, and severe delay in psychomotor development occur.

**Etiology** Karyotype of peripheral lymphocytes may be normal, but cultured fibroblasts and direct bone marrow analysis will show tetrasomy for 12p. All recorded cases have been sporadic.

**Epidemiology** Males and females are affected in equal numbers. Approximately 30 cases have been reported.

**Treatment—Standard** Prenatal diagnosis is made by amniocentesis or by cytogenetic studies of the bone marrow. Treatment of Pallister-Killian syndrome is symptomatic and supportive. Patients can benefit from early intervention programs for the mildly to moderately mentally retarded that emphasize educational, verbal, mobility, self-care, and social skills.

Surgical procedures, including plastic septum correction and functional septorhinoplasty, may be beneficial.

Genetic counseling is recommended for families of children with Pallister-Killian syndrome.

**Treatment—Investigational** Please contact the agencies listed under Resources, below, for the most current information. Addresses and telephone numbers of these agencies, as well as of individual experts and research centers, may be found in the Master Resources List.

**Resources**

**For more information on Pallister-Killian syndrome:** National Organization for Rare Disorders (NORD); NIH/National Institute for Child Health and Human Development; Pallister-Killian Family Support Group.

**For genetic information and genetic counseling referrals:** March of Dimes Birth Defects Foundation; Alliance of Genetic Support Groups.

**References**

Birth Defects Encyclopedia: M.L. Buyse, ed.-in-chief; Blackwell Scientific Publications, 1990, p. 1353.

Mosaicism in Pallister i(12p) Syndrome: S.L. Wenger, et al.; Am. J. Med. Genet., April 1990, vol. 35(4), pp. 523–525.

Prenatal Diagnosis of Pallister-Killian Syndrome: S. Soukup, et al.; Am. J. Med. Genet., April 1990, vol. 35(4), pp. 526–528.

Isochromosome 12p Mosaicism (Pallister Mosaic Aneuploidy or Pallister-Killian Syndrome): Report of 11 Cases: J.F. Reynolds, et al.; Am. J. Med. Genet., June 1987, vol. 27(2), pp. 257–274.

Mosaic Tetrasomy 12p: Four New Cases, and Confirmation of the Chromosomal Origin of the Supernumerary Chromosome in One of the Original Pallister-Mosaic Syndrome Cases: D. Warburton, et al.; Am. J. Med. Genet., June 1987, vol. 27(2), pp. 275–283.

Chromosomal Mosaicism in the Killian/Teschler-Nicola Syndrome: L.J. Raffel, et al.; Am. J. Med. Genet., August 1986, vol. 24(4), pp. 607–611.

# PALLISTER-W SYNDROME

**Description** Pallister-W syndrome is characterized by facial malformations and by seizures. Mental retardation, speech problems, and bone deformities are common.

**Synonyms**
> W Syndrome

**Signs and Symptoms** Apparent at birth, symptoms include ocular hypertelorism; a broad, flat nasal bridge; central clefting of the palate or upper lip; seizures; and mental retardation. There may also be bone abnormalities in the extremities. Cowlick, missing teeth, a high forehead, and slanting eyelids have also been noted.

**Etiology** The exact cause of Pallister-W syndrome is not known, but inheritance is thought to be either X-linked recessive or autosomal dominant.

**Epidemiology** Pallister-W syndrome affects males and females in equal numbers. However, males are more severely affected.

**Related Disorders** See *Oto-Palato-Digital Syndrome; Larsen Syndrome; Oral-Facial-Digital Syndrome.*

**Frontometaphyseal dysplasia** is a rare genetic disorder characterized by coarse facial features that include a wide nasal bridge, ocular hypertelorism, overgrowth of the bone over the eyes, micrognathia, and incomplete development of the sinuses. Multiple deformities of the teeth and bones may also be present. Occasionally mental retardation may occur.

**Treatment—Standard** Surgical repair of the palate and lip clefting and of the deformities of the extremities may be indicated. Antiseizure medication may be prescribed. Special education and related services are beneficial.

Genetic counseling is recommended for patients and their families. Other treatment is symptomatic and supportive.

**Treatment—Investigational** Researchers are studying a Teflon-glycerine paste that is applied to the rear of the pharynx in a minor surgical procedure. For further information, contact William N. Williams, D.D.S., University of Florida.

Please contact the agencies listed under Resources, below, for the most current information. Addresses and telephone numbers of these agencies, as well as of individual experts and research centers, may be found in the Master Resources List.

**Resources**

**For more information on Pallister-W syndrome:** National Organization for Rare Disorders (NORD); NIH/National Institute of Child Health and Human Development; Forward Face; National Craniofacial Foundation; FACES—National Association for the Craniofacially Handicapped; American Cleft Palate Cranial Facial Association; Children's Craniofacial Association; Craniofacial Family Association; AboutFace; National Foundation for Facial Reconstruction.

**For genetic information and genetic counseling referrals:** March of Dimes Birth Defects Foundation; Alliance of Genetic Support Groups.

**References**
Mendelian Inheritance in Man, 11th ed.: V.A. McKusick; The Johns Hopkins University Press, 1994, p. 2506.

Birth Defects Encyclopedia: M.L. Buyse, ed.-in-chief; Blackwell Scientific Publications, 1990, pp. 1354–1355.

# PARRY-ROMBERG SYNDROME

**Description** Parry-Romberg syndrome is characterized by unilateral soft tissue atrophy of the face. The syndrome can resolve spontaneously or worsen slowly and then stabilize.

**Synonyms**
> Facial Hemiatrophy
> Progressive Hemifacial Atrophy
> Romberg Syndrome
> Romberg Hemifacial Atrophy

**Signs and Symptoms** Parry-Romberg syndrome is characterized by abrupt unilateral atrophy of facial tissue, which can spread to the tongue, soft palate, and mucous membranes of the gums. Muscle and bone are rarely affected.

On the affected side there may be sensory impairment, hyperhidrosis, and tear duct dysfunction. Facial features may shift to the affected side, and the eye and cheek may become sunken. Some cases are accompanied by pain, similar to that which occurs with trigeminal neuralgia. Facial hair may turn white and fall out. Contralateral jacksonian (focal) epilepsy may occur.

**Etiology** The etiology of Parry-Romberg syndrome is not known. Possible causes include injury, irritation, neuritis in the peripheral sympathetic nervous system, or a trigeminal nerve lesion. Some cases may be a type of scleroderma. Nearly all cases have been sporadic.

**Epidemiology** Parry-Romberg syndrome is a rare disorder that affects males and females in equal numbers. Onset is usually during the 20s.

**Related Disorders** See *Scleroderma; Trigeminal Neuralgia; Horner Syndrome.*

**Treatment—Standard** Treatment of Parry-Romberg syndrome is by reconstructive or microvascular surgery. Some cases may respond to fat cell injection or silicone implantation. Muscle or bone grafts may also be helpful. Other treatment is symptomatic and supportive.

**Treatment—Investigational** Please contact the agencies listed under Resources, below, for the most current information. Addresses and telephone numbers of these agencies, as well as of individual experts and research centers, may be found in the Master Resources List.

**Resources**

**For more information on Parry-Romberg syndrome:** National Organization for Rare Disorders (NORD); FACES—National Association for the Craniofacially Handicapped; Society for the Rehabilitation of the Facially Disfigured; National Craniofacial Foundation; NIH/National Institute of Neurological Disorders and Stroke; NIH/National Institute of Dental Research.

**References**

Mendelian Inheritance in Man, 11th ed.: V.A. McKusick; The Johns Hopkins University Press, 1994, p. 621.

Progressive Hemifacial Atrophy (Parry-Romberg Disease): M.T. Miller, et al.; J. Pediatr. Ophthalmol. Strabismus, January–February 1987, vol. 24(1), pp. 27–36.

Liposuction Fat Grafts in Face Wrinkles and Hemifacial Atrophy: A. Chajchir, et al.; Aesthetic Plast. Surg., 1986, vol. 10(2), pp. 115–117.

The Use of Free Revascularized Grafts in the Amelioration of Hemifacial Atrophy: M.J. Jurkiewicz, et al.; Plast. Reconstr. Surg., July 1985, vol. 76(1), pp. 44–55.

Hemifacial Atrophy: A Review of an Unusual Craniofacial Deformity with a Report of a Case: D.D. Dedo; Arch. Otolaryngol., September 1978, vol. 104(9), pp. 538–541.

# PENTA X SYNDROME

**Description** A chromosomal disorder affecting females, penta X syndrome is characterized primarily by mental and growth deficiencies, upward slanting eyes with epicanthal folds, and patent ductus arteriosus.

**Synonyms**

49,XXXXX Syndrome

Pentasomy X

**Signs and Symptoms** Facial features include microcephaly, an unusually round face, hypertelorism, and the characteristic upwardly slanting eyes and epicanthal folds. A short neck, low hairline, low-set ears, dental abnormalities, and microcephaly are common. The hands of females with the syndrome are often small with simian creases and 5th-finger clinodactyly. Foot deformities include talipes equinovarus and overlapping toes. Multiple joint dislocations may affect the shoulder, elbow, hips, wrists, or fingers. Additionally, cardiac defects are common.

Mental deficiency is uniformly present. Affected children may fail to thrive and have growth deficiencies that can result in short stature.

**Etiology** The syndrome is caused by 3 successive nondisjunctions at maternal meiosis.

**Epidemiology** Only about 2 dozen cases have been reported.

**Related Disorders** See *Down Syndrome.*

**Treatment—Standard** Patent ductus arteriosus is dealt with surgically. Other treatment is symptomatic and supportive. Special education, physical therapy, and other medical, social, or vocational services may be beneficial, as may genetic counseling.

**Treatment—Investigational** Please contact the agencies listed under Resources, below, for the most current information. Addresses and telephone numbers of these agencies, as well as of individual experts and research centers, may be found in the Master Resources List.

**Resources**

**For more information on penta X syndrome:** National Organization for Rare Disorders (NORD); The Arc (a national organization on mental retardation); NIH/National Institute of Child Health and Human Development.

**For information about education of children with learning disabilities:** National Information Center for Handicapped Children and Youth.

**For genetic information and genetic counseling referrals:** March of Dimes Birth Defects Foundation; Alliance of Genetic Support Groups.

### References

Penta X Syndrome: A Case Report with Review of the Literature; R. Kassai, et al.; Am. J. Med. Genet., 1991, vol. 40, pp. 51–56.

Smith's Recognizable Patterns of Human Malformation, 4th ed.: K.L. Jones; W.B. Saunders Company, 1988, p. 73.

49,XXXXX Syndrome: R. Fragoso, et al.; Ann. Genet., 1982, vol. 25(3), pp. 145–148.

# PENTALOGY OF CANTRELL

**Description** Pentalogy of Cantrell is a congenital disorder of the thoracic cavity and abdominal wall.

**Synonyms**

Cantrell Syndrome

Cantrell-Haller-Ravich Syndrome

Cantrell Pentalogy

Pentalogy Syndrome

Peritoneopericardial Diaphragmatic Hernia

Thoracoabdominal Ectopia Cordis

Thoracoabdominal Syndrome

**Signs and Symptoms** Characteristics include the following: chest wall defects that include clefting; omphalocele; agenesis of the diaphragm muscles and location of the heart just under the skin; and an opening between the area of the body that contains the bowels, liver, and heart. Often the above defects impair the infant's breathing and heart functions and cause widespread infection of the abdominal cavity. It is thought that abnormal development of midline tissue originates 14 to 18 days after conception. Intelligence is usually normal.

**Etiology** Pentalogy of Cantrell can be transmitted by an X-linked gene, or it can arise sporadically.

**Epidemiology** Pentalogy of Cantrell affects 5.5 infants per 1 million live births. Males are affected more frequently and more severely than females. Approximately 50 cases have been identified in the medical literature.

**Treatment—Standard** The disorder is usually apparent at birth or shortly after. Ultrasound testing can determine if the condition is present in utero. A series of surgeries is required to repair the thoracoabdominal defects. Cardiac defects are repaired when the child is older.

Genetic counseling is recommended for families of affected children. Other treatment is symptomatic and supportive.

**Treatment—Investigational** Please contact the agencies listed under Resources, below, for the most current information. Addresses and telephone numbers of these agencies, as well as of individual experts and research centers, may be found in the Master Resources List.

**Resources**

**For more information on pentalogy of Cantrell:** National Organization for Rare Disorders (NORD); NIH/National Institute of Child Health and Human Development.

**For genetic information and genetic counseling referrals:** March of Dimes Birth Defects Foundation; Alliance of Genetic Support Groups.

### References

Mendelian Inheritance in Man, 11th ed.: V.A. McKusick; The Johns Hopkins University Press, 1994, p. 2545.

Nelson Textbook of Pediatrics, 14th ed.: R.E. Behrman, ed.-in-chief; W.B. Saunders Company, 1992, pp. 1032–1033.

Pentalogy of Cantrell and Ectopia Cordis: A Familial Developmental Field Complex: R.A. Marti; Am. J. Med. Genet., April 1992, vol. 42(6), pp. 839, 841.

Birth Defects Encyclopedia: M.L. Buyse, ed.-in-chief; Blackwell Scientific Publications, 1990, pp. 1375–1376.

Gastrointestinal Disease, Pathophysiology, Diagnosis, and Management, 4th ed.: M.H. Sleisenger, ed.; W.B. Saunders Company, 1989, pp. 1015–1017.

Prenatal Diagnosis of Pentalogy of Cantrell: A. Ghidini, et al.; J. Ultrasound Med., October 1988, vol. 7(10), pp. 567–572.

# PFEIFFER SYNDROME

**Description** Pfeiffer syndrome is an inherited disorder primarily characterized by coronal craniostenosis and abnormalities of the face as well as of the hands and feet.

**Synonyms**

Acrocephalosyndactyly V

**Signs and Symptoms** Craniofacial features include acrobrachycephaly, hypertelorism, and slightly slanted eyelid folds. Elevated intracranial pressure may occur, but intelligence is usually normal. An underdeveloped maxilla, high-arched palate, and prominent mandible may be apparent. Maleruption of the teeth may cause malocclusion. The facial appearance usually improves with age.

Partial syndactyly characterizes the toes and fingers, sometimes with broad, short thumbs and big toes. The small phalanges in the thumb may be either triangular or trapezoidal in shape and occasionally may be fused with the distal phalanx so that the thumb points away from the other fingers. A varus deformity may also be present. A mild hearing loss due to a defect in the middle ear may occur.

**Etiology** Pfeiffer syndrome is inherited as an autosomal dominant trait. Some patients have mutations of fibroblast growth factor receptor 1 **(FGFR1)**. More surprisingly, many patients have mutations of fibroblast growth factor receptor 2, which is the same gene involved in Crouzon disease and Jackson-Weiss syndrome.

**Epidemiology** This rare disorder affects males and females equally.

**Related Disorders** See *Apert Syndrome; Saethre-Chotzen Syndrome; Crouzon Disease; Jackson-Weiss Syndrome.*

**Treatment—Standard** Treatment is symptomatic and supportive. Early childhood interventions include surgery to relieve intracranial pressure and the Le Fort III advancement surgery to prevent progressive malformation of the upper jaw. Genetic counseling may be beneficial.

**Treatment—Investigational** Please contact the agencies listed under Resources, below, for the most current information. Addresses and telephone numbers of these agencies, as well as of individual experts and research centers, may be found in the Master Resources List.

**Resources**

**For more information on Pfeiffer syndrome:** National Organization for Rare Disorders (NORD); NIH/National Institute of Child Health and Human Development; FACES—National Association for the Craniofacially Handicapped; Forward Face; National Craniofacial Foundation; Society for the Rehabilitation of the Facially Disfigured; AboutFace.

**For genetic information and genetic counseling referrals:** March of Dimes Birth Defects Foundation; Alliance of Genetic Support Groups.

**References**

Mendelian Inheritance in Man, 11th ed.: V.A. McKusick; The Johns Hopkins University Press, 1994, pp. 21–22.
Smith's Recognizable Patterns of Human Malformation, 4th ed.: K.L. Jones; W.B. Saunders Company, 1988, pp. 368–369.
Maxillary Growth Following Le Fort III Advancement Surgery in Crouzon, Apert, and Pfeiffer Syndromes: D.I. Bachmayer, et al.; Am. J. Orthod. Dentofacial Orthop., November 1986, 90(5), pp. 420–430.
Hearing Loss in Pfeiffer's Syndrome: C.W. Cremers; Int. J. Pediatr. Otorhinolaryngol., December 1981, 3(4), pp. 343–353.
Variable Expression in Pfeiffer Syndrome: H.M. Sanchez, et al.; J. Med. Genet., February 1981, 18(1), pp. 73–75.

# PHOCOMELIA SYNDROME

**Description** The primary characteristic is deficient limb development, which is accompanied by growth and mental deficiencies and multiple other defects.

**Signs and Symptoms** Onset of growth deficiencies is both pre- and postnatal. The limb defects are variable. Commonly, the upper limbs are affected, and sections of the hands and arms may be malformed or missing. The legs and feet may also be involved. The hands and feet may be attached close to the body, or the limbs may be abnormally small.

The head may be small, with sparse, silvery-blond hair. Other characteristics include facial hemangioma, hypertelorism, cleft lip and possibly also cleft palate, micrognathia, and cryptorchidism.

Among the less common symptoms and signs are encephalocele, hydrocephalus, microphthalmia, corneal clouding, cataracts, hypospadias, a bicornuate uterus, thrombocytopenia, and kidney and heart abnormalities.

**Thalidomide syndrome,** a form of phocomelia syndrome caused by drugs, is usually the result of ingestion of thalidomide by a woman during pregnancy. Characteristics include limb defects of the arms or all of the limbs; abnormalities of the eyes and the ears, with possible deafness; paralysis of the face, with possible limited eye movements; heart defects; fistulas between the rectum, urethra, and vagina; abnormalities of internal organs; and cryptorchidism. A small percentage of individuals have spinal abnormalities and growth deficiencies. This type of phocomelia syndrome can also be caused by the acne drug Accutane.

**Roberts–SC phocomelia syndrome** is an inherited birth defect that may represent phocomelia syndrome in its mildest form. There have been a number of patients exhibiting overlap of symptoms between Roberts–SC syndrome and thalidomide syndrome.

**Etiology** Phocomelia syndrome is inherited as an autosomal recessive trait. Roberts–SC phocomelia syndrome also is inherited through recessive genes. The 2 disorders may be different expressions of a gene or represent variable severity of the same disorder.

The drug thalidomide, taken by a woman during pregnancy, caused a surge of infants born with phocomelia during the 1960s. The drug Accutane, taken for treatment of acne, can also cause phocomelia.

**Epidemiology** The hereditary form or forms are very rare, affecting only a dozen or more infants born each year. Males and females are affected in equal numbers. An upsurge of the number of phocomelia cases signals that certain drugs are causing the birth defect.

**Related Disorders** Many birth defects are associated with malformed or missing limbs. See *Thrombocytopenia–Absent Radius Syndrome.*

**Treatment—Standard** Treatment and rehabilitation of the limb deformities should be planned in infancy. Individual prostheses and ortheses may be needed. Genetic counseling will be helpful.

**Treatment—Investigational** Please contact the agencies listed under Resources, below, for the most current information. Addresses and telephone numbers of these agencies, as well as of individual experts and research centers, may be found in the Master Resources List.

**Resources**

**For more information on phocomelia syndrome:** National Organization for Rare Disorders (NORD); The Arc (a national organization on mental retardation); NIH/National Heart, Lung and Blood Institute Information Center; Association of Children's Prosthetic and Orthotic Clinics; National Rehabilitation Information Center; Thalidomide Society.

**For genetic information and genetic counseling referrals:** March of Dimes Birth Defects Foundation; Alliance of Genetic Support Groups.

**References**

Recognition of Thalidomide Defects: R.C. Smithells and C.G.H. Newman; J. Med. Genet., 1992, vol. 29, pp. 716–723.

Treatment and Rehabilitation of Dysmelic Children: L. Kullmann; Magy Traumatol. Orthop., 1989, vol. 32(2), pp. 99–106.

Roberts–SC Phocomelia Syndrome: Cytogenetic Findings and Clinical Variability in Three Brothers: G. Antinolo, et al.; An. Esp. Pediatr., September 1988, vol. 29(3), pp. 239–243.

Smith's Recognizable Patterns of Human Malformation, 4th ed.: K.L. Jones; W.B. Saunders Company, 1988, pp. 256–257.

Mendelian Inheritance in Man, 8th ed.: V.A. McKusick; The Johns Hopkins University Press, 1986, pp. 584, 907.

# PIERRE ROBIN SYNDROME

**Description** Pierre Robin syndrome is characterized by micrognathia, glossoptosis, and cleft soft palate. The latter 2 signs may be consequences of the underdevelopment of the jaw prior to 9 weeks' gestation.

**Synonyms**

Pierre Robin Anomalad
Pierre Robin Complex
Pierre Robin Sequence
Robin Anomalad
Robin Sequence
Robin Syndrome

**Signs and Symptoms** The placement of the tongue may obstruct normal breathing. This in turn can result in failure to thrive, dysphagia, and apneic spells. Cyanosis may be evident. Respiratory disturbances may lead to cor pulmonale, pulmonary hypertension, and possibly congestive heart failure. Infants may vomit and develop sleep disturbances that persist into adulthood.

**Etiology** The appearance of Pierre Robin syndrome with no underlying disorder may indicate autosomal recessive inheritance. The syndrome may also result from mechanical constraint of the fetus in the womb; e.g., the chin may be compressed in such a way as to limit its normal development. Recent research also suggests that the development of Pierre Robin syndrome may be influenced by drugs taken by a woman during pregnancy.

**Epidemiology** Pierre Robin syndrome affects males and females equally. In about one-third of cases it occurs as a feature in a multiple defect disorder, such as trisomy 18 syndrome, Stickler syndrome, or a number of other syndromes.

**Related Disorders** See *Stickler Syndrome; Cerebro-Costo-Mandibular Syndrome; Treacher Collins Syndrome.*

**Treatment—Standard** Pierre Robin syndrome can be detected in utero using ultrasound imaging.

Affected infants should be observed closely for breathing difficulties. Intubation or tracheostomy may be necessary.

Since spontaneous closure of the cleft soft palate may occur, surgical correction may be postponed for a few years. Surgery to improve the appearance of the jaw may be beneficial.

Genetic counseling may be helpful for patients and their families. Other treatment is symptomatic and palliative.

**Treatment—Investigational** Please contact the agencies listed under Resources, below, for the most current information. Addresses and telephone numbers of these agencies, as well as of individual experts and research centers, may be found in the Master Resources List.

**Resources**

**For more information on Pierre Robin syndrome:** National Organization for Rare Disorders (NORD); FACES—National Association for the Craniofacially Handicapped; National Craniofacial Foundation; Forward Face.

**For more information on cleft palate:** American Cleft Palate Cranial Facial Association; Let's Face It; NIH/National Institute of Child Health and Human Development.

**For genetic information and genetic counseling referrals:** March of Dimes Birth Defects Foundation; Alliance of Genetic Support Groups.

**References**

Smith's Recognizable Patterns of Human Malformation, 4th ed.: K.L. Jones; W.B. Saunders Company, 1988, pp. 196–199.

Glossoptosis-Apnea Syndrome in Infancy: F. Cozzi and A. Pierro; Pediatrics, May 1985, vol. 75(5), pp. 836–843.

The Pierre Robin Syndrome Reassessed in the Light of Recent Research: J.R. Edwards and D.R. Newall; Br. J. Plast. Surg., July 1985, vol. 38(3), pp. 339–342.

# POLAND SYNDROME

**Description** Poland syndrome is a congenital developmental disorder with variable unilateral involvement of chest muscles combined with syndactyly and other abnormalities of the hand, arm, and wrist.

**Synonyms**

Poland Anomaly

Poland Syndactyly

**Signs and Symptoms** Unilateral hypoplasia or absence of the pectoralis major muscle, along with ipsilateral syndactyly, characterizes the syndrome. In 75 percent of cases, the abnormality affects the right side of the body. Other chest muscles, the cartilage and ribs, and the breast and areola may be absent or abnormally developed on the affected side. Beside the ipsilateral syndactyly, other abnormalities of the hand, arm, forearm, and wrist may be present. Occasionally there are renal anomalies and hemivertebrae.

**Etiology** The cause of Poland syndrome is not known. Most cases are sporadic. An autosomal dominant mode of transmission is suggested in some instances.

**Epidemiology** Poland syndrome affects males 3 times as often as females. Incidence is about 1:30,000 births. Approximately 10 percent of patients with hand syndactyly may have Poland syndrome.

**Treatment—Standard** Reconstructive surgery is performed to replace absent chest muscles, correct hand abnormalities, and graft ribs into place.

**Treatment—Investigational** Please contact the agencies listed under Resources, below, for the most current information. Addresses and telephone numbers of these agencies, as well as of individual experts and research centers, may be found in the Master Resources List.

**Resources**

**For more information on Poland syndrome:** National Organization for Rare Disorders (NORD); NIH/National Arthritis and Musculoskeletal and Skin Diseases Information Clearinghouse.

**For genetic information and genetic counseling referrals:** March of Dimes Birth Defects Foundation; Alliance of Genetic Support Groups.

**References**

Mendelian Inheritance in Man, 11th ed.: V.A. McKusick; The Johns Hopkins University Press, 1994, pp. 1168–1169.

Smith's Recognizable Patterns of Human Malformation, 4th ed.: K.L. Jones; W.B. Saunders Company, 1988, pp. 260–261.

Early Correction of the Thoracic Deformity of Poland's Syndrome in Children with the Latissimus Dorsi Muscle Flap: Long Term Follow-up of Two Cases: H. Anderl, et al.; Br. J. Plast. Surg., April 1986, 39(2), pp. 167–172.

Poland's Syndrome: Correction of Thoracic Anomaly Through Minimal Incisions: P. Santi, et al.; Plast. Reconstr. Surg., October 1985, 76(4), pp. 639–641.

Early Reconstruction of Poland's Syndrome Using Autologous Rib Grafts Combined with a Latissimus Muscle Flap: J.A. Haller, Jr., et al.; J. Pediatr. Surg, August 1984, 19(4), pp. 423–429.

# PRADER-WILLI SYNDROME

**Description** Prader-Willi syndrome is a multisystem disorder diagnosed more often in males born after a prolonged gestation period, often in the breech position. The disease's primary features include infantile hypotonia, failure to thrive, hypogonadism, short stature, and impaired intellectual and behavioral functioning. Hyperphagia leads to obesity in early childhood.

**Synonyms**

> Hypogenital Dystrophy with Diabetic Tendency
> Hypotonia-Hypomentia-Hypogonadism-Obesity Syndrome
> Labhart-Willi Syndrome
> Prader-Labhart-Willi Syndrome
> Willi-Prader Syndrome

**Signs and Symptoms** Early symptoms include decreased fetal movement, low birth weight, hypotonia, sleepiness, weak cry, poor sucking ability, acromicria, narrow bifrontal forehead diameter, strabismus, almond-shaped palpebral fissures, and developmental delays in head control and ability to crawl. In 65 young infants with hypotonia of unknown origin, 29 of them proved to have Prader-Willi syndrome.

Hyperphagia develops between 1 and 3 years of age. If left uncontrolled, obesity can lead to life-threatening heart and lung complications.

Sexual development may begin early but stops before puberty. Cryptorchidism and micropenis occur frequently in boys, and hypoplastic labia are seen less frequently in girls. Patients are mentally retarded, most with IQs between 40 and 60. Patients tend to be fair and blue-eyed. They are sun-sensitive and frequently scratch or pick at sores and insect bites.

**Etiology** About 55 to 70 percent of persons with Prader-Willi syndrome have a cytogenetic deletion of chromosome 15q11.2–q12 when high-resolution techniques are used. The deletion always occurs on the paternally derived chromosome 15; these are sporadic de novo deletions, since the fathers of affected persons have normal chromosomes. There is less than 1:1,000 risk of recurrence when a cytogenetic deletion is found.

An identical cytogenetic deletion is seen in patients with Angelman syndrome, but the involved chromosome is always of maternal origin. These findings suggest that chromosomal imprinting may be critical in the expression of these 2 syndromes.

About 20 percent of patients with Prader-Willi syndrome who do not have a cytogenetic deletion have been found by DNA markers to have inherited both chromosomes from the mother (maternal uniparental disomy).

**Epidemiology** The prevalence is estimated to be 1:25,000 to 1:30,000.

**Treatment—Standard** High-resolution prometaphase chromosome analysis is recommended. Treatment is symptomatic. Physical therapy may be necessary to develop walking pattern and improve muscle size and tone. Extreme hyperphagia requires strict diet, nutrition, and exercise programs, including a 60 percent caloric intake reduction.

**Treatment—Investigational** Drs. Suzanne Cassidy and Robert Erickson at the University of Arizona Department of Pediatrics are studying the molecular genetics of Prader-Willi patients. George Bray, M.D., at the University of Southern California Medical Center, Los Angeles, is studying the association of diabetes and nutrition in Prader-Willi syndrome. Other research includes a study on human growth hormone (**HGH**) to help decrease fat and build muscle. For information about ongoing studies of Prader-Willi syndrome, contact NIH/National Institute of Child Health and Human Development.

Please contact the agencies listed under Resources, below, for the most current information. Addresses and telephone numbers of these agencies, as well as of individual experts and research centers, may be found in the Master Resources List.

**Resources**

**For more information on Prader-Willi syndrome:** National Organization for Rare Disorders (NORD); Prader-Willi Syndrome Association; NIH/National Institute of Child Health and Human Development.

**For genetic information and genetic counseling referrals:** March of Dimes Birth Defects Foundation; Alliance of Genetic Support Groups.

**References**

A Clinical, Cytogenetic, and Molecular Study of 40 Adults with Prader-Willi Syndrome: T. Webb; J. Med. Genet., 1995, vol. 32, pp. 181–185.

DNA Methylation-Based Testing of 450 Patients Suspected of Having Prader-Willi Syndrome: G. Gillessen-Kaesbach, et al.; J. Med. Genet., 1995, vol. 32, pp. 88–92.

Mendelian Inheritance in Man, 11th ed.: V.A. McKusick; The Johns Hopkins University Press, 1994, pp. 1208–1214.

Mutations of the P Gene in Oculocutaneous Albinism, Ocular Albinism, and Prader-Willi Syndrome Plus Albinism: S.T. Lee, et al.; N. Engl. J. Med., February 1994, vol. 8(330), pp. 529–534.

Cecil Textbook of Medicine, 19th ed.: J.B. Wyngaarden, et al., eds.; W.B. Saunders Company, 1992, p. 1146.

The Frequency of Uniparental Disomy in Prader-Willi Syndrome: Implications for Molecular Diagnosis: M.J. Mascari; N. Engl. J. Med., 1992, vol. 326, pp. 1599–1607.

Localization of the Gene Encoding the GABAA Receptor Beta 3 Subunit to the Angelman/Prader-Willi Region of Human Chromosome 15: J. Wagstaff, et al.; Am. J. Hum. Gen., August 1991, vol. 49(2), pp. 330–337.

Birth Defects Encyclopedia: M.L. Buyse, ed.-in-chief; Blackwell Scientific Publications, 1990, pp. 1408–1411.

Prader-Willi Syndrome: Current Understanding of Cause and Diagnosis: M.G. Butler; Am. J. Med. Genet., March 1990, vol. 35(3), pp. 319–332.

Smith's Recognizable Patterns of Human Malformation, 4th ed.: K.L. Jones; W.B. Saunders Company, 1988, pp. 170–173.

# PROTEUS SYNDROME

**Description** Proteus syndrome is a rare hereditary disorder characterized by abnormal, asymmetric growth in any system, and diverse abnormalities involving the skin, face, eyes, ears, lungs, muscles, and nerves.

**Signs and Symptoms** Although infants may appear normal at birth, symptoms become apparent during the first year. Hemihypertrophy, macrocephaly, and scoliosis are characteristic. Skin lesions resembling nevi may occur, as well as hemangiomas, lipomas, and lymphangiomas. Morbidity resulting in amputation is common. Areas of the tongue can become enlarged with longer-than-normal papillae. Abnormal growths in the abdominal cavity may occur in some cases. Infrequent abnormalities include mental deficiency, seizures, strabismus, myopia, external auditory canal hyperostosis, and pulmonary cystic malformations.

**Etiology** The cause is unknown; all instances have been sporadic. Joseph Merrick, the famous Elephant Man, is believed to have had this disorder rather than neurofibromatosis.

**Epidemiology** Proteus syndrome affects males and females in equal numbers.

**Related Disorders** See ***Klippel-Trenaunay Syndrome; Maffucci Syndrome; Neurofibromatosis.***

**Bannayan-Zonana syndrome** encompasses macrocephaly, multiple lipomas, and hemangiomas. The syndrome is hereditary.

**Cowden syndrome** is characterized by multiple nodules, hamartomas, lipomas, macrocephaly, thyroid nodules, and breast lesions.

**Nevus sebaceus of Jadassohn,** a port-wine lesion on the scalp or face, often enlarges during puberty or early adulthood. Rarely, it may be the precursor of other growths, including basal carcinoma.

**Treatment—Standard** Some growths and bone malformations can be removed or corrected surgically. Other treatment is symptomatic and supportive.

**Treatment—Investigational** Please contact the agencies listed under Resources, below, for the most current information. Addresses and telephone numbers of these agencies, as well as of individual experts and research centers, may be found in the Master Resources List.

**Resources**

**For more information on Proteus syndrome:** National Organization for Rare Disorders (NORD); International Center for Skeletal Dysplasia; NIH/National Arthritis and Musculoskeletal and Skin Diseases Information Clearinghouse.

**For genetic information and genetic counseling referrals:** March of Dimes Birth Defects Foundation; Alliance of Genetic Support Groups.

**References**

Mendelian Inheritance in Man, 11th ed.: V.A. McKusick; The Johns Hopkins University Press, 1994, pp. 1260–1261.

Smith's Recognizable Patterns of Human Malformation, 4th ed.: K.L. Jones; W.B. Saunders Company, 1988, pp. 458–459.

Proteus Syndrome: The Elephant Man Diagnosed: J.A.R. Tibbles, et al.; Br. Med. J., 1986, vol. 293, pp. 683–685.

Proteus Syndrome: Report of Two Cases with Pelvic Lipomatosis: T. Costa, et al.; Pediatrics, 1985, vol. 76, pp. 984–989.

Proteus Syndrome or Another Hamartosis?: B.G. Kousseff; J. Clin. Dysmorphol., 1984, 2(3), pp. 23–26.

The Proteus Syndrome: Partial Gigantism of the Hands and/or Feet, Nevi, Hemihypertrophy, Subcutaneous Tumors, Macrocephaly or Other Skull Anomalies and Visceral Afflictions: H.R. Wiedemann, et al.; Eur. J. Pediatr., 1983, vol. 140, pp. 5–12.

# PTERYGIUM SYNDROME, MULTIPLE

**Description** Multiple pterygium syndrome is characterized by webbing of the skin and an array of other abnormalities.

**Synonyms**

Escobar Syndrome
Pterygium Colli Syndrome
Pterygium Universale

**Signs and Symptoms** Primary characteristics are syndactyly; webbing of the neck, of the inside bend of the elbows, of the backs of the knees, and of the armpits; clinodactyly; short stature; rocker-bottom or clubbing of the feet; contractures of the joints; and epicanthal folds. Other symptoms include micrognathia, ptosis, a long philtrum, down-slanting eyes, low-set ears, fused neck vertebrae, cleft palate, and down-turned corners of the mouth. Males may have cryptorchidism and an abnormally small penis. Females may have underdeveloped or missing labia majora. Hernias, dislocated hips, and underdeveloped nipples are less common.

**Etiology** The majority of cases occur as isolated events. Affected siblings are thought to have inherited the disorder as an autosomal recessive trait. An autosomal dominant inheritance has also been reported.

**Epidemiology** Males and females are affected equally. Approximately 50 cases have been reported in Germany, France, and England.

**Related Disorders** See *Arthrogryposis Multiplex Congenita.*

**Treatment—Standard** Cleft lip can be corrected by surgery, beginning in the patient's infancy. Cleft palate may also be treated surgically or by a prosthesis. Plastic surgery may be of benefit to patients with webbed areas, fused fingers, and cleft palate. Extreme caution must be used to avoid major nerves and blood vessels in the areas that are too short to allow for full extension of the limbs. Physical therapy can help prevent the joints from becoming fixed. Genetic counseling may benefit families of patients with this disorder. Other treatment is symptomatic and supportive.

**Treatment—Investigational** Researchers are studying a paste that is applied to the rear of the pharynx in a minor surgical procedure to bring the pharynx and palate into proper relationship. For further information, contact William N. Williams, D.D.S., University of Florida.

Please contact the agencies listed under Resources, below, for the most current information. Addresses and telephone numbers of these agencies, as well as of individual experts and research centers, may be found in the Master Resources List.

**Resources**

**For more information on multiple pterygium syndrome:** National Organization for Rare Disorders (NORD); NIH/National Arthritis and Musculoskeletal and Skin Diseases Information Clearinghouse; International Center for Skeletal Dysplasia; American Cleft Palate Cranial Facial Association.

**For genetic information and genetic counseling referrals:** March of Dimes Birth Defects Foundation; Alliance of Genetic Support Groups.

**References**

Mendelian Inheritance in Man, 11th ed.: V.A. McKusick; The Johns Hopkins University Press, 1994, pp. 1279–1280, 2156–2157.

Birth Defects Encyclopedia: M.L. Buyse, ed.-in-chief; Blackwell Scientific Publications, 1990, pp. 1427–1428.

An Autosomal Dominant Multiple Pterygium Syndrome: C. M. McKeown, et al.; J. Med. Genet., February 1988, vol. 25(2), pp. 96–103.

Multiple Pterygium Syndrome: An Overview: J.C. Ramer, et al.; Am. J. Dis. Child., July 1988, vol. 142(7), pp. 794–798.

Smith's Recognizable Patterns of Human Malformation, 4th ed.: K.L. Jones; W.B. Saunders Company, 1988, p. 264.

Multiple Pterygium Syndrome: Evolution of the Phenotype: E.M. Thompson, et al.; J.. Med. Genet., December 1987, vol. 24(12), pp. 733–749.

# RIEGER SYNDROME

**Description** The syndrome is characterized by facial, dental, and eye abnormalities (**Rieger eye malformations** or **Rieger anomaly,** which may be present alone, or as a part of Rieger syndrome).

**Synonyms**

> Goniodysgenesis-Hypodontia
>
> Iridogoniodysgenesis with Somatic Anomalies

**Signs and Symptoms** The disorder can be detected during the first month of life when the eye defects may be visible. Otherwise, detection occurs in early childhood when the eye and dental defects become apparent.

Dental abnormalities include hypodontia, microdontia, and cone-shaped teeth.

Facial abnormalities include hypoplasia, a broad, flat bridge of the nose, and a protruding lower lip.

**Rieger eye malformations (Rieger anomaly)** include microcornea, an opaque ring around the outer edge of the cornea, adhesions in the front of the eye, off-center displacement of the pupil, and an underdeveloped iris.

Occasional features of Rieger syndrome include glaucoma, umbilical hernia, anal stenosis, and failure of the skin around the navel to decrease in size after birth (sometimes mistaken for umbilical hernia).

The following conditions have sometimes occurred in conjunction with Rieger syndrome, but it is uncertain whether they are separate entities in which the Rieger eye malformations are present: myotonic dystrophy, myotonia, conductive deafness, mental retardation.

**Etiology** The syndrome is inherited as an autosomal dominant trait.

**Epidemiology** Males and females are affected in equal numbers.

**Treatment—Standard** Treatment is symptomatic and supportive. Genetic counseling may benefit patients and their families.

**Treatment—Investigational** Please contact the agencies listed under Resources, below, for the most current information. Addresses and telephone numbers of these agencies, as well as of individual experts and research centers, may be found in the Master Resources List.

**Resources**

**For more information on Rieger syndrome:** National Organization for Rare Disorders (NORD); National Foundation for Ectodermal Dysplasia; Vision Foundation; National Association for Parents of the Visually Impaired; National Association for the Visually Handicapped; The Arc (a national organization on mental retardation); NIH/National Eye Institute.

**For genetic information and genetic counseling referrals:** March of Dimes Birth Defects Foundation; Alliance of Genetic Support Groups.

**References**

Mendelian Inheritance in Man, 11th ed.: V.A. McKusick; The Johns Hopkins University Press, 1994, pp. 1325–1326.

Birth Defects Encyclopedia: M.L. Buyse, ed.-in-chief; Blackwell Scientific Publications, 1990, p. 1497.

Smith's Recognizable Patterns of Human Malformation, 4th ed.: K.L. Jones; W.B. Saunders Company, 1988, pp. 532–533.

Diagnostic Recognition of Genetic Disease: W. Nyhan, et al.; Lea and Febiger, 1987, pp. 226–227.

The Rieger Syndrome and a Chromosome 13 Deletion: R.A. Stathacopoulos, et al.; J. Pediatr. Opthalmol. Strabismus, July–August 1987, vol. 24(4), pp. 198–203.

# ROBERTS SYNDROME

**Description** Roberts syndrome is a very rare genetic disorder characterized by severe defects in facial and limb development, growth deficiency, and mental retardation.

**Synonyms**

> Hypomelia–Hypotrichosis–Facial Hemangioma Syndrome
> Pseudothalidomide Syndrome

**Signs and Symptoms** Patients frequently are missing bones in their limbs. The bones that are present are often extremely short, and phocomelic.

A low birth weight, growth deficiency, and mental retardation are common, as are microbrachiocephaly; sparse, silvery hair; cleft lip with or without cleft palate; hypertelorism; malformed ears; micrognathia, and cryptorchidism. Less common signs include brain hernia, hydrocephaly, unusually small eyes, cataracts, clouding of the cornea, cardiac and renal anomalies, and thrombocytopenia.

**Etiology** Roberts syndrome is inherited as an autosomal recessive trait. Premature centromere separation is a common cytogenetic finding.

**Epidemiology** Males and females are affected in equal numbers.

**Related Disorders** See ***Thrombocytopenia–Absent Radius Syndrome.***

**Treatment—Standard** Individuals with Roberts syndrome may benefit from surgery for facial and limb defects. Prosthetic devices can also reduce problems associated with missing limbs. Other treatment is symptomatic and supportive. Genetic counseling may be helpful for patients and their families.

**Treatment—Investigational** Dr. Uta Francke of Howard Hughes Medical Institute, Stanford University School of Medicine, Stanford, CA, is studying the patients of Roberts syndrome, their parents, and asymptomatic siblings.

Please contact the agencies listed under Resources, below, for the most current information. Addresses and telephone numbers of these agencies, as well as of individual experts and research centers, may be found in the Master Resources List.

**Resources**

**For more information on Roberts syndrome:** National Organization for Rare Disorders (NORD); International Center for Skeletal Dysplasia; Association of Children's Prosthetic and Orthotic Clinics; FACES—National Association for the Craniofacially Handicapped; National Craniofacial Foundation; NIH/National Institute of Child Health and Human Development; AboutFace; Children's Craniofacial Association.

**For genetic information and genetic counseling referrals:** March of Dimes Birth Defects Foundation; Alliance of Genetic Support Groups.

**References**

Mendelian Inheritance in Man, 11th ed.: V.A. McKusick; The Johns Hopkins University Press, 1994, pp. 2180–2181.

Smith's Recognizable Patterns of Human Malformation, 4th ed.: K.L. Jones; W.B. Saunders Company, 1988, pp. 256–257.

# ROBINOW SYNDROME

**Description** The characteristic features of Robinow syndrome include a typical facies, short stature, and hypoplasia of the genitals.

**Synonyms**

Fetal Face Syndrome

**Signs and Symptoms** The forehead is bulging, and the child has a flattened profile. Hypertelorism, a prominent forehead, depressed nasal bridge, triangular mouth, and micrognathia are characteristic. The forearms and fingers are short, hemivertebrae may be present, and there is mild-to-moderate short stature. Males have micropenis and cryptorchidism; females, small clitoris and labia. Occasional symptoms include seizures, navel and inguinal hernias, cleft palate, other digital anomalies, and speech and walking difficulties.

**Etiology** Both autosomal dominant and autosomal recessive inheritances have been reported. The recessive type is said to be more severe, but the 2 forms usually cannot be separated.

**Epidemiology** Robinow syndrome affects males and females in equal numbers.

**Related Disorders** See *Aarskog Syndrome.*

**Treatment—Standard** Treatment for Robinow syndrome includes surgery to correct physical abnormalities. Genetic counseling may be beneficial. Other treatment is symptomatic and supportive.

**Treatment—Investigational** Please contact the agencies listed under Resources, below, for the most current information. Addresses and telephone numbers of these agencies, as well as of individual experts and research centers, may be found in the Master Resources List.

**Resources**

**For more information on Robinow syndrome:** National Organization for Rare Disorders (NORD); NIH/National Institute of Child Health and Human Development; Human Growth Foundation.

**For genetic information and genetic counseling referrals:** March of Dimes Birth Defects Foundation; Alliance of Genetic Support Groups.

**References**

Mendelian Inheritance in Man, 11th ed.: V.A. McKusick; The Johns Hopkins University Press, 1994, pp. 1330, 2182.

Craniofacial Pattern Similarities and Additional Orofacial Findings in Siblings with Robinow Syndrome: H. Israel, et al.; J. Craniofac. Genet. Dev. Biol., 1988, 8(1), pp. 63–73.

Smith's Recognizable Patterns of Human Malformation, 4th ed.: K.L. Jones; W.B. Saunders Company, 1988, pp. 112–113.

Robinow Syndrome: Report of Two Patients and Review of Literature: M. Butler, et al.; Clin. Genet., February 1987, 31(2), pp. 77–85.

# RUBINSTEIN-TAYBI SYNDROME

**Description** Rubinstein-Taybi syndrome is a rare genetic disorder associated with multiple abnormalities that include characteristic facial features and abnormally wide fingers and toes.

**Synonyms**

Rubinstein Syndrome

Broad Thumb-Hallux Syndrome

**Signs and Symptoms** The syndrome is present at birth. Craniofacial abnormalities include a small skull, narrow and prominent forehead, beaked nose, unusually high and narrow palate, low-set and abnormally shaped ears, and eye defects such as strabismus and blocked or missing tear ducts.

The fingertips and toes are typically broad. Other abnormalities include hirsutism, scoliosis, and congenital heart disease. In males, cryptorchidism and an angulated penis are present. A small, irregularly shaped pelvis, and kidney and lung defects may occur in some individuals.

Respiratory problems and eye and ear infections are common. Also typical are difficulties with feeding, such as regurgitation, gagging, and choking, as well as diarrhea and chronic constipation. These problems seem to improve for many children as they grow, after about 4 or 5 years of age.

Mental retardation of some degree is present.

**Etiology** The cause of Rubinstein-Taybi syndrome is not known. Most cases have been sporadic, although in some instances autosomal dominant or autosomal recessive inheritance is suggested. In about 25 percent of patients, a small deletion of chromosome 16p13.3 is found.

**Epidemiology** Since the syndrome was first described in 1963, more than 250 cases have been reported in the medical literature in the United States. According to one study, the disorder may affect approximately 1:300 to 1:500 institutionalized persons with mental retardation in the United States. There is no estimate for the prevalence among noninstitutionalized patients. Males and females are affected equally.

**Related Disorders** See *Hallermann-Streiff Syndrome; Seckel Syndrome; Treacher Collins Syndrome.*

**Treatment—Standard** Drugs or surgery may improve some associated symptoms, and antibiotics may be needed. Treatment otherwise is symptomatic and supportive. Patients may benefit from services for mentally retarded individuals. Speech therapy, sign language lessons, or an alternative method of communication should be taught as soon as possible. Genetic counseling will be beneficial.

**Treatment—Investigational** Please contact the agencies listed under Resources, below, for the most current information. Addresses and telephone numbers of these agencies, as well as of individual experts and research centers, may be found in the Master Resources List.

**Resources**

**For more information on Rubinstein-Taybi syndrome:** National Organization for Rare Disorders (NORD); Rubinstein-Taybi Parent Support Group; Rubinstein-Taybi Support Group; NIH/National Institute of Child Health and Human Development.

**For case documentation of Rubinstein-Taybi syndrome patients:** Jack H. Rubinstein, Director, Cincinnati Center for Developmental Disorders, Cincinnati, OH.

**For genetic information and genetic counseling referrals:** March of Dimes Birth Defects Foundation; Alliance of Genetic Support Groups.

**References**

Mendelian Inheritance in Man, 11th ed.: V.A. McKusick; The Johns Hopkins University Press, 1994, pp. 1332–1334.

Deletion of a Monosome 16p13.3 As a Cause of Rubinstein-Taybi Syndrome: Clinical Aspects: R.C.M. Hennekam, et al.; Am. J. Hum. Genet., 1993, vol. 52, pp. 258–262.

Rubinstein-Taybi Syndrome Caused by Submicroscopic Deletions Within 16p13.3: M.H. Breuning, et al.; Am. J. Hum. Genet., 1993, vol. 52, pp. 249–254.

Smith's Recognizable Patterns of Human Malformation, 4th ed.: K.L. Jones; W.B. Saunders Company, 1988, pp. 84–87.

Dominant Inheritance of a Syndrome Similar to Rubinstein-Taybi: P. Cotsirilos, et al.; Am. J. Med. Genet., January 1987, vol. 26(1), pp. 85–93.

Rubinstein-Taybi Syndrome in the Neonate: R. Gambon, et al.; Helv. Paediatr. Acta, August 1984, vol. 39(3), pp. 279–283.

# RUSSELL-SILVER SYNDROME

**Description** Russell-Silver syndrome is commonly thought of as a disorder of short stature, although some affected persons attain normal height in adulthood.

**Synonyms**

Russell Syndrome

Silver Syndrome

Silver-Russell Syndrome

**Signs and Symptoms** Full-term infants with Russell-Silver syndrome are usually small at birth, and many individuals remain short throughout life. Craniofacial features include a normal-sized head that may appear large in comparison to the rest of the body, a small triangular face with down-turned corners of the mouth, and a prominent forehead. Light-brown spots may occur on the skin. The arms are unusually short, 5th fingers may be short and inwardly curved, and there is syndactyly of the toes. Cryptorchidism as well as precocious puberty may occur. Intelligence is often normal; however, mental retardation is possible. Some developmental abnormalities tend to improve with age.

Lateral organ asymmetry may occur **(Silver syndrome).** When the organs are of equal size bilaterally, the disorder is sometimes termed **Russell syndrome.**

The syndrome can be diagnosed in utero.

**Etiology** The cause is unknown. Inheritance as either an X-linked or dominant trait with incomplete penetrance has been suggested, as has fetal disturbance at 6 to 7 weeks' gestation, or defects in the body's ability to manufacture or use human growth hormone.

**Epidemiology** Onset is in utero. Males and females are affected in equal numbers; however, males are usually more severely affected than females.

**Treatment—Standard** Some gains in overall body growth may occur with use of human growth hormone. Other treatment is symptomatic and supportive.

**Treatment—Investigational** Please contact the agencies listed under Resources, below, for the most current information. Addresses and telephone numbers of these agencies, as well as of individual experts and research centers, may be found in the Master Resources List.

**Resources**

**For more information on Russell-Silver syndrome:** National Organization for Rare Disorders (NORD); Association for Children with Russell-Silver Syndrome; NIH/National Arthritis and Musculoskeletal and Skin Diseases Information Clearinghouse; Human Growth Foundation; Parents of Dwarfed Children; Little People of America; International Center for Skeletal Dysplasia; Short Stature Foundation.

**For genetic information and genetic counseling referrals:** March of Dimes Birth Defects Foundation; Alliance of Genetic Support Groups.

### References
Mendelian Inheritance in Man, 11th ed.: V.A. McKusick; The Johns Hopkins University Press, 1994, pp. 1334, 2528.

Smith's Recognizable Patterns of Human Malformation, 4th ed.: K.L. Jones; W.B. Saunders Company, 1988, pp. 88–89.

Treatment of Silver-Russell Type Dwarfism with Human Growth Hormone: Effects on Serum Somatomedin-C Levels and on Longitudinal Growth Studied by Knemonetry: C.J. Partsch, et al.; Acta Endocrinol. [Suppl.] (Copenh.), 1986, vol. 279, pp. 139–146.

X-Linked Short Stature with Skin Pigmentation: Evidence for Heterogeneity of the Russell-Silver Syndrome: M.W. Partington; Clin. Genet., February 1986, vol. 29(2), pp. 151–156.

Reevaluation of Russell-Silver Syndrome: R.A. Pagon, et al.; J. Pediatr., November 1985, vol. 107(5), pp. 733–737.

# RUVALCABA SYNDROME

**Description** Ruvalcaba syndrome is a very rare malformation disorder whose major characteristics are short stature, unusual facial features, skeletal abnormalities, and varying degrees of mental retardation in over 50 percent of affected individuals.

### Synonyms
Mental Retardation–Osteodystrophy, Ruvalcaba Type

**Signs and Symptoms** Symptoms vary greatly among affected patients. Characteristic facial abnormalities are the most distinguishable expression of this disorder. Microcephaly with an oval face; down-slanting eyes; hooked or beaked nose; small, down-turned mouth; narrow, pointed jaw; low-set ears; and underdeveloped sides of the nose may be found in affected individuals. Short stature along with varying degrees of mental retardation has been found in over 50 percent of those affected by this disorder. Various skeletal abnormalities can be found in most affected individuals. A narrow chest, pectus carinatum, scoliosis, kyphosis, short limbs, short fingers and toes, clinodactyly, and small hands and feet may be present. Underdeveloped skin lesions ("onion skin"), underdeveloped reproductive organs, delayed puberty, and/or underdeveloped nostrils have been found in a few individuals with Ruvalcaba syndrome .

**Etiology** Ruvalcaba syndrome is thought to be inherited as an autosomal dominant trait.

**Epidemiology** Ruvalcaba syndrome affects males and females in equal numbers. There have been fewer than 20 cases of this disorder reported in North America, Japan, and Europe.

**Related Disorders** See *Hallermann-Streiff Syndrome; Seckel Syndrome.*

**Treatment—Standard** Treatment is symptomatic and supportive. Agencies that provide assistance for people with mental retardation may be helpful in those cases that include intellectual impairment. Genetic counseling may benefit patients and their families.

**Treatment—Investigational** Please contact the agencies listed under Resources, below, for the most current information. Addresses and telephone numbers of these agencies, as well as of individual experts and research centers, may be found in the Master Resources List.

### Resources
**For more information on Ruvalcaba syndrome:** National Organization for Rare Disorders (NORD); International Center for Skeletal Dysplasia; The Arc (a national organization on mental retardation); NIH/National Institute of Child Health and Human Development.

**For genetic information and genetic counseling referrals:** March of Dimes Birth Defects Foundation; Alliance of Genetic Support Groups.

### References
Mendelian Inheritance in Man, 11th ed.: V.A. McKusick; The Johns Hopkins University Press, 1994, pp. 1334–1335.

Birth Defects Encyclopedia: M.L Buyse, ed.-in-chief; Blackwell Scientific Publications, 1990, p. 1319.

Apparent Ruvalcaba Syndrome with Genitourinary Abnormalities: M.G. Bialer, et al.; Am. J. Med. Genet., July 1989, vol. 33(3), pp. 314–317.

Smith's Recognizable Patterns of Human Malformation, 4th ed.: K.L. Jones, ed.; W.B. Saunders Company, 1988, p. 226.

Ruvalcaba Syndrome: Autosomal Dominant Inheritance: Y. Sugio, et al.; Am. J. Med. Genet., December 1984, vol. 19(4), pp. 741–753.

# SAETHRE-CHOTZEN SYNDROME

**Description** Saethre-Chotzen syndrome is a congenital disorder characterized by various craniofacial and skeletal malformations. Short stature may be present, as well as skin abnormalities of the fingers and toes. Intelligence is usually normal, but mild-to-moderate mental retardation may develop.

**Synonyms**

> Acrocephalosyndactyly Type III
> Chotzen Syndrome

**Signs and Symptoms** The craniofacial abnormalities, some of which are related to the coronal craniostenosis characteristic of this disorder, include brachycephaly, skull asymmetry, hypertelorism, ptosis, and strabismus, as well as an unusually shaped ear with a prominent crus. Syndactyly is often present; brachydactyly and clinodactyly may occur. Some cardiac and renal problems can develop.

**Etiology** The syndrome is thought to be inherited as an autosomal dominant trait. The gene has been mapped to the 7p21–p22 region.

**Epidemiology** Both males and females can be affected.

**Related Disorders** See *Apert Syndrome; Pfeiffer Syndrome.*

**Treatment—Standard** Treatment is symptomatic and supportive. Patients should be monitored closely for cardiac or renal problems, and for signs of infection. A medical evaluation may be appropriate for family members because of the possibility of developing a milder, less debilitating form of the syndrome. Genetic counseling also may be worthwhile.

**Treatment—Investigational** Drs. Amy Feldman Lewanda and Ethylin Wang Jabs at Johns Hopkins Hospital in Baltimore are researching the genes responsible for craniofacial disorders.

Please contact the agencies listed under Resources, below, for the most current information. Addresses and telephone numbers of these agencies, as well as of individual experts and research centers, may be found in the Master Resources List.

**Resources**

**For more information on Saethre-Chotzen syndrome:** National Organization for Rare Disorders (NORD); National Craniofacial Foundation; FACES—National Association for the Craniofacially Handicapped; Society for the Rehabilitation of the Facially Disfigured; AboutFace; NIH/National Institute of Child Health and Human Development; Craniofacial Family Association.

**For genetic information and genetic counseling referrals:** March of Dimes Birth Defects Foundation; Alliance of Genetic Support Groups.

**References**

Mendelian Inheritance in Man, 11th ed.: V.A. McKusick; The Johns Hopkins University Press, 1994, pp. 20–21.

Smith's Recognizable Patterns of Human Malformation, 4th ed.: K.L. Jones; W.B. Saunders Company, 1988, pp. 364–367.

Dermatoglyphics in Saethre-Chotzen Syndrome: A Family Study: L. Borbolla, et al.; Acta Paediatr. Acad. Sci. Hung., 1983, vol. 24(3), pp. 269–279.

# SCHINZEL-GIEDION SYNDROME

**Description** Schinzel-Giedion syndrome is characterized by midface retraction and anomalies of the skeleton, kidney, hair, and brain.

**Signs and Symptoms** An obstructed ureter causes hydronephrosis. Growth delays are apparent at an early age. Hypertrichosis; ocular hypertelorism; a flat midface; low-set ears; a short, low-set nose; a short, wide neck with excessive skin; short lower arms and legs; widely spaced cranial sutures; epilepsy; and atrial septal defect are typical features. Vision and hearing problems, sleep apnea, and mental retardation are also common.

Less common are the following features: a high, protruding forehead; macroglossia; delayed eruption of teeth; choanal stenosis; underdeveloped nipples; abnormal nails of the fingers and toes; polydactyly; clubfoot; short penis; cryptorchidism; and interlabial sulcus.

**Etiology** Schinzel-Giedion syndrome is thought to be inherited as an autosomal recessive trait.

**Epidemiology** Males and females are affected in equal numbers. Approximately 10 cases have been reported.

**Related Disorders** See *Mucopolysaccharidosis.*

Infantile apnea and atrial septal defects may be associated with Schinzel-Giedion syndrome as secondary characteristics but are not necessary for a differential diagnosis.

**Treatment—Standard** Hydronephrosis may require temporary drainage of the urine. Surgery may be indicated when kidney function is compromised, or when pain or infection occurs.

The definitive treatment for atrial septal defects is surgical. The hole in the septum is either sutured shut or patched with a graft. The success rate is quite high. In ostim primum (endocardial cushion) defects, the atrioventricular valves may have to be repaired or replaced; the success rate is substantially lower in these more complex operations.

Anticonvulsant drugs are helpful in controlling epileptic seizures.

Genetic counseling may benefit patients and their families. Other treatment is symptomatic and supportive.

**Treatment—Investigational** Please contact the agencies listed under Resources, below, for the most current information. Addresses and telephone numbers of these agencies, as well as of individual experts and research centers, may be found in the Master Resources List.

**Resources**

**For more information on Schinzel-Giedion syndrome:** National Organization for Rare Disorders (NORD); The Arc (a national organization on mental retardation); NIH/National Institute of Child Health and Human Development.

**For genetic information and genetic counseling referrals:** March of Dimes Birth Defects Foundation; Alliance of Genetic Support Groups.

**References**

Mendelian Inheritance in Man, 11th ed.: V.A. McKusick; The Johns Hopkins University Press, 1994, p. 2188.

Birth Defects Encyclopedia: M.L. Buyse, ed.-in-chief; Blackwell Scientific Publications, 1990, p. 1513.

The Schinzel-Giedion Syndrome: A Case Report and Review of the Literature: M. Pul, et al.; Clin. Pediatr., April 1990, vol. 29(4), pp. 235–239.

Smith's Recognizable Patterns of Human Malformation, 4th ed.: K.L. Jones; W.B. Saunders Company, 1988, p. 188.

# SECKEL SYNDROME

**Description** Seckel syndrome is primarily characterized by marked intrauterine and postnatal growth failure, mental retardation, and a typical facies that gave rise to the adjective *bird-headed.*

**Synonyms**

Nanocephaly

**Signs and Symptoms** Craniofacial abnormalities include microcephaly and micrognathia and a resulting prominence of the midface and beaklike nose. The ears are low-set and malformed and the eyes large. Other congenital conditions include hypoplasia of the proximal radius, palmar simian crease, clinodactyly of the 5th finger, hip dislocation, hypoplasia of the proximal fibula, and cryptorchidism in the male. Among the abnormalities that are present in some cases are facial asymmetry, scoliosis, and hypoplastic external genitalia.

The height of affected persons reaches 3 to 3.5 ft (91 to 106 cm). Mental deficiency is moderate to severe.

**Etiology** Seckel syndrome is an inherited autosomal recessive trait.

**Epidemiology** Incidence is very slightly higher in females, but severity of the syndrome is equal in the sexes.

**Related Disorders** See *Anemia, Fanconi; Hallermann-Streiff Syndrome.*

**Treatment—Standard** Treatment of Seckel syndrome is symptomatic and supportive. Genetic counseling may be beneficial.

**Treatment—Investigational** Please contact the agencies listed under Resources, below, for the most current information. Addresses and telephone numbers of these agencies, as well as of individual experts and research centers, may be found in the Master Resources List.

**Resources**

**For more information on Seckel syndrome:** National Organization for Rare Disorders (NORD); International Center for Skeletal Dysplasia; Human Growth Foundation; Little People of America; Parents of Dwarfed Children; NIH/National Institute of Child Health and Human Development.

**For genetic information and genetic counseling referrals:** March of Dimes Birth Defects Foundation; Alliance of Genetic Support Groups.

**References**

Mendelian Inheritance in Man, 11th ed.: V.A. McKusick; The Johns Hopkins University Press, 1994, pp. 1666–1667.

Syndromes of the Head and Neck, 3rd ed.: R.J. Gorlin, et al.; Oxford University Press, 1990, pp. 313–316.

Smith's Recognizable Patterns of Human Malformation, 4th ed.: K.L. Jones; W.B. Saunders Company, 1988, pp. 100–101.

Microcephaly, Micrognathia, and Bird-Headed Dwarfism: Prenatal Diagnosis of a Seckel-like Syndrome: D.F. Majoor-Krakauer, et al.; Am. J. Med. Genet., May 1987, 27(1), pp. 183–188.

Seckel Syndrome: An Overdiagnosed Syndrome: E. Thompson, et al.; J. Med. Genet., June 1985, 22(3), pp. 192–201.

Pigmentary Changes in Seckel's Syndrome: A. Fathizadeh, et al.; J. Am. Acad. Dermatol., July 1979, 1(1), pp. 52–54.

# SEPTO-OPTIC DYSPLASIA

**Description** Septo-optic dysplasia is a birth defect characterized by hypoplastic optic disks and pituitary deficiencies. Often, the anterior horns of the brain's lateral ventricles are separated because of the absence of the septum pellucidum.

**Synonyms**

De Morsier Syndrome

**Signs and Symptoms** Features of septo-optic dysplasia are present at birth. The primary sign is visual impairment, including amblyopia and nystagmus. Pupil response to light may vary. Esotropia and exotropia sometimes occur.

Hypopituitarism of varying degree may be present early or develop later and, if not treated during childhood, will result in stunted growth. Jaundice occasionally occurs at birth. Mental retardation or learning disabilities may also occur.

**Etiology** The cause is not known.

**Epidemiology** Septo-optic dysplasia is rare. Affected children are often the firstborn of young mothers. Males and females are affected equally.

**Related Disorders Absent septum pellucidum with porencephaly** is a rare congenital disorder characterized by hemiatrophy, nystagmus, seizures, and short stature.

**Treatment—Standard** Therapy is symptomatic and supportive. Pituitary hormones deficiencies may be treated by hormone replacement therapy.

**Treatment—Investigational** Please contact the agencies listed under Resources, below, for the most current information. Addresses and telephone numbers of these agencies, as well as of individual experts and research centers, may be found in the Master Resources List.

**Resources**

**For more information on septo-optic dysplasia:** National Organization for Rare Disorders (NORD); NIH/National Institute of Neurological Disorders and Stroke.

**For genetic information and genetic counseling referrals:** March of Dimes Birth Defects Foundation; Alliance of Genetic Support Groups.

**References**

Absence of the Septum Pellucidum: Overlapping Clinical Syndromes: S.A. Morgan, et al.; Arch. Neurol., August 1985, vol. 42(8), pp. 769–770.

Hormonal, Metabolic, and Neuroradiologic Abnormalities Associated with Septo-Optic Dysplasia: S.A. Arslanian, et al.; Acta Endocrinol. (Copenh.), October 1984, vol. 107(2), pp. 282–288.

# SHORT SYNDROME

**Description** SHORT syndrome is an acronym for (**S**)hort stature, (**H**)yperextensibility, (**O**)cular depression, (**R**)ieger anomaly, and (**T**)eething delay.

**Synonyms**

Growth Retardation–Rieger Anomaly

Rieger Anomaly–Growth Retardation

**Signs and Symptoms** SHORT syndrome is characterized by low birth weight, lipoatrophy of the arms and face, inguinal hernias, a delay in teething and speech, recurrent viral infections, and Rieger anomaly, which can lead to glaucoma. Short stature and hyperextension are apparent at an early age. Craniofacial features include a triangular-shaped face, a wide nasal bridge, micrognathia, ears that protrude outward, sunken eyes, hypertelorism, and a down-turned mouth.

**Etiology** An autosomal recessive inheritance is suspected.

**Epidemiology** Males are affected more often than females.

**Related Disorders** See *Lipodystrophy; Rieger Syndrome; Russell-Silver Syndrome.*

**Treatment—Standard** A topical β-blocker is used to treat glaucoma. Laser surgery is reserved for cases refractory to medication. Other treatment is symptomatic and supportive. Genetic counseling is recommended for families of affected children.

**Treatment—Investigational** Please contact the agencies listed under Resources, below, for the most current information. Addresses and telephone numbers of these agencies, as well as of individual experts and research centers, may be found in the Master Resources List.

**Resources**

**For more information on SHORT syndrome:** National Organization for Rare Disorders (NORD); NIH/National Arthritis and Musculoskeletal and Skin Diseases Information Clearinghouse; NIH/National Eye Institute; Human Growth Foundation; Short Stature Foundation; Little People of America; Magic Foundation for Children's Growth; Parents of Dwarfed Children; Association for Research into Restricted Growth (U.K.).

**For genetic information and genetic counseling referrals:** March of Dimes Birth Defects Foundation; Alliance of Genetic Support Groups.

**References**

Mendelian Inheritance in Man, 11th ed.: V.A. McKusick; The Johns Hopkins University Press, 1994, p. 2193.

Birth Defects Encyclopedia: M.L. Buyse, ed.-in-chief; Blackwell Scientific Publications, 1990, pp. 1533–1534.

# SHPRINTZEN SYNDROME

**Description** Cleft palate, heart abnormalities, learning disabilities, and distinct physical features are all present in Shprintzen syndrome. The disorder is the most common syndrome related to cleft palate without cleft lip. Patients with this disorder probably have an expanded form of DiGeorge syndrome.

**Synonyms**

Velo-cardio-facial (VCF) Syndrome

**Signs and Symptoms** Affected persons have a mild form of cleft palate. Other craniofacial characteristics include microcephaly, retrognathia, tubular nose, flat cheeks, long philtrum, and outer ears that are small and asymmetric in size.

Patients are hypotonic, and are small and slender with tapered hands and fingers. Nasal-sounding speech is secondary to cleft palate. Cardiac abnormalities include right aortic arch anomalies and tetralogy of Fallot.

Mild intellectual delay is present in the majority of patients. The average IQ scores in high-school-age children are 69 to 87. Problems with abstraction and in reading and math comprehension are usually apparent at school age. Mental retardation is less frequent but may also be present.

Occasionally the following characteristics are present: an absent or underdeveloped thymus; absent or small adenoids or tonsils; hypocalcemia; scoliosis; inguinal or umbilical hernia; cryptorchidism; an abundance of scalp hair; hearing loss; and eye abnormalities that include small optic discs, cataract, microphthalmia, and twisted vessels in the optic disc. Newborns may have obstructed breathing secondary to the recessed jaw and hypotonia in the throat area.

**Etiology** The syndrome is caused by a deletion of chromosome 22q11, which is the same deletion found in patients with DiGeorge syndrome.

**Epidemiology** The syndrome is present in approximately 5 to 8 percent of children born with cleft palate (without cleft lip). Males and females are affected in equal numbers.

**Related Disorders** See *DiGeorge Syndrome.*

**Treatment—Standard** Most patients have mild impairments in speech, language development, and mathematics. This becomes apparent after entering school, and special class placement or supplementary educational services usually are required. Eventually most patients are mainstreamed and graduate from high school.

When obstructive apnea is present, a nasopharyngeal tube may improve respiration.

A pharyngeal flap can be created surgically to help eliminate the nasal sound when speaking. This procedure cannot be performed on patients with medial displacement of the carotid arteries. Those patients who cannot have the surgery may be fitted with a prosthetic speech device.

Rhinoplasty can be performed to remove the facial characteristics associated with this syndrome.

When congestion is causing the hearing impairment, the placement of tubes in the ears may be beneficial.

Genetic counseling may be useful for patients and their families.

**Treatment—Investigational** A Teflon-glycerine paste is being studied to improve cleft palate. The paste is applied to the rear of the pharynx in a minor surgical procedure. A rounder ledge or bump is formed, bringing the pharynx and palate into the proper relationship with each other. The hardened paste remains in place indefinitely; no side effects have been observed. Children as young as 8 years have been treated with this procedure. For further information, contact William N. Williams, D.D.S., University of Florida College of Dentistry.

A clinical database is being developed to help with chromosomal information on VCF patients. A DNA bank is being developed at Albert Einstein College of Medicine. Interested persons may contact Rosalie Goldberg, Genetic Counselor, or Robert J. Shprintzen, Ph.D., Director, Center for Craniofacial Disorders.

Please contact the agencies listed under Resources, below, for the most current information. Addresses and telephone numbers of these agencies, as well as of individual experts and research centers, may be found in the Master Resources List.

**Resources**

**For more information on Shprintzen syndrome:** National Organization for Rare Disorders (NORD); Velo-Cardio-Facial Syndrome Association; American Cleft Palate Cranial Facial Association; FACES—National Association for the Craniofacially Handicapped; National Foundation for Facial Reconstruction; American Heart Association; NIH/National Institute of Child Health and Human Development; NIH/National Institute of Dental Research.

**For genetic information and genetic counseling referrals:** March of Dimes Birth Defects Foundation; Alliance of Genetic Support Groups.

**References**

Mendelian Inheritance in Man, 11th ed.: V.A. McKusick; The Johns Hopkins University Press, 1994, pp. 1519–1520.

Deletions and Microdeletions of 22q11 in Velo-cardio-facial Syndrome: D.A. Driscoll, et al.; Am. J. Med. Genet., 1992, vol. 44, p. 261.

Velo-cardio-facial Syndrome Associated with Chromosome 22 Deletions Encompassing the DiGeorge Syndrome: P.J. Scambler, et al.; Lancet, 1992, vol. 339, p. 1138.

Birth Defects Encyclopedia: M.L. Buyse, ed.-in-chief; Blackwell Scientific Publications, 1990, pp. 1744–1745.
DiGeorge Anomaly and Velocardiofacial Syndrome: C.A. Stevens, et al.; Pediatrics, April 1990, vol. 85(4), pp. 526–530.
Smith's Recognizable Patterns of Human Malformation, 4th ed.: K.L. Jones, ed.; W.B. Saunders Company, 1988, p. 224.

# SIMPSON-GOLABI-BEHMEL SYNDROME

**Description** Simpson-Golabi-Behmel syndrome is an inherited disorder that includes pre- and postnatal overgrowth and distinctive facial features.

**Synonyms**

> Bulldog Syndrome
> Dysplasia Gigantism Syndrome, X-Linked
> Golabi-Rosen Syndrome
> Simpson Dysmorphia Syndrome

**Signs and Symptoms** An increase in birth weight and length, prognathism, a wide nasal bridge, hypertelorism, an upturned or broad nose, a large mouth, and a short neck are the primary manifestations.

Other signs include broad, short hands and fingers; hypoplastic or absent index fingernails; unilateral postaxial polydactyly; and bilateral syndactyly. Some individuals may have a grooved tongue or lower lip, an inferior alveolar ridge, macroglossia, a cleft palate or lip, an extra rib, additional nipples, Meckel diverticulum, cryptorchidism, bony appendages, skin tags, renal cysts, intestinal malrotation, and micro- or megalocephaly. Heart defects, such as cardiac arrhythmia in infants or cardiac arrest in adults, may be associated with the syndrome.

Intelligence is usually normal; however, mental retardation has been reported.

**Etiology** Simpson-Golabi-Behmel syndrome is inherited as an X-linked recessive trait. The gene responsible is located on the long arm of the X chromosome (Xq25–q27). Because some symptoms appear in female carriers of the gene, it may be an incomplete recessive trait.

**Epidemiology** Although the syndrome occurs mainly in males, it has been described in a female with an X-autosome translocation. About one dozen families with the disorder have been recorded.

**Related Disorders** See *Craniometaphyseal Dysplasia; Oro-Facial-Digital Syndrome; Oto-Palato-Digital Syndrome; Larsen Syndrome; Beckwith-Wiedemann Syndrome; Sotos Syndrome.*

**Treatment—Standard** Treatment of Simpson-Golabi-Behmel syndrome is symptomatic and supportive. Surgical repair of cleft lip is usually performed in a series of operations, beginning in the patient's infancy. Cleft palate may be repaired surgically or covered with a prosthesis.

Genetic counseling may benefit patients and their families.

**Treatment—Investigational** Researchers are studying a paste that is applied to the rear of the pharynx in a minor surgical procedure to bring the pharynx and palate into proper relationship. For further information, contact William N. Williams, D.D.S., University of Florida.

Please contact the agencies listed under Resources, below, for the most current information. Addresses and telephone numbers of these agencies, as well as of individual experts and research centers, may be found in the Master Resources List.

**Resources**

**For more information on Simpson-Golabi-Behmel syndrome:** National Organization for Rare Disorders (NORD); NIH/National Arthritis and Musculoskeletal and Skin Diseases Information Clearinghouse; National Craniofacial Foundation; FACES—National Association for the Craniofacially Handicapped; American Cleft Palate Cranial Facial Association.

**For genetic information and genetic counseling referrals:** March of Dimes Birth Defects Foundation; Alliance of Genetic Support Groups.

**References**

Mapping of the Simpson-Golabi-Behmel Syndrome to Xq25–q27: J.Y. Xuan, et al.; Hum. Mol. Genet., 1994, vol. 50, pp. 133–137.
Mendelian Inheritance in Man, 11th ed.: V.A. McKusick; The Johns Hopkins University Press, 1994, pp. 2530–2531.
Simpson-Golabi-Behmel Syndrome (SGBS) in a Female with an X-Autosome Translocation:. H.H. Purnett; Am. J. Med. Genet., 1994, vol. 50, pp. 391–393.
Report of Another Family with Simpson-Golabi-Behmel Syndrome and Review of the Literature: C.L. Garganta, et al.; Am. J. Med. Genet., 1992, vol. 44, pp. 129–135.
Simpson-Golabi-Behmel Syndrome with Severe Cardiac Arrhythmias: R. Konig et. al.; Am. J. Med. Genet., February–March 1991, vol. 38(2–3), pp. 244–247.
Birth Defects Encyclopedia: M.L. Buyse, ed.-in-chief; Blackwell Scientific Publications, 1990, pp. 1539–1540.
Dictionary of Medical Syndromes: S.I. Magalini, et al., eds.; J.B. Lippincott Company, 1990, p. 144.
The Golabi-Rosen Syndrome: Report of a Second Family: J.M. Opitz; Am .J .Med. Genet., January 1984, vol. 17(1), pp. 359–366.

# SIRENOMELIA SEQUENCE

**Description** Sirenomelia sequence is a congenital disorder characterized by a single lower extremity.

**Synonyms**

Mermaid Syndrome

**Signs and Symptoms** Abnormal development of the lower limbs results in a single lower extremity or 2 legs that are joined together. Accompanying spine and skeletal malformations, with either absent or defective vertebrae, commonly occur. The internal and external sex organs, rectum, kidneys, and bladder may also be missing or underdeveloped. An imperforate anus and other abnormalities of the lower gastrointestinal tract may be present. Ultrasonography can detect sirenomelia sequence during the 2nd trimester of pregnancy.

**Etiology** The cause of sirenomelia sequence is unknown, but irregularities in early embryonic vascular development produce the defects. Instead of the 2 umbilical arteries that normally branch out of the lower part of the aorta and carry blood to the caudal end of the embryo, a single large artery arises from high in the abdominal cavity. Referred to as a vitelline artery steal, this process diverts blood and nutrients away from the embryo's caudal region to the placenta.

**Epidemiology** Sirenomelia sequence occurs 1:60,000 to 1:100,000 births.

**Related Disorders** See *Caudal Regression Syndrome.*

**Treatment—Standard** Surgical separation of the joined legs has been successful. Prognosis depends on the involvement of the gastrointestinal system, vertebrae, and other structural deformities. Other treatment is symptomatic and supportive.

**Treatment—Investigational** Please contact the agencies listed under Resources, below, for the most current information. Addresses and telephone numbers of these agencies, as well as of individual experts and research centers, may be found in the Master Resources List.

**Resources**

**For more information on sirenomelia sequence:** National Organization for Rare Disorders (NORD); NIH/National Institute of Child Health and Human Development.

**For genetic information and genetic counseling referrals:** March of Dimes Birth Defects Foundation; Alliance of Genetic Support Groups.

**References**

Prenatal Diagnosis of Sirenomelia: M. Sitori, et al.; J. Ultrasound Med., February 1989, vol. 8(2), pp. 83–88.

Smith's Recognizable Patterns of Human Malformation, 4th ed.: K.L. Jones; W.B. Saunders Company, 1988, pp. 574–575.

Vascular Steal: The Pathogenetic Mechanism Producing Sirenomelia and Associated Defects of the Viscera and Soft Tissues: R.E. Stevenson, et al.; Pediatrics, September 1986, vol. 78(3), pp. 451–457.

Sirenomelia: Angiographic Demonstration of Vascular Anomalies: G. Malinger, et al.; Arch. Pathol. Lab. Med., July 1982, vol. 106(7), pp. 347–348.

# SMITH-LEMLI-OPITZ (SLO) SYNDROME

**Description** SLO syndrome is a hereditary developmental disorder characterized by craniofacial, limb, and genital abnormalities as well as failure to thrive and mental retardation. Two forms exist: type II is more severe than type I.

**Signs and Symptoms** In the severe form of the disorder, stillbirth is common; infants are often born in breech position and may not survive the neonatal period.

Physical characteristics of the less severe form include a small, abnormally long and narrow head; ptosis, epicanthal folds, and strabismus; a broad nasal tip with anteverted nostrils; and broad lateral ridges in the palate and a moderately small mandible. Palms and soles frequently have a simian crease; webbing often appears between the 2nd and 3rd toes. Fingertips frequently show whorl dermatoglyphic patterns. Cryptorchidism, hypospadias, and hypogonadism may be present. Many phenotypic patients are genotypically XY and have undergone sex-reversal.

Other characteristics include low birth weight and subsequent failure to thrive; vomiting in early infancy and tendency toward a shrill cry; moderate-to-severe mental retardation; and early hypotonia that later becomes hypertonic.

Occasional features of Smith-Lemli-Opitz syndrome include a broad nasal bridge, cleft palate, a clenched hand with the index finger overlying the 3rd finger, an asymmetric short thumb, and distal palmar axial triradius. The forefoot may deviate toward the metatarsus adductus, and a hip may be dislocated. The child may also have a deep sacral dimple, a pit anterior to the anus, nipples that are wide apart, inguinal hernia, pyloric stenosis, dilated renal calices, and a cardiac defect.

**Etiology** Smith-Lemli-Opitz syndrome is an autosomal recessive inherited disorder. Recent studies have established that a block in conversion of 7-dehydrocholesterol to cholesterol is the cause for the syndrome. The prevalence is 1:20,000 to 1:40,000.

**Epidemiology** Over 200 cases have been recorded.

**Treatment—Standard** Special education services, physical therapy, and genetic counseling are recommended. Research is under way in dietary treatment of the condition.

**Treatment—Investigational** Please contact the agencies listed under Resources, below, for the most current information. Addresses and telephone numbers of these agencies, as well as of individual experts and research centers, may be found in the Master Resources List.

**Resources**

**For more information on Smith-Lemli-Opitz syndrome:** National Organization for Rare Disorders (NORD); NIH/National Institute of Child Health and Human Development; SLO/RSH Advocacy Exchange; John M. Opitz, M.D., Shodar Children's Hospital, Helena, Montana.

**For genetic information and genetic counseling referrals:** March of Dimes Birth Defects Foundation; Alliance of Genetic Support Groups.

**References**

Cholesterol Metabolism in the Smith-Lemli-Opitz Syndrome: Summary of an NICHD Conference: J.M. Opitz and F. de la Cruz; Am. J. Med. Genet., 1994, vol. 50, pp. 326–338.

Defective Cholesterol Biosynthesis Associated with the Smith-Lemli-Opitz Syndrome: G.S. Tint, et al.; N. Engl. J. Med., January 1994, vol. 330(2), pp. 107–113.

SLO (Smith-Lemli-Opitz) Syndrome: Designing a High Cholesterol Diet for the SLO Syndrome: P.B. Acosta; Am. J. Med. Genet., 1994, vol. 50, pp. 358–363.

Smith's Recognizable Patterns of Human Malformation, 4th ed.: K.L. Jones; W.B. Saunders Company, 1988, pp. 104–105.

# SMITH-MAGENIS SYNDROME

**Description** Smith-Magenis syndrome is a chromosomal disorder characterized by unusual facial features, mental retardation, behavioral abnormalities, and speech problems.

**Synonyms**

Chromosome 17, Interstitial Deletion 17p-

**Signs and Symptoms** Severity depends on the amount of missing genetic material. Infants typically have unusual facial features that include a wide nose, a flat midface, and a prominent forehead and/or jaw. The head appears short and flat. A raspy or hoarse voice, speech delays, hearing loss, and short, wide fingers and toes also occur.

Growth delay, mental retardation, and hyperactivity may occur. Self-destructive behavior may include head-banging, wrist-biting, insertion of foreign bodies into body orifices, and pulling out fingernails and toenails. Myopia and strabismus occur frequently, detachment of the retina less often.

Difficulty falling asleep or remaining asleep is common. Some children experience a high pain threshold, burning sensations, peripheral neuropathy, amyotrophy, and absent or decreased reflexes.

Congenital heart defects may also occur.

**Etiology** Smith-Magenis syndrome usually occurs because of interstitial deletion on the short arm of chromosome 17 (p11.2). Some cases may occur de novo early in fetal development, as an autosomal dominant inheritance, or as isolated events.

**Epidemiology** Males and females are affected in equal numbers. Approximately 120 children worldwide have been diagnosed with this disorder.

**Related Disorders** See *Fraser Syndrome; Rubinstein-Taybi Syndrome; Marshall Syndrome.*

Self-mutilating behaviors may occur in other disorders, such as autism, Lesch-Nyhan syndrome, Tourette syndrome, and Rett syndrome. However, these children do not have the physical characteristics of those with Smith-Magenis syndrome.

**Therapies–Standard** Medication can alleviate hyperactivity and sleep difficulties. Special education may help in maximizing the potential of the child. Speech therapy and special classes for the hearing impaired may also be valuable. Counseling may be helpful for parents caring for a child with self-destructive behavioral problems.

Genetic counseling will benefit patients and their families. Other treatment is symptomatic and supportive.

**Treatment—Investigational** Please contact the agencies listed under Resources, below, for the most current information. Addresses and telephone numbers of these agencies, as well as of individual experts and research centers, may be found in the Master Resources List.

**Resources**

**For more information on Smith-Magenis syndrome:** National Organization for Rare Disorders (NORD);

Parents and Researchers Interested in Smith-Magenis Syndrome; Smith-Magenis Syndrome Contact Group; Chromosome Deletion Outreach; The Arc (a national organization on mental retardation); American Society for Deaf Children; Vision Foundation; NIH/National Institute of Child Health and Human Development.

**For genetic information and genetic counseling referrals:** March of Dimes Birth Defects Foundation; Alliance of Genetic Support Groups.

### References
Mendelian Inheritance in Man, 11th ed.: V.A. McKusick; The Johns Hopkins University Press, 1994, p. 1357.

Eye Abnormalities in the Smith-Magenis Contiguous Gene Deletion Syndrome: B.M. Finucane, et al.; Am. J. Med. Genet., February 1993, vol. 45(4), pp. 443–446.

Mosaicism for Deletion 17p11.2 in a Boy with the Smith-Magenis Syndrome: B.M. Finucane, et al.; Am. J. Med. Genet., February 1993, vol. 45(4), pp. 447–449.

Genetics in Medicine, 5th ed.: M.W. Thompson, et al.; W.B. Saunders Company, 1991, pp. 207–208.

Molecular Analysis of the Smith-Magenis Syndrome: A Possible Contiguous-Gene Syndrome Associated with Del (17) (p11): F. Greenberg, et al.; Am. J. Hum. Genet., December 1991, vol. 49(6), pp. 1207–1218.

Smith-Magenis Syndrome: A New Contiguous Gene Syndrome: Report of Three New Cases: A. Moncla, et al.; J. Med. Genet., September 1991, vol. 28(9), pp. 627–632.

Birth Defects Encyclopedia: M.L. Buyse, ed.-in-chief; Blackwell Scientific Publications, 1990, p. 380.

# SOTOS SYNDROME

**Description** Sotos syndrome is a rare hereditary disorder characterized by excessive growth over the 90th percentile during the first 2 to 3 years of life. Mild mental retardation may be present.

**Synonyms**

Cerebral Gigantism

**Signs and Symptoms** The primary symptoms of Sotos syndrome are large birth weight and excessive growth during the first 2 to 3 years of life. By 10 years of age, the patient reaches a height age of 14 or 15 years. Physical characteristics include a disproportionately large and long head with a slightly protrusive forehead, large hands and feet, hypertelorism, and down-slanting eyes. Not all of these features occur in every patient. Mild developmental retardation is common. Other characteristics include clumsiness and an awkward gait as well as unusual aggressiveness or irritability.

Persons with this disorder have abnormal dermatoglyphics. Bone and dental ages tend to be 2 to 4 and 1 to 2 years advanced, respectively.

Differential diagnosis should include XYY and fragile X syndromes. Endocrine evaluation usually reveals no abnormalities. Children should be tested for elevated growth hormone levels to rule out a growth-hormone–secreting pituitary tumor. Less than 5 percent of patients have developed benign or malignant tumors.

**Etiology** The great majority of cases are sporadic. A dominant hereditary pattern also has been documented in some cases. The disorder has been ascribed to impaired function of the hypothalamic-pituitary axis, but thus far all functional pituitary tests have been normal.

**Epidemiology** Sotos syndrome affects males and females equally.

**Related Disorders** See *Acromegaly.*

**Treatment—Standard** Initial abnormalities resolve as growth rate becomes normal after the first 2 to 3 years of life. Medical treatment is symptomatic and supportive.

**Treatment—Investigational** Please contact the agencies listed under Resources, below, for the most current information. Addresses and telephone numbers of these agencies, as well as of individual experts and research centers, may be found in the Master Resources List.

### Resources

**For more information on Sotos syndrome:** National Organization for Rare Disorders (NORD); Sotos Syndrome Support Association; Juan Sotos, M.D., Children's Hospital, Columbus, Ohio; Sotos Syndrome Support Group of Great Britain; NIH/National Institute of Child Health and Human Development.

**For genetic information and genetic counseling referrals:** March of Dimes Birth Defects Foundation; Alliance of Genetic Support Groups.

### References
Mendelian Inheritance in Man, 11th ed.: V.A. McKusick; The Johns Hopkins University Press, 1994, pp. 278–279.

Syndromes of the Head and Neck, 3rd ed.: R.J. Gorlin, et al.; Oxford University Press, 1990, pp. 332–336.

Smith's Recognizable Patterns of Human Malformation, 4th ed.: K.L. Jones; W.B. Saunders Company, 1988, pp. 128–129.

# SPLIT-HAND DEFORMITY

**Description** Split-hand deformity is a genetic disorder characterized by the absence of fingers or parts of fingers, often occurring with a cleft of the hand. When a cleft does occur, both hands and both feet usually are affected. Many types and combinations of deformities occur in this disorder.

**Synonyms**
> Ectrodactilia
> Ectrodactyly
> Ektrodactylie
> Karsch-Neugebauer Syndrome
> Lobster Claw Deformity

**Signs and Symptoms** There are 2 typical patterns of characteristics in split-hand deformity. In one type, in which the hand has a lobster-claw appearance, the 3rd digit is absent and replaced with a cone-shaped cleft that tapers toward the wrist, dividing the hand into 2 parts. The remaining fingers or parts of fingers on each side of the cleft are often joined or webbed. If the cleft is present, it generally is found on both hands, and the feet are usually similarly affected.

In the 2nd variety of split-hand deformity, only the 5th digit is present and there is no cleft. Severity varies between these types, and cases of each type occasionally are found in the same family.

Affected individuals usually have normal intelligence and live normal life spans, although with varying degrees of disability related to the severity of the deformity.

**Etiology** Split-hand deformity is an autosomal dominant inherited trait. Occasionally split-hand deformity will skip a generation.

**Epidemiology** Males and females are affected equally. Frequency is estimated at 1:90,000 births.

**Treatment—Standard** Reconstructive surgery when applicable may improve the deformity, and prosthetics are available to help achieve normal functioning. Genetic counseling may benefit patients and their families. Other treatment is symptomatic and supportive.

**Treatment—Investigational** Please contact the agencies listed under Resources, below, for the most current information. Addresses and telephone numbers of these agencies, as well as of individual experts and research centers, may be found in the Master Resources List.

**Resources**

**For more information on split-hand deformity:** National Organization for Rare Disorders (NORD); International Center for Skeletal Dysplasia; NIH/National Arthritis and Musculoskeletal and Skin Diseases Information Clearinghouse; Association of Children's Prosthetic and Orthotic Clinics.

**For genetic information and genetic counseling referrals:** March of Dimes Birth Defects Foundation; Alliance of Genetic Support Groups.

**References**

Mendelian Inheritance in Man, 11th ed.: V.A. McKusick; The Johns Hopkins University Press, 1994, pp. 1381–1382, 2534–2535.

Monodactylous Splithand-Splitfoot: A Malformation Occurring in Three Distinct Genetic Types: G. Bujdoso, et al.; Eur. J. Pediatr., May 1980, vol. 133(3), pp. 207–215.

# SPONDYLOEPIPHYSEAL DYSPLASIA CONGENITA

**Description** Congenital spondyloepiphyseal dysplasia is a rare hereditary disorder characterized by short stature, abnormal bone development, and ocular abnormalities.

**Signs and Symptoms** Symptom manifestations vary greatly. These include flat facial features, myopia or retinal detachment, short-trunk small stature, and barrel-chestedness. Knees tend to be misaligned, pointing either outward or inward, resulting in delayed onset of walking and a waddling gait. Hands and feet appear normal, and patients usually have normal intelligence. Patients may reach an adult height of 84 cm (33 inches) to 128 cm (50.4 inches).

In some cases complications ensue, e.g., retinal detachment resulting in severe vision impairment or blindness. Stress on the lax ligaments may cause spinal cord compression. Kyphoscoliosis, hyperextensible finger joints, and joint dislocation may also occur.

**Etiology** The disorder appears to be an autosomal dominant inherited trait. It is caused by a mutation of type II collagen gene (COL 2A1).

**Epidemiology** Incidence is about 1:100,000 live births. Males and females are equally affected.

**Related Disorders** See *Morquio Syndrome; Mucopolysaccharidosis; Spondyloepiphyseal Dysplasia Tarda.*

**Treatment—Standard** Treatment includes early symptomatic correction of clubfoot deformity, closure of the cleft palate, and prevention or treatment of retinal detachment. Lifelong orthopedic care is often necessary. Genetic counseling is recommended for further family planning.

**Treatment—Investigational** Please contact the agencies listed under Resources, below, for the most current information. Addresses and telephone numbers of these agencies, as well as of individual experts and research centers, may be found in the Master Resources List.

**Resources**

**For more information on congenital spondyloepiphyseal dysplasia:** National Organization for Rare Disorders (NORD); NIH/National Institute of Child Health and Human Development; Human Growth Foundation; Little People of America; Short Stature Foundation.

**For genetic information and genetic counseling referrals:** March of Dimes Birth Defects Foundation; Alliance of Genetic Support Groups.

**References**

Smith's Recognizable Patterns of Human Malformation, 4th ed.: K.L. Jones; W.B. Saunders Company, 1988, pp. 310–311.

# SPONDYLOEPIPHYSEAL DYSPLASIA TARDA

**Description** Spondyloepiphyseal dysplasia tarda is a hereditary disorder characterized by short stature and skeletal abnormalities.

**Synonyms**

X-Linked Spondyloepiphyseal Dysplasia

**Signs and Symptoms** Symptoms occur between 5 and 10 years of age, at which point spinal growth appears to stop. Shoulders become hunched, and kyphosis and scoliosis develop. The neck appears to shorten, and the chest broadens. During adolescence, skeletal abnormalities may cause pain in the back, hips, shoulders, knees, and ankles. Adult patients are short of stature; height usually ranges from 130 cm (51 inches) to 158 cm (62 inches). The trunk is short, the chest cage is large, and the limb length is relatively normal.

**Etiology** In most cases, the disorder is inherited as an X-linked recessive trait; the gene has been localized to Xp22.

**Epidemiology** Prevalence is approximately 1:100,000.

**Related Disorders** See *Morquio Syndrome; Mucopolysaccharidosis; Spondyloepiphyseal Dysplasia Congenita.*

**Multiple epiphyseal dysplasia** is characterized by development of a waddling gait in affected children between the ages of 2 and 5 years. Osteoarthritic joint changes cause pain. Patients have an almost normal body size, with disproportionately small hands and feet. Males and females are affected equally. The disorder is inherited as an autosomal dominant trait.

**Treatment—Standard** Treatment of spondyloepiphyseal dysplasia tarda is symptomatic and supportive. Physical therapy is recommended for joint stiffness and pain. Severely debilitating osteoarthritis of the hips may occur by age 60 and necessitate total hip replacement. Genetic counseling is recommended for further family planning.

**Treatment—Investigational** Please contact the agencies listed under Resources, below, for the most current information. Addresses and telephone numbers of these agencies, as well as of individual experts and research centers, may be found in the Master Resources List.

**Resources**

**For more information on spondyloepiphyseal dysplasia tarda:** National Organization for Rare Disorders (NORD); NIH/National Institute of Child Health and Human Development; Human Growth Foundation; Little People of America; Short Stature Foundation; Let's Face It.

**For genetic information and genetic counseling referrals:** March of Dimes Birth Defects Foundation; Alliance of Genetic Support Groups.

**References**

Smith's Recognizable Patterns of Human Malformation, 4th ed.: K.L. Jones; W.B. Saunders Company, 1988, pp. 328–329.

# SPRENGEL DEFORMITY

**Description** Sprengel deformity is a congenital upward displacement of the scapula.

**Synonyms**

High Scapula

Scapula Elevata

**Signs and Symptoms** An elevated, underdeveloped scapula is evident at birth, causing a lump at the posterior base of the neck and limiting arm movement. Bone, cartilage, or fiberlike tissue may form between the shoulder blade and adjacent vertebrae. Skeletal abnormalities and underdeveloped muscles are found in over half of patients.

Symptoms associated with Sprengel deformity include scoliosis, hemivertebrae, missing or fused ribs, ribs in the neck, abnormalities of the clavicle, underdeveloped or incomplete muscles of the shoulder girdle, abnormalities of the chest, displaced organs, spina bifida occulta, and cleft palate.

**Etiology** The majority of cases occur as isolated events. An autosomal dominant inheritance has been reported in some families.

**Epidemiology** Males and females are affected equally in autosomal dominant cases, and females twice as often as males in sporadic cases. Approximately 20 families have been reported with the inherited form.

**Related Disorders** See *Klippel-Feil Syndrome*.

**Treatment—Standard** Surgery may be performed in severe cases to improve mobility and cosmetic appearance. Treatment of cleft palate requires a team of specialists: pediatricians, dental specialists, surgeons, speech pathologists, and others. Cleft palate may be repaired by surgery or covered with a prosthesis.

Genetic counseling is beneficial for families of affected children. Other treatment is symptomatic and supportive.

**Treatment—Investigational** Researchers are studying a Teflon-glycerine paste that is applied to the rear of the pharynx in a minor surgical procedure to bring the pharynx and palate into proper relationship. For further information, contact William N. Williams, D.D.S., University of Florida.

Please contact the agencies listed under Resources, below, for the most current information. Addresses and telephone numbers of these agencies, as well as of individual experts and research centers, may be found in the Master Resources List.

**Resources**

**For more information on Sprengel deformity:** National Organization for Rare Disorders (NORD); NIH/National Arthritis and Musculoskeletal and Skin Diseases Information Clearinghouse; International Center for Skeletal Dysplasia.

**For genetic information and genetic counseling referrals:** March of Dimes Birth Defects Foundation; Alliance of Genetic Support Groups.

**References**

Mendelian Inheritance in Man, 11th ed.: V.A. McKusick; The Johns Hopkins University Press, 1994, p. 1387.

Birth Defects Encyclopedia: M.L. Buyse, ed.-in-chief; Blackwell Scientific Publications, 1990, pp. 1593–1594.

Sprengel Deformity: S.J. Leibovic, et al.; J. Bone Joint Surg., February 1990, vol. 72(2), pp. 192–197.

# STICKLER SYNDROME

**Description** Stickler syndrome is characterized by micrognathia, cleft palate, and congenital abnormalities of the eye. Bone abnormalities and degenerative changes in some joints may occur early in life. Expressivity of the syndrome may be mild, moderate, or severe. With early treatment the prognosis may be favorable.

**Synonyms**

Arthro-Ophthalmopathy

Epiphyseal Changes and High Myopia

Ophthalmoarthropathy

Weissenbacher-Zweymuller Syndrome

**Signs and Symptoms** Craniofacial abnormalities include a broad, flat, sunken bridge of the nose, giving a flattened appearance to the face, and cleft palate and small jaw (Pierre Robin syndrome). Both sensorineural and conductive deafness may develop. Ocular abnormalities may include severe myopia, astigmatism, and changes of the optic disk. Cataracts, detachment of the retina, and blindness may develop during the first decade of life. Glaucoma simplex may also occur.

Bony abnormalities are usually present in joints such as the ankles, knees, and wrists. Affected children may be stiff and sore after strenuous exercise. Sometimes swelling, redness, and warmth may be present and result in crepitation and temporary locking of joints. X-rays may show irregularities of the joint surfaces, especially in the vertebral column and the knees. Subluxation of the hips is another frequent finding. Abnormalities of the epiphyseal plate may occur, and cartilage fragments may be present within the joint. There may be hyperextensibility of the finger, knee, and elbow joints. Fingers may be tapered.

**Etiology** Stickler syndrome is inherited as an autosomal dominant and autosomal recessive trait. Very recently mutations have been found in the fibrillar collagen gene, COL 11A, on chromosome 6p21.

**Epidemiology** Both males and females are affected.

**Related Disorders** See *Spondyloepiphyseal Dysplasia Congenita.*

**Wagner syndrome** is inherited as an autosomal dominant disorder that may be mild, moderate, or severe. It is characterized by facial abnormalities, an underdeveloped jaw, saddle nose, cleft palate, and vision abnormalities. Hip deformities and joint hyperextensibility in the fingers, elbows, and knees may also occur. Differentiation from Stickler syndrome is difficult, and some experts believe they are the same condition.

**Treatment—Standard** Avoidance of excessive physical exertion including contact sports may prevent joint stiffness and soreness in the ankles, knees, and wrists. Detached retinas may be surgically corrected. Genetic counseling will be helpful to families of affected children.

**Treatment—Investigational** Please contact the agencies listed under Resources, below, for the most current information. Addresses and telephone numbers of these agencies, as well as of individual experts and research centers, may be found in the Master Resources List.

**Resources**

**For more information on Stickler syndrome:** National Organization for Rare Disorders (NORD); NIH/National Arthritis and Musculoskeletal and Skin Diseases Information Clearinghouse; NIH/National Eye Institute.

**References**

Autosomal Dominant and Recessive Osteochondrodysplasias Associated with the COL 11A2 Locus: M. Vikkula, et al.; Cell, 1995, vol. 30, pp. 431–437.

Mendelian Inheritance in Man, 11th ed.: V.A. McKusick; The Johns Hopkins University Press, 1994, pp. 166–167, 390.

Smith's Recognizable Patterns of Human Malformation, 4th ed.: K.L. Jones; W.B. Saunders Company, 1988, pp. 242–245.

Management of Retinal Detachment in the Wagner-Stickler Syndrome: B.M. Billington, et al.; Trans. Ophthalmol. Soc. UK, 1985, vol. 104(pt. 8), pp. 875–879.

Stickler's Syndrome or Hereditary Progressive Arthro-Ophthalmopathy: M. Vallat, et al.; J. Fr. Ophtalmol., 1985, vol. 8(4), pp. 301–307.

The Wagner-Stickler Syndrome—A Study of 22 Families: R.M. Liberfarb, et al.; J. Pediatrics, September 1981, vol. 99(3), pp. 394–399.

# STURGE-WEBER SYNDROME

**Description** Sturge-Weber syndrome is characterized by leptomeningeal angiomas, intracranial calcifications, and seizures. A facial nevus flammeus may be present. Intraocular angiomas may result in glaucoma.

**Synonyms**

Encephalofacial Angiomatosis
Encephalotrigeminal Angiomatosis
Leptomeningeal Angiomatosis
Meningeal Capillary Angiomatosis
Sturge-Kalischer-Weber Syndrome
Sturge-Weber Phakomatosis
Sturge-Weber-Dimitri Syndrome

**Signs and Symptoms** Usually, but not always, a unilateral nevus flammeus develops along the site of the trigeminal nerve. As the patient ages, the stain deepens and elevations may also develop. On the same side of the face as the nevus are leptomeningeal angiomas and intracranial calcifications.

Nevi are bilateral in about 37 percent of patients and unilateral in 50 percent. They involve the limbs and trunk in about 36 percent of patients, and lips and oral mucosa in about 25 percent.

Seizures, which are common, begin during the first year and worsen with age. Over half of patients experience mental deficiencies; and 30 percent, either hemiparesis or hemiplegia.

Ocular complications occur in about 40 percent of patients; they do not develop in individuals who do not have port-wine stains. The affected eye is always on the same side of the head as the nevus. Glaucoma and buphthalmos occur in about 30 percent of patients, often at birth; onset, however, may be anytime during the first 2 years. Other ocular complications include angiomas in the conjunctiva, choroid, and cornea; different-colored eyes; hydrophthalmos; hemianopia; lens opacification or displacement; retinal detachment; angioid streaks; optic atrophy; and cortical blindness.

Other syndromes that may occur in association with Sturge-Weber syndrome include Klippel-Trenaunay syndrome, tuberous sclerosis, and neurofibromatosis.

**Etiology** The etiology is unknown. Some cases are believed to be autosomal dominant in origin. Trauma sustained in utero may be the cause in others.

**Epidemiology** Only a few thousand cases have been reported in the United States. Males and females are equally affected.

**Related Disorders** See *Neurofibromatosis; Tuberous Sclerosis; von Hippel–Lindau Syndrome.*

**Treatment—Standard** Treatment is symptomatic and supportive. Until recently, the argon laser was used to try to remove or lighten the port-wine stain. This procedure was associated with crusting, scabbing, and scarring, and sufficient pain to require a local anesthetic. The flash pump dye laser has replaced the argon laser as a more effective means of removing or lessening the stain. Children as young as 1 month can be treated with this laser, because pain is minimal and skin is not damaged. Contact the Sturge-Weber Foundation (see Resources, below) for a list of institutions where this laser is used.

Anticonvulsant medications may be prescribed to control seizures; phenytoin, however, tends to aggravate oral tissue hypertrophy. Special education services, genetic counseling, and physical therapy may benefit patients and their families.

**Treatment—Investigational** Children under the age of 1 year with Sturge-Weber syndrome and seizures are being examined with the positron emission tomography (**PET**) scan by Harry T. Chugani, M.D., at the University of California at Los Angeles Medical Center, under a grant from the National Institutes of Health. Dr. Chugani is seeking to identify patients with controlled seizures who might benefit from hemispherectomy.

Research on port-wine stains is also being pursued by Dr. Odile Enjolras, Department of Dermatology, Hospital Tarnier, Paris, France.

Please contact the agencies listed under Resources, below, for the most current information. Addresses and telephone numbers of these agencies, as well as of individual experts and research centers, may be found in the Master Resources List.

**Resources**

For more information on Sturge-Weber syndrome: National Organization for Rare Disorders (NORD); Sturge-Weber Foundation; NIH/National Institute of Neurological Disorders and Stroke.

For genetic information and genetic counseling referrals: March of Dimes Birth Defects Foundation; Alliance of Genetic Support Groups.

**References**

Mendelian Inheritance in Man, 11th ed.: V.A. McKusick; The Johns Hopkins Press, 1994, p. 1395.
Syndromes of the Head and Neck, 3rd ed.: R.J. Gorlin, et al.; Oxford University Press, 1990, pp. 406–410.
Birth Defects Compendium, 2nd ed.: Daniel Bergsma; March of Dimes, 1979, 1987.

# SUMMITT SYNDROME

**Description** Summitt syndrome is an extremely rare genetic disorder characterized by malformations of the head, abnormalities of the hands and/or feet, and obesity. Summitt syndrome may be a variant of Carpenter syndrome (acrocephalopolysyndactyly type II). There are 4 types of acrocephalopolysyndactyly: Noack syndrome (type I), Carpenter syndrome (type II), Sakati syndrome (type III), and Goodman syndrome (type IV). All of these types are characterized by acrocephaly, polydactyly, and syndactyly.

**Synonyms**

Summitt Acrocephalosyndactyly

**Signs and Symptoms** Craniosynostosis causes the head to grow upward at an accelerated rate, resulting in a deformed skull that appears long, narrow, and pointed at the top. Affected individuals also have syndactyly and are usually obese. Other features include epicanthal folds, delayed tooth eruption, an abnormally narrow palate, coxa valga, and genu valgum. Males with Summitt syndrome may have gynecomastia. Intelligence is typically within normal limits.

**Etiology** Summitt syndrome is inherited as an autosomal recessive trait.

**Epidemiology** Three cases have been reported in the medical literature. Two of the affected individuals were brothers who were the children of closely related parents.

**Related Disorders** See *Carpenter Syndrome; Goodman Syndrome; Pfeiffer Syndrome; Antley-Bixler Syndrome.*

**Treatment—Standard** Surgical correction of malformations is the primary treatment. Early craniofacial surgery may be performed to correct craniosynostosis. Additional craniofacial surgery may be done later in life as well as surgery to correct deformities of the hands and/or feet.

Other treatment is symptomatic and supportive. Genetic counseling will benefit people with Summitt syndrome and their families.

**Treatment—Investigational** Please contact the agencies listed under Resources, below, for the most current information. Addresses and telephone numbers of these agencies, as well as of individual experts and research centers, may be found in the Master Resources List.

**Resources**

For more information on Summitt syndrome: National Organization for Rare Disorders (NORD); NIH/National Institute of Child Health and Human Development.

For information about craniofacial research and treatments: Forward Face; FACES—National Association for the Craniofacially Handicapped; Let's Face It; National Craniofacial Foundation; National Foundation for Facial Reconstruction; AboutFace; Craniofacial Family Association; Craniofacial Support Group.

**For genetic information and genetic counseling referrals:** March of Dimes Birth Defects Foundation; Alliance of Genetic Support Groups.

### References

Mendelian Inheritance in Man, 11th ed.: V.A. McKusick; The Johns Hopkins University Press, 1994, p. 2209.

Online Mendelian Inheritance in Man (OMIM): V.A. McKusick; last edit date 3/30/94, entry number 201000; last edit date 3/12/94, entry number 272350; last edit date 3/11/94, entry number 101120.

Carpenter's Syndrome (Acrocephalopolysyndactyly Type II) with Normal Intelligence: M.N. Jamil, et al.; Br. J. Neurosurg., 1992, vol. 6(3), pp. 243–247.

Birth Defects Encyclopedia: M.L Buyse, ed.-in-chief; Blackwell Scientific Publications, 1990, pp. 36–37.

Dictionary of Medical Syndromes, 3rd ed.: S.I. Magalini, et al. (eds.); J.B. Lippincott Company, 1990, p. 850.

Acrocephalopolysyndactyly Type II—Carpenter Syndrome: Clinical Spectrum and an Attempt at Unification with Goodman and Summitt Syndromes: D.M. Cohen, et al.; Am. J. Med. Genet., October 1987, vol. 28(2), pp. 311–324.

Carpenter Syndrome: Marked Variability of Expression to Include the Summitt and Goodman Syndromes: R. Gershoni-Baruch; Am. J. Med. Genet., February 1990, vol. 35(2), pp. 236–240.

# THROMBOCYTOPENIA–ABSENT RADIUS (TAR) SYNDROME

**Description** TAR syndrome is a genetic disorder characterized by thrombocytopenia and the absence or underdevelopment of the radius.

**Synonyms**
> Radial Aplasia–Amegakaryocytic Thrombocytopenia Syndrome
> Radial Aplasia–Thrombocytopenia Syndrome

**Signs and Symptoms** The thrombocytopenia is most severe during early infancy and may cause excessive bleeding from the skin or mucous membranes or intracranially. Other blood disorders, such as absent or underdeveloped megakaryocytes, eosinophilia, granulocytosis, and anemia may occur. Infants with TAR syndrome are said to be more likely to develop an intolerance to cow's milk.

The radius is absent or underdeveloped, usually bilaterally. Also present may be underdevelopment of the ulna and defects of the hands, legs, and feet.

Short stature, bowed legs, shortened humerus, underdeveloped shoulder girdle, and dislocation of the hip may occur, as well as spina bifida and kidney or heart defects. A nevus flammeus may be present on the forehead.

**Etiology** TAR syndrome is inherited as an autosomal recessive trait.

**Epidemiology** The disorder occurs at birth. Males and females are affected in equal numbers.

**Related Disorders** See ***Anemia, Fanconi.***

**Treatment—Standard** Early management is necessary for the various blood conditions of these patients. Braces and/or surgical correction may be required for related bone malformations. Genetic counseling is suggested for patients and their families. Other treatment is symptomatic and supportive.

**Treatment—Investigational** Please contact the agencies listed under Resources, below, for the most current information. Addresses and telephone numbers of these agencies, as well as of individual experts and research centers, may be found in the Master Resources List.

**Resources**

**For more information on thrombocytopenia–absent radius syndrome:** National Organization for Rare Disorders (NORD); Thrombocytopenia–Absent Radius Syndrome Association; NIH/National Institute of Child Health and Human Development.

**For genetic information and genetic counseling referrals:** March of Dimes Birth Defects Foundation; Alliance of Genetic Support Groups.

### References

Mendelian Inheritance in Man, 11th ed.: V.A. McKusick; The Johns Hopkins University Press, 1994, pp. 2229–2230.

Smith's Recognizable Patterns of Human Malformation, 4th ed.: K.L. Jones; W.B. Saunders Company, 1988, pp. 276.

Thrombocytopenia–Absent Radius Syndrome: A.G. Aledo, et al.; An. Esp. Pediatr., January 1982, vol. 16(1), pp. 82–87.

# TOOTH AND NAIL SYNDROME

**Description** Tooth and nail syndrome is characterized by absent teeth and poorly formed nails.

**Synonyms**
> Dysplasia of Nails with Hypodontia
> Witkop Tooth-Nail Syndrome

**Signs and Symptoms** Signs of tooth and nail syndrome include lack of mandibular incisors, second molars, maxillary canines, and other permanent teeth. Finger- and toenails are hypoplastic and slow-growing.

**Etiology** The syndrome appears to be inherited as an autosomal dominant trait in some families.

**Epidemiology** Males and females are affected equally.

**Treatment—Standard** Treatment is symptomatic and supportive; dentures may be helpful. Genetic counseling may be beneficial.

**Treatment—Investigational** Please contact the agencies listed under Resources, below, for the most current information. Addresses and telephone numbers of these agencies, as well as of individual experts and research centers, may be found in the Master Resources List.

**Resources**

**For more information on tooth and nail syndrome:** National Organization for Rare Disorders (NORD); National Foundation for Ectodermal Dysplasias; NIH/National Institute of Child Health and Human Development.

**For genetic information and genetic counseling referrals:** March of Dimes Birth Defects Foundation; Alliance of Genetic Support Groups.

**References**

Syndromes of the Head and Neck, 3rd ed.: R.J. Gorlin, et al.; Oxford University Press, 1990, pp. 863–864.

# TOWNES-BROCKS SYNDROME

**Description** Characteristics are present at birth and vary from person to person, both in type and severity. The major feature is an imperforate anus, in association with hand, foot, and ear abnormalities.

**Synonyms**

> Anus, Imperforate, with Hand, Foot, and Ear Anomalies
> Deafness, Sensorineural, with Imperforate Anus and Hypoplastic Thumbs
> Townes Syndrome

**Signs and Symptoms** Craniofacial abnormalities include hemifacial microsomia and poorly formed external ears that can be abnormally large or small, with preauricular protuberances or tags, and sometimes preauricular pits. Sensorineural hearing loss or deafness is present in some patients.

The thumbs may be hypoplastic or have the appearance more of a finger than a thumb. Other anomalies include triphalangeal thumb and hexadactyly. Syndactyly of fingers or toes may occur, as well as fusion of bones in the wrist. In the feet, the metatarsals may be fused and may be shorter than average. The 3rd toe may be hypoplastic. The 5th toe, or one or more fingers, may be malformed (clinodactyly).

Imperforate anus is present in most patients with Townes-Brocks syndrome. Fistulas, e.g., rectovaginal or rectoperineal, may occur. In some patients there may be abnormal placement and stenosis of the anus, as well as duodenal atresia.

Renal hypoplasia, other urorenal anomalies, and ureterovesical reflux can occur. Other characteristics include cardiac defects, cystic ovary, and hypospadias.

**Etiology** The syndrome is inherited as an autosomal dominant trait.

**Epidemiology** The disorder is extremely rare. Males and females are affected in equal numbers.

**Related Disorders** See *Holt-Oram Syndrome; Imperforate Anus; VACTERL Association.*

**Treatment—Standard** Treatment often includes surgery for malformations. Genetic counseling may be beneficial for patients and their families. Other treatment is symptomatic and supportive.

**Treatment—Investigational** Please contact the agencies listed under Resources, below, for the most current information. Addresses and telephone numbers of these agencies, as well as of individual experts and research centers, may be found in the Master Resources List.

**Resources**

**For more information on Townes-Brocks syndrome:** National Organization for Rare Disorders (NORD); NIH/National Institute of Child Health and Human Development; Hemifacial Microsomia Family Support Network.

**For genetic information and genetic counseling referrals:** March of Dimes Birth Defects Foundation; Alliance of Genetic Support Groups.

**References**

Mendelian Inheritance in Man, 11th ed.: V.A. McKusick; The Johns Hopkins University Press, 1994, p. 137.

Townes-Brocks Syndrome: Report of a Case and Review of the Literature: F.G. Ferraz, et al.; Ann. Genet., 1989, vol. 32(2), pp. 120–23.

A New Family with the Townes-Brocks Syndrome: M.A. de Vries-Van der Weerd, et al.; Clin. Genet., September 1988, vol. 34(3), pp. 195–200.

Smith's Recognizable Patterns of Human Malformation, 4th ed.: K.L. Jones; W.B. Saunders Company, 1988, pp. 218–219.

Townes Syndrome: A Distinct Multiple Malformation Syndrome Resembling VACTERL Association: J.H. Hersh, et al.; Clin. Pediatr. (Phila), February 1986, vol. 25(2), pp. 100–102.

# TREACHER COLLINS SYNDROME

**Description** Treacher Collins syndrome is a rare genetic disorder characterized by slanted eyes, dysphagia, deafness, and deformities of the maxilla, mandible, and ears.

**Synonyms**
> Francheschetti-Klein Syndrome
> Mandibulofacial Dysostosis

**Signs and Symptoms** Patients with Treacher Collins syndrome typically have an especially long face, a beaklike nose, and receding chin. Other characteristic features include slanted eyes and notching of the lower eyelids. Malar and maxillary as well as mandibular hypoplasia may cause dysphagia or respiratory problems for the newborn. The pinna and external acoustic meatus may be malformed, and the tympanic membrane may be replaced with a bony plate. Almost 50 percent of patients have conductive deafness.

**Etiology** The gene locus is the long arm of chromosome 5 (5q31.3–32). It is inherited as an autosomal dominant trait. A positive family history is found in fewer than half of new Treacher Collins patients. Thus, it is suspected that approximately 60 percent of cases represent new mutations.

**Epidemiology** Males and females are affected in equal numbers. The incidence is about 1:50,000 live births.

**Related Disorders** See *Goldenhar Syndrome; Oral-Facial-Digital Syndrome; Nager Syndrome.*

**Juberg-Hayward syndrome (oro-cranio-digital syndrome)** is a rare hereditary disorder also characterized by cleft lip and palate and by deformities of the thumbs as well as the toes. The head is microcephalic. Growth hormone deficiency resulting in short stature has been reported in one boy.

**Treatment—Standard** During infancy, insertion of feeding or breathing tubes may be required. Early hearing evaluation is indicated. The need for surgery or hearing aids will depend on the type of deafness present. Speech and language difficulties may require appropriate therapy. Surgery to improve the appearance of the jaw and ears may be appropriate.

The age of the child determines the type of surgical treatment. During infancy, attention is directed toward the upper airway. A tracheostomy may be needed. The notched lower eyelid can be repaired in the infant's first year, and slanting eyelids and flat cheek bones, during the preschool and early school years. Correction of the jaws and malocclusion is usually done in stages, with the final corrections being performed in teenage years, along with orthodontic therapy.

For external ear abnormalities, minor anomalies can be surgically corrected before the child starts school. If the major portion of the ear is missing, it is best to wait until age 6 so that sufficient rib cartilage is available for framework and grafting.

Genetic counseling may benefit patients and their families. Other treatment is symptomatic and supportive.

**Treatment—Investigational** Various surgical methods to improve the appearance of Treacher Collins patients are being studied. Most recently, the Tessier Integral procedure has been developed for correction of malformations of the eyes, maxilla, and mandible.

Drs. Amy Feldman Lewanda and Ethylin Wang Jabs at Johns Hopkins Hospital in Baltimore are researching the genes responsible for craniofacial disorders.

Please contact the agencies listed under Resources, below, for the most current information. Addresses and telephone numbers of these agencies, as well as of individual experts and research centers, may be found in the Master Resources List.

**Resources**

**For more information on Treacher Collins syndrome:** National Organization for Rare Disorders (NORD); Treacher Collins Family Foundation; NIH/National Institute of Child Health and Human Development; FACES— National Association for the Craniofacially Handicapped; National Craniofacial Foundation; Forward Face; American Society for Deaf Children; Deafness Research Foundation; Craniofacial Centre Children's Hospital.

**For genetic information and genetic counseling referrals:** March of Dimes Birth Defects Foundation; Alliance of Genetic Support Groups.

**References**

Mendelian Inheritance in Man, 11th ed.: V.A. McKusick; The Johns Hopkins University Press, 1994, pp. 912–913.

Familial Treacher Collins Syndrome: P.S. Murty, et al.; J. Laryngol. Otol., July 1988, vol. 102(7), pp. 620–622.

Smith's Recognizable Patterns of Human Malformation, 4th ed.: K.L. Jones; W.B. Saunders Company, 1988, pp. 210–211.

Psychosocial Adjustment of 20 Patients with Treacher Collins Syndrome Before and After Reconstructive Surgery: E.M. Arndt, et al.; Br. J. Plast. Surg., November 1987, vol. 40(6), pp. 605–609.

Anthropometric Evaluation of Dysmorphology in Craniofacial Anomalies: Treacher Collins Syndrome: J.C. Kolar, et al.; Am. J. Phys. Anthropol., December 1987, vol. 74(4), pp. 441–451.

# TRICHODENTOOSSEOUS SYNDROME (TDOS)

**Description** TDOS is one of the ectodermal dysplasias and primarily affects teeth, hair, and bones. Intelligence and life span are usually unaffected.

**Synonyms**

Curly Hair Osteosclerosis

**Signs and Symptoms** Infants are born with kinky hair that may straighten with age, and curly eyelashes. Nails are thin and likely to peel or break.

Dental abnormalities, including abscessed teeth during the first years of life, are a major feature of TDOS. Tooth enamel may become yellow-brown, thin, and pitted. X-rays reveal taurodontia and mild-to-moderate increased bone density. Since teeth may not grow appropriately during infancy, TDOS children may lose teeth and have delayed dentition.

Unlike most other ectodermal dysplasias, TDOS does not affect the respiratory tract.

**Etiology** TDOS is inherited as an autosomal dominant trait. Symptoms are caused by a defect in ectodermal cells involving the formation and structure of teeth, hair, and nails.

**Epidemiology** TDOS affects males and females equally and can occur in conjunction with other hereditary disorders.

**Treatment—Standard** Dental treatment involves early restoration of teeth with jacket crowns and/or prosthetic replacement. Genetic counseling may be beneficial.

**Treatment—Investigational** Please contact the agencies listed under Resources, below, for the most current information. Addresses and telephone numbers of these agencies, as well as of individual experts and research centers, may be found in the Master Resources List.

**Resources**

**For more information on trichodentoosseous syndrome:** National Organization for Rare Disorders (NORD); National Foundation for Ectodermal Dysplasias; NIH/National Institute of Dental Research.

**For genetic information and genetic counseling referrals:** March of Dimes Birth Defects Foundation; Alliance of Genetic Support Groups.

**References**

Mendelian Inheritance in Man, 11th ed.: V.A. McKusick; The Johns Hopkins University Press, 1994, p. 1478.

Smith's Recognizable Patterns of Human Malformation, 4th ed.: K.L. Jones; W.B. Saunders Company, 1988, pp. 482–483.

A Tricho-Odonto-Onychial Subtype of Ectodermal Dysplasia: H. Kresbach, et al.; Z. Hautkr., May 1984, 59(9), pp. 601–613.

Tricho-Dento-Osseous Syndrome: Heterogeneity or Clinical Variability: S.D. Shapiro, et al.; Am. J. Med. Genet., October 1983, 16(2), pp. 225–236.

# TRICHORHINOPHALANGEAL SYNDROME (TRPS)

**Description** TRPS occurs in 2 forms: types I and II. Type II (Langer-Giedion syndrome) is the more severe. Both types I and II are forms of ectodermal dysplasia, and are characterized by thin, brittle hair; a bulbous nose; cone-shaped epiphyses; and varying degrees of growth retardation. Fingers are abnormally developed and facial appearance is unusual.

**Synonyms**

Langer-Giedion Syndrome, Type II

**Signs and Symptoms TRPS type I** is characterized primarily by hair and bone abnormalities. Scalp hair is fine, brittle, and sparse. Some individuals may become completely bald. Eyebrows are thick near the nose but extremely thin nearer the temples. The tip of the nose is bulbous, and the upper lip is thin and the philtrum long. These facial abnormalities often subside at adolescence. Thin nails and extra teeth occur in some cases. Abnormalities of the skeletal system include cone-shaped epiphyses in some fingers and toes, pectus carinatum, and scoliosis. Intelligence is usually normal.

In **TRPS type II (Langer-Giedion syndrome),** facies, hair and epiphyseal abnormalities are similar to those of type I. Distinguishing features for Langer-Giedion syndrome are multiple exostoses, mild microcephaly, and mild-to-moderate mental retardation. The exostoses occur primarily near the ends of the tubular arm and leg bones and usually develop by age 3 or 4. Other bones may also be affected. Delayed onset of speech, and, less frequently, hearing loss have occurred. An increased susceptibility to respiratory infections and hip dislocations may be present. Clinical features overlap markedly in types I and II.

**Etiology** Visible cytogenic deletions, translocations, and insertions involve band 8q24.12 for TRPS type I. Type II (8q24.11–24.13) appears to be a true contiguous gene syndrome.

**Epidemiology** Both forms of trichorhinophalangeal syndrome are very rare.

**Treatment—Standard** Treatment is symptomatic and supportive. Surgery may correct limb deformities. Genetic counseling may be beneficial.

**Treatment—Investigational** Please contact the agencies listed under Resources, below, for the most current information. Addresses and telephone numbers of these agencies, as well as of individual experts and research centers, may be found in the Master Resources List.

**Resources**

**For more information on trichorhinophalangeal syndrome:** National Organization for Rare Disorders (NORD); National Foundation for Ectodermal Dysplasias; NIH/National Institute of Child Health and Human Development.

**For genetic information and genetic counseling referrals:** March of Dimes Birth Defects Foundation; Alliance of Genetic Support Groups.

**References**

Molecular Dissection of a Contiguous Gene Syndrome: Localization of the Genes Involved in the Langer-Giedeon Syndrome: L. Hermann-Josef, et al.; Hum. Mol. Genet., 1995, vol. 4, pp. 31–36.

Mendelian Inheritance in Man, 11th ed.: V.A. McKusick; The Johns Hopkins University Press, 1994, pp. 1479, 2242.

Syndromes of the Head and Neck, 3rd ed.: R.J. Gorlin, et al.; Oxford University Press, 1990, pp. 806–812.

Clinical and Scanning Electron Microscopic Findings in a Solitary Case of Trichorhinophalangeal Syndrome Type I: E.P. Prens, et al.; Acta Derm. Venereol. (Stockh.), 1984, vol. 64(3), pp. 2449–2453.

New Clinical Observations in the Trichorhinophalangeal Syndrome: R.M. Goodman, et al.; J. Craniofac. Genet. Dev. Biol., 1981, vol. 1(1), pp. 15–29.

Trichorhinophalangeal Dysplasia (Gideon Syndrome): A Case Report: G.B. Kuna, et al.; Clin. Pediatr. (Phila.), January 1978, vol. 17(1), pp. 96–98.

# TRIPLOID SYNDROME

**Description** Triploid syndrome is an extremely rare disorder in which a complete extra set of chromosomes is present. Affected infants usually are lost through early miscarriage. Some are stillborn or live only a few days, and a few infants have survived as long as 5 months. These infants have severely retarded fetal growth and many other prenatal abnormalities.

**Synonyms**

Chromosome Triploidy Syndrome

Triploidy

**Signs and Symptoms** Associated abnormalities include an unusually large placenta, lack of prenatal skeletal growth, and craniofacial characteristics such as ocular hypertelorism; low nasal bridge; low-set, malformed ears; and micrognathia. There may be syndactyly of the 3rd and 4th fingers, and simian creases of the hands. Congenital defects of the heart and sex organs may be present, as well as abnormal brain development and renal and adrenal hypoplasia. Less often there are an unusually shaped skull, cleft lip or palate, meningomyelocele, and hernias. There may also be liver and gallbladder deformities and twisted colon.

The pregnant mother may experience preeclampsia.

**Etiology** Triploid syndrome is caused by a complete extra set of chromosomes, i.e., 69 rather than 46. Triplication of the chromosomes is most often the result of double fertilization of an egg. The disorder is not inherited, and there is no evidence of increased risk of recurrence.

**Epidemiology** Parental age does not seem to be a factor. Males and females are affected in equal numbers.

**Related Disorders** See *Down Syndrome; Chromosome 11q- Syndrome; Chromosome 18p- Syndrome.*

**Treatment—Standard** Treatment of triploid syndrome is symptomatic and supportive.

**Treatment—Investigational** Please contact the agencies listed under Resources, below, for the most current information. Addresses and telephone numbers of these agencies, as well as of individual experts and research centers, may be found in the Master Resources List.

**Resources**

**For more information on triploid syndrome:** National Organization for Rare Disorders (NORD); NIH/National Institute of Child Health and Human Development.

**For genetic information and genetic counseling referrals:** March of Dimes Birth Defects Foundation; Alliance of Genetic Support Groups.

**References**

Syndromes of the Head and Neck, 3rd ed.: R.J. Gorlin, et al.; Oxford University Press, 1990, pp. 64–65.

Smith's Recognizable Patterns of Human Malformation, 4th ed.: K.L. Jones; W.B. Saunders Company, 1988, pp. 32–35.

Morphologic Anomalies in Triploid Liveborn Fetuses: N. Doshi, et al.; Hum. Pathol., August 1983, vol. 14(4), pp. 716–723.

Diplospermy II Indicated As the Origin of a Live Born Human Triploid (69, XXX): B.M. Page, et al.; J. Med. Genet., October 1981, vol. 18(5), pp. 386–389.

# TRISMUS PSEUDOCAMPTODACTYLY SYNDROME

**Description** Trismus pseudocamptodactyly syndrome is an inherited disorder of the tendons.

**Synonyms**

> Camptodactyly, Facultative Type
> Camptodactyly–Limited Jaw Excursion
> Camptodactyly-Trismus Syndrome
> Hecht Syndrome

**Signs and Symptoms** Trismus pseudocamptodactyly syndrome prevents normal development of the short muscle tendons. The severity of the disorder varies widely. A major feature is the limited ability to open the mouth, making chewing difficult for some. Short flexor tendons in the fingers causes irreducible flexion when the wrist is bent backward.

Some patients with trismus pseudocamptodactyly syndrome also have short flexor muscles of the feet, which results in talipes equinovarus, metatarsus adductus, pes planus, metatarsus varus, and/or calcaneovalgus.

Other symptoms may include short stature; a short gastrocnemius; short hamstrings, causing pelvic tilt; and/or spasmodic torticollis.

**Etiology** Trismus pseudocamptodactyly syndrome is inherited as an autosomal dominant genetic trait with varying severity.

**Epidemiology** Males and females are affected in equal numbers. Of the 35 cases reported, several have been traced to a Dutch girl who migrated to Tennessee, and 5 occurred in 3 generations of a Japanese family.

**Related Disorders** See *Gordon Syndrome; Spasmodic Torticollis.*

**Camptodactyly** may occur alone as an autosomal dominant trait or in association with another syndrome. Characteristics include flexion of fingers and in some cases toes. Typically, all the fingers are affected except the thumb. Males and females are affected equally.

**Treatment—Standard** Orthopedic care is indicated for foot deformities. Physical therapy may prove beneficial to some patients.

Genetic counseling will benefit patients and their families. Linkage analysis can identify carriers of the gene. Other treatment is symptomatic and supportive.

**Treatment—Investigational** Please contact the agencies listed under Resources, below, for the most current information. Addresses and telephone numbers of these agencies, as well as of individual experts and research centers, may be found in the Master Resources List.

**Resources**

**For more information on trismus pseudocamptodactyly syndrome:** National Organization for Rare Disorders (NORD); NIH/National Arthritis and Musculoskeletal and Skin Diseases Information Clearinghouse.

**For genetic information and genetic counseling referrals:** March of Dimes Birth Defects Foundation; Alliance of Genetic Support Groups.

**References**

Mendelian Inheritance in Man, 11th ed.: V.A. McKusick; The Johns Hopkins University Press, 1994, p. 953.

Birth Defects Encyclopedia: M.L. Buyse, ed.-in-chief; Blackwell Scientific Publications, 1990, pp. 257–258.

Smith's Recognizable Patterns of Human Malformation, 4th ed.: K.L. Jones; W.B. Saunders Company, 1988, p. 190.

Orthopedic Aspects of the Trismus Pseudocamptodactyly Syndrome: P.J. O'Brien, et al.; J. Pediatr. Orthop., August 1984, vol. 4(4), pp. 469–471.

Linkage Analysis with the Trismus-Pseudocamptodactyly Syndrome: R.D. Robertson, et al.; Am. J. Med. Genet., May 1982, vol. 12(1), pp. 115–120.

Trismus Pseudocamptodactyly Syndrome: Dutch-Kentucky Syndrome: C.C. Mabry, et al.; J. Pediatr., October 1974, vol. 85(4), pp. 503–508.

# TRISOMY

**Description** Trisomies are very rare genetic disorders in which an extra chromosome is added to one of the normal pairs. The triplication of the chromosome may be partial; i.e., either an extra short arm (p) or an extra long arm (q) is present. Defects are classified by the name of the abnormal chromosome pair and the portion of the chromosome affected. In general, the most common symptom of the trisomies is mental retardation. (There are, however, many causes of mental retardation; most are genetic anomalies that are not trisomies.)

**Synonyms**

> Chromosomal Triplication

**Signs and Symptoms** Following is a description of a few trisomy disorders not further discussed in PHYSICIANS' GUIDE TO RARE DISEASES. See also *Trisomy 13 Syndrome; Trisomy 18 Syndrome; Down Syndrome (Trisomy 21).*

**Partial trisomy 6p** is characterized by a triplicated section of the short arm of the 6th chromosome. Manifestations include mental retardation, multiple facial abnormalities, and malformations of the lungs and kidney. Two kidneys may be present on one side of the body, with crossed ureters.

**Trisomy 8** patients are typically slender and of normal height. The ears are low-set and malformed, and the eyes tend to be down-slanted. Bone and joint abnormalities may involve the ribs, spine, and kneecaps; joint contractures are common. Deep creases are seen in the palms of the hands and soles of the feet. Mental and motor retardation is mild to moderate, often associated with delayed and hard-to-understand speech. Most patients with trisomy 8 are chromosomal mosaics (i.e., they have 2 or more cell types that have different numbers of chromosomes).

**Trisomy 9p** is identified by an extra short arm of chromosome 9, leading to abnormalities in the hands, feet, and pelvic bones. The pattern of bone structures in x-rays of patients with trisomy 9p appears to be unique among patients with chromosomal abnormalities. Other typical features include down-turned corners of the mouth, a large rounded nose, slightly wide and deep-set slanted eyes, unusual fingerprints, and mental retardation.

**Trisomy 10q** is characterized by a triplication of part of the long arm of the 10th chromosome. Predominant manifestations include dolichocephaly, prominent forehead, and abnormally open seams and fontanelles on the skull at birth. A broad nose, cleft palate, ptosis, posteriorly rotated ears, congenital heart defects, and severe mental retardation also occur.

**Partial trisomy 22 (cat's-eye syndrome)** is characterized by coloboma of the iris and by anal atresia. Severe mental and physical retardation, wide-set slanted eyes, and preauricular tags or fistulas may develop. Congenital heart disease may occur. A few cases with full trisomy have been reported in patients with similar symptoms and signs, but micrognathia and hypotonia distinguish them from the partial trisomy.

**Etiology** The trisomies are inborn abnormalities of the chromosomes. In some cases the chromosomal abnormalities are related to advanced maternal or paternal age.

**Epidemiology** Some trisomies might affect a few hundred or a few thousand children per year; some only a handful of children in the United States. The most common trisomy is Down syndrome (trisomy 21), affecting approximately 7,000 newborn infants each year.

**Related Disorders** There are many partial trisomy disorders with a wide range of manifestations.

**Treatment—Standard** Genetic counseling will be helpful to families of patients with a trisomy disorder. Some genetic counselors suggest that pregnant women over the age of 35 should undergo amniocentesis, since many trisomies can be detected before birth.

Parent and infant education can begin immediately after birth. Children with mental retardation usually benefit from early intervention programs and special education. The individual child should receive direct service programming to develop learning, language, mobility, self-care, and socialization skills. Toddler and preschool programs can further enhance the acquisition of skills to enable persons with mental retardation to reach their maximum potential.

**Treatment—Investigational** Please contact the agencies listed under Resources, below, for the most current information. Addresses and telephone numbers of these agencies, as well as of individual experts and research centers, may be found in the Master Resources List.

**Resources**

**For more information on trisomy:** National Organization for Rare Disorders (NORD); Support Organization for Trisomy 18, 13 and Related Disorders; The Arc (a national organization on mental retardation); National Down Syndrome Congress.

**For genetic information and genetic counseling referrals:** March of Dimes Birth Defects Foundation; Alliance of Genetic Support Groups.

**References**

Smith's Recognizable Patterns of Human Malformation, 4th ed.: K.L. Jones; W.B. Saunders Company, 1988, pp. 10–79.

# TRISOMY 4P

**Description** Trisomy 4p is a chromosomal disorder in which there is an additional piece added to the short arm "p" of chromosome 4. The most frequent features of this disorder are facial abnormalities, slowed growth after birth, and psychomotor retardation.

**Synonyms**

Chromosome 4, Trisomy 4p

Chromosome 4, Partial Trisomy 4p

**Signs and Symptoms** The symptoms of trisomy 4p vary depending on the amount of genetic material duplicated on the short arm "p" of the 4th chromosome. There may be slowed growth with a tendency to become heavy, as well as psychomotor retardation. Mental retardation may range from moderate to severe. The head may be abnormally small, with a prominent forehead and ridges above the orbits of the eyes. The eyes may be widely spaced, and the nose may be bulbous, with a flat nasal bridge. The eyebrows may grow together (synophrys), and there is sometimes macroglossia. Abnormalities of the ears as well as a short neck and pointed chin are frequent features of trisomy 4p. Irregularities of the teeth, widely spaced nipples, and underdeveloped nails of the fingers and toes are found in many affected individuals. Clinodactyly may be present, and there may be abnormalities of the feet. Scoliosis as well as missing or additional ribs has also been present in patients with this disorder. In males there may be microphallus, hypospadias, and cryptorchidism. Other symptoms sometime encountered are eye abnormalities, malformed kidneys, congenital heart disease, and inguinal hernia.

**Etiology** The majority of cases of trisomy 4p are the result of a balanced translocation in one of the parents. The parent has no symptoms and is usually unaware that he or she has a chromosomal abnormality. When a balanced translocation is present, there is good chance of having a child with extra or missing chromosomal material.

Trisomy 4p has also been caused by a pericentric inversion in a few cases.

Several cases of trisomy 4p have been the result of a spontaneous duplication of the short arm of chromosome 4 during embryonic development. The parents of a child with a de novo duplication usually have normal chromosomes and a low probability of having another child with a chromosomal abnormality.

**Epidemiology** Trisomy 4p affects males and females in equal numbers. There have been approximately 35 cases of this disorder reported in the medical literature.

**Treatment—Standard** Trisomy 4p individuals with mental retardation usually benefit from early intervention programs and special education. Parent and infant education can begin immediately after birth. The child should receive direct service programming to develop learning, language, mobility, self-care, and socialization skills. Genetic counseling may benefit patients and their families. Other treatment is symptomatic and supportive.

**Treatment—Investigational** Please contact the agencies listed under Resources, below, for the most current information. Addresses and telephone numbers of these agencies, as well as of individual experts and research centers, may be found in the Master Resources List.

**Resources**

**For more information on trisomy 4p:** National Organization for Rare Disorders (NORD); The Arc (a national organization on mental retardation); NIH/National Institute of Child Health and Human Development.

**For genetic information and genetic counseling referrals:** March of Dimes Birth Defects Foundation; Alliance of Genetic Support Groups.

**References**

Nelson Textbook of Pediatrics, 14th ed.: R.E. Behrman, ed.-in-chief; W.B. Saunders Company, 1992, pp. 227–281.

Birth Defects Encyclopedia: M.L Buyse, ed.-in-chief; Blackwell Scientific Publications, 1990, p. 337.

Smith's Recognizable Patterns of Human Malformation, 4th ed.: K.L. Jones, ed.; W.B. Saunders Company, 1988, p. 36.

A Further Report on a Kindred with Cases of 4p Trisomy and Monosomy: J.G. Mortimer, et al.; Hum. Hered., 1980, vol. 30(1), pp. 58–61.

4p Trisomy Syndrome: Report of Four Additional Cases and Segregation Analysis of 21 Families with Different Translocations: J. Crane, et al.; Am. J. Med. Genet., 1979, vol. 4(3), pp. 219–298.

The Trisomy 4p Syndrome: Case Report and Review: C.H. Gonzalez, et al.; Am. J. Med. Genet., 1977, vol. 1(2), pp. 137–156.

# TRISOMY 13 SYNDROME

**Description** Trisomy 13 syndrome is a genetic disorder with varied characteristics that include gross defects of the brain; midline anomalies; cleft lip or cleft palate, or both; polydactyly; and cardiac defects.

**Synonyms**

> D Trisomy Syndrome
>
> Patau Syndrome
>
> Trisomy 13–15 Syndrome

**Signs and Symptoms** Prenatal diagnosis can be determined by amniocentesis and chorionic villus sampling. Chromosomal studies reveal an extra chromosome 13. Ultrasound studies reveal major developmental abnormalities. Newborns are usually small and have severe abnormalities: microcephaly and a sloping forehead; wide sutures and patent fontanelles; often a myelomeningocele (not quite one-half of cases); holoprosencephaly; and cleft lip and/or cleft palate. Other defects include capillary hemangiomas, especially on the forehead in the midline; dermal sinuses on the scalp; and loose folds of skin over the back of the neck. The ears are low-set and malformed. Infants are often apneic, appear to be deaf, and have severe mental retardation. Fetal hemoglobin is elevated in all cases.

Ocular anomalies frequently include microphthalmia, coloboma, and retinal dysplasia. Shallow supraorbital ridges and slanted palpebral fissures are characteristic. The hands are polydactylic, with flexed fingers that may or may not overlap; narrow, spherical fingernails; and a palmar simian crease. There may be polydactyly of the feet, and the heels are prominent.

Other common congenital anomalies include atrial and ventricular septal defects, a patent ductus arteriosus, defects of the pulmonary and aortic valves, and dextrocardia, as well as abnormal genitalia in both sexes, including cryptorchidism and bicornuate uterus.

**Etiology** An additional chromosome 13 causes the abnormalities. Some symptoms may be due to overexpression of certain genes on chromosome 13. Elevated levels of esterase D (the gene for which resides on 13q14.11) have been found in renal tissue of affected infants. More studies are needed to understand the role of esterase D in trisomy 13 syndrome.

**Epidemiology** Trisomy 13 syndrome occurs in 1:12,000 live births. Approximately 1 percent of all spontaneous abortions have trisomy 13. About half of affected infants die during the first months and about 90 percent during the first year. Studies have suggested an association between trisomy 13 syndrome and preeclampsia. Males and females of all nationalities and races are affected equally.

**Treatment—Standard** Treatment is symptomatic and supportive. Genetic counseling is of benefit for families of children with this disorder.

**Treatment—Investigational** Please contact the agencies listed under Resources, below, for the most current information. Addresses and telephone numbers of these agencies, as well as of individual experts and research centers, may be found in the Master Resources List.

**Resources**

**For more information on trisomy 13 syndrome:** National Organization for Rare Disorders (NORD); Support Organization for Trisomy 18, 13 and Related Disorders; NIH/National Institute of Child Health and Human Development; The Arc (a national organization on mental retardation); National Institute of Mental Retardation (Canada); In Touch (U.K.).

**For genetic information and genetic counseling referrals:** March of Dimes Birth Defects Foundation; Alliance of Genetic Support Groups.

**References**

Natural History of Trisomy 18 and Trisomy 13: I: Growth, Physical Assessment, Medical Histories, Survival, and Recurrence Risk: Natural History of Trisomy 18 and Trisomy 13: II: Psychomotor Development: B.J. Baty, et al.; Am. J. Med. Genet., January 1994, vol. 49(2), pp. 175–188, 189–194.

Holoprosencephaly-Polydactyly (Pseudotrisomy 13) Syndrome: Expansion of the Phenotypic Spectrum: I.W. Lurie, et al.; Am. J. Med. Genet., September 1993, vol. 47(3), pp. 405–509.

Overexpression of Esterase D in Kidney from Trisomy 13 Fetuses: S. Loughna, et al.; Am. J. Hum. Genet., October 1993, vol. 53(4), pp. 810–816.

The Ultrasound Markers for Chromosomal Disease: A Retrospective Study: P. Twining, et al.; Br. J. Radiol., May 1993, vol. 66(785), pp. 408–414.

Cecil Textbook of Medicine, 19th ed.: J.B. Wyngaarden, et al., eds.; W.B. Saunders Company, 1992, p. 139.

Fetal Growth in Aneuploid Conditions: S. Droste: Clin. Obstet. Gynecol., March 1992, vol. 35(1), pp. 119–125.

Nelson Textbook of Pediatrics, 14th ed.: R.E. Behrman, ed.-in-chief; W.B. Saunders Company, 1992, p. 286.

Pre-Eclampsia and Trisomy 13: J.F. Tuohy, et al.; Br. J. Obstet. Gynaecol., November 1992, vol. 99(11), pp. 891–894.

Harrison's Principles of Internal Medicine, 12th ed.: J.D. Wilson, et al.; McGraw-Hill, 1991, pp. 923, 925.

Pseudo-Trisomy 13 Syndrome: M.M. Cohen, et al.; Am. J. Med. Genet., June 1991, vol. 39(3), pp. 332–335, discussion pp. 336–337.

Birth Defects Encyclopedia: M.L. Buyse, ed.-in-chief; Blackwell Scientific Publications, 1990, pp. 368–369.

Dictionary of Medical Syndromes, 3rd ed.: S.I. Magalini, et al., eds.: J.B. Lippincott Company, 1990, p. 674.

Syndromes of the Head and Neck, 3rd ed.: R.J. Gorlin, et al.; Oxford University Press, 1990, pp. 40–43.

Smith's Recognizable Patterns of Human Malformation, 4th ed.: K.L. Jones; W.B. Saunders Company, 1988, pp. 20–25.

# TRISOMY 18 SYNDROME

**Description** Trisomy 18 syndrome is a genetic disorder with onset in utero. Infants have multiple congenital anomalies, appear thin and frail, have difficulty feeding, fail to thrive, and show generalized hypertonicity with rigidity in flexion of the limbs. Mental retardation also is present.

**Synonyms**

Edwards Syndrome

**Signs and Symptoms** Danger signals may occur in utero, with weak fetal activity and hydramnios. There is often just one umbilical artery and a small placenta, and the infant may be premature or small for gestational age, with a feeble cry and a lowered sound response. Skeletal muscle and subcutaneous fat are hypoplastic. The head is microcephalic, with a prominent occiput and small jaw and mouth, creating a pinched look. Epicanthal folds, cleft lip or cleft palate (or both), low-set and malformed ears, and redundant skin folds, especially over the back of the neck, are common. Mental retardation is usually severe.

The hand characteristically makes a clenched fist, the index finger overlapping the 3rd and 4th fingers; the fingernails are hypoplastic; and the thumbs are absent or hypoplastic. The distal crease on the 5th finger is often absent, and a low-arched dermal ridge fingertip pattern is common. Abnormalities of the feet include syndactyly, clubfeet, and a shortened and often dorsiflexed big toe.

Congenital anomalies often occur in the lungs and diaphragm; other frequent abnormalities include patent ductus arteriosus, ventricular and atrial septal defects, and pulmonary and aortic valve defects. The kidneys and ureters are often affected, and hernias, separation of the rectus muscles of the abdominal wall, and cryptorchidism are also common.

**Etiology** The syndrome is caused by the presence of a 3rd chromosome 18, which is responsible for the physical and mental abnormalities of this developmental disorder.

**Epidemiology** Female infants are 4 times more likely than male infants to have trisomy 18 syndrome. It occurs in 1:5,000 to 1:7,000 newborn infants. Maternal age is usually above average. About half of affected infants die by 2 months and fewer than 10 percent survive 1 year.

**Treatment—Standard** Treatment is symptomatic and supportive.

**Treatment—Investigational** Please contact the agencies listed under Resources, below, for the most current information. Addresses and telephone numbers of these agencies, as well as of individual experts and research centers, may be found in the Master Resources List.

**Resources**

**For more information on trisomy 18 syndrome:** National Organization for Rare Disorders (NORD); Support Organization for Trisomy 18, 13 and Related Disorders; NIH/National Institute of Child Health and Human Development; The Arc (a national organization on mental retardation); National Institute of Mental Retardation (Canada).

**For genetic information and genetic counseling referrals:** March of Dimes Birth Defects Foundation; Alliance of Genetic Support Groups.

**References**

Natural History of Trisomy 18 and Trisomy 13: I: Growth, Physical Assessment, Medical Histories, Survival, and Recurrence Risk: B.J. Baty, et al.; Am. J. Med. Genet., January 1994, vol. 49(2), pp. 175–188.

Molecular Studies of Trisomy 18: J.M. Fisher, et al.; Am. J. Hum. Genet., June 1993, vol. 52(6), pp. 1139–1144.

The Ultrasound Markers of Chromosomal Disease: A Retrospective Study: P. Twining, et al.; Br. J. Radiol., May 1993, vol. 66(785), pp. 408–414.

Cecil Textbook of Medicine, 19th ed.: J.B. Wyngaarden, et al., eds.; W.B. Saunders Company, 1992, p. 139.

Health Supervision and Anticipatory Guidance for Children with Genetic Disorder (Including Specific Recommendations for Trisomy 21, Trisomy 18, and Neurofibromatosis I): J.C. Carey; Pediatr. Clin. North Am., February 1992, vol. 39(1), pp. 25–53.

Nelson Textbook of Pediatrics, 14th ed.: R.E. Behrman, ed.-in-chief; W.B. Saunders Company, 1992, p. 286.

Harrison's Principles of Internal Medicine, 12th ed.: J.D. Wilson, et al.; McGraw-Hill, 1991, pp. 923, 925.

A Maternal Serum Screen for Trisomy 18: An Extension of Maternal Serum Screening for Down Syndrome: A.J. Staples, et al.; Am. J. Hum. Genet., November 1991, vol. 49(5), pp. 1025–1033.

Birth Defects Encyclopedia: M.L. Buyse, ed.-in-chief; Blackwell Scientific Publications, 1990, pp. 368–369.

Dictionary of Medical Syndromes, 3rd ed.: S.I. Magalini, et al., eds.: J.B. Lippincott Company, 1990, p. 674.

Ultrasonographic Detection of the Second-Trimester Fetus with Trisomy 18 and Trisomy 21: N. Ginsberg, et al.; Am. J. Obstet. Gynecol., October 1990, vol. 163(4 pt. 1), pp. 1186–1190.

Smith's Recognizable Patterns of Human Malformation, 4th ed.: K.L. Jones; W.B. Saunders Company, 1988, pp. 16–19.

# TURNER SYNDROME

**Description** Turner syndrome is a genetic disorder of females in which there is a lack of sexual development at puberty. Other characteristics include small stature, a webbed neck, heart defects, and various other abnormalities. About half of individuals have a 45,X karyotype; others are 45,X/46,XX mosaics or have other X chromosome defects.

**Synonyms**

45,X Syndrome
Bonnevie-Ulrich Syndrome
Gonadal Dysgenesis (45,X)
Monosomy X

**Signs and Symptoms** Affected individuals have female characteristics, but most do not undergo puberty or develop secondary sexual characteristics (breasts, and pubic and axillary hair) because they have immature (streak) ovaries and cannot produce estrogen.

Growth is slowed and adults are almost always under 5 feet tall. Intelligence is usually normal. Visual-spatial deficits may be present. Lowered self-esteem may occur during adolescence.

Congenital abnormalities may include a narrow, arched palate; small mandible; broad chest; and, at the nape of the neck, loose skin folds, webbing, and low hairline. Typical cardiac defects may include coarctation of the aorta and other left side anomalies. Urinary tract abnormalities include horseshoe kidney and double ureters. Patients with mosaicism (45,X/46,XX) have attenuated clinical manifestations. Some patients may develop breasts and even have menses for a short interval, but almost 100 percent are infertile.

**Etiology** The syndrome is caused by an absence or defect of the X chromosome. The karyotype is 45,X in 50 percent of cases, lacking one of the X chromosomes; in 30 to 40 percent, there is mosaicism (45,X/46,XX). In the remainder of cases, the 2nd X chromosome is present but shows a variety of abnormalities (isochromosomes, deletions, rings, etc.).

**Epidemiology** The disorder occurs in about 1:3,000 live-born females. The 45,X karyotype at conception is about 1.5 percent, but the majority are spontaneously aborted. Cystic hygroma is common in these aborted fetuses.

**Related Disorders** See *Noonan Syndrome.*

**Treatment—Standard** There is no cure, but certain measures can provide a more normal life. Growth hormone has proved helpful in many cases. At puberty, replacement therapy with estrogen allows normal development of breasts, labia, vagina, uterus, and fallopian tubes, although patients are infertile. In vitro fertilization with a donor egg and implanted pregnancy are possible.

**Treatment—Investigational** The National Institutes of Health request the cooperation of physicians in referring patients (age 4 to 12 years) with Turner syndrome. Patients will be offered enrollment in a long-term treatment protocol to assess the effect of treatment with low-dose estrogen and growth hormone on adult height. Referring physicians will receive a complete summary of all evaluations, and patients will continue to be followed in conjunction with their referring physicians. For more information, contact Gordon B. Cutler, Jr., M.D., National Institutes of Health, Bethesda, Maryland; or Judith Levine Ross, M.D., Jefferson Medical College, Philadelphia.

Ethinyl estradiol, a female hormone manufactured by Gynex, is being administered in small doses to stimulate development of secondary sexual characteristics. An increase in the predicted adult height without advancement of bone age is the objective. Optimal dosage and duration of therapy are under investigation.

To increase linear growth, researchers are evaluating the effectiveness of oxandrolone (Oxandrin; available from Gynex) on patients with Turner syndrome. In contrast to human growth hormone **(HGH)**, oxandrolone is taken orally and is less expensive.

To increase growth rate and adult height, many clinicians are using a combination of oxandrolone and HGH. The final consensus of such therapy is not yet at hand.

Please contact the agencies listed under Resources, below, for the most current information. Addresses and telephone numbers of these agencies, as well as of individual experts and research centers, may be found in the Master Resources List.

**Resources**

**For more information on Turner syndrome:** National Organization for Rare Disorders (NORD); Turner Syndrome Support Group of New England; Turner Syndrome Society of the United States; Turner Syndrome Society of Canada; NIH/National Institute of Child Health and Human Development.

**For genetic information and genetic counseling referrals:** March of Dimes Birth Defects Foundation; Alliance of Genetic Support Groups.

**References**

Combined Therapy with Growth Hormone and Oxandrolone in Adolescent Girls with Turner Syndrome: P.W. Ku, et al.; J. Paediatr. Child Health, February 1993, vol. 29(1) pp. 40–42.

Slow Baseline Growth and a Good Response to Growth Hormone (GH) Therapy Are Related to Elevated Spontaneous GH Pulse Frequency in Girls with Turner's Syndrome: G.A. Kamp, et al.; J. Clin. Endocrinol. Metab., June 1993, vol. 76(6), pp. 1604–1609.

Turner Syndrome Adolescents Receiving Growth Hormone Are Not Osteopenic: E.K. Neely; J. Clin. Endocrinol. Metab., April 1993, vol. 76(4), pp. 861–866.

Turner Syndrome: The Case of the Missing Sex Chromosome: A.R. Zinn, et al.; Trends Genet., March 1993, vol. 9(3), pp. 90–93.

Cecil Textbook of Medicine, 19th ed.: J.B. Wyngaarden, et al., eds.; W.B. Saunders Company, 1992, p. 139.

Nelson Textbook of Pediatrics, 14th ed.: R.E. Behrman, ed.-in-chief; W.B. Saunders Company, 1992, pp. 1460–1461.

Safety and Efficacy of Human Growth Hormone Treatment in Girls with Turner Syndrome: D.A. Price; Horm. Res., 1992 (39 suppl. 2), pp. 44–48.

Turner Syndrome: B. Lippe; Endocrinol. Metab. Clin. North Am., March 1991, vol. 20(1), pp. 121–152.

Birth Defects Encyclopedia: M.L. Buyse, ed.-in-chief; Blackwell Scientific Publications, 1990, pp. 1717–1719.

Dictionary of Medical Syndromes, 3rd ed.: S.I. Magalini, et al., eds.: J.B. Lippincott Company, 1990, p. 887.

Growth-Promoting Effect of Growth Hormone and Low Dose Ethinyl Estradiol in Girls with Turner's Syndrome: Vanderschueren-Lodeweyckx, et al.; J. Clin. Endocrinol. Metab., January 1990, vol. 70(1), pp. 122–126.

Serum Growth Hormone Levels Measured by Radioimmunoassay and Radioreceptor Assay: A Useful Diagnostic Tool in Children with Growth Disorders?: M.M. Ilondo, et al.; J. Clin. Endocrinol. Metab., May 1990, vol. 70(5), pp. 1445–1451.

Turner Syndrome: R.G. Rosenfeld and M.M. Grumbach, eds.; Marcel DeKles, 1989.

Smith's Recognizable Patterns of Human Malformation, 4th ed.: K.L. Jones; W.B. Saunders Company, 1988, pp. 75–79.

# VACTERL ASSOCIATION

**Description** VACTERL association is an acronym for (**V**)ertebral anomalies; (**A**)nal atresia; congenital (**C**)ardiac disease; (**T**)racheo(**E**)sophageal fistula; (**R**)enal anomalies; radial dysplasia and other (**L**)imb defects. These features can be combined in various ways, and can be manifestations of several recognized disorders. Related conditions such as the **REAR** syndrome (see below) and the **VATER** association, which have some of the same characteristics, have been expanded into the VACTERL association.

**Signs and Symptoms** The abnormalities of VACTERL association are present at birth.

Vertebral anomalies can include divided spinal disks, incomplete or half-developed spinal disks, and developmental abnormalities of the sacrum.

Anal atresia may be present, as may fistulas involving the rectum, urethra, and vagina.

The most common cardiac abnormality is ventricular septal defect (see ***Ventricular Septal Defects).***

Tracheoesophageal fistula can be present. Occasionally the esophagus may be absent.

The most common renal abnormality is agenesis; however, the renal tissue can be overdeveloped.

Radial limb dysplasia can include hypoplasia and triphalangism in the thumb, polydactyly, and absence of some of the fingers.

Some persons with VACTERL association may not grow at a normal rate, but mental development is usually normal.

**Etiology** The abnormalities of VACTERL association are presumed to be defects in the mesodermal layer of the embryo during fetal development. The developmental abnormalities are usually sporadic; however, some cases appear to be genetic. This multiple malformation syndrome appears to be a heterogeneous group of disorders.

**Epidemiology** VACTERL association is very rare. Males are affected in slightly greater numbers than females.

**Related Disorders** See ***Holt-Oram Syndrome; Townes-Brocks Syndrome.***

**REAR syndrome** is an acronym for (**R**)enal anomalies, deformed external (**E**)ars and perceptive deafness, (**A**)nal stenosis, and (**R**)adial dysplasia. Underdeveloped kidneys are the most common renal abnormalities. The external ears are malformed and deafness is present at birth. The anus is constricted or smaller than normal, and other anal abnormalities can occur. Abnormal tissue development is present in the area of the radius or humerus.

**Treatment—Standard** Treatment of VACTERL association by successive surgical rehabilitation of malformations is often useful. Other treatment is symptomatic and supportive.

**Treatment—Investigational** The Titanium Rib Project oversees the implantation of expandable ribs in children with disorders involving missing, underdeveloped, or malformed rib cages or chest walls. Contact Robert Campbell, M.D., at Santa Rosa Children's Hospital, San Antonio, Texas, for more information.

Please contact the agencies listed under Resources, below, for the most current information. Addresses and telephone numbers of these agencies, as well as of individual experts and research centers, may be found in the Master Resources List.

**Resources**

**For more information on VACTERL association:** National Organization for Rare Disorders (NORD); NIH/National Institute of Child Health and Human Development.

**For genetic information and genetic counseling referrals:** March of Dimes Birth Defects Foundation; Alliance of Genetic Support Groups.

**References**

Mendelian Inheritance in Man, 11th ed.: V.A. McKusick; The Johns Hopkins University Press, 1994, pp. 1518–1519, 2254, 2551.

Smith's Recognizable Patterns of Human Malformation, 4th ed.: K.L. Jones; W.B. Saunders Company, 1988, pp. 602–603.

Townes Syndrome: A Distinct Multiple Malformation Syndrome Resembling VACTERL Association: J.H. Hersh, et al.; Clin. Pediatr., February 1986, vol. 25(2), pp. 100–102.

Tracheal Agenesis and Associated Malformations: A Comparison with Tracheoesophageal Fistula and the VACTERL Association: J.A. Evans, et al.; Am. J. Med. Genet., May 1985, vol. 21(1), pp. 21–38.

A Population Study of the VACTERL Association: Evidence for Its Etiologic Heterogeneity: M.J. Khoury, et al.; Pediatrics, May 1983, vol. 71(5), pp. 815–820.

# VON HIPPEL–LINDAU SYNDROME

**Description** The von Hippel–Lindau syndrome is a hereditary tumor syndrome predisposing to renal cell carcinoma, pheochromocytoma, and pancreatic tumors, as well as to angiomas and hemangioblastoma of the cerebellum.

**Synonyms**

Angiomatosis Retina

Cerebelloretinal Hemangioblastomatosis

Retinocerebral Angiomatosis

**Signs and Symptoms** Onset usually is during young adulthood, but manifestations may appear as early as the age of 8. These include headaches, dizziness, ataxia, and behavioral abnormalities caused by neurologic disturbances. Retinal angiomas usually appear by the 3rd decade. Later in life, patients may develop angiomatous tumors in the cerebellum, spinal cord, lungs, liver, and elsewhere. Ophthalmoscopic examination reveals subretinal yellow spots and star-shaped material. Tumors of the retina may be associated with benign, slowly growing hemangioblastomas, usually located in the cerebellum. Other areas of the central nervous system are affected rarely.

Benign pheochromocytomas of the adrenal glands in about 15 percent of patients may cause chronic hypertension, headache, cold hands and feet, and excessive sweating. Blood pressure may return to normal as the patient ages. Renal cysts and tumors occur in about one-third of patients, and pancreatic cysts and tumors in one-fifth. There is marked clinical heterogeneity, with different families developing different constellations of manifestations.

**Etiology** The syndrome is inherited as an autosomal dominant trait. The defective gene has been mapped to chromosome 3p25–26, and the von Hippel–Lindau gene has been recently isolated. Germline mutations have been found in 85 of 114 unrelated families (75 percent). The mutations differ in families with pheochromocytoma from those families without.

**Epidemiology** Males and females are affected equally.

**Related Disorders** See *Neurofibromatosis; Sturge-Weber Syndrome; Tuberous Sclerosis.*

**Treatment—Standard** Laser and cryotherapy can destroy retinal lesions smaller than 2.5 cm. Larger lesions respond best to cryotherapy. Benign hemangioblastomas in asymptomatic patients with von Hippel–Lindau syndrome necessitate periodic neurologic evaluation. If neurologic symptoms are present, then surgery may be indicated. Pheochromocytomas usually necessitates surgical removal of tumor.

Early detection is the primary focus of medical evaluation. Ophthalmologic examinations should be made biannually for patients and annually for those at risk for the disease. Annual physical evaluation should include ultrasound, magnetic resonant imaging, or CT scan to detect tumors.

Genetic counseling may be of benefit; other treatment is symptomatic and supportive.

**Treatment—Investigational** The role of oncogenes in tumors from persons with von Hippel–Lindau syndrome is being investigated by Gary Skuse, M.D., and Peter Rowley, M.D., of the Division of Genetics, University of Rochester School of Medicine. They request notification of surgery for tumors in this condition so that arrangements can be made to receive tissue samples. Contact Barbara Kosciolek at the University of Rochester School of Medicine.

Please contact the agencies listed under Resources, below, for the most current information. Addresses and telephone numbers of these agencies, as well as of individual experts and research centers, may be found in the Master Resources List.

**Resources**

**For more information on von Hippel–Lindau syndrome:** National Organization for Rare Disorders (NORD); NIH/National Institute of Neurological Disorders and Stroke; NIH/National Eye Institute; Von Hippel–Lindau (VHL) Family Alliance; Von Hippel–Lindau Syndrome Foundation; VHL Patient and Relative Contact Group; NIH/National Cancer Institute Physician Data Query Phoneline.

**For genetic information and genetic counseling referrals:** March of Dimes Birth Defects Foundation; Alliance of Genetic Support Groups.

**References**

Germline Mutations in the von Hippel–Lindau Disease Tumor Suppressor Gene: Correlations with Phenotype: F. Chen, et al.; Hum. Mutat., 1995, vol. 5, pp. 66–75.

Mendelian Inheritance in Man, 11th ed.: V.A. McKusick; The Johns Hopkins University Press, 1994, pp. 1531–1534.

Conservative Renal Surgery for Renal Cell Carcinoma in Von Hippel–Lindau Disease: M. Frydenberg, et al.; J. Urol., March 1993, vol. 149(3), pp. 461–464.

Pheochromocytomas, Multiple Endocrine Neoplasia Type 2, and Von Hippel–Lindau Disease: H.P. Neumann, et al.; N. Engl. J. Med., November 1993, vol. 329(21), pp. 1531–1538.

Cecil Textbook of Medicine, 19th ed.: J.B. Wyngaarden, et al., eds.; W.B. Saunders Company, 1992, p. 2317.

Hemangioblastomas of the Central Nervous System: A 10-Year Study with Special Reference to Von Hippel–Lindau Syndrome: H.P. Neumann, et al.; J. Laryngol., May 1992, vol. 106(5), pp. 429–435.

Nelson Textbook of Pediatrics, 14th ed.: R.E. Behrman, ed.-in-chief; W.B. Saunders Company, 1992, pp. 1511–1512.

Textbook of Endocrinology, 8th ed.: J.D. Wilson and D.W. Foster, eds.; W.B. Saunders Company, 1992, pp. 672.

Neurotologic Manifestations of Von Hippel–Lindau Disease: S.F. Freeman, et al.; Ear Nose Throat J., December 1992, vol. 71(12), pp. 655–658.

Von Hippel–Lindau Disease: A Genetically Transmitted Multisystem Neoplastic Disorder: C.H. Martz; Semin. Oncol. Nurs., November 1992, vol. 8(4), pp. 281–287.

Central Nervous System Involvement in Von Hippel–Lindau Disease: M.R. Filling-Katz, et al.; Neurology, January 1991, vol. 41(1), pp. 41–46.

Pancreatic Lesions in the Von Hippel–Lindau Syndrome: H.P. Sigmund, et al.; Gastroenterology, August 1991, vol. 101(2), pp. 465–471.

Textbook of Uncommon Cancer: C.J. Williams, ed.; John Wiley and Sons, 1991, pp. 548, 753.

Von Hippel–Lindau Disease: A Genetic Study: E.R. Maher, et al.; J. Med. Genet., July 1991, vol. 28(7), pp. 443–447.

Birth Defects Encyclopedia: M.L. Buyse, ed.-in-chief; Blackwell Scientific Publications, 1990, pp. 1769–1770.

Clinical Features and Natural History of von Hippel–Lindau Disease: E.R. Maher, et al.; Q. J. Med., November 1990, vol. 77(283), pp. 1151–1163.

Clinical Ophthalmology, 2nd ed.; J.J. Kanski, ed.; Butterworth-Heinemann, 1990, p. 407.

Dictionary of Medical Syndromes, 3rd ed.: S.I. Magalini, et al., eds.: J.B. Lippincott Company, 1990, p. 914.

Islet-Cell Tumors in Von Hippel–Lindau Disease: Increased Prevalence and Relationship to the Multiple Endocrine Neoplasias: L.A. Binkovitz, et al.; Am. J. Roentgenol., September 1990, vol. 155(3), pp. 501–505.

The Abdominal Manifestation of Von Hippel–Lindau Disease and a Radiological Screening Protocol for an Affected Family: C.M. Jennings, et al.; Clin. Radiol., July 1988, vol. 39(4), pp. 363–367.

Smith's Recognizable Patterns of Human Malformation, 4th ed.: K.L. Jones; W.B. Saunders Company, 1988, p. 455.

# WAARDENBURG SYNDROME

**Description** Waardenburg syndrome is a hereditary disorder with characteristics that include abnormalities of the face and hair as well as deafness. The syndrome occurs in 2 forms: types I and II.

**Synonyms**

    Klein-Waardenburg Syndrome

    Van der Hoeve–Halbertsma–Waardenburg–Gualdi Syndrome

    Waardenburg-Klein Syndrome

**Signs and Symptoms Type I** is characterized by lateral displacement of the medial canthi and of the inferior lacrimal puncta. This leads to shortening of the eyelids and reduced visibility of the medial parts of the sclera, giving the impression of strabismus and hypertelorism. Other characteristics include partial or total heterochromia of the irides, a white forelock or premature graying of the hair, congenital sensorineural deafness, prominence of the medial portion of the eyebrows, synophrys, a thin nose, and full lips.

**Type II** is characterized by the pigmentary disorder and deafness, but lateral displacement of the medial canthi is absent.

Hirschsprung disease (aganglionic megacolon) has been reported in association with Waardenburg syndrome in several dozen patients (see *Hirschsprung Disease*).

**Etiology** Waardenburg syndrome is inherited through dominant genes with variable penetrance. Several mutations in PAX3, a gene on chromosome 2q35–37, have been identified, but mutations in a large number of patients remain unknown. The gene for Waardenburg syndrome type II maps to chromosome 3p12–p14.1. Recently, mutations in the microphthalmia **(MITF)** gene have been found in several families with type II.

**Epidemiology** The syndrome occurs in 1:4,000 live births. Males and females are affected equally.

**Related Disorders** See *Albinism; Vitiligo; Vogt-Koyanagi-Harada Syndrome.*

**Treatment—Standard** Recognition of the syndrome in infancy can lead to early detection of deafness.

Treatment is symptomatic and supportive. A hearing aid, sign language and lip-reading techniques, and special schooling may be helpful. Genetic counseling may aid families of affected children.

**Treatment—Investigational** Please contact the agencies listed under Resources, below, for the most current information. Addresses and telephone numbers of these agencies, as well as of individual experts and research centers, may be found in the Master Resources List.

**Resources**

    **For more information on Waardenburg syndrome:** National Organization for Rare Disorders (NORD); National Craniofacial Foundation; FACES—National Association for the Craniofacially Handicapped; Craniofacial Family Association; NIH/National Institute of Dental Research; NIH/National Eye Institute; Alexander Graham Bell Association for the Deaf; Self-Help for Hard-of-Hearing People; National Crisis Center for the Deaf; National Information Center on Deafness; National Association of the Deaf; Eye Research Institute of Retina Foundation; National Federation of the Blind; American Council of the Blind; American Foundation for the Blind; Council of Families with Visual Impairment; National Organization for Albinism and Hypopigmentation; National Vitiligo Foundation.

    **For genetic information and genetic counseling referrals:** March of Dimes Birth Defects Foundation; Alliance of Genetic Support Groups.

**References**

Further Elucidation of the Genomic Structure of PAX3, and Identification of Two Different Point Mutations Within the PAX3 Homeobox That Cause Waardenburg Syndrome Type 1 in Two Families: A.K. Lalwani, et al.; Am. J. Hum. Genet., 1995, vol. 56, pp. 75–83

Waardenburg Syndrome Type 2 Caused by Mutations in the Human Microphthalmia (MITF) Gene: M. Tarsabehji, et al.; Nat. Genet., 1994, vol. 8, pp. 251–255.

Syndromes of the Head and Neck, 3rd ed.: R.J. Gorlin, et al.; Oxford University Press, 1990, pp. 466–469.

Smith's Recognizable Patterns of Human Malformation, 4th ed.: K.L. Jones; W.B. Saunders Company, 1988, pp. 208–209.

# WEAVER SYNDROME

**Description** The syndrome is characterized by accelerated maturation of bone and physical growth accompanied by developmental delay and specific facial and bony abnormalities.

**Synonyms**
Weaver-Smith Syndrome

**Signs and Symptoms** Overgrowth is generally of prenatal onset but in some cases does not begin until the infant is a few months old. Hypertonia, progressive spasticity, and psychomotor retardation may occur. The child's cry is typically low-pitched and sounds hoarse.

Craniofacial features include a flat occiput, broad forehead, unusually large ears, a long philtrum, and micrognathia. Hypertelorism, epicanthal folds, and downward slanting palpebral fissures are commonly present.

The child's hair may be thin, and the skin appear somewhat loose. Nipples may be inverted. Inguinal or umbilical hernias may develop. Abnormalities of the hands include camptodactyly, broad thumbs, and prominent fingertip pads. Clinodactyly of the toes, pes cavus, talipes equinovarus or calcaneovalgus, and metatarsus adductus may be present. Elbow or knee extension may be restricted.

Abnormalities of the brain include hypervascularization, cerebral atrophy, and a cyst of the septum pellucidum.

**Etiology** The cause is unknown. Most cases have been sporadic, although autosomal dominant inheritance has been suggested.

**Epidemiology** Onset is usually prenatal. Although males are affected 3 times more often than females, there is as yet no explanation for that phenomenon.

**Related Disorders** See *Marshall-Smith Syndrome; McCune-Albright Syndrome; Sotos Syndrome.*

**Treatment—Standard** Treatment is symptomatic and supportive. An orthopedist can be consulted for correction of foot deformities. Genetic counseling may benefit patients and their families.

**Treatment—Investigational** Please contact the agencies listed under Resources, below, for the most current information. Addresses and telephone numbers of these agencies, as well as of individual experts and research centers, may be found in the Master Resources List.

**Resources**

**For more information on Weaver syndrome:** National Organization for Rare Disorders (NORD); Magic Foundation for Children's Growth; Human Growth Foundation; NIH/National Institute of Child Health and Human Development.

**For genetic information and genetic counseling referrals:** March of Dimes Birth Defects Foundation; Alliance of Genetic Support Groups.

**References**
Mendelian Inheritance in Man, 11th ed.: V.A. McKusick; The Johns Hopkins University Press, 1994, p. 2264.
Syndromes of the Head and Neck, 3rd ed.: R.J. Gorlin, et al.; Oxford University Press, 1990, pp. 338–340.
A New Autosomal Recessive Disorder Resembling Weaver Syndrome: A.S. Teebi, et al.; Am. J. Med. Genet., August 1989, vol. 33(4), pp. 479–482.
Weaver Syndrome: The Changing Phenotype in an Adult: F. Greenberg, et al.; Am. J. Med. Genet., May 1989, vol. 33(1), pp. 127–129.
Smith's Recognizable Patterns of Human Malformation, 4th ed.: K.L. Jones; W.B. Saunders Company, 1988, pp. 130–135.
A Girl with the Weaver Syndrome: E.M. Thompson; J. Med. Genet., April 1987, vol. 24(4), pp. 232–234.
Further Delineation of Weaver Syndrome: H.H. Ardinger, et al.; J. Pediatr., February 1986, vol. 108(2), pp. 228–235.
Weaver-Smith Syndrome. A Case Study with Long-Term Follow-Up: N. Amir, et al.; Am. J. Dis. Child., December 1984, vol.138(12), pp. 1113–1117.

# WEILL-MARCHESANI SYNDROME

**Description** The major features are short stature and a small, round lens of the eye.

**Synonyms**
Congenital Mesodermal Dysmorphodystrophy
Mesodermal Dysmorphodystrophy, Brachymorphic Type, Congenital
Spherophakia-Brachymorphia Syndrome

**Signs and Symptoms** Affected children and adults have a stocky build, tend to become overweight, and have limbs that are short and round. The face is full, with a wide skull, short neck, depressed nasal bridge, and pug nose. Eye abnormalities include a small, rounded lens that is prone to dislocation; shallow orbit; and myopia.

In some cases, the following are present: joint stiffness, with limited extension; acute glaucoma; ectopia lentis; blindness; mild maxillary hypoplasia; a narrow palate; malformed and malaligned teeth; and carpal tunnel syndrome.

**Etiology** The syndrome is thought to be inherited as an autosomal recessive trait with partial expression in the heterozygote. Dominant inheritance has also been suggested.

**Epidemiology** The average age for detection of the syndrome is 7 years, although symptoms and signs are usually apparent earlier in life. The disorder has been found worldwide and affects approximately 1:100,000 persons. Males and females are affected in equal numbers.

**Related Disorders** See *Kniest Dysplasia.*

**Ectopia lentis,** a congenital displacement of the lens of the eye, may occur alone, in which case it is inherited as an autosomal dominant trait, or as a part of other disorders. The lens dislocation may be present at birth or occur later. Some affected persons have no symptoms at all; others may have poor sight or double vision.

**Treatment—Standard** The specific individual associated disorders are treated appropriately.

**Treatment—Investigational** Please contact the agencies listed under Resources, below, for the most current information. Addresses and telephone numbers of these agencies, as well as of individual experts and research centers, may be found in the Master Resources List.

**Resources**

**For more information on Weill-Marshall syndrome:** National Organization for Rare Disorders (NORD); NIH/National Eye Institute; Magic Foundation for Children's Growth; Human Growth Foundation; Little People of America; Association for Repetitive Motion Syndrome; NIH/National Institute of Child Health and Human Development.

**For genetic information and genetic counseling referrals:** March of Dimes Birth Defects Foundation; Alliance of Genetic Support Groups.

**References**

Mendelian Inheritance in Man, 11th ed.: V.A. McKusick; The Johns Hopkins University Press, 1994, pp. 2264–2265.

Birth Defects Encyclopedia: M.L. Buyse, ed.-in-chief; Blackwell Scientific Publications, 1990, p. 1575.

The Weill-Marchesani Syndrome: Report of Two Cases and a Review: G.M. Haik, Sr., et al.; J. La. State Med. Soc., December 1990, vol. 142(12), pp. 25–28, 30–32.

Smith's Recognizable Patterns of Human Malformation, 4th ed.: K.L. Jones; W.B. Saunders Company, 1988, p. 397.

# WERNER SYNDROME

**Description** Werner syndrome is a form of premature aging that begins in adolescence or early adulthood and results in the appearance of old age by 30 to 40 years.

**Synonyms**

Progeria of Adulthood

**Signs and Symptoms** Affected individuals appear normal until adolescence or young adulthood. The syndrome progresses steadily. Stature typically is short. Facial characteristics include a nose that becomes beaked and thin, prominent eyes, and thinned eyebrows and lashes. Cataracts often develop by about age 25 to 30 years. By age 20 the patient may have graying hair, and baldness may ensue. The torso tends to be stocky, and the abdomen may protrude. Subcutaneous fat and muscle mass are lost, resulting in extreme thinness of the arms and legs. The hands and feet are small, and the fingers short and deformed.

The skin, especially on the face, legs, and feet, undergoes scleroderma-like changes that leave it taut and shiny. There may be ulcerations on the legs and feet. Hypogonadism may be present, and secondary sex characteristics, such as pubic, axillary, and facial hair, are absent or regress.

Diabetes mellitus, arteriosclerosis, and osteoporosis may develop. Calcification occurs in the extremities and the heart, particularly the valves and coronary arteries. Other potentially fatal complications include cerebral stroke and cancers.

Werner syndrome can occur in partial forms, exhibiting only a few of the symptoms described, and having a milder, slower course.

**Etiology** The syndrome appears to be hereditary, with an autosomal recessive mode of transmission. The gene responsible resides on the short arm of chromosome 8 (8p11.2–p12).

The biochemical defect or defects responsible for Werner syndrome are not known. Urinary hyaluronic acid has been found to be elevated.

**Epidemiology** Incidence in the United States appears to be between 1:1,000,000 and 20:1,000,000 cases. Males and females over the age of about 14 years are affected.

**Related Disorders** See *Hutchinson-Gilford Syndrome; Gottron Syndrome.*

**Treatment—Standard** Available treatments for Werner syndrome are supportive and symptomatic. They include surgery for cataracts and skin grafting for ulcerations.

**Treatment—Investigational** Please contact the agencies listed under Resources, below, for the most current information. Addresses and telephone numbers of these agencies, as well as of individual experts and research centers, may be found in the Master Resources List.

**Resources**

**For more information on Werner syndrome:** National Organization for Rare Disorders (NORD); New York State Institute for Basic Research in Developmental Disabilities; Progeria International Registry; NIH/National Institute on Aging.

**For genetic information and genetic counseling referrals:** March of Dimes Birth Defects Foundation; Alliance of Genetic Support Groups.

**References**

Mendelian Inheritance in Man, 11th ed.: V.A. McKusick; The Johns Hopkins University Press, 1994, pp. 2266–2277.
A Patient with Werner's Syndrome and Osteosarcoma Presenting As Scleroderma: J. Nakura, et al.; Gerontology, 1993, vol. 39(suppl. 1), pp. 11–15.
Cecil Textbook of Medicine, 19th ed.: J.B. Wyngaarden, et al., eds.; W.B. Saunders Company, 1992, p. 1141.
Nelson Textbook of Pediatrics, 14th ed.: R.E. Behrman, ed.-in-chief; W.B. Saunders Company, 1992, p. 407.
Birth Defects Encyclopedia: M.L. Buyse, ed.-in-chief; Blackwell Scientific Publications, 1990, pp. 1777–1778.
Dictionary of Medical Syndromes, 3rd ed.: S.I. Magalini, et al., eds.: J.B. Lippincott Company, 1990, p. 930.
Syndromes of the Head and Neck, 3rd ed.: R.J. Gorlin, et al.; Oxford University Press, 1990, pp. 485–487.
Smith's Recognizable Patterns of Human Malformation, 4th ed.: K.L. Jones; W.B. Saunders Company, 1988, pp. 120–121.

# WILDERVANCK SYNDROME

**Description** Wildervanck syndrome is a rare congenital disorder characterized by sensorineural deafness; fusion of cervical vertebrae and occasionally thoracic vertebrae, resulting in limited motion of the neck or upper spine *(Klippel-Feil Syndrome);* and limited movement of the eye, causing difficulty in focusing *(Duane Syndrome).*

**Synonyms**

Cervico-Oculo-Acoustic Syndrome

**Signs and Symptoms** The hearing loss is the result of a bony malformation of the inner ear, resulting in sensorineural deafness. In some cases the semicircular canals and nerve system of the inner ear may be absent or incompletely formed.

The symptoms of Klippel-Feil syndrome present in patients with Wildervanck syndrome are limited movement of the head, scoliosis, and a low hairline at the back of the head. Fusion of cervical vertebrae and thoracic vertebrae may be found in affected individuals, and hemivertebrae may be present. (See *Klippel-Feil Syndrome.)*

The symptoms of Duane syndrome present in patients with Wildervanck syndrome are restricted abduction and adduction of the affected eye, with difficulty in focusing. When the patient attempts to move the eye, the eyeball retracts inward. (See *Duane Syndrome.)*

**Etiology** Wildervanck syndrome appears to have polygenic inheritance, with limitations to females.

**Epidemiology** Wildervanck syndrome predominantly affects females. However, there have been a few reported cases of the disorder in males.

**Related Disorders** See *Klippel-Feil Syndrome; Duane Syndrome; Goldenhar Syndrome.*

**Treatment—Standard** Individuals with Wildervanck syndrome may derive some benefit from hearing aids.

Surgery may be considered when the affected eye is not straight in the primary position, causing the individual to tilt the head.

Genetic counseling may benefit patients and their families. Other treatment is symptomatic and supportive.

**Treatment—Investigational** Please contact the agencies listed under Resources, below, for the most current information. Addresses and telephone numbers of these agencies, as well as of individual experts and research centers, may be found in the Master Resources List.

**Resources**

**For more information on Wildervanck syndrome:** National Organization for Rare Disorders (NORD); Deafness Research Foundation; American Society for Deaf Children; Alexander Graham Bell Association for the Deaf; National Information Center on Deafness; NIH/National Eye Institute; NIH/National Arthritis and Musculoskeletal and Skin Diseases Information Clearinghouse.

**For genetic information and genetic counseling referrals:** March of Dimes Birth Defects Foundation; Alliance of Genetic Support Groups.

**References**

Mendelian Inheritance in Man, 11th ed.: V.A. McKusick; The Johns Hopkins University Press, 1994, p. 2552.
Diseases of the Nose, Throat, Ear, Head and Neck, 14th ed.: J.J. Ballenger; Lea and Febiger, 1991, pp. 1211.
Birth Defects Encyclopedia: M.L Buyse, ed.-in-chief; Blackwell Scientific Publications, 1990, pp. 306–307.

Clinical Ophthalmology, 2nd ed.: J.J. Kanski, ed.; Butterworth-Heinemann, 1990, pp. 431–432.

Hearing Loss in the Cervico-Oculo-Acoustic (Wildervanck) Syndrome: C.W. Cremers, et al.; Arch. Otolaryngol. Head Neck Surg., January 1984, vol. 110(1), pp. 54–57.

Wildervanck Syndrome—The External Appearance and Radiological Findings: J.A. Schilder, et al.; Int. J. Pediatr. Otorhinolaryngol., July 1984, vol. 7(3), pp. 305–310.

Wildervanck's Syndrome with Bilateral Subluxation of Lens and Facial Paralysis: P. Strisciuglio, et al.; J. Med. Genet., February 1983, vol. 20(1), pp. 72–73.

# WILLIAMS SYNDROME

**Description** Williams syndrome is a rare congenital disorder characterized by elfin facies, exceptionally sensitive hearing, developmental delays, short stature, and an impulsive, outgoing personality. Cardiovascular anomalies and/or infantile hypercalcemia are often present.

**Synonyms**

> Beuren Syndrome
> Hypercalcemia–Supravalvar Aortic Stenosis
> Infantile Hypercalcemia Syndrome, Idiopathic
> Williams-Beuren Syndrome

**Signs and Symptoms** Some children have a low birth weight and fail to thrive. Vomiting, gagging, diarrhea, and constipation are common in infancy. Blood calcium may be elevated; when this sign occurs, it persists only during the first year of life, then disappears.

The face at birth is characteristically elfin, with a small head, broad forehead, puffiness around the eyes, depressed nasal bridge, wide mouth, and full lips. Children whose eyes are blue or green (unlike those with brown eyes) may have a starlike pattern in the iris. Highly sensitive hearing often results in patients' overreacting to loud and high-pitched sounds. Motor development, e.g., sitting and walking, and gross and fine motor skills may be delayed. Language development, especially social use of language, is spared.

Heart disorders occur in 75 percent of cases. Most common findings are supravalvar aortic stenosis and pulmonary artery stenosis. Other vascular anomalies are common. Umbilical or inguinal hernias may occur.

The personality is friendly and talkative. Mild mental retardation may occur, but some children have average intelligence with severe learning disabilities. These children may exhibit attention-deficit behaviors but generally have good long-term memory.

**Etiology** Some patients have submicroscopic deletions within chromosome 7q11.23 and are hemizygous for the elastin locus. Using DNA technology, researchers have determined that 90 percent of patients have deletions of portions of the elastin gene.

**Epidemiology** Infants of both sexes and all races are affected. The disorder occurs in about 1:20,000 births.

**Related Disorders** See *Noonan Syndrome,* known to be an inherited disorder, which is also associated with pulmonary artery stenosis.

An elevated blood calcium in infancy, without a known cause or any other symptoms, may be due to **idiopathic infantile hypercalcemia.**

**Supravalvar aortic stenosis** (narrowing of the aorta above the aortic valve) may occur alone or in conjunction with other disorders.

**Treatment—Standard** To treat elevated blood calcium levels in affected infants, excessive vitamin D in the diet should be avoided and calcium should be restricted to 25 to 100 mg/day. For severe hypercalcemia, hydrocortisone analog therapy may be considered on a temporary basis. An endocrinologist should be consulted. After a child is a few months old, calcium levels will return to normal even in untreated patients.

For the physical and mental developmental deficiencies, centers for developmentally disabled children and special education services in schools may be needed. Medical help from specialists, speech and language therapy, occupational and physical therapy, and vocational training can all be beneficial.

**Treatment—Investigational** A collaborative effort to locate the genes responsible for Williams syndrome and supravalvular aortic stenosis is being made by the University of Nevada School of Medicine, the Indiana University School of Medicine, and the University of Utah School of Medicine. Researchers are collecting DNA from patients and their parents. Contact Dr. Colleen A. Morris at the University of Nevada School of Medicine for more information.

Please contact the agencies listed under Resources, below, for the most current information. Addresses and telephone numbers of these agencies, as well as of individual experts and research centers, may be found in the Master Resources List.

**Resources**

**For more information on Williams syndrome:** National Organization for Rare Disorders (NORD); Williams

Syndrome Association; Infantile Hypercalcaemia Foundation Ltd.; NIH/National Institute of Child Health and Human Development.

**For genetic information and genetic counseling referrals:** March of Dimes Birth Defects Foundation; Alliance of Genetic Support Groups.

### References

Deletions of the Elastin Gene at 7q11.23 Occur in ~90% of Patients with Williams Syndrome: E. Nickerson, et al.; Am. J. Hum. Genet., 1995, vol. 56, pp. 1156–1161.

Mendelian Inheritance in Man, 11th ed.: V.A. McKusick; The Johns Hopkins University Press, 1994, pp. 1547–1549.

The Elastin Gene I Disrupted by a Translocation Associated with Supravalvular Aortic Stenosis: M.E. Curran, et al.; Cell, 1993, vol. 73, pp. 159–168.

Hemizygosity at the Elastin Locus in a Development Disorder, Williams Syndrome: A.K. Ewart, et al.; Nat. Genet., 1993, vol. 5, pp. 11–16.

Smith's Recognizable Patterns of Human Malformation, 4th ed.: K.L. Jones; W.B. Saunders Company, 1988, pp. 106–107.

Facts About Williams Syndrome: Williams Syndrome Association.

# WINCHESTER SYNDROME

**Description** Winchester syndrome, believed to be closely related to the mucopolysaccharidoses, is characterized by short stature and arthritis-like symptoms, as well as by ocular and dermatologic problems.

**Synonyms**

      Winchester-Grossman Syndrome

**Signs and Symptoms** The syndrome becomes apparent at about 2 years of age, when the joints become stiff and painful with swelling and redness. The fingers, elbows, knees, and feet are affected most often. The skin darkens and becomes very thick and leathery, with excessive hair growth. The lips and gums are thickened, causing coarse facial features. As the child grows, short stature becomes apparent. During later childhood or adulthood, bones in the ankles and feet may weaken from loss of calcium. The eyes may develop corneal opacities, causing vision problems. The disorder leads to severe joint contractures, but mental functioning is not affected.

**Etiology** The syndrome is inherited as an autosomal recessive trait. Because oligosaccharide is lost in the urine of some patients, the disorder is thought to be a rare type of mucopolysaccharidosis. Tests have yet to prove this theory, however.

**Epidemiology** Males and females are affected in equal numbers. Fewer than 10 cases have been identified; the affected individuals are of Mexican, Indian, Puerto Rican, and Iranian descent. Other patients may be undiagnosed or misdiagnosed.

**Related Disorders** See *Mucopolysaccharidoses.*

    **Juvenile arthritis** is a relatively rare childhood disorder characterized by swollen and painful joints, fever, skin rash, swollen lymph glands, and hepatosplenomegaly.

**Treatment—Standard** Treatment of Winchester syndrome consists of physical therapy to help promote use of the affected limbs. The use of mobility devices may be required. Orthopedic procedures to decrease contractures may be of benefit. Genetic counseling may benefit patients and their families. Other treatment is symptomatic and supportive.

**Treatment—Investigational** Please contact the agencies listed under Resources, below, for the most current information. Addresses and telephone numbers of these agencies, as well as of individual experts and research centers, may be found in the Master Resources List.

**Resources**

    **For more information on Winchester syndrome:** National Organization for Rare Disorders (NORD); American Juvenile Arthritis Foundation; NIH/National Arthritis and Musculoskeletal and Skin Diseases Information Clearinghouse.

    **For genetic information and genetic counseling referrals:** March of Dimes Birth Defects Foundation; Alliance of Genetic Support Groups.

**References**

Mendelian Inheritance in Man, 11th ed.: V.A. McKusick; The Johns Hopkins University Press, 1994, p. 2271.

Birth Defects Encyclopedia: M.L. Buyse, ed.-in-chief; Blackwell Scientific Publications, 1990, p. 1781.

Two Cases of Winchester Syndrome with Increased Urinary Oligosaccharide Excretion: D.B. Dunger, et al.; Eur. J. Pediatr., November 1987, vol. 146(6), pp. 615–619.

Winchester Syndrome: Report of a Case from Iran: H. Nabai, et al.; J. Cutan. Pathol., October 1977, vol. 4(5), pp. 281–285.

The Skin in the Winchester Syndrome: A.H. Cohen, et al.; Arch. Dermatol., February 1975, vol. 111(2), pp. 230–236.

# WOLF-HIRSCHHORN SYNDROME (WHS)

**Description** Wolf-Hirschhorn syndrome is a chromosomal defect disorder with the manifestations discussed below.

**Synonyms**
> Chromosome 4p- Syndrome
> Chromosome Number 4 Short Arm Deletion Syndrome
> Wolf Syndrome

**Signs and Symptoms** The most frequently occurring features of the syndrome are low birth weight, hypotonia, physical and mental retardation, microcephaly, high forehead, wide nasal bridge with a broad or beaked nose, epicanthal folds, and hypertelorism. Cardiac and renal defects and seizures occur in about one-half of patients. Hypospadias and cryptorchidism are common in males; in females, the urethra may open into the vagina.

Other facial involvement includes strabismus, ptosis, coloboma of the eye, arched eyebrows, cleft lip, cleft palate, short philtrum, down-turned mouth, micrognathia, and low-set ears.

**Etiology** Wolf-Hirschhorn syndrome is a genetic disorder caused by a deletion of the 4p16 band of chromosome 4. Most instances are de novo defects, but in 10 to 15 percent the condition is inherited as a translocation defect.

**Epidemiology** Incidence has been reported to be 1:50,000. Females and males are affected in equal numbers. About one-third of patients die in the first 2 years of life. Long duration of life is possible, the oldest known patient being a 39-year-old man.

**Related Disorders** See *Cri du Chat Syndrome; Down Syndrome; Trisomy; Trisomy 13 Syndrome; Trisomy 18 Syndrome.*

**Treatment—Standard** Reconstructive surgery is indicated in some cases. Special education, physical therapy, vocational services, and genetic counseling may be beneficial. Other treatment is symptomatic and supportive.

**Treatment—Investigational** Gilbert N. Jones, III, and Susan A. Guckenberger at Southern Illinois University School of Medicine are studying genes associated with Wolf-Hirschhorn syndrome.

Please contact the agencies listed under Resources, below, for the most current information. Addresses and telephone numbers of these agencies, as well as of individual experts and research centers, may be found in the Master Resources List.

**Resources**

**For more information on Wolf-Hirschhorn syndrome:** National Organization for Rare Disorders (NORD); NIH/National Institute of Child Health and Human Development; Chromosome Deletion Outreach; Wolf-Hirschhorn Parent Contact Group.

**For genetic information and genetic counseling referrals:** March of Dimes Birth Defects Foundation; Alliance of Genetic Support Groups.

**References**
Mendelian Inheritance in Man, 11th ed.: V.A. McKusick; The Johns Hopkins University Press, 1994, p. 1557.
Syndromes of the Head and Neck, 3rd ed.: R.J. Gorlin, et al.; Oxford University Press, 1990, pp. 46–48.

# WOLFRAM SYNDROME

**Description** Wolfram syndrome is a rare, congenital, multisystem disorder in which diabetes insipidus, diabetes mellitus, and vision and hearing defects are the principal features.

**Synonyms**
> Diabetes Insipidus, Diabetes Mellitus, Optic Atrophy, Deafness

**Signs and Symptoms** Insulin-dependent diabetes mellitus (**IDDM**) usually occurs first, between 5 and 10 years of age. Decreased visual activity usually occurs between 8 and 20 years, finally leading to optic atrophy. Neurosensory hearing loss has its onset between 10 and 20 years. Diabetes insipidus occurs in about one-third of patients. The diabetes in these individuals differs from classic IDDM in that it is not HLA-related, it is not associated with islet cell antibodies, and it is not prone to ketosis.

In some patients dilatation of the urinary tract, megaloblastic anemia, sideroblastic anemia, neutropenia, thrombocytopenia, diabetic retinopathy, severe depression, and impulsive verbal and physical aggression may be present.

**Etiology** The syndrome is inherited as an autosomal recessive trait and is linked to markers on chromosome 4p. In other patients, the disorder is caused by a mitochondrial deletion and is associated with a severe myopathy.

**Epidemiology** Males and females are affected in equal numbers.

**Related Disorders** See *Granulomatous Disease, Chronic; Myelofibrosis-Osteosclerosis; Anemia, Pernicious.*

**Treatment—Standard** The various disease components are treated appropriately. When treated with thiamine, some patients appear to decrease their requirements for insulin, and blood findings such as anemia can return to normal. Genetic counseling may benefit patients and their families.

**Treatment—Investigational** For patients with neutropenia, colony-stimulating factor therapy is being tested. Granulocyte macrophage-colony stimulating factor **(GM-CSF),** a protein derived from bacteria, yeast, and mammalian cells, is being developed by Schering Plough and Sandoz Pharmaceuticals under the brand name Leucomax. Plasmapheresis is under investigation to analyze long-term effectiveness in treating neutropenia.

Please contact the agencies listed under Resources, below, for the most current information. Addresses and telephone numbers of these agencies, as well as of individual experts and research centers, may be found in the Master Resources List.

**Resources**

**For more information on Wolfram syndrome:** National Organization for Rare Disorders (NORD); Diabetes Insipidus and Related Disorders Network; American Diabetes Association, National Service Center; Juvenile Diabetes Foundation International; NIH/National Diabetes Information Clearinghouse; NIH/National Eye Institute; National Association for the Visually Handicapped; National Association for Parents of the Visually Impaired; Vision Foundation; NIH/National Heart, Lung and Blood Institute Information Center.

**For genetic information and genetic counseling referrals:** March of Dimes Birth Defects Foundation; Alliance of Genetic Support Groups.

**References**

Linkage of the Gene for Wolfram Syndrome to Markers on the Short Arm of Chromosome 4: M.H. Polymeropoulos, et al., Nat. Genet., 1994, vol. 8, pp. 95–97.

Mendelian Inheritance in Man, 11th ed.: V.A. McKusick; The Johns Hopkins University Press, 1994, pp. 1764–1765, 2601.

Deletion of Mitochondrial DNA in a Case of Early-Onset Diabetes Mellitus, Optic Atrophy, and Deafness (Wolfram Syndrome): A. Rotig, et al.; J. Clin. Invest., 1993, vol. 91, pp. 1095–1098.

Thiamine-Responsive Anemia in DIDMOAD Syndrome: B. Pignatti, et al.; J. Pediatr., March 1989, vol. 114(3), pp. 405–410.

Contrasting Features of Insulin Dependent Diabetes Mellitus Associated with Neuroectodermal Defects and Classical Insulin Dependent Diabetes Mellitus: P.P. Garcia-Luna, et al.; Acta Paediatr. Scand., 1988, vol. 77, pp. 413–418.

DIDMOAD Syndrome with Megacystis and Megaureter: P. Chu, et al.; Postgrad. Med. J., September 1986, vol. 62(731), pp. 859–863.

# XYY Syndrome

**Description** The salient features of this chromosomal disorder are tall stature and severe acne during adolescence. These characteristics are frequently not enough in themselves to distinguish the syndrome; hence diagnosis is often missed.

**Synonyms**

47,XYY Syndrome

**Signs and Symptoms** Affected persons are often very tall (the tall stature usually becoming apparent after ages 5 or 6) and develop severe cystic acne during adolescence. Adults with this disorder may be relatively impulsive, antisocial, and likely to break the law, but they are not especially aggressive. There may be some developmental disabilities.

Physical characteristics include an unusually long head with a slightly protruding forehead, long ears, large teeth, and long hands and feet. Pectoral and shoulder girdle muscle development is poor, and there may be mild pectus excavatum. Even though males with this syndrome are large, they tend to be weak and uncoordinated. Some may have a fine intentional tremor.

Less commonly, genital abnormalities (e.g., microphallus, hypospadias, cryptorchidism) occur, as well as synostosis of the proximal ends of the radius and ulna, causing joint stiffness.

Although aggressive behavior may form a part of the syndrome, linkage of the XYY karyotype to violent criminal behavior has been disputed as simplistic. More research is needed to understand the role of this chromosomal abnormality on behavior.

**Etiology** XYY syndrome is caused by the presence of an extra Y chromosome resulting from meiotic nondisjunction.

**Epidemiology** The disorder, which affects only males, is estimated to occur in approximately 1:1,000 live births.

**Related Disorders** See *Antisocial Personality Disorder; Klinefelter Syndrome; Marfan Syndrome; Sotos Syndrome.*

**Treatment—Standard** Therapy is symptomatic and supportive. Treatment of acne may help the patient's self-image. Counseling for behavioral problems may be of benefit.

**Treatment—Investigational** Anyone who had a prenatal diagnosis of XYY syndrome and is between the ages of 5 and 20 may wish to participate in a study being conducted to determine mental and behavioral outcomes connected with this syndrome. Interested persons may wish to contact John M. Graham, M.D., of the University of California, Los Angeles, School of Medicine.

Please contact the agencies listed under Resources, below, for the most current information. Addresses and telephone numbers of these agencies, as well as of individual experts and research centers, may be found in the Master Resources List.

### Resources

**For more information on XYY syndrome:** National Organization for Rare Disorders (NORD); National Mental Health Association; National Alliance for the Mentally Ill; National Mental Health Consumer Self-Help Clearinghouse; NIH/National Institute of Mental Health.

**For genetic information and genetic counseling referrals:** March of Dimes Birth Defects Foundation; Alliance of Genetic Support Groups.

### References

Cecil Textbook of Medicine, 18th ed.: J.B. Wyngaarden and L.H. Smith, Jr., eds.; W.B. Saunders Company, 1988, p. 167.

Sex Chromosome Anomalies, Hormones, and Sexuality: R.C. Schiavi, et al.; Arch. Gen. Psychiatry, January 1988, vol. 45(1), pp. 19–24.

Smith's Recognizable Patterns of Human Malformation, 4th ed.: K.L. Jones; W.B. Saunders Company, 1988, pp. 64–65.

Sperm Chromosome Complements in a 47,XYY Man: J. Benet and R.H. Martin; Hum. Genet., April 1988, vol. 78(4), pp. 313–315.

# 2 | INBORN ERRORS OF METABOLISM
### By Jess G. Thoene, M.D.

The human genome comprises more than 100,000 genes and is susceptible to mutation at each locus. Interruption in the DNA sequence coding for an enzyme leads to failure of the chemical reaction mediated by that enzyme to proceed at the proper rate. This produces adverse consequences resulting from underproduction of an essential metabolite, accumulation of unmetabolized precursors, or overproduction of compounds that normally exist in minute amounts. Coined by Archibald Garrod in the first decade of this century, the term *inborn errors of metabolism* applies to several hundred separate diseases, each resulting in a defect in a specific enzymatic pathway involved in human metabolism. The standard reference text in this area, *The Metabolic and Molecular Basis of Inherited Disease*, now occupies three volumes arranged in more than 150 separate subdivisions. The clinical impact resulting from mutations in these pathways varies widely, ranging from relatively asymptomatic findings, such as in cystathioninuria, to a modest impairment of fitness, such as in cystinuria with renal stones, to diseases with a catastrophic impact, such as defects in the urea cycle, which are lethal in the newborn period if not properly diagnosed.

Most inborn errors of metabolism are rare, with an incidence of 1:100,000 in the general population. Most are inherited via an autosomal recessive pattern. This means that both parents of the affected individual are carriers (obligate heterozygotes) but usually are clinically unaffected. The risk of two carriers' having another such affected (homozygous) individual is 1:4 for each pregnancy. A few inborn errors are inherited as X-linked traits. In X-linked conditions, half of a carrier female's daughters will also be carriers, half of her sons will be affected (hemizygotes), and half of her sons and daughters will be unaffected. Typical X-linked traits include Lesch-Nyhan syndrome, ornithine transcarbamylase deficiency (**OTC**), and Hunter syndrome.

The understanding of human inheritance recently became complicated by the knowledge that mitochondrial DNA, which replicates separately from nuclear DNA, also sustains mutations and can lead to inborn errors of metabolism. The complicating feature arises because all mitochondria are inherited from the maternal lineage and not from the paternal. Oocytes contain all the mitochondria that become incorporated in the developing embryo, and the mitochondria replicate within each cell, leading in some instances to tissue-specific segregation of mitochondrial mutations. There is also a high somatic mutation rate in mitochondria, resulting in increasing effect with age. All of these factors combine to produce diseases with variable expressivity throughout the life span and with pedigrees that in no way resemble classical Mendelian inheritance. Examples of conditions known to result from mutations in the mitochondrial genome include Leber hereditary optic neuropathy, MERRF syndrome, MELAS syndrome, a group of mitochondrial myopathies, and some cardiomyopathies. Sporadic cases of Leigh disease have been identified as the result of mitochondrial mutations, although nuclear mutations also can produce this clinical syndrome. Kearns-Sayre syndrome is also the result of mitochondrial mutations. See individual disease entries for additional details.

The diagnosis of inborn errors of metabolism requires access to a laboratory skilled in the analysis of body fluids for the metabolites of interest, such as assays for amino acids and organic acids in plasma and urine. The diagnosis of storage disorders usually requires direct tissue assay of the suspected defective enzyme, e.g., lysosomal enzymes. Disorders of carbohydrate metabolism, heavy metals, steroid metabolism, and other disorders may require shipping samples to specific reference laboratories as well. The physician can determine a center able to provide the required analysis by querying the resource agencies listed at the end of each rare disease discussion in this chapter. The preferred test for the initial diagnosis of most inborn errors of metabolism is urinalysis. Urine samples are readily obtained and disclose more information about disease states than plasma (Table 2.1).

The infant with catastrophic, overwhelming illness is a frequent dilemma in neonatal intensive care units. Although most of the time these infants' illnesses derive from sepsis or disorders of the respiratory or cardiovascular system, some are due to an inborn error of metabolism. The diagram accompanying this chapter (Figure 2.1) shows an approach to sorting out the various diagnostic possibilities. It is essential to remember to measure the infant's electrolytes and bicarbonate initially. Demonstration of an increased anion gap (the sum of the sodium and potassium minus the sum of the chloride and bicarbonate >18 mEq/L) is a strong indication of the presence of an organic aciduria. In this case, analysis of urine for organic acids is essential.

Finding abnormalities in urinary organic acids should lead directly to a diagnosis. Some of these are listed in Figure 2.1. Among them are maple syrup urine disease (**MSUD**), β-ketothiolase deficiency, propionic and methylmalonic aciduria, isovaleric acidemia (**IVA**), medium-chain acyl-CoA dehydrogenase deficiency (**MCAD**), glutaricaciduria I, glutaricaciduria II, oxoprolinuria, and a number of other rare disorders. Other clinical signs suggesting an organic acidemia in the newborn period include thrombocytopenia and/or neutropenia, elevations of plasma lactate, or a peculiar odor. Several organic acidemias such as MSUD and IVA result in an excretion of compounds that are very pungent.

If the organic acids are normal and an increased anion gap is present, then plasma lactate should be measured. Urinary lactate is unstable and may not be detected by a urinary organic acid determination. Elevation in plasma lactate above 2 mM suggests either primary or secondary lactate acidosis. Secondary lactic acidosis may be the result of shock or a number of inborn errors of metabolism, including the glycogen storage diseases, tyrosinemia, galactosemia, and nonmetabolic diseases, such as coarctation of the aorta. Primary lactic acidoses include defects in the enzymes pyruvate carboxylase and pyruvate dehydrogenase complex, as well as mitochondrial oxidative-phosphorylation defects.

**Table 2.1  Choice of Sample to Submit to a Screening Laboratory to Detect Inborn Errors of Metabolism**

| Disease Category | First | Second | Third |
|---|---|---|---|
| Urea cycle disorders | urine | plasma | liver bx |
| Amino acidopathies | urine | plasma | CSF (nonketotic hyperglycemia) |
| Organic aciduria | urine | —— | fibroblasts, liver bx |
| Mucopolysaccharidoses | urine | WBC for enzyme panel | —— |
| CHO disorders | urine | WBC/fibroblasts | Liver |
| Miscellaneous | ——Consult specific disease entry—— | | |

**Figure 2.1 An approach to diagnosis of infants with inborn errors of metabolism.**

**Clinical Presentation**
1) Lethargy, coma, seizures
2) Vomiting
3) Odor

$HCO_3^-$ → NORMAL → $NH_4^+$ → $NH_4^+$ → NKH / AAA'uria / PKU / Non-Metabolic

$<16$ → GC/MS → ORGANIC ACIDS

$NH_4^+$ >200μM → Citrulline

$NH_4^+$ Normal

Citrulline: 0 / <200μM / >1000μM → Citrullinemia

Orotate 0 → CPS / OTC
ASA → ASA'uria

NORMAL → LACTATE > 2.0mM

ABNORMAL

$1^2$ Lactic Acidosis — PC Def, PDHC Def

$2^2$ Lactic Acidosis — Glycogen St., Tyrosinemia, Galactosemia, CoArct Ao, Other

Proprionic, Methylmalonic, ß-Keto-thiolase, MSUD, Isovaleric, MCAD, Glutaric I & II, Oxoprolinuria

| | |
|---|---|
| AAA | = Alpha-aminoadipic acid |
| ASA | = Argininosuccinic acid |
| CoArct Ao | = Coarctation of the aorta |
| CPS | = Carbamoyl phosphate synthetase |
| GC/MS | = Gas chromatography/mass spectrometry |
| $HCO_3^-$ | = Bicarbonate |
| MCAD | = Medium-chain acyl-CoA dehydrogenase |
| MSUD | = Maple syrup urine disease |
| $NH_4^+$ | = Ammonium |
| NKH | = Nonketotic hyperglycinemia |
| OTC | = Ornithine transcarbamylase |
| PC def | = Pyruvate carboxylase defect |
| PDHC def | = Pyruvate dehydrogenase complex defect |
| PKU | = Phenylketonuria |

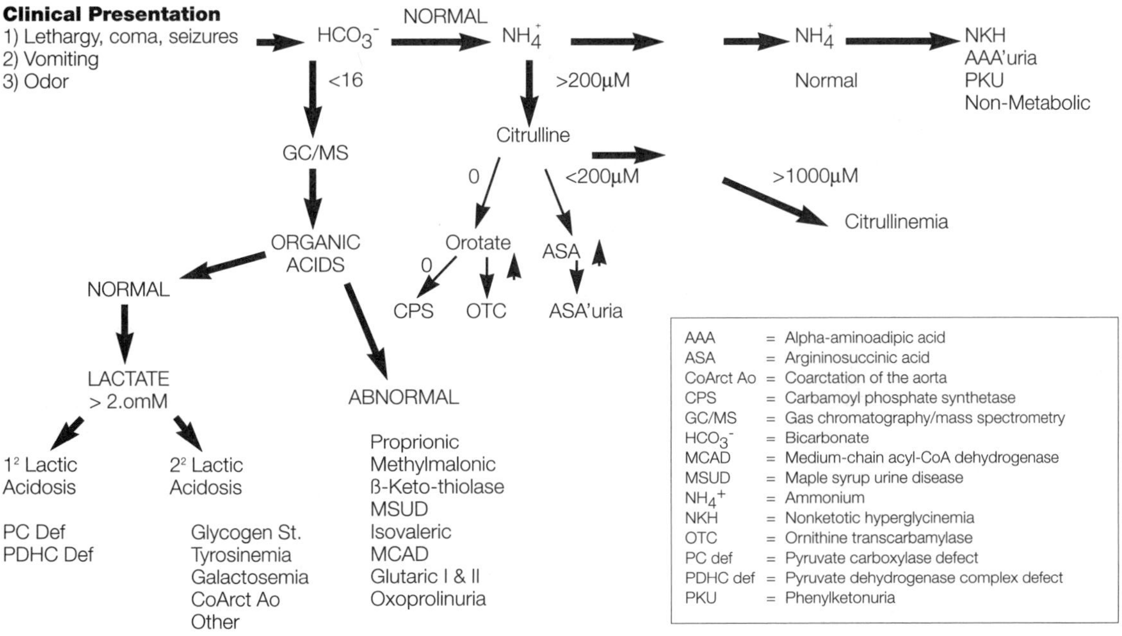

(Expanded from Urea Cycle Enzymes, Figure 20-4, p. 640, by S.W. Brusilow and A.L. Horwich; *in* The Metabolic Basis of Inherited Disease, 6th ed.: C.R. Scriver, et al., eds. Copyright McGraw-Hill, 1989. Used with permission.)

If the acid-base balance is normal and the ammonia is elevated, then plasma citrulline should be determined. This distinguishes the various disorders in the urea cycle, including carbamoyl phosphate synthetase **(CPS)** deficiency, ornithine transcarbamylase **(OTC)** deficiency, argininosuccinic aciduria **(ASA),** and citrullinemia. If both the organic acids and ammonia are normal, then only a few inborn errors of metabolism are likely to produce this clinical picture, including nonketotic hyperglycinemia **(NKH)** and α-aminoadipic aciduria.

Mucopolysaccharidoses may be detected by finding an increase in the urinary excretion of mucopolysaccharides. Other storage disorders do not produce excretion of characteristic metabolites in the urine. These patients require either skin biopsy or other measurement of tissue enzyme deficiency for diagnosis.

The physical examination is usually normal in patients with disorders of amino acid metabolism and urea cycle defects, except for neurologic symptoms. Findings suggestive of a storage disorder include ocular changes, with retinal pigmentation, cherry-red spots, or cataracts. Coarse facies, enlargement of liver and spleen, abnormal thickening of the skin, joint limitation, and bony abnormalities also are hallmarks of a number of storage disorders.

For many years, inborn errors were diagnosable but lacked any effective treatment. With the delineation of PKU in the midpart of the century, diet therapy became established as one means of dealing with an interrupted metabolic pathway. Patients diagnosed in the first few months of life and maintained on a diet with strict limitation of phenylalanine intake have an outcome that produces a mean IQ of approximately 100. Subsequently, diet therapy has been introduced for galactemia, maple syrup urine disease, and tyrosinemia, but with diminished efficacy. Although their lives may be preserved, patients with galactemia and tyrosinemia continue to manifest difficulties that require additional interventions.

Effective therapy for many disorders of amino acid metabolism and of carbohydrate metabolism as well as some other inborn errors is becoming available. Most disorders of amino acid metabolism can be partially treated by limiting intake of the offending metabolite. These children may not be able to tolerate more than 1 gm/kg/day of dietary protein, which may still permit adequate growth and development. Although most infants in America are fed a diet containing between 2 and 3 gm/kg/day of protein, many infants in the Third World thrive on much less than that. This dietary limitation can be ameliorated to some extent by increasing the amount of dietary amino acids that are not metabolized via the defective metabolic pathway. Many special infant formulas with specific amino acids deleted are available.

A second means to treat inborn errors of metabolism arose with the innovative treatment provided by Saul Brusilow at Johns Hopkins, who devised alternative means of waste nitrogen disposition. These compounds are described under the specific urea cycle defect entries and provide a pharmacologic means to permit the body to compensate for its inability to synthesize urea from ammonia. Also in the category of alternative paths is cysteamine treatment of nephropathic cystinosis. In this disease, cystine is unable to leave lysosomes, resulting in an elevated accumulation of lysosomal cystine, the renal Fanconi syndrome, followed by progressive renal failure resulting in end-stage renal disease by 10 years of age. Cysteamine (Cystagon, manufactured by Mylan Laboratories, Inc.) was granted new drug approval by the Food and Drug Administration in 1994. This compound reacts inside the lysosomes of cystinotic patients to produce a compound that can leave the lysosomes. Clinical studies demonstrated that long-term administration of Cystagon to persons with nephropathic cystinosis results in preservation of renal function and enhanced linear growth. Another pharmacotherapy is provided by NTBC treatment of tyrosinemia type I. This catastrophic disease leads to nodular cirrhosis and hepatocellular carcinoma. NTBC blocks the production of the toxic metabolites that lead to the pathologic process observed in the liver, and clinical studies to date demonstrate significant biochemical and clinical improvement.

Disorders of organic acid metabolism may respond to vitamin therapy. Many enzymes require cofactors (vitamins) for catalytic activity. In rare instances, the genetic defect involves the region of the enzyme that binds the cofactor. In these cases it is sometimes possible to achieve some improvement in enzyme function by treating the patient with pharmacologic doses of the specific vitamin cofactor needed by that enzyme. An example is B12 therapy in vitamin B12–responsive methylmalonic aciduria.

Plasma carnitine should be measured in patients with metabolic acidosis, particularly if organic acids are abnormal. If the carnitine is low, therapy with carnitine can be instituted, with good effect in many instances. Carnitine is required for the oxidation of fatty acids within mitochondria, since fatty acids are conjugated to carnitine prior to their transport into mitochondria. Many organic acidemias result in secondary carnitine deficiency because of the urinary excretion of acylcarnitines, which are the conjugation product between the organic acids that accumulate in the disorder and the body's endogenous carnitine stores. Secondary carnitine deficiency then augments the debility caused by the organic acidemia, since failure to oxidize fatty acids completely in the mitochondria leads to accumulation of ketone bodies and hypoglycemia as well as metabolic acidosis and enhanced lactate production.

Clearly, the long-term hope for persons with genetic diseases is gene therapy. An ideal protocol would introduce the gene of interest to the tissue that lacks it via a vector that integrates, producing stable, long-term expression of the desired gene product without deleterious side effects. Some studies have been undertaken to treat diseases like adenosine deaminase deficiency, cystic fibrosis, and LDL receptor deficiency. The results of these studies to date have been to demonstrate the feasibility of the methodology and to encourage further investigation. Sadly, because these are orphan diseases, it appears that the major efforts in gene therapy will be directed toward the more prevalent diseases, at least in the near term, rather than the classic orphan diseases represented by inborn errors of metabolism.

A high index of suspicion coupled with rapid referral to an appropriate diagnostic laboratory or tertiary care center will result in ameliorating illness and saving lives for patients with these diseases.

**References**

The Metabolic and Molecular Basis of Inherited Disease, 7th ed.: C.R. Scriver, et al., eds.; McGraw-Hill, 1995.

Disorders of Amino Acid Metabolism: J.G. Thoene; *in* Internal Medicine, 4th ed.: J.H. Stein, ed.-in-chief; C.V. Mosby Company, 1994, pp. 1462–1472.

# INBORN ERRORS OF METABOLISM

*Listings in This Section*

# 5-Oxoprolinuria

**Description** 5-Oxoprolinuria is caused by an inborn error of glutathione metabolism, which may result in central nervous system impairment.

**Synonyms**
>  Pyroglutamicaciduria

**Signs and Symptoms** Massive amounts of 5-oxoproline (pyroglutamic acid) are excreted in the urine, and abnormally high levels of this acid and lactic acid are found in the blood and cerebrospinal fluid. Metabolic acidosis usually is present. Without treatment, mental retardation, impaired muscle coordination (cerebellar ataxia), and seizures may occur.

**Etiology** 5-Oxoprolinuria, inherited as an autosomal recessive trait, is the result of a deficiency of the enzyme glutathione synthetase.

**Epidemiology** The disorder is very rare. It can be present at birth, and affects males and females equally.

**Related Disorders** The inborn **5-oxoprolinase deficiency** is characterized by excretion of a moderate amount of 5-oxoproline in the urine, and by higher than normal blood levels of this substance. There usually are no other symptoms related to the enzyme deficiency.

**Glutathionuria (γ-glutamyl transpeptidase deficiency)** is a very rare, possibly hereditary metabolic disorder. Concentrations of glutathione in blood and urine are excessive. Mild mental retardation and behavioral problems may be present.

**Treatment—Standard** Bicarbonate therapy is used to compensate for metabolic acidosis. Genetic counseling is recommended for families of affected children.

**Treatment—Investigational** Please contact the agencies listed under Resources, below, for the most current information. Addresses and telephone numbers of these agencies, as well as of individual experts and research centers, may be found in the Master Resources List.

**Resources**
   **For more information on 5-oxoprolinuria:** National Organization for Rare Disorders (NORD); The Arc (a national organization on mental retardation); NIH/National Institute of Neurological Disorders and Stroke; William Rhead, M.D., University of Iowa Hospital and Clinics; Research Trust for Metabolic Diseases in Children.

   **For genetic information and genetic counseling referrals:** March of Dimes Birth Defects Foundation; Alliance of Genetic Support Groups.

**References**
The Metabolic and Molecular Basis of Inherited Disease, 7th ed.: C.R. Scriver, et al., eds.; McGraw-Hill, 1995, pp. 1465–1470.

Ophthalmological, Psychometric and Therapeutic Investigation in Two Sisters with Hereditary Glutathione Synthetase Deficiency (5-Oxoprolinuria): A. Larsson, et al.; Neuropediatrics, August 1985, vol. 16(3), pp. 131–136.

Neonatal 5-Oxoprolinuria: Difficult-to-Diagnose?: I.S. Mendelson, et al.; J. Inherit. Metab. Dis., 1983, vol. 6(1), pp. 44–48.

The Cerebral Lesions in a Patient with Generalized Glutathione Deficiency and Pyroglutamic Aciduria (5-Oxoprolinuria): K. Skullerud, et al.; Acta Neuropathol. (Berlin), 1980, vol. 52(3), pp. 235–238.

# Acidemia, Isovaleric (IVA)

**Description** IVA is a hereditary metabolic disorder that usually begins in infancy and occurs in both an acute and a chronic intermittent form.

**Synonyms**
>  Isovaleric Acid–CoA Dehydrogenase Deficiency
>  Isovalericacidemia
>  Isovaleryl-CoA Carboxylase Deficiency

**Signs and Symptoms** Onset may be as early as a few days of age or as late as 1 year. The acute form of IVA is characterized by attacks of vomiting, lack of appetite, and listlessness. Infants become increasingly lethargic, have increased neuromuscular irritability, and are often hypothermic. Usually there is a strong odor, like that of sweaty feet.

Intermittent episodes are most often triggered by upper respiratory infections or excessive consumption of high-protein foods. Severe acidity and ketoacidosis follow, and coma may ensue. Ketoacidotic episodes tend to occur often in early infancy and young childhood, but their frequency usually diminishes as the patient grows older. Children with IVA often have a natural aversion to protein foods, even at a young age.

IVA can be diagnosed prenatally by measuring the amounts of isovalerylglycine in amniotic fluid.

**Etiology** IVA is inherited as an autosomal recessive trait, as are all known organic acidemias. IVA symptoms are the result of a deficiency of the enzyme isovaleryl CoA dehydrogenase, which is needed for the oxidation of the amino acid leucine.

Many of the adverse effects of the organic acidemias are worsened as a result of secondary carnitine depletion.

**Epidemiology** Males and females are affected equally.

**Related Disorders** See *Acidemia, Methylmalonic; Acidemia, Propionic; Glutaricaciduria II; Maple Syrup Urine Disease; Nonketotic Hyperglycinemia.*

**Treatment—Standard** IVA is treated with moderate dietary restriction of the amino acid leucine and supplementation of L-carnitine. Oral administration of glycine at 150 to 300 mg/kg/day is lifesaving and may permit normal growth and development. Other treatment is symptomatic and supportive. Genetic counseling is recommended for families of affected children.

With treatment and a low-protein diet, the disorder becomes chronically intermittent, and a nearly normal life is possible.

**Treatment—Investigational**

Please contact the agencies listed under Resources, below, for the most current information. Addresses and telephone numbers of these agencies, as well as of individual experts and research centers, may be found in the Master Resources List.

**Resources**

**For more information on isovaleric acidemia:** National Organization for Rare Disorders (NORD); Organic Acidemia Association; British Organic Acidemia Association; The Arc (a national organization on mental retardation); NIH/National Digestive Diseases Information Clearinghouse; Research Trust for Metabolic Diseases in Children.

**For genetic information and genetic counseling referrals:** March of Dimes Birth Defects Foundation; Alliance of Genetic Support Groups.

**References**

The Metabolic and Molecular Basis of Inherited Disease, 6th ed.: C.R. Scriver, et al., eds.; McGraw-Hill, 1989, pp. 795–798.

The Response to L-Carnitine and Glycine Therapy in Isovaleric Acidaemia: C. de Sousa, et al.; Eur. J. Pediatr., February 1986, vol. 144(5), pp. 451–456.

Stable Isotope Dilution Analysis of Isovalerylglycine in Amniotic Fluid and Urine and Its Application for the Prenatal Diagnosis of Isovaleric Acidemia: D.G. Hine, et al.; Pediatr. Res., March 1986, vol. 20(3), pp. 222–226.

# ACIDEMIA, METHYLMALONIC

**Description** The methylmalonic acidemias are caused by an enzymatic defect in the oxidation of amino acids. The resultant metabolic acidosis causes the symptoms described below.

**Synonyms**

Methylmalonic Aciduria

**Signs and Symptoms** The onset of symptoms usually is during the first few months of life. Acutely, drowsiness, coma, and seizures may occur, with mental retardation a long-term consequence. Symptoms may also include lethargy, failure to thrive, recurrent vomiting, dehydration, respiratory distress, diminished muscle tone, and an enlarged liver.

Laboratory findings include an abnormally high amount of methylmalonic acid in the blood and urine. Metabolic acidosis is present. The blood or urine may show elevated levels of ketone as well as excessive amounts of the amino acid glycine. Hyperammonemia may also occur. White blood cell count may be lower than normal. Hypoglycemia may occur.

**Etiology** The methylmalonic acidemias, which segregate into 4 complementation groups, all inherited as autosomal recessive traits, are caused by defects in the enzyme methylmalonyl-CoA mutase, or in adenosylcobalamin synthetic enzymes.

Many of the effects of the organic acidemias are worsened because of secondary carnitine depletion.

**Related Disorders** See *Acidemia, Propionic.*

**Epidemiology** The incidence of methylmalonic acidemia is approximately 1:50,000 to 1:100,000 live births.

**Treatment—Standard** The diet must be carefully controlled. Treatment includes a low-protein regimen and/or restriction of the amino acids isoleucine, valine, and threonine. To ensure a balanced diet, certain medical foods must be fed to affected children. Pharmacologic doses of vitamin B12 are indicated in the B12-responsive variants.

Carnitine supplementation at 100 to 300 mg/kg/day is recommended for associated carnitine deficiency.

Genetic counseling is recommended for the families of affected children. The recurrence risk is 25 percent.

**Treatment—Investigational** Please contact the agencies listed under Resources, below, for the most current information. Addresses and telephone numbers of these agencies, as well as of individual experts and research centers, may be found in the Master Resources List.

**Resources**

**For more information on the methylmalonic acidemias:** National Organization for Rare Disorders (NORD); Organic Acidemia Association; British Organic Acidemia Association; The Arc (a national organization on mental retardation); Research Trust for Metabolic Diseases in Children.

**For genetic information and genetic counseling referrals:** March of Dimes Birth Defects Foundation; Alliance of Genetic Support Groups.

**References**

The Metabolic Basis of Inherited Disease, 6th ed.: C.R. Scriver, et al., eds.; McGraw-Hill, 1989, pp. 832–840.

Clinical Heterogeneity in Cobalamin C Variant of Combined Homocystinuria and Methylmalonic Aciduria: G.A. Mitchell, et al.; J. Pediatr., March 1986, vol. 108(3), pp. 410–415.

# ACIDEMIA, PROPIONIC

**Description** Propionic acidemia is an inherited disorder caused by a deficiency of the biotin-requiring enzyme propionyl-CoA carboxylase (**PCC**) and usually results in catastrophic illness beginning in the newborn period.

**Synonyms**

Hyperglycinemia with Ketoacidosis and Leukopenia

Ketotic Hyperglycinemia

Propionyl-CoA Carboxylase (PCC) Deficiency

**Signs and Symptoms** The initial signs in affected infants are protein intolerance, vomiting, failure to thrive, lethargy, and profound metabolic acidosis. Intercurrent infections may prove fatal.

Other characteristics may include diminished muscle tone, leukopenia, and liver abnormalities. The blood exhibits an elevated concentration of glycine and a massive amount of propionate. EEG abnormalities are possible, and affected patients may experience slowed development and mental retardation.

Amniocentesis to test for PCC activity in amniocytes is possible. An alternative is to measure the concentration of methylcitrate in the amniotic fluid.

When the disorder is suspected in patients and relatives of patients who may be carriers, definitive diagnosis requires measurement of PCC activity in leukocytes or fibroblasts.

Without treatment, the acidosis and ketosis cause dehydration, lethargy, and vomiting. Brain damage, including coma, generalized seizures, and death result if the disorder is left untreated.

**Etiology** Propionic acidemia is an autosomal recessive disorder, one of the organic acidemias. The parents of affected patients may show consanguinity.

Symptoms and signs are due to metabolic acidosis caused by a deficiency of PCC, which is needed for metabolism of the amino acids isoleucine, valine, threonine, and methionine.

Many of the adverse effects of organic acidemia are due to secondary carnitine depletion.

**Epidemiology** Males and females are affected equally. The incidence is estimated at 1:100,000 live births.

**Related Disorders** See *Acidemia, Methylmalonic.*

**Treatment—Standard** Treatment requires fluid and electrolyte therapy. Sodium bicarbonate is used to resolve the acidosis. This also can be accomplished by either peritoneal dialysis or hemodialysis. Treatment must begin as soon as acidosis is recognized.

Long-term treatment involves maintenance of a diet low in protein through use of special formulas low in the amino acids isoleucine, valine, threonine, and methionine. On these restricted diets, patients can experience good metabolic control with acceptable growth and development if adequate general nutrition is maintained through use of medical foods.

Patients with propionic acidemia develop secondary carnitine deficiency because of loss of propionyl-carnitine and other acyl-carnitines in the urine. In **carnitine deficiency syndromes,** the transport of fatty acids into mitochondria for oxidation and energy production is impaired. Because large amounts of glucose must be used to meet the patient's metabolic requirements, hypoglycemia often results.

**Treatment—Investigational** It is possible that patients with propionic acidemia can respond to biotin treatment. A therapeutic trial of this coenzyme of PCC can be performed.

Please contact the agencies listed under Resources, below, for the most current information. Addresses and telephone numbers of these agencies, as well as of individual experts and research centers, may be found in the Master Resources List.

### Resources
**For more information on propionic acidemia:** National Organization for Rare Disorders (NORD); Organic Acidemia Association; British Organic Acidemia Association; Research Trust for Metabolic Diseases in Children; The Arc (a national organization on mental retardation); NIH/National Digestive Diseases Information Clearinghouse.

**For genetic information and genetic counseling referrals:** March of Dimes Birth Defects Foundation; Alliance of Genetic Support Groups.

### References
Mendelian Inheritance in Man, 9th ed.: V.A. McKusick; The Johns Hopkins University Press, 1990, pp. 1211–1213.
The Metabolic Basis of Inherited Disease, 6th ed.: C.R. Scriver, et al., eds.; McGraw-Hill, 1989, pp. 821–845.

# ADRENOLEUKODYSTROPHY (ALD)

**Description** ALD is characterized by cerebral demyelination and adrenal atrophy. The disease has 2 inheritance patterns and appears in 3 different forms categorized by age of onset (X-linked, occurring as adult-onset and childhood-onset; and autosomal recessive, with neonatal onset).

**Synonyms**
> Addison Disease with Cerebral Sclerosis
> Addison-Schilder Disease
> Adrenomyeloneuropathy
> Encephalitis Periaxialis Diffusa
> Flatau-Schilder Disease
> Myelinoclastic Diffuse Sclerosis
> Schilder Disease
> Schilder Encephalitis
> Siewerling-Creutzfeldt Disease
> Sudanophilic Leukodystrophy

**Signs and Symptoms** All forms of ALD, including 85 percent of heterozygotes, are characterized by greatly increased plasma and tissue levels of very long-chain fatty acids **(VLCFAs),** which accumulate in the cerebral white matter and the adrenal glands. A few persons with elevated VLCFA levels may have mild symptoms or none at all. In others, the disease may progress very slowly.

Women who are heterozygotic for childhood or adult-onset ALD but are not symptomatic during childhood may have elevated levels of VLCFAs. At age 30 years, symptoms and signs may begin; these may include progressive spastic paraparesis, ataxia, hypertonia, mild peripheral neuropathy, abnormal reflexes of the plantar extensors, and urinary problems. There are no adrenal symptoms, however, and mental and sensory functions are unimpaired.

**Childhood ALD,** the most common form of the disorder, affects only males. The first symptoms appear between the ages of 4 and 8 years. Females may be carriers of childhood ALD but are asymptomatic. Behavioral changes such as poor memory, deteriorating school work, increasing loss of emotional control, and dementia may be the first signs. A spastic gait, hyperreflexia, hemiparesis, speech disorders, hearing loss, and vision problems including visual agnosia are also seen in children with this disorder.

Manifestations of decreased adrenal gland function usually appear later than the neurologic features. These adrenocortical symptoms and signs can include hypotension, weakness, fatigue, dehydration, weight loss, microcardia, increased skin pigmentation, and decreased secretion of adrenal hormones in response to adrenocorticotropic hormone **(ACTH).** More advanced neurologic signs can include a progressive optic atrophy and brain demyelination. Magnetic resonance imaging **(MRI)** shows lesions in the posterior occipital and parietal lobe white matter. In the adrenal cortex, distended cells can be found in the inner and the thick middle layers.

**Adolescent or adult-onset ALD (adrenomyeloneuropathy)** may affect the spinal cord. It, too, affects only males, although females can be carriers. Symptoms and signs, which usually first appear between the ages of 21 and 35, may include progressive leg stiffness, spastic paraparesis of the lower extremities, and ataxia. Sensory changes indicate that involvement of the spinal tracts and peripheral nerves has occurred. Decreased function of the adrenal cortex and testes may be present. ALD should be suspected, even in the absence of neurologic manifestations, in males who have decreased adrenal function with a family history of Addison disease (see *Addison Disease).* Although adult-onset ALD progresses more slowly than the childhood form, it too can ultimately result in deterioration of brain function.

**Neonatal ALD** is inherited as an autosomal recessive disorder, and therefore both males and females are affected. It has different pathologic findings. Symptoms and signs appear in the newborn period and include mental retardation, facial abnormalities, seizures, polymicrogyria, retinal degeneration, hypotonia, hepatomegaly, and adrenal insufficiency. In addition to demyelination of the brain's white matter, there may also be gray matter involvement. Hepatic peroxisomes are decreased or absent, and plasma pipecolic acid may be increased. This form of ALD tends to be quickly progressive. Persons who are heterozygotic for neonatal ALD exhibit no neurologic or adrenal symptoms.

CT scan or MRI shows changes in the brain. Laboratory tests for VLCFAs are the most definitive diagnostic procedures. Female carriers and newborn infants at high risk for ALD are detected by measuring the level of long-chain fatty acids in plasma or fibroblast cultures. Prenatal diagnosis can be made through amniocentesis and culture of amniotic cells or by study of cultured chorionic villus biopsy.

**Etiology** Abnormal or absent peroxisomes lead to the accumulation of VLCFAs in these conditions, but the precise enzyme deficiency preventing breakdown of VLCFAs is not known. The excess of saturated and unsaturated fatty acid chains is distributed throughout the tissues of the entire body, but tends to accumulate more in the brain's white matter and the adrenal cortex.

**Epidemiology** Childhood ALD usually begins before age 10 (most often around 7 years). Onset of adult ALD is usually between ages 21 and 35. Female heterozygotes for ALD rarely have manifestations of the disorder, but if these do occur they commonly appear after the age of 30 years.

**Related Disorders** See *Addison Disease; Leukodystrophy, Canavan; Leukodystrophy, Metachromatic; Refsum Syndrome; Zellweger Syndrome.*

**Treatment—Standard** Adrenal steroids are given for the adrenocortical deficiency symptoms of ALD, which are the same as those of Addison disease. Treatment for neurologic symptoms associated with ALD is symptomatic and supportive. Seizures usually respond well to anticonvulsants. The severe discomfort of spasticity has been managed with some success with baclofen.

Physical therapy, psychological support, special education, and visiting nurse services are often required to help the patient and family cope with the effects of childhood ALD. Genetic counseling for families affected by the disorder is suggested.

**Treatment—Investigational** Current research is directed toward the identification of the gene that causes ALD.

Hugo W. Moser, M.D., at the Kennedy-Krieger Institute at Johns Hopkins University, has been awarded a grant from the Office of Orphan Products Development, Food and Drug Administration, for research in treating ALD with glycerol trioleate. A recent modification in which dietary VLCFA restriction is combined with oral glycerol trioleate does lower VLCFA levels. Its clinical efficacy is being tested.

Lorenzo's oil (erucic acid) is being tested in conjunction with triolein oil as a possible treatment for patients with rapidly progressive childhood ALD. Because of the possible toxicity of this agent, careful monitoring is required.

Bone-marrow transplantation also is being tested as a treatment for childhood ALD; this procedure, however, is not recommended for patients with relatively advanced neurologic symptoms.

β-Interferon and thalidomide are being tested at the Clinical Research Center at The Johns Hopkins Hospital as possible treatments for ALD.

Please contact the agencies listed under Resources, below, for the most current information. Addresses and telephone numbers of these agencies, as well as of individual experts and research centers, may be found in the Master Resources List.

**Resources**

**For more information on adrenoleukodystrophy:** National Organization for Rare Disorders (NORD); National Adrenal Diseases Foundation; United Leukodystrophy Foundation; ALD Project, Hugo W. Moser, M.D. Kennedy-Krieger Institute, Johns Hopkins University; The Arc (a national organization on mental retardation); NIH/National Institute of Neurological Disorders and Stroke; Association Européenne contre les Leucodystrophies; Research Trust for Metabolic Diseases in Children.

**For genetic information and genetic counseling referrals:** March of Dimes Birth Defects Foundation; Alliance of Genetic Support Groups.

**References**

Adrenoleukodystrophy (X-Linked): H.W. Moser and A.B. Moser; *in* Metabolic and Molecular Basis of Inherited Disease, 7th ed.: C.R. Scriver, et al., eds.; McGraw-Hill, 1995, p. 2326.

Mendelian Inheritance in Man, 10th ed.: V.A. McKusick; The Johns Hopkins University Press, 1992, pp. 1199, 1769–1772.

Birth Defects Encyclopedia: M.L Buyse, ed.-in-chief; Blackwell Scientific Publications, 1990, pp. 61–62.

Disorders of Peroxisome Biogenesis: P.B. Lazarow and H.W. Moser; *in* Metabolic Basis of Inherited Disease, 6th ed.: C.R. Scriver, et al., eds.; McGraw-Hill, 1989, pp. 1479–1509.

Principles of Neurology, 4th ed.: R.D. Adams and M. Victor, eds.: McGraw-Hill, 1989, pp. 811–812.

Adrenoleukodystrophy: Extracts from "Adrenoleukodystrophy in Children and Adults—Diagnosis and Genetic Counseling": H.W. Moser; Newsletter of Research Trust for Metabolic Diseases in Children, 1986, pp. 5–7.

Adrenoleukodystrophy: Survey of 303 Cases: Biochemistry, Diagnosis, and Therapy: H.W. Moser, et al.; Ann. Neurol., December 1984, vol. 16(6), pp. 628–641.

# ALCAPTONURIA

**Description** Patients with alcaptonuria excrete large amounts of dark-colored urine, the result of spontaneous oxidation of homogentisic acid, which also accumulates in the tissues. In normal functioning, the amino acid tyrosine is metabolized into homogentisic acid, and further into maleylacetoacetic acid. In alcaptonuria, the pathway is not completed because of a deficiency of the enzyme homogentisic acid oxidase, and further metabolism of homogentisic acid is prevented. Accumulation of the acid leads to severe degeneration of the cartilage of the spine and other major joints, and osteoarthritis.

**Synonyms**
> Alcaptonuric Ochronosis
> Hereditary Alcaptonuria
> Homogentisicaciduria

**Signs and Symptoms** In their late 20s or 30s, patients develop discoloration of the nose and sclera of the eye. The urine may be dark or may darken upon standing. Somewhat later, patients develop stiffness, pain, and restricted motion in the hips, knees, and shoulders. Still later, symptoms include more severely restricted motion of the spine, thickened ear cartilages, and darkened middle and inner ear structures.

Patients with alcaptonuria who also have kidney disease, and thus an impaired excretion of homogentisic acid, become symptomatic earlier and symptoms tend to be more severe.

**Etiology** Deficiency of the enzyme homogentisic acid oxidase is inherited as an autosomal recessive trait.

**Epidemiology** Males and females are affected in equal numbers, although symptoms tend to be more severe in males. Alcaptonuria is unusually prevalent in Czechoslovakia and the Dominican Republic.

**Treatment—Standard** Occupations that place stress on the large joints should be avoided. Attempts to prevent symptoms through diets low in tyrosine or high in ascorbic acid have had no effect. Other treatment is symptomatic and supportive.

**Treatment—Investigational** Please contact the agencies listed under Resources, below, for the most current information. Addresses and telephone numbers of these agencies, as well as of individual experts and research centers, may be found in the Master Resources List.

**Resources**

**For more information on alcaptonuria:** National Organization for Rare Disorders (NORD); NIH/National Arthritis and Musculoskeletal and Skin Diseases Information Clearinghouse; Bert N. La Du, M.D., Department of Pharmacology, University of Michigan School of Medicine; Research Trust for Metabolic Diseases in Children.

**For genetic information and genetic counseling referrals:** March of Dimes Birth Defects Foundation; Alliance of Genetic Support Groups.

**References**

The Metabolic and Molecular Basis of Inherited Disease, 7th ed.: C.R. Scriver, et al., eds.; McGraw-Hill, 1995, pp. 1371–1386.
Internal Medicine, 3rd ed.: J.H. Stein, ed.-in-chief; Little, Brown and Company, 1990, pp. 2301–2310.

# ANDERSEN DISEASE

**Description** Andersen disease, one of the glycogen storage diseases, is characterized by cirrhosis and, possibly, liver failure.

**Synonyms**
> Amylopectinosis
> Andersen Glycogenosis
> Brancher Deficiency
> Glycogen Storage Disease IV
> Glycogenosis Type IV

**Signs and Symptoms** A newborn with Andersen disease appears to be normal. However, within a few months the infant fails to thrive, with little weight gain, a lack of muscle tone, and nonspecific gastrointestinal problems. The liver and spleen progressively enlarge. The course of Andersen disease is marked by progressive cirrhosis of the liver, edema, and sometimes ascites. Besides the hypotonia, neurologic abnormalities include muscular atrophy and decreased tendon reflexes.

Diagnosis can be made prenatally.

**Etiology** The disease is inherited as an autosomal recessive trait. Symptoms are caused by lack of the brancher enzyme amyl-transglucosidase, and by abnormal glycogen.

**Epidemiology** Andersen disease is one of the rarest of the glycogen storage diseases, affecting less than 5 percent of all patients with these conditions. It usually begins during infancy and affects males and females in equal numbers. All glycogen storage diseases together affect fewer than 1:40,000 persons in the United States.

**Related Disorders** See *von Gierke Disease; Glycogen Storage Disease III; Hers Disease.*

**Treatment—Standard** Treatment primarily focuses on managing the cirrhosis and associated problems. A low-protein diet and salt restriction can be helpful for edema or ascites. Further treatment is symptomatic and supportive. Genetic counseling for families of affected children is essential.

**Treatment—Investigational** Liver transplantation has been used experimentally in the treatment of Andersen disease. More research is needed before this procedure can be recommended as a useful therapy, since other tissues are involved.

Please contact the agencies listed under Resources, below, for the most current information. Addresses and telephone numbers of these agencies, as well as of individual experts and research centers, may be found in the Master Resources List.

**Resources**

**For more information on Andersen disease:** National Organization for Rare Disorders (NORD); NIH/National Digestive Diseases Information Clearinghouse; Association for Glycogen Storage Diseases; Research Trust for Metabolic Diseases in Children.

**For genetic information and genetic counseling referrals:** March of Dimes Birth Defects Foundation; Alliance of Genetic Support Groups.

**References**

The Metabolic and Molecular Basis of Inherited Disease, 7th ed.: C.R. Scriver, et al., eds.; McGraw-Hill, 1995, pp. 950–951.

Liver Transplantation for Type IV Glycogen Storage Disease: R. Selby, et al.; N. Engl. J. Med., January 3, 1991, vol. 324(1), pp. 39–42.

A Juvenile Variant of Glycogenosis IV (Andersen Disease): A.S. Guerra, et al.; Eur. J. Pediatr., August 1986, vol. 145(3), pp. 179–181.

Liver-Spleen Scintigraphy in Glycogen Storage Disease (Glycogenoses): S. Heyman; Clin. Nucl. Med., December 1985, vol. 10(12), pp. 839–843.

Nervous System Involvement in Type IV Glycogenosis: K.R. McMaster, et al.; Arch. Pathol. Lab. Med., March 1979, vol. 103(3), pp. 105–111.

# ARGINASE DEFICIENCY

**Description** Arginase deficiency is 1 of the 6 urea cycle disorders, caused by a deficiency of one of the biosynthetic enzymes needed for the conversion of ammonia to urea, which is then normally excreted in the urine. These enzymatic deficiencies cause an excess of ammonia in the blood and body tissues.

**Synonyms**

Argininemia
Inborn Errors of Urea Synthesis
Urea Cycle Disorder

**Signs and Symptoms** The onset of symptoms may be at birth, but in some cases symptoms may not be noticeable until the infant is several weeks or months of age. The disorder is characterized in infants by progressive mental retardation, seizures, and spasticity. Symptoms also include lack of appetite, vomiting, and hepatomegaly. If left untreated, the disorder may progress to serious and permanent central nervous system dysfunction. A life-threatening elevation of ammonia in the blood is rare, however.

The diagnosis is suspected in the presence of an elevated level of arginine in the blood with concomitant hyperammonemia, and normal plasma concentrations of other amino acids.

**Etiology** Arginase deficiency has an autosomal recessive inheritance.

**Epidemiology** The deficiency is rare, with fewer than 1,000 known cases in the United States. Males and females are affected equally.

**Related Disorders** See *Reye Syndrome.*

The following urea cycle disorders are all characterized by deficiencies of enzymes that are needed for different steps in the synthesis of urea from ammonia. See *N-Acetyl Glutamate Synthetase (NAGS) Deficiency; Ornithine Transcarbamylase (OTC) Deficiency; Carbamyl Phosphate Synthetase (CPS) Deficiency; Citrullinemia; Argininosuccinic Aciduria.* The symptoms of all urea cycle disorders include hyperammonemia, in different degrees of severity.

**Treatment—Standard** Diagnostic testing should be done immediately when a urea cycle disorder is suspected. Tests should include measurement of plasma levels of ammonia, amino acids, and bicarbonate.

Treatment should be started when hyperammonemia is noted, to prevent coma and brain damage. The orphan drug benzoate/phenylacetate (Ucephan, manufactured by McGaw Laboratories) was approved in 1988 for use in the prevention and treatment of hyperammonemia in patients with urea cycle enzymopathy due to enzyme deficiencies.

Arginase deficiency may respond to restriction of dietary protein, and to Ucephan therapy.

Genetic counseling is vital for families of children with urea cycle disorders.

**Treatment—Investigational** A new investigational drug, sodium phenylbutyrate, which does not have an offensive smell, is being developed by Saul Brusilow, M.D., at Johns Hopkins Hospital. This drug is intended to enhance waste nitrogen excretion and prevent ammonia buildup in the blood.

An investigative regimen consisting of acute hemodialysis followed by a restricted intake of protein, plus sodium benzoate, sodium phenylacetate, and arginine or citrulline, is being used on an experimental basis for the treatment of hyperammonemia.

Please contact the agencies listed under Resources, below, for the most current information. Addresses and telephone numbers of these agencies, as well as of individual experts and research centers, may be found in the Master Resources List.

**Resources**

**For more information on arginase deficiency:** National Organization for Rare Disorders (NORD); National Urea Cycle Disorders Foundation; NIH/National Digestive Diseases Information Clearinghouse; Research Trust for Metabolic Diseases in Children; Saul Brusilow, M.D., Johns Hopkins Hospital; Stephen Cederbaum, M.D., UCLA Medical School.

**For genetic information and genetic counseling referrals:** March of Dimes Birth Defects Foundation; Alliance of Genetic Support Groups.

**References**

Urea Cycle Enzymes: S.W. Brusilow and A.L. Horwich; *in* The Metabolic and Molecular Basis of Inherited Disease, 7th ed.: C.R. Scriver, et al., eds.; McGraw-Hill, 1995, pp. 1187–1232.

Disorders of the Urea Cycle: S.W. Brusilow; Hosp. Pract., October 15, 1985, vol. 305, pp. 65–72.

Symptomatic Inborn Errors of Metabolism in the Neonate: S.W. Brusilow and D.L. Vallee; *in* Current Therapy in Neonatal-Perinatal Medicine, Marcel Decker, 1985, pp. 207–212.

# ARGININOSUCCINIC ACIDURIA

**Description** Argininosuccinic aciduria is 1 of 6 hereditary urea cycle disorders, which are caused by deficiency of the enzymes required for the synthesis of urea from ammonia. The deficiencies result in an excess of ammonia in the blood and body tissues.

**Synonyms**

Argininosuccinase Deficiency

Inborn Errors of Urea Synthesis

Urea Cycle Disorder

**Signs and Symptoms** Argininosuccinic aciduria is characterized by hyperammonemia in early infancy. The onset usually is at birth, but symptoms and signs may not be noticeable for days or weeks. Manifestations include lethargy, lack of appetite, vomiting, seizures, and coma. Hepatomegaly may be present. The plasma level of citrulline is moderately elevated (about 100 $\mu$M). The markedly increased plasma concentration of argininosuccinic acid is the basis for the diagnosis (see Figure 2.1 in the introduction to this chapter). Immediate treatment after diagnosis in newborns is imperative. If the disorder is left untreated, brain damage, coma, and death will occur.

**Etiology** The disorder has an autosomal recessive inheritance. Deficiency of the enzyme argininosuccinase causes the accumulation of excess ammonia.

**Epidemiology** Argininosuccinic aciduria is rare, affecting fewer than 100 persons in the United States. Males and females are affected equally.

**Related Disorders** The symptoms of all urea cycle disorders result from hyperammonemia, in different degrees of severity. See *N-Acetyl Glutamate Synthetase (NAGS) Deficiency; Ornithine Transcarbamylase (OTC) Deficiency; Carbamyl Phosphate Synthetase (CPS) Deficiency; Citrullinemia; Arginase Deficiency.*

**Organic acidemias** may be accompanied by hyperammonemia associated with metabolic acidosis, with an increased anion gap and/or ketonuria. These disorders are also of genetic origin and affect the urea cycle as a secondary phenomenon.

See also *Reye Syndrome.*

**Treatment—Standard** Diagnostic testing should be done immediately when a urea cycle disorder is suspected. Tests should include measurement of plasma levels of ammonia, amino acids, and bicarbonate. Before the results of these tests are available, however, treatment of hyperammonemia should begin, to prevent coma or brain damage.

The drug benzoate/phenylacetate (Ucephan, manufactured by McGaw Laboratories) has been approved for use in the prevention and treatment of hyperammonemia in patients with urea cycle enzymopathy due to enzyme deficiencies.

Genetic counseling is imperative for children with argininosuccinic aciduria and their families.

**Treatment—Investigational** A regimen being used on an experimental basis consists of acute hemodialysis followed by a restricted intake of protein and administration of sodium benzoate, sodium phenylacetate, and arginine or citrulline.

Two investigational drugs, sodium benzoate and sodium phenylacetate, are used to enhance waste nitrogen excretion and thus prevent toxic ammonia buildup in the blood. These orphan drugs have been developed by Saul Brusilow, M.D., of Johns Hopkins Hospital.

Please contact the agencies listed under Resources, below, for the most current information. Addresses and telephone numbers of these agencies, as well as of individual experts and research centers, may be found in the Master Resources List.

**Resources**

**For more information on argininosuccinic aciduria:** National Organization for Rare Disorders (NORD); National Urea Cycle Disorders Foundation; NIH/National Digestive Diseases Information Clearinghouse; National Kidney Foundation; American Kidney Fund; Research Trust for Metabolic Diseases in Children; Saul Brusilow, M.D., Johns Hopkins Hospital.

**For genetic information and genetic counseling referrals:** March of Dimes Birth Defects Foundation; Alliance of Genetic Support Groups.

**References**

Urea Cycle Enzymes, S.W. Brusilow and A.L. Horwich *in* The Metabolic and Molecular Basis of Inherited Disease, 7th ed.: C.R. Scriver, et al., eds.; McGraw-Hill, 1995, pp. 1187–1232.

Disorders of the Urea Cycle: S.W. Brusilow; Hosp. Pract., October 15, 1985, vol. 305, pp. 65–72.

Symptomatic Inborn Errors of Metabolism in the Neonate: S.W. Brusilow and D.L. Vallee; *in* Current Therapy in Neonatal-Perinatal Medicine, Marcel Decker, 1985, pp. 207–212.

# ASPARTYLGLUCOSAMINURIA

**Description** Aspartylglucosaminuria is a lysosomal storage disease that is found most commonly in persons of Finnish descent. The disorder is caused by a defect in aspartylglucosaminidase.

**Synonyms**

AGA

AGU

Aspartylglycosaminuria

**Signs and Symptoms** Aspartylglucosaminuria is characterized by abnormal development beginning after the first few months of life. There are recurrent infections and diarrhea, and progressive coarsening of facial features. Mild skeletal abnormalities may occur, and the ocular lens may develop crystalline deposits. Mental deterioration may begin to occur after age 5, and behavior problems are common. Lung, heart, and hematologic problems tend to occur in later years. The patient may exhibit mental retardation and uneven development of the head and face, with sagging cheeks, a wide nose, and a broad face. Scoliosis may be present, and the neck may be unusually short. Adult stature is usually below normal.

**Etiology** Aspartylglucosaminuria is inherited as an autosomal recessive trait. The gene responsible for this disorder is located on the long arm of the 4th chromosome at 4q21. A deficiency of aspartylglucosaminidase causes accumulation of aspartylglucosamine, resulting in disorders in the various body systems. Persons of Finnish ancestry are most often affected by this disorder. However, aspartylglucosaminuria can occur in people of all heritages.

**Epidemiology** Aspartylglucosaminuria is a rare disorder that affects males and females in equal numbers. However, in Finland, where the majority of cases are reported, there are an estimated 130 cases in 4.5 million persons. In the rest of the world, the condition is extremely rare.

**Related Disorders** See *Mucopolysaccharidosis; Mucolipidosis III; Mucolipidosis II.*

**Treatment—Standard** Treatment of aspartylglucosaminuria is symptomatic and supportive. Genetic counseling of affected families is essential.

**Treatment—Investigational** Enzyme replacement therapy is being investigated as a treatment for aspartylglucosaminuria.

Please contact the agencies listed under Resources, below, for the most current information. Addresses and telephone numbers of these agencies, as well as of individual experts and research centers, may be found in the Master Resources List.

**Resources**

**For more information on aspartylglucosaminuria:** National Organization for Rare Disorders (NORD); The Arc (a national organization on mental retardation); NIH/National Institute of Diabetes, Digestive and Kidney Diseases; Research Trust for Metabolic Diseases in Children.

**For genetic information and genetic counseling referrals:** March of Dimes Birth Defects Foundation; Alliance of Genetic Support Groups.

### References

The Metabolic and Molecular Basis of Inherited Disease, 7th ed.: C.R. Scriver, et al., eds.; McGraw-Hill, 1995, pp. 2546–2548.

Aspartylglycosaminuria in a Non-Finnish Patient Caused by a Donor Splice Mutation in the Glycoasparaginase Gene: I. Mononen, et al.; J. Biol. Chem., February 15, 1992, vol. 267(5), pp. 3196–3199.

Aspartylglycosaminuria in the Finnish Population: Identification of Two Point Mutations in the Heavy Chain of Glycoasparaginase: I. Mononen, et al.; Proc. Natl. Acad. Sci. USA, April 1, 1991, vol. 88(7), pp. 2941–2945.

High Prevalence of Aspartylglycosaminuria Among School-Age Children in Eastern Finland: T. Mononen, et al.; Hum. Genet., July 1991, vol. 87(3), pp. 266–268.

Two Japanese Cases with Aspartylglycosaminuria: Clinical and Morphological Features: K. Yoshida, et al.; Clin. Genet., October 1991, vol. 40(4), pp. 318–325.

Birth Defects Encyclopedia: M.L Buyse, ed.-in-chief; Blackwell Scientific Publications, 1990, pp. 198–199.

Mendelian Inheritance in Man, 9th ed.: V.A. McKusick; The Johns Hopkins University Press, 1990, p. 1047.

# BLUE DIAPER SYNDROME

**Description** Blue diaper syndrome is a metabolic disorder characterized by digestive disturbances, fever, bluish urine, and visual difficulties. Kidney disease may eventually develop in some cases.

**Synonyms**
> Drummond Syndrome
> Hypercalcemia
> Indicanuria Syndrome

**Signs and Symptoms** The syndrome is generally detected in infants only when their urine stains their diapers blue. Other general findings include irritability, failure to thrive, constipation, poor appetite, and vomiting. Infections and fevers are frequent. The child typically has poor vision resulting from ocular abnormalities.

Because blood levels of calcium are elevated, nephrocalcinosis develops, which may lead to eventual kidney failure.

**Etiology** Blue diaper syndrome has an autosomal recessive mode of inheritance. The biochemical nature of the defect remains uncertain, although it is thought to relate to a defect in the intestinal absorption of tryptophan. Intestinal bacteria convert the excessive tryptophan into indican and related derivatives; it is these substances that color the urine blue.

**Epidemiology** Blue diaper syndrome is a very rare disorder, affecting males and females equally.

**Treatment—Standard** Ingestion of calcium should be kept to a relatively low level to prevent kidney damage. The use of antibiotics for intestinal bacteria, and administration of nicotinic acid may be beneficial.

**Treatment—Investigational** Please contact the agencies listed under Resources, below, for the most current information. Addresses and telephone numbers of these agencies, as well as of individual experts and research centers, may be found in the Master Resources List.

**Resources**

**For more information on blue diaper syndrome:** National Organization for Rare Disorders (NORD); National Kidney Foundation; American Kidney Fund; NIH/National Digestive Diseases Information Clearinghouse; Research Trust for Metabolic Diseases in Children.

**For genetic information and genetic counseling referrals:** March of Dimes Birth Defects Foundation; Alliance of Genetic Support Groups.

### References

Mendelian Inheritance in Man, 10th ed.: V.A. McKusick; The Johns Hopkins University Press, 1992, pp. 1255–1256.

Nelson Textbook of Pediatrics, 14th ed.: R.E. Behrman, ed.-in-chief; W.B. Saunders Company, 1992, pp. 316, 984.

The Kidney, 4th ed.: B.M. Brenner and F.C. Rector, Jr., eds.: W.B. Saunders Company, 1991, p. 1601.

Birth Defects Encyclopedia: M.L Buyse, ed.-in-chief; Blackwell Scientific Publications, 1990, p. 1712.

Dictionary of Medical Syndromes, 3rd ed.: S.I. Magalini, et al., eds.; J.B. Lippincott Company, 1990, p. 262.

The Metabolic Basis of Inherited Disease, 6th ed.: C.R. Scriver, et al., eds.; McGraw-Hill, 1989, p. 2519.

# CARBAMYL PHOSPHATE SYNTHETASE (CPS) DEFICIENCY

**Description** In CPS deficiency, 1 of 6 hereditary urea cycle disorders, the enzyme lacking is carbamyl phosphate synthetase, needed for the synthesis of urea from ammonia. The result is an excess of ammonia in the blood and body tissues. If untreated, brain damage, coma, and death may ensue.

**Synonyms**

>Hyperammonemia
>Inborn Errors of Urea Synthesis
>Urea Cycle Disorder

**Signs and Symptoms** Onset of the symptoms occurs at birth. Manifestations in infants are hyperammonemia, lethargy, coma, and seizures. Other symptoms and signs include vomiting and hepatomegaly. The diagnosis is based on severe hyperammonemia with normal citrulline in plasma, and absent orotate in the urine (see Figure 2.1 in the introduction to this chapter). For these infants, immediate treatment after diagnosis is imperative.

**Etiology** This condition is inherited as an autosomal recessive trait.

**Epidemiology** The disorder is very rare; fewer than 1,000 persons in the United States are affected, males and females equally.

**Related Disorders** See *Reye Syndrome.*

The symptoms of all urea cycle disorders result from hyperammonemia, in varying degrees of severity. See *N-Acetyl Glutamate Synthetase (NAGS) Deficiency; Ornithine Transcarbamylase (OTC) Deficiency; Citrullinemia; Argininosuccinic Aciduria; Arginase Deficiency.*

**Organic acidemias** may be accompanied by hyperammonemia associated with metabolic acidosis, with an increased anion gap and/or ketonuria. These disorders are also of genetic origin and affect the urea cycle as a secondary phenomenon.

**Treatment—Standard** Diagnostic testing should be done as soon as a urea cycle disorder is suspected. Tests should include measurement of plasma levels of ammonia, amino acids, and bicarbonate.

Treatment should be started as soon as possible to prevent coma or brain damage. As soon as hyperammonemia due to CPS deficiency is diagnosed in a newborn, dialysis or exchange transfusion should be started.

The drug benzoate/phenylacetate (Ucephan, manufactured by McGaw Laboratories) has been approved for use in the prevention and treatment of hyperammonemia in patients with urea cycle enzymopathy due to enzyme deficiencies.

Genetic counseling is imperative for the family of children with CPS deficiency.

**Treatment—Investigational** A regimen being used on an experimental basis consists of acute hemodialysis followed by a restricted intake of protein, plus sodium benzoate, sodium phenylacetate, and arginine or citrulline.

Two investigational drugs, sodium benzoate and sodium phenylacetate, are used to enhance waste nitrogen excretion. These orphan drugs have been developed by Saul Brusilow, M.D., Johns Hopkins Hospital.

Please contact the agencies listed under Resources, below, for the most current information. Addresses and telephone numbers of these agencies, as well as of individual experts and research centers, may be found in the Master Resources List.

**Resources**

**For more information on carbamyl phosphate synthetase deficiency:** National Organization for Rare Disorders (NORD); National Urea Cycle Disorders Foundation; NIH/National Digestive Diseases Information Clearinghouse; National Kidney Foundation; American Kidney Fund; Research Trust for Metabolic Diseases in Children; Saul Brusilow, M.D., Johns Hopkins Hospital.

**For genetic information and genetic counseling referrals:** March of Dimes Birth Defects Foundation; Alliance of Genetic Support Groups.

**References**

Urea Cycle Enzymes: S.W. Brusilow and A.L. Horwich; *in* The Metabolic and Molecular Basis of Inherited Disease, 7th ed.: C.R. Scriver, et al., eds.; McGraw-Hill, 1995, pp. 1187–1232.

Disorders of the Urea Cycle: S.W. Brusilow; Hosp. Pract., October 15, 1985, vol. 305, pp. 65–72.

Symptomatic Inborn Errors of Metabolism in the Neonate: S.W. Brusilow and D.L. Vallee; *in* Current Therapy in Neonatal-Perinatal Medicine, Marcel Decker, 1985, pp. 207–212.

# CARNITINE DEFICIENCY SYNDROMES, HEREDITARY

**Description** A deficiency in carnitine, which is normally synthesized in the liver and kidneys, results in muscle weakness and other manifestations described below.

**Signs and Symptoms** Muscle weakness is the primary symptom. Intermittent shortages of energy supply in muscle tissue may result in rhabdomyolyis. Urinary myoglobin loss may also be associated.

Systemic carnitine deficiency differs from myopathic carnitine deficiency by the presence of low carnitine concentrations in tissues other than muscle, as well as in blood and urine. Central nervous system, hepatic, and myocardial involvement may be present. Degenerative encephalopathy may lead to episodes of vomiting, confusion, and stupor, progressing to coma.

Carnitine deficiency may also be associated with hypoglycemia, and damage to the heart muscle may result in chronic cardiomyopathy.

**Etiology** Excessive urinary loss of acylcarnitines is the cause of carnitine deficiency in most individuals. Carnitine deficiency usually occurs in conjunction with organic acidemias, such as isovaleric, methylmalonic, and propionic acidemias. It may also rarely be present where there is severe liver disease or renal tubular dysfunction.

**Epidemiology** Males and females are equally affected. Individuals with any of the organic acidemias, severe liver disease, or renal tubular dysfunction are at risk of developing the deficiency.

**Related Disorders** See *Acidemia, Isovaleric; Acidemia, Propionic; Acidemia, Methylmalonic.*

**Treatment—Standard** Carnitine deficiency may be corrected by oral L-carnitine and, to some degree, by certain changes in diet. Consumption of foods high in carnitine content, such as red meat and dairy products, should be encouraged. High oral doses of L-carnitine may cause an extremely unpleasant fishlike body odor; this disappears with dosage reduction. Diarrhea may occasionally occur in some patients.

Synthetic L-carnitine is available in tablet and liquid form.

**Treatment—Investigational** Please contact the agencies listed under Resources, below, for the most current information. Addresses and telephone numbers of these agencies, as well as of individual experts and research centers, may be found in the Master Resources List.

**Resources**

For more information on hereditary carnitine deficiency syndromes: National Organization for Rare Disorders (NORD); Association for Babies and Children with Carnitine Deficiency; Organic Acidemia Association; Research Trust for Metabolic Diseases in Children.

For genetic information and genetic counseling referrals: March of Dimes Birth Defects Foundation; Alliance of Genetic Support Groups.

**References**

Cecil Textbook of Medicine, 19th ed.: J.B. Wyngaarden, et al., eds.; W.B. Saunders Company, 1992, p. 2259.

Mendelian Inheritance in Man, 10th ed.: V.A. McKusick; The Johns Hopkins University Press, 1992, pp. 92–94.

Birth Defects Encyclopedia: M.L Buyse, ed.-in-chief; Blackwell Scientific Publications, 1990, p. 1200.

Carnitine Deficiency Syndromes: G.N. Breningstall; Pediatr. Neurol., 1990, vol. 6, pp. 75–81.

Carnitine: Metabolism And Clinical Chemistry: N. Siliprandi, et al.; Clin. Chim. Acta, July 31, 1989, vol. 183(1), pp. 3–11.

The Metabolic Basis of Inherited Disease, 6th ed.: C.R. Scriver, et al., eds.; McGraw-Hill, 1989, pp. 894–898.

Transport of Carnitine into Cells in Hereditary Carnitine Deficiency: B.O. Eriksson, et al.; J. Inherit. Metab. Dis., 1989, vol. 12(2), pp. 108–111.

Decreased Fasting Free Fatty Acids with L-Carnitine in Children with Carnitine Deficiency: W.F. Schwenk, et al.; Pediatr. Res., May 1988, vol. 23(5), pp. 491–494.

# CARNITINE PALMITYLTRANSFERASE (CPT) II DEFICIENCY

**Description** CPT II deficiency is a very rare disorder of lipid metabolism that affects the muscle's ability to function properly. Strenuous exercise leads to the breakdown of muscle tissue and the appearance of myglobin in the urine. Major symptoms may include myalgia, fatigue, and the excretion of reddish-brown urine.

**Synonyms**

Myopathy with Deficiency of Carnitine Palmityltransferase

Myopathy, Metabolic, Carnitine Palmityltransferase Deficiency

**Signs and Symptoms** CPT II deficiency is characterized by easy fatigability during prolonged exertion, disabling myalgia that sometimes lasts for days, and lipid levels in the muscles that usually remain the same or increase only slightly. Destruction of skeletal muscles (rhabdomyolysis) and the resultant passage of reddish-brown urine (myoglobinuria) may follow prolonged exercise, viral illness, sleep and food deprivation, and overexposure to cold, especially in diabetic patients or persons on a high-fat diet. The combination of these conditions may sometimes become life-threatening. Between attacks, the patient is usually asymptomatic.

CPT II deficiency is diagnosed by enzymatic studies and muscle biopsy. As a precaution, siblings of CPT II deficiency patients should be tested for the disorder to help prevent development of symptoms.

**Etiology** CPT II deficiency is inherited as an autosomal recessive trait. The gene responsible for the disorder is assigned to chromosome 1 in the region of 1q12–1pter.

**Epidemiology** CPT II deficiency occurs in males more often than females. It usually becomes apparent in adulthood. However, a more serious form may affect children. The disorder is more apparent in diabetics and in patients with malnutrition.

**Related Disorders** See *Eaton-Lambert Syndrome; Scapuloperoneal Myopathy.*

**Fibromyalgia** is a chronic disorder characterized by pain throughout much of the body. The pain may begin gradually or have a sudden onset. Other symptoms are muscle spasms, fatigue, muscle stiffness, and nonrestorative sleep. The exact cause of this disorder is unknown.

**Treatment—Standard** CPT II patients, especially those who are diabetic, should exercise in moderation, eat adequate amounts of food, avoid stress and high-fat foods, and keep warm. Dietary carnitine supplementation is not usually helpful in CPT II deficiency. Genetic counseling may be of benefit for patients and their families. Other treatment is symptomatic and supportive.

**Treatment—Investigational** Enzyme replacement therapy is being investigated as a treatment for CPT II deficiency.

Please contact the agencies listed under Resources, below, for the most current information. Addresses and telephone numbers of these agencies, as well as of individual experts and research centers, may be found in the Master Resources List.

**Resources**

**For more information on carnitine palmityltransferase II deficiency**: National Organization for Rare Disorders (NORD); NIH/National Institute of Diabetes, Digestive and Kidney Diseases; Research Trust for Metabolic Diseases in Children.

**For genetic information and genetic counseling referrals:** March of Dimes Birth Defects Foundation; Alliance of Genetic Support Groups.

**References**

Carnitine Palmityltransferase in Human Erythrocyte Membrane: Properties and Malonyl-CoA Sensitivity: R.R. Ramsay, et al.; Biochem. J., May 1, 1991, vol. 275(3), pp. 685–688.

Birth Defects Encyclopedia: M.L Buyse, ed.-in-chief; Blackwell Scientific Publications, 1990, pp. 1200–1201.

Mendelian Inheritance in Man, 9th ed.: V.A. McKusick; The Johns Hopkins University Press, 1990, p. 1365.

Chronic Myopathy with a Partial Deficiency of the Carnitine Palmityltransferase Enzyme: R.I. Kieval, et al.; Arch. Neurol., May 1989, vol. 46(5), pp. 575–576.

Fatal Rhabdomyolysis Following Influenza Infection in a Girl with Familial Carnitine Palmityltransferase Deficiency: K.J. Kelly, et al.; Pediatrics, August 1989, vol. 84(2), pp. 312–316.

The Metabolic Basis of Inherited Disease, 6th ed.: C.R. Scriver, et al., eds.; McGraw-Hill, 1989, pp. 388, 889, 911.

Regulation of Carnitine Palmityltransferase in Vivo by Glucagon and Insulin: P.S. Brady, et al.; Biochem. J., March 15, 1989, vol. 258(3), pp. 677–682.

# CARNOSINEMIA

**Description** Patients with carnosinemia, a hereditary metabolic disorder, may display neurologic abnormalities such as severe mental retardation and myoclonic seizures. However, a causal relationship between symptoms and enzymatic deficiency has not been established.

**Synonyms**

Carnosinase Deficiency

Homocarnosinosis

**Signs and Symptoms** In some patients with carnosinemia, seizures occur at less than 1 year of age. Growth and motor and mental development are slow. As neurologic damage progresses, myoclonic jerks involving the head and limbs occur. By the age of 2 years, signs of mental retardation may be apparent. Other patients with low serum carnosinase are normal.

**Etiology** Carnosinemia is an autosomal recessive metabolic disorder. The biochemical mechanisms are not clear. There is defective metabolism of carnosine (β-alanyl-L-histidine), a dipeptide usually found in muscle tissue, by the enzyme carnosinase. Patients usually have carnosinuria and deficient serum carnosinase.

**Epidemiology** Carnosinemia is a very rare disorder that affects males and females equally.

**Treatment—Standard** Treatment is symptomatic and supportive.

**Treatment—Investigational** Please contact the agencies listed under Resources, below, for the most current information. Addresses and telephone numbers of these agencies, as well as of individual experts and research centers, may be found in the Master Resources List.

**Resources**

**For more information on carnosinemia:** National Organization for Rare Disorders (NORD); The Arc (a national organization on mental retardation); NIH/National Institute of Child Health and Human Development; Research Trust for Metabolic Diseases in Children.

**For genetic information and genetic counseling referrals:** March of Dimes Birth Defects Foundation; Alliance of Genetic Support Groups.

**References**

The Metabolic and Molecular Basis of Inherited Disease, 7th ed.: C.R. Scriver, et al., eds.; McGraw-Hill, 1995, pp. 1350–1351.

Cecil Textbook of Medicine, 19th ed.: J.B. Wyngaarden, et al., eds.; W.B. Saunders Company, 1992, p. 1098.

Mendelian Inheritance in Man, 10th ed.: V.A. McKusick; The Johns Hopkins University Press, 1992, p. 1267.

Birth Defects Encyclopedia: M.L Buyse, ed.-in-chief; Blackwell Scientific Publications, 1990, pp. 285–286.

Dictionary of Medical Syndromes, 3rd ed.: S.I. Magalini, et al., eds.; J.B. Lippincott Company, 1990, p. 161.

# CITRULLINEMIA

**Description** Citrullinemia is 1 of 6 hereditary urea cycle disorders that are caused by a deficiency of one of the enzymes needed for the synthesis of urea from ammonia. In citrullinemia, the deficient enzyme is argininosuccinic acid synthetase. Untreated citrullinemia is characterized by hyperammonemia, which leads to brain damage, coma, and death.

**Synonyms**
>       Argininosuccinic Acid Synthetase Deficiency
>       Urea Cycle Disorder
>       Inborn Errors of Urea Synthesis

**Signs and Symptoms** The onset of symptoms usually is in the newborn period. The hyperammonemia is accompanied by lack of appetite, vomiting, listlessness, seizures, and coma. Diagnosis is based on hyperammonemia plus the absence of argininosuccinate and its anhydrides in plasma, and a plasma concentration of citrulline greater than 1,000 µM (markedly elevated). The disorder must be treated immediately upon diagnosis. If the patient is left untreated, brain damage, coma, and death occur in the first weeks of life.

**Etiology** Citrullinemia is an autosomal recessive disorder. Deficient activity of argininosuccinic acid synthetase causes an accumulation of excess ammonia in blood and body tissues.

**Epidemiology** The disorder is rare, affecting fewer than 100 persons in the United States. Males and females are affected equally.

**Related Disorders** The urea cycle disorders are all characterized by deficiencies of enzymes needed for steps in the synthesis of urea from ammonia. See *N-Acetyl Glutamate Synthetase (NAGS) Deficiency; Ornithine Transcarbamylase (OTC) Deficiency; Carbamyl Phosphate Synthetase (CPS) Deficiency; Argininosuccinic Aciduria; Arginase Deficiency.*

**Organic acidemias** may be accompanied by hyperammonemia associated with metabolic acidosis, with an increased anion gap and/or ketonuria. These disorders are also of genetic origin and affect the urea cycle as a secondary phenomenon.

**Treatment—Standard** Diagnostic testing should be done as soon as a urea cycle disorder is suspected. Tests should include measurement of plasma levels of ammonia, amino acids, and bicarbonate.

Treatment of hyperammonemia should be started as soon as possible to prevent coma or brain damage. The drug benzoate/phenylacetate (Ucephan, manufactured by McGaw Laboratories) has been approved for use in preventing and treating hyperammonemia in patients with urea cycle enzymopathy due to enzyme deficiencies.

Genetic counseling is imperative for the family of children with citrullinemia.

**Treatment—Investigational** Two investigational drugs, sodium benzoate and sodium phenylacetate, are being used to enhance waste nitrogen excretion, and prevent toxic ammonia buildup in the blood. These orphan drugs have been developed by Saul Brusilow, M.D., Johns Hopkins Hospital, who is also developing sodium phenylbutyrate, which does not have an offensive smell. One experimental regimen consists of acute hemodialysis followed by a restricted intake of protein, plus administration of sodium benzoate, sodium phenylbutyrate, and arginine.

Please contact the agencies listed under Resources, below, for the most current information. Addresses and telephone numbers of these agencies, as well as of individual experts and research centers, may be found in the Master Resources List.

**Resources**

**For more information on citrullinemia:** National Organization for Rare Disorders (NORD); National Urea Cycle Disorders Foundation; NIH/National Digestive Diseases Information Clearinghouse; National Kidney Foundation; American Kidney Fund; Research Trust for Metabolic Diseases in Children; Saul Brusilow, M.D., Johns Hopkins Hospital.

**For genetic information and genetic counseling referrals:** March of Dimes Birth Defects Foundation; Alliance of Genetic Support Groups.

**References**
Urea Cycle Enzymes: S.W. Brusilow and A.L. Horwich; *in* The Metabolic and Molecular Basis of Inherited Disease, 7th ed.: C.R. Scriver, et al., eds.; McGraw-Hill, 1995, pp. 1187–1232.

Disorders of the Urea Cycle: S.W. Brusilow; Hosp. Pract., October 15, 1985, vol. 305, pp. 65–72.

Symptomatic Inborn Errors of Metabolism in the Neonate: S.W. Brusilow and D.L. Vallee; *in* Current Therapy in Neonatal-Perinatal Medicine, Marcel Decker, 1985, pp. 207–212.

# CYSTINOSIS

**Description** Cystinosis is an inherited disorder of lysosomal cystine transport characterized by the intralysosomal accumulation of cystine. Clinically, 3 forms of the disease are recognized. **Infantile nephropathic cystinosis,** in which symptoms and signs can appear as early as 6 to 12 months of life, is the most severe form of the disease, leading to renal failure by 10 years of age if untreated. In **benign** (or **adult**) **cystinosis,** cystine crystals accumulate in the cornea. In the **intermediate** form (also termed **juvenile** or **adolescent cystinosis**), renal manifestations become significant in the patients' teens or twenties.

One of the major manifestations of cystinosis is the renal **Fanconi syndrome**.

**Synonyms**

      Cystine Storage Disease

      Fanconi II

      Lignac-Fanconi Syndrome

**Signs and Symptoms** Cystine accumulates in the lysosomes of all tissues. Early clinical manifestations involve the kidneys and eyes. Hexagonal or rectangular crystals are present in marrow aspirates, leukocytes, and rectal mucosa, as well as in the cornea and conjunctiva. In heterozygotes for this disorder, intracellular cystine is elevated, but no clinical manifestations are found. Cystine accumulation in the kidney results in renal tubular acidosis, hypokalemia, polyuria, polydipsia, hypophosphatemia. The accumulation of cystine crystals in the cornea and conjunctiva causes photophobia, headache, and itching and burning of the eyes. The crystals are visible by slit-lamp examination of the cornea.

Infantile nephropathic cystinosis becomes apparent before the age of 1 year. Ocular findings include patchy depigmentation of the retina and photophobia. Hypophosphatemic (vitamin D–resistant) rickets occurs, as well as poor linear growth, and the child is pale and thin and fails to thrive. Rickets appears as the child grows older. Untreated cystinosis leads to glomerular failure by 10 years of age.

Renal manifestations of intermediate, or juvenile, cystinosis resemble those of the infantile form, although the course is milder. Rickets may occur if treatment is inadequate.

The adult form of cystinosis is typically benign. This form is characterized by corneal crystals. Renal function remains intact.

**Etiology** The mode of inheritance for all forms of cystinosis is autosomal recessive.

**Related Disorders Fanconi syndrome** is characterized by abnormal renal proximal tubular function, particularly involving excessive excretion of glucose, phosphates, amino acids, bicarbonate, water, potassium, calcium, sodium, and carnitine. This syndrome may be associated with other hereditary metabolic conditions including tyrosinemia, galactosemia, fructose intolerance, glycogen storage disease type I, Wilson disease, familial nephrosis, and Lowe syndrome. Fanconi syndrome also is associated with iatrogenic and environmental causes, including the use of certain aminoglycosides or outdated tetracycline; and poisoning by heavy metals or other chemicals.

See **Wilson Disease; Lowe Syndrome.**

**Treatment—Standard** Benign forms of cystinosis require no treatment.

Nephropathic cystinosis is treated symptomatically with fluids and electrolytes to prevent dehydration. Sodium bicarbonate or sodium citrate is administered to maintain normal electrolyte balance. Phosphate and vitamin D are required to correct hypophosphatemia and prevent rickets.

The cystine-depleting agent cysteamine (Cystagon, manufactured by Mylan Laboratories) has been approved by the Food and Drug Administration for treatment of nephropathic cystinosis.

Hemodialysis or renal transplantation is required in end-stage renal disease. Renal transplantation is successful in this condition, although little improvement in growth accompanies renal transplantation. Corneal transplantation has been successfully performed using living related donors.

Cystinosis can be detected prenatally by amniocentesis, or via chorionic villus sampling.

**Treatment—Investigational** Cystamine and cysteamine eyedrops are being investigated to treat the ocular manifestations of this disease by William A. Gahl, M.D., Ph.D., NIH/National Insitute of Child Health and Human Development; Jerry A. Schneider, M.D., University of California, San Diego; and Jess G. Thoene, M.D., University of Michigan.

Please contact the agencies listed under Resources, below, for the most current information. Addresses and telephone numbers of these agencies, as well as of individual experts and research centers, may be found in the Master Resources List.

**Resources**

**For more information on cystinosis:** National Organization for Rare Disorders (NORD); Cystinosis Foundation; NIH/National Kidney and Urologic Diseases Information Clearinghouse; Research Trust for Metabolic Diseases in Children.

**For genetic information and genetic counseling referrals:** March of Dimes Birth Defects Foundation; Alliance of Genetic Support Groups; Jess G. Thoene, M.D., University of Michigan School of Medicine.

### References

Lysosomal Transport Defects: J. Thoene; *in* A Physician's Guide to Laboratory Diagnosis of Inherited Metabolic Disease: N. Blau, et al., eds.; Chapman and Hall, 1995.

The Metabolic and Molecular Basis of Inherited Disease, 7th ed.: C.R. Scriver, et al., eds.; McGraw-Hill, 1995, pp. 3763–3797.

Mendelian Inheritance in Man, 10th ed.: V.A. McKusick; The Johns Hopkins University Press, 1992, pp. 92–94.

NIH Conference: Cystinosis: Progress in a Prototypic Disease; W.A. Gahl, et al.; Ann. Intern. Med., October 1988, vol. 109(7), pp. 557–569.

Abnormalities in Amino Acid Metabolism in Clinical Medicine: W.L. Nyhan; Appleton-Century-Crofts, 1984.

# CYSTINURIA

**Description** Cystinuria is marked by abnormal intestinal and kidney transport of the amino acids cystine, lysine, arginine, and ornithine. Excessive cystinuria causes formation of calculi in the kidney, bladder, and ureter. Four types of cystinuria are recognized. In **type I** cystinuria, there is a defect in the active transport of cystine and the dibasic amino acids lysine, arginine, and ornithine in the kidneys and small intestine. Carriers of the defective gene are generally asymptomatic. In **type II** cystinuria, cystine and lysine transport is severely impaired in the kidney and only moderately in the intestines. In **type III** cystinuria, renal transport of cystine and lysine is defective; intestinal transport is normal. Carriers of the defective gene for this variant of the disease typically have slightly elevated levels of cystine and lysine in the urine. In **hypercystinuria,** there is moderate elevation of urinary cystine excretion but normal intestinal absorption of cystine and the dibasic amino acids.

**Signs and Symptoms** Urinary excretion of cystine is excessively high, exceeding the solubility limit of cystine. Also excreted in massive amounts in the urine are the amino acids lysine, arginine, and ornithine; these, however, are much more soluble in urine than cystine, and produce no associated symptoms.

The initial symptom of cystinuria is usually acute renal colic. Other findings include hematuria, obstruction, and infections of the urinary tract. Frequent recurrences ultimately may lead to kidney damage.

The calculi are usually small, with a jagged crystalline surface. These may be accompanied by urinary "gravel," which consists of yellowish-brown hexagonal crystals.

All patients with urinary calculi should be screened for cystinuria.

**Etiology** Cystinuria is an autosomal recessive disorder caused by abnormal transport of cystine and the dibasic amino acids.

**Epidemiology** Onset of cystinuria symptoms generally is between ages 10 and 30, although elevated cystine excretion is found from infancy. The disorder occurs in approximately 1:7,000 to 1:10,000 persons; the prevalence varies by country. The disease occurs in both sexes.

**Related Disorders** In **dibasic aminoaciduria,** transport of lysine, arginine, and ornithine is impaired, resulting in increased urinary levels of these amino acids. In **lysinuria,** lysine transport alone is defective, with ensuing large amounts of urinary lysine. Disease carriers tend to have increased levels of the relevant amino acids.

See also *Cystinosis.*

**Treatment—Standard** The primary objective is reduction of cystine concentration in the urine. Consumption of large amounts of fluid both day and night maintains a high volume of urine and reduces cystine concentration. Alkalinization of the urine increases the solubility of cystine and therefore helps prevent stone formation. Agents used include sodium bicarbonate, citrate, and acetazolamide.

Another approach is administration of D-penicillamine, although there is some risk of side effects with this drug. D-Penicillamine promotes mixed-disulfide formation, which is more soluble in the urine and is excreted. Side effects may include fever and rash, and other allergic reactions.

The orphan drug α-mercaptopropionylglycine (Thiola, manufactured by Mission Pharmacal of San Antonio, Texas) has been approved by the Food and Drug Administration as a treatment for cystinuria. This agent also lowers the level of urinary cystine.

Kidney and bladder surgery sometimes becomes necessary, but calculi commonly recur. Small stones may be removed by endoscopic basket extraction, and laser techniques and ultrasound have been used to dissolve stones.

**Treatment—Investigational** Meso-2,3-dimercaptosuccinic acid (Succimer) is being tested as a treatment for cystinuria. This drug may be useful in preventing the formation of cystine calculi.

The orphan drug 2,3-dimercaptosuccinic acid (CHEMET, manufactured by McNeil), is also being tested as a treatment for cystinuria. This drug may prevent kidney damage in those patients prone to recurring calculi.

Please contact the agencies listed under Resources, below, for the most current information. Addresses and telephone numbers of these agencies, as well as of individual experts and research centers, may be found in the Master Resources List.

## Resources

**For more information on cystinuria:** National Organization for Rare Disorders (NORD); Cystinuria Support Network; National Kidney Foundation; American Kidney Fund; Charles Y.C. Pak, M.D., University of Texas Health Science Center at Dallas.

**For genetic information and genetic counseling referrals:** March of Dimes Birth Defects Foundation; Alliance of Genetic Support Groups.

## References

The Metabolic and Molecular Basis of Inherited Disease, 7th ed.: C.R. Scriver, et al., eds.; McGraw-Hill, 1995, pp. 3581–3601.

Cecil Textbook of Medicine, 19th ed.: J.B. Wyngaarden, et al., eds.; W.B. Saunders Company, 1992, pp. 603–608.

Mendelian Inheritance in Man, 10th ed.: V.A. McKusick; The Johns Hopkins University Press, 1992, p. 1322.

The Kidney, 4th ed.: B.M. Brenner and F.C. Rector, Jr., eds.: W.B. Saunders Company, 1991, pp. 1602–1604.

Birth Defects Encyclopedia: M.L Buyse, ed.-in-chief; Blackwell Scientific Publications, 1990, pp. 483–484.

Percutaneous Catheter Dissolution of Cystine Calculi: S.P. Dretler, et al.; J. Urol., February 1984, vol. 131(2), pp. 216–219.

# ERDHEIM-CHESTER DISEASE

**Description** Erdheim-Chester disease is a lipid storage disorder of the long bones. The heart, lungs, peritoneum, and kidneys can also be affected.

**Synonyms**

>Lipid Granulomatosis
>Lipid Storage Disease
>Polyostotic Sclerosing Histiocytosis
>Visceral Xanthogranulomatosis
>Xanthogranulomatosis, Generalized

**Signs and Symptoms** Lipid granulomatous histiocytes infiltrate the bones, causing growth abnormalities. Abnormal deposits of granulomatous material in the heart result in cardiomyopathy; in the lungs, severe lung disease; and in the kidneys, chronic renal failure. Blindness can result if the eyes are affected. In addition, the liver, spleen, thyroid, skin, and gums may be infiltrated. If left untreated, the disorder can be life-threatening.

**Etiology** The cause is unknown.

**Epidemiology** Males and females are affected in equal numbers. Approximately 30 cases have been reported.

**Related Disorders** See *Histiocytosis-X; Wegener Granulomatosis; Granulomatous Disease, Chronic; Lymphomatoid Granulomatosis.*

**Cerebrotendinous xanthomatosis** is an extremely rare congenital lipid storage disease characterized by xanthomatosis in many tissues. Affected children may have difficulty walking, developmental delays, and/or mental retardation. Arteriosclerosis may develop during young adulthood.

**Treatment—Standard** Erdheim-Chester disease is usually treated with corticosteroids and chemotherapy (vinblastine and doxorubicin). The diagnosis is made through bone biopsy, and through x-ray or magnetic resonance imaging scans.

**Treatment—Investigational** Please contact the agencies listed under Resources, below, for the most current information. Addresses and telephone numbers of these agencies, as well as of individual experts and research centers, may be found in the Master Resources List.

## Resources

**For more information on Erdheim-Chester disease:** National Organization for Rare Disorders (NORD); NIH/National Arthritis and Musculoskeletal and Skin Diseases Information Clearinghouse.

## References

Cecil Textbook of Medicine, 19th ed.: J.B. Wyngaarden, et al., eds.; W.B. Saunders Company, 1992, pp. 1022–1023, 1286–1287.

Erdheim-Chester Disease: Case Report with Autopsy Findings: M.G. Fink, et al.; Arch. Pathol. Lab. Med., June 1991, vol. 115(6), pp. 619–623.

Orbital and Eyelid Involvement with Erdheim-Chester Disease: A Report of Two Cases: J.A. Shields, et al.; Arch. Ophthalmol., June 1991, vol. 109(6), pp. 850–854.

Premature Alveolar Bone Loss in Erdheim-Chester Disease: I.H. Valdez, et al.; Oral Surg. Oral Med. Oral Pathol., September 1990, vol. 70(3), pp. 294–296.

Erdheim-Chester Disease: Case Report and Review of the Literature: R.L. Miller, et al.; Am. J. Med., June 1986, vol. 80 (6), pp. 1230–1236.

# FABRY DISEASE

**Description** Fabry disease is a disorder of lipid metabolism in which products of glycolipids accumulate in various tissues.

**Synonyms**

>Angiokeratoma Corporis Diffusum
>α-Galactosidase Deficiency
>Glycolipid Lipidosis
>Hemorrhagic Nodular Purpura

**Signs and Symptoms**

Wartlike angiokeratomas typically appear over the lower trunk. Abdominal pain may develop, similar to that seen in appendicitis. There may be pain in the extremities (acroparesthesia) that lasts minutes to days, and episodic fever. Manifestations in the eyes include glycolipid deposits and contortion and dilation of the blood vessels. Symptomatic episodes increase with age, and kidney failure and cardiac or cerebral complications may develop as the patient ages.

The milder form of Fabry disease that develops in women is characterized by corneal opacities.

Prenatal diagnosis by amniocentesis is possible.

**Etiology** Fabry disease is inherited as an X-linked recessive trait with variable penetrance. The gene that causes this disease is located on the long arm of the X chromosome (Xq21.33–Xq22). The condition is caused by α-galactosidase-A deficiency, which produces an accumulation of glycolipid products, particularly glycosphingolipid, in various tissues of the body.

**Epidemiology** Fabry disease primarily affects males but also may affect heterozygous females in a milder form. Prevalence in the United States is estimated at 2,500 persons. Individuals of any race may be affected, but most cases have been persons of Western European descent.

**Related Disorders Schindler disease (α-N-acetylgalactosaminidase deficiency)** is a rare inborn error of metabolism that usually appears during infancy. Symptoms may include developmental delays, loss of previously acquired intellectual skills, seizures, muscular weakness, lack of coordination, blindness, and/or deafness. In the rarer adult-onset form of the disease, angiokeratomas similar to those of Fabry disease appear. Affected adults may develop coarse facial features and experience angina.

See also ***Gaucher Disease; Raynaud Disease and Phenomenon.***

**Treatment—Standard** Daily oral doses of phenytoin (Dilantin) or low doses of diphenylhydantoin or carbamazepin may help to alleviate chronic pain in the hands and feet. Dexamethasone may also help to relieve acute symptoms. Angiokeratomas may be successfully removed with laser therapy. Replacement of the deficient enzyme by transfusion has been tried but is not generally practical on a long-term basis. Treatment is otherwise symptomatic and supportive.

**Treatment—Investigational** A biotechnology process is being developed to manufacture the orphan drug ceramide trihexosidase/α-galactosidase-A as a treatment for Fabry disease. For more information, contact Dr. D. Calhoune, Department of Chemistry, City College of New York.

Enzyme replacement therapy using the orphan drug Fabrase is being developed by Genzyme Corporation.

Please contact the agencies listed under Resources, below, for the most current information. Addresses and telephone numbers of these agencies, as well as of individual experts and research centers, may be found in the Master Resources List.

**Resources**

**For more information on Fabry disease:** National Organization for Rare Disorders (NORD); National Lipid Diseases Foundation; National Tay-Sachs and Allied Diseases Association; NIH/National Institute of Neurological Disorders and Stroke; Research Trust for Metabolic Diseases in Children; Dr. Robert Desnick, International Center for Fabry Disease, Mount Sinai School of Medicine.

**For genetic information and genetic counseling referrals:** March of Dimes Birth Defects Foundation; Alliance of Genetic Support Groups.

**References**

The Metabolic and Molecular Basis of Inherited Disease, 7th ed.: C.R. Scriver, et al., eds.; McGraw-Hill, 1995, pp. 2741–2784.

Angiokeratomas in Fabry's Disease and Fordyce's Disease: Successful Treatment with Copper Vapour Laser: J. Lapins, et al.; Acta Derm. Venereol., April 1993, vol. 73(2), pp. 133–135.

Psychiatric Disorder in Patients with Fabry's Disease: R.P. Grewal; Int. J. Psychiatry Med., 1993, vol. 23(3), pp. 307–312.

Cecil Textbook of Medicine, 19th ed.: J.B. Wyngaarden, et al., eds.; W.B. Saunders Company, 1992, pp. 1090–1091.

Fabry Disease: Immunocytochemical Characterization of Neuronal Involvement: G.A. deVeber, et al.; Ann. Neurol., April 1992, vol. 31(4), pp. 409–415.

Fabry's Disease: H. Kato, et al.; Intern. Med., May 1992, vol. 31(5), pp. 682–685.

Joint Manifestations of Fabry's Disease: S.O. Paira, et al.; Clin. Rheumatol., December 1992, vol. 11(4), pp. 562–565.

Mendelian Inheritance in Man, 10th ed.: V.A. McKusick; The Johns Hopkins University Press, 1992, pp. 1788–1790.

Nelson Textbook of Pediatrics, 14th ed.: R.E. Behrman, ed.-in-chief; W.B. Saunders Company, 1992, pp. 348–349.

Harrison's Principles of Internal Medicine, 12th ed.: J.D. Wilson, et al., eds.; McGraw-Hill, 1991, pp. 1186, 1848–1849.

Birth Defects Encyclopedia: M.L Buyse, ed.-in-chief; Blackwell Scientific Publications, 1990, pp. 670–671.

Dictionary of Medical Syndromes, 3rd ed.: S.I. Magalini, et al., eds.; J.B. Lippincott Company, 1990, pp. 298–299.

# FARBER DISEASE

**Description** Farber disease is characterized by the inability to produce lysosomal acid ceramidase, causing painful and progressive articular deformities.

**Synonyms**

> Acid Ceramidase Deficiency
>
> Farber Lipogranulomatosis

**Signs and Symptoms** There are a number of variants. In the most severe, symptoms typically appear before 4 months of age. The first signs are swollen joints and a hoarse cry, skin that is sensitive to the touch, and finger flexion. Difficulty in breathing and swallowing, vomiting, and fever may also develop. Cardiac involvement occurs because of nodular growth around the valves. Nodules also are often found in the spleen, intestines, lymph nodes, kidney, tongue, thymus, gallbladder, and liver. The central nervous system is usually involved, and intelligence may or may not be normal. Death occurs in infancy. Other forms present later and permit survival into the teenage years. Central nervous system involvement is variable.

**Etiology** The disease is due to deficiency of lysosomal acid ceramidase and is inherited as an autosomal recessive trait.

**Epidemiology** Farber disease affects males and females equally.

**Related Disorders** Symptoms of juvenile rheumatoid arthritis may be similar to those of Farber disease and should be considered in the differential diagnosis.

**Treatment—Standard** Treatment is symptomatic and supportive. Corticosteroids may provide some relief for joint pain. Tracheostomy may be necessary if breathing passages become blocked by nodular growths. Cosmetic surgery may be desirable for growths in the facial area.

Genetic counseling is appropriate for patients and their families. Prenatal diagnosis by amniocentesis is possible.

**Treatment—Investigational** Please contact the agencies listed under Resources, below, for the most current information. Addresses and telephone numbers of these agencies, as well as of individual experts and research centers, may be found in the Master Resources List.

**Resources**

For more information on **Farber disease:** National Organization for Rare Disorders (NORD); Arthritis Foundation; NIH/National Arthritis and Musculoskeletal and Skin Diseases Information Clearinghouse; Research Trust for Metabolic Diseases in Children; Hugo Moser, M.D., Kennedy-Krieger Institute, Johns Hopkins University.

For genetic information and genetic counseling referrals: March of Dimes Birth Defects Foundation; Alliance of Genetic Support Groups.

**References**

The Metabolic and Molecular Basis of Inherited Disease, 7th ed.: C.R. Scriver, et al., eds.; McGraw-Hill, 1995, pp. 2589–2599.

Farber's Disease (Lysosomal Acid Ceramidase Deficiency): R.A. Jameson, et al., Ann. Rheum. Dis., July 1987, vol. 46(7), pp. 559–561.

Internal Medicine, 2nd ed.: J.H. Stein, ed.; Little, Brown and Company, 1987, pp. 2073.

Diagnosis of Lipogranulomatosis (Farber's Disease) by Use of Cultured Fibroblasts: J.T.Dulaney, et al.; J. Pediatr., July 1976, vol. 89(1), pp. 59–61.

# FRUCTOSE INTOLERANCE, HEREDITARY

**Description** Hereditary fructose intolerance is an inherited disorder characterized by an inability to metabolize fructose or its precursors. The metabolic error results from a deficiency of the enzyme fructose-1-phosphate aldolase.

**Synonyms**

> Fructose-1-Phosphate Aldolase Deficiency
>
> Fructosemia

**Signs and Symptoms** Manifestations of the disease begin shortly after birth. Addition of fructose to the diet of an affected infant will produce prolonged vomiting, failure to thrive, coma, jaundice, and hepatomegaly. A bleeding tendency occurs because of a deficiency in clotting factors. Blood levels of glucose and phosphate are lowered, and levels of fructose in the blood and urine are increased. Patients with hereditary fructose intolerance usually develop an aversion for fruit and sweets.

Early recognition is important to avoid damage to the liver, kidney, and small intestine. There may be intellectual impairment.

**Etiology** Hereditary fructose intolerance is caused by a deficiency of the enzyme fructose-1-phosphate aldolase. It is inherited as an autosomal recessive trait.

**Epidemiology** Hereditary fructose intolerance occurs equally in males and females.

**Related Disorders** See *Fructosuria*.

**Treatment—Standard** As long as patients with hereditary fructose intolerance do not ingest fructose or fructose-containing sugars, such as sucrose, they can remain asymptomatic.

**Treatment—Investigational** Please contact the agencies listed under Resources, below, for the most current information. Addresses and telephone numbers of these agencies, as well as of individual experts and research centers, may be found in the Master Resources List.

**Resources**

**For more information on hereditary fructose intolerance:** National Organization for Rare Disorders (NORD); NIH/National Digestive Diseases Information Clearinghouse.

**For genetic information and genetic counseling referrals:** March of Dimes Birth Defects Foundation; Alliance of Genetic Support Groups.

**References**

The Metabolic and Molecular Basis of Inherited Disease, 7th ed.: C.R. Scriver, et al., eds.; McGraw-Hill, 1995, pp. 399, 905–934.

# FRUCTOSURIA

**Description** Fructosuria, characterized by urinary excretion of fructose, is caused by a deficiency of hepatic fructokinase, which is needed for the synthesis of glycogen from fructose.

**Synonyms**

> Essential Fructosuria
> Hepatic Fructokinase Deficiency
> Levulosuria

**Signs and Symptoms** Fructosuria is marked only by the presence of fructose in the urine, which is the basis for the diagnosis. It is a benign heritable trait that causes no symptoms.

**Etiology** The disorder is inherited as an autosomal recessive trait.

**Epidemiology** Fructosuria affects approximately 1:130,000 persons in the United States. It occurs equally in males and females.

**Related Disorders** Because fructose in the urine may be mistaken for glucose, fructosuria should be differentiated from diabetes mellitus.

**Treatment—Standard** Treatment is not required.

**Treatment—Investigational** Please contact the agencies listed under Resources, below, for the most current information. Addresses and telephone numbers of these agencies, as well as of individual experts and research centers, may be found in the Master Resources List.

**Resources**

**For more information on fructosuria:** National Organization for Rare Disorders (NORD); NIH/National Digestive Diseases Information Clearinghouse; Research Trust for Metabolic Diseases in Children.

**For genetic information and genetic counseling referrals:** March of Dimes Birth Defects Foundation; Alliance of Genetic Support Groups.

**References**

Disorders of Fructose Metabolism: R. Gitzelmann, et al.; *in* The Metabolic and Molecular Basis of Inherited Disease, 5th ed.: C.R. Scriver, et al., eds.; McGraw-Hill, 1995, pp. 905–934.

Mendelian Inheritance in Man, 7th ed.: V.A. McKusick; The Johns Hopkins University Press, 1986, p. 978.

# GALACTOSEMIA, CLASSIC

**Description** Classic galactosemia is a disorder of galactose metabolism causing symptoms in the newborn period. If untreated, severe hepatic and neurologic dysfunction occurs.

**Synonyms**

 Galactose-1-Phosphate Uridyl Transferase Deficiency

**Signs and Symptoms** Clinical manifestations appear early in the newborn period and include vomiting, jaundice, hepatomegaly, hypoglycemia, irritability, listlessness, aminoaciduria, ascites, mental retardation, and cataracts. If treatment is not begun when the symptoms first appear, hepatic cirrhosis, severe mental retardation, growth deficiency, and overwhelming infection can ensue. Girls with galactosemia may develop impaired ovarian function even when treated appropriately. Some cases of classic galactosemia are mild, with few symptoms and without severe impairment.

Galactosemia can be diagnosed at birth by determining the enzyme activity level in red blood cells.

**Etiology** Classic galactosemia is inherited as an autosomal recessive trait. Deficiency of the enzyme galactose-1-phosphate uridyl transferase results in the infant's inability to metabolize galactose and leads to accumulation of galactose-1-phosphate.

**Epidemiology** The incidence is about 1:50,000. Males and females are affected in equal numbers.

**Treatment—Standard** After birth, an affected infant's diet should consist of galactose and lactose-free milk substitutes and foods, such as casein hydrolysates and soybean products. Dietary galactose restriction should be maintained as long as possible. Appropriate treatment may be necessary to control intercurrent infections. Emotional effects of the strict diet may require attention throughout childhood. Genetic counseling is recommended for families of galactosemia patients.

Liver and kidney failure, brain damage, and cataracts can be prevented through avoidance of galactose. Children treated with this special diet usually show satisfactory general health and growth, and can make reasonable, though often not optimal, intellectual progress.

**Treatment—Investigational** Please contact the agencies listed under Resources, below, for the most current information. Addresses and telephone numbers of these agencies, as well as of individual experts and research centers, may be found in the Master Resources List.

**Resources**

**For more information on galactosemia:** National Organization for Rare Disorders (NORD); Parents of Galactosemic Children; NIH/National Digestive Diseases Information Clearinghouse; Research Trust for Metabolic Diseases in Children.

**For genetic information and genetic counseling referrals:** March of Dimes Birth Defects Foundation; Alliance of Genetic Support Groups.

**References**

The Metabolic and Molecular Basis of Inherited Disease, 7th ed.: C.R. Scriver, et al., eds.; McGraw-Hill, 1995, pp. 399, 967–1000.
Galactosemia: How Does Long-Term Treatment Change the Outcome?: R. Gitzelmann, et al.; Enzyme, 1984, vol. 32(1), pp. 37–46.

# GAUCHER DISEASE

**Description** Gaucher disease is the most common of the lipid storage diseases, which include Tay-Sachs, Fabry, and Niemann-Pick diseases. There are 3 forms of Gaucher disease: type I (nonneuronopathic); type II (acute neuronopathic, or infantile cerebral); type III (subacute neuronopathic).

**Synonyms**

 Cerebroside Lipidosis
 Familial Splenic Anemia
 Gaucher-Schlagenhaufer
 Glucosyl Ceramide Lipidosis

**Signs and Symptoms** In **type I** Gaucher disease, bone deterioration is a prominent finding. Other symptoms and signs include hepatomegaly, splenomegaly, and anemia. Rare manifestations may include renal and pulmonary involvement, but the central nervous system is spared.

In **type II,** symptoms and signs include hepatomegaly or splenomegaly and severe neurologic manifestations, such as neck rigidity, apathy, catatonia, strabismus, increased deep reflexes, laryngeal spasm, and death before age 2 years.

In **type III,** symptoms and signs are similar to those of type II but are milder and later in onset.

A diagnostic assay is available to detect affected persons and carriers, and the condition can also be diagnosed with amniocentesis.

**Etiology** All types of Gaucher disease are inherited as autosomal recessive traits and are caused by failure to produce the enzyme glucocerebrosidase. All are characterized by the presence of Gaucher (lipid-laden) cells in the bone marrow and other organs, e.g., the spleen and liver. The defective gene that causes Gaucher disease and controls the enzyme glucocerebrosidase is thought to be located at the q21–q31 region of chromosome 1. It is believed that different mutations in this gene are associated with the different types of Gaucher disease.

**Epidemiology Type I** affects both men and women, with onset at any age, although most patients are in their late teens. A high proportion of Ashkenazic Jews are affected.

**Type II** is a rare form of the disease with onset usually in the first few months of life. Both sexes are affected, with a slight prevalence in males. There is no racial prevalence.

**Type III,** the rarest form of Gaucher disease, may be variable in its age of onset but usually begins during childhood and adolescence. Both sexes are affected.

All types of Gaucher disease together affect between 20,000 and 40,000 people worldwide.

**Related Disorders** See *Sandhoff Disease; Hajdu-Cheney Syndrome; Hepatic Fibrosis; Osteonecrosis.*

**Treatment—Standard** Treatment is symptomatic and supportive. When circumstances warrant, total or partial splenectomy and joint replacement may be considered.

The orphan drug Ceredase (glucocerebrosidase/β-glucosidase) was approved by the Food and Drug Administration in April 1991 for use in type I Gaucher disease. For further information, contact Genzyme Corporation.

**Treatment—Investigational** The National Institutes of Health **(NIH)** have established a program to study neurogenetic and lysosomal storage disorders. Patients included in these studies may be evaluated at the NIH through the Interinstitute Medical Genetics Clinic as well as the Molecular Neurogenetics Unit, Clinical Neuroscience Branch, National Institute of Mental Health (NIMH); and the Human Genetics Branch, National Institute of Child Health and Human Development (NICHHD). For further information, please contact Patient Care Coordinator, Human Genetics Branch, NIH/National Institute of Child Health and Human Development, Bethesda, Maryland 20892; (301) 496-7661.

For research on replacement enzymes in bone marrow transplantations, contact Robert Desnick, M.D., Division of Medical Genetics, Mount Sinai Hospital.

Robert E. Lee, M.D., is compiling a database dealing with the disease. He can be contacted at the University of Pittsburgh Medical School.

The NIH and Massachusetts General Hospital are conducting a joint 2-year study to examine the effects of Ceredase on bone structure and metabolism and to learn whether the response can be enhanced by vitamin supplements. Eligible patients must be between the ages of 18 and 43, have undergone a splenectomy, and not be currently on enzyme replacement therapy. For more information, contact Mrs. Connie Kreps at the NIH or Ramnik Xavier at Massachusetts General Hospital.

A clinical trial is under way to evaluate the effectiveness of recombinant human glucocerebrosidase modified by polyethylene glycol **(PEG).** The study is being coordinated by Dr. Ellen Sidransky and Dr. Edward Ginns of the Clinical Neuroscience Branch of the National Institutes of Health. PEG-glucocerebrosidase is being developed by Enzon and has received orphan drug designation by the Food and Drug Administration. Because of the PEG modification, the drug may be administered by injection rather than by intravenous infusion. The first phase of the clinical trial will include moderately to severely affected individuals, with or without spleens, who have depressed blood counts. For more information, contact Ms. Elizabeth Alzona, Clinical Neuroscience Branch, National Institutes of Health.

Please contact the agencies listed under Resources, below, for the most current information. Addresses and telephone numbers of these agencies, as well as of individual experts and research centers, may be found in the Master Resources List.

**Resources**

**For more information on Gaucher disease:** National Organization for Rare Disorders (NORD); National Gaucher Foundation; Tay-Sachs and Allied Diseases Association; The Arc (a national organization on mental retardation); NIH/National Institute of Neurological Disorders and Stroke.

**For genetic information and genetic counseling referrals:** March of Dimes Birth Defects Foundation; Alliance of Genetic Support Groups.

**References**

The Metabolic and Molecular Basis of Inherited Diseases, 7th ed.: C.R. Scriver, et al., eds.; McGraw-Hill, 1995, pp. 2641–2670.

Cecil Textbook of Medicine, 19th ed.: J.B. Wyngaarden, et al., eds.; W.B. Saunders Company, 1992, pp. 1091–1092.

Gaucher's Disease: New Molecular Approaches to Diagnosis and Treatment: E. Buetler; Science, May 1992, vol. 256(5058), pp. 794–799.

Birth Defects Encyclopedia: M.L Buyse, ed.-in-chief; Blackwell Scientific Publications, 1990, pp. 769–770.

Mendelian Inheritance in Man, 9th ed.: V.A. McKusick; The John Hopkins University Press, 1990, pp. 1200–1204.

# GLUTARICACIDURIA I (GA I)

**Description** GA I is an enzyme deficiency disorder characterized by dystonia and dyskinesia. Mental retardation also may occur.

**Synonyms**

> Glutaricacidemia I
> Glutaryl-CoA Dehydrogenase Deficiency

**Signs and Symptoms** Affected individuals may have macrocephaly at birth. During the first year of life, disease manifestations appear suddenly after a period of apparent normal development and include vomiting, metabolic acidosis, hypotonia, and central nervous system degeneration. Opisthotonus, dystonia, and chronic athetotic and choreic movements are observed in some patients. Mental retardation may be present, and some patients have unusual facies.

Concentrations of glutaric acid and 3-hydroxyglutaric acid are elevated in the urine. The excretion of glutaric acid may exceed 1 gm per day. Glutaric acid concentrations are also elevated in blood serum, cerebrospinal fluid, and body tissues.

Glutaricaciduria can be diagnosed by the finding of excessive glutaric acid in the urine, or by analysis of the deficient enzyme in leukocytes. Fetal detection is possible by testing amniocytes for the enzyme glutaryl-CoA dehydrogenase.

**Etiology** Glutaricaciduria, one of the organic acidemias, is inherited as an autosomal recessive trait. The gene associated with the disorder has been mapped to chromosome 19 (19p13.2). The condition is caused by a deficiency of the enzyme glutaryl-CoA dehydrogenase. Accumulation of 5-carbon dicarboxylic acids may secondarily impair synthesis of γ-aminobutyric acid **(GABA),** which functions as a neurotransmitter in the brain, inhibiting nerve excitation.

Many of the adverse effects of the organic acidemias are due to carnitine depletion.

**Epidemiology** Males and females are affected equally. There are fewer than 100 cases of this type of organic aciduria known in the United States.

**Related Disorders** See *Glutaricaciduria II.*

**Treatment—Standard** See as in *Glutaricaciduria II.*

Peritoneal dialysis or hemodialysis may be necessary. The usefulness of dietary restriction of lysine (which is oxidized via glutaric acid) has not been established. Acute episodes of metabolic acidosis and dehydration are treated with intravenous fluids and bicarbonate.

Patients with suspected secondary carnitine deficiency should have plasma carnitine measured. If a deficiency is present, supplementation with 100 to 300 mg/kg/day of oral L-carnitine is recommended.

Genetic counseling is mandatory for families of children with glutaricaciduria.

**Treatment—Investigational** An experimental regimen for the treatment of glutaricaciduria involves a low-protein or low-lysine diet and the administration of riboflavin and baclofen, a GABA analog. Diet and riboflavin have had inconsistent effects on the clinical symptoms. Urinary excretion of glutaric acid markedly decreased with this treatment. Some neurologic symptoms improved during treatment with baclofen. Long-term effects of this therapy are unknown.

Please contact the agencies listed under Resources, below, for the most current information. Addresses and telephone numbers of these agencies, as well as of individual experts and research centers, may be found in the Master Resources List.

**Resources**

**For more information on glutaricaciduria I:** National Organization for Rare Disorders (NORD); Lactic Acidosis Support Group; Lactic Acidosis Support Trust; The Arc (a national organization on mental retardation); Organic Acidemia Association; British Organic Acidemia Association; Research Trust for Metabolic Disorders in Children; Stephen Goodman, M.D., University of Colorado Health Science Center, Denver.

**For genetic information and genetic counseling referrals:** March of Dimes Birth Defects Foundation; Alliance of Genetic Support Groups.

**References**

The Metabolic and Molecular Basis of Inherited Diseases, 7th ed.: C.R. Scriver, et al., eds.; McGraw-Hill, 1995, pp. 1451–1460.

Human Genetics Disorders: J. NIH Res., August 1994, vol. 6(8), pp. 115–134.

Treatment of Glutaryl-CoA Dehydrogenase Deficiency (Glutaric Aciduria): Experience with Diet, Riboflavin, and GABA Analog: N.J. Brandt, et al.; J. Pediatr., April 1979, vol. 94(4), pp. 669–673.

# GLUTARICACIDURIA II (GA II)

**Description** GA II, one of the organic acidemias, manifests itself in 3 forms. The more serious neonatal form, with or without congenital anomalies, is characterized by large amounts of glutaric and other acids in the blood and urine. Severe disease may cause newborn death within a few weeks. The milder later-onset form is associated with metabolic acidosis, and hypoglycemia without ketosis.

**Synonyms**

> Electron Transfer Flavoprotein (ETF) Deficiency
> Multiple Acyl-CoA Dehydrogenation Deficiency

**Signs and Symptoms** The neonatal form of GA II, the more severe condition, may or may not be associated with congenital anomalies.

In newborns with congenital anomalies, the onset of severe hypoglycemia, metabolic acidosis, hypotonia, hepatomegaly, and, often, the odor of sweaty feet is within the first days of life. Congenital anomalies include hypoplastic midface, hypertelorism, low-set ears, abdominal wall defects, and hypospadias. The organic acids glutaric, lactic, butyric, isobutyric, 2-methylbutyric, ethylmalonic, adipic, and isovaleric are produced during oxidation of amino acids and accumulate in the plasma in very high amounts. These infants may not survive their first week.

Initial symptoms and signs and disease course seen in newborns without congenital anomalies are similar to those described above. In some instances, manifestations are milder, and infants survive for a longer period.

In the later-onset form, initial manifestations may first occur anywhere between a few weeks or years of life to adulthood. One patient with this form presented with vomiting, hypoglycemia, and acidosis at 7 weeks of age. Others are symptom-free until adulthood, when vomiting, severe hypoglycemia, and fatty infiltration of the liver are seen. One sibling of a woman with GA II had only nausea and a stale odor to her breath, but then developed hypoglycemic coma. Another sibling of this patient had jaundice, hepatomegaly, and hypoglycemia. Excessive amounts of glutaric and ethylmalonic acids were excreted in the urine of the latter 3 related patients.

GA II can be diagnosed by the findings of excessive glutaric, ethylmalonic, 2-hydroxyglutaric, and lactic acids in the urine, or by analysis of the deficient enzyme in leukocytes. Fetal detection is possible by testing for acyl-CoA dehydrogenase; otherwise, it is imperative that testing be done as soon after birth as possible.

**Etiology** Each form of GA II is inherited as an autosomal recessive trait, and each is caused by deficiency of an element (electron transfer flavoprotein [**ETF**], or electron transfer flavoprotein ubiquinone oxidoreductase [**ETF-QO**]) common to all 3 acyl-CoA dehydrogenase enzymes.

Many of the adverse effects of organic acidemias are due to secondary carnitine depletion.

**Related Disorders** See *Glutaricaciduria I; Medium-Chain Acyl-CoA Dehydrogenase Deficiency.*

**Treatment—Standard** GA II is usually fatal for newborns having immediate signs of severe disease, even when there are no congenital anomalies. The usefulness of restricting the amino acids lysine, hydroxylysine, and tryptophan (which generate glutaric acid) has not been established. Acute metabolic acidosis and dehydration are treated with fluids and bicarbonate.

For patients with milder disease, dietary restriction of protein and fat together with administration of riboflavin and carnitine has had some success.

Patients with secondary carnitine depletion should have plasma carnitine measured. If it is deficient, a supplement of 100 to 300 mg/kg/day of oral L-carnitine should be started.

Genetic counseling is recommended for families of patients with glutaricaciduria II.

**Treatment—Investigational** Please contact the agencies listed under Resources, below, for the most current information. Addresses and telephone numbers of these agencies, as well as of individual experts and research centers, may be found in the Master Resources List.

**Resources**

**For more information on glutaricaciduria II:** National Organization for Rare Disorders (NORD); Lactic Acidosis Support Group; Lactic Acidosis Support Trust; National Urea Cycle Disorders Foundation; Organic Acidemia Association; British Organic Acidemia Association; Research Trust for Metabolic Disorders in Children; Stephen Goodman, M.D., University of Colorado Health Science Center, Denver.

**For genetic information and genetic counseling referrals:** March of Dimes Birth Defects Foundation; Alliance of Genetic Support Groups.

**References**

The Metabolic and Molecular Basis of Inherited Disease, 7th ed.: C.R. Scriver, et al., eds.; McGraw-Hill, 1995, pp. 1501–1502.

Symptomatic Inborn Errors of Metabolism in the Neonate: S.W. Brusilow and D.L. Vallee; *in* Current Therapy in Neonatal-Perinatal Medicine: Marcel Decker, 1985, pp. 24–27.

# Glycogen Storage Disease III (GSD III)

**Description** GSD III, a glycogen storage disease, is caused by a lack of the enzyme amylo-1,6-glucosidase. Excessive amounts of glycogen are accumulated in the liver and muscles, and cardiac involvement is seen in some cases.

**Synonyms**
      Amylo-1,6-Glucosidase Deficiency
      Cori Disease
      Forbes Disease
      Glycogenosis Type III
      Limit Dextrinosis

**Signs and Symptoms** During the first 4 to 6 years of life, manifestations of GSD III may be indistinguishable from those of von Gierke disease, although the latter tends to be more severe. The amount of glycogen in the liver and muscles is abnormally high. The liver is enlarged and the abdomen protrudes. The muscles are often flaccid.

Other findings include hypoglycemia that does not respond to glucagon administration, and hyperlipemia.

Some patients show only the protruding abdomen and enlarged liver. In these patients, the liver decreases in size progressively through adolescence, and the symptoms disappear. Growth is slow during childhood, and puberty may be delayed, but adult height is usually normal.

Diagnosis is made by detection of elevated glycogen on liver biopsy. White blood cells or fibroblasts can be used to assay for amylo-1,6-glucosidase deficiency.

**Etiology** GSD III is inherited as an autosomal recessive trait. Without activity of amylo-1,6-glucosidase, stored glycogen is only partially metabolized, and the resulting limit dextrin accumulates in liver and muscle tissues, producing the impaired glycemic response.

**Epidemiology** All glycogen storage diseases together affect fewer than 1:40,000 persons in the United States. GSD III usually begins during childhood, and males are found to be affected more often than females.

**Related Disorders** See *von Gierke Disease; Andersen Disease; Hers Disease.*

**Treatment—Standard** Treatment is aimed at prevention of hypoglycemia, with frequent small servings of carbohydrates and a high protein diet advised during the day. Continuous nighttime tube feeding of hydrolyzed protein, amino acid, or carbohydrate solutions may be needed to promote normal childhood growth.

Genetic counseling is required for families of children with GSD III and other glycogen storage diseases. Affected individuals can expect to live a normal life span, but muscle and skeletal disorders may develop with age.

**Treatment—Investigational** Please contact the agencies listed under Resources, below, for the most current information. Addresses and telephone numbers of these agencies, as well as of individual experts and research centers, may be found in the Master Resources List.

**Resources**

**For more information on glycogen storage disease III:** National Organization for Rare Disorders (NORD); NIH/National Digestive Diseases Information Clearinghouse; Association for Glycogen Storage Diseases; Research Trust for Metabolic Diseases in Children.

**For genetic information and genetic counseling referrals:** March of Dimes Birth Defects Foundation; Alliance of Genetic Support Groups.

**References**

The Metabolic and Molecular Basis of Inherited Disease, 7th ed.: C.R. Scriver, et al., eds.; McGraw-Hill, 1995, pp. 949–951.

Neuromuscular Involvement in Glycogen Storage Disease Type III: S.W. Moses, et al.; Acta Paediatr. Scand., March 1986, vol. 75(2), pp. 289–296.

Myopathy and Growth Failure in Debrancher Enzyme Deficiency: Improvement with High-Protein Nocturnal Enteral Therapy: A.E. Slonim, et al.; J. Pediatr., December 1984, vol. 105(6), pp. 906–911.

# Glycogen Storage Disease VII (GSD VII)

**Description** GSD VII is characterized by a deficiency of the enzyme phosphofructokinase-I in muscle and a partial deficiency of the enzyme in red blood cells. This deficiency prevents the metabolism of glucose into available energy during exercise.

**Synonyms**
      Glycogen Disease of Muscle
      Glycogenosis Type VII
      Muscle Phosphofructokinase Deficiency
      Phosphofructokinase Deficiency
      Tarui Disease

**Signs and Symptoms** Patients experience easy fatigability, and, on strenuous exercise, muscular pain and cramps and myoglobinuria, which is usually not severe. Hyperuricemia accompanies exercise, and other manifestations include gout and recurrent jaundice.

**Etiology** GSD VII is inherited as an autosomal recessive trait.

**Epidemiology** Onset is in childhood, and males and females are affected in equal numbers.

**Related Disorders** See *McArdle Disease; Pompe Disease; Glycogen Storage Disease III.*

**Treatment—Standard** Treatment of GSD VII is symptomatic and supportive. Avoidance of strenuous exercise prevents muscle pain and cramps.

**Treatment—Investigational** Please contact the agencies listed under Resources, below, for the most current information. Addresses and telephone numbers of these agencies, as well as of individual experts and research centers, may be found in the Master Resources List.

**Resources**

For more information on GSD VII: National Organization for Rare Disorders (NORD); Association for Glycogen Storage Diseases; NIH/National Digestive Diseases Information Clearinghouse; Research Trust for Metabolic Diseases in Children.

For genetic information and genetic counseling referrals: March of Dimes Birth Defects Foundation; Alliance of Genetic Support Groups.

**References**

The Metabolic and Molecular Basis of Inherited Disease, 7th ed.: C.R. Scriver, et al., eds.; McGraw-Hill, 1995, pp. 954–955.

Excess Purine Degradation in Exercising Muscles of Patients with Muscle Glycogen Storage Disease Types V and VII: I. Mineo, et al.; J. Clin. Invest., August 1985, vol. 76(2), pp. 556–560.

# HARTNUP DISEASE

**Description** Hartnup disease is a rare metabolic disorder that involves an error of neutral amino acid transport. Intermittent episodes of skin rash and ataxia are the primary clinical features.

**Synonyms**

Pellagra–Cerebellar Ataxia–Renal Aminoaciduria Syndrome

**Signs and Symptoms** The disease is characterized by a red, scaly rash that typically occurs after exposure to sunlight. Sudden attacks of ataxia, double vision, and fainting may occur. If the disorder is left untreated, retarded mental development, short stature, emotional instability, and dementia may develop. Mild arrhythmias may also occur in untreated cases but are extremely rare.

**Etiology** Hartnup disease is an inborn error of renal and intestinal amino acid transport involving tryptophan and the other neutral amino acids. The condition is inherited as an autosomal recessive trait. Genetic evaluation of children born to mothers affected by Hartnup disease suggests that the abnormal metabolism of amino acids in this disorder does not have an adverse effect on the fetus.

**Epidemiology** Hartnup disease usually begins in childhood and continues into adulthood; males and females seem to be affected equally. The condition occurs in approximately 1:24,000 newborns.

**Related Disorders Pellagra** results from a deficiency of nicotinic acid. Generalized manifestations of pellagra include anorexia, diarrhea, constipation, weakness, and emotional instability. Cutaneous manifestations of the disorder include burning or stinging after exposure to the sun, scaliness or roughness, and reddish-brown coloration. There also may be soreness of the oral cavity. Pellagra tends to occur in countries where corn is the staple food, and is very rare in the United States.

**Treatment—Standard** Symptomatic episodes of Hartnup disease can be minimized with good nutrition and 50 to 300 mg/day of nicotinamide. Avoidance of the sun and sulfonamide drugs is also indicated. Treatment of episodes is symptomatic and supportive. Genetic counseling may be appropriate for affected families.

**Treatment—Investigational** Please contact the agencies listed under Resources, below, for the most current information. Addresses and telephone numbers of these agencies, as well as of individual experts and research centers, may be found in the Master Resources List.

**Resources**

For more information on Hartnup disease: National Organization for Rare Disorders (NORD); The Arc (a national organization on mental retardation); NIH/National Digestive Diseases Information Clearinghouse; Research Trust for Metabolic Diseases in Children.

For genetic information and genetic counseling referrals: March of Dimes Birth Defects Foundation; Alliance of Genetic Support Groups.

**References**

The Metabolic and Molecular Basis of Inherited Disease, 7th ed.: C.R. Scriver, et al., eds.; 1995, pp. 3629–3642.

Maternal Hartnup Disorder: B.E. Mahon, et al.; Am. J. Med. Genet., July 1986, vol. 24(3), pp. 513–518.
Occurrences of Methylmalonic Aciduria and Hartnup Disorder in the Same Family: V.E. Shih, et al.; Clin. Genet., September 1984, vol. 26(3), pp. 216–220.

# HERS DISEASE

**Description** Hers disease is a hereditary glycogen storage disease manifested by milder symptoms than most other glycogen storage diseases. Characteristics include hepatomegaly and ketosis, and moderate hypoglycemia and growth retardation. Symptoms and signs may not be apparent during childhood, and affected individuals can often lead normal lives. In some cases, however, symptoms are more severe.

**Synonyms**

>Glycogen Storage Disease VI
>Glycogenosis Type VI
>Hepatophosphorylase Deficiency Glycogenosis
>Liver Phosphorylase Deficiency
>Phosphorylase *b* Kinase Deficiency

**Signs and Symptoms** The mild-to-moderate hypoglycemia of Hers disease can cause faintness, weakness, hunger, and nervousness. Other findings may include hepatomegaly caused by accumulation of glycogen in the liver, and slowing of the growth rate. In many instances, affected individuals can adapt to the hypoglycemia and remain asymptomatic for long periods.

The specific diagnosis can be established by liver biopsy and assay for phosphorylase activity.

**Etiology** Hers disease is heterogeneous, and the enzyme subunits are coded on both autosomes and the X chromosome. Symptoms result from deficiency of phosphorylase *b* kinase, which leads to hepatic accumulation of glycogen, and hypoglycemia.

**Epidemiology** All glycogen storage diseases together affect fewer than 1:40,000 persons in the United States. Manifestations of Hers disease may not be noticed until adulthood.

**Related Disorders** See *von Gierke Disease; Glycogen Storage Disease III; Andersen Disease.*

**Treatment—Standard** Symptoms of Hers disease are generally mild, and the patient usually requires no specific treatment. Avoidance of prolonged fasting, and regular monitoring by a physician are recommended. Genetic counseling is mandatory.

**Treatment—Investigational** Please contact the agencies listed under Resources, below, for the most current information. Addresses and telephone numbers of these agencies, as well as of individual experts and research centers, may be found in the Master Resources List.

**Resources**

For more information on Hers disease: National Organization for Rare Disorders (NORD); Association for Glycogen Storage Diseases; Research Trust for Metabolic Diseases in Children; NIH/National Digestive Diseases Information Clearinghouse.

For genetic information and genetic counseling referrals: March of Dimes Birth Defects Foundation; Alliance of Genetic Support Groups.

**References**

The Metabolic and Molecular Basis of Inherited Disease, 7th ed.: C.R. Scriver, et al., eds.; McGraw-Hill, 1995, pp. 953–954.
Cecil Textbook of Medicine, 18th ed.: J.B. Wyngaarden and L.H. Smith, Jr., eds.: W.B. Saunders Company, 1988, p. 425.

# HISTIDINEMIA

**Description** Deficiency of the enzyme histidase, required for oxidation of the amino acid histidine, results in elevated concentrations of histidine in the blood, and excessive amounts of histidine, imidazole pyruvic acid, and other imidazole metabolism products excreted in the urine. Mental retardation and a speech defect have been thought to be associated with some cases of histidinemia, although this is now believed to be an artifact of ascertainment.

**Synonyms**

>Histidase Deficiency

**Signs and Symptoms** Early cases of histidinemia were identified by such features as mental retardation, speech defects, seizures, unusual behavior, and learning disabilities. It is now known, however, that histidinemia occurs in clinically normal persons.

**Etiology** The disorder is inherited as an autosomal recessive trait.

**Epidemiology** Histidinemia occurs in about 1:20,000 births, with males and females affected equally.

**Related Disorders Histidinuria,** characterized by abnormally high amounts of histidine in the urine, is due to a defect of histidine reabsorption in the renal distal tubules. The disorder is inherited as an autosomal recessive trait, and is very rare.

**Treatment—Standard** Benign cases of histidinemia require no treatment. Speech therapy can be helpful, if appropriate, and genetic counseling is beneficial.

**Treatment—Investigational** Please contact the agencies listed under Resources, below, for the most current information. Addresses and telephone numbers of these agencies, as well as of individual experts and research centers, may be found in the Master Resources List.

**Resources**

**For more information on histidinemia:** National Organization for Rare Disorders (NORD); NIH/National Digestive Diseases Information Clearinghouse; The Arc (a national organization on mental retardation); Research Trust for Metabolic Diseases in Children.

**For genetic information and genetic counseling referrals:** March of Dimes Birth Defects Foundation; Alliance of Genetic Support Groups.

**References**

The Metabolic and Molecular Basis of Inherited Disease, 7th ed.; C.R. Scriver, et al., eds.; McGraw-Hill, 1995, pp. 1107–1123.

# HOMOCYSTINURIA

**Description** Homocystinuria is a metabolic disorder characterized by abnormal amounts of homocystine and methionine in blood, cerebrospinal fluid, and urine.

**Synonyms**

Homocystinemia

Cystathionine β-Synthase Deficiency

**Signs and Symptoms** Manifestations of homocystinuria include ectopia lentis, zonal cataracts, osteoporosis, seizures, mental retardation, pulmonary embolism, and coronary occlusion. Patients may have the signs and symptoms of Marfan syndrome (e.g., elongated body and extremities, pectus excavatum, and cardiovascular defects— see *Marfan Syndrome*).

**Etiology** Homocystinuria is inherited as an autosomal recessive trait. Symptoms are caused by an inborn error of amino acid metabolism resulting from deficiency of the enzyme cystathionine β-synthase.

**Epidemiology** Onset is at birth. Males and females are affected in equal numbers. Like other inborn errors of metabolism, homocystinuria is a very rare disorder, affecting 1:200,000 live births.

**Related Disorders** See *Marfan Syndrome.*

**Treatment—Standard** Treatment for homocystinuria consists of a methionine-restricted diet supplemented with cystine. Pharmacologic doses of pyridoxine may also be beneficial. Genetic counseling will be helpful for families of affected children.

**Treatment—Investigational** Betaine treatment for homocystinuria is being investigated.

Please contact the agencies listed under Resources, below, for the most current information. Addresses and telephone numbers of these agencies, as well as of individual experts and research centers, may be found in the Master Resources List.

**Resources**

**For more information on homocystinuria:** National Organization for Rare Disorders (NORD); NIH/National Digestive Diseases Information Clearinghouse; The Arc (a national organization on mental retardation).

**For genetic information and genetic counseling referrals:** March of Dimes Birth Defects Foundation; Alliance of Genetic Support Groups.

**References**

The Metabolic and Molecular Basis of Inherited Disease, 7th ed.: C.R. Scriver, et al., eds.; McGraw-Hill, 1995, pp. 1279–1327.

# HUNTER SYNDROME

**Description** Hunter syndrome (mucopolysaccharidosis type II—**MPS II**) occurs in 2 forms, mild and severe, both with the same enzymatic deficiency of iduronate sulfatase.

**Synonyms**

Mucopolysaccharidosis Type II

**Signs and Symptoms** Onset of symptoms in patients with the severe form usually is from ages 2 to 4 years, with progressive mental and physical deterioration thereafter. Facial features become coarsened, and a short neck, widely spaced teeth, and hearing loss are also often present. Whitish nodular skin lesions may occur on the arms or back. Hydrocephalus is commonly seen after 4 years of age. Recurrent upper respiratory infections, diarrhea, hepatomegaly, joint stiffness, growth failure, and mental retardation are typical features of the severe form of Hunter syndrome. The syndrome is often fatal between 7 and 10 years of age, usually from neurologic and cardiopulmonary disease.

In the mild form of Hunter syndrome, mental function is usually normal and physical deterioration is greatly reduced. Complications include coronary and valvular disease and hearing impairment. Carpal tunnel syndrome and joint stiffness can result in loss of hand function. Some patients succumb to cardiopulmonary disease as young adults, while others survive into their 70s.

Hunter syndrome can be diagnosed prenatally.

**Etiology** The syndrome is inherited as an X-linked recessive trait. Deficiency of the enzyme iduronate sulfatase results in an inability to metabolize mucopolysaccharides. The accumulation of large, undegraded mucopolysaccharides in the cells of the body causes the physical and mental deterioration.

**Epidemiology** Only males are affected. The disorder occurs in 1:100,000 live births.

**Related Disorders** See *Hydrocephalus.*

The severe form of Hunter syndrome has features similar to those of Hurler syndrome except for the lack of corneal clouding and slower progression of physical involvement and mental retardation. See *Hurler Syndrome.*

The mucolipidoses are a family of similar disorders, producing symptoms very much like those of the mucopolysaccharidoses. See *Mucopolysaccharidosis; Mucolipidosis II; Mucolipidosis III; Mucolipidosis IV.*

**Treatment—Standard** Treatment of Hunter syndrome is symptomatic and supportive. Hernias may require surgical intervention. Implantation of a ventricular shunt may be needed for hydrocephalus. Hearing devices, physical therapy, and genetic counseling services may be helpful for patients and their families.

**Treatment—Investigational** Treatments aimed at checking early development of Hunter syndrome are now being studied. Approaches include enzyme replacement therapy, bone marrow transplantation, and gene therapy.

Please contact the agencies listed under Resources, below, for the most current information. Addresses and telephone numbers of these agencies, as well as of individual experts and research centers, may be found in the Master Resources List.

**Resources**

**For more information on Hunter syndrome:** National Organization for Rare Disorders (NORD); Joseph Muenzer, M.D., Ph.D., University of North Carolina; National Mucopolysaccharidoses Society; Society of Mucopolysaccharide Diseases; Society of MPS Diseases; The Arc (a national organization on mental retardation); NIH/National Digestive Diseases Information Clearinghouse.

**For genetic information and genetic counseling referrals:** March of Dimes Birth Defects Foundation; Alliance of Genetic Support Groups.

**References**

The Metabolic and Molecular Basis of Inherited Disease, 7th ed.: C.R. Scriver, et al., eds.; McGraw-Hill, 1995, pp. 2472–2474.

# HURLER SYNDROME

**Description** Hurler syndrome (mucopolysaccharidosis type I—**MPS I**) appears in 3 forms of varying severity. Hurler syndrome (**MPS I-H**) is the most severe; Scheie syndrome (**MPS I-S**) is milder; and Hurler/Scheie syndrome (**MPS I-H/S),** is considered to be the intermediate form.

**Synonyms**

Mucopolysaccharidosis Type I

**Signs and Symptoms** Newborns with Hurler syndrome (**MPS I-H**) usually appear normal, although inguinal and umbilical hernias may be present. Onset of symptoms is from 6 months to 2 years of age. Craniofacial abnormalities occurring at this time include coarse facial features, a prominent forehead, macroglossia, misaligned teeth, and clouding of the cornea. Also evident are recurrent upper respiratory infections, noisy breathing, and a persistent nasal discharge. Hydrocephalus appears after 2 to 3 years of age. Developmental delay becomes apparent from 1 to 2 years of age. The child is short of stature, and mental retardation is progressive thereafter. Joint stiffness is severe, resulting in claw hand, and kyphoscoliosis and hepatomegaly may develop.

Hurler/Scheie syndrome (**MPS I-H/S),** the intermediate form, is characterized by normal intelligence but progressive physical involvement that is milder than in Hurler syndrome. Corneal clouding, joint stiffness, deafness, and valvular heart disease can develop by the early to mid teens.

In Scheie syndrome (**MPS I-S),** the mild form, stature, intelligence, and life expectancy are normal. Onset of symptoms such as stiff joints, clouding of the cornea, and aortic valvular disease and/or stenosis usually occurs after 5 years of age, but diagnosis often is not made until the patient is 10 to 20 years of age.

Diagnosis can be made prenatally.

**Etiology** The 3 forms of Hurler syndrome described above are autosomal recessive, and all are due to α-L-iduronidase deficiency.

**Epidemiology** Males and females tend to be affected equally. Incidence is approximately 1:100,000 live births.

**Related Disorders** See *Hydrocephalus; Mucopolysaccharidosis.*

The mucolipidoses are a family of similar disorders, producing symptoms very much like those of MPS. Mucolipidosis II resembles Hurler syndrome; the 2 disorders are very difficult to distinguish (see *Mucolipidosis II).*

**Treatment—Standard** Treatment is symptomatic and supportive. Physical therapy and medical and genetic counseling services may be useful to patient and family.

**Treatment—Investigational** Treatment approaches for checking early development of MPS are under study. These include enzyme replacement therapy, bone marrow transplantation, and gene therapy.

Please contact the agencies listed under Resources, below, for the most current information. Addresses and telephone numbers of these agencies, as well as of individual experts and research centers, may be found in the Master Resources List.

**Resources**

**For more information on Hurler syndrome:** National Organization for Rare Disorders (NORD); National Mucopolysaccharidoses Society; The Arc (a national organization on mental retardation); NIH/National Digestive Diseases Information Clearinghouse; Society of Mucopolysaccharide Diseases; Society of MPS Diseases.

**For genetic information and genetic counseling referrals:** March of Dimes Birth Defects Foundation; Alliance of Genetic Support Groups.

**References**

The Metabolic and Molecular Basis of Inherited Disease, 7th ed.: C.R. Scriver, et al., eds.; McGraw-Hill, 1995, pp. 2471–2472.

# HYPERCHYLOMICRONEMIA

**Description** Hyperchylomicronemia is a rare hereditary inborn error of metabolism caused by the absence of the enzyme lipoprotein lipase. The disorder is characterized by a massive accumulation of chylomicrons in blood plasma following consumption of dietary fats, and a corresponding increase of the blood plasma concentration of triglycerides (greater than 2,000 mg/dl). The concentration of very low density lipoprotein (**VLDL**) is normal, distinguishing type I from type V chylomicronemia.

**Synonyms**

Familial Lipoprotein Lipase Deficiency

Mixed Hyperlipemia

Type V Hyperlipidemia

**Signs and Symptoms** The disorder initially is characterized by eruptive xanthomas, which are raised whitish-yellow nodules containing a milky fluid, on a red base. These lesions may vary from 0.1 to 0.3 inches in diameter, but may cluster and form large plaques. The number of nodules can range from few to hundreds. They are generally located on the buttocks, shoulders, and extremities, although sometimes they are also found on the face and mucous membranes. These eruptive xanthomas are neither painful nor itchy, and the patient may mistake them for acne. The nodules typically appear with an increased level of triglycerides in the blood, and disappear when the triglyceride level decreases.

Some patients also experience gastrointestinal symptoms, including anorexia, nausea, abdominal distension, diarrhea, and abdominal pain. Pancreatitis, sometimes with bleeding, often occurs when triglyceride levels are excessively high. Hepatomegaly and splenomegaly may occur, particularly in infants and children. Macrophages that have incorporated chylomicrons are sometimes seen in the spleen and bone marrow of these patients.

Ocular findings include a milky or "tomato juice" appearance in the retinal blood vessels; and the fundus may appear pale pink upon ophthalmologic examination. The retina may contain white fatty deposits, and circulation may be disturbed, with narrowing of the blood vessels and bleeding. Vision can be adversely affected.

**Etiology** The disorder is transmitted as an autosomal recessive trait. The specific metabolic error is a deficiency of the enzyme lipoprotein lipase.

**Epidemiology** Hyperchylomicronemia is present at birth and affects males and females in equal numbers. It is estimated to affect 20,000 adults in the United States.

**Related Disorders Familial apolipoprotein C-II deficiency** is a rare autosomal recessive hereditary disorder characterized by a deficiency of apolipoprotein C-II, which is needed for the enzyme lipoprotein lipase to function. An accumulation of chylomicrons and elevated VLDL occurs in blood plasma. Attacks of pancreatitis may recur.

**Treatment—Standard** Restriction of dietary fat is the most effective management approach. However, adequate intake of essential fatty acids must be maintained, and an increase in carbohydrates will be required. If the patient can tolerate medium-chain-triglyceride supplements, dietary management may be simplified.

Use of alcohol should be discouraged, and drugs such as estrogens that affect triglyceride synthesis should be avoided. During pregnancy, strict dietary control and monitoring will be required, and genetic counseling is recommended for afflicted families.

**Treatment—Investigational** Please contact the agencies listed under Resources, below, for the most current information. Addresses and telephone numbers of these agencies, as well as of individual experts and research centers, may be found in the Master Resources List.

**Resources**

**For more information on hyperchylomicronemia:** National Organization for Rare Disorders (NORD); NIH/National Digestive Diseases Information Clearinghouse; Research Trust for Metabolic Diseases in Children.

**For genetic information and genetic counseling referrals:** March of Dimes Birth Defects Foundation; Alliance of Genetic Support Groups.

**References**

The Metabolic and Molecular Basis of Inherited Disease, 7th ed.: C.R. Scriver, et al., eds.; McGraw-Hill, 1995, pp. 1913–1980.

Mendelian Inheritance in Man, 9th ed.: V.A. McKusick; The Johns Hopkins University Press, 1990, pp. 1256–1257.

# HYPEROXALURIA, PRIMARY (PH)

**Description** PH is an inherited disorder characterized by excessive urinary excretion of oxalic acid, which forms oxalate crystals and urine stones. Two forms are presently recognized, PH type I and PH type II.

**Synonyms**

Oxalosis

Oxaluria

**Signs and Symptoms** The 2 forms of PH are distinguished by excessive urinary glycolic excretion (**PH type I**) or glyceric acid (**PH type II**).

In **PH type I,** clinical manifestations usually first appear in childhood, but the onset of symptoms can occur during infancy or occasionally in adulthood. Calcium oxalate crystals and stones can cause renal colic, urinary tract obstruction, and hematuria. The small crystals collect in the kidneys, causing nephrocalcinosis and leading to progressive kidney damage and eventual renal failure. Some patients present in end-stage renal disease with oliguria or anuria. Calcium oxalate deposition (oxalosis) can occur in the eyes, bones, joints, heart, and other organs.

In **PH type II,** the symptoms are limited to those resulting from urolithiasis.

Prenatal diagnosis has been obtained by fetal liver biopsy during the 17th week of pregnancy.

**Etiology PH type I,** the more common form of the disorder, is inherited as an autosomal recessive trait. PH type I is due to a deficiency of peroxisomal alanine: glyoxalate aminotransferase.

**PH type II,** also autosomal recessive, is due to a deficiency of D-glycerate dehydrogenase.

**Epidemiology** Males and females are affected in equal numbers.

**Treatment—Standard** The principal treatment for PH type I and PH type II consists of high fluid intake, large daily doses of pyridoxine (vitamin B6), and supplements of phosphate and magnesium.

In patients who still have kidney function, a greatly increased fluid intake helps keep the kidneys flushed out and limits crystal formation. In patients who have lost kidney function, aggressive dialysis is an appropriate treatment until kidney transplantation can be performed. This should be done as soon as possible, since dialysis does not adequately remove oxalate. Previously, kidney transplants were considered inappropriate for patients with PH, but transplantation with therapy to help prevent recurrence is now a successful method of treatment.

Genetic counseling is helpful to families. However, the severity of the disease may be impossible to predict because it varies widely, even in the same family.

**Treatment—Investigational** For PH type I, liver transplantation provides the normal enzyme and corrects the metabolic defect. Combined liver and kidney transplantation has been performed on more than 25 patients with type PH type I. Liver transplantation alone has been performed on one patient with adequate residual kidney function.

Please contact the agencies listed under Resources, below, for the most current information. Addresses and telephone numbers of these agencies, as well as of individual experts and research centers, may be found in the Master Resources List.

**Resources**

**For more information on primary hyperoxaluria:** National Organization for Rare Disorders (NORD); Oxalosis and Hyperoxaluria Foundation; NIH/National Digestive Diseases Information Clearinghouse; Research Trust for Metabolic Diseases in Children.

**For genetic information and genetic counseling referrals:** March of Dimes Birth Defects Foundation; Alliance of Genetic Support Groups.

### References

The Metabolic and Molecular Basis of Inherited Disease, 7th ed.: C.R. Scriver, et al., eds.; McGraw-Hill, 1995, pp. 2385–2424.

Understanding Oxalosis and Hyperoxaluria: Treatment of Renal Failure in the Primary Hyperoxalurias: R.W.E. Watts; Nephron, 1990, vol. 56, pp. 1–5.

Oxalate Metabolism in Relation to Urinary Stone: G.A. Rose, ed.; Springer-Verlag, 1988.

# HYPERPROLINEMIA TYPE I

**Description** Hyperprolinemia type I is a very rare hereditary disorder characterized by an excessive elevation of proline in the blood and urine. The high level of this amino acid is caused by a deficiency in the metabolic activity of the enzyme proline oxidase.

**Synonyms**

Proline Dehydrogenase Deficiency

Proline Oxidase Deficiency

**Signs and Symptoms** Diagnosis is established by measurement of plasma proline. The proline concentration in the plasma is between 500 and 2,000 μM. Other findings associated with hyperprolinemia type I include abnormally high urinary levels of hydroxyproline and glycine. Renal disturbances have also been reported in association with this condition, but are not thought to be causally related.

**Etiology** Hyperprolinemia type I is transmitted as an autosomal recessive trait.

**Epidemiology** The disorder is present at birth. Males and females are affected in equal numbers.

**Related Disorders** See *Hyperprolinemia Type II.*

**Treatment—Standard** No therapy is indicated.

**Resources**

**For more information on hyperprolinemia type I:** National Organization for Rare Disorders (NORD); NIH/National Digestive Diseases Information Clearinghouse; Research Trust for Metabolic Diseases in Children.

**For genetic information and genetic counseling referrals:** March of Dimes Birth Defects Foundation; Alliance of Genetic Support Groups.

### References

Mendelian Inheritance in Man, 9th ed.: V.A. McKusick; The Johns Hopkins University Press, 1990, pp. 1261–1262.

The Metabolic Basis of Inherited Disease, 6th ed.: C.R. Scriver, et al., eds.; McGraw-Hill, 1989, pp. 587–588.

# HYPERPROLINEMIA TYPE II

**Description** Hyperprolinemia type II is a very rare hereditary disorder characterized by excessive plasma and urinary proline. The high level of this amino acid results from a deficiency of the enzyme Δ1 pyrroline-5-carboxylic acid dehydrogenase.

**Synonyms**

Pyrroline Carboxylate Dehydrogenase Deficiency

**Signs and Symptoms** The abnormally high plasma level of proline (greater than 2,000 μM) is the primary feature of the disorder. In some cases, mental retardation and seizures have been reported and are now thought to be causally related. It is distinguished from hyperprolinemia type I by the elevation in plasma Δ1 pyrroline-5-carboxylate, which is found only in hyperprolinemia type II.

**Etiology** Hyperprolinemia type II is transmitted as an autosomal recessive trait.

**Epidemiology** The disorder is present at birth. Males and females are affected in equal numbers.

**Related Disorders** See *Hyperprolinemia Type I.*

**Treatment—Standard** No therapy is indicated.

**Resources**

**For more information on hyperprolinemia type II:** National Organization for Rare Disorders (NORD); The Arc (a national organization on mental retardation); NIH/National Digestive Diseases Information Clearinghouse; Research Trust for Metabolic Diseases in Children.

**For genetic information and genetic counseling referrals:** March of Dimes Birth Defects Foundation; Alliance of Genetic Support Groups.

### References

The Metabolic and Molecular Basis of Inherited Disease, 7th ed.: C.R. Scriver, et al., eds.; McGraw-Hill, 1995, pp. 1125–1146.

Mendelian Inheritance in Man, 9th ed.: V.A. McKusick; The Johns Hopkins University Press, 1990, p. 1262.

# KEARNS-SAYRE SYNDROME

**Description** Kearns-Sayre syndrome is a rare myopathy associated with mitochondrial dysfunction, cardiomyopathy, neuropathy, and ophthalmoplegia and retinal disease.

**Synonyms**
Oculocraniosomatic Neuromuscular Disease

**Signs and Symptoms** Cardiomyopathy and cardiac dilatation accompanied by arrhythmias and heart block may occur. The eye muscles become progressively weaker, causing ophthalmoplegia and ptosis; an associated retinal degeneration may result in impaired vision. Muscle function in the arms and legs also may be diminished, and growth may be retarded. Mental retardation, cerebellar ataxia, deafness, and short stature frequently occur.

**Etiology** The cause is usually a mitochondrial deletion, but some cases are due to a point mutation in a nuclear gene.

**Epidemiology** Both sexes are affected. The onset typically is before age 20 years.

**Related Disorders** See **Retinitis Pigmentosa.**

**Treatment—Standard** Treatment of reduced muscle function is symptomatic and supportive. Associated heartbeat irregularities may be treated with various antiarrhythymic drugs or by installing a pacemaker.

**Treatment—Investigational** Coenzyme Q10, a new compound being investigated, appears to improve the production of energy by muscle mitochondria. This treatment also may improve heart, vision, and neurologic symptoms. The long-term safety and effectiveness of Coenzyme Q10 is yet to be determined.

Please contact the agencies listed under Resources, below, for the most current information. Addresses and telephone numbers of these agencies, as well as of individual experts and research centers, may be found in the Master Resources List.

**Resources**

**For more information on Kearns-Sayre syndrome:** National Organization for Rare Disorders (NORD); Mitochondrial Disorders Foundation of America; Education and Support Exchange; American Heart Association; Foundation Fighting Blindness; NIH/National Eye Institute; NIH/National Arthritis and Musculoskeletal and Skin Diseases Information Clearinghouse.

**References**

The Metabolic and Molecular Basis of Inherited Disease, 7th ed.: C.R. Scriver, et al., eds.; McGraw-Hill, 1995, pp. 1571–1583.

The Fine Structure of the Intramitochondrial Crystalloids in Mitochondrial Myopathy: T.M. Mukherjee, et al.; J. Submicrosc. Cytol., July 1986, vol. 18(3), pp. 595–604.

Heart Involvement in Progressive External Ophthalmoplegia (Kearns-Sayre Syndrome): Electrophysiologic, Hemodynamic and Morphologic Findings: B. Schwartzkopff, et al.; Z. Kardiol., March 1986, vol. 75(3), pp. 161–169.

Treatment of Kearns-Sayre Syndrome with Coenzyme Q10: S. Ogasahara, et al.; Neurology, January 1986, vol. 36(1), pp. 45–53.

# LEIGH DISEASE

**Description** Leigh disease is a genetic metabolic disorder characterized by lesions of the brain, spinal cord, and optic nerve. Serum levels of lactic acid, pyruvate, and alanine are elevated. Some cases have been associated with a defect in the enzyme pyruvate dehydrogenase phosphatase.

**Synonyms**
Ataxia with Lactic Acidosis II
Encephalomyelopathy
Leigh Necrotizing Encephalopathy
Pyruvate Dehydrogenase Phosphatase
Subacute Necrotizing Encephalopathy

**Signs and Symptoms** The diagnosis is generally made in infancy (between the ages of 3 months and 2 years). Prominent features include low body weight, growth retardation, and seizures. If onset is in early infancy, loss of head control and poor sucking ability may be the first noticeable symptoms. These may be accompanied by profound anorexia, vomiting, irritability, continuous crying, and seizures. If onset occurs later in infancy (2 years), affected children may experience dysarthria, ataxia, and loss of previously acquired intellectual skills. Episodes of lactic acidosis and hypercapnia may occur. Progressive neurologic deterioration follows, with mental retardation and death.

Symptoms of some forms of Leigh disease resemble those of Wernicke encephalopathy, a thiamine deficiency disorder. Respiratory problems (e.g., apnea, dyspnea, hyperventilation), visual problems (e.g., optic atrophy, nystagmus, strabismus), and cardiac problems (e.g., cardiomegaly, hypertrophic cardiomyopathy, asymmetric septal hypertrophy) may develop in some cases.

The adult-onset form of the disease (subacute necrotizing encephalomyelopathy) occurs very infrequently, beginning during adolescence or early adulthood. Initial symptoms are usually visual (e.g., central scotoma, color blindness, bilateral optic atrophy). Neurologic deterioration progresses slowly. By age 50, affected individuals may experience ataxia, spastic paresis, clonic jerks, grand mal seizures, and varying degrees of dementia.

Diagnosis may be confirmed through MRI and CT scans of the brain and measurement of lactic acid, pyruvate, alanine, and glucose.

**Etiology** In most case, Leigh disease is inherited as an autosomal recessive trait and has been linked to a genetic defect in 1 of 2 enzymes, pyruvate dehydrogenase or pyruvate carboxylase. Other genetically based enzyme deficiencies (e.g., NADH-CoQ and cytochrome C oxidase) have also been implicated as the cause of some cases of autosomal recessive Leigh disease. In addition to autosomal recessive inheritance, there is evidence that Leigh disease may also be inherited as the result of mitochondrial mutation. (See the introduction to this chapter for a description of mitochondrial inheritance.)

**Epidemiology** In 80 percent of known cases, the disease develops in infants and affects both sexes equally.

**Related Disorders Wernicke encephalopathy,** a degenerative brain disorder associated with a deficiency of thiamine, is marked by ataxia and apathy, confusion, disorientation, or delirium. Various vision dysfunctions may also develop. This disorder often occurs in conjunction with ***Korsakoff Syndrome,*** which involves a thiamine deficiency that is usually caused by alcoholism. Wernicke encephalopathy can be severely disabling and life-threatening if it is not recognized and treated early.

See ***Tay-Sachs Disease; Sandhoff Disease; Kufs Disease; Batten Disease; Niemann-Pick Disease; Alpers Disease; MELAS Syndrome; MERFF Syndrome.***

**Treatment—Standard** Administration of thiamine or thiamine derivatives may cause temporary symptomatic improvement and slow the progression of the disease. In those patients who also have a deficiency of pyruvate dehydrogenase enzyme complex, a high-fat, low-carbohydrate diet may be recommended. Intravenous or oral sodium bicarbonate is used to correct acidosis. Intravenous infusion of tris-hydroxymethyl aminomethane (**THAM**) may also help to control acute episodes of acidosis without resulting in sodium overload, which may be associated with the administration of sodium bicarbonate.

Genetic counseling is recommended for families. Services that benefit visually impaired people may be helpful, if needed.

**Treatment—Investigational** Please contact the agencies listed under Resources, below, for the most current information. Addresses and telephone numbers of these agencies, as well as of individual experts and research centers, may be found in the Master Resources List.

**Resources**

For more information on **Leigh disease:** National Organization for Rare Disorders (NORD); National Leigh Disease Foundation; Mitochondrial Disorders Foundation of America; Lactic Acidosis Support Group; Lactic Acidosis Support Trust; The Arc (a national organization on mental retardation); NIH/National Institute of Neurological Disorders and Stroke; Children's Brain Diseases Foundation for Research; Research Trust for Metabolic Diseases in Children.

For information relating to vision problems: NIH/National Eye Institute; American Council of the Blind; American Foundation for the Blind; American Printing House for the Blind; National Association for Parents of the Visually Impaired; Research Trust for Metabolic Diseases in Children.

For genetic information and genetic counseling referrals: March of Dimes Birth Defects Foundation; Alliance of Genetic Support Groups.

**References**

The Metabolic and Molecular Basis of Inherited Disease, 7th ed.: C.R. Scriver, et al., eds.; McGraw-Hill, 1995, pp. 1479–1498.

Mendelian Inheritance in Man, 11th ed.: V.A. McKusick; The Johns Hopkins University Press, 1994, pp. 1000, 2057, 2441, 2583–2584.

Online Mendelian Inheritance in Man (OMIM): V.A. McKusick; last edit date 8/19/94, entry number 256000; last edit date 6/7/94, entry number 308930; last edit date 7/1/87, entry number 161700.

Disorders of Movement in Leigh Syndrome: A. Macaya, et al.; Neuropediatrics, April 1993, vol. 24(2), pp. 60–67.

Infant Onset Subacute Necrotizing Encephalomyelopathy (Leigh's Disease): S.A. Morris, et al.; J. Paediatr. Child Health, October 1993, vol. 29(5), pp. 363–367.

Maternally Inherited Leigh Syndrome: E. Ciafaloni, et al.; J. Pediatr., March 1993, vol. 122(3), pp. 419–422.

Molecular Genetic Characterization of an X-Linked Form of Leigh's Syndrome: P.M. Matthews, et al.; Ann. Neurol., June 1993, vol. 33(6), pp. 652–655.

The Mutation at nt8993 of Mitochondrial DNA Is a Common Cause of Leigh's Syndrome: F.M. Santorelli, et al.; Ann. Neurol., December 1993, vol. 34(6), pp. 827–834.

Principles of Neurology, 5th ed.: R.D. Adams and M. Victor, eds.; McGraw-Hill, 1993, pp. 812–813.

Cecil Textbook of Medicine, 19th ed.: J.B. Wyngaarden, et al., eds.; W.B. Saunders Company, 1992, p. 2260.

Heteroplasmic mtDNA Mutation (T—G) at 8993 Can Cause Leigh Disease When the Percentage of Abnormal mtDNA Is High: Y. Tatch, et al.; Am. J. Hum. Genet., April 1992, vol. 50(4), pp. 852–858.

Nelson Textbook of Pediatrics, 14th ed.: R.E. Behrman, ed.-in-chief; W.B. Saunders Company, 1992, pp. 136, 364–365, 1517.

Harrison's Principles of Internal Medicine, 12th ed.: J.D. Wilson, et al., eds.; McGraw-Hill, 1991, pp. 2045–2046.

Birth Defects Encyclopedia: M.L Buyse, ed.-in-chief; Blackwell Scientific Publications, 1990, pp. 615–617.

Dictionary of Medical Syndromes, 3rd ed.: S.I. Magalini, et al., eds.; J.B. Lippincott Company, 1990, pp. 527–528.

MR Findings in Patients with Subacute Necrotizing Encephalomyelopathy (Leigh's Syndrome): Correlation with Biochemical Defect: L. Medina, etal.; Am. J. Roentgenol., June 1990, vol. 154(6), pp. 1269–1274.

Diagnostic Criteria in Classical Infantile Subacute Necrotizing Encephalomyelopathy (Leigh's Disease): W. Sperl, et al.; Klin. Padiatr., March–April 1989, vol. 210(2), pp. 86–92.

Subacute Necrotizing Encephalomyelopathy (Leigh Disease): CT Study: H.J. Paltiel, et al.; Radiology, January 1987, vol. 162(1 pt. 1), pp. 115–118.

# LESCH-NYHAN SYNDROME

**Description** Lesch-Nyhan syndrome, a metabolic disorder caused by deficiency of hypoxanthine-guanine phosphoribosyltransferase **(HPRT),** is characterized by hyperuricemia and severe neurologic disturbances.

**Synonyms**

>   Hereditary Hyperuricemia
>   Hyperuricemia–Choreoathetosis–Self-Mutilation Syndrome
>   Hyperuricemia-Oligophrenia
>   Juvenile Gout–Choreoathetosis–Mental Retardation Syndrome
>   Nyhan syndrome

**Signs and Symptoms** Clinical manifestations are first seen at 3 to 6 months of age. Hyperuricemia is usually present, and orange crystals may occasionally be seen in the diapers. Neurologic signs and symptoms begin within the first year with athetosis, or with hypotonia leading to difficulty in holding the head. Mental retardation is usually present and moderate, although evaluation may be difficult because of dysarthria. Nephrolithiasis may develop.

The striking feature of Lesch-Nyhan syndrome, seen in 85 percent of cases, is self-mutilation. The characteristic is quite variable: it can first appear at 1 year of age or in the mid-teens; can involve biting of lips, fingers, and hands, and beating of the head against hard objects; and can occur for periods of time ranging from days to months.

The syndrome can be detected prenatally by amniocentesis or chorionic villus biopsy.

**Etiology** Lesch-Nyhan syndrome is an X-linked hereditary disorder that results from deficiency of HPRT, which is located in the human genome at Xq26–q27.

**Epidemiology** Only males are known to be affected.

**Treatment—Standard** Allopurinol is used to treat the symptoms related to hyperuricemia. There is no present effective, sustained treatment for the neurologic sequelae, although success has been reported with carbidopa/levodopa as well as behavior modification techniques for the self-mutilating behavior; and diazepam, phenobarbital, and haloperidol for chorea.

**Treatment—Investigational** Applications of gene replacement therapy are being investigated.

Please contact the agencies listed under Resources, below, for the most current information. Addresses and telephone numbers of these agencies, as well as of individual experts and research centers, may be found in the Master Resources List.

**Resources**

**For more information on Lesch-Nyhan syndrome:** National Organization for Rare Disorders (NORD); Lesch-Nyhan Syndrome Registry; International Lesch-Nyhan Disease Association; The Arc (a national organization on mental retardation); NIH/National Institute of Neurological Disorders and Stroke; William L. Nyhan, M.D., University of California School of Medicine, San Diego; Research Trust for Metabolic Diseases in Children.

**For genetic information and genetic counseling referrals:** March of Dimes Birth Defects Foundation; Alliance of Genetic Support Groups.

**References**

The Metabolic and Molecular Basis of Inherited Disease, 7th ed.: C.R. Scriver, et al., eds.; McGraw-Hill, 1995, pp. 1679–1706.

# LOWE SYNDROME

**Description** Lowe syndrome is a rare, inherited metabolic disorder characterized by ocular and renal abnormalities and mental retardation.

**Synonyms**

>   Cerebrooculorenal Dystrophy
>   Lowe-Bickel Syndrome

Lowe-Terry-Machlachlan Syndrome
Oculocerebrorenal Syndrome

**Signs and Symptoms** Manifestations usually are first seen in early infancy, in males. These signs and symptoms include hydrophthalmos, cataracts and glaucoma, epicanthal folds, areflexia, joint hypermobility, rickets, underdeveloped testes, excess fatty tissue, and wide-ranging weight and temperature fluctuations. Hyperactivity and mental retardation are commonly found. Female carriers sometimes have opacities in the lens of the eye.

Aminoaciduria and phosphaturia may be present, and renal tubular acidosis may develop. Microscopic studies may show abnormalities in the kidneys, testes, eyes, and brain.

DNA probes are available for carrier and prenatal detection.

**Etiology** Lowe syndrome is transmitted through an X-linked recessive gene, which has been localized to the Xq25–q26 region. This gene controls production of inositol-polyphosphate-5-phosphatase; symptoms may develop because of a lack of this enzyme.

**Epidemiology** The syndrome is very rare and affects only males.

**Related Disorders Renal tubular acidosis** is a disorder in which renal secretion of hydrogen and reabsorption of bicarbonate are deficient. Sequelae may be chronic metabolic acidosis and potassium depletion, osteomalacia, or rickets.

See *Cystinosis.*

**Treatment—Standard** Treatment consists of appropriate medications to reduce or alleviate symptoms and to correct behavioral and renal problems. The low blood level of phosphorus is treated with oral replacement of phosphorus alone, or phosphorus in combination with vitamin D to prevent rickets. Electrolyte replacement and alkalinization therapy are required to correct the metabolic and electrolyte imbalance. Surgery or drugs may be used to treat eye problems such as cataracts and glaucoma; the cataractous lens can be removed in infancy. Eyeglasses or contact lenses may be necessary. Genetic counseling may be beneficial.

**Treatment—Investigational** Please contact the agencies listed under Resources, below, for the most current information. Addresses and telephone numbers of these agencies, as well as of individual experts and research centers, may be found in the Master Resources List.

**Resources**

**For more information on Lowe syndrome:** National Organization for Rare Disorders (NORD); Lowe Syndrome Association; The Arc (a national organization on mental retardation); NIH/National Institute of Child Health and Human Development.

**For genetic information and genetic counseling referrals:** March of Dimes Birth Defects Foundation; Alliance of Genetic Support Groups.

**References**

The Metabolic and Molecular Basis of Inherited Disease, 7th ed.: C.R. Scriver, et al., eds.; McGraw-Hill, 1995, pp. 3705–3716.

Recent Developments in Certain X-Linked Genetic Eye Disorders: B.S. Shastry; Biochem. Biophys. Acta, September 1993, vol. 1182(2), pp. 119–127.

Cecil Textbook of Medicine, 19th ed.: J.B. Wyngaarden, et al., eds.; W.B. Saunders Company, 1992, p. 1100.

The Lowe's Oculocerebrorenal Syndrome Gene Encodes a Protein Highly Homologous to Inositol Polyphosphate-5-Phosphatase: O. Attree, et al.; Nature, July 1992, vol. 358(6383), pp. 239–242.

Mendelian Inheritance in Man, 10th ed.: V.A. McKusick; The Johns Hopkins University Press, 1992, pp. 1895–1896.

Nelson Textbook of Pediatrics, 14th ed.: R.E. Behrman, ed.-in-chief; W.B. Saunders Company, 1992, pp. 1346, 1579, 1756.

Clinical and Laboratory Findings in the Oculocerebrorenal Syndrome of Lowe, with Special Reference to Growth and Renal Function: L.R. Charnas, et al.; N. Engl. J. Med., May 9, 1991, vol. 324(19), pp. 1318–1325.

Lowe Oculocerebrorenal Syndrome in a Female with a Balanced X;20 Translocation: Mapping of the X Chromosome Breakpoint: P.R. Papenhausen, et al.; Am. J. Hum. Genet., October 1991, vol. 49(4), pp. 804–810.

The Oculocerebral Syndrome of Lowe: L. Charnas and W. Gahl; National Institutes of Health, Institute of Child Health and Human Development, Bethesda, MD, 1991.

Birth Defects Encyclopedia: M.L. Buyse, ed.-in-chief; Blackwell Scientific Publications, 1990, pp. 1275–1276.

Dictionary of Medical Syndromes, 3rd ed.: S.I. Magalini, et al., eds.; J.B. Lippincott Company, 1990, pp. 550–551.

Ophthalmology: Principles and Concepts, 7th ed.: J.J. Kanski, ed.; Butterworth-Heinemann, 1990, pp. 235, 258.

Oral Carnitine Therapy in Children with Cystinosis and Renal Fanconi Syndrome: W. Gahl, et al.; J. Clin. Invest., February 1988, vol. 81(2), pp. 549–560.

Smith's Recognizable Patterns of Human Malformation, 4th ed.: K.L. Jones; W.B. Saunders Company, 1988, pp. 180–181.

# α-MANNOSIDOSIS

**Description** α-Mannosidosis is a genetic disorder characterized by a defect in the degradation of glycoproteins, the end result of which is a lysosomal accumulation of oligosaccharides, and progressive mental and physical deterioration. Two forms occur, primarily differentiated by degree of severity.

**Synonyms**

> Lysosomal α-D-Mannosidase Deficiency

**Signs and Symptoms** Symptoms of **type I** α-mannosidosis, the more severe form, begin within the first year of life. Findings include rapidly progressive mental retardation, hepatosplenomegaly, and skeletal abnormalities. This form of α-mannosidosis may be fatal before the child reaches 10 years of age.

The milder form of the disorder, **type II,** develops between 1 year and 4 years of age. Mild-to-moderate mental retardation usually is noticed in childhood or adolescence.

Other findings in types I and II may vary in degree, and include a prominent forehead and jaw, flattening of the nose, widely spaced teeth, and thick tongue and lips. Corneal opacities, cataracts, and hearing loss may develop. Abdominal distention results from the hepatosplenomegaly. Articular and spinal abnormalities may develop, and growth is impaired. Immune system compromise may lead to susceptibility to infection, particularly bacterial infection of the respiratory tract.

**Etiology** α-Mannosidosis is inherited as an autosomal recessive trait. The lysosomal enzyme, α-mannosidase, responsible for the condition is located on chromosome 19p13.2–q12.

**Epidemiology** α-Mannosidosis probably affects only a few hundred persons, both males and females, in the United States.

**Related Disorders** See *Mucopolysaccharidosis; Mucolipidosis II; Mucolipidosis III.*

**Treatment—Standard** Treatment of α-mannosidosis is symptomatic and supportive. Genetic counseling may be beneficial.

**Treatment—Investigational** Enzyme replacement by means of bone marrow transplantation is under investigation for treatment of the lysosomal storage disorders, including α-mannosidosis.

Please contact the agencies listed under Resources, below, for the most current information. Addresses and telephone numbers of these agencies, as well as of individual experts and research centers, may be found in the Master Resources List.

**Resources**

**For more information on α-mannosidosis:** National Organization for Rare Disorders (NORD); The Arc (a national organization on mental retardation); NIH/National Digestive Diseases Information Clearinghouse; Research Trust for Metabolic Diseases in Children.

**For genetic information and genetic counseling referrals:** March of Dimes Birth Defects Foundation; Alliance of Genetic Support Groups.

**References**

The Metabolic and Molecular Basis of Inherited Disease, 7th ed.: C.R. Scriver, et al., eds.; McGraw-Hill, 1995, pp. 2529–2561.

# MAPLE SYRUP URINE DISEASE

**Description** Maple syrup urine disease, a hereditary condition that derives its name from the odor of the patient's urine and sweat, is caused by abnormal metabolism of the branched chain amino acids, leucine, isoleucine, and valine. Catastrophic illness in the newborn period with metabolic acidosis, seizures, coma, and death occur in the untreated patient.

**Synonyms**

> Branched Chain Ketonuria
> Ketoaciduria

**Signs and Symptoms** Newborns begin to develop symptoms and signs several days after birth. Findings include the characteristic sweet odor of the sweat and urine, along with poor feeding, lethargy, and coma. Seizures also may occur. If the infant survives longer than a few months, mental retardation becomes apparent.

An **intermittent form** of the disease occurs after the neonatal period in previously healthy children who are exposed to stress, such as surgery or infections. Symptoms include vomiting, sweet-smelling urine and sweat, ataxia, lethargy, and coma.

In the **mild form** of the disease, occurring in children after the neonatal period, symptoms are similar to but milder than those characteristic of the classic form of the disease.

A rare form of the disorder, **thiamine-responsive maple syrup urine disease,** is characterized by mild or occasional symptoms in children, whose conditions improve when large doses of thiamine are administered.

Blood tests reveal high levels of leucine, isoleucine, and valine.

**Etiology** The disease is transmitted as an autosomal recessive trait due to defective branched chain keto-acid dehydrogenase. Their excessive accumulation causes severe metabolic acidosis and neurologic damage.

**Epidemiology** The disease is extremely rare. Incidence in the United States white population is estimated at 1:200,000; the disease is more common among Mennonite populations. Males and females are equally affected.

**Related Disorders** See *Acidemia, Isovaleric; Acidemia, Proprionic; Nonketotic Hyperglycinemia.*

**Treatment—Standard** Treatment should begin as soon as possible after birth. Acidosis is treated by intravenous bicarbonate, peritoneal dialysis, or exchange transfusions. Children with this disorder must stay on a strict diet established by a physician, limiting the dietary intake of the branched chain amino acids. In thiamine-responsive maple syrup urine disease, there may be improvement or, occasionally, complete resolution of symptoms in patients treated with large doses of thiamine.

Genetic counseling is necessary for the families of maple syrup urine disease patients.

**Treatment—Investigational** Please contact the agencies listed under Resources, below, for the most current information. Addresses and telephone numbers of these agencies, as well as of individual experts and research centers, may be found in the Master Resources List.

**Resources**

**For more information on maple syrup urine disease:** National Organization for Rare Disorders (NORD); Families with Maple Syrup Urine Disease; Research Trust for Metabolic Diseases in Children; NIH/National Digestive Diseases Information Clearinghouse.

**For genetic information and genetic counseling referrals:** March of Dimes Birth Defects Foundation; Alliance of Genetic Support Groups.

**References**

The Metabolic and Molecular Basis of Inherited Disease, 7th ed.: C.R. Scriver, et al., eds.; McGraw-Hill, 1995, pp. 1239–1277.

Nutrient Intakes of Adolescents with Phenylketonuria and Infants and Children with Maple Syrup Urine Disease on Semisynthetic Diets: S.S. Gropper, et al.; J. Am. Coll. Nutr., April 1993, vol. 12(2), pp. 108–114.

Cecil Textbook of Medicine, 19th ed.: J.B. Wyngaarden, et al., eds.; W.B. Saunders Company, 1992, pp. 1096, 1105.

Maple Syrup Urine Disease: Interrelations Between Branched Chain Amino-, Oxo- and Hydroxyacids; Implications for Treatment; Associations with CNS Dysmyelination: E. Treacy, et al.; J. Inherit. Metab. Dis., 1992, vol. 15(1), pp. 121–135.

Mendelian Inheritance in Man, 10th ed.: V.A. McKusick; The Johns Hopkins University Press, 1992, pp. 1513–1516.

Nelson Textbook of Pediatrics, 14th ed.: R.E. Behrman, ed.-in-chief; W.B. Saunders Company, 1992, pp. 316–319.

Acute Illness in Maple Syrup Urine Disease: Dynamics of Protein Metabolism and Implications for Management: G.N. Thompson, et al.; J. Pediatr., July 1991, vol. 119(1 pt. 1), pp. 35–41.

Continuous Venovenous Hemofiltration in the Management of Acute Decompensation in Inborn Errors of Metabolism: G.N. Thompson, et al.; J. Pediatr., June 1991, vol. 118(6), pp. 879–884.

Intellectual Outcome in Children with Maple Syrup Urine Disease: P. Kaplan, et al.; J. Pediatr., July 1991, vol. 119(1 pt. 1), pp. 46–50.

Birth Defects Encyclopedia: M.L Buyse, ed.-in-chief; Blackwell Scientific Publications, 1990, pp. 1102–1103.

Clearance of Branched Chain Amino Acids by Peritoneal Dialysis in Maple Syrup Urine Disease: Y. McMahon, et al.; Adv. Perit. Dial., 1990, vol. 6, pp. 31–34.

Dictionary of Medical Syndromes, 3rd ed.: S.I. Magalini, et al., eds.; J.B. Lippincott Company, 1990, p. 565.

Evidence for Both a Regulatory Mutation and a Structural Mutation in a Family with Maple Syrup Urine Disease: B. Zhang, et al.; J. Clin. Invest., April 1989, vol. 83(4), pp. 1425–1429.

Principles of Neurology, 4th ed.: R.D. Adams and M. Victor, eds.: McGraw-Hill, 1989, pp. 780, 793, 801, 858.

# MAROTEAUX-LAMY SYNDROME

**Description** There are 3 clinical variants of Maroteaux-Lamy syndrome (mucopolysaccharidosis type VI—**MPS VI):** severe, intermediate, and mild. The severe form of this condition is similar to the severe form of Hurler syndrome, except for the preservation of intelligence in patients with Marotaux-Lamy syndrome.

**Synonyms**

Arylsulfatase B Deficiency

Mucopolysaccharidosis Type VI

Polydystrophic Dwarfism

**Signs and Symptoms** Macrocephaly and a prominent sternum may be present at birth. Other manifestations of Maroteaux-Lamy syndrome usually appear between the 2nd and 3rd year. The most common findings are coarse facial features and short stature. Corneal opacities may be present. Bone abnormalities including stubby fingers, joint restrictions and claw hand, lumbar lordosis, and pain in the hip generally occur after age 3 or 4. Carpal tunnel syndrome may develop, as well as a wobbly gait that is the result of inwardly pointed knees and toes. Other typical findings include noisy and strained breathing, deafness, hepatosplenomegaly, and aortic valvular dysfunction. Blindness and hydrocephalus may be complications. The intellect is usually normal.

**Etiology** The syndrome has an autosomal recessive inheritance. A deficiency of the enzyme arylsulfatase B (N-acetylgalactosamine-4-sulfatase) causes an excess of dermatan sulfate in the urine. The enzyme deficiency results in an inability to metabolize mucopolysaccharides. Accumulation of these large undegraded mucopolysaccharides in body cells causes the physical symptoms and abnormalities.

**Epidemiology** The incidence is unknown. Maroteaux-Lamy syndrome affects males and females equally.

**Related Disorders** See *Mucopolysaccharidosis.*

The mucolipidoses are a family of disorders that produce symptoms very much like those of the mucopolysaccharidoses. See *Mucolipidosis II; Mucolipidosis III; Mucolipidosis IV.*

**Treatment—Standard** Treatment is symptomatic and supportive. Hernias may require surgery. Physical therapy and hearing aids may benefit the patient. Genetic counseling may be helpful to patient and family. Prenatal diagnosis is now possible.

**Treatment—Investigational** Treatment approaches aimed at checking early development of Maroteaux-Lamy syndrome include enzyme replacement therapy and bone marrow transplantation. The latter procedure was used to treat a young girl with the syndrome, and greatly decreased the size of her enlarged liver and spleen and improved her cardiopulmonary function, joint mobility, and visual acuity. The successful outcome of bone marrow transplantation in this case demonstrates that toxic compounds that accumulate in the tissues can be removed and metabolized by transplanted cells. However, more research is needed before this treatment becomes available for general use.

Please contact the agencies listed under Resources, below, for the most current information. Addresses and telephone numbers of these agencies, as well as of individual experts and research centers, may be found in the Master Resources List.

**Resources**

**For more information on Maroteaux-Lamy syndrome:** National Organization for Rare Disorders (NORD); National Mucopolysaccharidoses Society; Society of Mucopolysaccharide Diseases; Society of MPS Diseases; NIH/National Digestive Diseases Information Clearinghouse.

**For genetic information and genetic counseling referrals:** March of Dimes Birth Defects Foundation; Alliance of Genetic Support Groups.

**References**

The Metabolic and Molecular Basis of Inherited Disease, 7th ed.: C.R. Scriver, et al., eds.; McGraw-Hill, 1995, pp. 2465–2494.

# MCARDLE DISEASE

**Description** McArdle disease is a rare glycogen storage disease associated with a deficiency of muscle phosphorylase, normally utilized in the degradation of glycogen to glucose in muscle tissue. Painful cramps occur after strenuous exercise, and kidney failure can rarely develop.

**Synonyms**

Glycogen Storage Disease Type V
Glycogenosis Type V
Muscle Phosphorylase Deficiency
Myophosphorylase Deficiency

**Signs and Symptoms** Symptoms of the disease usually do not appear before age 10 years, and development is normal. Muscle function is normal while at rest or during moderate exercise. Painful muscle cramps occur after vigorous exercise, at which time myoglobin can often be detected in the urine. Diagnosis is confirmed by failure to see a rise in blood lactate after exercise. The diagnosis can also be confirmed by muscle biopsy; phosphorylase activity will be reduced or absent in affected patients.

**Etiology** McArdle disease is caused by deficiency of the enzyme myophosphorylase. It is inherited as an autosomal recessive trait. The defect that causes the disorder is found in genes located on chromosome 11q13–qter.

**Epidemiology** All glycogen storage diseases together affect fewer than 1:40,000 persons in the United States, with males and females being affected in equal numbers.

**Related Disorders** See *Pompe Disease; Glycogen Storage Disease III; Glycogen Storage Disease VII.*

**Treatment—Standard** Treatment usually consists of avoidance of strenuous exercise. Oral glucose and fructose supplements have been used but with varied results.

**Treatment—Investigational** Please contact the agencies listed under Resources, below, for the most current information. Addresses and telephone numbers of these agencies, as well as of individual experts and research centers, may be found in the Master Resources List.

**Resources**

**For more information on McArdle disease:** National Organization for Rare Disorders (NORD); Association for Glycogen Storage Diseases; NIH/National Digestive Diseases Information Clearinghouse; Research Trust for Metabolic Diseases in Children.

**For genetic information and genetic counseling referrals:** March of Dimes Birth Defects Foundation; Alliance of Genetic Support Groups.

**References**

The Metabolic and Molecular Basis of Inherited Disease, 7th ed.: C.R. Scriver, et al., eds.; McGraw-Hill, 1995, pp. 951–953.
Cecil Textbook of Medicine, 18th ed.: J.B. Wyngaarden and L.H. Smith, Jr., eds.; W.B. Saunders Company, 1988, p. 1135.

# MEDIUM-CHAIN ACYL-COA DEHYDROGENASE (MCAD) DEFICIENCY

**Description** This metabolic disorder, caused by an inherited enzyme deficiency, is characterized by recurrent episodes of metabolic acidosis, hypoglycemia, lethargy, and coma.

**Synonyms**
> Acyl-CoA Dehydrogenase Deficiency, Medium-Chain
> Dicarboxylicaciduria

**Signs and Symptoms** Onset of symptoms is in infancy or early childhood. Intermittent hypoglycemia and metabolic acidosis are characteristic after fasting. Coma sometimes ensues. During episodes of hypoglycemia, tests usually show excessive amounts of dicarboxylic acids in the urine (6 to 8 carbon atoms in length). Fatty changes in the liver may also occur. Detection of the compounds suberylglycine and phenylpropionylglycine in the urine appears to be diagnostic for this condition.

**Etiology** MCAD is due to deficiency of the enzyme medium-chain acyl-CoA dehydrogenase, which is needed for the oxidation of medium-chain fatty acids. This enzyme plays a central role in the metabolism of fats.

Many of the effects of organic acidemias are attributed to secondary carnitine depletion.

**Epidemiology** Incidence is about 1:50,000 live births. Males and females are affected in equal numbers.

**Related Disorders** See *Glutaricaciduria II.*

**Treatment—Standard** Prevention of fasting for prolonged periods will help prevent symptoms. This may require awakening the child at night for feeding, or nighttime intravenous or enteral feeding. Acute episodes of acidosis and dehydration are treated with fluids and bicarbonate.

Patients with carnitine deficiency should be given a supplement of 100 to 300 mg/kg/day of oral L-carnitine. Other treatment is symptomatic and supportive.

**Treatment—Investigational** Please contact the agencies listed under Resources, below, for the most current information. Addresses and telephone numbers of these agencies, as well as of individual experts and research centers, may be found in the Master Resources List.

**Resources**

**For more information on medium-chain acyl-CoA dehydrogenase deficiency:** National Organization for Rare Disorders (NORD); Medium-Chain Acyl-CoA Dehydrogenase Family Support Group; Organic Acidemia Association; British Organic Acidemia Association; NIH/National Digestive Diseases Information Clearinghouse; Research Trust for Metabolic Diseases in Children.

**For genetic information and genetic counseling referrals:** March of Dimes Birth Defects Foundation; Alliance of Genetic Support Groups.

**References**

The Metabolic and Molecular Basis of Inherited Disease, 7th ed.: C.R. Scriver, et al., eds.; McGraw-Hill, 1995, pp. 1501–1533.

Catalytic Defect of Medium-Chain Acyl-Coenzyme A Dehydrogenase Deficiency: Lack of Both Cofactor Responsiveness and Biochemical Heterogeneity in Eight Patients: B.A. Amendt, et al.; J. Clin. Invest., 1985, vol. 76, pp. 963–969.

Dicarboxylic Aciduria: Deficient 1-(14)C-Octanoate Oxidation and Medium-Chain Acyl-CoA Dehydrogenase in Fibroblasts: W.J. Rhead, et al.; Science, 1983, vol. 221, pp. 73–75.

# MELAS SYNDROME

**Description** MELAS ([**M**]itchondrial [**E**]ncephalopathy, [**L**]actic [**A**]cidosis, [**S**]troke) syndrome is one of a group of rare mitochondrial encephalomyopathies that include Kearns-Sayre syndrome and MERRF syndrome. Defects in mitochondria, as well as the presence of ragged-red fibers in muscle tissue on microscopic examination, are present in all 3 disorders.

**Synonyms**
> Mitochondrial Myopathy, Encephalopathy, Lactic Acidosis, and Strokelike Episodes
> Myopathy, Mitochondrial–Encephalopathy–Lactic Acidosis–Stroke

**Signs and Symptoms** The distinguishing feature in MELAS syndrome is recurring strokelike episodes characterized by sudden headaches, followed by vomiting and seizures. Hemiparesis, cortical blindness, and hemianopsia may also occur. Lactic acidosis, progressive dementia, and short stature may also be present. Onset of symptoms is usually between the ages of 5 and 15 years.

Studies have shown that milder forms of MELAS syndrome may be found in relatives of affected individuals. In some cases, the affected relatives have no apparent symptoms.

The overlapping symptoms of Kearns-Sayre syndrome, MERRF syndrome, and MELAS syndrome can make it difficult to diagnose MELAS syndrome in some cases.

**Etiology** MELAS syndrome is a rare mitochondrial disorder resulting from a mutation in mitochondrial tRNA$^{Leu}$. Inheritance patterns are therefore complicated because of the nature of mitochondrial inheritance and expression.

**Epidemiology** MELAS syndrome affects males and females in equal numbers.

**Related Disorders** See *Kearns-Sayre Syndrome; MERFF Syndrome.*

**Treatment—Standard** Anticonvulsant drugs are used to help control seizures associated with MELAS syndrome. Genetic counseling may be of benefit for patients and their families. Other treatment is symptomatic and supportive.

**Treatment—Investigational** The role of mitochondrial DNA (**mtDNA**) mutations in adult-onset hereditary neuromuscular disease is being investigated at Emory University by Dr. Douglas C. Wallace.

The molecular genetic basis of mitochondrial myopathies is being investigated at John Hopkins University by Donald R. Johns, M.D.

Please contact the agencies listed under Resources, below, for the most current information. Addresses and telephone numbers of these agencies, as well as of individual experts and research centers, may be found in the Master Resources List.

**Resources**

**For more information on MELAS syndrome:** National Organization for Rare Disorders (NORD); Education and Support Exchange; Mitochondrial Disorders Foundation of America; Lactic Acidosis Support Group; NIH/National Institute of Neurological Disorders and Stroke; Epilepsy Foundation of America; Research Trust for Metabolic Diseases in Children.

**References**

The Metabolic and Molecular Basis of Inherited Disease, 7th ed.: C.R. Scriver, et al., eds.; McGraw-Hill, 1995, pp. 1562–1564.
Cecil Textbook of Medicine, 19th ed.: J.B. Wyngaarden, et al., eds.; W.B. Saunders Company, 1992, p. 2260.
MELAS: An Original Case and Clinical Criteria for Diagnosis: M. Hirano, et al.; Neuromuscul. Disord., 1992, vol. 2(2), pp. 125–135.
MELAS: Clinical Features, Biochemistry, and Molecular Genetics: E. Ciafaloni, et al.; Ann. Neurol., April 1992, vol. 31(4), pp. 391–398.
Mendelian Inheritance in Man, 10th ed.: V.A. McKusick; The Johns Hopkins University Press, 1992, p. 1543.
Mitochondrial Myopathy, Encephalopathy, Lactic Acidosis, and Stroke-Like Episodes (MELAS): A Correlative Study of the Clinical Features and Mitochondrial DNA Mutation: Y. Goto, et al.; Neurology, March 1992, vol. 42(3 pt. 1), pp. 545–550.
Nelson Textbook of Pediatrics, 14th ed.: R.E. Behrman, ed.-in-chief; W.B. Saunders Company, 1992, p. 1517.
The Other Human Genome: J. Palca; Science, September 7, 1990, vol. 249, pp. 1104–1105.
Principles of Neurology, 4th ed.: R.D. Adams and M. Victor, eds.; McGraw-Hill, 1989, p. 1144.
Advances in Contemporary Neurology: F. Plum, ed.; F.A. Davis Company, 1988, pp. 95–133.
MELAS Syndrome Involving a Mother and Two Children: P.F. Driscoll, et al.; Arch. Neurol., September 1987, vol. 44(9), pp. 971–973.

# MENKES DISEASE

**Description** Menkes disease is a genetic disturbance of intestinal copper absorption resulting in deficient copper levels in many body tissues. Structural changes occur in the hair, brain, bones, liver, and arteries. The disease is most often fatal by 2 years of age.

**Synonyms**

    Kinky Hair Disease
    Steely Hair Disease
    Trichopoliodystrophy
    X-Linked Copper Deficiency
    X-Linked Copper Malabsorption

**Signs and Symptoms** Affected individuals are often born prematurely, and hypothermia and hyperbilirubinemia may be present. Neonates appear normal, some with characteristic pudgy cheeks. At about 6 weeks of age, the fine neonatal hair loses pigment and eventually becomes kinky, tangled, and sparse. Neurologic deficit is evident by 1 to 3 months of age, with hypertonia, irritability, feeding difficulties, convulsions, and subdural hematoma or cranial thrombosis, with eventual spastic dementia and seizures. At this time developmental delay is apparent. On x-ray, osteoporosis and wormian bones may be seen. Fractures occur often, and the combination of these seen with subdural hematoma has led to the incorrect diagnosis of child abuse.

Other findings in Menkes disease include emphysema, bladder abnormalities, and ocular irregularities.

**Etiology** Menkes disease is inherited as an X-linked recessive trait and maps to Xq13. The defect in copper absorption results in very low serum copper and ceruloplasmin concentrations.

**Epidemiology** An Australian study of Menkes disease from 1966 to 1971 suggested an incidence of 1:35,500 live births. A 1980 study modified this figure to 1:90,000 live births. Other estimates place the number of cases at 1:50,000 and 1:100,000. As in all X-linked traits, the disease primarily affects males.

**Related Disorders** See *Wilson Disease; Primary Biliary Cirrhosis.*

**Indian childhood cirrhosis** is a familial and probably genetically determined disease. In this condition, an extremely large amount of copper accumulates in the liver, and the clinical picture is similar to that of Menkes disease.

**Treatment—Standard** Copper supplementation corrects hepatic and serum copper levels, but cerebral deterioration continues. Other treatment is symptomatic and supportive.

**Treatment—Investigational** Copper histidine is being investigated a possible treatment for Menkes disease. For more information, please contact Dr. Steven Kaler at the National Institutes of Health.

Please contact the agencies listed under Resources, below, for the most current information. Addresses and telephone numbers of these agencies, as well as of individual experts and research centers, may be found in the Master Resources List.

**Resources**

**For more information on Menkes disease:** National Organization for Rare Disorders (NORD); Corporation for Menkes Disease; NIH/National Institute of Neurological Disorders and Stroke.

**For genetic information and genetic counseling referrals:** March of Dimes Birth Defects Foundation; Alliance of Genetic Support Groups.

**References**

The Metabolic and Molecular Basis of Inherited Disease, 7th ed.: C.R. Scriver, et al., eds.; McGraw-Hill, 1995, pp. 2211–2235.

Mendelian Inheritance in Man, 9th ed.: V.A. McKusick; The Johns Hopkins University Press, 1990, pp. 1665–1668.

Life-Span and Menkes Kinky Hair Syndrome: Report of a 13-Year Course of This Disease: C. Sander, et al.; Clin. Genet., March 1988, vol. 33(3), pp. 228–233.

Menkes Syndrome in a Girl with X-Autosome Translocation: S. Kapur, et al.; Am. J. Med. Genet., February 1987, vol. 26(2), pp. 503–510.

Metallothionein Gene Regulation in Menkes Syndrome: D.H. Hamer; Arch. Dermatol., October 1987, vol. 123(10), pp. 1384a–1385a.

# MERRF Syndrome

**Description** MERRF ([**M**]yoclonus [**E**]pilepsy associated with [**R**]agged-[**R**]ed [**F**]ibers) syndrome is one of a group of rare mitochondrial encephalomyopathies that include Kearns-Sayre syndrome and MELAS syndrome. Defects in mitochondria, as well as the presence of ragged-red fibers in muscle tissue on microscopic examination, are present in all 3 disorders.

**Synonyms**

Fukuhara Syndrome

Myoclonus Epilepsy Associated with Ragged-Red Fibers

Myoencephalopathy Ragged-Red Fiber Disease

**Signs and Symptoms** The distinguishing feature in MERRF syndrome is myoclonic seizures. Lactic acidosis, ataxia, muscle weakness, dysarthria, optic atrophy, and nystagmus may also be found in affected individuals. Short stature and hearing loss are other common symptoms. Slowly progressive dementia may also be present. Symptoms begin in childhood or early adult life and worsen over time.

Studies have shown that milder forms of MERRF syndrome may be found in some affected individuals. The overlapping symptoms of Kearns-Sayre syndrome, MELAS syndrome, and MERRF syndrome can make it difficult to diagnose MERRF syndrome in some cases.

**Etiology** MERRF syndrome is a rare mitochondrial disorder due to a mutation in the mitochondrial gene for tRNA$^{Lys}$. Pedigrees are complicated by the nature of mitochondrial gene inheritance.

**Epidemiology** MERRF syndrome affects males and females in equal numbers.

**Related Disorders** See *Kearns-Sayre Syndrome; MELAS Syndrome.*

**Treatment—Standard** Anticonvulsant drugs are used to help control seizures associated with MERRF syndrome. Genetic counseling may be of benefit for patients and their families. Other treatment is symptomatic and supportive.

**Treatment—Investigational** The role of mitochondrial DNA (**mtDNA**) mutations in adult-onset hereditary neuromuscular disease is being investigated at Emory University by Dr. Douglas C. Wallace.

The molecular genetic basis of mitochondrial myopathies is being investigated at John Hopkins University by Dr. Donald R. Johns.

Please contact the agencies listed under Resources, below, for the most current information. Addresses and telephone numbers of these agencies, as well as of individual experts and research centers, may be found in the Master Resources List.

**Resources**
   **For more information on MERRF syndrome:** National Organization for Rare Disorders (NORD); Education and Support Exchange; Mitochondrial Disorders Foundation of America; Lactic Acidosis Support Group; NIH/National Institute of Neurological Disorders and Stroke; Epilepsy Foundation of America; Research Trust for Metabolic Diseases in Children.

**References**
   The Metabolic and Molecular Basis of Inherited Disease, 7th ed.: C.R. Scriver, et al., eds.; McGraw-Hill, 1995, pp. 1560–1562.
   Cecil Textbook of Medicine, 19th ed.: J.B. Wyngaarden, et al., eds.; W.B. Saunders Company, 1992, pp. 2279–2280.
   Mendelian Inheritance in Man, 10th ed.: V.A. McKusick; The Johns Hopkins University Press, 1992, p. 1573.
   Nelson Textbook of Pediatrics, 14th ed.: R.E. Behrman, ed.-in-chief; W.B. Saunders Company, 1992, p. 1517.
   A tRNA (Lys) Mutation in the mtDNA Is the Causal Genetic Lesion Underlying Myoclonic Epilepsy and Ragged-Red Fibers (MERRF) Syndrome: A.S. Noer, et al.; Am. J. Hum. Gen. October 1991, vol. 49(4), pp. 715–722.
   The Other Human Genome: J. Palca; Science, September 7, 1990, vol. 249, pp. 1104–1105.
   Myoclonus Epilepsy and Ragged-Red Fibers (MERRF): A Clinical Pathological, Biochemical, Magnetic Resonance Spectrographic and Positron Emission Tomographic Study: S.F. Berkovic, et al.; Brain, October 1989, vol. 112(5), pp. 1231–1260.
   Principles of Neurology, 4th ed.; R.D. Adams and M. Victor, eds.; McGraw-Hill, 1989, p. 810.
   Advances in Contemporary Neurology: F. Plum, ed.; F.A. Davis Company, 1988, pp. 95–133.

# MORQUIO SYNDROME

**Description** Morquio syndrome (mucopolysaccharidosis type IV—**MPS IV**) manifests itself in 2 forms, A and B. Both forms are due to enzyme deficiency, which leads to an accumulation of keratan sulfate. Bony abnormalities of the head, chest, hands, knees, and spine may result. Intellect is preserved. Each form has mild and severe phenotypes.

**Synonyms**
      Morquio Disease
      Mucopolysaccharidosis Type IV

**Signs and Symptoms** Both forms are characterized by short stature with a short trunk and a unique spondyloepiphyseal dysplasia.

   The first signs may be detected from 12 months to 3.5 years of age. These include macrocephaly, a broad mouth, small nose, short neck, corneal clouding, and widely spaced and thinly enameled teeth. Other early features are retarded growth, genu valgum, kyphosis, and a short trunk. The child may have a tendency to fall. As development continues, a short barrel chest and disproportionately long arms are evident, along with enlarged and possibly hyperextensible wrists and stubby hands. The misaligned knees and knobby joints may cause a wobbly gait. Joint laxity and bony abnormalities of the spine can result in spinal cord compression. Further findings include hepatomegaly, thoracic kyphoscoliosis, aortic regurgitation, and hearing loss.

**Etiology** The syndrome is autosomal recessive. **Type A** results from a deficiency of galactose-6-sulfatase; **type B,** from deficient β-galactosidase. Both deficiencies lead to an inability to metabolize mucopolysaccharides. The accumulation of these large undegraded mucopolysaccharides in body cells, and the resultant accumulation of keratan sulfate in the urine, cause the physical symptoms and abnormalities.

**Epidemiology** Males and females are affected in equal numbers. In the general population, prevalence is fewer than 1:100,000 live births. In the French-Canadian population, Morquio syndrome is the most common type of mucopolysaccharidosis.

**Related Disorders** See *Mucopolysaccharidosis.*

   The mucolipidoses are a family of similar disorders that produce symptoms very much like those of the mucopolysaccharidoses. See *Mucolipidosis II; Mucolipidosis III; Mucolipidosis IV.*

**Treatment—Standard** When spinal cord compression is present, surgery to stabilize the upper cervical spine, usually by spinal fusion, can be lifesaving. Treatment is otherwise symptomatic and supportive. Physical therapy and special educational services may be useful, and genetic counseling may be helpful to the parents of patients.

**Treatment—Investigational** Treatments aimed at checking early development of Morquio syndrome are under study. These include enzyme replacement therapy and bone marrow transplantation.

   Please contact the agencies listed under Resources, below, for the most current information. Addresses and telephone numbers of these agencies, as well as of individual experts and research centers, may be found in the Master Resources List.

**Resources**
   **For more information on Morquio syndrome:** National Organization for Rare Disorders (NORD); National Mucopolysaccharidoses Society; NIH/National Digestive Diseases Information Clearinghouse; Society of Mucopolysaccharide Diseases; Society of MPS Diseases.

**For genetic information and genetic counseling referrals:** March of Dimes Birth Defects Foundation; Alliance of Genetic Support Groups.

**References**
The Metabolic and Molecular Basis of Inherited Disease, 7th ed.: C.R. Scriver, et al., eds.; McGraw-Hill, 1995, pp. 2465–2494.

# MUCOLIPIDOSIS II (ML II)

**Description** ML II is a hereditary metabolic disorder caused by enzyme deficiency. Mucolipids and mucopolysaccharides accumulate in body tissues, resulting in facial and skeletal abnormalities and physical and mental retardation. The disorder is similar to Hurler syndrome, but without mucopolysaccharide excretion. It usually occurs earlier in life and is more severe.

**Synonyms**
> I-Cell Disease
> Inclusion Cell Disease
> Leroy Disease

**Signs and Symptoms** Many features of ML II may be apparent at birth, but onset of manifestations often occurs from 6 to 10 months of age. Craniofacial abnormalities include depression of the nasal bridge, a long and narrow head, and a high forehead. Skeletal features include kyphoscoliosis, gibbus, anterior beaking and wedging of vertebrae, widening of the ribs, and proximal pointing of the metacarpals. Physical and mental retardation may be severe. Inguinal and umbilical hernias and hepatomegaly accompanied by a protruding abdomen are often seen. Other clinical problems include frequent respiratory infections, gingival hyperplasia, corneal opacities, and severe joint contractures.

Increased urinary excretion of glycosaminoglycans has not been observed with this condition.

Prenatal detection is possible.

**Etiology** ML II is autosomal recessive. A variety of lysosomal enzymes are deficient in body cells but are strikingly elevated in the blood. The primary defect is in lysosomal phosphotransferase.

**Epidemiology** Males and females are affected equally.

**Related Disorders** See *Hurler Syndrome; Mucolipidosis III; Mucopolysaccharidosis.*

**Treatment—Standard** Treatment is symptomatic and supportive. Antibiotics are often prescribed for respiratory infections, and orthopedic complications are managed as they arise. Genetic counseling is advised for families with this disorder.

**Treatment—Investigational** Treatments under study for checking early development of ML II include enzyme replacement therapy and bone marrow transplantation.

Please contact the agencies listed under Resources, below, for the most current information. Addresses and telephone numbers of these agencies, as well as of individual experts and research centers, may be found in the Master Resources List.

**Resources**
**For more information on mucolipidosis II:** National Organization for Rare Disorders (NORD); Society of Mucopolysaccharide Diseases; Society of MPS Diseases; The Arc (a national organization on mental retardation); NIH/National Digestive Diseases Information Clearinghouse.

**For genetic information and genetic counseling referrals:** March of Dimes Birth Defects Foundation; Alliance of Genetic Support Groups.

**References**
The Metabolic and Molecular Basis of Inherited Disease, 7th ed.: C.R. Scriver, et al., eds.; McGraw-Hill, 1995, pp. 2495–2508.

# MUCOLIPIDOSIS III (ML III)

**Description** The enzyme deficiencies in ML III result in the accumulation of mucopolysaccharides and mucolipids in body tissues without excess of mucopolysaccharides in the urine. Although this form of mucolipidosis is less severe than ML II (I-cell disease), most individuals do not survive past age 30 years.

**Synonyms**
> Gangliosidosis GM1 Type I
> Pseudo-Hurler Polydystrophy
> Pseudopolydystrophy

**Signs and Symptoms** Clinical manifestations appear from 2 to 4 years of age. Joint stiffness is one of the first symptoms and is progressive, with the child developing scoliosis and claw-hand deformity by age 6. Short stature is also evident by then. Hip joint deterioration and carpal tunnel syndrome develop. Other characteristics include corneal opacities and minimal-to-moderate coarseness of facial features. Aortic valve disease is common, and aortic regurgitation may be present. Mild mental retardation, easy fatigability, congestive heart failure, and dysostosis multiplex may occur.

**Etiology** ML III is inherited as an autosomal recessive trait. The disorder is due to defective mannose-6-phosphate lysosomal recognition markers, resulting in excess accumulations of ganglioside; these affect the central nervous system, liver, spleen, renal glomerular epithelium, and bone tissue.

**Epidemiology** Males and females are affected equally.

**Related Disorders** See *Mucolipidosis II; Marotaux-Lamy Syndrome.*

**Treatment—Standard** Treatment is symptomatic and supportive. Physical therapy may be beneficial. It is suggested that hip replacement be performed after puberty. Genetic counseling is recommended for further family planning.

**Treatment—Investigational** Please contact the agencies listed under Resources, below, for the most current information. Addresses and telephone numbers of these agencies, as well as of individual experts and research centers, may be found in the Master Resources List.

**Resources**

**For more information on mucolipidosis III:** National Organization for Rare Disorders (NORD); Society of Mucopolysaccharide Diseases; Society of MPS Diseases; The Arc (a national organization on mental retardation); NIH/National Digestive Diseases Information Clearinghouse.

**For genetic information and genetic counseling referrals:** March of Dimes Birth Defects Foundation; Alliance of Genetic Support Groups.

**References**

The Metabolic and Molecular Basis of Inherited Disease, 7th ed.: C.R. Scriver, et al., eds.: McGraw-Hill, 1995, pp. 2495–2508.

# MUCOLIPIDOSIS IV (ML IV)

**Description** ML IV is a metabolic disorder due to ganglioside sialidase deficiency. It is associated with psychomotor deterioration, retinal degeneration, and blindness.

**Synonyms**

Sialolipidosis

**Signs and Symptoms** Manifestations generally are seen at birth or during early infancy. The initial finding usually is clouding of the cornea. Retinal degeneration is sometimes seen in the first year. Retardation of physical and mental development usually is not evident until the end of the first year and progresses gradually. Although a few patients may slowly improve their psychomotor skills, most affected children are severely retarded, physically and mentally. Patients with this condition do not develop hepatomegaly, splenomegaly, or mucopolysacchariduria, and have no skeletal involvement. Cultured fibroblasts show abnormal lysosomal inclusions.

The condition can be detected prenatally through amniocentesis.

**Etiology** ML IV is transmitted as an autosomal recessive trait.

**Epidemiology** Children of both sexes are affected. Approximately 50 percent of reported patients are of Ashkenazic Jewish extraction, with ancestors from eastern Europe, especially southern Poland. Fewer than 20 patients have been reported in the medical literature, but the exact incidence is unknown.

**Treatment—Standard** Treatment is symptomatic and supportive. Genetic counseling is advised for families affected by the disorder.

**Treatment—Investigational** Treatments involving enzyme replacement therapy and bone marrow transplantation may be beneficial but have not been attempted for ML IV.

Please contact the agencies listed under Resources, below, for the most current information. Addresses and telephone numbers of these agencies, as well as of individual experts and research centers, may be found in the Master Resources List.

**Resources**

**For more information on mucolipidosis IV:** National Organization for Rare Disorders (NORD); ML 4 Foundation; Children's Association for Research on Mucolipidosis IV; The Arc (a national organization on mental retardation); NIH/National Digestive Diseases Information Clearinghouse.

**For genetic information and genetic counseling referrals:** March of Dimes Birth Defects Foundation; Alliance of Genetic Support Groups.

**References**

The Metabolic and Molecular Basis of Inherited Disease, 7th ed.: C.R. Scriver, et al., eds.; McGraw-Hill, 1995, p. 374.

# MUCOPOLYSACCHARIDOSIS (MPS)

**Description** The mucopolysaccharidoses are a group of hereditary disorders of lysosomal storage in which enzyme deficiencies result in deposition of undegraded mucopolysaccharides in body tissues and organs. Each deficient enzyme will produce fairly specific clinical manifestations, so that diagnosis rests both on clinical and enzymatic assessment.

**Signs and Symptoms** The clinical manifestations and degree of severity of the various MPS disorders are varied, but some characteristics are shared by all: unusual facies; a progressive, chronic, and disabling course; multisystem involvement with organ enlargement; and dysostosis multiplex. Newborns may appear normal. However, in severe cases, signs of growth and mental retardation are evident at about 12 months of age. Growth may appear to stop after the age of 3 or 4 years. In mild forms of MPS, patients have normal stature. In many patients vision and hearing are impaired, as are joint mobility and cardiovascular and respiratory function. Hepatosplenomegaly occurs in most patients, and the central nervous system and brain may be affected.

For individual discussions of the following mucopolysaccharidosis disease subdivisions, see *Hurler Syndrome; Hunter Syndrome; Sanfilippo Syndrome; Morquio Syndrome; Marotaux-Lamy Syndrome; Sly Syndrome.*

| | |
|---|---|
| **MPS I-H** | Hurler Syndrome—severe form of MPS I |
| **MPS I-S** | Scheie Syndrome—mild form of MPS I |
| **MPS I-H/S** | Hurler/Scheie Syndrome |
| **MPS II (severe)** | Hunter Syndrome—severe form of MPS II |
| **MPS II (mild)** | Hunter Syndrome—mild form of MPS II |
| **MPS III-A III-B III-C III-D** | Sanfilippo Syndrome |
| **MPS IV-A IV-B** | Morquio Syndrome |
| **MPS V** | No longer used—formerly, Scheie Syndrome |
| **MPS VI** | Maroteaux-Lamy—severe, intermediate, mild |
| **MPS VII** | Sly Syndrome |

**Etiology** All the mucopolysaccharidoses have autosomal recessive inheritance except for Hunter syndrome, which is X-linked recessive. Each MPS disorder is caused by deficiency of a specific lysosomal enzyme necessary for the metabolism of dermatan sulfate, heparan sulfate, and/or keratan sulfate. These undegraded mucopolysaccharides accumulate in tissues and organs and are also excreted in the urine.

**Epidemiology** Males and females are affected equally in the mucopolysaccharidoses except for the X-linked Hunter syndrome, which only affects males.

**Related Disorders** The mucolipidoses are a family of disorders that produce symptoms and signs very much like those of MPS. See *Mucolipidosis II; Mucolipidosis III; Mucolipidosis IV.*

**Treatment—Standard** Treatment of all the mucopolysaccharidoses is symptomatic and supportive. If hernias, hydrocephalus, and vision problems occur, corrective surgery may be indicated. Physical therapy may be helpful for joint contractures. Genetic counseling will benefit families of affected patients.

**Treatment—Investigational** Treatments that are being investigated are enzyme replacement therapy and bone marrow transplantation.

Please contact the agencies listed under Resources, below, for the most current information. Addresses and telephone numbers of these agencies, as well as of individual experts and research centers, may be found in the Master Resources List.

**Resources**

**For more information on mucopolysaccharidosis:** National Organization for Rare Disorders (NORD); National Mucopolysaccharidoses Society; Society of MPS Diseases; Society of Mucopolysaccharide Diseases; The Arc (a national organization on mental retardation); NIH/National Digestive Diseases Information Clearinghouse; Joseph Muenzer, M.D., Ph.D., University of North Carolina.

**For genetic information and genetic counseling referrals:** March of Dimes Birth Defects Foundation; Alliance of Genetic Support Groups.

**References**

The Metabolic and Molecular Basis of Inherited Disease, 7th ed.: C.R. Scriver, et al., eds.; McGraw-Hill, 1995, pp. 2465–2494.

The Mucopolysaccharidoses and Anaesthesia: A Report of Clinical Experience: I.A. Herrick, et al.; Can. J. Anaesth., January 1988, vol. 35(1), pp. 67–73.

Mucopolysaccharidoses and Anaesthetic Risks: P. Sjögren, et al.; Acta Anaesthesiol. Scand., April 1987, vol. 31(3), pp. 214–218.

Electroretinographic Findings in the Mucopolysaccharidoses: R.C. Caruso, et al.; Ophthalmology, December 1986, vol. 93(12), pp. 1612–1616.

# MULTIPLE CARBOXYLASE DEFICIENCY

**Description** Multiple carboxylase deficiency results from impaired activity of 3 enzymes that are dependent on the vitamin biotin: propionyl CoA carboxylase, β-methylcrotonyl CoA carboxylase, and pyruvate carboxylase. This impairment causes defective organic acid metabolism. The disorder is treatable.

**Synonyms**
>Biotinidase Deficiency

**Signs and Symptoms** Multiple carboxylase deficiency is characterized by the development of an erythematous rash, ataxia, alopecia, seizures, neuroirritability, and lactic acidosis. Other symptoms and signs that may occur are hypotonia and immune system impairment. Additionally, poor muscle coordination associated with ataxia and impaired physical development are seen. Hearing loss also may develop.

Multiple carboxylase deficiency is diagnosed by testing the urine for metabolites that indicate deficiency in the carboxylase enzymes.

**Etiology** Multiple carboxylase deficiency is an autosomal recessive hereditary disorder caused by a defect in the enzyme biotinidase, which has been mapped to chromosome 3p25.

**Epidemiology** The onset of multiple carboxylase deficiency usually occurs at about 3 months of age. Males and females are affected in equal numbers.

**Treatment—Standard** Treatment is with oral biotin supplements. *It is imperative that treatment be started as soon as the diagnosis is made.* With biotin treatment, symptoms of the disorder disappear.

Genetic counseling is recommended for families of affected children.

**Treatment—Investigational** Please contact the agencies listed under Resources, below, for the most current information. Addresses and telephone numbers of these agencies, as well as of individual experts and research centers, may be found in the Master Resources List.

**Resources**
>**For more information on multiple carboxylase deficiency:** National Organization for Rare Disorders (NORD); NIH/National Digestive Diseases Information Clearinghouse; Research Trust for Metabolic Diseases in Children.

**References**
Disorders of Biotin Metabolism: B. Wolf; *in* The Metabolic and Molecular Basis of Inherited Disease, 7th ed.: C.R. Scriver, et al., eds.; McGraw-Hill, 1995, pp. 3151–3177.

Disorders of Amino Acid Metabolism: J. Thoene; *in* Internal Medicine, 4th ed.: J. Stein, ed.-in-chief; C.V. Mosby Company, 1994, p. 1469.

# MULTIPLE SULFATASE DEFICIENCY

**Description** Multiple sulfatase deficiency is a very rare hereditary metabolic disorder characterized by impairment of several sulfatase enzymes, leading to ichthyosis and corneal opacities, with severe neurologic and skeletal abnormalities also occurring.

**Synonyms**
>Mucosulfatidosis
>Sulfatidosis, Juvenile, Austin Type

**Signs and Symptoms** Manifestations of multiple sulfatase deficiency usually become apparent during the 1st or 2nd year of life. Development of walking and speech are abnormal. Other characteristics include a depressed bridge of the nose, large head circumference, deafness, pectus excavatum, and spinal abnormalities. The sella turcica may be J-shaped, and the phalanges broader than normal. Hepatomegaly and splenomegaly are often seen, and ichthyosis is a common finding.

Laboratory tests show abnormal bone marrow cells and white blood cells. The levels of urinary dermatan sulfate and heparan sulfate are elevated, and deficiencies of various other sulfatase enzymes are observed.

**Etiology** The disorder is transmitted as an autosomal recessive trait. The metabolic error is deficiency of arylsulfatases A, B, and C; 2 steroid sulfatases; and 4 other sulfatases required for the metabolism of mucopolysaccharides. Possibly the disease results from a mutual post-translational modification of all the affected enzymes.

**Epidemiology** Multiple sulfatase deficiency is present at birth, although symptoms typically only become noticeable during the first 2 years of life. The disorder affects males and females in equal numbers.

**Related Disorders** See *Maroteaux-Lamy Syndrome; Leukodystrophy, Metachromatic; Ichthyosis.*

**Treatment—Standard** Orthopedic management is recommended for spinal abnormalities. Dermatologic symptoms can be alleviated by the application of emollients such as petroleum jelly after bathing. Twelve percent ammonium lactate lotion has also been used effectively to treat the skin lesions.

**Treatment—Investigational** Please contact the agencies listed under Resources, below, for the most current information. Addresses and telephone numbers of these agencies, as well as of individual experts and research centers, may be found in the Master Resources List.

**Resources**

**For more information on multiple sulfatase deficiency:** National Organization for Rare Disorders (NORD); NIH/National Institute of Neurological Disorders and Stroke; National Tay-Sachs and Allied Diseases Association; Research Trust for Metabolic Diseases in Children; Association Européenne contre les Leucodystrophies.

**For genetic information and genetic counseling referrals:** March of Dimes Birth Defects Foundation; Alliance of Genetic Support Groups.

**References**

The Metabolic and Molecular Basis of Inherited Disease, 7th ed.: C.R. Scriver, et al., eds.; McGraw-Hill, 1995, pp. 2693–2739.

Therapeutic Activity of Lactate 12% Lotion in the Treatment of Ichthyosis: Active Versus Vehicle and Active Versus a Petroleum Cream: M. Buxman, et al.; J. Am. Acad. Dermatol., December 1986, vol. 15(6), pp. 1253–1258.

# N-ACETYL GLUTAMATE SYNTHETASE (NAGS) DEFICIENCY

**Description** NAGS deficiency is the most recently described and rarest of the hereditary urea cycle disorders. These disorders are caused by a deficiency of one of the enzymes needed for the synthesis of urea from ammonia. The deficiencies result in hyperammonemia. Untreated, this disorder leads to brain damage, coma, and eventually death.

**Synonyms**

Inborn Errors of Urea Synthesis

Urea Cycle Disorder

**Signs and Symptoms** NAGS deficiency is characterized in infants by hyperammonemia. Manifestations include anorexia, vomiting, and hepatomegaly. The diagnosis is suspected if hyperammonemia is present, if citrulline is absent in plasma, and if there is a low level of orotic acid in the urine. Confirmation requires measurement of the enzyme in the liver. Immediate treatment after diagnosis in newborns is imperative.

**Etiology** This condition is inherited as an autosomal recessive hereditary disorder in which the activity of N-acetyl glutamate synthetase is deficient. Its product, N-acetyl-L-glutamate, is required for activation of the enzyme carbamyl phosphate synthetase. This secondary deficiency causes an accumulation of excess ammonia in blood and body tissues.

**Epidemiology** Fewer than 100 individuals in the United States are known to have this disorder. Males and females are affected equally.

**Related Disorders** The symptoms of all urea cycle disorders result from hyperammonemia, in varying degrees of severity. See *Carbamyl Phosphate Synthetase (CPS) Deficiency; Ornithine Transcarbamylase (OTC) Deficiency; Citrullinemia; Argininosuccinic Aciduria; Arginase Deficiency.*

See also *Reye Syndrome.*

**Organic acidemias** may be accompanied by hyperammonemia associated with metabolic acidosis, with an increased anion gap and/or ketonuria. These disorders are also of genetic origin and affect the urea cycle as a secondary phenomenon.

**Treatment—Standard** Diagnostic testing should begin as soon as a urea cycle disorder is suspected. These tests should include measurement of pH and determination of plasma levels of ammonia, amino acids, and bicarbonate. Treatment of hyperammonemia should be started before test results are available, to prevent coma or brain damage.

Immediate dialysis or exchange transfusion to treat hyperammonemia due to N-acetyl glutamate synthetase deficiency in the newborn is imperative.

The orphan drug benzoate/phenylacetate (Ucephan, manufactured by McGaw Laboratories) has been approved for use in the prevention and treatment of hyperammonemia in patients with urea cycle enzymopathy due to enzyme deficiencies.

Hemodialysis or exchange transfusion should also be initiated. Two new investigational drugs—sodium benzoate and sodium phenylacetate—are used to enhance nitrogen excretion.

**Treatment—Investigational** Saul Brusilow, M.D., of Johns Hopkins Medical School is developing sodium phenyl-butyrate, which does not have the offensive smell of phenylacetate.

Please contact the agencies listed under Resources, below, for the most current information. Addresses and telephone numbers of these agencies, as well as of individual experts and research centers, may be found in the Master Resources List.

**Resources**

**For more information on N-acetyl glutamate synthetase deficiency:** National Organization for Rare Disorders (NORD); National Urea Cycle Disorders Foundation; NIH/National Digestive Diseases Information Clearinghouse; Saul Brusilow, M.D., Johns Hopkins Hospital; National Kidney Foundation; American Kidney Fund; Research Trust for Metabolic Diseases in Children.

**For genetic information and genetic counseling referrals:** March of Dimes Birth Defects Foundation; Alliance of Genetic Support Groups.

**References**

The Metabolic and Molecular Basis of Inherited Disease, 7th ed.: C.R. Scriver, et al., eds.; McGraw-Hill, 1995, pp. 1206–1207.

Disorders of the Urea Cycle: S.W. Brusilow; Hosp. Pract., October 15, 1985, vol. 305, pp. 65–72.

Symptomatic Inborn Errors of Metabolism in the Neonate: S.W. Brusilow and D.L. Vallee; *in* Current Therapy in Neonatal-Perinatal Medicine, Marcel Decker, 1985, pp. 207–212.

# NIEMANN-PICK DISEASE

**Description** Niemann-Pick disease is characterized by the accumulation of sphingomyelin and lipids in many organs. A recent classification divides the group into 2 major categories based on etiology: type A and type B. Both disorders result from acid sphingomyelinase deficiency.

**Synonyms**

Lipid Histiocytosis

Sphingomyelin Lipidosis

**Signs and Symptoms** Certain characteristics are shared by both types A and B: different degrees of hepatosplenomegaly and formation of foam cells in bone marrow; and disparate, increased amounts of sphingomyelin, cholesterol, glycosphingolipids, and bis(monoacylglycero)-phosphate in the large thoracic and abdominal organs.

The acute form, or **type A,** is the more common. Prenatal lipid storage has occurred. Sphingomyelinase activity is deficient, and hepatosplenomegaly and nervous system abnormalities are evident in patients ranging in age from 6 months to 1 year. Other characteristics include vomiting, diarrhea, failure to thrive, pyrexia, bright red spots in the macula, and skin discoloration. Progression is rapid in type A, with death usually occurring before age 5 years.

**Type B** has minimal central nervous system involvement and permits survival to adulthood, albeit with pulmonary complications.

**Etiology** The inheritance of all forms of Niemann-Pick disease appears to be autosomal recessive. Acid sphingomyelinase is located on chromosome 11p15.1–11p15.4.

**Epidemiology** This group of diseases is rare. It has been identified in persons of all races, but the incidence of type A appears to be greater in families of Jewish ancestry.

**Related Disorders** See *Refsum Syndrome; Tay-Sachs Disease; Sandhoff Disease; Gaucher Disease; Batten Disease; Leigh Disease; Kufs Disease.*

**Treatment—Standard** Treatment is supportive and symptomatic.

**Treatment—Investigational** Bone marrow transplantation is being investigated for some forms of Niemann-Pick disease.

Please contact the agencies listed under Resources, below, for the most current information. Addresses and telephone numbers of these agencies, as well as of individual experts and research centers, may be found in the Master Resources List.

**Resources**

**For more information on Niemann-Pick disease:** National Organization for Rare Disorders (NORD); National Tay-Sachs and Allied Diseases Association; National Lipid Diseases Foundation; NIH/National Institute of Neurological Disorders and Stroke; Research Trust for Metabolic Diseases in Children.

**For genetic information and genetic counseling referrals:** March of Dimes Birth Defects Foundation; Alliance of Genetic Support Groups.

**References**

The Metabolic and Molecular Basis of Inherited Disease, 7th ed.: C.R. Scriver, et al., eds.; McGraw-Hill, 1995, pp. 2601–2624.

Adult Onset Niemann-Pick Disease Type C Presenting with Dementia and Absent Organomegaly: C.M. Hulette, et al.; Clin. Neuropathol., November–December 1992, vol. 11(6), pp. 293–297.

Bone Marrow Transplantation for Niemann-Pick Type 1A Disease: E. Bayever, et al.; J. Inherit. Metab. Dis., 1992, vol. 15(6), pp. 919–928.

Cecil Textbook of Medicine, 19th ed.: J.B. Wyngaarden, et al., eds.; W.B. Saunders Company, 1992, pp. 1093–1094.

Identification and Expression of a Common Missense Mutation (L302P) in the Acid Sphingomyelinase Gene of Ashkenazi Jewish Type A Niemann-Pick Disease Patients: O. Levran, et al.; Blood, October 1992, vol. 80(8), pp. 2081–2087.

Mendelian Inheritance in Man, 10th ed.: V.A. McKusick; The Johns Hopkins University Press, 1992, pp. 1597–1600.

Nelson Textbook of Pediatrics, 14th ed.: R.E. Behrman, ed.-in-chief; W.B. Saunders Company, 1992, pp. 347–348.

Ophthalmologic Manifestations of Type B Niemann-Pick Diseases: M.R. Filling-Katz, et al.; Metab. Pediatr. Syst. Ophthalmol., 1992, vol. 15(1–3), pp. 16–20.

Prenatal Diagnosis of Niemann-Pick Type C Disease: Current Strategy from an Experience of 37 Pregnancies at Risk: M.F. Peyrat, et al., Am. J. Hum. Genet., July 1992, vol. 51(1), pp. 111–122.

Birth Defects Encyclopedia: M.L Buyse, ed.-in-chief; Blackwell Scientific Publications, 1990, pp. 1252–1253.

# Nonketotic Hyperglycinemia

**Description** Nonketotic hyperglycinemia is a genetic disorder characterized by a defect in glycine metabolism. Severe illness usually occurs soon after birth and may be fatal. Surviving patients become mentally retarded and may develop seizures.

**Synonyms**

Nonketotic Glycinemia

**Signs and Symptoms** Affected newborns may appear normal for the first day or two, after which they become listless and may have seizures. Progression is rapid. The neonate feeds poorly. In some cases vomiting occurs, and the patient fails to thrive. Apnea is fatal without support, and most infants die in these early days. Patients who survive this early period usually develop seizures (generally myoclonic, sometimes grand mal) and are severely mentally retarded, although some patients have a milder course. Other manifestations include opisthotonos and hiccuping.

The amount of glycine in plasma, urine, and cerebrospinal fluid is extremely high (approximately 1,000 µM in plasma).

**Etiology** Nonketotic hyperglycinemia is an autosomal recessive disorder caused by a defective glycine cleavage enzyme. The enzyme is coded for by genes located on both chromosome 9p13 and 3p21.2–p21.1.

**Epidemiology** Males and females are affected in equal numbers.

**Related Disorders** See *Acidemia, Isovaleric; Acidemia, Methylmalonic; Acidemia, Propionic; Glutaricaciduria II; Maple Syrup Urine Disease.*

**Treatment—Standard** Sodium benzoate can sometimes be effective in improving the clinical condition. Other treatment is symptomatic and supportive. Genetic counseling is recommended for families of affected children.

**Treatment—Investigational** Please contact the agencies listed under Resources, below, for the most current information. Addresses and telephone numbers of these agencies, as well as of individual experts and research centers, may be found in the Master Resources List.

**Resources**

**For more information on nonketotic hyperglycinemia:** National Organization for Rare Disorders (NORD); Organic Acidemia Association; British Organic Acidemia Association; The Arc (a national organization on mental retardation); NIH/National Digestive Diseases Information Clearinghouse; Research Trust for Metabolic Diseases in Children.

**For genetic information and genetic counseling referrals:** March of Dimes Birth Defects Foundation; Alliance of Genetic Support Groups.

**References**

The Metabolic and Molecular Basis of Inherited Disease, 7th ed.: C.R. Scriver, et al., eds.; McGraw-Hill, 1995, pp. 1337–1348.

The Effectiveness of Benzoate in the Management of Seizures in Nonketotic Hyperglicinemia: J.A. Wolff, et al.; Amer. J. Dis. Child, June 1986, vol. 140(6), pp. 596–602.

Nonketotic Hyperglycinemia: Treatment with Diazepam–A Competitor for Glycine Receptors: R. Matalon, et al.; Pediatrics, April 1983, vol. 71(4), pp. 581–584.

# ORNITHINE TRANSCARBAMYLASE (OTC) DEFICIENCY

**Description** OTC deficiency is 1 of 6 hereditary urea cycle disorders that are caused by a deficiency of one of the enzymes needed for the synthesis of urea from ammonia. The deficiencies cause an excess of ammonia in the blood and body tissues.

**Synonyms**

> Hyperammonemia Type II
> Inborn Errors of Urea Synthesis
> Ornithine Carbamoyl Transferase Deficiency
> Ornithine Carbamyl Transferase Deficiency
> Urea Cycle Disorder

**Signs and Symptoms** The disorder is characterized by hyperammonemia, anorexia, vomiting, drowsiness, seizures, and coma. Hepatomegaly may be present. Diagnosis is based on finding a high level of orotate in the urine, which distinguishes OTC deficiency from carbamyl phosphate synthetase deficiency. Citrulline is absent in the plasma.

Immediate treatment after diagnosis is imperative. If left untreated, brain damage and coma usually occur, and death may ensue.

**Etiology** OTC deficiency is an X-linked hereditary disorder at locus Xp2.1. Affected males (hemizygotes) have catastrophic symptoms, whereas heterozygotic females have a much milder course. Approximately one-third of cases may be due to a new mutation in the gene responsible for the deficiency. Deficiency of ornithine transcarbamylase results in an accumulation of excess ammonia in blood and body tissues.

**Epidemiology** Fewer than 100 persons in the United States have the disorder; it occurs in approximately 1:25,000 births. Onset of symptoms in males is during the first few days of life. Females who carry the mutant gene are usually asymptomatic. Some women who are OTC carriers may not experience hyperammonemia until during pregnancy or delivery.

**Related Disorders** The symptoms of all urea cycle disorders result from hyperammonemia, in varying degrees of severity. See *N-Acetyl Glutamate Synthetase (NAGS) Deficiency; Carbamyl Phosphate Synthetase (CPS) Deficiency; Citrullinemia; Argininosuccinic Aciduria; Arginase Deficiency.*

See also *Reye Syndrome.*

**Organic acidemias** may be accompanied by hyperammonemia associated with metabolic acidosis, with an increased anion gap and/or ketonuria. These disorders are also of genetic origin and affect the urea cycle as a secondary phenomenon.

**Treatment—Standard** Diagnostic testing should begin as soon as a urea cycle disorder is suspected. These tests should include measurement of pH and determination of plasma levels of ammonia, amino acids, and bicarbonate. Treatment of hyperammonemia should be started before test results are available, to prevent coma or brain damage.

Immediate dialysis or exchange transfusion after diagnosis of OTC deficiency in male newborns is imperative.

The orphan drug benzoate/phenylacetate (Ucephan, manufactured by McGaw Laboratories) has been approved for use in the prevention and treatment of hyperammonemia in patients with urea cycle enzymopathy due to enzyme deficiencies.

Genetic counseling is imperative for the family of children with OTC Deficiency.

**Treatment—Investigational** Saul Brusilow, M.D., Johns Hopkins Hospital, is developing sodium (or calcium) phenylbutyrate, which does not have the offensive smell of the other drugs used.

Please contact the agencies listed under Resources, below, for the most current information. Addresses and telephone numbers of these agencies, as well as of individual experts and research centers, may be found in the Master Resources List.

**Resources**

**For more information on ornithine transcarbamylase deficiency:** National Organization for Rare Disorders (NORD); National Urea Cycle Disorders Foundation; NIH/National Digestive Diseases Information Clearinghouse; Saul Brusilow, M.D., Johns Hopkins Hospital; National Kidney Foundation; British Organic Acidemia Association; Research Trust for Metabolic Diseases in Children.

**For genetic information and genetic counseling referrals:** March of Dimes Birth Defects Foundation; Alliance of Genetic Support Groups.

**References**

The Metabolic and Molecular Basis of Inherited Disease, 7th ed.: C.R. Scriver, et al., eds.; McGraw-Hill, 1995, pp. 1187–1232.
Allopurinol Challenge Test in Children: A.B. Burlina; J. Inherit. Metab. Dis., 1992, vol. 15(5), pp. 707–712.
Cecil Textbook of Medicine, 19th ed.: J.B. Wyngaarden, et al., eds.; W.B. Saunders Company, 1992, pp. 1105, 1118.
Mendelian Inheritance in Man, 10th ed.: V.A. McKusick; The Johns Hopkins University Press, 1992, pp. 1937–1942.
A Case Study: Urea Cycle Disorder: M.M. Gallagher; Neonatal Netw., September 1991, vol. 10(2), pp. 35–44.
Birth Defects Encyclopedia: M.L Buyse, ed.-in-chief; Blackwell Scientific Publications, 1990, pp. 1307–1308.

# PEPCK Deficiency, Mitochondrial and Cytosolic

**Description** PEPCK is present as distinct isoforms in both ctysol and mitochondria. Deficiency in either enzyme results in an extremely rare disorder of carbohydrate metabolism characterized by failure of gluconeogenesis and lactic acidosis.

**Synonyms**

Phosphoenolpyruvate Carboxykinase Deficiency, Mitochondrial or Cytosolic

**Signs and Symptoms** Major symptoms are lactic acidosis, hypotonia, hypoglycemia, hepatomegaly, and failure to thrive. The course of this disorder can be very rapid. One patient with mitochondrial PEPCK deficiency was reported to have peripheral edema, hepatic dysfunction, and fever. It is not known whether these symptoms are related to the disorder.

Diagnosis of PEPCK deficiency can be made shortly after birth by biochemical analysis of fibroblasts.

**Etiology** Mitochondrial PEPCK deficiency is inherited as an autosomal recessive trait.

**Epidemiology** Mitochondrial PEPCK deficiency affects males and females in equal numbers.

**Related Disorders** See *Korsakoff Syndrome; Leigh Disease; Pyruvate Carboxylase Deficiency; Pyruvate Dehydrogenase (PDH) Deficiency.*

**Treatment—Standard** Treatment is symptomatic and supportive. Genetic counseling may be of benefit for patients and their families.

**Treatment—Investigational** Treatment of severe lactic acidosis with dichloroacetate appears to improve certain laboratory tests but does not result in improvement of symptoms.

Please contact the agencies listed under Resources, below, for the most current information. Addresses and telephone numbers of these agencies, as well as of individual experts and research centers, may be found in the Master Resources List.

**Resources**

**For more information on mitochondrial and cytosolic PEPCK deficiency:** National Organization for Rare Disorders (NORD); Mitochondrial Disorders Foundation of America; Lactic Acidosis Support Group; Research Trust for Metabolic Diseases in Children; NIH/National Digestive Diseases Information Clearinghouse.

**For genetic information and genetic counseling referrals:** March of Dimes Birth Defects Foundation; Alliance of Genetic Support Groups.

**References**

Controlled Clinical Trial of Dichloroacetate for Treatment of Lactic Acidosis in Adults: P.W. Stacpoole, et al.; N. Engl. J. Med., November 26, 1992, vol. 327(22), pp. 1564–1569.

Mendelian Inheritance in Man, 9th ed.: V.A. McKusick; The Johns Hopkins University Press, 1990, p. 1421.

The Metabolic Basis of Inherited Disease, 6th ed.: C.R. Scriver, et al., eds.; McGraw-Hill, 1989, pp. 878–879.

# Phenylketonuria (PKU)

**Description** PKU is a metabolic disorder caused by a deficiency of the enzyme phenylalanine hydroxylase. The interrupted metabolism of dietary phenylalanine results in accumulation of the amino acid in body fluids, resulting in progressive, severe, irreversible mental retardation.

**Synonyms**

Fölling Disease

Phenylalaninemia

Phenylpyruvic Oligophrenia

**Signs and Symptoms** Infants are normal at birth, and phenylpyruvic acid, a phenylalanine metabolite, may not be found in the urine during the first days of life. Some neonates may be lethargic and feed poorly. Other manifestations in infants include vomiting, irritability, an eczematoid skin rash, and a musty or mousy body odor that is caused by phenylacetic acid in the urine and perspiration.

In untreated children, retarded development may be evident at several months of age, and patients are often short for their age. Because high concentrations of phenylalanine interfere with melanin production, affected individuals are almost always light-haired with a fair complexion. Craniofacial abnormalities in untreated children include microcephaly, prominent maxilla, widely spaced teeth, and impaired development of dental enamel. Skin coarsening may occur. Occasionally bone decalcification, syndactyly, and flat feet are present.

It is not understood why high levels of phenylalanine cause severe mental retardation in children. The average IQ of untreated children is less than 50, and these patients have to be institutionalized as adults. Heterozygotic children of women with PKU often have severe mental retardation.

Neurologic findings are present only in some patients, and vary. Seizures occur in about 25 percent of older children, and EEG abnormalities in 80 percent. Spasticity, hypertonicity, and increased deep tendon reflexes are among the most frequent neurologic manifestations; about 5 percent of children thus affected become physically disabled. Athetosis and tremors have been seen. Nervous system myelinization seems to be delayed but not absent.

In adulthood, the sperm count of affected males may be low. Females often have spontaneous abortions and intrauterine growth retardation. Children of women with PKU may have microcephaly and congenital heart disease, as well as the mental retardation mentioned above. There appears to be some correlation between the severity of these manifestations and the mother's plasma level of phenylalanine.

**Laboratory findings:** Plasma levels of phenylalanine are 10 to 60 times normal; plasma tyrosine is low; and levels of phenylalanine metabolites such as phenylpyruvic acid and other phenolic acids excreted in the urine are high. Substances such as dopamine, serotonin, and melanin are reduced.

Many studies demonstrate that PKU patients who are treated with a low-phenylalanine diet before 3 months of age do well, with mean IQs of 100 (see Treatment—Standard, below).

There are several variants of PKU **(hyperphenylalaninemias),** which are characterized by elevated plasma phenylalanine levels that are not so high as those in classical PKU. For example, in tetrahydrobiopterin deficiency, neurologic deterioration occurs even when phenylalanine levels are controlled (see Etiology, below).

Prenatal diagnosis is available, and routine neonatal screening is required by law in all 50 states and in virtually all hospitals in developed countries.

**Etiology** PKU has an autosomal recessive inheritance. The defective gene that causes the disorder is located at 12q22–24.1. The condition is caused by a defect of phenylalanine hydroxylase, a liver enzyme that catalyses the hydroxylation of phenylalanine to tyrosine. The other forms of hyperphenylalaninemia, which are clinically and biochemically distinct from PKU, result from an enzyme complex, of which varying members may be deficient.

The mechanism of mental retardation in PKU is not known. Normal brain development may be disturbed by a high phenylalanine concentration. Impairment of brain myelinization has been suggested, as well as disturbed neuronal migration in the first 6 months of life.

High plasma phenylalanine levels may also be caused by tetrahydrobiopterin deficiency, possibly resulting from insufficient amounts of either biopterin or dihydropterin reductase. Since tetrahydrobiopterin is involved in the production of serotonin, dopamine, and norephrine, for example, a deficiency of these neurotransmitters may be the reason for the continued neurologic deterioration in spite of controlled plasma phenylalanine. (See also *Tetrahydrobiopterin Deficiencies.)*

**Epidemiology** Phenylketonuria occurs in 1:11,600 live births in the United States. Males and females are affected equally. The disorder is found in most racial groups, although it is rarer in blacks and Ashkenazic Jews.

**Related Disorders** Phenylketonuria belongs to the group of disorders caused by defective amino acid metabolism.

**Treatment—Standard** The goal of treatment, to keep plasma phenylalanine levels within the normal range, can be achieved through diet. Limiting the child's intake of phenylalanine, however, must be done cautiously, because it is an essential amino acid. A carefully maintained dietary regimen can prevent mental retardation and neurologic, behavioral, dermatologic, and EEG abnormalities. Treatment must be started at a very young age (under 3 months), however, or some degree of mental retardation may be expected. If it is begun after the age of 2 or 3 years, only hyperactivity and seizures may be controlled. If patients are subsequently allowed to stop controlling their phenylalanine intake, neurologic changes occur in adolescence and adulthood. Their IQs may decline after a peak at the end of the controlled diet periods. Other problems that may appear and become severe once the patient is off the diet include academic and behavioral problems, poor visual-motor coordination, poor problem-solving skills, low developmental age, and the onset of EEG abnormalities.

There is some controversy over the age at which dietary treatment can be discontinued, but it begins to be clear that high phenylalanine levels continue to harm even after brain myelinization is complete. Phenylalanine intake should therefore probably be limited indefinitely, with possibly some relaxation of dietary control.

Since phenylalanine occurs in almost all natural proteins, maintaining proper nutrition is impossible on a low-phenylalanine diet. Dietary use of special phenylalanine-free preparations is therefore essential. These include Lofenalac (for a low-phenylalanine diet) and Phenyl-Free, both from Mead Johnson. Low-protein foods such as fruits, vegetables, and some cereals are allowed.

As mentioned above, phenylalanine intake must not be too severely limited or phenylalanine deficiency may develop, resulting in anorexia, fatigue, aggressive behavior, and sometimes anemia. Both the child's behavior and plasma levels of phenylalanine and its metabolites must be monitored regularly.

Mild forms of PKU appear to require no treatment. See also *Tetrahydrobiopterin Deficiencies.*

**Treatment—Investigational** See also *Tetrahydrobiopterin Deficiencies.*

Attempts are being made to develop improved medical foods for affected adults.

Tetrahydro-L-biopterin dihydrochloride is available for the experimental treatment. Please contact Joseph Muenzer, M.D., Ph.D., University of North Carolina.

Please contact the agencies listed under Resources, below, for the most current information. Addresses and telephone numbers of these agencies, as well as of individual experts and research centers, may be found in the Master Resources List.

**Resources**

**For more information on phenylketonuria:** National Organization for Rare Disorders (NORD); Phenylketonuria Parents; National Phenylketonuria Foundation; NIH/National Institute of Child Health and Human Development; The Arc (a national association on mental retardation); National Institute on Mental Retardation.

**For genetic information and genetic counseling referrals:** March of Dimes Birth Defects Foundation; Alliance of Genetic Support Groups.

**References**
The Metabolic and Molecular Basis of Inherited Disease, 7th ed.: C.R. Scriver, et al., eds.; McGraw-Hill, 1995, pp. 1015–1075.
Cecil Textbook of Medicine, 19th ed.: J.B. Wyngaarden, et al., eds.; W.B. Saunders Company, 1992, pp. 1101–1102.
Mendelian Inheritance in Man, 10th ed.: V.A. McKusick; The Johns Hopkins University Press, 1992, pp. 1629–1638.
Nelson Textbook of Pediatrics, 14th ed.: R.E. Behrman, ed.-in-chief; W.B. Saunders Company, 1992, pp. 307–309.
Birth Defects Encyclopedia: M.L Buyse, ed.-in-chief; Blackwell Scientific Publications, 1990, pp. 1382–1383.
Biochemical and Neuropsychological Effects of Elevated Plasma Phenylalanine in Patients with Treated PKU: W. Krause, et al.; J. Clin. Inv., January 1985, vol. 75(1), pp. 40–48.
Loss of Intellectual Function in Children with Phenylketonuria After Relaxation of Dietary Phenylalanine Restriction: M. Seashore, et al.; Pediatrics, February 1985, vol. 75(2), pp. 226–232.
Abnormalities in Amino Acid Metabolism in Clinical Medicine: W.L. Nyhan; Appleton-Century-Crofts, 1984.
Tetrahydrobiopterin Deficiencies: Preliminary Analysis from an International Survey: J.L. Dhondt; J. Pediatr., April 1984, vol. 104(4), pp. 501–508.
Phenylketonuria and Its Variants: S. Kaufman; Adv. Hum. Genet., 1983, vol. 13, pp. 217–297.
Diet Termination in Children with Phenylketonuria. A Review of Psychological Assessments Used to Determine Outcome: S.E. Waisbren, et al.; J. Inherit. Metab. Dis., 1980, vol. 3(4), pp. 149–153.

# PHOSPHOGLYCERATE KINASE DEFICIENCY

**Description** Phosphoglycerate kinase deficiency is an extremely rare X-linked metabolic disorder characterized by chronic anemia, neurologic impairment, and muscle dysfunction.

**Synonyms**
Anemia, Hemolytic
Erythrocyte Phosphoglycerate Kinase Deficiency
Phosphoglycerokinase

**Signs and Symptoms** Symptoms are especially severe in males and include mild-to-severe neurologic dysfunction, including possible mental retardation, paralysis, seizures, kinetic disorders, behavioral problems, and severe anemia. Patients may even lapse into a coma during a crisis. Muscles may be painful, and rhabdomyolisis may occur, resulting in myoglobinuria. Weakness, fatigue, and exertional stress may also occur.

The disorder is diagnosed by measuring the amount of phosphoglycerate kinase in the erythrocytes.

**Etiology** Phosphoglycerate kinase deficiency is an X-linked inborn error of metabolism. The gene is located on the long arm of the X chromosome at Xq13.

**Epidemiology** Phosphoglycerate kinase deficiency affects both males and females. Males have the more serious form of the disorder. Approximately 12 cases have been noted in the medical literature.

**Related Disorders** See *Anemia, Hemolytic, Warm-Antibody; Anemia, Sideroblastic; Anemia, Aplastic; Anemia, Hemolytic, Cold-Antibody.*

**Treatment—Standard** Treatment consists of iron supplements and blood transfusions when needed. When there is evidence that muscle breakdown has taken place, the avoidance of strenuous exercise is very important. Special care is needed during neurologic crisis to avoid life-threatening situations. Genetic counseling may be of benefit for patients and their families. Other treatment is symptomatic and supportive.

**Therapies–Investigational** Enzyme replacement therapy is being investigated as a possible treatment for phosphoglycerate kinase deficiency.

Please contact the agencies listed under Resources, below, for the most current information. Addresses and telephone numbers of these agencies, as well as of individual experts and research centers, may be found in the Master Resources List.

**Resources**

**For more information on phosphoglycerate kinase deficiency:** National Organization for Rare Disorders (NORD); NIH/National Heart, Lung and Blood Institute Information Center; The Arc (a national organization on mental retardation); Research Trust for Metabolic Diseases in Children.

**For genetic information and genetic counseling referrals:** March of Dimes Birth Defects Foundation; Alliance of Genetic Support Groups.

**References**

The Metabolic and Molecular Basis of Inherited Disease, 7th ed.: C.R. Scriver, et al., eds.; McGraw-Hill, 1995, pp. 3496–3497.

Clonality in Myeloproliferative Disorders: Analysis by Means of the Polymerase Chain Reaction: D.G. Gilliland, et al.; Proc. Natl. Acad. Sci. USA, August 1, 1991, vol. 88(15), pp. 6848–6852.

X-Linked Sideroblastic Anemia and Ataxia: Linkage to Phosphoglycerate Kinase at Xq13: W.H. Raskind, et al.; Am. J. Hum. Genet., February 1991, vol. 48(2), pp. 335–341.

Birth Defects Encyclopedia: M.L Buyse, ed.-in-chief; Blackwell Scientific Publications, 1990, p. 127.

Hematology, 4th ed.: W.J. Williams, et al., eds.; McGraw-Hill, 1990, p. 359.

Mendelian Inheritance in Man, 9th ed.: V.A. McKusick; The Johns Hopkins University Press, 1990, pp. 1422, 1704.

Red Cell Enzymopathies of the Glycolytic Pathway: K.R. Tanaka, et al.; Semin. Hematol., April 1990, vol. 27(2), pp. 165–185.

# POMPE DISEASE

**Description** Pompe disease is a glycogen storage disease in which excessive glycogen accumulates in tissue lysosomes, particularly in the muscles. In the infantile form, the clinical result is hypotonia, with death due to respiratory and cardiac failure in the first year of life. Other, less severe, variants are known.

**Synonyms**

Acid Maltase Deficiency

Cardiomegalia Glycogenica Diffusa

Generalized Glycogenosis

α-1,4-Glucosidase Deficiency

Glycogenosis Type II

Lysosomal α-Glucosidase Deficiency

**Signs and Symptoms** Pompe disease occurs in different degrees of severity, depending on the age at onset.

In the **infantile form,** symptoms onset usually is at 2 to 5 months of age, but can occur at birth. There are problems with respiration, and severe muscle weakness without muscle wasting is noted. Cardiomegaly, hepatomegaly, and macroglossia also occur. Progressive cardiac deterioration follows, and the condition is usually fatal by 12 to 18 months of age.

In the **childhood form,** symptoms begin in late infancy or early childhood, and progression is slower than in the early infantile form. The extent of organ involvement varies. Skeletal muscle weakness is usually present, while cardiac involvement is minimal. Children usually survive into their teens.

The **adult form** usually begins in the 2nd to 4th decade, with muscle weakness typical of other chronic muscle disorders. This form of the disorder is slowly progressive and without cardiac involvement, and life expectancy is usually normal.

Prenatal diagnosis of Pompe disease is possible with amniocentesis. Diagnosis after birth can be made by measuring the level of enzyme activity in white blood cells, and by determining the glycogen content of muscle cells.

**Etiology** Pompe disease is inherited as an autosomal recessive trait. The metabolic error is an inborn lack of the enzyme acid α-1,4-glucosidase.

**Epidemiology** Pompe disease and all other glycogen storage disorders together affect fewer than 1:40,000 persons in the United States. Males and females are affected in equal numbers, and the infantile and childhood forms are more common than the adult form.

**Related Disorders** See *McArdle Disease; Glycogen Storage Disease VII; Glycogen Storage Disease III; Andersen Disease; Werdnig-Hoffmann Disease.*

**Treatment—Standard** Treatment of Pompe disease is symptomatic and supportive. Attempts at enzyme replacement have thus far not been successful. Genetic counseling may be helpful for the families of children with the disease.

**Treatment—Investigational** Please contact the agencies listed under Resources, below, for the most current information. Addresses and telephone numbers of these agencies, as well as of individual experts and research centers, may be found in the Master Resources List.

**Resources**

For more information on **Pompe disease:** National Organization for Rare Disorders (NORD); Association for Glycogen Storage Diseases; Research Trust for Metabolic Diseases in Children; NIH/National Digestive Diseases Information Clearinghouse.

For genetic information and genetic counseling referrals: March of Dimes Birth Defects Foundation; Alliance of Genetic Support Groups.

**References**

The Metabolic and Molecular Basis of Inherited Disease, 7th ed.: C.R. Scriver, et al., eds.; McGraw-Hill, 1995, pp. 935–965.

Cecil Textbook of Medicine, 18th ed.: J.B. Wyngaarden and L.H. Smith, Jr., eds.; W.B. Saunders Company, 1988, pp. 361, 1134.

# PORPHYRIA

**Description** The porphyrias are a group of disorders characterized by an overproduction of porphyrin or its precursors. The porphyrias are generally classified as hepatic or erythropoietic according to the site of porphyrinogenesis. The main clinical manifestations of these disorders are cutaneous or neurologic.

**Etiology** Four of the major porphyrias are inherited as autosomal dominant traits; 1 (porphyria cutanea tarda) can be both inherited (autosomal dominant) and acquired; and 3 are autosomal recessive. Various environmental factors, such as drugs, chemicals, food, and exposure to the sun, can precipitate acute attacks.

**Epidemiology** It is unlikely that more than one form of porphyria will occur in the same family, or that someone with one type of porphyria will develop another.

**Related Disorders** See the separate discussions of the following porphyrias: *Porphyria, Acute Intermittent; Porphyria, ALA-D; Porphyria, Congenital Erythropoietic; Porphyria Cutanea Tarda; Porphyria, Erythropoietic Protoporphyria; Porphyria, Hereditary Coproporphyria; Porphyria, Variegate.*

**Treatment—Standard** Acute attacks are treated by intravenous fluids and the administration of hematin.

In general, drugs that trigger acute attacks in persons with acute intermittent porphyria, variegate porphyria, and hereditary coproporphyria include the barbiturates, some tranquilizers and sedatives, sulfonamides, griseofulvin, antiepileptic agents, and contraceptive pills.

**Treatment—Investigational** Dr. Karl E. Anderson of the University of Texas Medical Branch has received orphan drug designation for Histrelin to treat various types of porphyria. Dr. Anderson is also conducting clinical trials on the Finnish product heme arginate (Normasang).

The orphan product hemin and zinc mesoporphyrin (HEMEX) is being used for treatment of acute porphyric syndromes. For more information, please contact Herbert L. Bonkovsky, M.D., University of Massachusetts Medical Center.

Please contact the agencies listed under Resources, below, for the most current information. Addresses and telephone numbers of these agencies, as well as of individual experts and research centers, may be found in the Master Resources List.

**Resources**

**For more information on porphyria:** National Organization for Rare Disorders (NORD); American Porphyria Foundation; NIH/National Digestive Diseases Information Clearinghouse.

**For genetic information and genetic counseling referrals:** March of Dimes Birth Defects Foundation; Alliance of Genetic Support Groups.

**References**

The Metabolic and Molecular Basis of Inherited Disease, 7th ed.: C.R. Scriver, et al., eds.; McGraw-Hill, 1995, pp. 2103–2159.

# PORPHYRIA, ACUTE INTERMITTENT (AIP)

**Description** AIP is one of the hereditary hepatic porphyrias. The enzymatic defect is a lack of porphobilinogen deaminase **(PBG-D;** uroporphyrinogen I-synthase), but other factors, such as drugs, hormones, and dietary changes, contribute to acute attacks.

**Synonyms**

Pyrroloporphyria

Swedish Porphyria

**Signs and Symptoms** The manifestations of AIP are varied and can mimic those of numerous other conditions. The finding of an increased level of urinary δ-aminolevulinic acid indicates that an acute porphyria is present; a deficiency of PBG-D in red blood cells usually establishes the diagnosis of AIP (although false positive results can occur).

Severe abdominal pain is a common symptom of the acute attack, with nausea, vomiting, and constipation. There may be pain in the back, arms, and legs, and muscle weakness. Urinary retention may occur, but urinary symptoms may also include frequency, incontinence, dysuria, and urine the color of port wine. Both hypertension and hyponatremia (from the vomiting) may occur during an acute attack. Central nervous system involvement may include confusion, hallucinations, and seizures. Neuropathy is a common symptom, and motor neuropathy may result in respiratory deficiency. The patient may feel depressed, anxious, and paranoid; porphyria has been misdiagnosed as psychosis.

The course of AIP varies; it may be chronic with few acute attacks, or there may be periods of remission alternating with acute attacks. Not all individuals who inherit this condition become symptomatic. The prognosis greatly depends on early detection and careful preventive measures.

**Etiology** AIP is inherited as an autosomal dominant trait. Environmental factors that contribute to precipitation of the acute attack include certain drugs, chemicals, and diet. These factors can greatly influence the severity of symptoms. PBG-D maps to chromosome 11q23–qter.

**Epidemiology** Symptomatic AIP is estimated to affect approximately 5:100,000 to 10:100,000 persons, most frequently those of Scandinavian, Anglo-Saxon, or German ancestry. Women are affected more often than men; in both, the disorder generally occurs after puberty.

**Related Disorders** See *Porphyria; Porphyria, ALA-D.* See also the separate discussions of the following porphyrias: *Porphyria, Congenital Erythropoietic; Porphyria Cutanea Tarda; Porphyria, Erythropoietic Protoporphyria; Porphyria, Hereditary Coproporphyria; Porphyria, Variegate.*

**Treatment—Standard** The orphan drug hematin (Panhematin) is effective in suppressing acute attacks of AIP. Newer agents such as heme arginate and Sn-protoporphyrin appear promising.

Diagnosis is essential before medications are given, since the effects of many commonly used drugs are unknown or unclear in some types of porphyria. Advice from a center specializing in porphyria is recommended regarding drug administration to these patients. A list of these institutions may be obtained from the American Porphyria Foundation. If a person is diagnosed as having acute intermittent porphyria while taking long-term medications such as tranquilizers, antiseizure drugs, or birth control pills, specialist monitoring or withdrawal of the drug may be needed.

Because acute attacks can occur with carbohydrate restriction, patients should be advised not to restrict carbohydrate and caloric intake. If weight loss is desired, consultation with a nutritionist is recommended.

Some women report premenstrual attacks of AIP that resolve with the onset of menstruation. Exogenous steroids have been used in some such cases.

Genetic counseling is recommended for individuals with AIP. Only 50 percent of an affected person's offspring will carry the gene, and many of those with the disease will remain latent for most of their lives. If the condition is identified early, preventive measures can be taken and treatment can successfully control symptoms in most cases.

Patients with symptomatic AIP should wear a Medic Alert bracelet.

**Treatment—Investigational** Dr. Karl E. Anderson of the University of Texas Medical Branch has received orphan drug designation for Histrelin to treat various types of porphyria. Dr. Anderson is also conducting clinical trials on the Finnish product heme arginate (Normasang).

The orphan product hemin and zinc mesoporphyrin (HEMEX) is being used for treatment of acute porphyric syndromes. For more information, please contact Herbert L. Bonkovsky, M.D., University of Massachusetts Medical Center.

Researchers at the Mount Sinai School of Medicine are developing a genetic test to help identify AIP patients. Blood samples from AIP patients are needed to help diagnose different genetic lesions. Please contact Dr. Cecilia Warner at the Division of Medical and Molecular Genetics.

Please contact the agencies listed under Resources, below, for the most current information. Addresses and telephone numbers of these agencies, as well as of individual experts and research centers, may be found in the Master Resources List.

**Resources**

**For more information on acute intermittent porphyria:** National Organization for Rare Disorders (NORD); American Porphyria Foundation; NIH/National Digestive Diseases Information Clearinghouse.

**For genetic information and genetic counseling referrals:** March of Dimes Birth Defects Foundation; Alliance of Genetic Support Groups.

**References**

The Metabolic and Molecular Basis of Inherited Disease, 7th ed.: C.R. Scriver, et al., eds.; McGraw-Hill, 1995, pp. 2103–2159.

# PORPHYRIA, ALA-D

**Description** ALA-D porphyria is a recently described, very rare acute hepatic porphyria. The enzymatic defect is a lack of δ-aminolevulinic acid dehydratase.

When a patient is diagnosed as having ALA-D, relatives should be examined as well, so that individuals with latent disease can avoid precipitating agents.

**Signs and Symptoms** Symptoms resemble those of acute intermittent porphyria. Severe abdominal pain is a common symptom of the acute attack, with nausea, vomiting, and constipation. Pain may also affect the extremities, and generalized muscle weakness may be present. There may be paralysis of the extremities and of the muscles of the respiratory system.

Determination of elevated urinary ALA indicates that an acute porphyria is present; if the level of erythrocyte

ALA-D is deficient in red blood cells, the diagnosis of ALA-D porphyria is usually established (although false positive and equivocal results do occur).

**Etiology** The disorder is inherited as an autosomal recessive trait. Environmental factors that contribute to precipitation of acute attacks may include certain drugs, chemicals, reduced carbohydrate intake, ingestion of alcohol, exposure to the sun, and stress. These factors can greatly influence the severity of symptoms.

**Epidemiology** ALA-D porphyria is extremely rare. There are only a few known cases.

**Related Disorders** See *Porphyria; Porphyria, Acute Intermittent.* See also the separate discussions of the following porphyrias: *Porphyria, Congenital Erythropoietic; Porphyria Cutanea Tarda; Porphyria, Erythropoietic Protoporphyria; Porphyria, Hereditary Coproporphyria; Porphyria, Variegate.*

**Treatment—Standard** Because the disorder is so rare, therapeutic experience is not extensive. ALA-D porphyria is similar to acute intermittent porphyria, and treatment should cautiously be the same: elimination of precipitating factors, routine carbohydrate intake, administration of glucose, and use of hematin. For treatment information, see *Porphyria, Acute Intermittent.*

**Treatment—Investigational** The orphan product hemin and zinc mesoporphyrin (HEMEX) is being used for treatment of acute porphyric syndromes. For more information, please contact Herbert L. Bonkovsky, M.D., University of Massachusetts Medical Center.

Please contact the agencies listed under Resources, below, for the most current information. Addresses and telephone numbers of these agencies, as well as of individual experts and research centers, may be found in the Master Resources List.

**Resources**

**For more information on ALA-D porphyria:** National Organization for Rare Disorders (NORD); American Porphyria Foundation; NIH/National Digestive Diseases Information Clearinghouse.

**For genetic information and genetic counseling referrals:** March of Dimes Birth Defects Foundation; Alliance of Genetic Support Groups.

**References**

The Metabolic and Molecular Basis of Inherited Disease, 7th ed.: C.R. Scriver, et al., eds.; McGraw-Hill, 1995, pp. 2103–2159.

# PORPHYRIA, CONGENITAL ERYTHROPOIETIC (CEP)

**Description** CEP is one of the hereditary erythropoietic porphyrias; the deficient enzyme is uroporphyrinogen III cosynthase. Levels of porphyrins are markedly increased in bone marrow, red blood cells, plasma, urine, and feces, and may also be deposited in the teeth and bones.

**Synonyms**

>    Congenital Porphyria
>    Günther Porphyria

**Signs and Symptoms** As is characteristic of the erythropoietic porphyrias, symptoms usually begin during early infancy, although cases of adult onset have been reported. The initial sign in infancy may be pink to brown diaper staining resulting from reddish urine. Skin photosensitivity may also be an early characteristic; bullae may result in bacterial infection and scarring of the damaged skin. Facial features and fingers may be lost over time. Erythrodontia, hypertrichosis, and alopecia are common. Red blood cells have a shortened life span, and anemia often results. Splenomegaly may be present.

**Etiology** CEP is inherited as an autosomal recessive trait. The metabolic error is a faulty conversion of porphobilinogen (**PBG**) to uroporphyrinogen in the erythroid cells of the bone marrow. Environmental factors that may aggravate the symptoms or provoke an acute attack include drugs, chemicals, diet, and sun exposure. These factors can greatly influence the severity of symptoms.

**Epidemiology** CEP is extremely rare, with fewer than 200 cases reported worldwide. No gender or racial predilections have been established.

**Related Disorders** See *Porphyria.* See also the separate discussions of the following porphyrias: *Porphyria, Acute Intermittent; Porphyria, ALA-D; Porphyria Cutanea Tarda; Porphyria, Erythropoietic Protoporphyria; Porphyria, Hereditary Coproporphyria; Porphyria, Variegate.*

**Treatment—Standard** Sunlight and trauma to the skin from infection and injury should be avoided. Transfusions with packed erythrocytes and splenectomy have been performed. These procedures have short-term effects on the hemolysis and porphyrin excretion but must be used with caution. Intravenous hematin and oral charcoal have also been used.

Consultation with a medical center specializing in porphyria is advisable concerning the use of drugs by these patients. Genetic counseling may be useful when appropriate.

**Treatment—Investigational** Please contact the agencies listed under Resources, below, for the most current information. Addresses and telephone numbers of these agencies, as well as of individual experts and research centers, may be found in the Master Resources List.

**Resources**

**For more information on congenital erythropoietic porphyria:** National Organization for Rare Disorders (NORD); American Porphyria Foundation; NIH/National Digestive Diseases Information Clearinghouse.

**For genetic information and genetic counseling referrals:** March of Dimes Birth Defects Foundation; Alliance of Genetic Support Groups.

**References**

The Metabolic and Molecular Basis of Inherited Disease, 7th ed.: C.R. Scriver, et al., eds.; McGraw-Hill, 1995, pp. 2103–2159.

# Porphyria Cutanea Tarda (PCT)

**Description** PCT results from an inherited or acquired deficiency of the enzyme uroporphyrinogen decarboxylase. The disorder occurs in both children and adults.

**Synonyms**

Idiosyncratic Porphyria

Porphyria Cutanea Symptomatica

**Signs and Symptoms** Initial symptoms of both inherited and acquired PCT are cutaneous, with blistering on the hands, face, and arms after exposure to sunlight or minor trauma. Hyper- and hypopigmentation, and hirsutism as well as alopecia may develop. Neurologic and abdominal symptoms are not characteristic of PCT. Liver function abnormalities are common but are generally mild.

**Etiology** PCT may be inherited as an autosomal dominant trait, or it may be acquired. The metabolic error in either case is a deficiency of the enzyme uroporphyrinogen decarboxylase (**URO-D**). In the inherited form, the enzyme is lacking in all body tissues; when acquired, the deficiency is present only in the liver. Environmental factors may include estrogens, chlorinated hydrocarbons, iron, alcohol, and of course, exposure to the sun.

**Epidemiology** PCT is the most common of the porphyrias. The inherited form generally is first seen in childhood. Acquired PCT most often occurs in adults and is more prevalent in males, although the number of affected females is increasing. In males, onset is usually in the 4th decade of life.

**Related Disorders** See *Porphyria.* See also the separate discussions of the following porphyrias: ***Porphyria, Acute Intermittent; Porphyria, ALA-D; Porphyria, Congenital Erythropoietic; Porphyria, Erythropoietic Protoporphyria; Porphyria, Hereditary Coproporphyria; Porphyria, Variegate.***

**Treatment—Standard** Precipitating factors (see Etiology, above) must be avoided. Phlebotomy or, alternatively, chloroquine has been used to treat PCT.

**Treatment—Investigational** Dr. Karl E. Anderson of the University of Texas Medical Branch has received a grant from the Food and Drug Administration for investigation of the orphan drug erythropoietin in the treatment of PCT in patients on long-term hemodialysis.

The orphan product hemin and zinc mesoporphyrin (HEMEX) is being used for treatment of acute porphyric syndromes. For more information, please contact Herbert L. Bonkovsky, M.D., University of Massachusetts Medical Center.

Please contact the agencies listed under Resources, below, for the most current information. Addresses and telephone numbers of these agencies, as well as of individual experts and research centers, may be found in the Master Resources List.

**Resources**

**For more information on porphyria cutanea tarda:** National Organization for Rare Disorders (NORD); American Porphyria Foundation; NIH/National Digestive Diseases Information Clearinghouse.

**For genetic information and genetic counseling referrals:** March of Dimes Birth Defects Foundation; Alliance of Genetic Support Groups.

**References**

The Metabolic and Molecular Basis of Inherited Disease, 7th ed.: C.R. Scriver, et al., eds.; McGraw-Hill, 1995, pp. 2103–2159.

# Porphyria, Erythropoietic Protoporphyria (EPP)

**Description** EPP is characterized by a deficiency of ferrochelatase, which leads to an accumulation of protoporphyrin in the plasma, in red blood cells, and sometimes in the liver. Excess protoporphyrin is excreted by the liver into the bile, which in turn enters the intestine and is excreted in the feces. There are no urinary abnormalities associated with EPP.

**Synonyms**
> Erythrohepatic Protoporphyria
> Protoporphyria

**Signs and Symptoms** Symptoms begin in childhood and are mostly related to photosensitivity. After exposure to artificial light as well as sunlight, patients may experience burning, itching, edema, and erythema. Occasionally, the skin problems occur only after extended sunlight exposure. In some cases lesions occur that persist for days or weeks and leave a scar. Severe sequelae such as bullae, hyperpigmentation, and mutilation are not common. The cutaneous manifestations of EPP tend to be more severe in the summer and can recur throughout life.

Other manifestations of this type of porphyria include gallstones containing protoporphyrin, and, occasionally, the development of severe hepatic complications. Some carriers of the genetic abnormality remain asymptomatic and have normal porphyrin levels.

The diagnosis is established by identification of increased protoporphyrin in the red blood cells, plasma, and feces.

**Etiology** EPP is inherited as an autosomal dominant trait. The ferrochelatase gene has been mapped to chromosome 18q.

**Epidemiology** Erythropoietic protoporphyria usually begins in childhood, affecting males and females in equal numbers.

**Related Disorders** See *Porphyria*. See also the separate discussions of the following porphyrias: ***Porphyria, Acute Intermittent; Porphyria, ALA-D; Porphyria, Congenital Erythropoietic; Porphyria Cutanea Tarda; Porphyria, Hereditary Coproporphyria; Porphyria, Variegate.***

**Treatment—Standard** Exposure to the sun and some artificial light, especially theater lighting, should be avoided. Beta-carotene may improve sunlight tolerance. Cholestyramine may be photoprotective to some extent and reduces hepatic protoporphyrin.

Hepatic deposits of protoporphyrin may lead to liver abnormalities in patients with EPP. Although hepatic involvement is not common, when it occurs it is severe, and avoidance of hepatotoxic agents is recommended.

It is advisable to consult with a center specializing in the treatment of porphyria before administering any drug to a patient with EPP. Genetic counseling may be useful, since pregnancy is tolerated much better than was formerly believed.

**Treatment—Investigational** The orphan product L-cysteine (manufactured by Tyson and Associates) is being tested for the prevention and lessening of photosensitivity in EPP.

Please contact the agencies listed under Resources, below, for the most current information. Addresses and telephone numbers of these agencies, as well as of individual experts and research centers, may be found in the Master Resources List.

**Resources**
**For more information on erythropoietic protoporphyria porphyria:** National Organization for Rare Disorders (NORD); American Porphyria Foundation; NIH/National Digestive Diseases Information Clearinghouse.

**For genetic information and genetic counseling referrals:** March of Dimes Birth Defects Foundation; Alliance of Genetic Support Groups.

**References**
The Metabolic and Molecular Basis of Inherited Disease, 7th ed.: C.R. Scriver, et al., eds.; McGraw-Hill, 1995, pp. 2139–2141.

# Porphyria, Hereditary Coproporphyria (HCP)

**Description** HCP, an inherited hepatic porphyria, is due to deficiency of coproporphyrinogen oxidase, and is similar to acute intermittent porphyria **(AIP),** but with milder symptoms and with the additional characteristic in some patients of photosensitivity.

**Signs and Symptoms** Although the patient is sensitive to sunlight, skin disease is rarely severe in HCP. The characteristic features of AIP are present here in milder form and include pain in the abdomen, arms, and legs; generalized weakness that may result in respiratory paralysis; urinary retention; vomiting; constipation; increased heart rate; confusion; hallucinations; psychosis; and seizures.

The diagnosis is established by identification of excess coproporphyrin in urine and stool.

**Etiology** HCP is inherited as an autosomal dominant trait. Symptoms are the result of a deficiency of coproporphyrinogen oxidase. Drugs such as barbiturates, tranquilizers, anticonvulsants, and estrogens may precipitate an attack, as may diet and sun exposure.

**Epidemiology** HCP is the least common of the hepatic porphyrias. Onset may be at any age. Males and females are affected in equal numbers.

**Related Disorders** See *Porphyria; Porphyria, Acute Intermittent.* See also the separate discussions of the following porphyrias: *Porphyria, ALA-D; Porphyria, Congenital Erythropoietic; Porphyria Cutanea Tarda; Porphyria, Erythropoietic Protoporphyria; Porphyria, Variegate.*

**Treatment—Standard** Precipitating factors must be avoided. For treatment information, see *Porphyria, Acute Intermittent.*

**Treatment—Investigational** Dr. Karl E. Anderson of the University of Texas Medical Branch has received orphan drug designation for Histrelin to treat various types of porphyria. Dr. Anderson is also conducting clinical trials on the Finnish product heme arginate (Normasang).

The orphan product hemin and zinc mesoporphyrin (HEMEX) is being used for treatment of acute porphyric syndromes. For more information, please contact Herbert L. Bonkovsky, M.D., University of Massachusetts Medical Center.

Please contact the agencies listed under Resources, below, for the most current information. Addresses and telephone numbers of these agencies, as well as of individual experts and research centers, may be found in the Master Resources List.

**Resources**

**For more information on hereditary coproporphyria porphyria:** National Organization for Rare Disorders (NORD); American Porphyria Foundation; NIH/National Digestive Diseases Information Clearinghouse.

**For genetic information and genetic counseling referrals:** March of Dimes Birth Defects Foundation; Alliance of Genetic Support Groups.

**References**

The Metabolic and Molecular Basis of Inherited Disease, 7th ed.: C.R. Scriver, et al., eds.; McGraw-Hill, 1995, pp. 2135–2137.

# PORPHYRIA, VARIEGATE (VP)

**Description** VP, a hepatic porphyria produced by a deficiency in protoporphyrinogen oxidase, is characterized by neurologic abnormalities or photosensitivity, or both.

**Synonyms**

> Protocoproporphyria
> Royal Malady
> South African Genetic Porphyria

**Signs and Symptoms** The neurologic and visceral features of VP are similar to those seen in acute intermittent porphyria and hereditary coproporphyria. The cutaneous features are identical to those seen in porphyria cutanea tarda **(PCT).** Differential diagnosis must be made, because the treatment used for PCT is not successful in variegate porphyria. Plasma porphyrin fluorescence is usually seen in VP. When only cutaneous symptoms are present, the urinary 8- and 7-carboxylic porphyrins and isocoproporphyrin seen in porphyria cutanea tarda will differentiate that disorder from variegate porphyria.

Cutaneous symptoms and signs include burning, blistering, and scarring of sun-exposed areas; hyperpigmentation; hypertrichosis; and skin fragility (see *Porphyria Cutanea Tarda).*

The neurovisceral symptoms and signs include severe abdominal pain, vomiting, and neuropathy (see *Porphyria, Acute Intermittent).*

**Etiology** VP is inherited as an autosomal dominant trait. Symptoms are due to an inborn deficiency of protoporphyrinogen oxidase. Factors that may trigger acute neurovisceral attacks are the same as for acute intermittent porphyria and hereditary coproporphyria, and include barbiturates, estrogens, and reduced carbohydrate ingestion. Precipitating factors for the cutaneous symptoms and signs are the same as for porphyria cutanea tarda.

**Epidemiology** VP may begin between the ages of 10 and 30 years. It is more common in the white population of South Africa than elsewhere in the world. The disorder affects males and females in equal numbers.

**Related Disorders** See *Porphyria; Porphyria, Acute Intermittent; Porphyria, Hereditary Coproporphyria; Porphyria Cutanea Tarda.* See also the separate discussions of the following porphyrias: *Porphyria, ALA-D; Porphyria, Congenital Erythropoietic; Porphyria, Erythropoietic Protoporphyria.*

**Treatment—Standard** Precipitating factors must be eliminated. For treatment of acute attacks, see *Porphyria, Acute Intermittent.*

**Treatment—Investigational** Dr. Karl E. Anderson of the University of Texas Medical Branch has received orphan drug designation for Histrelin to treat various types of porphyria. Dr. Anderson is also conducting clinical trials on the Finnish product heme arginate (Normasang).

The orphan product hemin and zinc mesoporphyrin (HEMEX) is being used for treatment of acute porphyric syndromes. For more information, please contact Herbert L. Bonkovsky, M.D., University of Massachusetts Medical Center.

Please contact the agencies listed under Resources, below, for the most current information. Addresses and telephone numbers of these agencies, as well as of individual experts and research centers, may be found in the Master Resources List.

**Resources**

**For more information on variegate porphyria:** National Organization for Rare Disorders (NORD); American Porphyria Foundation; NIH/National Digestive Diseases Information Clearinghouse.

**For genetic information and genetic counseling referrals:** March of Dimes Birth Defects Foundation; Alliance of Genetic Support Groups.

**References**

The Metabolic and Molecular Basis of Inherited Disease, 7th ed.: C.R. Scriver, et al., eds.; McGraw-Hill, 1995, pp. 2137–2139.

# PSEUDOCHOLINESTERASE DEFICIENCY

**Description** Pseudocholinesterase deficiency is a rare genetic disorder characterized by a deficiency or absence of the plasma enzyme pseudocholinesterase, which can cause respiratory difficulty during surgery if the muscle-relaxant succinylcholine is used.

**Synonyms**

Succinylcholine Sensitivity

**Signs and Symptoms** Individuals with pseudocholinesterase deficiency have difficulty reversing the effects of succinylcholine (also called suxamethonium, or anectine) when administered during surgery. The ensuing paralysis of respiratory muscles may cause the patient to stop breathing for an extended period of time. Mechanical ventilation may be necessary until the succinylcholine is eliminated from the body and the patient is able to resume breathing. Individuals who are never exposed to succinylcholine may never know that they have pseudocholinesterase deficiency.

**Etiology** Pseudocholinesterase deficiency is inherited as an autosomal recessive trait. The gene is located at 3q26.

**Epidemiology** Pseudocholinesterase deficiency is present at birth and occurs in approximately 1:2,500 people in the United States. It seems to affect white Americans, Alaskan Eskimos, Greeks, Yugoslavs, and East Indians more often than other populations. In white Americans, it seems to affect males almost twice as often as females.

**Related Disorders** See *Apnea, Sleep; Malignant Hyperthermia.*

**Treatment—Standard** Testing can be done to determine the presence of plasma pseudocholinesterase deficiency before surgery is performed. When the enzyme deficiency is identified, succinylcholine is not prescribed and other muscle relaxants can be used instead. If testing for pseudocholinesterase deficiency has not been done beforehand, and the patient stops breathing for a prolonged period of time during surgery, mechanical ventilation can be performed until the patient is able to resume normal breathing.

People with pseudocholinesterase deficiency should warn their relatives to be tested before surgery. People who have relatives who have died for unknown reasons during surgery should be screened for pseudocholinesterase deficiency prior to undergoing surgery.

**Treatment—Investigational** Please contact the agencies listed under Resources, below, for the most current information. Addresses and telephone numbers of these agencies, as well as of individual experts and research centers, may be found in the Master Resources List.

**Resources**

**For more information on pseudocholinesterase deficiency:** National Organization for Rare Disorders (NORD); Malignant Hyperthermia Association of the United States.

**For genetic information and genetic counseling referrals:** March of Dimes Birth Defects Foundation; Alliance of Genetic Support Groups.

**References**

Mendelian Inheritance in Man, 11th ed.: V.A. McKusick; The Johns Hopkins University Press, 1994, pp. 1273–1277.

Textbook of Critical Care, 2nd ed.: W.C. Shoemaker, et al.; W.B. Saunders Company, 1989, pp. 109–114.

An Alternative Approach to the Prevention of Succinyldicholine-Induced Apnoea: M. Panteghini, et al.; J. Clin. Chem. Biochem., February 1988, vol. 26(2), pp. 85–90.

Plasma Cholinesterase Genetic Variants Phenotyped Using a Cobas-Fara Centrifugal Analyser: A. Brock; J. Clin. Chem. Biochem., December 1988, vol. 26(12), pp. 873–875.

AMA Drug Evaluation, 6th ed., 1986, p. 321.

Prolonged Apnea of an Oral Surgery Patient After Administration of Succinylcholine: T. Gerosky, et al.; J. Oral Surg., June 1979, vol. 37(6), pp. 428–431.

Transient Respiratory Depression of the Newborn: Its Occurrence After Succinylcholine Administration to the Mother: D. Hoefnagel, et al.; Am. J. Dis. Child., August 1979, vol. 133(8), pp. 825–826.

# PYRUVATE CARBOXYLASE DEFICIENCY

**Description** Pyruvate carboxylase deficiency is one cause of primary lactic acidosis. This deficiency blocks the conversion of pyruvate to oxaloacetate, impairing gluconeogenesis and resulting in lactic acidosis.

**Synonyms**
> Ataxia with Lactic Acidosis

**Signs and Symptoms** Pyruvate carboxylase deficiency symptoms may be apparent at birth and include metabolic acidosis, failure to thrive, ataxia, hypotonia, seizures, vomiting, spasticity, and unusual eye motion.

**Etiology** Pyruvate carboxylase deficiency is inherited as an autosomal recessive trait. The gene responsible for the disease is located on the long arm of chromosome 11.

**Epidemiology** Pyruvate carboxylase deficiency is a very rare metabolic disorder that affects males and females in equal numbers.

**Related Disorders** See **_Leigh Disease; Pyruvate Dehydrogenase (PDH) Deficiency; Korsakoff Syndrome._**

**Treatment—Standard** Treatment consists of dietary limitation of protein and carbohydrate. Since this enzyme requires biotin as a cofactor, some cases may respond to pharmacologic doses of biotin. Other treatment is symptomatic and supportive. Genetic counseling benefits affected families.

**Treatment—Investigational** Dichloroacetate is being investigated as an experimental treatment for congenital lactic acidosis.

Please contact the agencies listed under Resources, below, for the most current information. Addresses and telephone numbers of these agencies, as well as of individual experts and research centers, may be found in the Master Resources List.

**Resources**

**For more information on pyruvate carboxylase deficiency:** National Organization for Rare Disorders (NORD); Lactic Acidosis Support Group; Peter W. Stacpoole, Ph.D., M.D., University of Florida College of Medicine; NIH/National Institute of Neurological Disorders and Stroke; Children's Brain Diseases Foundation for Research; Research Trust for Metabolic Diseases in Children.

**For genetic information and genetic counseling referrals:** March of Dimes Birth Defects Foundation; Alliance of Genetic Support Groups.

**References**

Mendelian Inheritance in Man, 11th ed.: V.A. McKusick; The Johns Hopkins University Press, 1994, p. 2164.

Controlled Clinical Trial of Dichloroacetate for Treatment of Lactic Acidosis in Adults: P.W. Stacpoole, et al.; N. Engl. J. Med., November 26, 1992, vol. 327(22), pp. 1564–1569.

Birth Defects Encyclopedia: M.L Buyse, ed.-in-chief; Blackwell Scientific Publications, 1990, pp. 1449–1450.

Determination of U-13c Glucose Turnover into Various Metabolite Pools for the Differential Diagnosis of Lactic Acidemias: Kassel, D.B., et al.; Anal. Biochem., February 1, 1989, vol. 176(2), pp. 382–389.

The Metabolic Basis of Inherited Disease, 6th ed.: C.R. Scriver, et al., eds.; McGraw-Hill, 1989, pp. 872–878.

Pyruvate Carboxylase Deficiency: Acute Exacerbation After ACTH Treatment of Infantile Spasms: Rutledge, S.L., et al.; Pediatr. Neurol., July–August 1989, vol. 5(4), pp. 249–252.

# PYRUVATE DEHYDROGENASE (PDH) DEFICIENCY

**Description** Pyruvate dehydrogenase deficiency is a disorder of carbohydrate metabolism that results in persistent or recurrent lactic acidosis, mental retardation, and other neurologic symptoms and signs. The enzyme complex is made up of 5 separate subunits coded on both autosomes and the X chromosome.

**Synonyms**
> Alaninuria
>
> Intermittent Ataxia with Pyruvate Dehydrogenase Deficiency
>
> Lactic and Pyruvate Acidemia with Carbohydrate Sensitivity
>
> Lactic and Pyruvate Acidemia with Episodic Ataxia and Weakness

**Signs and Symptoms** Biochemical abnormalities of PDH deficiency may vary from severe acidosis (due to abnormally high levels of lactic acid) appearing shortly after birth, to mildly elevated levels following a meal high in carbohydrates. Elevation of blood lactate levels and alaninuria may occur only during acute episodes. Diagnosis can be made postnatally by biochemical assay in fibroblast cells.

Recurrent episodes of ataxia are seen, often with upper respiratory infection or other minor stress. The growth rate may be slowed in affected children, and varying degrees of neurologic deficits and mental retardation may occur.

**Etiology** The disorder may be inherited as either an autosomal recessive or an X-linked dominant trait, depending on which subunit is mutated. A deficiency of the enzyme pyruvate dehydrogenase causes defective oxidation of pyruvate and lactic acidosis.

**Epidemiology** Males are affected in slightly higher numbers than females.

**Related Disorders** See *Leigh Disease.*

**Treatment—Standard** Symptoms of this disorder can be controlled to some extent by avoiding carbohydrates and increasing fat in the diet. Avoidance of infection and undue stress is also recommended. Some cases may respond to treatment with thiamine (vitamin B1) or lipoic acid.

Genetic counseling is appropriate for families of affected children.

**Treatment—Investigational** A clinical trial of dichloroacetate (**DCA**) in infants and children with congenital lactic acidosis is under way. More research is needed to determine the long-term safety and efficacy of this drug in the treatment of PDH deficiency. For further information, please contact Peter W. Stacpoole, Ph.D., M.D., University of Florida College of Medicine.

Please contact the agencies listed under Resources, below, for the most current information. Addresses and telephone numbers of these agencies, as well as of individual experts and research centers, may be found in the Master Resources List.

**Resources**

**For more information on pyruvate dehydrogenase deficiency:** National Organization for Rare Disorders (NORD); Lactic Acidosis Support Group; Lactic Acidosis Support Trust; Organic Acidemia Association; British Organic Acidemia Association; Research Trust for Metabolic Diseases in Children; The Arc (a national organization on mental retardation); NIH/National Institute of Neurological Disorders and Stroke.

**For genetic information and genetic counseling referrals:** March of Dimes Birth Defects Foundation; Alliance of Genetic Support Groups.

**References**
The Metabolic and Molecular Basis of Inherited Disease, 7th ed.: C.R. Scriver, et al., eds.; McGraw-Hill, 1995, pp. 1479–1499.
Mendelian Inheritance in Man, 10th ed.: V.A. McKusick; The Johns Hopkins University Press, 1992, pp. 1237–1238, 1951–1952.

# PYRUVATE KINASE DEFICIENCY

**Description** Pyruvate kinase deficiency, a hereditary blood disorder, is characterized by a deficiency of the enzyme pyruvate kinase and is associated with hemolytic anemia.

**Signs and Symptoms** The chronic hemolytic anemia that occurs varies from mild to severe. Jaundice, splenomegaly, gallstones, or leg ulcers may develop. The anemia tends to worsen after infections. Onset of anemia and jaundice is usually in infancy or early childhood. If symptoms are first seen in adulthood, the disorder is generally less severe.

**Etiology** Pyruvate kinase deficiency is inherited as an autosomal recessive trait.

**Epidemiology** The disorder is rare, with a distribution that appears to be worldwide. Males and females are affected in equal numbers.

**Related Disorders** See the discussion of **Glucose-6-phosphatase dehydrogenase (G6PD) deficiency** in *Anemia, Hemolytic, Hereditary Nonspherocytic.*

**Treatment—Standard** The anemia of pyruvate kinase deficiency is usually treated with blood transfusions. In severe cases among infants and young children, splenectomy may be needed. Other treatment is symptomatic and supportive.

**Treatment—Investigational** Please contact the agencies listed under Resources, below, for the most current information. Addresses and telephone numbers of these agencies, as well as of individual experts and research centers, may be found in the Master Resources List.

**Resources**

**For more information on pyruvate kinase deficiency:** National Organization for Rare Disorders (NORD); NIH/National Heart, Lung and Blood Institute Information Center.

**For genetic information and genetic counseling referrals:** March of Dimes Birth Defects Foundation; Alliance of Genetic Support Groups.

**References**
The Metabolic Basis of Inherited Disease, 6th ed.: C.R. Scriver, et al., eds.; McGraw-Hill, 1989, pp. 2342–2348.
Hemolytic Anemias and Erythrocyte Enzymopathies: W.N. Valentine, et al.; Ann. Intern. Med., August 1985, vol. 103(2), pp. 245–257.

# REFSUM SYNDROME

**Description** Refsum syndrome is a slowly progressive disorder of lipid metabolism characterized by the accumulation of phytanic acid in blood and tissues and associated with neurologic disorders.

**Synonyms**

> Heredopathia Atactica Polyneuritiformis
> Hypertrophic Neuropathy of Refsum
> Phytanic Acid Storage Disease

**Signs and Symptoms** The 4 major features of the syndrome are retinitis pigmentosa, peripheral neuropathy, ataxia, and elevated protein in cerebrospinal fluid without pleocytosis. Other characteristics include nystagmus, anosmia, ichthyosis, and epiphyseal dysplasia.

**Etiology** The syndrome is inherited as an autosomal recessive trait. Deficiency of phytanic acid α-oxidase leads to an accumulation of phytanic acid in the blood plasma and tissues of the body.

**Epidemiology** Onset is from early childhood to age 50, but symptoms and signs are most often first seen by age 20. Persons of Scandinavian descent are most frequently affected. Males and females are affected in equal numbers.

**Treatment—Standard** Dietary restriction of foods containing phytanic acid lowers its plasma concentration. This reduction, however, may not be seen for months, leading to the conclusion that phytanate body stores are being used. With adherence to the diet, peripheral neuropathy is eventually arrested and ichthyosis disappears. It appears that while eye and ear symptoms do not regress, progression is arrested. Foods containing phytanic acid include dairy products; tunafish, cod, and haddock; lamb and stewed beef; white bread, white rice, and boiled potatoes; and egg yolk.

Plasmapheresis as a supplement to a dietary regimen has been effective in providing a positive initial response.

**Treatment—Investigational** Plasmapheresis as a treatment for Refsum syndrome is being tested and appears to hold promise for alleviating the neurologic problems associated with this disorder.

Please contact the agencies listed under Resources, below, for the most current information. Addresses and telephone numbers of these agencies, as well as of individual experts and research centers, may be found in the Master Resources List.

**Resources**

**For more information on Refsum syndrome:** National Organization for Rare Disorders (NORD); United Leukodystrophy Foundation; Foundation Fighting Blindness; NIH/National Institute of Neurological Disorders and Stroke; Association Européenne contre les Leucodystrophies; Research Trust for Metabolic Diseases in Children.

**For genetic information and genetic counseling referrals:** March of Dimes Birth Defects Foundation; Alliance of Genetic Support Groups.

**References**

The Metabolic and Molecular Basis of Inherited Disease, 7th ed.: C.R. Scriver, et al., eds.; McGraw-Hill, 1995, pp. 2351–2369.

Heredopathia Atactica Polyneuritiformis (Refsum's Disease) Treated by Diet and Plasma-Exchange: F.B. Gibberd, et al.; Lancet, 1986, vol. 1(8116), pp. 575–578.

# SANDHOFF DISEASE

**Description** Sandhoff disease is a progressive, inherited, lipid storage disorder that leads to the eventual destruction of the central nervous system as well as involvement of the larger viscera. It is a severe form of Tay-Sachs disease and is not restricted to any particular ethnic group.

**Synonyms**

> Gangliosidosis GM2 Type II

**Signs and Symptoms** Initial manifestations usually are seen in the 3rd to 6th month of life and include feeding problems, lethargy, and a marked startle response to sound. Cherry-red macular spots are usually seen. Motor and mental deterioration may be progressive, and symptoms and signs include motor weakness, spasticity, heart murmurs, myoclonic and generalized seizures, blindness, and splenomegaly. A positive Babinski sign is typical, and the outer toes spread after the side of the sole of the foot has been stroked.

**Etiology** Sandhoff disease is transmitted as an autosomal recessive condition. It is caused by hexosaminidase β-subunit deficiency. GM2 ganglioside accumulates in the brain and large viscera. The Hex B subunit maps to chromosome 5.

**Epidemiology** The disorder is very rare and is found in persons of all ethnic backgrounds. Males and females are affected equally.

**Related Disorders** See *Tay-Sachs Disease; Gaucher Disease; Niemann-Pick Disease; Batten Disease; Leigh Disease; Kufs Disease.*

**Treatment—Standard** Treatment is symptomatic and supportive. Genetic counseling will benefit families of affected persons.

**Treatment—Investigational** Enzyme replacement therapy is being tested as a possible treatment for Sandhoff disease, but more research is needed to determine the safety and efficacy of this procedure.

Please contact the agencies listed under Resources, below, for the most current information. Addresses and telephone numbers of these agencies, as well as of individual experts and research centers, may be found in the Master Resources List.

**Resources**

**For more information on Sandhoff disease:** National Organization for Rare Disorders (NORD); National Tay-Sachs and Allied Diseases Association; NIH/National Institute of Neurological Disorders and Stroke.

**For genetic information and genetic counseling referrals:** March of Dimes Birth Defects Foundation; Alliance of Genetic Support Groups.

**References**

The Metabolic and Molecular Basis of Inherited Disease, 7th ed.: C.R. Scriver, et al., eds.; McGraw-Hill, 1995, pp. 2839–2879.

Mendelian Inheritance in Man, 10th ed.: V.A. McKusick; The Johns Hopkins University Press, 1992, pp. 1687–1688.

Nelson Textbook of Pediatrics, 14th ed.: R.E. Behrman, ed.-in-chief; W.B. Saunders Company, 1992, p. 1526.

Birth Defects Encyclopedia: M.L. Buyse, ed.-in-chief; Blackwell Scientific Publications, 1990, p. 760.

Internal Medicine, 3rd ed.: J.H. Stein, ed.-in-chief; Little, Brown and Company, 1990, p. 2320.

# SANFILIPPO SYNDROME

**Description** Sanfilippo syndrome (mucopolysaccharidosis type III—**MPS III**) is characterized by severe mental deterioration but only mild physical disease, and urinary excretion of heparan sulfate. The 4 forms of the syndrome are classified according to the specific enzyme lack in the process of eliminating heparan sulfate. Types A and B are the most common.

MPS III-A lacks heparan N-sulfatase.

MPS III-B lacks $\alpha$-N-acetylglucosaminidase.

MPS III-C lacks acetyl-CoA: $\alpha$-glucosaminide acetyltransferase.

MPS III-D lacks N-acetylglucosamine 6-sulfatase.

**Synonyms**

Mucopolysaccharidosis Type III

**Signs and Symptoms** Children appear normal at birth; onset of symptoms and signs is between 2 and 6 years of age. Initial manifestations include hyperactivity, hirsutism, developmental delay (generally evident by 2 to 3 years of age), and mild hepatosplenomegaly. An unexplained diarrhea may occur but usually disappears in later childhood. There may be mild dysostosis multiplex and mild joint stiffness.

Signs of mental retardation are usually first seen at ages 3 to 5 years, and neurologic deterioration is evident from 6 to 10 years. Between the ages of 3 and 6 years, behavioral disturbances and intellectual decline usually are first seen. Sleep disturbance may be present, and seizures may occur. Speech is often delayed, and some children never acquire the ability to speak. Deafness may be profound in even the moderately affected patient. The child may be able to start school but will often have behavioral problems, with temper tantrums and aggressiveness increasing as dementia progresses.

**Etiology** All types of Sanfilippo syndrome are autosomal recessive. Deficiency of the enzymes specific to the syndrome results in an inability to metabolize mucopolysaccharides. The accumulation of these large, undegraded mucopolysaccharides in the cells of the body causes the physical symptoms and abnormalities.

**Epidemiology** The syndrome occurs in about 1:50,000 live births. Males and females are affected equally.

**Related Disorders** Patients with MPS Type III are more similar to those with MPS Type II (see *Hunter Syndrome*) than to those with other forms.

**Treatment—Standard** Treatment is symptomatic and supportive. Genetic counseling may be helpful to the parents of affected patients. Prenatal diagnosis is now possible for this disorder.

**Treatment—Investigational** Treatments aimed at checking early development of Sanfilippo syndrome are now under study. These include enzyme replacement therapy and bone marrow transplantation.

Please contact the agencies listed under Resources, below, for the most current information. Addresses and telephone numbers of these agencies, as well as of individual experts and research centers, may be found in the Master Resources List.

**Resources**

**For more information on Sanfilippo syndrome:** National Organization for Rare Disorders (NORD); National Mucopolysaccharidoses Society; Society of Mucopolysaccharide Diseases; Society of MPS Diseases; The Arc (a national organization on mental retardation); NIH/National Digestive Diseases Information Clearinghouse.

**For genetic information and genetic counseling referrals:** March of Dimes Birth Defects Foundation; Alliance of Genetic Support Groups.

**References**

The Metabolic and Molecular Basis of Inherited Disease, 7th ed.: C.R. Scriver, et al., eds.; McGraw-Hill, 1995, pp. 2474–2476.

# SIALIDOSIS

**Description** Sialidosis, previously called **mucolipidosis I,** is caused by a deficiency in the degradation of glycoproteins due to an inherited defect in the enzyme α-neuraminidase. Findings include normal urinary mucopolysaccharides and elevated urinary oligosaccharides containing sialic acid.

Two forms of sialidosis are known: **type I,** characterized by myoclonus and neuropathy; and **type II,** typified by myoclonus plus mild coarsening of the facial features, skeletal changes, and mild mental retardation.

**Synonyms**

Mucolipidosis I

**Signs and Symptoms Type I** symptoms and signs, usually first seen in the teens, include an ocular cherry-red spot, impaired vision, night blindness, myoclonus, and, possibly, ataxia, tremor, nystagmus, and seizures.

**Type II** is characterized by the visual abnormalities of type I plus other manifestations, such as a coarse facies, hepatosplenomegaly, dysostosis multiplex, and mental retardation. Time of onset is variable, but affected infants who appear normal at birth progress to the full type II syndrome.

Carriers of sialidosis can be detected by an enzyme assay in cultured fibroblasts, making prenatal diagnosis possible.

**Etiology** Sialidosis is an autosomal recessive inherited disorder in which the activity of the enzyme α-neuraminidase is deficient.

**Epidemiology** The disorder is very rare. Males and females are affected equally.

**Treatment—Standard** Treatment is symptomatic and supportive. Genetic counseling is advised for families affected by this disorder.

**Treatment—Investigational** Please contact the agencies listed under Resources, below, for the most current information. Addresses and telephone numbers of these agencies, as well as of individual experts and research centers, may be found in the Master Resources List.

**Resources**

**For more information on sialidosis:** National Organization for Rare Disorders (NORD); Society of Mucopolysaccharide Diseases; Society of MPS Diseases; The Arc (a national organization on mental retardation); NIH/National Digestive Diseases Information Clearinghouse; International Tremor Foundation.

**For genetic information and genetic counseling referrals:** March of Dimes Birth Defects Foundation; Alliance of Genetic Support Groups.

**References**

The Metabolic and Molecular Basis of Inherited Disease, 7th ed.: C.R. Scriver, et al., eds.; McGraw-Hill, 1995, pp. 2529–2561.

# SLY SYNDROME

**Description** Sly syndrome (mucopolysaccharidosis type VII—**MPS VII**) is a metabolic disorder in which there is an excess of urinary dermatan sulfate. Symptomatology is similar to that seen in Hurler syndrome (see ***Hurler Syndrome).*** Mental retardation, short stature, and skeletal, intestinal, and corneal abnormalities are characteristic.

**Synonyms**

β-Glucuronidase Deficiency

Mucopolysaccharidosis Type VII

**Signs and Symptoms** Moderate and nonprogressive mental retardation initially appearing at about 3 years of age seems to be a common feature of Sly syndrome. Patients have unusual facies. Corneal opacities develop at about 8 years of age. Short stature is a common characteristic, and the dysostosis multiplex seen in the mucopolysaccharidoses may be severe and includes joint contractures, dislocated hips, and spinal malformations. Other findings include hepatosplenomegaly, inguinal and umbilical hernias, and aortic regurgitation.

A severe neonatal form exists, with the newborns presenting with hydrops fetalis and dysostosis multiplex.

Prenatal diagnosis is possible for Sly syndrome.

**Etiology** The syndrome is inherited as an autosomal recessive trait. The enzyme β-glucuronidase is deficient.

**Epidemiology** Fewer than 25 cases have been identified worldwide. Males and females are affected equally.

**Related Disorders** See *Mucopolysaccharidosis.*

The mucolipidoses are a family of disorders that produce symptoms very similar to those of the mucopolysaccharidoses. See *Mucolipidosis II; Mucolipidosis III; Mucolipidosis IV.*

**Treatment—Standard** Treatment of Sly syndrome is symptomatic and supportive. Surgical intervention may be required to correct orthopedic problems, hernias, and ocular and cardiovascular abnormalities. Genetic counseling may be helpful to both patient and family.

**Treatment—Investigational** Treatments aimed at checking early development of Sly syndrome include enzyme replacement therapy and bone marrow transplantation.

Please contact the agencies listed under Resources, below, for the most current information. Addresses and telephone numbers of these agencies, as well as of individual experts and research centers, may be found in the Master Resources List.

**Resources**

**For more information on Sly syndrome:** National Organization for Rare Disorders (NORD); National Mucopolysaccharidoses Society; Society of Mucopolysaccharide Diseases; Society of MPS Diseases; The Arc (a national organization on mental retardation); NIH/National Digestive Diseases Information Clearinghouse.

**For genetic information and genetic counseling referrals:** March of Dimes Birth Defects Foundation; Alliance of Genetic Support Groups.

**References**
The Metabolic and Molecular Basis of Inherited Disease, 7th ed.: C.R. Scriver, et al., eds.; McGraw-Hill, 1995, pp. 2465–2494.

# TANGIER DISEASE

**Description** Tangier disease is a slowly progressive inherited metabolic disease marked by decreased or absent plasma concentrations of high density lipoproteins, low plasma cholesterol levels, and accumulation of cholesterol esters in certain body tissues.

**Synonyms**
> An–Lipoproteinemia
> Familial α-Lipoprotein Deficiency
> Familial High-Density Lipoprotein Deficiency
> α-High-Density Lipoprotein Deficiency
> α-Lipoproteinemia

**Signs and Symptoms** Initial characteristics are severely decreased plasma high density lipoproteins, low plasma cholesterol levels, normal or elevated triglycerides, and large, yellow-orange tonsils and adenoids. The rectum may also have the same color. As the disease progresses, neuropathy, hepatomegaly, splenomegaly, corneal deposits, and coronary artery disease may develop. In some cases, small, solid papules may appear.

**Etiology** The cause seems to be autosomal recessive inheritance of a defective gene controlling high density lipoprotein production. The absence of normal amounts of high density lipoproteins in the blood causes the symptoms.

**Epidemiology** Tangier disease is thought to be present at birth, but symptoms become apparent only during later childhood or adulthood. The disease is very rare; probably fewer than 50 persons are affected worldwide.

**Treatment—Standard** Treatment of Tangier disease is symptomatic and supportive. Splenectomy may become necessary in some cases. Genetic counseling of affected families may be beneficial.

**Treatment—Investigational** Please contact the agencies listed under Resources, below, for the most current information. Addresses and telephone numbers of these agencies, as well as of individual experts and research centers, may be found in the Master Resources List.

**Resources**

**For more information on Tangier disease:** National Organization for Rare Disorders (NORD); NIH/National Institute of Neurological Disorders and Stroke; National Tay-Sachs and Allied Diseases Association.

**For genetic information and genetic counseling referrals:** March of Dimes Birth Defects Foundation; Alliance of Genetic Support Groups.

**References**
The Metabolic and Molecular Basis of Inherited Disease, 7th ed.: C.R. Scriver, et al., eds.; McGraw-Hill, 1995, p. 2053–2072.

Analytical Capillary Isotachophoresis: A Routine Technique for the Analysis of Lipoproteins and Lipoprotein Subfractions in Whole Serum: U. Borgmann, et al.; J. Chromotogr., February 22, 1985, vol. 320(1), pp. 253–262.

Tangier Disease: A Histological and Ultrastructural Study: P. Dechelotte, et al.; Pathol. Res. Pract., October 1985, vol. 180(4), pp. 424–430.

Japanese Adult Siblings with Tangier Disease and Statistical Analysis of Reported Cases: K. Fujii, et al.; Tokai J. Exp. Clin. Med., December 1984, vol. 9(5–6), pp. 379–387.

# TAY-SACHS DISEASE

**Description** Tay-Sachs disease, a GM2 gangliosidosis, results in progressive destruction of the central nervous system. The disease is generally found in children of Jewish heritage.

**Synonyms**

> GM2 Gangliosidosis, Type I
>
> Hexosaminidase α-Subunit Deficiency (Variant B)

**Signs and Symptoms** Mild motor weakness is usually the initial manifestation, with onset around 3 to 5 months of age. An abnormal startle response and myoclonic jerk may also be seen at this time. Between 6 and 10 months of age, further signs appear, i.e., feeding difficulties, hypotonia, weakness, restlessness, and vision abnormalities, such as staring episodes, unusual eye movements, and cherry-red macular spots. By the end of the first year, there is increasing loss of vision.

After 12 months of age, the child begins to regress, losing learned skills and coordination. Seizures begin, and deterioration continues, ending with the child flaccid, unresponsive, and paralyzed.

Tay-Sachs disease can be detected prenatally through amniocentesis, and prospective parents can be tested to determine their carrier status.

**Etiology** Tay-Sachs is inherited as an autosomal recessive trait and results in deficient hexosaminidase A activity. Hex A maps to chromosome 15. This deficiency leads to storage of GM2 gangliosides in the central nervous system.

**Epidemiology** The disease primarily affects persons of Jewish ancestry, especially those of eastern European Ashkenazic descent. It also is often found in some communities of Italian descent, in Irish Catholics, and in non-Jewish Canadians.

**Related Disorders** See **Sandhoff Disease,** which is clinically indistinguishable from Tay-Sachs but is found in the general population.

See also **Alpers Disease; Kufs Disease; Leigh Disease.**

**Treatment—Standard** Treatment is symptomatic.

**Treatment—Investigational** Please contact the agencies listed under Resources, below, for the most current information. Addresses and telephone numbers of these agencies, as well as of individual experts and research centers, may be found in the Master Resources List.

**Resources**

**For more information on Tay-Sachs disease:** National Organization for Rare Disorders (NORD); National Tay-Sachs and Allied Diseases Association; NIH/National Institute of Child Health and Human Development; NIH/National Institute of Neurological Disorders and Stroke; National Foundation for Jewish Genetic Diseases; Tay-Sachs and Allied Diseases Association; Dr. Roy Gravel, Montreal Children's Hospital; Research Trust for Metabolic Diseases in Children.

**For genetic information and genetic counseling referrals:** March of Dimes Birth Defects Foundation; Alliance of Genetic Support Groups.

**References**

The Metabolic and Molecular Basis of Inherited Disease, 7th ed.: C.R. Scriver, et al., eds.; McGraw-Hill, 1995, pp. 2839–2879.

Biochemistry and Genetics of Tay-Sachs Disease: Can. J. Neurol. Sci., August 1991, vol. 18(3 suppl.), pp. 419–423.

Mendelian Inheritance in Man, 9th ed.: V.A. McKusick; The Johns Hopkins University Press, 1990, pp. 1492–1497.

Cecil Textbook of Medicine, 18th ed.: J.B. Wyngaarden and L.H. Smith, Jr., eds.; W.B. Saunders Company, 1988, pp. 149, 157, 174.

# TETRAHYDROBIOPTERIN DEFICIENCIES

**Description** Tetrahydrobiopterin deficiency is a rare genetic neurologic disorder present at birth. When the coenzyme tetrahydrobiopterin is deficient, an abnormally high blood level of the amino acid phenylalanine occurs and low levels of neurotransmitters result. To avoid irreversible neurologic damage, diagnosis and treatment of this progressive disorder are essential early in life.

**Synonyms**

> Atypical Hyperphenylalaninemia
>
> BH4 Deficiency
>
> Malignant Hyperphenylalaninemia

**Signs and Symptoms** Symptoms of tetrahydrobiopterin deficiencies usually include neurologic disturbances, muscle tone and coordination abnormalities, seizures, and delayed motor development.

**Etiology** Tetrahydrobiopterin deficiencies are inherited as autosomal recessive traits.

**Epidemiology** Tetrahydrobiopterin deficiencies occur worldwide and are estimated to affect 1 to 3 percent of infants diagnosed with phenylketonuria **(PKU)** at birth. PKU occurs in 1:11,600 live births in the United States.

**Related Disorders** See *Phenylketonuria.*

**Hyperphenylalaninemia** is identified by the presence of abnormally high blood levels of the amino acid phenylalanine in newborns, which may or may not be associated with elevated levels of tyrosine. This disorder may be a type of PKU or it may be associated with short-term deficiencies of phenylalanine hydroxylase or *p*-hydroxyphenylpyruvic acid oxidase.

**Treatment—Standard** Treatment should be started as early as possible to prevent the potentially severe neurologic disturbances. A low-phenylalanine diet does not control the metabolic imbalance but may be necessary to keep phenylalanine levels within normal range. Treatment with tetrahydrobiopterin **(BH4)** is mandatory to normalize blood phenylalanine levels by restoring liver phenylalanine hydroxylase activity.

Genetic counseling is essential for patients and their families.

**Treatment—Investigational** Treatments being tested for tetrahydrobiopterin deficiencies include administration of L-dopa and 5-hydroxytryptophan. High-dosage tetrahydrobiopterin administration is used, with dynamic improvement occurring in some patients. Synthetic forms of tetrahydrobiopterin are also under study.

The Food and Drug Administration has awarded a research grant to Joseph Muenzer, M.D., Ph.D., University of North Carolina, for studies on tetrahydrobiopterin as a treatment for this disorder.

Please contact the agencies listed under Resources, below, for the most current information. Addresses and telephone numbers of these agencies, as well as of individual experts and research centers, may be found in the Master Resources List.

**Resources**

**For more information on tetrahydrobiopterin deficiencies:** National Organization for Rare Disorders (NORD); NIH/National Institute of Neurological Disorders and Stroke; The Arc (a national organization on mental retardation); National Institute of Mental Retardation; Children's Brain Diseases Foundation for Research; Research Trust for Metabolic Diseases in Children.

**For genetic information and genetic counseling referrals:** March of Dimes Birth Defects Foundation; Alliance of Genetic Support Groups.

**References**

The Metabolic and Molecular Basis of Inherited Disease, 7th ed.: C.R. Scriver, et al., eds.; McGraw-Hill, 1995, p. 1049.

Differential Diagnosis of Tetrahydrobiopterin Deficiency: A. Neiderweiser, et al.; J. Inherit. Metab. Dis., 1985, vol. 8(suppl. 1), pp. 34–38.

Hyperphenylalaninaemia Caused by Defects in Biopterin Metabolism: S. Kaufman; J. Inherit. Metab. Dis., 1985, vol. 8(suppl. 1), pp. 20-27.

Hyperphenylalaninaemia Due to Impaired Dihydrobiopterin Biosynthesis: Leukocyte Function and Effect of Tetrahydrobiopterin Therapy: K. Fukuda, et al.; J. Inherit. Metab. Dis., 1985, vol. 8(2), pp. 49–52.

# TRIMETHYLAMINURIA

**Description** Trimethylaminuria is a very rare metabolic disorder that occurs when there is an impairment in the ability of the liver enzyme trimethylamine-N-oxide synthetase to break down trimethylamine from choline and trimethylamine oxide in the diet. When trimethylamine is not properly metabolized, it is excreted in the urine, sweat, and breath, causing a strong fishy odor. The disorder may be either inherited or acquired.

**Synonyms**

Fish Odor Syndrome

Flavin Containing Monooxygenase 2

FMO2

FMO, Adult Liver Form

Stale Fish Syndrome

**Signs and Symptoms** The accumulation of trimethylamine in the body results in a characteristic fishy odor to sweat, urine, and breath. The odor may become stronger after puberty, possibly causing psychological and social problems.

Trimethylaminuria may be acquired as a result of large oral doses of the amino acid derivative L-carnitine (levocarnitine). Symptoms disappear as the dosage is lowered. L-Carnitine is used in the treatment of carnitine deficiency syndromes and is sometimes used by athletes who believe it enhances physical strength.

A urinalysis after oral administration of 600 mg of trimethylamine may be useful in detecting possible carriers of trimethylaminuria.

**Etiology** Trimethylaminuria may be inherited as an autosomal dominant genetic trait or occur as the result of treatment with large doses of the drug L-carnitine.

**Epidemiology** Trimethylaminuria affects males and females in equal numbers. Approximately 18 cases of the inherited form of trimethylaminuria have been reported in the medical literature. The symptoms can occur at any age, depending on the ingestion of foods that contain choline and trimethylamine oxide.

**Treatment—Standard** In most cases symptoms are relieved when a low-protein, low-lysine diet is prescribed.

**Treatment—Investigational** Please contact the agencies listed under Resources, below, for the most current information. Addresses and telephone numbers of these agencies, as well as of individual experts and research centers, may be found in the Master Resources List.

**Resources**

**For more information on trimethylaminuria:** National Organization for Rare Disorders (NORD); Research Trust for Metabolic Diseases in Children; NIH/National Institute of Diabetes, Digestive and Kidney Diseases.

**For genetic information and genetic counseling referrals:** March of Dimes Birth Defects Foundation; Alliance of Genetic Support Groups.

**References**

Mendelian Inheritance in Man, 10th ed.: V.A. McKusick; The Johns Hopkins University Press, 1992, p. 398.

Birth Defects Encyclopedia: M.L Buyse, ed.-in-chief; Blackwell Scientific Publications, 1990, p. 1710.

The Metabolic Basis of Inherited Disease, 6th ed.: C.R. Scriver, et al., eds.; McGraw-Hill, 1989, p. 894.

Trimethylaminuria: The Detection of Carriers Using Trimethylamine Load Test: M. Al-Waiz, et al.; J. Inherit. Metab. Dis., 1989, vol. 12(1), pp. 80–85.

Trimethylaminuria (Fish Odor Syndrome): A Study of an Affected Family: M. Al-Waiz, et al.; Clin. Sci., March 1988, vol. 73(3), pp. 231–236.

Trimethylaminuria: M.A. Brewster, et al.; Ann. Clin. Lab. Sci., January–February 1983, vol. 13(1), pp. 20–24.

Trimethylaminuria: E. Spellacy, et al.; J. Inherit. Metab. Dis., 1980, vol. 2(4), pp. 85–88.

# TYROSINEMIA I

**Description** Tyrosinemia I is a metabolic disorder caused by a lack of the enzyme fumarylacetoacetate hydrolyase, yielding elevated levels of tyrosine and its metabolites. Clinically, acute and chronic forms are seen.

**Synonyms**

Tyrosinemia, Hereditary, Hepatorenal Type

Tyrosyluria

**Signs and Symptoms Acute tyrosinemia I** is present at birth. Within weeks or months the infant fails to thrive. Typical findings include vomiting, diarrhea, and a cabbagelike odor. Other frequent symptoms and signs include hepatomegaly, edema, ascites, melena, and hemorrhagic diathesis. This form, if untreated, is fatal in the first year of life.

**Chronic tyrosinemia I** is milder, with symptoms that include rickets, a mild cirrhosis, renal tubular dysfunction, hypertension, and neurologic abnormalities. Hepatoma may develop.

The diagnosis is established by testing for succinylacetone in the urine and for fumarylacetoacetate hydrolyase in tissues. Prenatal diagnosis of tyrosinemia I can be done by identification of amniotic cells that show a reduction in activity of fumarylacetoacetase, or by detection of succinylacetone in amniotic fluid.

**Etiology** Tyrosinemia I is inherited as an autosomal recessive trait. The genetic abnormality results in deficiency of the enzyme fumarylacetoacetate hydrolyase. This enzyme maps to chromosome 15.

**Epidemiology** Tyrosinemia I in the acute form affects approximately 1:100,000 newborns in the United States, with both sexes being affected equally. The chronic form of this disorder affects far fewer patients. Both forms may be found in the same family.

**Treatment—Standard** Treatment is by dietary restriction of phenylalanine, tyrosine, and methionine. Liver transplantation has been helpful for severely affected patients. Other treatment is symptomatic and supportive. Genetic counseling is recommended.

**Treatment—Investigational** A new drug, NTBC (manufactured by ICI), is being studied by Dr. Lindstedt of Gothenburg University in Sweden as a treatment for tyrosinemia I. It shows promise for producing improvement both clinically and biochemically.

Please contact the agencies listed under Resources, below, for the most current information. Addresses and telephone numbers of these agencies, as well as of individual experts and research centers, may be found in the Master Resources List.

**Resources**

**For more information on tyrosinemia I:** National Organization for Rare Disorders (NORD); Research Trust for Metabolic Diseases in Children; The Arc (a national organization on mental retardation); NIH/National Digestive Diseases Information Clearinghouse; Jess G. Thoene, M.D., University of Michigan School of Medicine.

**For genetic information and genetic counseling referrals:** March of Dimes Birth Defects Foundation; Alliance of Genetic Support Groups.

### References

The Metabolic and Molecular Basis of Inherited Disease, 7th ed.: C.R. Scriver, et al., eds.; McGraw-Hill, 1995, pp. 1077–1106.

A Single Mutation of the Fumarylacetoacetate Hydrolase Gene in French Canadians with Hereditary Tyrosinemia Type I: M. Grompe, et al.; N. Engl. J. Med., August 11, 1994, vol. 331(6), pp. 353–357.

Neurologic Crises in Hereditary Tyrosinemia: G. Mitchell, et al.; N. Engl. J. Med., February 15, 1990, vol. 322(7), pp. 432–437.

Prenatal Diagnosis of Hereditary Tyrosinemia by Determination of Fumarylacetoacetase in Cultured Amniotic Fluid Cells: E.A. Kvittingen, et al.; Pediatr. Res., April 1985, vol. 19(4), pp. 334–337.

# VALINEMIA

**Description** Valinemia is a very rare metabolic disorder characterized by elevated levels of the amino acid valine in the blood and urine resulting from a deficiency of valine transaminase.

**Synonyms**

> Hypervalinemia
> Valine Transaminase Deficiency

**Signs and Symptoms** Typical findings include poor appetite, frequent vomiting, and failure to thrive. Hypotonia, excessive drowsiness, and hyperactivity may also be seen.

**Etiology** Valinemia is thought to be inherited as an autosomal recessive trait.

**Epidemiology** The disorder is very rare, occurring in fewer than 200 persons in the United States. It is present at birth.

**Treatment—Standard** Valine is restricted in the diet.

**Treatment—Investigational** Please contact the agencies listed under Resources, below, for the most current information. Addresses and telephone numbers of these agencies, as well as of individual experts and research centers, may be found in the Master Resources List.

**Resources**

**For more information on valinemia:** National Organization for Rare Disorders (NORD); NIH/National Digestive Diseases Information Clearinghouse; Research Trust for Metabolic Diseases in Children.

**For genetic information and genetic counseling referrals:** March of Dimes Birth Defects Foundation; Alliance of Genetic Support Groups.

**References**

Mendelian Inheritance in Man, 9th ed.: V.A. McKusick; The Johns Hopkins University Press, 1990, p. 1524.

The Metabolic Basis of Inherited Disease, 6th ed.: C.R. Scriver, et al., eds.; McGraw-Hill, 1989, p. 678.

# VITAMIN E DEFICIENCY

**Description** Vitamin E deficiency, which occurs most often in infants with impaired bile flow, may lead to progressive neuromuscular dysfunction characterized in part by areflexia and loss of balance.

**Synonyms**

> Tocopherol Deficiency

**Signs and Symptoms** The first sign of vitamin E deficiency is usually areflexia, which may progress to ataxia, loss of balance, and peripheral muscle weakness. There may be difficulties with walking, such as stumbling and staggering (titubation), and abnormal posturing. Ophthalmoplegia and bradykinesia may occur, and sensations of pain, vibration, and position may be impaired.

Vitamin E deficiency in premature and low-birth-weight infants also may cause hemolytic anemia.

**Etiology** Rarely is vitamin E deficiency caused by dietary deficiency. It usually is associated with an underlying disease, such as fat malabsorption, liver disease, or disorders of bile secretion (see ***Acanthocytosis).*** Recent research suggests that vitamin E deficiency with no underlying disease may derive from an inherited defect of vitamin E storage.

**Epidemiology** Vitamin E deficiency with no underlying disorder is extremely rare. The disease is more common in infants, children, and young adults than in adults. Males and females are affected in equal numbers except when an underlying disorder affects one sex more readily.

Approximately 1:5,000 infants has impaired bile flow due to liver diseases such as hepatitis or biliary atresia. In these infants, the vitamin deficiency causes degenerative progressive neuromuscular disease.

**Related Disorders** Symptoms of the following disorders can be similar to the neurologic symptoms of vitamin E deficiency. See ***Ataxia, Friedreich; Ataxia, Marie; Charcot-Marie-Tooth Disease; Olivopontocerebellar Atrophy.***

**Treatment—Standard** Any causative underlying disorder must be corrected. Supplementation with vitamin E, α-tocopherol, α-tocopheryl acetate, and α-tocopheryl succinate has not been successful.

**Treatment—Investigational** Intramuscular injection of an investigational form of vitamin E (*dl*-α-tocopherol) has, in some cases, stabilized or reversed the neurologic symptoms caused by vitamin E deficiency. This experimental drug is manufactured by Hoffmann–La Roche.

A water-soluble form of Vitamin E (*d*-α-tocopheryl polyethylene glycol-1000 succinate, or TPGS), which does not require bile for intestinal absorption, is being investigated under a grant from the National Organization for Rare Disorders (NORD). Preliminary studies indicate that this approach may stabilize or reverse neurologic dysfunction in infants with bile duct obstruction. Participants in this study must be older than 6 months and under 20 years of age, and their vitamin E deficiency must be caused by some form of cholestatic hepatobiliary liver disease. For information, contact Ronald J. Sokol, M.D., University of Colorado School of Medicine.

Please contact the agencies listed under Resources, below, for the most current information. Addresses and telephone numbers of these agencies, as well as of individual experts and research centers, may be found in the Master Resources List.

**Resources**

**For more information on vitamin E deficiency:** National Organization for Rare Disorders (NORD); NIH/National Digestive Diseases Information Clearinghouse; American Liver Foundation; United Liver Association; Children's Liver Foundation.

**References**

Intramuscular Vitamin E Repletion in Children with Chronic Cholestrasis: D.H. Perlmutter, et al.; Am. J. Dis. Child, February 1987, vol. 141(2), pp. 170–174.

Vitamin E Deficiency and Neurologic Disease in Adults with Cystic Fibrosis: M.D. Sitrin, et al.; Ann. Intern. Med., July 1987, vol. 107(1), pp. 51–54.

Vitamin E Deficiency Linked to Liver Disease in Children: C. Pierce; Research Resources Reporter, October 1986; National Institutes of Health, pp. 7–9.

# VON GIERKE DISEASE

**Description** An inborn lack of the enzyme glucose-6-phosphatase is responsible for von Gierke disease, a glycogen storage disease. The enzyme is required for the conversion of glycogen into glucose. A deficiency causes deposits of excess glycogen in liver and kidney cells.

**Synonyms**

Glycogen Storage Disease I
Glycogenosis Type I
Hepatorenal Glycogenosis

**Signs and Symptoms** Manifestations of von Gierke disease are usually noticed during the first year of life. Findings include persistent hunger, fatigue, and irritability. Hepatomegaly, weight loss, and a slow growth rate are also seen. Hypoglycemia and lactic acidosis develop if food is withheld, and seizures may occur if the hypoglycemia is severe. The diagnosis can be confirmed with a glucose test and glucagon tolerance test, and by enzymatic assay.

Other findings seen during childhood include easy bruisability and frequent nosebleeds, lipidemia, xanthomas, and hyperuricemia. Microscopic glycogen deposits may be seen in liver cells and throughout the kidneys. Although the disease may be severe at times, symptoms tend to improve with age and with appropriate dietary control.

**Etiology** The disease is inherited as an autosomal recessive trait.

**Epidemiology** This and other glycogen storage diseases together affect about 1:40,000 persons in the United States. Males and females are affected in equal numbers.

**Related Disorders** See ***Glycogen Storage Disease III; Andersen Disease.***

**Treatment—Standard** A nearly normal blood glucose level can be maintained through frequent small daily meals of carbohydrates plus a nighttime nasogastric infusion of glucose. An alternative to the nasogastric feeding is the use of uncooked cornstarch in the daily diet. A high-protein diet should be maintained. This regimen will promote a normal childhood growth rate.

The uric acid concentration in the blood must be carefully monitored to prevent the development of gouty arthritis during adolescence or adulthood. Allopurinol may be needed if symptoms of gout-like arthritis develop.

**Treatment—Investigational** Yuan-Tsong Chen, M.D., Ph.D., of Duke University was awarded a grant in 1988 for his work using cornstarch as a treatment for von Gierke disease.

Please contact the agencies listed under Resources, below, for the most current information. Addresses and telephone numbers of these agencies, as well as of individual experts and research centers, may be found in the Master Resources List.

### Resources

**For more information on von Gierke disease:** National Organization for Rare Disorders (NORD); Association for Glycogen Storage Diseases; NIH/National Digestive Diseases Information Clearinghouse; Research Trust for Metabolic Diseases in Children.

**For genetic information and genetic counseling referrals:** March of Dimes Birth Defects Foundation; Alliance of Genetic Support Groups.

### References

The Metabolic and Molecular Basis of Inherited Disease, 7th ed.: C.R. Scriver, et al., eds.; McGraw-Hill, 1995, pp. 935–965.

Optimal Rate of Enteral Glucose Administration in Children with Glycogen Storage Disease Type I: W.F. Schwenk, et al.; N. Engl. J. Med., March 13, 1986, vol. 314(11), pp. 682–685.

Glycogen Storage Disease Type I: Results of Treatment with Frequent Daytime Feeding, Combined with Nocturnal Intragastric Feeding and with Administration of an Alpha-Glucosidase Inhibitor: H. Grube, et al.; Eur. J. Pediatr., April 1983, vol. 140(2), pp. 102–104.

# WILSON DISEASE

**Description** Wilson disease is a rare genetic disorder characterized by excess copper stored in various body tissues, particularly the liver, brain, and corneas. Eventual developments include hepatic disease and central nervous system dysfunction. Early diagnosis and treatment can prevent serious long-term disability.

### Synonyms

> Hepatolenticular Degeneration
> Lenticular Degeneration, Progressive

**Signs and Symptoms** The usual presentation of Wilson disease is with hepatic or neurologic disturbances, or both. Symptoms of liver disease usually appear after 6 years of age and include jaundice and vomiting. Neurologic symptoms are first seen between the ages of 12 and 32 years. Findings include drooling, dysarthria, dysphagia, lack of coordination, tremor, spasticity, muscle rigidity, and double vision. Other presenting signs and symptoms include renal stones, joint disorders, acute hemolytic crisis, and cardiomyopathy.

The Kayser-Fleischer ring, a rusty-brown deposit in the cornea that may not be present in the early stages of Wilson disease, is an important sign that appears in almost all patients and in 100 percent of those with neurologic involvement.

Neurologic signs and symptoms that may appear later in the course of the disease include decreased mentation and behavioral disturbances. Joint and bone involvement includes osteoporosis, the appearance of osteophytes at large joints, and reduced spinal and extremity joint spaces. Kidney involvement includes renal tubular damage.

The psychiatric manifestations of Wilson disease vary from patient to patient, and may be confused with psychiatric disorders, ranging from depression to schizophrenia. Accurate diagnosis is crucial; phenothiazines can aggravate the neurologic and psychiatric symptoms of Wilson disease. The side effects of these drugs also may appear similar to symptoms of Wilson disease. Most patients with psychiatric symptoms deriving from Wilson disease also have neurologic disease and Kayser-Fleischer rings in their eyes.

In adolescent females, menstruation may not begin until the disease is treated, because of the general disturbances in metabolism.

**Etiology** Wilson disease is inherited as an autosomal recessive trait located on chromosome 13q14, which prevents the liver from adequately excreting copper in the bile. The resulting gradual accumulation of copper in the body is toxic.

**Epidemiology** Males and females are affected in equal numbers, and the disease is found in all races and ethnic groups. The incidence is approximately 1:100,000 worldwide, with about 2,000 diagnosed cases in the United States. Many cases are misdiagnosed, however, usually as mental illness, and the true incidence may actually be higher.

**Related Disorders** See *Sydenham Chorea; Primary Biliary Cirrhosis; Heavy Metal Poisoning; Huntington Disease; Tourette Syndrome; Cerebral Palsy.*

**Treatment—Standard** The standard treatment for Wilson disease is D-penicillamine. Treatment must be lifelong, but some patients cannot tolerate long-term penicillamine therapy. The orphan drug trientine (Syprine, manufactured by Merck Sharp and Dohme) has been found effective for patients who are unable to tolerate penicillamine.

Foods high in copper content, such as chocolate, nuts, and shellfish, should be avoided. Dietary information is available from the Wilson Disease Association.

Physical therapy and speech therapy may be useful for neurologic involvement. In cases of severe liver disease, transplantation has been effective.

**Treatment—Investigational** The orphan drug zinc acetate is being tested as maintenance therapy for Wilson disease. This is a common nutritional substance, but it must be taken in certain doses at specific times during the day in order to affect copper metabolism. Careful monitoring is therefore necessary. For more information, please contact either George J. Brewer, M.D., University of Michigan Medical School, or the manufacturer, Lemmon Company.

Please contact the agencies listed under Resources, below, for the most current information. Addresses and telephone numbers of these agencies, as well as of individual experts and research centers, may be found in the Master Resources List.

**Resources**

**For more information on Wilson disease:** National Organization for Rare Disorders (NORD); Wilson's Disease Association; American Liver Foundation; United Liver Association; Children's Liver Foundation; NIH/National Institute of Neurological Disorders and Stroke; We Move, Mount Sinai Medical Center.

**For genetic information and genetic counseling referrals:** March of Dimes Birth Defects Foundation; Alliance of Genetic Support Groups.

**References**

The Metabolic and Molecular Basis of Inherited Disease, 7th ed.: C.R. Scriver, et al., eds.; McGraw-Hill, 1995, pp. 2211–2235.
Cecil Textbook of Medicine, 19th ed.: J.B. Wyngaarden, et al., eds.; W.B. Saunders Company, 1992, pp. 1132–1133.
Mendelian Inheritance in Man, 10th ed.: V.A. McKusick; The Johns Hopkins University Press, 1992, pp. 1756–1757.
Wilson's Disease: Current Status: J.C. Yarse, et al.; Am. J. Med., June 1992, vol. 92(6), pp. 643–654.
Pathophysiology and Treatment of Wilson's Disease: R.M. Tankanow; Clin. Pharm., November 1991, vol. 10(11), pp. 839–849.
Wilson's Disease: S.E. Woods; Am. Fam. Physician, July 1989, vol. 40(1), pp. 171–178.

# ZELLWEGER SYNDROME

**Description** Zellweger syndrome is a rare hereditary disorder characterized by failure to import proteins into peroxisomes of liver, kidney, and brain cells. Manifestations include facial dysmorphology, ophthalmologic and neurologic abnormalities, hepatomegaly, and unusual problems in prenatal development.

**Signs and Symptoms** Affected newborns have a typical flat facies, with a high forehead, shallow supraorbital ridges, hypertelorism, and epicanthal folds. The neonate also has profound hypotonia, feeding difficulty, seizures, cardiac defects, hepatomegaly, and vision abnormalities, such as clouding of the cornea and cataracts. Jaundice and gastrointestinal bleeding may develop because of a deficient coagulation factor in the blood. Pneumonia or respiratory distress may develop if infections are not prevented and controlled. The syndrome is usually fatal within 12 months.

**Etiology** Zellweger syndrome is inherited as an autosomal recessive trait. Symptoms result from a deficiency or absence of peroxisomes in brain, liver, and kidney tissues. The cause of the peroxisomal deficiency is not known.

**Epidemiology** An Australian study indicated that the syndrome may occur 1:100,000 live births, but it is possible that some cases have gone undiagnosed.

**Related Disorders** See *Adrenoleukodystrophy; Refsum Syndrome.*

**Treatment—Standard** Treatment is symptomatic and supportive. Genetic counseling is of benefit to families of patients with this disorder.

**Treatment—Investigational** Use of the antihyperlipidemic agent, clofibrate, has been tried but has not proved effective in treating Zellweger syndrome.

Please contact the agencies listed under Resources, below, for the most current information. Addresses and telephone numbers of these agencies, as well as of individual experts and research centers, may be found in the Master Resources List.

**Resources**

**For more information on Zellweger syndrome:** National Organization for Rare Disorders (NORD); United Leukodystrophy Foundation; Muscular Dystrophy Association; The Arc (a national organization on mental retardation); NIH/National Institute of Neurological Disorders and Stroke; Association Européenne contre les Leucodystrophies;.

**For genetic information and genetic counseling referrals:** March of Dimes Birth Defects Foundation; Alliance of Genetic Support Groups.

**References**

The Metabolic and Molecular Basis of Inherited Disease, 7th ed.: C.R. Scriver, et al., eds.; McGraw-Hill, 1995, pp. 2287–2324.
Smith's Recognizable Patterns of Human Malformation, 4th ed.: K.L. Jones; W.B. Saunders Company, 1988, pp. 178–179.
Zellweger Syndrome: Diagnostic Assays, Syndrome Delineation, and Potential Therapy: G.N. Wilson, et al.; Am. J. Med. Genet., May 1986, vol. 24(1), pp. 69–82.
Unsuccessful Attempts to Induce Peroxisomes in Two Cases of Zellweger Disease by Treatment with Clofibrate: I. Bjorkhem, et al.; Pediatr. Res., June 1985, vol. 19(6), pp. 590–593.

# 3 | NEUROLOGIC AND PSYCHIATRIC DISORDERS
## By Melvin H. Van Woert, M.D.

The diagnosis of a neurologic disease requires the anatomic localization of the lesion on the basis of symptomatology, physical signs, and special laboratory and imaging techniques. For example, the loss of normal movement of an extremity may be due to an abnormality in one or several different parts of the central or peripheral nervous system. Some of the regions that regulate motor function and could produce this symptom include the motor cortex; spinal motor neurons; peripheral nerves; vestibular, red, and medullary reticular nuclei; basal ganglia; cerebellum; and accessory motor cortex. Accurate diagnosis requires the identification of the involved areas of the nervous system. A similar complexity in anatomic localization applies to other neurologic symptoms, such as visual disturbances, sensory loss, tremor, impairment of balance, and pain. In some cases, the office neurologic examination will identify the abnormal neuronal pathways producing the symptoms. More frequently, special neurologic procedures will be necessary to confirm clinical impressions.

The anatomic localization may suggest the etiologic diagnosis immediately. In other cases, medical facts such as age of onset, family history, and evolution of symptoms, and sometimes specific laboratory tests will be necessary. Based upon etiology, neurologic diseases are divided into categories such as inflammations; neoplasms; vascular disorders; demyelination; trauma; and degenerative, congenital, and metabolic disorders. Some of these categories, particularly degenerative, congenital, and metabolic disorders, contain a significant number of genetic diseases.

Psychiatric diagnosis relies predominantly upon observation of the patient and critical evaluation of the patient's statements and opinions. There are rarely any objective signs, as in most neurologic disorders. Interpretation of the patient's behavior and response to questions can reveal symptoms such as hallucinations, delusions, or impaired memory, which form the basis for a psychiatric diagnosis. Psychiatric diagnoses have been divided into categories that have been precisely classified in the American Psychiatric Association's *Diagnostic and Statistical Manual of Mental Disorders, 3rd Edition, Revised (DSM-III-R)*. These diagnostic categories include, for example, personality disorders, mood disorders, schizophrenia, anxiety disorders, and disorders first evident in infancy, childhood, or adolescence. Formal personality tests, such as the Minnesota Multiphasic Personality Inventory, can be used to obtain scores on conditions such as anxiety, mania, depression, schizophrenia, paranoia, and hypochondriasis. Intelligence tests (Wechsler Adult Intelligence Scale—Revised and Wechsler Intelligence Scale for Children–Revised) and neuropsychological testing for specific cognitive functions, such as memory, attention, and fluency of thinking, are particularly useful in evaluating organic mental diseases.

Although older diagnostic procedures such as cerebrospinal fluid examinations, electroencephalography, electromyography, and stimulus-induced evoked potential and arteriographic examinations remain very useful, particularly in neurologic disorders, major advances in neuroradiology and genetic studies have recently resulted in even earlier and more accurate assessment of many pathologic processes in the central nervous system. The introduction of computerized tomography **(CT)** and magnetic resonance imaging **(MRI)** has produced dramatic improvements in the diagnosis of neurologic diseases and has greatly diminished the need for risky invasive diagnostic procedures. In addition, CT and MRI have been used in psychiatry to rule out organic diseases (e.g., multi-infarct dementia or subdural hematoma) as causes of symptoms such as memory impairment, personality changes, delusions, or depression. However, as patients with different psychiatric disorders are examined by CT, abnormalities are being detected in some of these mental conditions. For example, the ventricles of schizophrenic patients tend to be larger than those of normal individuals. This ventricular enlargement in patients with schizophrenia has been confirmed by MRI studies. MRI has also detected decreased temporal lobe size in schizophrenic patients, and cerebellar abnormalities in children with autism.

Positron emission tomography **(PET)** offers a new dimension in neuroradiologic sophistication by allowing studies of biochemical, physiological, and pharmacologic processes to be carried out in patients. Abnormal patterns of glucose utilization in the brain, detected by PET studies, have been observed in stroke, Alzheimer disease, seizures, and tumors, and in psychiatric disorders such as schizophrenia, bipolar depression, and obsessive-compulsive disorder. Dementia also is known to occur with progressive supranuclear palsy, and studies of regional glucose metabolism by PET scanning have found a decreased glucose uptake in the prefrontal cortex. Other PET studies can detect neuroreceptor abnormalities in basal ganglia diseases such as Parkinson disease.

Molecular genetic techniques are rapidly being applied to hereditary neurologic and psychiatric diseases to localize abnormal genes. One method is to digest deoxyribonucleic acid **(DNA)** with an enzyme called restriction endonuclease, which splits the DNA at specific sites to form multiple segments known as restriction fragment length polymorphisms **(RFLPs).** The variation in fragment lengths of these segments is a genetic characteristic, and it may be possible to localize an abnormal disease-producing gene within an RFLP in an afflicted family. Lymphocytic DNA from family members is scanned to determine whether a specific variation in restriction fragment length is linked to the disease in family members. This RFLP linkage technique was used to establish that chromosome 4 contained the abnormal gene for Huntington disease; this information led to a diagnostic test for individuals at risk for this condition. Applied to psychiatric disorders, the same technique showed a close linkage between bipolar illness and the X chromosome marker for color blindness. Significant progress also has been made in identifying gene alterations and their chromosomal localization for familial Alzheimer disease, Machado-Joseph disease, dominantly inherited ataxia, Charcot-Marie-Tooth disease, myotonic muscular dystrophy, Duchenne muscular dystrophy, familial amyotrophic lateral sclerosis, and neurofibromatosis. Further research should enable identification of the abnormal genotype of at-risk persons and at-risk pregnancies for these diseases and eventual metabolic or gene therapy.

The localization of the gene for Duchenne muscular dystrophy on the short arm of the X chromosome led to the cloning of the gene and its translocation to reveal the protein produced by that gene. The protein is called dystrophin, and it provides the strength and stability to the sarcolemmal membrane. A deficiency of dystrophin results in rupture of the sarcolemmal membrane and death of the muscle fiber. Possibly, the functional gene could be transplanted into the muscle of patients with Duchenne muscular dystrophy in some form of vehicle to correct this genetic defect.

There are approximately 1,000 genetic disorders that can impair neurologic or mental function.

Specific therapy for these conditions is uncommon. However, dietary treatment has been successful in patients with phenylketonuria, maple syrup urine disease, galactosemia, and Refsum syndrome, by limiting the intake of a precursor that may have a toxic accumulation. In Wilson disease, the toxic accumulation of copper in the body can be prevented by chelation therapy with penicillamine and triethylene tetramine. As the site and product of the abnormal genes present in hereditary diseases of the nervous system are identified, new therapeutic approaches are expected.

Advances in neuroimmunology have greatly improved diagnosis and treatment of diseases such as Guillain-Barré syndrome, myasthenia gravis, and multiple sclerosis.

The identification of multiple neurotransmitters in the brain has led to the association of abnormalities of these chemical messengers with various disease states. Impetus has thus been provided for pharmaceutical companies to research and develop drugs that alter neurotransmitter metabolism for the treatment of central nervous system diseases. The development of therapy for Parkinson disease is an excellent example. In the early 1960s, concentration of the neurotransmitter dopamine was found to be markedly depleted in the striatum of the parkinsonian brain because of degeneration of the dopaminergic nigro-striatal neuronal pathway. L-Dopa, which is converted to dopamine in the brain, was observed to produce dramatic clinical improvement. This observation stimulated continued research along the same lines, which led to the marketing of antiparkinsonian dopaminergic agonists (e.g., bromocriptine, pergolide) and the monoamine oxidase B inhibitor selegiline (Eldepryl—see the Directory on Orphan Drugs).

Neural transplants or grafting has yielded some promising results in Parkinson disease and is being considered for other neurologic disorders in which critical neurons are insufficient or their function is impaired. In Parkinson disease, fetal dopamine-producing neurons have been transplanted into the striatum, in an attempt to restore the impaired dopaminergic function. Huntington disease is another potential target for neural grafting, since there is intrinsic loss of striatal neurons. Theoretically, grafting of striatal neurons might produce functional improvement. Cholinergic neuronal replacement in Alzheimer disease also has been considered.

Neurotrophic growth factors (e.g., nerve growth factor, brain-derived neurotrophic factor, neurotrophins 3, 4, or 5) also have been considered for the treatment of neurodegenerative diseases such as Parkinson disease and Alzheimer disease. These agents may slow degenerative processes and enable the remaining neurons to compensate for degenerating neurons. Clinical trials of nerve growth factor in Alzheimer disease and Parkinson disease are in progress.

Abnormalities of cholinergic, serotonergic, peptidergic, GABA-ergic, and noradrenergic systems are being identified in other neurologic and psychiatric diseases. Certain types of myoclonic disorders appear to be due to diminished serotonin metabolism; and the serotonin precursor, L-5-hydroxytryptophan, has been demonstrated to have a beneficial effect. The loss of cholinergic input to the cerebral cortex has been observed in the Alzheimer patient's brain, and clinical trials of drugs that increase brain acetylcholine levels are producing some encouraging results. Neuropharmacologic manipulation of neurotransmitters in various regions of the brain also has been successfully applied to the development of drugs for the treatment of psychiatric disorders such as anxiety and depression.

There have been several recent breakthroughs in the pharmacologic treatment of neurologic diseases. Betaseron (interferon beta-1b) has been approved for the treatment of mild-to-moderate relapsing-remitting multiple sclerosis. The mechanism of action of Betaseron is unknown, but it may be due to its antiviral, antiproliferative, or immunomodulating effects. Betaseron increases T-suppressor-cell activity, blocks synthesis of interferon-g, and decreases T-cell proliferation. Subcutaneous injections of Betaseron decrease both the number and severity of relapses in patients with multiple sclerosis.

The cholinergic cell loss in Alzheimer disease is thought to be related to the pathogenesis of Alzheimer disease. Cognex (tacrine, tetrahydroaminoacridine) is a reversible acetylcholinesterase inhibitor that prevents the degradation of endogenously released acetylcholine. Cognex theoretically optimizes the action of the remaining intact cholinergic neurons and has been approved for the treatment of Alzheimer disease.

Since 1993, three new antiepileptic drugs have been marketed in the United States. The first one, felbamate (Felbatol), has very limited use because of an unexpected high incidence of aplastic anemia observed after it had been in general use for only a short period of time. Gabapentin (Neurotin) is structurally related to the neurotransmitter γ-aminobutyric acid **(GABA),** but it does not affect GABA-ergic neurotransmission. Its mechanism of anticonvulsant action is unknown. Clinical studies demonstrate that gabapentin is effective in the treatment of partial seizures and in reducing the frequency of secondary generalized tonic-clonic seizures. Lamotrigine (Lamictal), a drug that blocks voltage-dependent sodium channels resulting in decreased release of stimulatory neurotransmitters such as glutamate and aspartate, also has been found to be effective in treating partial seizures and the refractory generalized seizures associated with Lennox-Gastaut syndrome.

### References

Handbook of Clinical Neurology, vols. 1–58: P.J. Vinken, G.W. Bruyn, and H.L. Klawans, eds.; Elsevier Science Publishers, 1990.

Merritt's Textbook of Neurology, 8th ed.: L.P. Rowland, ed.; Lea and Febiger, 1989.

Principles of Neurology, 4th ed.: R.D. Adams and M. Victor; McGraw-Hill, 1989.

Treatments of Psychiatric Disorders: Task Force Report of the American Psychiatric Association, vols. 1–3: American Psychiatric Association, 1989.

Diagnostic and Statistical Manual of Mental Disorders, 3rd ed., revised: R.L. Spitzer, et al., eds.; American Psychiatric Association, 1987.

# NEUROLOGIC AND PSYCHIATRIC DISORDERS
*Listings in This Section*

# ACOUSTIC NEUROMA

**Description** An acoustic neuroma is a benign tumor of the 8th cranial nerve. This nerve lies within the internal auditory canal.

**Synonyms**

> Acoustic Neurilemoma
> Bilateral Acoustic Neuroma
> Cerebellopontine Angle Tumor
> Fibroblastoma, Perineural
> Neurinoma
> Neurofibroma
> Schwannoma

**Signs and Symptoms** The early manifestations of an acoustic neuroma include tinnitus, hearing loss, or both; these symptoms arise from pressure on the 8th cranial nerve.

Other nerves also may be affected by an acoustic neuroma. Compression of the facial nerve (7th cranial nerve) produces facial muscle weakness. The trigeminal nerve (5th cranial nerve) is responsible for sensation on the skin of the face and the surface of the eye. Tumor involvement of this nerve may lead to facial numbness.

The direction of tumor growth determines symptom development. Tumor growth in the direction of the brain stem may push toward the cerebellum, causing ataxia of the arms and legs, and nystagmus. Downward expansion of the tumor can produce numbness in the mouth, dysphagia, and hoarseness.

With increasing intracranial pressure, personality changes and impaired cognition may develop, and as pressure increases on the facial nerve, facial twitching and asymmetry may result. Sudden expansion of the tumor may be caused by hemorrhage or edema. MRI with gadolinium enhancement will detect even small tumors.

**Etiology** The cause of acoustic neuroma is unknown, although there appears to be a hereditary predisposition in a small group of patients with bilateral involvement.

**Epidemiology** Small asymptomatic acoustic neuromas have been found on autopsy in 2.4 percent of the general population. Estimates of occurrence of symptomatic acoustic neuroma range from 1:3,500 persons to 5:1,000,000, with women being affected more often than men. An unusually large concentration of cases have been found in Humboldt County, California. Most surgical procedures for acoustic neuroma are performed on individuals between 30 and 60 years of age.

**Related Disorders** See *Neurofibromatosis,* which discusses the acoustic neuromas seen in NF 2.

**Treatment—Standard** At the present time, the only curative treatment is surgical removal of the tumor. The location and size of the tumor determine whether the approach is suboccipital or translabyrinthine. Postoperative problems can include headache, cerebrospinal fluid leak, meningitis, and decreased mental alertness due to development of a blood clot or obstruction of flow of cerebrospinal fluid. Large acoustic neuromas may have to be resected in stages.

Removal of an acoustic neuroma is a complex and delicate process, and complications relating to the cranial nerves may develop after surgery.

Hearing is often lost, partially or completely, with medium or large tumors, particularly if the tumor protrudes into the brain. It may be possible to preserve hearing, however, with tumors smaller than 0.6 inches. Monitoring of hearing function during surgery may lessen the possibility of hearing loss.

Tinnitus may persist after surgery, and occasionally only begins after surgery.

The facial nerve may be damaged during the procedure, and in some cases, portions of it are removed. Temporary or permanent facial paralysis may result and may lead to eventual dental problems. Nerve regeneration may take up to 1 year. If the paralysis persists, hypoglossal facial nerve anastomosis may bring improvement.

Ocular complications develop in approximately 50 percent of patients following surgical removal of an acoustic neuroma. Diplopia may occur if there is pressure on the 6th nerve, and there may be impairment of the eyelid muscles. Artificial tears or eye lubricants are often needed by these patients.

Because the vestibular portion of the 8th nerve is often removed during surgery, dizziness and unsteadiness are common until the vestibular apparatus in the normal ear can compensate. Unsteadiness in the dark may be permanent.

**Treatment—Investigational** Surgical techniques are improving dramatically, and research is continuing on the development of safer and more effective procedures and rehabilitation.

A new type of treatment, developed in Sweden, involves a special form of radiation therapy. The long-term benefits and side effects are not known, however.

The National Institute on Deafness and Other Communication Disorders is conducting research on hereditary acoustic neuroma.

Please contact the agencies listed under Resources, below, for the most current information. Addresses and telephone numbers of these agencies, as well as of individual experts and research centers, may be found in the Master Resources List.

**Resources**

**For more information on acoustic neuroma:** National Organization for Rare Disorders (NORD); Acoustic Neuroma Association; Alexander Graham Bell Association for the Deaf; Deafness Research Foundation; International Association of Parents of the Deaf; National Information Center on Deafness; NIH/National Institute on Deafness and Other Communication Disorders.

**For acoustic neuroma associated with neurofibromatosis:** National Neurofibromatosis Foundation; Neurofibromatosis.

**For genetic information and genetic counseling referrals:** March of Dimes Birth Defects Foundation; Alliance of Genetic Support Groups.

**References**

Human Genetics Disorders: J. NIH Res., August 1994, vol. 6(8), pp. 115–134.

Cecil Textbook of Medicine, 19th ed.: J.B. Wyngaarden, et al., eds.: W.B. Saunders Company, 1992, pp. 2108, 2112, 2219.

Conservative Management of Acoustic Neuromas: J.M. Nedzelski; Otolaryngol. Clin. North Am., June 1992, vol. 25(2), pp. 691–705.

Mendelian Inheritance in Man, 9th ed.: V.A. McKusick; The Johns Hopkins University Press, 1990, pp. 12–13.

# ADIE SYNDROME

**Description** Tonicity of pupillary eye muscles results in the major symptoms of Adie syndrome. The disorder is not progressive or life-threatening.

**Synonyms**

Adie's Tonic Pupil
Holmes-Adie Syndrome
Papillotonic Psuedotabes
Tonic Pupil Syndrome

**Signs and Symptoms** Usually, only the pupil of one eye is affected; occasionally both eyes are involved. In most patients the affected pupil is always dilated, constricting very little or not at all in response to light, and very slowly when focusing on objects close to view. Headache, facial pain, blurred vision, and emotional fluctuations may occur.

Pupil dilation may be caused by other factors than disease, e.g., certain drugs including transdermal scopolamine.

Diagnosis is made by using dilute pilocarpine to test the pupil's reaction to light. The Adie syndrome pupil will have a supersensitive response to dilute pilocarpine.

**Etiology** The cause is unknown. The disorder may be inherited as an autosomal dominant trait. Neuronal loss in the ciliary ganglion has been found in patients with Adie syndrome.

**Epidemiology** Females between the ages of 25 to 45 are affected more often than males, but the disorder is seen in both sexes.

**Related Disorders** See *Peripheral Neuropathy.*

**Treatment—Standard** Corrective lenses are prescribed for blurred vision. Dilute pilocarpine may improve stereoacuity in some patients. Genetic counseling is useful. Other treatment is symptomatic and supportive.

**Treatment—Investigational** Please contact the agencies listed under Resources, below, for the most current information. Addresses and telephone numbers of these agencies, as well as of individual experts and research centers, may be found in the Master Resources List.

**Resources**

**For more information on Adie syndrome:** National Organization for Rare Disorders (NORD); NIH/National Eye Institute; NIH/National Institute of Neurological Disorders and Stroke.

**For genetic information and genetic counseling referrals:** March of Dimes Birth Defects Foundation; Alliance of Genetic Support Groups.

**References**

Accommodative Fluctuations in Adie's Syndrome: K. Ukai and S. Ishikawa; Ophthalmic Physiol. Opt., January 1989, vol. 9(1), pp. 76–78.

Miotic Adie's Pupils: M. L. Rosenberg; J. Clin. Neuro. Ophthalmol., March 1989, vol. 9(1), pp. 43–45.

Cecil Textbook of Medicine, 18th ed.: J.B. Wyngaarden and L.H. Smith, Jr., eds.; W.B. Saunders Company, 1988, p. 2284.

On the Cause of Hyporeflexia in the Holmes-Adie Syndrome: J. M. Miyasaki, et al.; Neurology, February 1988, vol. 38(2), pp. 262–265.

Mendelian Inheritance in Man, 8th ed.: V.A. McKusick; The Johns Hopkins University Press, 1986, pp. 506, 893, 1090–1091.

The Therapy of Adie's Syndrome with Dilute Pilocarpine Hydrochloride Solutions: A.J. Flach and B.J. Dolan; J. Ocul. Pharmacol., Winter 1985, vol. 1(4), pp. 353–362.

# AGENESIS OF THE CORPUS CALLOSUM (ACC)

**Description** ACC is a rare congenital abnormality involving a partial or complete absence of the transverse fibers that connect the 2 cerebral hemispheres. In some cases mental retardation may result, but other cases may be asymptomatic and intelligence normal. ACC is diagnosed during the first 2 years of life in 90 percent of cases. Affected patients can expect a normal life span.

**Synonyms**
> Agenesis of Commissura Magna Cerebri
> Asymptomatic Callosal Agenesis
> Corpus Callosum, Agenesis

**Signs and Symptoms** The initial manifestation may be the onset of grand mal or jacksonian epileptic seizures. This may occur during the first weeks or within the first 2 years of life.

Hydrocephalus and impairment of mental and physical development also occur in some patients in the early stages of ACC. Neurologic evaluation may reveal nonprogressive mental retardation, impaired hand-eye coordination, and visual or auditory memory impairment.

In some mild cases, symptoms may not appear for many years, and the disorder is diagnosed when an older patient develops seizures.

**Etiology** ACC is usually inherited as an X-linked recessive trait, but it may also be caused by an intrauterine infection during pregnancy leading to developmental disturbance in the fetal brain.

**Epidemiology** ACC is a very rare condition that usually produces symptoms during the first 2 years of life.

**Related Disorders** See *Aicardi Syndrome; Spina Bifida.*

**Andermann syndrome** is a genetic disorder characterized by a combination of ACC, mental retardation, and progressive neuropathy. All known cases of this disorder originate from Charlevois County and the Saguenay-Lac St. Jean area of Quebec, Canada. The exact mode of inheritance is unknown.

**Treatment—Standard** Treatment is symptomatic and supportive, involving anticonvulsive medications, special education, and physical therapy. The pressure of hydrocephalus may be relieved with a surgical shunt. Genetic counseling is recommended for families with this disorder.

**Treatment—Investigational** Please contact the agencies listed under Resources, below, for the most current information. Addresses and telephone numbers of agencies, as well as of individual experts and research centers, may be found in the Master Resources List.

**Resources**

**For more information on agenesis of the corpus callosum:** National Organization for Rare Disorders (NORD); NIH/National Institute of Neurological Disorders and Stroke.

**For more information on shunts:** Association for Brain Tumor Research.

**For genetic information and genetic counseling referrals:** March of Dimes Birth Defects Foundation; Alliance of Genetic Support Groups.

**References**

Mendelian Inheritance in Man, 9th ed.: V.A. McKusick; The Johns Hopkins University Press, 1990, pp. 1111–1112, 1581.

Anatomical and Behavioral Study of a Case of Asymptomatic Callosal Agenesis: R. Bruyer, et al.; Cortex, September 1985, vol. 21(3), pp. 417–430.

Aicardi's Syndrome: Agenesis of the Corpus Callosum, Infantile Spasms, and Ocular Anomalies; S. Dinani, et al.; J. Ment. Defic. Res., June 1984, vol. 28(pt. 2), pp. 143–149.

The Andermann Syndrome: Agenesis of the Corpus Callosum Associated with Mental Retardation and Progressive Sensorimotor Neuronopathy: A. Larbrisseau, et al.; Can. J. Neurol. Sci., May 1984, vol. 11(2), pp. 257–261.

# AGNOSIA, PRIMARY VISUAL

**Description** Primary visual agnosia is characterized by the total or partial loss of the ability to recognize and identify familiar objects and people by sight. This occurs without loss of vision.

**Synonyms**
> Agnosis
> Visual Amnesia
> Monomodal Visual Amnesia

**Signs and Symptoms** Affected persons may have one or several impairments in visual recognition without impairment of intelligence, motivation, or attention. Vision is almost always intact and the mind is clear. In object agnosia, for instance, the individual can see a familiar object but is unable to name it. However, objects can be identified by touch, sound, or smell.

In other cases, familiar persons cannot be identified (**prosopagnosia**). The patient can see and describe, but cannot name, the individual. When the identification problem is associated with surroundings, familiar places, or buildings, the condition is termed **loss-of-environmental-familiarity agnosia.** Affected individuals may be able to describe a familiar environment from memory and point to it on a map.

**Simultanagnosia** is characterized by the inability to read and the inability to view one's surroundings as a whole. The affected individual can see parts of the surrounding scene, but not the whole. There is an inability to comprehend more than one part of a visual scene at a time or to coordinate the parts.

In rare cases, patients may not be able to recognize or point to various parts of the body (**autotopagnosia**). Symptoms may also include loss of the ability to distinguish left from right.

Testing to distinguish primary visual agnosia from primary perceptual disorders includes a number of sophisticated perceptual tests (e.g., visual adaptation, perceptions of pattern, and a flicker-fusion test). Brain damage may be identified through imaging techniques such as CT, PET, and MRI.

**Etiology** The disorder results from damage to areas of the brain associated with visual memory. In most cases of primary visual agnosia, lesions occur unilaterally in the occipital lobe. In the form associated with the loss of environmental familiarity, the damage usually is to the right side of the brain. However, some affected individuals, especially those with prosopagnosia, have bilateral occipitotemporal lesions.

Lesion causes include traumatic brain injury, stroke, or overexposure to environmental toxins. Secondary visual agnosia may also occur in association with other underlying disorders, such as Alzheimer disease, agenesis of the corpus callosum, and other conditions that result in progressive dementia.

In some cases, the cause of the brain damage may not be known.

**Epidemiology** The disorder is very rare. Males and females are affected in equal numbers.

**Related Disorders** See *Alzheimer Disease; Pick Disease.*

**Treatment—Standard** Treatment is symptomatic and supportive. For persons with visual object agnosia, moving the object into more familiar surroundings may be helpful, as may touching or smelling the object. In cases of secondary visual agnosia, further brain damage should be treated and prevented, if possible.

**Treatment—Investigational** Please contact the agencies listed under Resources, below, for the most current information. Addresses and telephone numbers of these agencies, as well as of individual experts and research centers, may be found in the Master Resources List.

**Resources**

For more information on primary visual agnosia: National Organization for Rare Disorders (NORD); NIH/National Institute of Neurological Disorders and Stroke; Brain Injury Association; Brain Research Foundation.

**References**

Cecil Textbook of Medicine, 19th ed.: J.B. Wyngaarden, et al., eds.; W.B. Saunders Company, 1992, pp. 2071–2073.

Impaired Drawing from Memory in a Visual Agnosic Patient: L. Trojano, et al.; Brain Cogn., November 1992, vol. 20(2), pp. 149–170.

A Historic Case of Visual Agnosia Revisited After 40 Years: S.A. Sparr, et al.; Brain, April 1991, vol. 114(pt. 2), pp. 789–800.

Simultanagnosia: A Defect of Sustained Attention Yields Insights on Visual Information Processing: M. Rizzo, et al.; Neurology, March 1990, vol. 40(3 pt. 1), pp. 447–455.

# AICARDI SYNDROME

**Description** Aicardi syndrome is an extremely rare congenital disorder in which the corpus callosum has failed to develop. The absence of this structure's linking the 2 cerebral hemispheres is associated with frequent seizures, marked abnormalities of the chorionic and retinal layers of the eye, and severe mental retardation.

**Synonyms**

> Callosal Agenesis
> Chorioretinal Anomalies
> Corpus Callosum Agenesis
> Infantile Spasms
> Spasm in Flexion

**Signs and Symptoms** Infantile spasms, beginning between birth and 4 months of age, are the first manifestations of the syndrome. The diagnostic sign is the presence of many cream-colored lacunae in the fundus. Subsequent findings include epilepsy, mental retardation, hypotonia, microcephaly, microphthalmia, colobomas, and abnormalities of the ribs and vertebrae. CT scans or autopsy reveal that the corpus callosum is missing.

Patients with this disorder tend to deteriorate with age. Children as old as 4 years may be unable to achieve normal standing posture. Mortality is unusually high, although some patients survive to adulthood.

**Etiology** The cause of Aicardi syndrome is unknown. A single dominant gene on the X chromosome may be involved.

**Epidemiology** Aicardi syndrome is extremely rare. Only females are affected; males are thought to die in utero.

**Treatment—Standard** Drug therapy includes corticosteroids, anticonvulsants, and adrenocorticotropic hormone. Treatment, otherwise, is symptomatic and supportive.

**Treatment—Investigational** Please contact the agencies listed under Resources, below, for the most current information. Addresses and telephone numbers of these agencies, as well as of individual experts and research centers, may be found in the Master Resources List.

**Resources**

**For more information on Aicardi syndrome:** National Organization for Rare Disorders (NORD); Aicardi Syndrome Newsletter; NIH/National Institute of Neurological Disorders and Stroke; Richard Allen, M.D., Pediatric Neurology Service, University of Michigan Medical Center.

**For genetic information and genetic counseling referrals:** March of Dimes Birth Defects Foundation; Alliance of Genetic Support Groups.

**References**

Mendelian Inheritance in Man, 10th ed.: V.A. McKusick; The Johns Hopkins University Press, 1992, pp. 1808–1809.

Birth Defects Encyclopedia: M.L. Buyse, ed.-in-chief; Blackwell Scientific Publications, 1990, pp. 66–68.

Principles of Neurology, 4th ed.: R.D. Adams and M. Victor, eds.; McGraw-Hill, 1989, pp. 971–973.

Aicardi's Syndrome: Agenesis of the Corpus Callosum, Infantile Spasms, and Ocular Anomalies; S. Dinani, et al.; J. Ment. Defic. Res., June 1984, vol. 28(pt. 2), pp. 143–149.

A New Syndrome: Spasms in Flexion, Callosal Agenesis, Ocular Abnormalities: J. Aicardi, et al.; Electroencephalography and Clinical Neurology, 1965, vol. 19, pp. 609–610.

# ALEXANDER DISEASE

**Description** Alexander disease is one of the rarest of the dystrophies, a group of progressive metabolic neurologic disorders, frequently inherited. Histologically the disease is characterized by demyelination and the formation of Rosenthal fibers in the white matter of the brain, especially around blood vessels and on the surface of the brain. Onset typically is in infancy and is associated with mental retardation and spastic quadriparesis. Juvenile- and adult-onset forms are recognized but occur infrequently.

**Synonyms**

> Dysmyelogenic Leukodystrophy–Megalobarencephaly
> Fibrinoid Degeneration of Astrocytes
> Leukodystrophy with Rosenthal Fibers
> Megalencephaly with Hyaline Inclusion
> Megalencephaly with Hyaline Panneuropathy

**Signs and Symptoms** Early symptoms of Alexander disease in infants include muscle spasticity and mental and physical retardation associated with megalencephaly. With progression of the disease, seizures may occur. Juvenile-onset Alexander disease has a longer course (average, 8 years). In adult-onset cases, intermittent ataxia and spastic quadriparesis usually occur, and the clinical picture can resemble multiple sclerosis. CT scanning can confirm the presence of a leukodystrophy.

**Etiology** An autosomal recessive inheritance has been postulated. The precise metabolic defect has not been identified.

**Epidemiology** Males and females are equally affected.

**Related Disorders** Alexander disease must be distinguished from other leukodystrophies and from brain or metabolic disorders producing similar symptoms. See *Astrocytoma, Malignant; Astrocytoma, Benign; Hydrocephalus; Adrenoleukodystrophy; Leukodystrophy, Canavan; Leukodystrophy, Krabbe; Leukodystrophy, Metachromatic; Pelizaeus-Merzbacher Brain Sclerosis; Refsum Syndrome; Multiple Sclerosis.*

**Treatment—Standard** Treatment is symptomatic and supportive.

**Treatment—Investigational** Current research is focused on identifying the exact composition of the Rosenthal fibers and the factors responsible for their formation and growth. Recently, 2 compounds present in Rosenthal fibers have been identified.

Please contact the agencies listed under Resources, below, for the most current information. Addresses and telephone numbers of these agencies, as well as of individual experts and research centers, may be found in the Master Resources List.

**Resources**

**For more information on Alexander disease:** National Organization for Rare Disorders (NORD); United Leukodystrophy Foundation; NIH/National Institute of Neurological Disorders and Stroke; Children's Brain Diseases Foundation for Research; The Arc (a national organization on mental retardation).

**For genetic information and genetic counseling referrals:** March of Dimes Birth Defects Foundation; Alliance of Genetic Support Groups.

**References**

Mendelian Inheritance in Man, 10th ed.: V.A. McKusick; The Johns Hopkins University Press, 1992, pp. 1207–1208.

Birth Defects Encyclopedia: M.L. Buyse, ed.-in-chief; Blackwell Scientific Publications, 1990, pp. 83–84.

Merrit's Textbook of Neurology, 8th ed.: L.P. Rowland, ed.; Lea and Febiger, 1989.

The Metabolic Basis of Inherited Disease, 6th ed.: C.R. Scriver, et al., eds.; McGraw-Hill, 1989, pp. 1699–1705.

Progressive Fibrinoid Degeneration of Fibrillary Astrocytes Associated with Mental Retardation in a Hydrocephalic Infant: W.S. Alexander; Brain, vol. 1949(72), pp. 373–381.

# ALPERS DISEASE

**Description** Alpers disease is a progressive neurologic condition affecting infants and children. It is characterized by degeneration of the cerebral gray matter, resulting in motor disturbances, seizures, and dementia. Liver disease is often associated.

**Synonyms**

Alpers Diffuse Degeneration of Cerebral Gray Matter with Hepatic Cirrhosis

Alpers Progressive Infantile Poliodystrophy

Poliodystrophia Cerebri Progressiva

Progressive Poliodystrophy

**Signs and Symptoms** Characteristic features include motor retardation, partial paralysis, spasticity, myoclonus, liver damage, blindness, and growth retardation. Intractable seizures and progressive mental deterioration may also occur. Symptoms of the disease may be intensified by stress or other illnesses.

**Etiology** The cause is unknown in most cases. A familial form has been identified.

**Epidemiology** Males and females are affected equally.

**Related Disorders** See *Leigh Disease; Batten Disease; Tay-Sachs Disease.*

**Treatment—Standard** Treatment is symptomatic and supportive.

**Treatment—Investigational** Please contact the agencies listed under Resources, below, for the most current information. Addresses and telephone numbers of these agencies, as well as of individual experts and research centers, may be found in the Master Resources List.

**Resources**

**For more information on Alpers disease:** National Organization for Rare Disorders (NORD); Association for Neurometabolic Disorders; Children's Brain Diseases Foundation for Research; NIH/National Institute of Neurological Disorders and Stroke.

**References**

Mendelian Inheritance in Man, 9th ed.: V.A. McKusick; The Johns Hopkins University Press, 1990, p. 1023–1024.

Progressive Neuronal Degeneration of Childhood with Liver Disease (Alpers Disease): Characteristic Neurophysiological Features: S.G. Boyd, et al.; Neuropediatrics, May 1986, vol. 17(2), pp. 75–80.

Progressive Poliodystrophy (Alpers Disease) with a Defect in Cytochrome aa3 in Muscle: A Report of Two Unrelated Patients: M.J. Prick, et al.; Clin. Neurol. Neurosurg., 1983, vol. 85(1), pp. 57–70.

Progressive Infantile Poliodystrophy (Alpers Disease) with a Defect in Citric Acid Cycle Activity in Liver and Fibroblasts: M.J. Prick, et al.; Neuropediatrics, May 1982, vol. 13(2), pp. 108–111.

# ALZHEIMER DISEASE

**Description** Alzheimer disease is a progressive degenerative condition of the brain affecting memory, thought, and language. The degenerative changes lead to plaques and neurofibrillary tangles, as well as a loss of cholinergic innervation in the brain.

**Synonyms**

Presenile Dementia

Senility

**Signs and Symptoms** The early behavioral changes of Alzheimer disease may be barely noticeable, but with disease progression memory losses increase, and personality, mood, and behavior change. Disturbances of judgment, concentration, and speech occur, along with confusion and restlessness. The type, severity, sequence, and progression of mental changes vary widely. Long periods with little change are common, although in some cases the disease is rapidly progressive.

Persons with Alzheimer disease should be given regular physical examinations to detect other organic disorders that may develop, because these patients may be unable to communicate clearly regarding the development of new or unrelated symptoms.

**Etiology** At least 10 percent of cases are inherited through a dominant gene. Alzheimer disease frequently occurs in individuals with Down syndrome who live past 35 years of age. Chromosome 21 abnormalities are common to both Down syndrome patients and some of the familial Alzheimer patients.

Some studies suggest that the disease may not be a single illness and that several factors may be involved. Researchers at the UCLA Medical School found that 100 percent of men with early Alzheimer disease (before age 60) had the protein HLA-A2 on the surface of their white blood cells, compared to 30 percent of healthy men under 60, and 40 percent of men with late-onset disease. It is suggested that HLA-A2–positive men under 60 may be at higher risk of early-onset Alzheimer disease.

Researchers at Johns Hopkins University are studying brain tissue of deceased Alzheimer patients and have found neuronal degeneration at the nucleus basalis. These neurons are believed to contain the neurotransmitter acetyl-choline, and some patients had lost 90 percent of these cells. There appear to be abnormally low levels of acetyl-choline in the brains of Alzheimer disease patients.

Recent studies suggest that at least 3 chromosomes carry genes that can lead to the development of Alzheimer disease. A gene located on the long arm of chromosome 14 (14q) is believed to be responsible for the early onset form of the condition. Another gene, known as the B-amyloid precursor protein gene **(APPPP),** is located on the long arm of chromosome 21 (21q) and is believed to cause a small percentage of persons about age 50 years to become affected. The presence of a specific defective gene on the long arm of chromosome 19 (19q) is an impor-tant risk factor for the development of late-onset Alzheimer disease. The apolipoprotein E **(ApoE)** gene has 3 vari-eties: E2, E3, and E4. Studies have shown that a patient with one copy of the E4 gene has double the risk that a person with no E4 gene has of developing Alzheimer disease. Individuals with 2 such alleles have 8 times the risk.

**Epidemiology** Alzheimer disease occurs in 2 percent to 3 percent of the general population over 60 years of age. Approximately 2.5 million people in the United States are affected. The disease affects females more than males and blacks more than whites.

**Related Disorders** See *Binswanger Disease; Creutzfeldt-Jakob Disease; Pick Disease.*

**Treatment—Standard** Treatment is symptomatic and supportive. Tranquilizers may decrease agitation, anxiety, and behavioral disturbances. Depression accompanying the illness can be treated with various antidepressant drugs. Other helpful general measures include proper diet and fluid intake, and exercise and physical therapy. Alcoholic beverages should be avoided. The daily routine of a patient should be maintained as normal as possible, with con-tinuation of social activities.

The drug tetrahydroaminoacridine (tacrine, Cognex) is available for treatment of patients with mild-to-moder-ate Alzheimer disease. Tacrine increases levels of acetylcholine in the brain by inhibiting its breakdown.

**Treatment—Investigational** Diagnosed Alzheimer disease patients who have one or more relatives (living or deceased) also diagnosed with the disease may participate in a clinical research study being conducted at the National Insti-tute of Neurological Disorders and Stroke. Please contact Linda Nee, M.S.W., or Ronald Polinsky, M.D.

The National Institute of Mental Health and the Neuropsychiatric Research Hospital are studying early-onset dementia occurring as a result of Alzheimer disease. This study includes a thorough neuropsychological evalua-tion, state-of-the-art brain imaging, and evaluation using newly developed biochemical assay techniques. Partici-pants in this study must be under 45 years of age and should not require special medical care. For information, contact Denise Juliano, M.S.W., Coordinator of Admissions, Neuropsychiatric Research Hospital, Washington, DC.

The narcotic antagonist drug naltrexone is being tested for treatment of senile dementia of the Alzheimer type.

The drug Desferal, administered IM twice daily, is being investigated as a treatment for Alzheimer disease. The drug is manufactured by Ciba-Geigy.

New drugs being developed include Velnacrine (Metane), Suronacrine (HP 128), HP 749, Ebiratide (HOE 427), HOE 065, and CAS 493.

The drug linopirine is being tested on Alzheimer disease patients. Du Pont Merck Pharmaceutical Co. is the manufacturer.

Other drugs in development include Capoten, SQ 29852, HP290, Nimotop, Guanfacine, Zacopride, Milacemide, Alcar, Oxiracetam, Avan, and Cognex.

Please contact the agencies listed under Resources, below, for the most current information. Addresses and tele-phone numbers of these agencies, as well as of individual experts and research centers, may be found in the Mas-ter Resources List.

**Resources**

**For more information on Alzheimer disease:** National Organization for Rare Disorders (NORD); Alzheimer's Disease Education and Referral Center; NIH/National Institute of Neurological Disorders and Stroke; NIH/Nation-al Institute on Aging.

**For genetic information and genetic counseling referrals:** March of Dimes Birth Defects Foundation; Alliance of Genetic Support Groups.

**References**

Genetic Mistakes Point the Way for Alzheimer's Disease: J. Hardy; J. NIH Res., November 1993, vol. 5, pp. 45–49.

Cecil Textbook of Medicine, 19th ed.: J.B. Wyngaarden, et al., eds.: W.B. Saunders Company, 1992, pp. 2075–2079.

A Double-Blind, Placebo-Controlled Multicenter Study of Tacrine for Alzheimer's Disease: K..L. Davis, et al.; N. Engl. J. Med., October 29, 1992, vol. 327(22), pp. 1253–1259.

Mendelian Inheritance in Man, 10th ed.: V.A. McKusick; The Johns Hopkins University Press, 1992, pp. 57–61.

Therapeutic Frontiers in Alzheimer's Disease: S.W. Miller, et al.; Pharmacotherapy 1992, vol. 12(3), pp. 217–231.

Drug Treatment of Alzheimer's Disease: J.K. Cooper; Arch. Intern. Med., February 1991, vol. 151(2), pp. 245–249.

# AMYOTROPHIC LATERAL SCLEROSIS (ALS)

**Description** ALS is a disease of the motor neurons that innervate skeletal muscles. It generally affects both upper and lower motor neurons and results in progressive wasting and weakness of involved muscles. Several variant forms of ALS exist.

Disease forms and related disease entities include slow motor neuron disease, focal motor neuron disease, spinal muscular atrophy (Kugelberg-Welander disease, juvenile spinal muscular atrophy), progressive bulbar palsy, benign focal amyotrophy, primary lateral sclerosis, infantile spinal muscular atrophy (Werdnig-Hoffmann disease), Wohlfart-Kugelberg-Welander disease, and floppy infant syndrome.

**Synonyms**

> Aran-Duchenne Muscular Atrophy
> Lou Gehrig's Disease
> Motor Neuron Disease
> Progressive Bulbar Paralysis
> Progressive Muscular Atrophy
> Pseudobulbar Palsy

**Signs and Symptoms** Early symptoms include slight, patchy muscular weakness; clumsy hand movements; difficulty in performing fine motor tasks; leg weakness, often resulting in tripping; slowed speech; dysphagia; bulbar symptoms; and nocturnal leg cramps, often in calf or thigh muscles. In weeks or months, the disease involves more muscles. Other signs and symptoms may include muscle fasciculations, leg stiffness, hyperactive deep tendon reflexes, and coughing. Severe weight loss occurs in 5 percent of cases. As mobility impairment progresses, the patient is at increased risk of respiratory failure and anoxia, aspiration pneumonia, or inadequate nutrition.

**Etiology** The cause is unknown. Allergic, infectious, and viral causes have been proposed. Five to 10 percent of all cases are familial. Research on a possible defective glutamate absorption process for affected persons is ongoing.

The defective gene associated with the inherited form of ALS has been found (superoxide diamitase-1 gene); it is inherited as an autosomal dominant trait and is located on the long arm of chromosome 21. The symptoms of the sporadic and familial form of ALS are the same. It is not yet known if the gene causes ALS or predisposes a person toward the disease.

**Epidemiology** ALS is estimated to affect about 2,500 persons in the United States, mainly between the ages of 40 and 70. Sixty percent of cases involve men; 40 percent, women.

**Related Disorders** It is unclear whether the following disorders are separate disease entities or are variants of ALS.

See ***Kugelberg-Welander Syndrome; Primary Lateral Sclerosis; Werdnig-Hoffmann Disease.***

**Focal motor neuron disease** affects only one area of the body, most commonly the shoulder girdle. The disease progresses over several months, leaving the patient with a fixed deficit. Some patients later develop more extensive motor neuron disease. If focal motor neuron disease is considered as a diagnosis, care should be taken to exclude other causes of focal atrophy.

**Progressive bulbar palsy** is a variant of ALS characterized by weakness and atrophy of the muscles innervated by the cranial nerves.

**Benign focal amyotrophy** is a variant in which muscle weakness and atrophy are limited to a single limb. The onset may resemble that of classical ALS.

**Treatment—Standard** Medical management generally requires a team approach that involves physical therapists, speech pathologists and therapists, pulmonary therapists, medical social workers, and nurses.

Several drugs may be useful in controlling symptoms. Baclofen may reduce spasticity. Patients troubled by leg cramps may benefit from quinine compounds. Fasciculations, which may interfere with sleep, can be treated with agents such as diazepam.

Maintaining proper nutrition is essential, but vitamin therapy has not been shown to affect the course of ALS. Soft foods should be carefully chosen for patients with dysphagia.

Physical therapy, consisting of daily range-of-motion exercises, is very important. The exercises can help maintain joint flexibility and prevent fixation of muscle contractions.

Communication devices can be useful for patients with dysarthria. Aids to communication include codes involving extraocular movement, artificial speech articulation utilizing small computers, the use of written messages, and other methods that can help to combat feelings of isolation.

Respiratory aids are often needed in advanced stages.

**Treatment—Investigational** Extensive ALS research is directed toward nerve growth factors, axonal transport, androgen receptors in motor neurons, alterations in DNA and RNA, and metabolic studies of the neuromuscular junction.

Some evidence suggests that defective metabolism of the amino acid glutamate may be responsible for degeneration of the nerve cells in ALS. The effects of branched chain amino acids, particularly L-leucine, L-isoleucine, and L-valine, are being studied to determine whether these substances will prevent the toxic effects of glutamate.

Other research (Rup Tandan, M.D., of the University of Vermont) focuses on the orphan drug L-threonine and branched chain amino acids.

Orphan drugs being tested for treatment in ALS are human ciliary neurotrophic factor; Riluzole; and Neurotrophin-1.

Please contact the agencies listed under Resources, below, for the most current information. Addresses and telephone numbers of these agencies, as well as of individual experts and research centers, may be found in the Master Resources List.

**Resources**

**For more information on amyotrophic lateral sclerosis:** National Organization for Rare Disorders (NORD); Amyotrophic Lateral Sclerosis Association; NIH/National Institute of Neurological Disorders and Stroke.

**For information on the childhood form of motor neuron disease:** Families of Spinal Muscular Atrophy.

**References**

Mendelian Inheritance in Man, 10th ed.: V.A. McKusick; The Johns Hopkins University Press, 1992, pp. 71–72.

L-Threonine As a Symptomatic Treatment for Amyotrophic Lateral Sclerosis (ALS): J.B. Roufs; Med. Hypotheses., January 1991, vol. 34(1), pp. 20–23.

Motor Neuron Disease (Amyotrophic Lateral Sclerosis): D.B. Williams; Mayo Clin. Proc.; January 1991, vol. 66(1), pp. 54–82.

Birth Defects Encyclopedia: M.L. Buyse, ed.-in-chief; Blackwell Scientific Publications, 1990, pp. 110–111.

Principles of Neurology, 4th ed.: R.D. Adams and M. Victor, eds.; McGraw-Hill, 1989, pp. 953–954.

Cecil Textbook of Medicine, 18th ed.: J.B. Wyngaarden and L.H. Smith, Jr., eds.: W.B. Saunders Company, 1988, pp. 2154–2157, 2254.

# ANOREXIA NERVOSA

**Description** Anorexia nervosa is an illness of self-starvation associated with a disturbed sense of body image and extreme anxiety about weight gain.

**Synonyms**

> Apepsia Hysterica
> Eating Disorder
> Magersucht

**Signs and Symptoms** Persons suffering from anorexia nervosa have an extreme preoccupation with food and usually consider themselves to be fat when in reality that is not the case. Periods of self-starvation often alternate with periods of binge eating **(bulimia).** A 20- to 25-percent body weight loss is typical. Females with anorexia nervosa usually experience amenorrhea, and hyperactivity combined with depression is seen in many patients.

**Etiology** Anorexia nervosa is currently considered to be a psychiatric condition, possibly associated with a stressful life situation. Many individuals are described as having been perfectionists and model children. A biological cause has not been established.

**Epidemiology** Approximately 95 percent of affected persons are female. Onset of the disorder is usually in early to late adolescence. A 1989 study of the disorder's prevalence in South Australia found that the condition affected 1.05 out of 1,000 female secondary school students.

**Related Disorders** See *Bulimia.*

**Treatment—Standard** Treatment begins with correction of the malnutrition. Psychotherapy is usually essential, and family therapy can be most helpful toward provision of a calm, supportive, stable environment.

**Treatment—Investigational** Please contact the agencies listed under Resources, below, for the most current information. Addresses and telephone numbers of these agencies, as well as of individual experts and research centers, may be found in the Master Resources List.

**Resources**

**For more information on anorexia nervosa:** National Organization for Rare Disorders (NORD); American Anorexia and Bulimia Association; Anorexia Nervosa and Associated Disorders; Anorexia Nervosa and Related Eating Disorders; Bulimia, Anorexia Self-Help; NIH/National Institute of Mental Health; National Mental Health

Association; National Alliance for the Mentally Ill; National Mental Health Consumer Self-Help Clearinghouse.

**References**

Pathogenesis of Anorexia: D.M. Garner; Lancet, June 1993, vol. 341(8861), pp. 1631–1635.

Treatment of Anorexia Nervosa: P.J.V. Beumont, et al.; Lancet, June 1993, vol. 341(8861), pp. 1635–1640.

The Prevalence of Anorexia Nervosa: D.I. Ben-Tovim, et al.; N. Engl. J. Med., March 16, 1989, vol. 320(11), pp. 736–737.

Diagnostic and Statistical Manual of Mental Disorders, 3rd ed., revised: R.L. Spitzer, et al., eds.; American Psychiatric Association, 1987, pp. 65–67.

# ANTISOCIAL PERSONALITY (ASP) DISORDER

**Description** ASP disorder is a mental illness that is usually observed before the age of 15 and is characterized by antisocial behavior and a lack of concern for the rights of others.

**Signs and Symptoms** Signs in early childhood include behavior such as lying, stealing, fighting, truancy, and resisting authority. In adolescence, there may be excessive drinking, drug use, and aggressive sexual behavior. The behavioral difficulties usually persist throughout life, with markedly impaired capacity to sustain lasting, responsible relationships with family, friends, or sexual partners. In many cases, individuals with ASP disorder are unable to be consistently self-sufficient, and problems with legal authorities are common. Affected individuals tend to be irritable and aggressive, which results in physical fights, assaults, and criminality.

**Etiology** The cause is unknown. There may be association with a single-parent home, absence of parental discipline, extreme poverty, or removal from the home. Lack of educational achievement and the use of drugs may contribute. Predisposing factors may include childhood disturbances such as attention deficit hyperactivity disorder and conduct disorder.

**Epidemiology** ASP disorder affects approximately 3 percent of American males and 1 percent of American females. Males are affected at a much earlier age than females, with behavioral difficulties beginning in childhood.

**Related Disorders**

**Attention deficit hyperactivity disorder** is characterized by a very short attention span, impulsiveness, and hyperactivity. Symptoms usually occur to varying degrees depending on environmental factors, becoming worse in situations requiring sustained attention and improving when the affected person receives frequent reinforcement or is in a very structured, non-distracting setting. Onset usually is before age 4 years.

**Substance abuse** refers to the maladaptive behavior associated with regular or excessive use of a substance that can modify mood or behavior, such as alcohol or drugs. Social, occupational, psychological, or physical problems may result. Symptoms of addiction must persist for at least 1 month or occur repeatedly over a longer period of time in order to be diagnosed as a substance abuse disorder.

**Treatment—Standard** Psychological counseling is required for antisocial personality disorder, and in serious cases hospitalization and drug therapy may be necessary. Other treatment is symptomatic and supportive.

**Treatment—Investigational** Please contact the agencies listed under Resources, below, for the most current information. Addresses and telephone numbers of these agencies, as well as of individual experts and research centers, may be found in the Master Resources List.

**Resources**

**For more information on antisocial personality disorder:** National Organization for Rare Disorders (NORD); National Mental Health Association; NIH/National Institute of Mental Health.

**References**

Diagnostic and Statistical Manual of Mental Disorders, 3rd ed., revised: R.L. Spitzer, et al., eds.; American Psychiatric Association, 1987, pp. 342–346, 165–185.

Genetic and Environmental Factors in Alcohol Abuse and Antisocial Personality: R.J. Cadoret, et al.; J. Stud. Alcohol, January 1987, vol. 48(1), pp. 1–8.

Parental Behavior in the Cycle of Aggression: J. McCord; Psychiatry, February 1988, vol. 51(1), pp. 14–23.

The Relationship Between Attention Problems in Childhood and Antisocial Behavior Eight Years Later: J.L. Wallander; J. Child Psychol., Psychiatry, January 1988, vol. 29(1), pp. 53–61.

# APNEA, INFANTILE

**Description** Apnea ("without breath") denotes the temporary cessation of breathing as a result of neural arrest of respiration and consequent inhibition of air flow through the air passages. Mechanical, neurologic, and traumatic events may contribute in varying degrees to the different subdivisions of apnea. Infantile apnea, defined as apnea occurring in children less than 1 year old, may be related to some cases of infant death syndrome. Episodes of apnea may decrease with age.

**Synonyms**

> Central Apnea (Diaphragmatic Apnea)
> Mixed Apnea
> Obstructive Apnea (Upper Airway Apnea)
> Sleep Apnea

**Signs and Symptoms** The clinical picture of apnea includes a temporary cessation of breathing, accompanied by cyanosis and bradycardia. The precise physiologic derangements leading to cessation of breathing vary. In central or diaphragmatic apnea, there are no chest movements and no air passes through the mouth or nostrils. When there are diaphragmatic and thoracic movements but no airflow into the lungs, the disorder is known as obstructive apnea. Central apnea followed by or mixed with obstructive apnea is called mixed apnea.

**Etiology** The cause of infantile apnea is not known.

**Epidemiology** Infantile apnea by definition occurs in children less than 1 year old.

**Related Disorders** See *Apnea, Sleep.*

**Treatment—Standard** Respiratory stimulants such as theophylline or caffeine may be prescribed. Parents and caretakers should be knowledgeable in cardiopulmonary resuscitation. Home monitoring devices may be purchased and used under the advice of a physician.

**Treatment—Investigational** Please contact the agencies listed under Resources, below, for the most current information. Addresses and telephone numbers of these agencies, as well as of individual experts and research centers, may be found in the Master Resources List.

**Resources**

 **For more information on infantile apnea:** National Organization for Rare Disorders (NORD); National Sudden Infant Death Syndrome Resource Center; NIH/National Institute of Neurological Disorders and Stroke; Center for Research in Sleep Disorders.

**References**

Online Mendelian Inheritance in Man (OMIM): V.A. McKusick; The Johns Hopkins University; last edit date 3/31/93, entry number 107640.

Neurology in Clinical Practice, vol. II.: The Neurological Disorders: W.G. Bradley, et al., eds.: Butterworth-Heinemann, 1991, p. 1493.

Cecil Textbook of Medicine, 18th ed.: J.B. Wyngaarden and L.H. Smith, Jr., eds.; W.B. Saunders Company, 1988, p. 2079.

# APNEA, SLEEP

**Description** Sleep apnea syndrome is characterized by temporary, recurrent interruptions of respiration during sleep. Nocturnal wakefulness, daytime sleepiness, and obesity are typical features. The disorder occurs in 3 forms. **Obstructive sleep apnea (upper airway apnea),** the most common, results from blockage of the respiratory passages. Respiratory drive is normal. In the rarer **central sleep apnea,** there is little brain respiratory activity; breathing stops until the oxygen-starved brain sends impulses that activate the diaphragm and thorax. The **pickwickian syndrome** is a combination of obstructive apnea and obesity.

**Signs and Symptoms** The most common manifestations of sleep apnea are daytime sleepiness and loud nocturnal snoring. In obstructive apnea, the labored breathing is interrupted by airway constriction. The episode ends when the muscles of the diaphragm and the chest build up sufficient pressure to force the airway open. Partial awakening then occurs, as the person gasps for air; sleep is resumed as breathing begins again. This cycle may be repeated several times during the night and may lead to sleep deprivation if the person is unable to return to sleep quickly.

 Complications associated with untreated sleep apnea include hypertension, arrhythmias, abnormal blood levels of oxygen and carbon dioxide, and peripheral edema. Other complications include sleepwalking, blackouts, automatic robotlike behavior, intellectual deterioration, hallucinations, anxiety, irritability, aggressiveness, jealousy, suspiciousness, and irrational behavior. Loss of interest in sex, morning headaches, and bedwetting may also occur with time.

 Diagnosis of sleep apnea may require evaluation at a sleep disorder center. The patient fills out a questionnaire or a sleep/wake diary, and overnight examination or daytime sleep tests may be undertaken.

**Etiology** Several conditions are often associated with obstructive sleep apnea. These include obesity and a short thick neck, and reduction in muscle tone of the soft palate, the uvula, and the pharynx. The upper airway may be narrowed by enlarged tonsils or adenoids, a deviated nasal septum, nasal polyps, or congenital abnormalities. At high altitudes, sleep disruption may occur because of low oxygen concentration.

 The unstable brain respiratory control in central apnea may be associated with elevated partial pressure carbon dioxide or with decreased metabolic rate during sleep. Central sleep apnea may be produced by lesions of the region of the primary respiratory neurons of the medulla or of the descending pathways in the cervical cord.

**Epidemiology** About 2.5 million people in the United States suffer from sleep apnea, with males outnumbering premenopausal females 30 to 1. Many affected individuals are at least 20 percent above ideal body weight.

**Related Disorders** See *Apnea, Infantile; Narcolepsy; Ondine's Curse.*

**Treatment—Standard** Treatment of mild cases of obstructive sleep apnea usually consists of elevating the head with pillows, sleeping in a recliner chair, or elevating the bed's headposts by 6 to 8 inches. Elevation of the head can keep the tongue from falling backward and blocking the upper airway. In some cases drugs are used, including theophylline, protriptyline, clomipramine, pemoline, thioridazine, or nicotine.

When positional apnea is diagnosed (occurring when the patient sleeps in positions that predispose to breathing obstruction), sewing a bulky object in the back of the sleeping garment can make the supine position so uncomfortable that the person turns over.

Many patients with either central or obstructive sleep apnea have responded well to treatment with continuous positive airway pressure **(CPAP).** The device is effective in approximately 85 percent of obstructive sleep apnea patients.

A surgical technique being used increasingly is uvulo-palato-pharyngoplasty **(UPPP).** Loose tissues are tightened in the back of the mouth and top of the throat, and excess tissues that block the airway in those areas are trimmed away. UPPP has been helpful in about 55 percent of patients with obstructive sleep apnea.

**Treatment—Investigational** John Elefteriades, M.D., at Yale University School of Medicine, is conducting clinical trials to study diaphragm pacing for persons with sleep apnea who do not respond to other treatments.

Please contact the agencies listed under Resources, below, for the most current information. Addresses and telephone numbers of these agencies, as well as of individual experts and research centers, may be found in the Master Resources List.

**Resources**

**For more information on sleep apnea:** National Organization for Rare Disorders (NORD); American Sleep Apnea Association; Awake Network; Narcolepsy and Cataplexy Foundation of America; Narcolepsy Network; NIH/National Institute of Neurological Disorders and Stroke.

**References**

Cecil Textbook of Medicine, 19th ed.: J.B. Wyngaarden, et al., eds.; W.B. Saunders Company, 1992, pp. 454–455, 2066–2067.

Mechanisms of Obstructive Sleep Apnea: D.W. Hudgel; Chest, February 1992, vol. 101(2), pp. 541–549.

Mendelian Inheritance in Man, 10th ed.: V.A. McKusick; The Johns Hopkins University Press, 1992, pp. 71–72.

Clinical Features and Treatment of Obstructive Sleep Apnea: R.J. Kimoff, et al.; Can. Med. Assoc. J., March 1991, vol. 144(6), pp. 689–695.

Diseases of the Nose, Throat, Ear, Head and Neck, 14th ed.: J.J. Ballenger; Lea and Febiger, 1991, pp. 246–247.

Principles of Neurology, 4th ed.: R.D. Adams and M. Victor, eds.; McGraw-Hill, 1989, pp. 953–954.

# APRAXIA

**Description** Apraxia is a disorder of brain function in which a person is unable to carry out familiar movements, even though the desire is there and the physical ability exists.

**Synonyms**

Wieacker Syndrome

**Signs and Symptoms** When intended movement does occur, it may be clumsy, uncontrolled, and inappropriate. Some patients with apraxia are unable to dress themselves. Movement may also occur unintentionally. Apraxia is sometimes accompanied by aphasia.

**Constructional apraxia** refers to the inability to draw or construct simple configurations. Persons with **buccofacial apraxia** are not able to lick their lips, whistle, cough, or wink, and those with **oculomotor apraxia** find it difficult to move their eyes, although eye reflex movement can occur.

**Etiology** The lesion that causes apraxia may be the result of metabolic or structural diseases that involve several different regions of the brain. It may be caused by stroke, with symptoms usually appearing during the acute phase and diminishing within weeks of onset. Head injuries and degenerative dementia may result in apraxia. Some cases are the result of congenital malformations of the central nervous system.

**Related Disorders Aphasia** is a disturbance in the ability to comprehend or use language, usually resulting from injury to the cerebral cortex. Affected individuals may select the wrong words in conversing and may have difficulties interpreting verbal messages.

**Treatment—Standard** Treatment involves relearning limb gestures in conjunction with physical and occupational therapy. When apraxia is a symptom of another neurologic disorder, the underlying condition must be treated.

**Treatment—Investigational** Please contact the agencies listed under Resources, below, for the most current information. Addresses and telephone numbers of these agencies, as well as of individual experts and research centers, may be found in the Master Resources List.

**Resources**

**For more information on apraxia:** National Organization for Rare Disorders (NORD); NIH/National Institute of Neurological Disorders and Stroke.

**References**

Harrison's Principles of Internal Medicine, 12th ed.: J.D. Wilson, et al., eds.; McGraw-Hill, 1991, pp. 159–160.

The Relationship Between Limb Apraxia and the Spontaneous Use of Communicative Gesture in Aphasia: J.C. Borod, et al.; Brain Cogn., May 1989, vol. 10(1), pp. 121–131.

Cecil Textbook of Medicine, 18th ed.: J.B. Wyngaarden and L.H. Smith, Jr., eds.; W.B. Saunders Company, 1988, pp. 2082, 2087.

On the Cerebral Localization of Constructional Apraxia: K. Ruessman et al.; Int. J. Neurosci., September 1988, vol. 42(1–2), pp. 59–62.

Apraxia and the Supplementary Motor Area: R.T. Watson, et al.; Arch. Neurol., August 1986, vol. 43(8), pp. 787–792.

# ARACHNOID CYSTS

**Description** Arachnoid cysts occur on the arachnoid membrane covering the brain and spinal cord. The cysts may expand into the subarachnoid space but do not usually appear within the cerebrum or the ventricles.

**Signs and Symptoms** Arachnoid cysts may be present at birth and cause no symptoms throughout an individual's life. They are often discovered when a person seeks medical attention for headaches or seizures. When the cysts increase in size over time, symptoms may appear, especially if the cysts press against a cranial nerve, the brain, or the spinal cord. Symptoms are determined by the location of the cyst on the membrane.

Principal signs and symptoms include macrocephaly, disorders of hearing or vision, headaches, vertigo, psychomotor retardation, epileptic seizures, and premature sexual development. Other characteristics include nausea, olfactory loss, ataxia in the arms and legs, and paraplegia. In children, macrocephaly, continuous bobbing of the head, skin hypersensitive to touch, and mental retardation may be present.

Arachnoid cysts of the posterior fossa may cause vague symptoms, such as dizziness and headache, which are often associated with inner ear problems. Individuals with long-standing complaints related to the ear, and who have normal hearing tests, should be referred for CT scan or MRI.

Complications can occur when a cyst is damaged because of trauma; when fluid within a cyst leaks into other areas (e.g., subarachnoid space); when intracystic hemorrhage results from surface blood vessels bleeding into the cyst, increasing its size; or when hematoma results from bleeding outside of the cyst. In the cases of intracystic hemorrhage and hematoma, the individual may have symptoms of increased pressure within the cranium and signs of compression of nearby neural tissue.

Premature sexual development may occur secondary to a suprasellar arachnoid cyst. Symptoms of this type of cyst include head nodding, abnormal gait, and abnormalities of vision.

**Etiology** The cause of arachnoid cysts is unknown. Some are congenital, perhaps occurring as a result of developmental disturbances of the meninges; or they may develop in response to prenatal meningeal inflammation. It has been reported that in some families the cysts appear to be familial. In a few rare cases, intracranial arachnoid cysts may be inherited as an autosomal recessive trait.

There are several reports in the medical literature of arachnoid cysts and intramedullary spinal cord cysts occurring together in persons who have had spinal surgery or spinal cord trauma.

**Epidemiology** Arachnoid cysts may occur at any age and have been found in all races and geographic locations. The cysts are not rare in the general population, but they rarely occur in certain areas of the central nervous system. It has been thought that males and females are affected equally, but some reports indicate that incidence is more frequent in males.

**Related Disorders** See *Acoustic Neuroma; Arachnoiditis; Dandy-Walker Syndrome; Empty Sella Syndrome.*

**Bobble-head doll syndrome** is a rare disorder that appears in childhood and is characterized by hydrocephalus and/or obesity. Symptoms include a continuous bobbing of the head, rhythmic bending and straightening of the head and arms, a generalized fine tremor, skin that is very sensitive to touch, mental retardation, and impaired vision. The syndrome can be caused by any obstruction that results in the enlargement of the 3rd ventricle of the brain. Draining the fluid from the cyst, removal of the cyst, and/or insertion of a shunt are standard therapies.

**Hyperprolactinemia** has been associated with the extension of arachnoid cysts into the suprasellar cistern. Symptoms in women include amenorrhea and galactorrhea. Symptoms in men have been reported to include impotence and abnormally decreased function of the testes.

**Panhypopituitarism** is a rare disorder characterized by a generalized reduction or cessation of pituitary gland function. This can result when an expanding intrasellar arachnoid cyst causes the pituitary gland to become flattened. Such a cyst can be mistaken for a pituitary tumor. A CT scan or MRI may be necessary for diagnosis.

**Porencephaly** is a major congenital malformation of the brain characterized by cysts or cavitations within the brain. Symptoms usually include mental retardation, spastic paralysis, mild ophthalmoplegia, and epilepsy. Porencephaly can be diagnosed by CT scan examination.

**Treatment—Standard** If it is decided that treatment is necessary, it usually consists of surgical removal and/or drainage of the cyst. A shunt may be necessary.

If the subarachnoid space has become blocked by an arachnoid cyst, it may also be necessary to place a shunt between a ventricle and the peritoneal cavity. This will bypass the blockage and provide an adequate passageway for cerebrospinal fluid to circulate.

**Treatment—Investigational** In one study, 3 individuals who had bilateral hearing loss as a result of arachnoid cysts were treated with diuretics. This therapy resulted in improvement in symptoms, with no evidence of enlargement of the cysts during several years of follow-up.

Please contact the agencies listed under Resources, below, for the most current information. Addresses and telephone numbers of these agencies, as well as of individual experts and research centers, may be found in the Master Resources List.

**Resources**

**For more information on arachnoid cysts:** National Organization for Rare Disorders (NORD); NIH/National Institute of Neurological Disorders and Stroke; Brain and Pituitary Foundation of America.

**References**

Mendelian Inheritance in Man, 10th ed.: V.A. McKusick; The Johns Hopkins University Press, 1992, pp. 696–698, 1030, 1226.

Textbook of Endocrinology, 8th ed.: J.D. Wilson and D.W. Foster, eds.; W.B. Saunders Company, 1992, pp. 1191–1192.

Textbook of Uncommon Cancer: C.J. Williams, ed.; John Wiley and Sons, Ltd., 1991, pp. 573–579.

Birth Defects Encyclopedia: M.L. Buyse, ed.-in-chief; Blackwell Scientific Publications, 1990, pp. 236–239.

Diagnosis and Treatment of Arachnoid Cysts of the Posterior Fossa: T.J. Haberkamp, et al.; Otolaryngol. Head Neck Surg., October 1990, vol. 103(4), pp. 610–614.

Dictionary of Medical Syndromes, 3rd ed.: S.I. Magalini, et al., eds.; J.B. Lippincott Company, 1990, pp. 123, 216–217.

# ARACHNOIDITIS

**Description** Arachnoiditis is a progressive inflammatory disorder of the arachnoid membrane, with possible involvement of the brain and spinal cord.

**Synonyms**

Arachnitis

Cerebral Arachnoiditis

Chronic Adhesive Arachnoiditis

Serous Circumscribed Meningitis

Spinal Arachnoiditis

**Signs and Symptoms** Initially, the patient experiences gradual loss of sensations and movement of the legs; as the condition progresses, muscle atrophy, weakness, and involuntary twitching of muscles are seen. Cerebral involvement leads to symptoms such as severe headaches, visual disturbances, dizziness, nausea, and vomiting. Spinal involvement may cause pain, weakness, and paralysis. In the most severe cases, loss of vision and paralysis may develop. Ossification of the arachnoid membrane also may occur.

**Etiology** Arachnoiditis can be a complication of meningitis, trauma, or subarachnoid hemorrhage, or may develop following local injections of anesthetic agents or testing dyes. An immune deficiency may also contribute.

**Epidemiology** Males and females are affected in equal numbers. Individuals who have had spinal surgery or injuries to the spine or head may be at greater risk.

**Related Disorders** See *Pseudotumor Cerebri.*

**Leptomeningitis** is characterized by inflammation of the soft membranes surrounding the brain and spinal cord, including the pia mater and arachnoid membrane. This disorder is thought to be a complication of chronic meningitis.

**Epiduritis** is characterized by inflammation of the dura mater.

**Treatment—Standard** Treatment consists of a combination of surgery and drug therapy. Surgical removal of adhesions and accumulated fluids may be helpful in some cases, especially if pressure develops. Cyclophosphamide and nitrogen mustard may improve headaches and vision loss, and anti-inflammatory drugs may also be used. Other treatment is symptomatic and supportive.

**Treatment—Investigational** For arachnoiditis caused by a parasitic infection (a rare cause in the United States), the drug praziquinatel has been used with some success.

Please contact the agencies listed under Resources, below, for the most current information. Addresses and telephone numbers of these agencies, as well as of individual experts and research centers, may be found in the Master Resources List.

**Resources**

**For more information on arachnoiditis:** National Organization for Rare Disorders (NORD); Arachnoiditis Information and Support Network; NIH/National Institute of Neurological Disorders and Stroke; American Paraplegia Society; Spinal Cord Society; National Spinal Cord Injury Hotline; National Spinal Cord Injury Association.

**References**

Spinal Arachnoiditis Due to *Aspergillus* Meningitis in a Previously Healthy Patient: F.A. Van de Wyngaert, et al.; J. Neurol., February 1986, vol. 233(1), pp. 41–43.

Pathogenesis of Postmyelographic Arachnoiditis: J.C. Garancis, et al.; Invest. Radiol., January–February 1985, vol. 20(1), pp. 85–89.

Spinal Ossifying Arachnoiditis: Case Report: F. Tomasello, et al.; J. Neurosurg. Sci., October–December 1985, vol. 29(4), pp. 335–340.

# ARNOLD-CHIARI SYNDROME

**Description** Arnold-Chiari syndrome is characterized by displacement of the distal brain stem (medulla) through the foramen magnum, where it becomes impacted in the upper cervical canal. Infantile Arnold-Chiari syndrome is usually associated with myelomeningocele. Hydrocephalus is commonly present, as well as other malformations of the brain and spinal cord.

**Synonyms**

Arnold-Chiari Malformation

Cerebellomedullary Malformation Syndrome

**Signs and Symptoms** In infants, vomiting, mental impairment, head and facial muscle weakness, and difficulties with swallowing may be present. The extremities may be paralyzed.

In adults and adolescents, the malformation may be asymptomatic until gradual signs and symptoms of cerebellar, lower cranial nerve, and pyramidal dysfunction occur. Downbeat nystagmus is characteristic. Dizziness, headache, vomiting, diplopia, deafness, weakness of the legs, ataxia, and occipital neuralgia may occur.

Symptoms may also simulate those produced by tumors near the foramen magnum or by multiple sclerosis.

**Etiology** Because of the complexity and associated defects, the cause is uncertain; it appears to be due to a failure of normal development of the brain stem and upper cervical region.

**Epidemiology** Arnold-Chiari syndrome is usually found in infants but may occur in adolescents and adults.

**Related Disorders** Hydrocephalus is frequently found with this syndrome. In addition, myelomeningocele, stenosis of the aqueduct, platybasia, syringobulbia, and syringomyelia are often associated with Arnold-Chiari syndrome. See *Hydrocephalus; Spina Bifida; Syringobulbia; Syringomyelia.*

**Treatment—Standard** Surgical repair of an existing meningocele and ventricular shunting procedures for relief of hydrocephalus are necessary. Prognosis is poor for infants with extensive defects.

In adults, surgical enlargement of the foramen magnum and decompression of the cervicomedullary junction may prove beneficial.

**Treatment—Investigational** Please contact the agencies listed under Resources, below, for the most current information. Addresses and telephone numbers of these agencies, as well as of individual experts and research centers, may be found in the Master Resources List.

**Resources**

**For more information on Arnold-Chiari syndrome:** National Organization for Rare Disorders (NORD); Arnold-Chiari Family Network; NIH/National Institute of Neurological Disorders and Stroke; American Syringomyelia Alliance Project.

**For genetic information and genetic counseling referrals:** March of Dimes Birth Defects Foundation; Alliance of Genetic Support Groups.

**References**

Mendelian Inheritance in Man, 9th ed.: V.A. McKusick; The Johns Hopkins University Press, 1990, p. 1043.

Cecil Textbook of Medicine, 18th ed.: J.B. Wyngaarden and L.H. Smith, eds.; W.B. Saunders Company, 1988, p. 2258.

# ASPERGER SYNDROME

**Description** Asperger syndrome is a neuropsychiatric disorder whose major manifestation is an inability to understand how to interact socially. Other features include poor verbal and motor skills, single-mindedness, and social withdrawal. The syndrome has similarities to autism.

**Signs and Symptoms** Symptoms of Asperger syndrome are not usually recognized until a child reaches 30 months of age. The child displays little interest or pleasure in other persons, and imaginative play may be absent or repetitious.

Speech begins at the normal age but is unusual, with the child talking at length on a single subject. Grammar may eventually be understood, but the child has difficulty with pronouns, referring to himself or herself in the 2nd or 3rd person. Speaking usually is monotonous or, contrarily, exaggerated. Many children with Asperger syndrome have excellent rote memory and musical ability.

Nonverbal communication is also affected. The face is usually expressionless unless the child feels strong emotions. Bodily movement may be limited or inappropriate, and walking may be delayed. Lack of coordination results in difficulties with running, ball throwing, and other games, as well as with writing and drawing.

The lack of social and communicative skills results in a feeling of being different and an inability to understand and participate in social interaction, leading to withdrawal from society. These difficulties reach a peak during adolescence. A young man with Asperger syndrome and a strong sex drive, wanting to be normal but with no understanding, may show inappropriate behavior towards the opposite sex.

**Etiology** The cause is unclear. Some affected children and adults have had a history of pre-, peri-, or postnatal problems. Cerebral damage has been postulated; almost 50 percent of those studied suffered lack of oxygen at birth. An organic deficiency of brain function has also been suggested as a cause. Possible hereditary aspects of Asperger syndrome have not been well investigated.

**Epidemiology** Males are affected more often than females.

**Treatment—Standard** Intensive, highly structured, skill-oriented training on a continual basis is most useful for both children and adults with this syndrome. Other treatment is symptomatic and supportive.

**Treatment—Investigational** Please contact the agencies listed under Resources, below, for the most current information. Addresses and telephone numbers of these agencies, as well as of individual experts and research centers, may be found in the Master Resources List.

**Resources**

**For more information on Asperger syndrome:** National Organization for Rare Disorders (NORD); NIH/National Institute of Neurological Disorders and Stroke; Learning Disabilities Association of America; NIH/National Society for Children and Adults with Autism; Martha Dencklau, M.D., Johns Hopkins School of Medicine.

**References**

Asperger's Syndrome: Diagnosis, Treatment and Outcome: Szatmari, P.; Psychiatr. Clin. North Am., March 1991, vol. 14, pp. 81–92.

Asperger's Syndrome: To Be or Not to Be: Kerbeshian, et al.; Brit. J. Psychiatry, May 1990, vol. 156, pp. 721–725.

Is Asperger's a Syndrome?: J. Green; Dev. Med. Child Neur., August 1990, vol. 32(8), pp. 743–747.

Left Temporal Lobe Damage in Asperger's Syndrome: P. Jones, et al.; Brit. J. Psychiatry, April 1990, vol. 156, pp. 570–572.

Non-Autistic Pervasive Developmental Disorders: F. Volkmar, et al.; Psychiatry, 1990, vol. 2(ch. 27), pp. 1–10.

Developmental Cortical Anomalies in Asperger's Syndrome: Neurological Findings in Two Patients: M.L. Besthier, et al.; J. Neuropsychiatry Clin. Neurosci., Spring 1990, vol. 2(2), pp. 197–201.

# ASTROCYTOMA, BENIGN

**Description** Benign astrocytomas, tumors composed of glial cells (astrocytes), can occur anywhere in the brain or spinal cord. The subcortical white matter is the most common location in adults, and the optic nerve, cerebellum, and brain stem are the most common locations in children.

**Synonyms**

> Astrocytoma Grade I
> Astrocytoma Grade II
> Brain Tumor
> Intracranial Neoplasm
> Intracranial Tumor

**Signs and Symptoms** Manifestations of a benign astrocytoma depend on its size, location, and rate of growth. Onset may be sudden or gradual.

Recurrent headache, usually resulting from pressure on blood vessels, cranial nerves, or pain-sensitive tissue, is the initial symptom in 50 percent of cases. Seizures are the initial manifestation in 20 percent of cases and are typically the result of slow-growing astrocytomas.

Gradual-onset symptoms include mental changes, such as increased irritability, emotional instability, forgetfulness, and loss of initiative or spontaneity. With increased tumor size, symptoms may progress to confusion, lethargy, and stupor.

Other manifestations may include nausea, vomiting, bradycardia, incontinence, astereognosis, paralysis, ataxia, aphasia, nystagmus, and facial pain or numbness.

**Etiology** The cause is not known.

**Epidemiology** Benign astrocytomas may occur in anyone at any age, but white males between the ages of 40 and 70 are most commonly affected.

**Related Disorders** See *Astrocytoma, Malignant; Multiple Sclerosis.*

**Treatment—Standard** Benign astrocytomas are generally detected by CT scan or MRI; biopsy is then performed to determine the optimal treatment approach.

Preoperative treatment attempts to control fluid accumulation with corticosteroids or a shunt; anticonvulsant agents are given to prevent seizures. Surgical removal of the astrocytoma may be successful if the tumor is accessible. Laser microsurgery can remove local infiltrates with minimal tissue damage. Surgery is usually followed by radiation therapy.

Radiation is used as primary therapy in some instances, followed by chemotherapy.

**Treatment—Investigational** Various experimental approaches are being used as treatment for astrocytomas. Brachytherapy involves surgical implantation of radioactive pellets of iodine, iridium, or gold isotopes. This procedure can be used for a tumor that is less than 2.5 inches in diameter and is confined to one side of the brain. Other investigational therapies include use of cell radiosensitizers that can increase the effectiveness of radiation, hyperthermia and photoradiation, intraoperative radiation, and hyperfractionation.

A multitude of new drugs, drug combinations, and drug delivery systems are being tested for effectiveness against astrocytomas. Agents being used to boost the immune system include interferon, levamisole, interleukin-2, thymosine, and bacille Calmette-Guérin.

A new orphan drug and delivery system being tested uses a biodegradable wafer containing a cytotoxic agent that is implanted at the site of the tumor. As the wafer dissolves over a period of many weeks, the drug is slowly released. For more information contact Nova Pharmaceutical Corporation.

Please contact the agencies listed under Resources, below, for the most current information. Addresses and telephone numbers of these agencies, as well as of individual experts and research centers, may be found in the Master Resources List.

**Resources**

**For more information on benign astrocytoma:** National Organization for Rare Disorders (NORD); NIH/National Institute of Neurological Disorders and Stroke; American Brain Tumor Association.

**References**

Benign Astrocytic and Oligodendrocytic Tumors of the Cerebral Hemispheres in Children: J.F. Hirsch, et al.; J. Neurosurg., April 1989, vol. 70(4), pp. 568–572.

Long-Term Follow-up After Surgical Treatment of Cerebellar Astrocytomas in 100 Children: S. Undjian, et al.; Childs Nerv. Syst., April 1989, vol. 5(2), pp. 99–101.

Low-Grade Astrocytomas: Treatment with Unconventionally Fractionated External, Beam Stereotactic Radiation Therapy: F. Pozza, et al.; Radiology, May 1989, vol. 171(2), pp. 565–569.

Cecil Textbook of Medicine, 18th ed.: J.B. Wyngaarden and L.H. Smith, Jr., eds.; W.B. Saunders Company, 1988, pp. 2229–2235.

Low-Grade Astrocytomas: Treatment Results and Prognostic Variables: C.A. Medbery 3rd, et al.; Int. J. Radiat. Oncol. Biol. Phys., October 1988, vol. 15(4), pp. 837–841.

# ASTROCYTOMA, MALIGNANT

**Description** A malignant astrocytoma is an infiltrating primary brain tumor composed of astrocytes. Typical onset is in late middle age. Tentacles from the tumor invade normal tissue, spreading through the white matter of the cerebral hemispheres in a butterfly pattern. Occasionally the dura or ventricles (reached through the spinal fluid) are involved. Familial cases have been identified, and an association with exposure to industrial chemicals is recognized. About one-third of cases are fatal in the first year.

**Synonyms**

> Anaplastic Astrocytoma
> Astrocytoma, Grades III and IV
> Giant Cell Glioblastoma
> Spongioblastoma Multiforme

**Signs and Symptoms** The earliest symptom typically is headache, caused by increased intracranial pressure. The headache is generalized, worse in the morning, and accompanied by vomiting. Personality changes may accompany or precede the headache.

Other symptoms are referable to the particular area of brain affected. Frontal lobe tumors are associated with memory loss, intellectual impairment, and a flat affect; these symptoms may be accompanied by contralateral convulsions or paralysis. Parietal lobe tumors result in agraphia, paresthesias, loss of proprioception, and occasionally seizures. Symptoms of temporal lobe tumors are less marked initially but eventually include seizures, muscle incoordination, and difficulty in language use and interpretation.

Sixty-five to 70 percent of patients are alive 1 year after diagnosis; 40 percent survive for 2 years.

**Etiology** The cause of malignant astrocytoma is unknown. Because of an apparent familial predilection, a hereditary component has been postulated but not proved. A viral etiology has also been postulated. Some cases have been linked to exposure to industrial chemicals, such as polyvinyl chloride and agricultural pesticides.

**Epidemiology** Malignant astrocytoma commonly affects individuals between the ages of 48 and 60 years, although it has also occurred in children. The prevalence is higher in men than in women, especially men with type A blood, and higher in whites than in nonwhites.

**Related Disorders** See *Glioblastoma Multiforme.*

**Treatment—Standard** Open surgery or laser microsurgery is the preferred treatment for astrocytomas. Surgery is followed by irradiation of the whole brain, and chemotherapy. For inoperable tumors, a subtotal decompressive resection may be performed to reduce the number of tumor cells and increase the effectiveness of radiation therapy and chemotherapy.

**Treatment—Investigational** Brachytherapy has been tried experimentally, primarily for small recurrences. The mode, fraction schedule, and time of delivery of conventional radiation therapy have been manipulated in various trials. The use of cell radiosensitizers may increase the effectiveness of radiation.

Immunotherapy drugs may be administered to stimulate the body's defenses against the tumor. Techniques under investigation include the intra-arterial delivery of various drugs, and disruption of the blood-brain barrier to facilitate drug entry into the brain.

A new orphan drug and delivery system is being tested for treatment of astrocytoma and glioblastoma. During surgery to remove the tumor, a biodegradable wafer containing BCNU is implanted at the site. James Kenealy, M.D., of Nova Pharmaceutical Corporation in Baltimore, can be contacted.

Please contact the agencies listed under Resources, below, for the most current information. Addresses and telephone numbers of these agencies, as well as of individual experts and research centers, may be found in the Master Resources List.

**Resources**

**For more information on malignant astrocytoma:** National Organization for Rare Disorders (NORD); American Brain Tumor Association; American Cancer Society; NIH/National Institute of Neurological Disorders and Stroke; NIH/National Cancer Institute Physician Data Query Phoneline.

**References**

About Glioblastoma Multiforme and Malignant Astrocytoma: D.P. Hesser, et al., eds.; Association for Brain Tumor Research, 1985.

# ATAXIA, FRIEDREICH

**Description** Friedreich ataxia is a progressive, hereditary spinocerebellar degeneration disorder that typically manifests in childhood or adolescence. Slow degenerative changes of the spinal cord and brain affect speech and motor coordination, producing numbness or weakness of the arms and legs, secondary lateral scoliosis, and lower limb paralysis. Although the disorder is progressive and treatment is symptomatic only, spontaneous remissions of 5 to 10 years in duration have been reported.

**Synonyms**

Familial Ataxia
Friedreich Disease
Friedreich Tabes
Hereditary Ataxia
Spinocerebellar Ataxia

**Signs and Symptoms** Ataxia denotes a failure of muscle coordination that typically results in an unsteady gait. The hallmark of Friedreich ataxia is progressive weakness of the legs, reflected in a staggering, lurching gait, or trembling when the subject is standing still. Partial loss of the sense of touch or sensitivity to pain and temperature may occur. With time, a high-arched foot may develop. Involvement of the throat muscles leads to impaired swallowing and choking and may result in difficulty eating. The intellect and emotions are rarely affected. Scoliosis, diabetes mellitus, or cardiomyopathy may occur but are not necessary for a diagnosis. The average age at death is about 35 to 40 years.

**Etiology** Friedreich ataxia is usually inherited as an autosomal recessive trait involving chromosome 9. A variant form is inherited as a dominant trait; its gene has been located on chromosome 6.

Symptoms are caused by degeneration of nerve cells in the dorsal root ganglia, spinal cord, and brain.

**Epidemiology** Although Friedreich ataxia can be present at birth, symptoms usually first appear between the ages of 8 and 15 years. Estimates of prevalence in the United States range from 2,000 to 3,000 cases to as many as 20,000.

A more precise estimate is difficult to render, as many cases are likely misdiagnosed. The syndrome is the most common of the various forms of hereditary ataxia.

**Related Disorders** Ataxia is common to several disorders and may take many forms, not all hereditary in origin. See **Ataxia, Marie; Charcot-Marie-Tooth Disease; Ataxia Telangiectasia; Olivopontocerebellar Atrophy.**

**Treatment—Standard** Treatment is symptomatic and supportive. Therapy includes medication, physiotherapy, orthotic support, and surgery. Propranolol may be effective against the static tremors of Friedreich ataxia and, less often, against intention tremors. Dantrolene sodium may help some patients with muscle spasms of the legs. Use of these drugs must be monitored in the individual patient to avoid toxicity. Physiotherapy to promote remaining muscle function is frequently helpful, and orthopedic surgery or braces may be prescribed to correct scoliosis and abnormalities of the feet.

Continuous medical supervision is necessary to avoid complications involving the heart, lungs, skeleton, and muscles. Preventing pneumonia in advanced stages of Friedreich ataxia is a medical challenge. Medication may be used to treat the cardiomyopathy and diabetes mellitus associated with Friedreich ataxia. These secondary problems may increase the patient's susceptibility to infection, leading to the need for further drug therapy.

Genetic and psychological counseling can assist many patients and families affected by one of the hereditary ataxias. Prenatal diagnosis is available for pregnant women.

**Treatment—Investigational** Epidural spinal electrostimulation (**ESES**) with a multiprogrammable spinal cord stimulator is currently being evaluated in the treatment of motor dysfunction. The device, which can be implanted surgically over the spine, may provide therapeutic benefit in some types of ataxia when other measures have failed.

Please contact the agencies listed under Resources, below, for the most current information. Addresses and telephone numbers of these agencies, as well as of individual experts and research centers, may be found in the Master Resources List.

**Resources**

**For more information on Friedreich ataxia:** National Organization for Rare Disorders (NORD); National Ataxia Foundation; NIH/National Institute of Neurological Disorders and Stroke; International Tremor Foundation.

**For information on clinical services for persons with Friedreich ataxia, including provision of orthopedic aids, recreation at summer and winter camps, and transportation assistance:** Muscular Dystrophy Association.

**For more information on scoliosis:** National Scoliosis Foundation.

**For more information on diabetes:** American Diabetes Association.

**For genetic information and genetic counseling referrals:** March of Dimes Birth Defects Foundation; Alliance of Genetic Support Groups.

**References**

Cecil Textbook of Medicine, 19th ed.: J.B. Wyngaarden, et al., eds.; W.B. Saunders Company, 1992, p. 2138.

Birth Defects Encyclopedia: M.L. Buyse, ed.-in-chief; Blackwell Scientific Publications, 1990, pp. 203–204.

The Friedreich Ataxia Gene Is Assigned to Chromosome 9q13–q21 by Mapping of Tightly Linked Markers and Shows Linkage Disequilibrium with D9S15: A. Hanauer, et al.; Am. J. Hum. Genet., January 1990, vol. 46(1), pp. 131–137.

Mendelian Inheritance in Man, 9th ed.: V.A. McKusick; The Johns Hopkins University Press, 1990, pp. 1184–1186.

# ATAXIA, MARIE

**Description** Marie ataxia is a hereditary cerebellar disorder that affects muscle coordination, producing an early symptom of unsteady gait. Progressive spinal nerve degeneration leads to muscle atrophy in the limbs and head and neck area. The condition appears to have 2 peaks of onset: the 1st in early adulthood, and the 2nd in middle age. Persons first affected in middle age are more likely to have mild cases.

**Synonyms**

> Cerebellar Syndrome
> Hereditary Cerebellar Ataxia
> Nonne Syndrome
> Pierre-Marie Disease

**Signs and Symptoms** Marie ataxia typically manifests first with lower limb motor deficits that are noticed as the afflicted person walks up or down stairs or over uneven ground. The likelihood of falls increases with progression of the disease. The uncoordination and muscle tremors eventually involve the arms and head. When muscles of the head and neck are affected, speech may be difficult to produce, and choking becomes a major concern. Because the ability to clear secretions from the lungs is also affected, patients are more susceptible to pneumonia and other respiratory tract diseases. Extraocular and facial muscle weakness and tongue atrophy may occur. Vision abnormalities are a late development.

A set of manifestations rarely found with other ataxias may occur in Marie ataxia; these include abnormal reflexes, muscle contractions, and diminished perception of pain or touch. The patient usually retains good bladder control and sexual function.

**Etiology** Marie ataxia is inherited as a dominant trait. Atrophy of the cerebellum and spinal cord is believed responsible for the symptoms.

**Epidemiology** Some 7,000 cases of Marie ataxia have been diagnosed in the United States, although the total may be higher as a result of misdiagnosis and underreporting.

**Related Disorders** Ataxia, or failure of muscle coordination with a notable early symptom of unsteady gait, occurs in many disorders. There are as well many forms of ataxia, some inherited, others acquired, frequently secondary to another disorder. See *Ataxia, Friedreich; Ataxia Telangiectasia; Olivopontocerebellar Atrophy.*

**Treatment—Standard** Treatment is directed at controlling symptoms. Propranolol can be effective for control of some tremors, and dantrolene sodium may be of limited help for patients with leg muscle spasms, but these drugs must be monitored for side effects. Physiotherapy and daily walking, assisted as necessary, will promote remaining muscle function. Surgery, prescription lenses, or drugs may be used to address vision problems. The patient is advised to avoid foods that could precipitate choking spells. Prevention of pneumonia is a challenge that may be met with a combination of antibiotics and postural drainage.

**Treatment—Investigational** The multiprogrammable spinal cord stimulator, an implantable device that delivers epidural spinal electrostimulation **(ESES),** may aid in the treatment of ataxias and other neuromuscular disorders refractory to medical treatment by improving mobility and alleviating spasticity and pain.

The orphan drug physostigmine salicylate (Antilirium) is being studied in the treatment of the inherited ataxias.

Please contact the agencies listed under Resources, below, for the most current information. Addresses and telephone numbers of these agencies, as well as of individual experts and research centers, may be found in the Master Resources List.

**Resources**

**For more information on Marie ataxia:** National Organization for Rare Disorders (NORD); National Ataxia Foundation; NIH/National Institute of Neurological Disorders and Stroke.

**For information on clinical services for persons with ataxia, including provision of orthopedic aids, recreation at summer and winter camps, and transportation assistance:** Muscular Dystrophy Association.

**For genetic information and genetic counseling referrals:** March of Dimes Birth Defects Foundation; Alliance of Genetic Support Groups.

**References**

Spinocerebellar Ataxia Associated with Localized Amyotrophy of the Hands, Sensorineural Deafness and Spastic Paraparesis in Two Brothers: F. Gemignani; J. Neurogenet., March 1986, vol. 3(2), pp. 125–133.

Treatment of Patients with Degenerative Diseases of the Central Nervous System by Electrical Stimulation of the Spinal Cord: D.M. Dooley, et al.; Contin. Neurol., 1981, vol. 44(1–3), pp. 71–76.

Otoneurologic Symptomatology in Hereditary Cerebellar Ataxia (Pierre-Marie disease): Ila Kalinovskaia, et al.; Zh. Nevropatol. Psikhiatr., 1980, vol. 80(3), pp. 367–372.

# ATAXIA TELANGIECTASIA

**Description** Ataxia telangiectasia is a severe inherited cerebellar ataxia characterized by progressive loss of motor coordination in the limbs and head, vascular oculocutaneous lesions, heightened susceptibility to sinopulmonary disease and neoplasms, and, frequently, premature aging. In some cases the disorder is associated with IgA or IgE immunodeficiency. Mental development may be normal in the early stages of the disease, but progressive dementia can occur during the 2nd decade of life. The clinical presentation may resemble that of Friedreich ataxia; however, the telangiectasia distinguishes ataxia telangiectasia.

**Synonyms**

Louis-Bar Syndrome

Cerebello-Oculocutaneous Telangiectasia

Immunodeficiency with Ataxia Telangiectasia

**Signs and Symptoms** The signs and symptoms of ataxia telangiectasia are wide-ranging and affect many distinct systems. Manifestations usually begin in infancy; some may not appear until the child is school age. An early sign is impaired muscle coordination, which usually becomes evident when walking is attempted. Coordination of the head and neck muscles is also impaired, and tremors may occur. Mental development may be delayed or regress as the disorder advances.

When the patient is 3 to 6 years of age, the hallmark telangiectasia appears in the eyes, followed by involvement of the face and roof of the mouth. Other symptoms, especially those linked to growth and development, become more prominent at this age. Impaired neuromuscular function in the head and neck area leads to abnormal eye movements, faulty speech production, dysphagia, choking, and poor cough reflexes. Abnormal development or nondevelopment of thymus, adenoids, tonsils, and peripheral lymph nodes is a component in some cases of ataxia telangiectasia. A variety of tics, jerks, and other irregular involuntary movements may accompany the disorder. Diminished immune system function and cell-mediated immunity make patients increasingly susceptible to sinopulmonary infections at about 3 years.

Premature aging occurs in 90 percent of cases, typically against a background of growth retardation. Incomplete sexual development and other endocrine abnormalities affect children of both sexes.

Persons with ataxia telangiectasia have a higher-than-normal incidence of carcinoma and lymphoma, first noticeable in adulthood. Exposure to X-irradiation may trigger the development of tumors.

**Etiology** Ataxia telangiectasia is believed to be inherited as an autosomal recessive trait. Various mechanisms have been postulated to account for the multiplicity of symptoms in this disorder. Neuromuscular symptoms may be due to degenerative central nervous system changes. A thymus gland deficiency has been linked to the immunologic abnormalities. The disorder has also been attributed variously to a defect in early fetal development and to a genetic defect in ability to repair damaged cells.

**Epidemiology** Ataxia telangiectasia has a familial tendency, frequently affecting more than one sibling. No sex predominance has been discerned. Approximately 1:40,000 newborns in the United States are affected.

**Related Disorders** See ***Ataxia, Friedreich; Ataxia, Marie; Charcot-Marie-Tooth Disease; Olivopontocerebellar Atrophy.***

**Treatment—Standard** Medication and physiotherapy are the mainstays of the symptomatic treatment of ataxia telangiectasia. Rigorous medical supervision is necessary to prevent infections or reduce their impact. Antibiotics, gammaglobulin, and postural drainage may be prescribed for respiratory tract infections. The neuromuscular effects, such as slurred speech and muscle contractions, may improve with diazepam. Reducing exposure to sunlight will help prevent the spread of lesions. Physiotherapy promotes muscle strength and may delay the onset of limb contractures.

**Treatment—Investigational** Specific diagnostic and therapeutic efforts directed toward the immunologic and endocrinologic components of ataxia telangiectasia are under way. The drugs under investigation in these research protocols include levamisole, interleukin-2, and interferon, for their immune effects, and various chemotherapeutic agents. The orphan drug physostigmine salicylate (Antilirium) is in clinical trial for the treatment of the inherited ataxias. For more information, contact Forest Pharmaceuticals in St. Louis, Missouri.

Please contact the agencies listed under Resources, below, for the most current information. Addresses and telephone numbers of these agencies, as well as of individual experts and research centers, may be found in the Master Resources List.

**Resources**

**For more information on ataxia telangiectasia:** National Organization for Rare Disorders (NORD); NIH/National Institute of Neurological Disorders and Stroke; National Ataxia Foundation; Ataxia Telangiectasia Research Foundation; International Tremor Foundation.

**For more information on tumors:** American Cancer Society; NIH/National Cancer Institute Physician Data Query Phoneline.

**For genetic information and genetic counseling referrals:** March of Dimes Birth Defects Foundation; Alliance of Genetic Support Groups.

**References**

Cancer Incidences in Families with Ataxia Telangiectasia: M. Swift, et al.; N. Engl. J. Med., December 26, 1991, vol. 325(26), pp. 12831–12836.
Vascular Disorders: The Genodermatoses : A.S. Paller; Dermatol. Clin., February 1987, vol. 5(1), pp. 239–250.
Ataxia-Telangiectasia of Louis-Bar Syndrome: S.L. Conerly, et al.; J. Am. Acad. Dermatol., April 1985, vol. 12(4), pp. 681–696.

# AUTISM

**Description** Autism is a lifelong, nonprogressive neurologic disorder characterized by onset usually before age 30 months, language and communication disorders, withdrawal from social contacts, and extreme reactions to changes in the immediate environment. About 75 percent of autistic children have low scores on standardized intelligence tests. The prognosis for independent living may be improved with intensive training but is generally poor. Life span is normal.

**Synonyms**

Infantile Autism

Kanner Syndrome

**Signs and Symptoms** Autism generally manifests before age 3. Among the earliest symptoms are lack of response to other persons and a marked preference for passive, solitary activity. The child does not watch others and avoids physical contact. Toddlers tend to form stronger attachments to objects than to people. Slight rearrangement of the objects in the physical environment, such as furniture, may provoke a violent and extreme reaction. Autistic children's response to aural and visual stimuli is unpredictable, ranging from seeming indifference to violent emotion. Hyperactivity is common and may lead to sleeping and eating disorders. Tantrums may occur if the child feels confused or is hindered in the pursuit of some activity. Autistic children may spend hours rocking rhythmically or engaged in some other solitary, repetitive activity; the child appears self-absorbed. Motor development is frequently delayed.

Delayed acquisition of language skills is prominent among the communication disorders observed in autistic children. When speech does develop, it is characterized by echophrasia and lack of grammar. Voluntary statements are often inappropriate in pitch, rhythm, or inflection. Some children stop speaking for years. Although hearing is intact, autistic children often appear deaf. Proposed deficits in information processing by the brain at the level of synthesis and abstraction may account for the difficulties in acquiring and using language.

Emotional lability and a preference for solitude remain prominent as the autistic child grows up. Play has a strong ritualistic, repetitive component. Unusual mannerisms develop, and bodily posture or limb movements may be contorted. Oral expression may pass into a stage of tooth grinding and muttering in place of speech. Reading and writing are learned with great difficulty. A few children exhibit unusual ability in aspects of music, mathematics, or rote memory.

Clinically, electroencephalographic abnormalities occur in some autistic patients.

Behavior usually improves around school age. Nevertheless, only a small proportion of autistic people ever adjust to independent living, even with intensive social and educational training. Most remain fully dependent and in need of sheltered homes for life.

**Etiology** Earlier theories proposing a psychogenic basis for autism have been superseded by the theory that the condition is an organic brain disorder. Several of the defects in autism can be traced to a central nervous system incapacity to process and respond to informational input, particularly auditory and visual stimuli. A deficit in information-processing capability could account for the impaired interpretive and conceptualizing skills exhibited by the autistic person.

A familial or genetic cause for some types of autism has been postulated, in part because of the higher incidence of the disorder in siblings. Autism may be inherited through autosomal recessive genes. A genetic component is also suggested by the greater number of boys than girls with infantile autism.

The role of metabolic, infectious, genetic, and environmental influences pre- and perinatally is under investigation. Defective tryptophan processing has been proposed as a metabolic factor. More research is needed to confirm a genetic origin and to elucidate the contribution of prenatal events to the development of autism.

**Epidemiology** About 5:10,000 children have the fully expressed syndrome; some 15:10,000 children have 2 or more of the cardinal features of autism. Nearly 4,000 American families have 2 or more autistic children. Boys are affected 4 times more frequently than girls.

**Related Disorders** Other childhood disorders, such as epilepsy, metabolic diseases, congenital rubella, and mental retardation of other cause, may have an autistic component. The autistic syndrome must be differentiated from other conditions in which impaired language reception and use or schizophrenia are prominent symptoms. See *Asperger Syndrome; Phenylketonuria; Rett Syndrome; Rubella, Congenital.*

**Treatment—Standard** Treatment is primarily educational. Highly structured programs initiated early in life and providing around-the-clock care and oversight will maximize the child's chances of normal adaptation. Parental education programs and support groups benefit families considerably. Institutionalization is not recommended. Major tranquilizers such as trifluoperazine or haloperidol may be used to control hyperactivity or emotional lability.

**Treatment—Investigational** Fenfluramine is being studied investigationally as treatment for a subcategory of autistic people.

Brain opioid levels may be unusually high in autism. Naltrexone, a drug manufactured for the treatment of opioid drug abuse, is being studied as therapy for autism on the theory that it will block brain cell receptors for natural opioids and secondarily decrease the effects of these neurochemicals in autistic persons.

Please contact the agencies listed under Resources, below, for the most current information. Addresses and telephone numbers of these agencies, as well as of individual experts and research centers, may be found in the Master Resources List.

**Resources**

**For more information on autism:** National Organization for Rare Disorders (NORD); Autism Society of America; National Mental Health Association; National Alliance for the Mentally Ill; National Mental Health Consumer Self-Help Clearinghouse; NIH/National Institute of Neurological Disorders and Stroke; NIH/National Institute of Mental Health.

**For genetic information and genetic counseling referrals:** March of Dimes Birth Defects Foundation; Alliance of Genetic Support Groups.

**References**

Nelson Textbook of Pediatrics, 14th ed.: R.E. Behrman, ed.-in-chief; W.B. Saunders Company, 1992, p. 72.
Mendelian Inheritance in Man, 9th ed.: V.A. McKusick; The Johns Hopkins University Press, 1990, pp. 1058–1059.

# BALÓ DISEASE

**Description** Baló disease is a childhood condition of brain demyelination characterized by progressive spastic paralysis and other neurologic symptoms, depending on which parts of the brain are affected. The areas of demyelination can be localized in any part of the brain (e.g., the cerebral hemispheres, the cerebellum, and the brain stem); the lesions consist of irregular patches in concentric circles. The disease may progress rapidly over several weeks, or over 2 to 3 years.

**Synonyms**

Concentric Sclerosis
Encephalitis Periaxialis Concentrica
Leukoencephalitis Periaxialis Concentrica

**Signs and Symptoms** The child gradually becomes spastic and paralyzed. Other neurologic, intellectual, and physiologic abnormalities may also develop, depending on the area of the brain affected.

**Etiology** The cause is unknown. There may be involvement of autoimmune factors or a slow virus. The disorder has been considered to be a variant of multiple sclerosis.

**Epidemiology** Baló disease affects children of both sexes.

**Related Disorders** See *Adrenoleukodystrophy; Alexander Disease; Leukodystrophy, Canavan; Leukodystrophy, Metachromatic; Leukodystrophy, Krabbe; Multiple Sclerosis.*

**Schilder disease,** a more severe form of brain demyelinization, appears to differ in its progression. Baló disease and Schilder disease may be related.

**Treatment—Standard** There is no specific treatment. Care is supportive and symptomatic.

**Treatment—Investigational** Please contact the agencies listed under Resources, below, for the most current information. Addresses and telephone numbers of these agencies, as well as of individual experts and research centers, may be found in the Master Resources List.

**Resources**

**For more information on Baló disease:** National Organization for Rare Disorders (NORD); United Leukodystrophy Foundation; NIH/National Institute of Neurological Disorders and Stroke.

**References**

Dictionary of Medical Syndromes, 3rd ed.: S.I. Magalini, et al.; J.B. Lippincott Company, 1990, p. 84.
Principles of Neurology, 4th ed.: R.D. Adams and M. Victor, eds.; McGraw-Hill, 1989, pp. 768–769.

# BATTEN DISEASE

**Description** Batten disease is the juvenile form of a group of inherited progressive neurologic diseases known as **neuronal ceroid lipofuscinoses.** It is characterized by accumulation of lipopigment in the brain and other tissues, leading to rapidly progressive optic atrophy, seizures, and intellectual impairment. Age at onset is 5 to 10 years.

**Synonyms**

Amaurotic Familial Idiocy, Juvenile type
Batten-Mayou Syndrome
Batten-Spielmeyer-Vogt Disease
Batten-Vogt Syndrome
Neuronal Ceroid Lipofuscinosis
Spielmeyer-Vogt Disease
Spielmeyer-Vogt-Batten Syndrome
Stengel Syndrome
Stengel-Batten-Mayou-Spielmeyer-Vogt-Stock Disease

**Signs and Symptoms** The major findings are ocular atrophy with pigmentary degeneration, intellectual deterioration, and seizures. Other manifestations include kyphoscoliosis, twitching, spasticity, and ataxia.

The diagnosis of Batten disease requires blood tests and rectal, skin, or conjunctival punch biopsy for biochemical and ultrastructural studies. Other useful information may be derived from an electroencephalogram, electroretinogram, and visual evoked response test, as well as from magnetic resonance imaging and computed tomography. A biochemical evaluation is also performed to determine the urinary level of dolichol, which is elevated in patients with Batten disease.

**Etiology** Batten disease is transmitted as an autosomal recessive trait. It is suspected that an enzyme deficiency leads to accumulation of lipopigments in nerves and other tissues.

**Epidemiology** In the United States, all forms of neuronal ceroid lipofuscinoses occur in approximately 3:100,000 live births. It is seen more commonly in families of Scandinavian ancestry, particularly Swedish.

**Related Disorders** Symptoms of all the neuronal ceroid lipofuscinoses are similar; they are mainly differentiated by age of onset.

**Treatment—Standard** Treatment is usually symptomatic and supportive. Regular ophthalmic evaluation and services that benefit persons with visual impairment are beneficial. Genetic counseling may be useful.

**Treatment—Investigational** Clinical, pathologic, biochemical, and genetic research on the neuronal ceroid lipofuscinoses began in 1987.

The National Institute of Neurological Disorders and Stroke and the National Institute of Mental Health support 2 national human brain specimen banks that supply tissue for investigation into neurologic and psychiatric diseases. Prospective donors are asked to contact Wallace W. Tourtellotte, M.D., at the V.A. Wadsworth Medical Center in Los Angeles, or Edward D. Bird, M.D., at McLean Hospital in Belmont, Massachusetts.

Michael Bennett, M.D., and associates at Baylor University Medical Center are studying cultured fibroblasts of children with chromosome-16–linked juvenile Batten disease.

Please contact the agencies listed under Resources, below, for the most current information. Addresses and telephone numbers of these agencies, as well as of individual experts and research centers, may be found in the Master Resources List.

**Resources**

**For more information on Batten disease:** National Organization for Rare Disorders (NORD); Batten's Disease Support and Research Association; New York State Institute for Basic Research in Developmental Disabilities; NIH/National Institute of Neurological Disorders and Stroke; National Tay-Sachs and Allied Diseases Association; National Lipid Diseases Foundation; Children's Brain Diseases Foundation for Research; Research Trust for Metabolic Disease in Children.

**For genetic information and genetic counseling referrals:** March of Dimes Birth Defects Foundation; Alliance of Genetic Support Groups.

**References**

Mendelian Inheritance in Man, 9th ed.: V.A. McKusick; The Johns Hopkins University Press, 1990, pp. 1026–1027, 1028, 1382.

# BELL'S PALSY

**Description** Bell's palsy is a nonprogressive facial nerve disorder characterized by sudden onset of facial paralysis. The paralysis results from ischemia and compression of the 7th cranial nerve.

**Synonyms**

> Facial Nerve Palsy
> Facial Paralysis
> Refrigeration Palsy

**Signs and Symptoms** Early symptoms include pain behind the ear, a stiff neck, and unilateral facial weakness and stiffness. Onset can be rapid, over several hours, and sometimes follows exposure to cold temperatures or a draft. Part or all of the face may be affected on one side.

In most cases, only muscle weakness is involved, and the facial paralysis is temporary. Occasionally, only the upper or lower half of the face is affected. In severe cases, the facial muscles on the affected side are completely paralyzed, causing that side of the face to become smooth, expressionless, and immobile. Often the palpebral fissure is enlarged, remaining open even during sleep, with the result that the eyes cannot be closed. Corneal reflex also may be absent. If the lesion is proximal to the nerve branching, there may be decreased salivation and lacrimation, ipsilateral loss of the sense of taste, and hyperacusis. In some cases, pinprick sensation behind the ear also is decreased.

Recovery depends on the extent and severity of nerve damage. If the facial paralysis is only partial, complete recovery can be expected. The affected muscles usually regain their original function within 1 to 2 months. If, as recovery proceeds, the nerve fibers regrow to muscles other than the ones they originally innervated, there may be synkinesia. Crocodile tears (inappropriate lacrimation) associated with facial muscular contractions occasionally develop in the aftermath of Bell's palsy.

**Etiology** Ischemia and compression of the facial nerve within the canal occur as the result of nerve swelling and hyperemia of the nerve sheath. Although the cause is unknown, viral and immune diseases often are implicated. There also appears to be an inherited tendency toward developing this disorder.

**Related Disorders** See *Acoustic Neuroma; Melkersson-Rosenthal Syndrome; Myasthenia Gravis.*

Other disorders of the 7th cranial nerve and nucleus include mastoid and middle ear infections, Ramsay Hunt syndrome (geniculate ganglion herpes), pontine tumors, and nerve invasion by carcinoma. Supranuclear lesions from stroke or tumor are characterized by weakness only below the eyes. Unilateral myasthenia gravis may present similar clinical findings.

**Treatment—Standard** About 85 percent of patients with Bell's palsy will make a complete recovery without treatment. Massage and mild electrical stimulation of the paralyzed muscles maintain muscle tone and prevent atrophy. Treatment with oral corticosteroids, such as prednisone, has been more successful than surgical attempts to widen the facial canal. Methylcellulose drops, eyeglasses or goggles, temporary patching, or, in extreme cases, tarsorrhaphy, can help protect the exposed eye. If permanent paralysis has resulted, the peripheral facial nerve can be surgically anastomosed with the spinal accessory or hypoglossal nerves to allow some eventual return of muscle function.

**Treatment—Investigational** The orphan drug acyclovir (Zovirax) is being used to treat some cases of Bell's palsy, alone or in combination with prednisone.

Please contact the agencies listed under Resources, below, for the most current information. Addresses and telephone numbers of these agencies, as well as of individual experts and research centers, may be found in the Master Resources List.

**Resources**

**For more information on Bell's palsy:** National Organization for Rare Disorders (NORD); NIH/National Institute of Neurological Disorders and Stroke.

**References**

Cecil Textbook of Medicine, 19th ed.: J.B. Wyngaarden, et al., eds.; W.B. Saunders Company, 1992, pp. 1774, 2248.

Mendelian Inheritance in Man, 10th ed.: V.A. McKusick; The Johns Hopkins University Press, 1992, p. 376.

Medical Management of Idiopathic (Bell's) Palsy: K.K. Adour; Otolaryngol. Clin. North Am., June 1991, vol. 24(3), pp. 663–673.

Bell's Palsy: G.J. Petruzzeli; Postgrad. Med., August 1990, vol. 90(2), pp. 115–118, 121–122, 125–127.

Bell's Palsy: Ensuring the Best Outcome: J.D. Morgenlander; October 1990, vol. 88(5), pp. 157–161, 164.

Principles of Neurology, 4th ed.: R.D. Adams and M. Victor, eds.; McGraw-Hill, 1989, pp. 953–954.

# BENIGN ESSENTIAL BLEPHAROSPASM (BEB)

**Description** BEB is a disorder in which the orbiculares oculi muscles do not function properly and there is intermittent involuntary contraction or spasm of the musculature around the eyes. Although the eyes themselves are unaffected, the patient may eventually become functionally blind because of inability to open the eyes.

**Synonyms**

> Blepharospasm
> Secondary Blepharospasm

**Signs and Symptoms** In the early stages, BEB is characterized by unusually frequent or forceful blinking, as well as by occasional short episodes of involuntary eye closure. Over a period of several years, the episodes increase in frequency and duration. Ultimately, the eyes may be closed 75 percent of the time.

Approximately two-thirds of patients also have a general lack of facial muscle tone, and one-third experience tremor. Episodes may be provoked by bright light, emotional stress, motion (such as riding in a car), and reading.

**Etiology** The disorder results from dysfunction of the 7th cranial nerve, but the underlying cause is not known. BEB is frequently but incorrectly considered to be a problem of psychological origin.

**Epidemiology** Females are affected more often than males in an approximate ratio of 3:2. Most patients are older than 50, but onset may be as early as the 2nd decade. All types of blepharospasm together are estimated to affect approximately 150,000 individuals in the United States.

**Related Disorders Tetany** is a mineral imbalance characterized by spasms of the voluntary muscles.

**Tetanus** is a bacterial infection characterized by spasms of the voluntary muscles and especially the muscles of the jaw.

See *Meige Syndrome; Tardive Dyskinesia; Tourette Syndrome; Wilson Disease.*

**Treatment—Standard** Anticholinergic drugs and dopamine depleters have been administered with moderate but often temporary effect.

Two surgical approaches are in use, but also with limited success. Following neurectomy, paralysis of the entire upper face may result, with nerve regeneration after a period of months or years. The second procedure, a protractor myectomy, involves the destruction of the eyelid muscles themselves.

The orphan drug botulinum A toxin (Oculinum) has been approved by the Food and Drug Administration as a treatment for blepharospasm. Small amounts of this agent are injected into the orbicularis oculi, paralyzing these muscles for several months. The procedure must then be repeated. These injections have been very helpful for some, but not all, patients with blepharospasm. The drug is available from Allergan, Irvine, California, and financial assistance is available.

**Treatment—Investigational** Please contact the agencies listed under Resources, below, for the most current information. Addresses and telephone numbers of these agencies, as well as of individual experts and research centers, may be found in the Master Resources List.

**Resources**

**For more information on benign essential blepharospasm:** National Organization for Rare Disorders (NORD); Benign Essential Blepharospasm Research Foundation; NIH/National Institute of Neurological Disorders and Stroke; Dystonia Medical Research Foundation; We Move.

**References**

Cecil Textbook of Medicine, 19th ed.: J.B. Wyngaarden, et al., eds.; W.B. Saunders Company, 1992, p. 2135.

Clinical Doxorubicin Chemomyectomy: An Experimental Treatment for Benign Essential Blepharospasm and Hemifacial Spasm: J.D. Wirtschafter; Ophthalmology, March 1991, vol. 98(3), pp. 357–366.

Facial Dystonias, Essential Blepharospasm and Hemifacial Spasm: J.B. Hold; Am. Fam. Physician, June 1991, vol. 43(6), pp. 2113–2120.

A Genetic Study of Idiopathic Focal Dystonias: H.M. Waddy, et al.; Ann. Neurol., March 1991, vol. 29(3), pp. 320–324.

Ophthalmology: Principles and Concepts, 7th ed.: F.W. Newell; Mosby Year Book, 1991, p. 194.

# BENIGN ESSENTIAL TREMOR SYNDROME

**Description** Benign essential tremor is a disorder of unknown etiology primarily affecting the hands and head. The disease may be slowly progressive, eventually affecting other parts of the body.

**Synonyms**

> Hereditary Benign Tremor
> Presenile Tremor Syndrome

**Signs and Symptoms** The primary characteristic is a fine or coarse rhythmic tremor, with a frequency of 4 to 12 times per second when the affected part is in movement or voluntarily held in one position. This is in contrast to Parkinson disease tremors, which usually diminish or disappear entirely with purposeful movement (see *Parkinson Disease).* The tremors mainly affect the upper extremities and are aggravated by stress, anxiety, fatigue, and cold. Speech involvement and hyperhidrosis may be seen.

**Etiology** The disorder may occur spontaneously, in which case the cause is unknown, or be inherited as an autosomal dominant trait.

**Epidemiology**. Onset may be in childhood or old age, but middle-aged adults are affected most frequently. The mean age of onset is 45. Males and females are affected in equal numbers, but males may experience symptoms at an earlier age than females.

**Treatment—Standard** Tremors may be diminished or controlled by the use of phenobarbital, lorazepam, alprazolam, propranolol, or primidone. Methazolamide may be effective, especially in those individuals with head and voice tremors. Rest may be helpful. Alcohol can relieve the symptoms but should be used with care because of its potential for abuse.

**Treatment—Investigational** The surgical procedures thalamotomy and pallidotomy have been used to treat rare, severely disabling cases of benign essential tremor. High-frequency thalamic stimulation procedures are also being tested.

Please contact the agencies listed under Resources, below, for the most current information. Addresses and telephone numbers of these agencies, as well as of individual experts and research centers, may be found in the Master Resources List.

**Resources**

**For more information on benign essential tremor syndrome:** National Organization for Rare Disorders (NORD); International Tremor Foundation; NIH/National Institute of Neurological Disorders and Stroke.

**For genetic information and genetic counseling referrals:** March of Dimes Birth Defects Foundation; Alliance of Genetic Support Groups.

**References**

Cecil Textbook of Medicine, 19th ed.: J.B. Wyngaarden, et al., eds.; W.B. Saunders Company, 1992, pp. 2133–2134.

Mendelian Inheritance in Man, 10th ed.: V.A. McKusick; The Johns Hopkins University Press, 1992, p. 1108.

The Symptomatic and Functional Outcome of Stereotactic Thalamotomy for Medically Intractable Essential Tremor: M.S. Goldman, et al.; J. Neurosurg., June 1992, vol. 76(6), pp. 924–928.

Clinicopathologic Observations in Essential Tremor: Report of Six Cases: A.H. Rajput, et al.; Neurology, February 1991, vol. 41(2 pt. 1), pp. 1422–1424.

Essential Tremor: Clinical Correlates in 350 Patients: J.S. Lou, et al.; Neurology, February 1991, vol. 41(2 pt. 1), pp. 234–238.

Treatment of Essential Tremor with Methazolamide: M.D. Muenter, et al.; Mayo Clin. Proc., October 1991, vol. 66(10), pp. 991–997.

Birth Defects Encyclopedia: M.L. Buyse, ed.-in-chief; Blackwell Scientific Publications, 1990, p. 1696.

Principles of Neurology, 4th ed.: R.D. Adams and M. Victor, eds.; McGraw-Hill, 1989, p. 81.

# Benign Paroxysmal Positional Vertigo (BPPV)

**Description** BPPV is characterized by extreme dizziness on certain movements of the head, and by nystagmus.

**Synonyms**
> Cupulolithiasis
> Postural Vertigo

**Signs and Symptoms** Episodes of violent dizziness occur without warning, triggered by movements such as turning the head from side to side, by lying on the right or left ear, and by moving to a sitting position. The dizziness (vertigo) is often accompanied by nausea and vomiting, and nystagmus usually also occurs. The symptoms may last only a few weeks or months and may disappear spontaneously.

**Etiology** Head trauma, ear infection, and ear surgery are among the causes of BPPV. In many cases the cause is unknown.

**Epidemiology** BPPV primarily affects females during middle or late adulthood.

**Related Disorders** See *Meniere Disease.*

**Vestibular neuronitis of Dix and Hallpike** is characterized by dizziness, nausea, and vomiting; symptoms may worsen with head movement. Hearing is usually not impaired. Onset is abrupt in young adulthood, and the disorder may continue through the 40s. Etiology is unknown, although there is often an association with upper respiratory tract infection and fever.

**Treatment—Standard** Patients learn to avoid the precipitating positions. Medications can be used to decrease dizziness and to control nausea or vomiting. If bacterial infection is present in the ear, antibiotics are appropriate.

**Treatment—Investigational** A Jannetta procedure may be helpful in some cases of BPPV. For more information on this type of experimental surgery, contact Margareta Moller, M.D., Presbyterian University Hospital, Pittsburgh, Pennsylvania.

Please contact the agencies listed under Resources, below, for the most current information. Addresses and telephone numbers of these agencies, as well as of individual experts and research centers, may be found in the Master Resources List.

**Resources**

**For more information on benign paroxysmal positional vertigo:** National Organization for Rare Disorders (NORD); E.A.R. Foundation; NIH/National Institute of Neurological Disorders and Stroke; Vestibular Disorders Association.

**References**

Internal Medicine, 3rd ed.: J.H. Stein, ed.-in-chief; Little, Brown and Company, 1990, p. 1929.

# Binswanger Disease

**Description** Binswanger disease is a form of senile dementia associated with lesions of the deep white matter in the brain resulting from small-vessel arteriosclerotic changes.

**Synonyms**
> Binswanger Encephalopathy
> Ischemic Periventricular Leukoencephalopathy
> Multi-Infarct Dementia
> Subcortical Arteriosclerotic Encephalopathy

**Signs and Symptoms** Progressive loss of recent memory, difficulty coping with unusual events, self-centeredness, and childish behavior are typical findings. Urinary incontinence, difficulty walking, parkinsonian-type tremors, and depression are also prominent features of the disease.

**Etiology** Binswanger disease is a form of chronic cerebrovascular disease. Hypertension and diabetes may predispose to this condition. A history of repeated small strokes is commonly obtained.

**Epidemiology** Males are affected more often than females. Disease onset is generally after 60 years of age.

**Related Disorders** Many neurologic disorders can cause dementia and memory disturbances. See ***Alzheimer Disease; Pick Disease; Creutzfeldt-Jakob Disease.***

**Treatment—Standard** Treatment is symptomatic and supportive, relying on antihypertensive and antidepressant agents.

**Treatment—Investigational** Please contact the agencies listed under Resources, below, for the most current information. Addresses and telephone numbers of these agencies, as well as of individual experts and research centers, may be found in the Master Resources List.

**Resources**

**For more information on Binswanger disease:** National Organization for Rare Disorders (NORD); Alzheimer's Disease and Related Disorders Association; NIH/National Institute of Neurological Disorders and Stroke; NIH/National Institute on Aging; International Tremor Foundation.

**References**

Reversible Depression in Binswanger Disease: N. Venna, et al.; J. Clin. Psychiatry, January 1988, vol. 49(1), pp. 23–26.

Senile Dementia of the Binswanger Type: A Vascular Form of Dementia in the Elderly: G.C. Roman; JAMA, October 1987, vol. 258(13), pp. 1782–1788.

White Matter Lucencies on Computed Tomography, Subacute Arteriosclerotic Encephalopathy (Binswanger Disease), and Blood Pressure: B.A. McQuinn, et al.; Stroke, September–October 1987, vol. 18(5), pp. 900–905.

Subcortical Arteriosclerotic Encephalopathy (Binswanger Disease): Computed Tomographic, Nuclear Magnetic Resonance, and Clinical Correlations: W.R. Kinkel, et al.; Arch. Neurol., October 1985, vol. 42(10), pp. 951–959.

# BROWN-SÉQUARD SYNDROME

**Description** The spinal cord is affected unilaterally in this spinal cord injury.

**Synonyms**

> Hemisection of the Spinal Cord
> Partial Spinal Sensory Syndrome

**Signs and Symptoms** Symptoms most often appear after trauma to the neck or back. Ipsilateral loss of touch and proprioception and contralateral loss of pain and temperature occur below the level of the lesion. Bladder and bowel function may be gone. Paralysis ipsilateral to the wound often occurs and may be permanent if diagnosis is delayed.

**Etiology** Aside from the most common cause (injury to the back or neck), the syndrome can be the result of viral or bacterial disease, an arachnoid cyst, or epidural hematoma. Blunt trauma, such as occurs in a fall or automobile accident, may also rarely cause the disorder, if there is vascular damage.

**Epidemiology** The syndrome is very rare; approximately 500 cases have been reported to date. Males and females are affected in equal numbers.

**Related Disorders** See ***Primary Lateral Sclerosis.***

**Motor neuron disease,** a degenerative condition, may affect the upper or lower motor neurons. **Progressive spinal muscular atrophy** is a slowly progressive motor neuron disease. Muscle weakness and wasting may begin in the hands and eventually affect the arms, shoulders, legs, and the rest of the body. Muscle twitching may occur in the limbs and tongue.

**Treatment—Standard** Treatment involves drugs that control muscle symptoms: baclofen to relieve spasticity, quinine for cramping, and diazepam for muscular contractions.

Devices that help the patient continue daily activities, such as braces, hand splints, limb supports, or a wheelchair, are important. Various other aids may be necessary if the patient has difficulty breathing or swallowing. Other treatment is symptomatic and supportive.

**Treatment—Investigational** Human ciliary neurotrophic factor, recombinant, and insulin-like growth factor-1 (Myotrophin) are orphan products being tested for treatment of motor neuron diseases.

Please contact the agencies listed under Resources, below, for the most current information. Addresses and telephone numbers of these agencies, as well as of individual experts and research centers, may be found in the Master Resources List.

**Resources**

**For more information on Brown-Séquard syndrome:** National Organization for Rare Disorders (NORD); NIH/National Institute of Neurological Disorders and Stroke; Amyotrophic Lateral Sclerosis Association.

**For information about motor neuron disease that occurs during childhood:** Families of Spinal Muscular Atrophy.

**References**

Blunt Cervical Spine Brown-Séquard Injury: A Report of Three Cases: D.W. Oller, et al.; Am. Surg., June 1991, vol. 57(6), pp. 361–365.

Brown Séquard Syndrome Caused by Borrelia Burgdorferi: P. Berlit, et al.; Eur. Neurol., 1991, vol. 31(1), pp. 18–20.

Brown-Séquard Syndrome Following Cervical Spine Compression Fracture: P.J. Zorn; Del. Med. J., September 1991, vol. 9, pp. 549–553.
Brown-Séquard Syndrome Associated with Posttraumatic Cervical Epidural Hematoma: Case Report and Review of the Literature: G.M. Zupruk, et al.; Neurosurgery, August 1989, vol. 25(2), pp. 278–280.
Principles of Neurology, 4th ed.: R.D. Adams and M. Victor, eds.; McGraw-Hill, 1989, pp. 50, 129–130, 722, 740, 743.

# BULIMIA

**Description** Bulimia is a psychiatric disorder characterized by binge eating followed by self-induced vomiting or purging with laxatives or diuretics.

**Signs and Symptoms** The alternating bingeing and purging or fasting typical of the patient with bulimia can lead to significant weight fluctuations. Menstrual irregularities also may be seen. Many patients fear they cannot stop eating voluntarily.

**Etiology** The cause is unknown.

**Epidemiology** Approximately 95 percent of bulimic persons are female. Onset is usually during adolescence or early adulthood.

**Related Disorders** See *Anorexia Nervosa.*

**Treatment—Standard** Treatment attempts to improve self-image and stabilize eating patterns through provision of a calm, supportive, stable environment and psychotherapy.

**Treatment—Investigational** Please contact the agencies listed under Resources, below, for the most current information. Addresses and telephone numbers of these agencies, as well as of individual experts and research centers, may be found in the Master Resources List.

**Resources**

**For more information on bulimia:** National Organization for Rare Disorders (NORD); Bulimia, Anorexia Self-Help; American Anorexia and Bulimia Association; Anorexia Nervosa and Associated Disorders; Anorexia Nervosa and Related Eating Disorders; NIH/National Institute of Mental Health; National Mental Health Association; National Anorexic Aid Society; National Alliance for the Mentally Ill; National Mental Health Consumer Self-Help Clearinghouse.

**References**
Cecil Textbook of Medicine, 18th ed.: J.B. Wyngaarden and L.H. Smith, Jr., eds.; W.B. Saunders Company, 1988, pp. 656, 1218–1219.
Diagnostic and Statistical Manual of Mental Disorders, 3rd ed., revised: R.L. Spitzer, et al., eds.; American Psychiatric Association, 1987, pp. 67–69.

# CENTRAL CORE DISEASE

**Description** Central core disease, characterized by muscle weakness beginning in the neonatal period, is one of the diseases contributing to floppy baby syndrome. The legs are usually most severely involved. The disease derives its name from the characteristic biopsy finding of an abnormal core in each muscle fiber.

**Synonyms**

Muscle Core Disease

Nonprogressive Congenital Myopathy

**Signs and Symptoms** The muscles of the upper arm are hypotonic, weak, and somewhat underdeveloped. Infants find it difficult to learn to sit and to walk. By about 6 years of age, however, most affected children can walk, and as adults, the disease often is experienced only as slight weakness in the legs. Persons with central core disease seem to be unusually susceptible to malignant hyperthermia in response to anesthesia. Creatine kinase blood levels may be increased.

**Etiology** Families with central core disease usually demonstrate dominant gene inheritance. The gene that causes central core disease has been located on the long arm of chromosome 19 (19q12–q13.2). Some studies have linked this disease with a specific gene at this location known as the ryanodine receptor gene **(RYR1)**, but the biochemical abnormality causing muscular weakness and the presence of the core in the muscle fibers is not known. Absence of mitochondria and certain oxidative enzymes is observed in the involved muscle fibers.

**Epidemiology** Males and females are affected in equal numbers.

**Related Disorders** See *Centronuclear Myopathy; Muscular Dystrophy, Batten Turner; Fiber Type Disproportion, Congenital; Leukodystrophy, Canavan; Muscular Dystrophy, Limb-Girdle; Nemaline Myopathy.*

It has been suggested that *Malignant Hyperthermia* and central core disease are caused by defects in the same gene.

**Treatment—Standard** Treatment of central core disease is symptomatic and supportive.

**Treatment—Investigational** Please contact the agencies listed under Resources, below, for the most current information. Addresses and telephone numbers of these agencies, as well as of individual experts and research centers, may be found in the Master Resources List.

**Resources**

**For more information on central core disease:** National Organization for Rare Disorders (NORD); NIH/National Institute of Neurological Disorders and Stroke; Muscular Dystrophy Association; Malignant Hyperthermia Association of the United States.

**For genetic information and genetic counseling referrals:** March of Dimes Birth Defects Foundation; Alliance of Genetic Support Groups.

**References**

Refined Genetic Localization for Central Core Disease: J.C. Mulley, et al.; Am. J. Hum. Genet., February 1993, vol. 52(2), pp. 398–405.
Cecil Textbook of Medicine, 19th ed.: J.B. Wyngaarden, et al., eds.; W.B. Saunders Company, 1992, p. 2256.
Mendelian Inheritance in Man, 10th ed.: V.A. McKusick; The Johns Hopkins University Press, 1992, p. 206.
Birth Defects Encyclopedia: M.L. Buyse, ed.-in-chief; Blackwell Scientific Publications, 1990, p. 1192.
Principles of Neurology, 4th ed.: R.D. Adams and M. Victor, eds.; McGraw-Hill, 1989, pp. 995, 1143.

# CEREBELLAR AGENESIS

**Description** Affected persons are born with partial formation or total absence of the cerebellum.

**Synonyms**

> Cerebellar Aplasia
> Cerebellar Hemiagenesis
> Cerebellar Hypoplasia

**Signs and Symptoms** Patients with partial formation of the cerebellum may have few or no symptoms. When the cerebellum is absent, problems include ataxia, hypotonia, and nystagmus. Mental retardation occurs in some patients.

**Etiology** Cerebellar agenesis is thought to be inherited as an autosomal recessive trait.

**Epidemiology** The disorder is very rare; cases from approximately 7 families have been documented in the medical literature. Males and females are affected in equal numbers.

**Related Disorders** See *Arnold-Chiari Syndrome; Joubert Syndrome.*

**Treatment—Standard** Treatment is symptomatic and supportive. Special education services and physical therapy may be beneficial. Genetic counseling will benefit both patient and family.

**Treatment—Investigational** Please contact the agencies listed under Resources, below, for the most current information. Addresses and telephone numbers of these agencies, as well as of individual experts and research centers, may be found in the Master Resources List.

**Resources**

**For more information on cerebellar agenesis:** National Organization for Rare Disorders (NORD); Children's Brain Diseases Foundation for Research; The Arc (a national organization on mental retardation); NIH/National Institute of Neurological Disorders and Stroke.

**For genetic information and genetic counseling referrals:** March of Dimes Birth Defects Foundation; Alliance of Genetic Support Groups.

**References**

Birth Defects Encyclopedia: M.L. Buyse, ed.-in-chief; Blackwell Scientific Publications, 1990, p. 298.
Mendelian Inheritance in Man, 9th ed.: V.A. McKusick; The Johns Hopkins University Press, 1990, p. 1082.

# CEREBELLAR DEGENERATION, SUBACUTE

**Description** Subacute cerebellar degeneration may involve not only the cerebellum but also the medulla oblongata, the cerebral cortex, and possibly the brain stem. Two subtypes exist: **paraneoplastic cerebellar degeneration** and **alcoholic/nutritional cerebellar degeneration.** The former is associated with and often may precede the development of several types of cancer. It occurs most often in patients with lung cancer (especially small cell carcinoma), but may also occur in patients with cancers of the ovary, breast, stomach, or uterus, as well as in patients with Hodgkin disease.

**Synonyms**

> Subacute Cerebellar Degeneration

**Signs and Symptoms** Characteristics of subacute cerebellar degeneration include ataxia, dysarthria (especially noticeable in the paraneoplastic subtype), dysphagia, dementia (occurring in approximately half of patients with paraneoplastic cerebellar degeneration), nystagmus, diplopia, vertigo, and ophthalmoplegia. In alcoholic cerebellar degeneration, the ataxia predominantly involves the lower extremities; dysarthria and nystagmus are unusual.

In subacute cerebellar degeneration, a loss of Purkinje cells occurs throughout the cerebellum. A CT scan may show enlargement of the 4th ventricle as well as progressive cerebellar atrophy with prominent cerebellar folia. Examination of cerebrospinal fluid is usually normal except that it may show elevated lymph cells, an elevated protein level, and increased IgG concentration.

**Etiology** Paraneoplastic cerebellar degeneration is thought to be an autoimmune disorder. Alcoholic/nutritional cerebellar degeneration is associated with a thiamine deficiency. Antibodies reacting to Purkinje cells have been found in the serum and cerebrospinal fluid of some patients with paraneoplastic cerebellar degeneration associated with gynecologic cancers (ovarian, uterine, breast).

**Epidemiology** In the paraneoplastic subtype, the average age of onset is 50, with males affected more often than females. This form of cerebellar degeneration may precede cancer. The alcoholic or nutritional subtype, affecting those with thiamine deficiency, is not related to cancer and is more common.

**Related Disorders** See *Hodgkin Disease; Korsakoff Syndrome; Multiple Sclerosis.*

**Wernicke encephalopathy,** a degenerative brain disorder associated with a deficiency of thiamine and alcoholism, is marked by ataxia and apathy, confusion, disorientation, or delirium. Various visual dysfunctions may also develop. This disorder often occurs in conjunction with *Korsakoff Syndrome.* Wernicke encephalopathy can be severely disabling and life-threatening if it is not recognized and treated early.

**Treatment—Standard** Paraneoplastic cerebellar degeneration may improve after successful treatment of the underlying cancer. Plasmapheresis has been reported to be beneficial in a few cases of paraneoplastic cerebellar degeneration. For alcoholic/nutritional cerebellar degeneration, thiamine is given along with other B vitamins, usually relieving the condition if the patient stops drinking alcohol and resumes a normal diet.

**Treatment—Investigational** Please contact the agencies listed under Resources, below, for the most current information. Addresses and telephone numbers of these agencies, as well as of individual experts and research centers, may be found in the Master Resources List.

**Resources**

**For more information on subacute cerebellar degeneration:** National Organization for Rare Disorders (NORD); American Cancer Society; NIH/National Institute of Neurological Disorders and Stroke; NIH/National Cancer Institute.

**For genetic information and genetic counseling referrals:** March of Dimes Birth Defects Foundation; Alliance of Genetic Support Groups.

**References**

Characterization of a CDNA Encoding a 34-Kda Purkinje Neuron Protein Recognized by Sera from Patients with Paraneoplastic Cerebellar Degeneration: H.M. Furneaux, et al.; Proc. Natl. Acad. Sci. USA, April 1989, vol. 86(8), pp. 2873–2877.

Internal Medicine, 2nd ed.: J.H. Stein, ed.-in-chief; Little, Brown and Company, 1987, pp. 997, 999, 2250.

A Quantitative Histological Study of the Cerebellar Vermis in Alcoholic Patients: S.C. Phillips, et al.; Brain, April 1987, vol. 110(pt. 2), pp. 301–314.

Mendelian Inheritance in Man, 8th ed.: V.A. McKusick; The Johns Hopkins University Press, 1986, p. 1262.

# CEREBRAL PALSY

**Description** Cerebral palsy is a neuromuscular disorder resulting from injury to the brain during early fetal development or at birth. Affected individuals typically exhibit a lack of muscle control and coordination. The disorder is not progressive.

**Synonyms**

Cerebral Diplegia

Infantile Cerebral Paralysis

Little's Disease

Palsy

**Signs and Symptoms** Infants with cerebral palsy may exhibit developmental delay during the 1st or 2nd year, and may have muscle weakness and abnormal muscle tone.

As the child grows, typical findings include drooling, difficulty gaining bladder or bowel control, convulsive seizures, hand tremors, and the inability to identify objects by touch. Poor vision is found more often in these patients than in the general population. The intellect may be average or above average, or there may be impairment ranging from mild to severe.

Cerebral palsy is classified according to which limbs are affected and to the quality of the movement disturbance. If both legs are affected, the condition is called diplegia; if both arms and legs are affected, quadriplegia.

**Spastic cerebral palsy** is characterized by involuntary contraction of the muscles and a scissor gait. The lower legs may turn in and cross at the ankle. In some cases, the extensor leg muscles are so tightly contracted that the heels do not touch the floor and the child walks on tiptoe.

**Athetoid cerebral palsy** is characterized by athetosis that may be accompanied by facial grimacing, abnormal tongue movements, and drooling. Involuntary flailing or jerky motions may also occur.

In **ataxic cerebral palsy,** the principal disturbance in movement is a lack of balance and coordination. The person may sway when standing, have trouble maintaining balance, and may walk with the feet spread wide apart to avoid falling.

**Etiology** Cerebral palsy is caused by injury to the brain during the early stages of fetal development or at birth. The injury may result from maternal-fetal infection, bleeding into the brain, or lack of oxygen at birth. Premature infants are especially susceptible.

Cerebral palsy also may be acquired postnatally. Head injuries, infections such as meningitis, and other forms of brain damage occurring in the first months of life are the main causes.

**Epidemiology** The United Cerebral Palsy Association estimates that between 1:1,000 and 3:1,000 infants develop cerebral palsy each year, or about 9,000 new cases. Severity can range from mild to very severe.

**Related Disorders** See *Kernicterus; Phenylketonuria.*

**Treatment—Standard** Treatment relies on physical therapy, biofeedback, occupational therapy, and vocational training. In some cases, a surgical procedure will lengthen and transfer tendons in patients with severe muscle contractions; this can be done in several body areas, including the elbows, shoulders, and back of the heel.

Certain drugs are useful in treating cerebral palsy. Anticonvulsant drugs are usually prescribed to treat associated seizures. Diazepam and other muscle relaxants can sometimes relieve spasticity. In patients who experience difficulty with urinary control because of uncontrolled bladder contractions, administration of anticholinergic drugs may help.

**Treatment—Investigational** Local electrical stimulation of nerves important for motor coordination and control is under investigation as a possible treatment. A surgical procedure being tested for selected cerebral palsy patients involves rhizotomy. Improvement has been seen in certain patients with severe diplegia, but the procedure is used only on an experimental basis when conservative measures have proved ineffective.

The orphan drug flunarizine (Sibelium) is being tested as a treatment for hemiplegia associated with cerebral palsy. The orphan drug botulinum toxin type A (Botox) is being tested for treatment of spastic muscles. The orphan drug baclofen is under investigation as a treatment for muscle spasticity that does not respond to other drugs. Dantrolene (Dantrium) testing is under way; it may reduce spastic muscle contractions.

Please contact the agencies listed under Resources, below, for the most current information. Addresses and telephone numbers of these agencies, as well as of individual experts and research centers, may be found in the Master Resources List.

**Resources**

**For more information on cerebral palsy:** National Organization for Rare Disorders (NORD); United Cerebral Palsy Association; NIH/National Institute of Neurological Disorders and Stroke; National Easter Seal Society; March of Dimes Birth Defects Foundation.

**References**

Nelson Textbook of Pediatrics, 14th ed.: R.E. Behrman, ed.-in-chief; W.B. Saunders Company, 1992, p. 1516.

Neurosurgical Treatment of Spasticity: Selective Posterior Rhizotomy and Intrathecal Baclofen: A.L. Albright; Stereotact. Funct. Neurosurg., 1992, vol. 58(1–4), pp. 3–13.

Selective Functional Posterior Rhizotomy for Treatment of Spastic Cerebral Palsy in Children: Review of 50 Consecutive Cases: P. Steinbok; Pediatr. Neurosurg., 1992, vol. 18(1), pp. 24–42.

Birth Defects Encyclopedia: M.L. Buyse, ed.-in-chief; Blackwell Scientific Publications, 1990, pp. 300–301.

Cerebral Palsy: Management of the Upper Extremity: L.A. Koman, et al.; Clin. Orthop., April 1990, vol. 235, pp. 62–74.

Principles of Neurology, 4th ed.: R.D. Adams and M. Victor, eds.; McGraw-Hill, 1989, pp. 471–474.

Submandibular Gland Resection and Bilateral Parotid Duct Ligation As a Management for Chronic Drooling in Cerebral Palsy: S.R. Brundage, et al.; Plast. Reconstr. Surg., March 1989, vol. 83(3), pp. 443–446.

Cervical Spinal Cord Stimulation for Spasticity in Cerebral Palsy: H. Hugenholtz et al.; Neurosurgery, April 1988, vol. 22(4), pp. 707–714.

# CEREBRO-OCULO-FACIO-SKELETAL (COFS) SYNDROME

**Description** COFS syndrome is a degenerative disorder of the brain and spinal cord characterized by craniofacial and skeletal abnormalities, hypotonia, and diminished or absent reflexes. The white matter of the brain is reduced, with gray mottling.

**Synonyms**
> Pena Shokeir II Syndrome

**Signs and Symptoms** Craniofacial characteristics include microcephaly and micrognathia; small eyes, cataracts, and blepharophimosis; and large ears and a long philtrum. Kyphosis and osteoporosis may be present. There may be camptodactyly, flexion contractures, and rocker-bottom feet.

The child fails to thrive and is highly vulnerable to respiratory infections. Death may occur within 5 years.

**Etiology** COFS syndrome is inherited as an autosomal recessive trait.

**Epidemiology** The syndrome is present at birth and is seen in infants of diverse ethnic heritage.

**Related Disorders** See *Cockayne Syndrome; Neu-Laxova Syndrome; Seckel Syndrome.*

**Potter syndrome (bilateral renal agenesis)** is a rare condition characterized by a flattened face with a "parrot-beak" nose, hypertelorism and abnormalities of the eyelids, micrognathia, and low-set floppy ears. The skin appears dehydrated. A kidney is absent or underdeveloped. Skeletal abnormalities such as clubfoot and contracted joints occur frequently.

**Treatment—Standard** Treatment is symptomatic and supportive. Genetic counseling is recommended for families of affected children.

**Treatment—Investigational** Please contact the agencies listed under Resources, below, for the most current information. Addresses and telephone numbers of these agencies, as well as of individual experts and research centers, may be found in the Master Resources List.

**Resources**

**For more information on cerebro-oculo-facio-skeletal syndrome:** National Organization for Rare Disorders (NORD); NIH/National Institute of Neurological Disorders and Stroke; FACES—National Association for the Craniofacially Handicapped; National Craniofacial Foundation; Society for the Rehabilitation of the Facially Disfigured; AboutFace; Forward Face; Children's Craniofacial Association; Craniofacial Family Association.

**For genetic information and genetic counseling referrals:** March of Dimes Birth Defects Foundation; Alliance of Genetic Support Groups.

**References**

Smith's Recognizable Patterns of Human Malformation, 4th ed.: K.L. Jones; W.B. Saunders Company, 1988, pp. 146–147.

The Neu-Cofs (Cerebro-Oculo-Facio-Skeletal) Syndrome: Report of a Case: M.C. Silengo, et al.; Clin. Genet., February 1984, vol. 25(2), pp. 201–204.

# CHARCOT-MARIE-TOOTH DISEASE

**Description** Charcot-Marie-Tooth disease is a progressive, hereditary motor and sensory neuropathy characterized by weakness and atrophy, primarily in the peroneal and distal leg muscles.

**Synonyms**
> Hereditary Sensory Motor Neuropathy
> Peroneal Muscular Atrophy

**Signs and Symptoms** Symptoms of Charcot-Marie-Tooth disease type I (**CMT1**) manifest in middle childhood or the teenage years, with pes cavus and slowly progressive weakness and atrophy of peroneal muscle groups, producing a "stork-leg" deformity. Eventually, impairment spreads to the upper extremities, with a stocking-glove pattern of decrease in sensitivity to vibration, pain, and temperature. Nerve conduction responses become slower over time, deep tendon reflexes are absent, and enlarged peripheral nerves may be palpable.

Charcot-Marie-Tooth disease type II (**CMT2**) symptoms develop later in life, and the disorder progresses more slowly. Individuals affected by both types I and II have normal life spans.

**Etiology** The disease is usually inherited as an autosomal dominant trait. It may also be inherited through a recessive hereditary mechanism or sex-linked recessive inheritance.

CMT1 has been discovered to be a multigene disorder located on chromosome 17p at 11.1p12. CMT1 has been linked to mutations in the protein genes PMP-22 (peripheral membrane protein 22), Po (myelin protein zero), and Cx32 (connexin 32). The most common form of CMT1 occurs when one or both of the original copies of the PMP-22 gene are duplicated.

**Epidemiology** Males and females are affected in equal numbers. The disorder occurs worldwide at a rate of 1:2,500. About 125,000 persons in the United States have Charcot-Marie-Tooth disease.

**Related Disorders** See *Dejerine-Sottas Disease;* the age of onset, clinical findings, and prognosis are similar to those of Charcot-Marie-Tooth disease. See also *Refsum Syndrome,* in which peripheral neuropathy is present. See also *Neuropathy, Hereditary Sensory, Type I.*

**Familial amyloid neuropathy** is characterized by accumulation of amyloid in peripheral nerves. This rare disorder is inherited as an autosomal dominant trait.

**Treatment—Standard** Bracing to correct foot drop, or orthopedic surgery to stabilize the foot are appropriate therapeutic options. Vocational counseling may also be helpful.

**Treatment—Investigational** Please contact the agencies listed under Resources, below, for the most current information. Addresses and telephone numbers of these agencies, as well as of individual experts and research centers, may be found in the Master Resources List.

**Resources**

   **For more information on Charcot-Marie-Tooth disease:** National Organization for Rare Disorders (NORD); Charcot-Marie-Tooth Association; Charcot-Marie-Tooth Disease/Peroneal Muscular Atrophy Association; NIH/National Institute of Neurological Disorders and Stroke.

   **For genetic information and genetic counseling referrals:** March of Dimes Birth Defects Foundation; Alliance of Genetic Support Groups.

**References**

Cecil Textbook of Medicine, 18th ed.: J.B. Wyngaarden and L.H. Smith, Jr., eds.: W.B. Saunders Company, 1988, pp. 2264, 2155.

Mendelian Inheritance in Man, 8th ed.: V.A. McKusick; The Johns Hopkins University Press, 1986, pp. 140–143, 860, 1262.

Scientific American MEDICINE: E. Rubinstein and D. Federman, eds.; Scientific American, 1978–1991, pp. 11:II:1–2.

# CHRONIC HICCUPS

**Description** Hiccups are involuntary spasms of the diaphragm that occur suddenly and repeatedly, usually a few times per minute. Most episodes are transient, lasting only a few minutes. When hiccups persist, the possibility of underlying illness must be investigated.

**Synonyms**

   Singultus

**Signs and Symptoms** Chronic hiccups may last hours or days, and may recur frequently with only a few hours of relief between spasms. Lack of sleep, exhaustion, and weight loss may result if chronic hiccups are not controlled.

**Etiology** The characteristic "hic" sound is caused by intake of air into the larynx.

   Hiccups develop in response to irritation of afferent or efferent nerves, or of the medullary centers in the brain that control the diaphragm muscle. Chronic hiccups can occur idiopathically, although a persistent form may suggest the presence of such underlying conditions as brain lesions or tumors, pancreatitis, or intestinal, hepatic, or renal disease. Pregnancy, pleurisy of the diaphragm, pneumonia, and alcoholism have also been associated. Surgery or anesthesia can cause hiccups.

**Epidemiology** Males are affected more frequently than females. The occurrence of ordinary, transient hiccups is common; the occurrence of chronic hiccups is very rare.

**Related Disorders** Many disorders involving the autonomic nervous system control unconscious activities of the body such as breathing, sweating, heartbeat, hiccups, and coughing.

**Treatment—Standard** Since ordinary hiccups tend to be self-limited, they do not require treatment.

   Chronic hiccups may be controlled with drugs such as chlorpromazine, metoclopramide, anticonvulsants, quinidine, or carbamazepine. Ephedrine or ketamine are the drugs of choice if hiccups develop during anesthesia and surgery. Hypnosis and acupuncture have been successful in treating some patients. For unresponsive cases, small amounts of procaine solution may be injected into the phrenic nerve to block stimulation of the diaphragm. Surgery to sever the phrenic nerve in the neck has been used in cases where all other therapies have failed.

**Treatment—Investigational** In research at Walter Reed Hospital, nifedipine (Adalat or Procardia) was found to be successful in stopping chronic hiccuping in 5 of 7 patients treated. The long-term efficacy of nifedipine for this purpose is being evaluated.

   In a report of a study in England, it was noted that baclofen was effective in stopping the chronic hiccups of one patient. The patient's relatives also had attacks of the disorder.

   Please contact the agencies listed under Resources, below, for the most current information. Addresses and telephone numbers of these agencies, as well as of individual experts and research centers, may be found in the Master Resources List.

**Resources**

   **For more information on chronic hiccups:** National Organization for Rare Disorders (NORD); NIH/National Heart, Lung and Blood Institute.

**References**

Hiccups and Esophageal Dysfunction: G. Triadafilopoulos; Am. J. Gastroenterol., February 1989, vol. 84(2), pp. 164–169.

Sleep Hiccup: J.J. Askenasy; Sleep, April 1988, vol. 11(2), pp. 187–194.

Chronic Hiccups: M.S. Lipsky; Am. Fam. Physician, November 1986, vol. 34(5), pp. 173–177.

# CHRONIC INFLAMMATORY DEMYELINATING POLYNEUROPATHY (CIDP)

**Description** In CIDP, nerve roots become swollen and there is extensive destruction of the myelin sheath of peripheral nerves. Typically, there is no preceding viral infection and no family history of other similar disorders or polyneuropathy.

**Signs and Symptoms** The patient may experience weakness, paralysis, and impairment in motor function, especially of the limbs. Sensory loss may also be present, causing numbness and tingling. Tendon reflexes may be absent or reduced, and facial and intercostal muscles may be weak. The motor and sensory impairments are usually symmetrical, and the degree of severity can vary. The course of CIDP may also vary. Some patients may follow a slow steady pattern of symptoms, while others may have symptoms that wax and wane and increase in severity after many months or 1 year or more.

CIDP can be difficult to diagnose. Characteristic features must be present for at least 1 month, and typically there is no preceding ailment.

**Etiology** The cause is not known. An immune system defect has been suggested but not proved.

**Epidemiology** The disorder is very rare. Any age group can be affected, and onset may occur at any time in the life span.

**Related Disorders** See *Ataxia, Friedreich; Charcot-Marie-Tooth Disease; Dejerine-Sottas Disease; Guillain-Barré Syndrome; Multiple Sclerosis.*

**Treatment—Standard** Glucocorticoid drugs have been effective in treating patients with CIDP, but often the side effects discourage long-term therapy. Intravenous immunoglobulin (**IVIG**) is frequently used in treatment, generally in very high initial doses. Azathioprine and cyclophosphamide have been helpful for some patients.

**Treatment—Investigational** Plasmapheresis may be of benefit in CIDP, but the procedure is still under investigation and can presently only be suggested for use in the most severe cases.

Please contact the agencies listed under Resources, below, for the most current information. Addresses and telephone numbers of these agencies, as well as of individual experts and research centers, may be found in the Master Resources List.

**Resources**

**For more information on chronic inflammatory demyelinating polyneuropathy:** National Organization for Rare Disorders (NORD); American Autoimmune Related Diseases Association; NIH/National Institute of Neurological Disorders and Stroke.

**References**

Cecil Textbook of Medicine, 19th ed.: J.B. Wyngaarden, et al., eds.; W.B. Saunders Company, 1992, p. 2262.

Consensus Statement—NIH Consensus Development Conference: Chronic Inflammatory Demyelinating Polyneuropathy: May 21–23, 1990, vol. 8(5).

High-Dose Intravenous Human Immunoglobulin in Chronic Inflammatory Demyelinating Polyneuropathy: J.M. Faed, et al.; Neurology, 1989, vol. 39, pp. 422–425.

# CHRONIC SPASMODIC DYSPHONIA (CSD)

**Description** CSD is a speech disorder that resembles stuttering and is caused by vigorous adduction or abduction of the vocal cords. The voice sounds hoarse, soft, and strained, and the breathing pattern is abnormal.

**Synonyms**

Abductor Spasmodic Dysphonia
Adductor Spasmodic Dysphonia
Dysphonia Spastica

**Signs and Symptoms** Chronic spasmodic dysphonia is characterized by uncontrolled vocal spasms, conscious effort in order to speak, tightness in the throat, and intermittent hoarseness.

Symptoms gradually progress over the first 2 years and then generally stabilize. The disorder usually remains chronic without marked changes over a period of years, although symptoms may worsen with stress.

In the most severe form of CSD, patients may experience aphonia. Coughing, laughing, and sometimes singing may be less affected than speaking.

A milder subtype of CSD is characterized by difficulty controlling speech after certain sounds (e.g., "P," "T," and "K").

Diagnosis of chronic spasmodic dysphonia usually includes laryngoscopy to rule out vocal cord structural abnormalities, such as nodules, polyps, or tumors.

**Etiology** The cause is not known. It is possible that the adduction or abduction of the vocal cords may relate to brain stem dysfunction. In about 60 percent of patients, symptoms onset follows a severe upper respiratory tract infection with laryngitis. The disorder may also occur after head injury or prolonged use of phenothiazines. Some patients may have associated movement disorders, such as tardive dyskinesia, oral-facial dystonia, torticollis, or essential tremor.

**Epidemiology** The disorder occurs most often in those who use their voices a great deal and who have had voice training. Onset usually is between 20 and 60 years of age, and over 70 percent of affected persons are female.

**Related Disorders** In **chronic stuttering** there is an abnormal speech pattern characterized by repetitions, prolongations, unusual hesitations, and pauses that disrupt rhythmic flow of speech. The disorder usually appears before age 12 and is often familial.

**Essential voice tremor** is an involuntary movement of the vocal cords produced by rhythmic alternate contractions of opposing laryngeal muscles (see **Benign Essential Tremor Syndrome**).

**Vocal cord polyps** may be caused by voice abuse, chronic allergies affecting the larynx, or irritation of the vocal cords by industrial fumes or cigarette smoke. Vocal cord polyps typically result in hoarseness and breathiness.

**Vocal cord nodules (singer's, teacher's, or screamer's nodules)** are concentrations of connective tissue on the vocal cords. These nodules may be due to chronic voice abuse, or unnatural lowering of the voice. Hoarseness and a breathy voice quality result.

**Vocal cord paralysis** may result from lesions in several locations in the brain, the 10th cranial nerve (nervus vagus), laryngeal nerves, or neck or thoracic lesions; neurotoxins such as lead; infections such as diphtheria; or viral illness. Vocal cord paralysis usually results in loss of vocal cord abduction or adduction, and may affect speech, respiration, and swallowing.

If the vocal cord paralysis is unilateral, the voice is hoarse and breathy. If the paralysis is bilateral, the voice is very soft but of good quality. Breathing difficulty with wheezing may occur on moderate exertion.

**Squamous cell carcinoma of the larynx** is the most common malignant laryngeal tumor. The earliest symptom is usually hoarseness. Early treatment with radiation or cordectomy usually results in a cure rate of 85 to 95 percent.

**Treatment—Standard** In 40 percent of cases, the symptoms of chronic spasmodic dysphonia improve with severance of one of the recurrent laryngeal nerves. However, the nerve can grow back 3 to 9 months after surgery, resulting in return of symptoms. Another 40 percent of patients may benefit from treatment with propranolol. Speech therapy also can be helpful.

**Treatment—Investigational** Researchers at 12 treatment centers including the National Institute on Deafness and Other Communication Disorders are currently treating adults who suffer from chronic spasmodic dysphonia with the orphan drug botulinum A toxin (Oculinum). The drug is injected into the thyroarytenoid cartilage at intervals of several weeks. To date, this procedure has been beneficial in all test cases, with varying degrees of hoarseness and swallowing difficulties as side effects, depending on dosage. Symptoms usually return after 2 to 3 months, and reinjections are required.

Adults over 18 years of age who have had dysphonia for more than 2 years may contact the following persons if they wish to participate in research projects on spasmodic dysphonia: Christy Ludlow, Ph.D., NIH/National Institute on Deafness and Other Communication Disorders, or Andrew Blitzer, M.D., College of Physicians and Surgeons, Columbia University.

For information concerning research on spasmodic dysphonia as well as other debilitating communicative disorders, contact Sandra Chapman, M.D., Callier Center for Communicative Disorders, Dallas Center for Vocal Motor Control, Dallas, Texas.

Botulinum toxin is available from Alan Scott, M.D., Smith-Kettlewell Eye Research Foundation, San Francisco, California.

For information on an epidemiologic study on spastic dysphonia, contact Clarence T. Sasaki, M.D., Yale University School of Medicine.

Please contact the agencies listed under Resources, below, for the most current information. Addresses and telephone numbers of these agencies, as well as of individual experts and research centers, may be found in the Master Resources List.

**Resources**

**For more information on chronic spasmodic dysphonia:** National Organization for Rare Disorders (NORD); National Spasmodic Dysphonia Association; Voluntary Organization for Communication and Language; NIH/National Institute on Deafness and Other Communication Disorders Information Clearinghouse; Andrew Blitzer, M.D., College of Physicians and Surgeons, Columbia University; Sandra Chapman, M.D.; Dystonia Clinical Research Center at Columbia Presbyterian Hospital; Dystonia Medical Research; We Move.

**References**

Diagnostic and Statistical Manual of Mental Disorders, 3rd ed.: American Psychiatric Association, 1980, p. 79.

# CLUSTER HEADACHE

**Description** Cluster headaches are a rare disabling neuralgia characterized by profound unilateral, nonthrobbing pain, and accompanied by rhinorrhea and lacrimation. Attacks usually last 15 to 30 minutes and may recur several times daily. Onset occurs during sleep. Cyclic and chronic forms of cluster headache are recognized.

**Synonyms**
> Histamine Cephalalgia
> Vasogenic Facial Pain

**Signs and Symptoms** The patient with cluster headaches may awake from sleep with deep, agonizing, nonthrobbing pain in the face, eye, temple, or forehead, on one side of the head. When the pain passes, the patient falls into a deep sleep, only to be aroused again by another attack in the same site. The eyelid over an affected eye may droop, and an involved eye or nostril may water copiously.

Attacks occur in groups of 1 to 4 headaches, daily or more often, and may continue for weeks to months. The cyclic variant is characterized by a headache-free period of variable duration; a remission for several years may be followed by a new onslaught of cluster headaches. When the headaches recur regularly without intervening headache-free periods, the condition is considered chronic. Alcohol ingestion appears to trigger the attacks in some patients.

**Etiology** The cause of cluster headaches is unknown. The condition has been speculatively linked to hormonal imbalances, spasms, edema, and carotid artery inflammation.

**Epidemiology** Cluster headaches have a strong male sex predominance. Young to middle-aged males can be affected, but incidence is most common in the 5th, 6th, or 7th decade of life. Women are rarely affected.

**Related Disorders** Severe headache is a feature of many disorders, particularly neuralgias, cerebrovascular syndromes, and brain tumors. Like cluster headaches, **migraine headaches** typically are unilateral. The headaches may be accompanied by gastrointestinal upset (nausea, vomiting, constipation, or diarrhea), irritability, and visual problems, such as photosensitivity or double vision. Affected individuals appear to have a genetic predisposition. Migraine headache has been attributed to constriction of the cranial arteries, but the cause of the constriction is unknown.

See *Tolosa-Hunt Syndrome; Trigeminal Neuralgia; Arteritis, Giant Cell.*

**Treatment—Standard** Inhalation of ergotamine and oxygen may speed recovery from an attack. Methysergide, lithium carbonate, prednisone, verapamil, and nifedipine may be prescribed to help prevent recurrences. Alcohol ingestion should be avoided.

**Treatment—Investigational** Various surgical procedures have been proposed for extreme cases of cluster headache unresponsive to medication. Sphenopalatine ganglion neurectomy has been tried experimentally to relieve pain when medical treatment has failed. The safety and efficacy of this procedure are unknown.

Please contact the agencies listed under Resources, below, for the most current information. Addresses and telephone numbers of these agencies, as well as of individual experts and research centers, may be found in the Master Resources List.

**Resources**

**For more information on cluster headache:** National Organization for Rare Disorders (NORD); NIH/National Institute of Neurological Disorders and Stroke; National Migraine Foundation.

**References**

Unilateral Impairment of Pupillary Response to Trigeminal Nerve Stimulation in Cluster Headache: M. Fanciullacci, et al.; Pain, February 1989, vol. 36(2), pp. 185–191.

Cluster Headache Pain vs. Other Vascular Headache Pain: Differences Revealed with Two Approaches to the McGill Pain Questionnaire: A. Jerome, et al.; Pain, July 1988, vol. 34(1), pp. 35–42.

Cluster Headaches: J.P. McKenna; Am. Fam. Physician, April 1988; vol. 37(4), pp. 173–178.

Internal Medicine, 2nd ed.: J.H. Stein, ed.-in-chief; Little, Brown and Company, 1987, pp. 2180–2185.

Vasogenic Facial Pain (Cluster Headache): L.R. Eversole, et al.; Int. J. Oral Maxillofac. Surg., February 1987; vol. 16(1), pp. 25–35.

# CONVERSION DISORDER

**Description** Conversion disorder is a psychological, neurotic condition involving physical symptoms that develop out of emotional conflicts or needs, without any physiological basis and without any intention for effect. The physical symptoms usually appear suddenly during times of extreme psychological stress. Conversion disorder can be distinguished from other physiological disorders by the associated inappropriate lack of concern over debilitating symptoms *(la belle indifférence)*.

### Synonyms

Hysterical Neurosis, Conversion Type

**Signs and Symptoms** Common symptoms of conversion disorder, which often resemble neurologic diseases, include paralysis, seizures, aphonia, dyskinesia, and temporary blindness. Patients usually exhibit only one symptom, and an episode tends to appear and disappear suddenly. With recurrent episodes, the symptom may appear in a different location or with varying severity.

The conversion symptoms are thought to be symbolic resolutions to psychological conflicts, i.e., vomiting may represent revulsion and disgust, or blindness may portray an inability to accept witnessing a traumatic event. Organic disease must be ruled out before establishing a diagnosis of conversion disorder.

**Etiology** The source of this disorder is an inner conflict that creates extreme psychological stress. Conversion symptoms arise as a means to partially resolve the inner conflict. For example, a soldier who subconsciously wishes to avoid firing a gun may develop a paralyzed hand.

**Epidemiology** Onset is usually in the teens and 20s, but can be later in life. Individuals with previous physical disorders and individuals who are exposed to persons with real physical symptoms are susceptible to developing this disorder. A large number of the known cases of conversion disorder have appeared in military settings, particularly during wartime. One particular symptom, globus hystericus, is more common in females.

**Related Disorders** Physical disorders with vague somatic symptoms may initially be misdiagnosed as conversion disorder; these include multiple sclerosis, Wilson disease, and demyelinating polyneuropathy.

**Treatment—Standard** Treatment is individualized and can include psychoanalysis, family therapy, or specific life changes. Antidepressant and antipsychotic drugs can be helpful in reducing some symptoms. Although hypnosis may eliminate certain specific symptoms, often a substitute symptom arises. Temporary paralysis may be treated by electromyographic biofeedback.

**Treatment—Investigational** Please contact the agencies listed under Resources, below, for the most current information. Addresses and telephone numbers of these agencies, as well as of individual experts and research centers, may be found in the Master Resources List.

### Resources

**For more information on conversion disorder:** National Organization for Rare Disorders (NORD); National Mental Health Association; NIH/National Institute of Mental Health; National Alliance for the Mentally Ill; National Mental Health Consumer Self-Help Clearinghouse.

### References

The Utility of Electromyographic Biofeedback in the Treatment of Conversion Paralysis: D.A. Fishbain, et al.; Am. J. Psychiatry, December 1988, vol. 145(12), pp. 1572–1575.

Diagnostic and Statistical Manual of Mental Disorders, 3rd ed., revised: R.L. Spitzer, et al., eds.; American Psychiatric Association, 1987, pp. 257–259.

Globus Hystericus Syndrome Responsiveness to Antidepressants: I.H. Bangash, et al.; Am. J. Psychiatry, July 1986, vol. 143(7), pp. 917–918.

# CORTICOBASAL DEGENERATION

**Description** Corticobasal degeneration is a rare progressive neurologic disorder characterized by cell atrophy in the cerebral cortex and substantia nigra. Affected individuals may have sufficient muscle power for manual tasks but often have difficulty directing their movements appropriately.

### Synonyms

Cortico-Basal Ganglionic Degeneration

**Signs and Symptoms** Initial features typically appear in persons in their 60s, and may include muscle rigidity, apraxia (e.g., difficulty buttoning a shirt), and difficulty pantomiming actions. Muscle rigidity may cause awkward or uncomfortable postures (e.g., a tightly flexed hand), and the affected person may be unaware of the movement of a limb. Symptoms and signs usually are unilateral initially, but both sides may be affected as the disease progresses.

Other features include postural or action tremor, bradykinesia, and akinesia. Sudden involuntary muscle spasms may occur. Dysarthria, dysphagia, gaze palsy, an inability to control eyelid blinking, and an ataxic gait may also be present.

Cognitive impairment occurs in some patients; e.g., anosognosia and dementia, usually late in the course. Visual-spatial impairments may also be present.

Diagnosis is suspected if neurologic symptoms occur in the absence of a stroke, tumor, or other neurologic lesion. CT and MRI may reveal atrophy, usually most pronounced in the cerebral cortex and substantia nigra. Some scientists feel that the pattern of nerve cell loss associated with corticobasal degeneration combined with neurologic symptoms is sufficient to confirm the diagnosis. PET and SPECT may support the diagnosis.

**Etiology** The cause is not known. Symptoms develop because of progressive tissue deterioration in different areas of the brain, most typically the cerebral cortex and substantia nigra. The severity and type of symptoms depend on the area of the brain affected by the disease.

Studies have shown a decreased blood flow and glucose metabolism in the affected areas of the brain, with a greater reduction in metabolism contralateral to body symptoms. One study identified corticobasal inclusions in the substantia nigras of 3 affected individuals, although the role of these inclusions is not known.

**Epidemiology** Symptoms onset is between the ages of 50 and 70. Although fewer than 50 cases have been documented in the medical literature, the disorder may be underdiagnosed because its symptoms are similar to those of other neurologic disorders. Females are affected slightly more often than males.

**Related Disorders** *See Alzheimer Disease; Creutzfeldt-Jakob Disease; Joseph Disease; Parkinson Disease.*

**Treatment—Standard** Treatment includes physical, speech, and occupational therapy to help maintain joint and muscle mobility. Other treatment is symptomatic and supportive.

**Treatment—Investigational** Please contact the agencies listed under Resources, below, for the most current information. Addresses and telephone numbers of these agencies, as well as of individual experts and research centers, may be found in the Master Resources List.

**Resources**

**For more information on corticobasal degeneration:** National Organization for Rare Disorders (NORD); NIH/National Institute of Neurological Disorders and Stroke; International Tremor Foundation.

**References**

Clinically Diagnosed Corticobasal Degeneration (CBD): T. Nagao, et al.; Rinsho Shinkeigaku, January 1993, vol. 33(1), pp. 45–49.

Principles of Neurology, 5th ed.: R.D. Adams and M. Victor, eds.; McGraw-Hill, 1993, pp. 397, 974.

Corticobasal Degeneration: Decreased and Asymmetrical Glucose Consumption As Studied with PET: J. Blin, et al.; Mov. Disord., October 1992, vol. 7(4), pp. 348–354.

Three-Dimensional Surface Display with 123i-Imp in Corticobasal Degeneration: B. Okuda, et al.; Rinsho Shinkeigaku, July 1992, vol. 32(7), pp. 774–776.

Corticobasal Degeneration: A Unique Pattern of Regional Cortical Oxygen Hypometabolism and Striatal Fluorodopa Uptake Demonstrated by Positron Emission Tomography: G.V. Sawle, et al.; Brain, February 1991, vol. 114(pt. 1B), pp. 541–556.

Focal Reflex Myoclonus in Corticobasal Degeneration: F. Caracella, et al.; Funct. Neurol., April–June 1991, vol. 6(2), pp. 165–170.

The Metabolic Landscape of Cortico-Basal Ganglionic Degeneration: Regional Asymmetries Studies with Positron Emission Tomography: D. Eidelberg, et al.; J. Neurol. Neurosurg. Psychiatry, October 1991, vol. 54(10), pp. 856–862.

Cortical-Basal Ganglionic Degeneration: D.E. Riley, et al.; Neurology, August 1990, vol. 40(8), pp. 1203–1212.

# CREUTZFELDT-JAKOB DISEASE

**Description** Creutzfeldt-Jakob disease is a rare, fatal, transmissible spongiform encephalopathy occurring in middle life and characterized by progressive degeneration of the central nervous system and by neuromuscular disturbances.

**Synonyms**

Corticostriatal-Spinal Degeneration

Jakob-Creutzfeldt Disease

Spastic Pseudosclerosis

Subacute Spongiform Encephalopathy

**Signs and Symptoms** The early stages are marked by memory failures, behavioral changes, difficulty in concentration and coordination, or visual disturbances. Myoclonus, extensor plantar reflexes, and hyperreflexia may be seen. The illness progresses to pronounced mental deterioration, hemiparesis, sensory disturbances, and progressive muscular atrophy; mutism, akinesia, seizures, and semicoma may ensue. Death generally occurs within 1 year and may take place after only a few months.

The disease can produce characteristic changes in the electroencephalograph (**EEG**). CT scan can demonstrate atrophy of the brain.

**Etiology** The etiologic agent in Creutzfeldt-Jakob disease is believed to be a prion (protein infectious agent). The mode of transmission is not completely understood. About 10 percent of reported cases are familial.

**Epidemiology** Creutzfeldt-Jakob disease affects both males and females, with peak incidence of the disorder occurring in the late 50s.

**Related Disorders** See *Alzheimer Disease.*

**Treatment—Standard** Treatment is symptomatic and supportive. Patients should be guarded against infection.

**Treatment—Investigational** The following investigators have expressed an interest in receiving biopsy and autopsy tissue, blood, and cerebrospinal fluid from patients with Creutzfeldt-Jakob and related diseases: Stephen DeArmond, M.D., and Stanley Prusiner, M.D., University of California; Clarence J. Gibbs, M.D., and D. Carleton Gajdusek, M.D., NIH/National Institute of Neurological Disorders and Stroke; Elias Manuelidis, M.D., Yale University School of Medicine.

A study of early-onset dementia occurring as a result of Creutzfeldt-Jakob disease is being conducted by the National Institute of Mental Health and the Neuropsychiatric Research Hospital. Participants in this study must be under 45 years of age and not require special medical care. Please contact Denise Juliano.

An epidemiologic study of Creutzfeldt-Jakob disease is being conducted at Loma Linda University under the supervision of Carey G. Smoak.

Please contact the agencies listed under Resources, below, for the most current information. Addresses and telephone numbers of these agencies, as well as of individual experts and research centers, may be found in the Master Resources List.

### Resources

**For more information on Creutzfeldt-Jakob disease:** National Organization for Rare Disorders (NORD); Alzheimer's Disease and Related Disorders Association; NIH/National Institute of Neurological Disorders and Stroke.

**For more information on long-term care facilities:** National Hospice Organization.

### References

Cecil Textbook of Medicine, 19th ed.: J.B. Wyngaarden, et al., eds.; W.B. Saunders Company, 1992, pp. 2191–2193.

Mendelian Inheritance in Man, 10th ed.: V.A. McKusick; The Johns Hopkins University Press, 1992, pp. 281–282, 927–929.

Creutzfeldt-Jakob Disease in Pituitary Growth Hormone Recipients in the United States: R. Thomson; JAMA, February 1991, vol. 20(265), pp. 880–884.

Molecular Biology of Prion Diseases: S.B. Prusiner; Science, June 1991, vol. 252(5012), pp. 1515–1522.

Human Growth Hormone and Creutzfeldt-Jakob Disease: S. Zekauskas; J. Okla. State Med. Assoc., September 1990, vol. 83(9), pp. 447–448.

Principles of Neurology, 4th ed.: R.D. Adams and M. Victor, eds.; McGraw-Hill, 1989, pp. 609–611.

# CYCLIC VOMITING SYNDROME

**Description** Cyclic vomiting syndrome is assumed to be a rare form of "abdominal migraine" in children.

**Synonyms**

    Abdominal Migraine

    Chronic Vomiting in Childhood

**Signs and Symptoms** The condition is characterized by recurrent periods of nausea and vomiting. Midline abdominal pain is often accompanied by headaches, loss of appetite, and upset stomach. Recurrent vomiting can last several hours, a week, or more, and may recur several times a week or once a year. Many times the child is aware of being excited or under stress, or having a cold or flu before the beginning of an attack of cyclic vomiting.

**Etiology** The cause is not known. Diagnosis can be made only after other causes of recurrent vomiting in children have been ruled out. No underlying disease has been detected, and no diagnostic procedures have been found to predict the syndrome. However, affected children tend to get migraine headaches when they grow to adulthood.

**Epidemiology** Cyclic vomiting syndrome usually occurs in children aged 3 and up, although infants have been seen to exhibit symptoms of the disorder. Onset after puberty is rare. Patients may be prone to migraine headaches in later years. The number of children affected by this disorder is unknown, but it is probably massively un- or misdiagnosed.

### Related Disorders

The development of projectile vomiting immediately after eating or when the stomach is filled is one of the first symptoms of **pyloric stenosis**. Constipation is a frequent complication, as is failure of the infant to gain weight. The disorder is usually apparent during the first few months of life, but may also occur in adults. Adult signs and symptoms are similar to those in the infant.

The intense pain of **migraine headaches** can last several hours or even days and may be accompanied by nausea, vomiting, and extreme sensitivity to light. Migraine headaches can begin in childhood or middle age, but onset often is in adolescence. Girls are affected more often than boys, and there is frequently a strong family history. Frequency is increased by stress. Triggers include foods such as chocolate, red wine, and certain cheeses.

**Treatment—Standard** No known treatment prevents or shortens attacks of cyclic vomiting.

**Treatment—Investigational** Research on this disorder is being conducted by David Fleisher, M.D., at the University of Missouri School of Medicine, Columbia, Missouri.

Please contact the agencies listed under Resources, below, for the most current information. Addresses and telephone numbers of these agencies, as well as of individual experts and research centers, may be found in the Master Resources List.

### Resources

**For more information on cyclic vomiting syndrome:** National Organization for Rare Disorders (NORD); Cyclic Vomiting Syndrome Association; NIH/National Digestive Diseases Information Clearinghouse; National Headache/Migraine Foundation.

### References

Idiopathic Gastroparesis in Patients with Unexplained Nausea and Vomiting: D. Wengrower, et al.; Dig. Dis. Sci., September 1991, vol. 36(9), pp. 1255–1258.

Reversible Quantitative EEG Changes in a Case of Cyclic Vomiting: Evidence for Migraine Equivalent: S.A. Jernigan, et al.; Dev. Med. Child Neurol., January 1991, vol. 33(1), pp. 80–85.

Testing the Psychogenic Vomiting Diagnosis: Four Pediatric Patients: J. Gonzales-Heydrich, et al.; Am. J. Dis. Child, August 1991, vol. 145(8), pp. 913–916.

Value of Ultrasound in Differentiating Causes of Persistent Vomiting in Infants: M.D. Rollins, et al.; Gut, June 1991, vol. 32(6), pp. 612–614.

Abdominal Migraine: A Childhood Syndrome Defined: D.N. Symon, et al.; Cephalalgia, December 1986, vol. 6(4), pp. 223–228.

The Periodic Syndrome in Pediatric Migraine Sufferers: G. Lanzi, et al.; Cephalalgia, August 3, 1983, suppl. 1, pp. 91–93.

# DANDY-WALKER SYNDROME

**Description** Dandy-Walker syndrome is characterized by congenital hydrocephalus resulting from obstruction of the foramina of Magendie and Luschka.

**Synonyms**

Dandy-Walker Cysts

Obstructive Hydrocephalus

**Signs and Symptoms** The hydrocephalus is accompanied by headache, vomiting, irritability, convulsions, abnormal reflexes, bradypnea, bradycardia, and ataxia. Transient visual disturbances, nystagmus, papilledema, and impaired hearing may be present.

Prenatal diagnosis can be made by ultrasound, and confirmed in the newborn by clinical evaluation and ultrasound, CT scan, and MRI.

**Etiology** The syndrome is inherited as an autosomal recessive trait. The disorder is caused by a developmental malformation in which the 4th ventricle of the brain is malformed.

**Epidemiology** Dandy-Walker syndrome is very rare. Males appear to be affected more often than females.

**Related Disorders** See *Arnold-Chiari Syndrome; Hydrocephalus; Walker-Warburg Syndrome.*

**Treatment—Standard** Dandy-Walker syndrome may be treated with a ventriculo-peritoneal shunt procedure.

**Treatment—Investigational** Please contact the agencies listed under Resources, below, for the most current information. Addresses and telephone numbers of these agencies, as well as of individual experts and research centers, may be found in the Master Resources List.

### Resources

**For more information on Dandy-Walker syndrome:** National Organization for Rare Disorders (NORD); Hydrocephalus Parent Support Group; National Hydrocephalus Foundation; NIH/National Institute of Neurological Disorders and Stroke.

**For genetic information and genetic counseling referrals:** March of Dimes Birth Defects Foundation; Alliance of Genetic Support Groups.

### References

Principles of Neurology, 5th ed.: R.D. Adams and M. Victor, eds.; McGraw-Hill, 1993, p. 1020.

Cecil Textbook of Medicine, 19th ed.: J.B. Wyngaarden, et al., eds.; W.B. Saunders Company, 1992, pp. 2223–2224.

The Dandy-Walker Syndrome: The Value of Antenatal Diagnosis: E. Cornford, et al.; Clin. Radiol, March 1992, vol. 45(3), pp. 172–174.

Dandy-Walker Variant: Prenatal Sonographic Features and Clinical Outcome: J.A. Estroff, et al.; Radiology, December 1992, vol. 185(3), pp. 755–758.

Mendelian Inheritance in Man, 10th ed.: V.A. McKusick; The Johns Hopkins University Press, 1992, pp. 1325–1326.

Nelson Textbook of Pediatrics, 14th ed.: R.E. Behrman, ed.-in-chief; W.B. Saunders Company, 1992, pp. 1488–1489.

Birth Defects Encyclopedia: M.L. Buyse, ed.-in-chief; Blackwell Scientific Publications, 1990, pp. 887–888.

Dictionary of Medical Syndromes, 3rd ed.: S.I. Magalini, et al., eds.; J.B. Lippincott Company, 1990, p. 226.

Dandy-Walker Syndrome: A Review of Fifteen Cases Evaluated by Prenatal Sonography: P.D. Ross, et al.; An. J. Obstet. Gynecol., August 1989, vol. 161(2), pp. 401–406.

# DEJERINE-SOTTAS DISEASE

**Description** Dejerine-Sottas disease is an irregularly progressive, hereditary hypertrophic demyelinating neuropathy that affects motor function of the legs and, in later stages, muscle strength and coordination in the hands and forearms. Enlargement of the peripheral nerves, accompanied by recurrent loss of myelin, is the cause of the muscle weakness.

**Synonyms**

> Hereditary Motor Sensory Neuropathy Type III
> Hypertrophic Interstitial Neuropathy
> Onion-Bulb Neuropathy

**Signs and Symptoms** The patient with Dejerine-Sottas disease first notices weakness in the back of the leg that then spreads to the front of the leg. Walking becomes difficult and painful; eventually the leg muscles atrophy. Reflexes and heat sensitivity may be lost. As the disease progresses, the hands and forearms are affected.

**Etiology** Dejerine-Sottas disease usually is inherited as a recessive trait. The cause of the recurrent loss of myelin is not known.

**Epidemiology** Onset usually occurs between ages 10 and 30 years, but may occur in infancy. Males and females are believed to be equally affected.

**Related Disorders** See *Charcot-Marie-Tooth Disease; Neuropathy, Hereditary Sensory, Type I.*

**Treatment—Standard** The cornerstones of treatment are physiotherapy, which promotes remaining muscle function, and orthopedic supports, which help stabilize involved joints. Surgery may be necessary. Patients and their families may benefit from genetic and occupational counseling.

**Treatment—Investigational** Please contact the agencies listed under Resources, below, for the most current information. Addresses and telephone numbers of these agencies, as well as of individual experts and research centers, may be found in the Master Resources List.

**Resources**

  **For more information on Dejerine-Sottas disease:** National Organization for Rare Disorders (NORD); Muscular Dystrophy Association; NIH/National Institute of Neurological Disorders and Stroke.

  **For genetic information and genetic counseling referrals:** March of Dimes Birth Defects Foundation; Alliance of Genetic Support Groups.

**References**

Abnormal Auditory Evoked Potentials in Dejerine-Sottas Disease: Report of Two Cases with Central Acoustic and Vestibular Impairment: F. Baiocco, et al.; J. Neurol., 1984, vol. 231(1), pp. 46–49.

The Importance of Quantitative Electron Microscopy in Studying Hypertrophic Neuropathies: A Comparison Between a Case of Dejerine-Sottas Disease (HMSN III) and a Case of the Hypertrophic Form of Charcot-Marie-Tooth Disease (HMSN I): G. Tredici, et al.; Int. J. Tissue React., 1984, vol. 6(3), pp. 267–274.

# DEPERSONALIZATION DISORDER

**Description** Depersonalization disorder is marked by persistent or recurring episodes of loss of the sense of self or reality.

**Synonyms**

> Depersonalization Neurosis

**Signs and Symptoms** During an episode of depersonalization disorder, a person's perception of self is altered, so that there is a feeling of detachment from and lack of control over his or her own reality, i.e., actions, thoughts, and physical self. Symptoms may be aggravated by mild anxiety or depression.

  The condition usually begins during adolescence or early adulthood, and is chronic with periods of remissions and exacerbations.

**Etiology** The specific cause of depersonalization disorder is unknown, although attacks may be precipitated by severely stressful situations, anxiety, or depression. Psychoactive drug use also is associated with the disorder.

**Epidemiology** The prevalence and sex distribution of depersonalization disorder are unknown. Brief periods involving feelings of depersonalization may be fairly common during adolescence.

**Related Disorders** See *Panic-Anxiety Syndrome.*

  **Agoraphobia** is an intense fear of finding oneself among other persons in public areas where one might have an attack of panic and be humiliated, or be unable to get to a safe place. The anxiety associated with attacks causes many individuals with agoraphobia to be unwilling to leave their homes.

**Treatment—Standard** Treatment of depersonalization disorder involves psychotherapy. The antidepressant drug desipramine may be beneficial. Other treatment is symptomatic and supportive.

**Treatment—Investigational** Please contact the agencies listed under Resources, below, for the most current information. Addresses and telephone numbers of these agencies, as well as of individual experts and research centers, may be found in the Master Resources List.

**Resources**

**For more information on depersonalization disorder:** National Organization for Rare Disorders (NORD); NIH/National Institute of Mental Health; National Mental Health Association; National Alliance for the Mentally Ill; National Mental Health Consumer Self-Help Clearinghouse.

**References**

Desipramine: A Possible Treatment for Depersonalization Disorder: R. Noyes, Jr., et al.; Can. J. Psychiatry, December 1987, vol. 32(9), pp. 782–784.

Diagnostic and Statistical Manual of Mental Disorders, 3rd ed., revised: R.L. Spitzer, et al., eds.; American Psychiatric Association, 1987, pp. 275–277.

Depersonalization and Agoraphobia Associated with Marijuana Use: C. Moran; Br. J. Med. Psychol., June 1986, vol. 59(pt. 2), pp. 187–196.

Depersonalization in a Nonclinical Population: D. Trueman; J. Psychol., January 1984, vol. 116(1st half), pp. 107–112.

# DEVIC DISEASE

**Description** Devic disease is a rare nerve condition characterized by demyelination of the optic nerve and the nerves in the spinal cord.

**Synonyms**

Neuromyelitis Optica

Ophthalmoneuromyelitis

Retrobulbar Neuropathy

**Signs and Symptoms** The initial symptoms are slight fever, sore throat, or head cold. The inflammation and demyelination of the optic nerve lead to swelling and pain within the eye and eventual loss of clear vision. The ocular findings initially may be unilateral but may become bilateral. Spinal cord abnormalities associated with mild paraparesis of the lower limbs and loss of bowel and bladder control develop later. Deep tendon reflexes are diminished or absent, and variable sensory loss occurs. With time there may be improvement of both paraparesis and ocular symptoms; but this may be followed by worsening.

**Etiology** The cause is not known. Some research indicates that Devic disease may be an autoimmune or genetic disorder. The disease may occur spontaneously, usually following a fever, or in conjunction with multiple sclerosis or systemic lupus erythematosus.

**Epidemiology** Males and females are affected in equal numbers.

**Related Disorders** See **Guillain-Barré Syndrome.** See also **Multiple Sclerosis** and **Systemic Lupus Erythematosus,** disorders that may precede the development of Devic disease.

**Acute disseminated encephalomyelitis (postinfectious encephalitis),** a central nervous system disorder characterized by inflammation of the brain and spinal cord caused by damage to the myelin sheath, can occur spontaneously but more commonly follows a viral infection or inoculation, e.g., of a bacterial or viral vaccine.

**Treatment—Standard** Early treatment using adrenocorticotropic hormone or corticosteroid drugs may successfully control inflammation of the optic nerve and spinal cord. Other treatment is symptomatic and supportive.

**Treatment—Investigational** Lymphocytoplasmapheresis is being investigated as a possible treatment for patients with Devic disease.

Please contact the agencies listed under Resources, below, for the most current information. Addresses and telephone numbers of these agencies, as well as of individual experts and research centers, may be found in the Master Resources List.

**Resources**

**For more information on Devic disease:** National Organization for Rare Disorders (NORD); NIH/National Eye Institute; NIH/National Institute of Neurological Disorders and Stroke.

**References**

Lymphocytoplasmapheresis in Devic's Syndrome: A.J. Aguilera, et al.; Transfusion, January–February 1985, vol. 25(1), pp. 54–56.

Devic's Syndrome and Systemic Lupus Erythematosus: A Case Report with Necropsy: E.L. Kinney, et al.; Arch. Neurol., October 1979, vol. 36(10), pp. 643–644.

# DIENCEPHALIC SYNDROME

**Description** The syndrome, normally seen in infancy or early childhood, is characterized principally by failure to thrive, emaciation, and normal linear growth.

**Synonyms**

      Russell Diencephalic Cachexia

**Signs and Symptoms** Severe emaciation is the most prominent feature. The eyes are often affected; the infant or child may have strabismus, nystagmus, or papilledema. There may be a tumor of the optic nerve that can result in vision loss. Increased intracranial pressure is often present. Although unusually sleepy, the child behaves in a normal, happy manner that is not in keeping with the physical appearance. Height is normal or even above average. Growth hormone plasma levels may be elevated.

    Diagnosis is made by CT or MRI scans. Without immediate medical attention, the disorder has serious consequences.

**Etiology** The syndrome usually results from development of a brain tumor, often a glioma or astrocytoma, or, rarely, a brain cyst. The tumor invades the anterior 3rd ventricle of the brain, the optic nerve (chiasm), or the hypothalamus, resulting in elevated pressure in the skull. Eye problems and emaciation result from tumor growth.

**Epidemiology** Usually the patient is a young infant or child; however, some cases have been reported in older children and even adults. Males and females are affected in equal numbers. The syndrome occurs worldwide.

**Related Disorders** See *Hydrocephalus; Tolosa-Hunt Syndrome.*

**Treatment—Standard** Treatment includes surgery, radiation, and chemotherapy. Radiation of very young infants and children may affect their growth and physical development.

**Treatment—Investigational** Several experimental drugs are being investigated for the treatment of brain tumors. These include interferon alfa-2b, serratia marcescens extract (polyribosomes), adenosine, borolife (sodium monomercaptoundecahydro-closo-dodecaborate), liposome encapsulated recombinant interleukin-2, and recombinant human interferon beta.

    Biodegradable carmustine (biodel), a polymer implant for treatment of malignant glioma, and photon therapy, a high beam form of radiation therapy, are being tested as treatments for brain tumors.

    Please contact the agencies listed under Resources, below, for the most current information. Addresses and telephone numbers of these agencies, as well as of individual experts and research centers, may be found in the Master Resources List.

**Resources**

    **For more information on diencephalic syndrome:** National Organization for Rare Disorders (NORD); NIH/National Cancer Institute Physician Data Query Phoneline; American Cancer Society.

**References**

Cecil Textbook of Medicine, 19th ed.: J.B. Wyngaarden, et al., eds.; W.B. Saunders Company, 1992, p. 2062.

Nelson Textbook of Pediatrics, 14th ed.: R.E. Behrman, ed.-in-chief; W.B. Saunders Company, 1992, p. 1534.

Chemotherapeutic Treatment of the Diencephalic Syndrome: A Case Report: M.C. Chamberlain, et al.; Cancer, May 1, 1989, vol. 63(9), pp. 1681–1684.

Principles of Neurology, 4th ed.: R.D. Adams and M. Victor, eds.; McGraw-Hill, 1989, p. 453.

The Paramedian Diencephalic Syndrome: A Dynamic Phenomenon: I. Meissner, et al.; Stroke, March–April 1987, vol. 18(2), pp. 380–385.

# DYSLEXIA

**Description** Dyslexia is the inability to interpret written language by a person with normal vision and hearing and no mental impairment or cultural deprivation. The condition is usually noted in childhood.

**Synonyms**

      Congenital Word Blindness
      Developmental Reading Disorder
      Primary Reading Disability
      Specific Reading Disability

**Signs and Symptoms** The perceptual confusion of letters may lead to difficulties in other areas of symbolic processing, such as arithmetic; however, spelling is not necessarily impaired. The child may not be able to tell right from left. Sensory perception and gross neurologic status are usually normal. Facility with mirror reading or mirror writing is common.

    When asked to read, a dyslexic child may make up a story to fit a picture in the text, or may substitute other words for those that are not understood. Reading is hesitant and slow. The inevitable frustration with classroom performance may lead to behavioral problems, such as delinquency, aggression, and poor social relations with parents and peers.

To forestall or interrupt development of a pattern of failure, early diagnosis is important. Audiometric and vision testing as well as psychological and neurologic examinations are advised.

**Etiology** An autosomal dominant inheritance has been suggested for some cases. There may be a central nervous system defect in the ability to organize graphic symbols. Dyslexia can also result from injury to the cerebral cortex.

**Epidemiology** Dyslexia is usually noticed between ages 6 and 9 years. Prevalence among school children appears to be between 2 and 8 percent.

**Related Disorders** Inability to understand written language may follow injury to the language-processing centers in the cerebral cortex (**alexia**).

**Treatment—Standard** The treatment of dyslexia entails remedial education for children and various self-checking strategies for adults.

**Treatment—Investigational** Please contact the agencies listed under Resources, below, for the most current information. Addresses and telephone numbers of these agencies, as well as of individual experts and research centers, may be found in the Master Resources List.

**Resources**

**For more information on dyslexia:** National Organization for Rare Disorders (NORD); NIH/National Institute of Neurological Disorders and Stroke; Orton Dyslexia Society; Learning Disabilities Association of America; National Network of Learning-Disabled Adults; HEATH Resource Center (Higher Education and the Handicapped).

**For genetic information and genetic counseling referrals:** March of Dimes Birth Defects Foundation; Alliance of Genetic Support Groups.

**References**

Mendelian Inheritance in Man, 9th ed.: V.A. McKusick; The Johns Hopkins University Press, 1990, pp. 275–276.

Diagnostic and Statistical Manual of Mental Disorders, 3rd ed., revised: R.L. Spitzer, et al., eds.; American Psychiatric Association, 1987, pp. 43–44.

# Eaton-Lambert Syndrome (ELS)

**Description** ELS is an immune-mediated neuromuscular disorder characterized generally by weakness and fatigue, especially of the pelvic and thigh muscles. There is a strong association with small cell carcinoma of the lungs.

**Synonyms**

Lambert-Eaton Myasthenic Syndrome
Lambert-Eaton Syndrome
Myasthenic Syndrome of Lambert-Eaton

**Signs and Symptoms** Principal characteristics are limb weakness and fatigue. Lower extremities are affected more often than upper limbs, resulting in a slow and waddling gait. Other features include dryness of the mouth, diplopia, dysarthria, ptosis, altered reflexes of the pupils of the eyes, impotence, hypohidrosis, and orthostatic hypotension.

Diagnosis of ELS is made by electromyogram (**EMG**) and electron microscopy. The EMG initially shows a reduced amplitude of electrical activity in the muscle. After stimulation or exercise, the activity increases. Electron microscopy may show changes in the postsynaptic membranes and nerve cell terminals.

**Etiology** The syndrome results from autoimmune-mediated reduction of nerve-evoked quantal release of acetylcholine at the motor end-plate. Cancer, usually a small cell carcinoma of the lung, is associated in two-thirds of cases. The syndrome may occur up to 3 years before a tumor is detected, or may not appear until after cancer diagnosis.

**Epidemiology** Of those affected with ELS who are over 40 years of age, 70 percent of men and 30 percent of women will have a malignant tumor. However, in one-third of Eaton-Lambert patients, the syndrome is not related to cancer and may occur at any age. There are approximately 400 known cases in the United States.

**Related Disorders** See *Guillain-Barré Syndrome; Myasthenia Gravis.*

**Treatment—Standard** Initial treatment is directed at any cancer present, which may result in relief of ELS symptoms as well.

Symptoms are often relieved or improved with guanidine, which increases the release of acetylcholine in the muscles. Immunosuppressive drugs such as prednisone and azathioprine may also be helpful. Other treatment is symptomatic and supportive.

**Treatment—Investigational** The Food and Drug Administration has approved the orphan drug dynamine for testing as treatment for ELS.

Clinical trials are under way to study the orphan drug 3,4-diaminopyridine for improvement of strength in patients with the syndrome.

Plasmapheresis is used in treating some cases of ELS.

Please contact the agencies listed under Resources, below, for the most current information. Addresses and telephone numbers of these agencies, as well as of individual experts and research centers, may be found in the Master Resources List.

**Resources**

**For more information on Eaton-Lambert syndrome:** National Organization for Rare Disorders (NORD); Myasthenia Gravis Foundation; NIH/National Institute of Neurological Disorders and Stroke; Muscular Dystrophy Association.

**References**

3,4-Diaminopyridine in the Treatment of Lambert-Eaton Myasthenic Syndrome: K.M. McEvoy; N. Engl. J. Med. 1989, vol. 321, pp. 1567–1571.

Autonomic Dysfunction in Lambert-Eaton Myasthenic Syndrome: R.K. Khurana, et al.; J. Neurol. Sci., May 1988, vol. 85(1), pp. 77–86.

Cecil Textbook Of Medicine, 18th Ed.: J.B. Wyngaarden and L.H. Smith, Jr., eds.; W.B. Saunders Company, 1988, pp. 1106, 1633, 2285, 2287.

Eaton-Lambert Syndrome As a Harbinger of Recurrent Small-Cell Carcinoma of the Cervix with Improvement After Combination Chemotherapy: G.P. Sutton, et al.; Obstet. Gynecol., September 1988, vol. 72(3 pt. 2), pp. 516–518.

Internal Medicine, 2nd ed.: J.H. Stein, ed.-in-chief; Little, Brown and Company, 1987, pp. 999–1000.

# EMPTY SELLA SYNDROME

**Description** Empty sella syndrome is a rare brain disorder in which the sella turcica appears as an extension of the subarachnoid space and is filled with cerebrospinal fluid. This results from a defect in the diaphragma sellae. Alternatively, the syndrome may be primary or secondary to a pituitary tumor or to irradiation or surgery on the pituitary gland.

**Synonyms**

Empty Sella Turcica

**Signs and Symptoms** The clinical picture is dominated by headaches, impaired vision, and obesity. In some cases these findings are accompanied by hypertension and cold intolerance. Sex-specific differences may be seen: hirsutism in women, and gynecomastia and reduced libido in men.

Computed tomography may show a vestigial diaphragma sellae, a diffusely enlarged sella, and an apparently empty pituitary fossa. Other diagnostic studies include hormone assays and neurologic examination. Pituitary function is normal.

**Etiology** The primary form of empty sella syndrome is inherited as an autosomal dominant trait. Secondary cases develop as a result of birth defects, pituitary adenomas, and irradiation or surgery on the pituitary gland.

**Epidemiology** Empty sella syndrome predominantly develops in obese middle-aged women, although men and, rarely, children may also be affected.

**Related Disorders** The syndrome must be distinguished from tumors of the brain or optic nerve, especially in the setting of diabetes and visual deficits. Thus, the entity must be distinguished from ***Achard-Thiers Syndrome, Meningioma,*** and optic glioma, a slow-growing optic nerve tumor that occasionally extends to the 3rd ventricle.

**Treatment—Standard** Treatment is symptomatic and supportive.

**Treatment—Investigational** Please contact the agencies listed under Resources, below, for the most current information. Addresses and telephone numbers of these agencies, as well as of individual experts and research centers, may be found in the Master Resources List.

**Resources**

**For more information on empty sella syndrome:** National Organization for Rare Disorders (NORD); NIH/National Institute of Neurological Disorders and Stroke.

**For genetic information and genetic counseling referrals:** March of Dimes Birth Defects Foundation; Alliance of Genetic Support Groups.

**References**

Mendelian Inheritance in Man, 8th ed.: V.A. McKusick; The Johns Hopkins University Press, 1988, p. 226.

MRI and CT of Sellar and Parasellar Disorders: M.H. Naheedy, et al.; Radiol. Clin. North Am., July 1987, vol. 25(4), pp. 819–847.

Subarachnoid Hemorrhage with Normal Cerebral Angiography: A Prospective Study on Sellar Abnormalities and Pituitary Function: P. Bjerre, et al.; Neurosurgery, December 1986, vol. 19(6), pp. 1012–1015.

The "Empty Sella" in Childhood: D.C. Costigan, et al.; Clin. Pediatr., August 1984, vol. 23(8), pp. 437–440.

# ENCEPHALOCELE

**Description** Encephalocele is a form of neural tube defect, producing an opening in the skull, through which meningeal and other brain tissues protrude.

**Synonyms**

    Cranial Meningoencephalocele

    Craniocele

    Cranium Bifidum

**Signs and Symptoms** The defect is usually in the midline, most often in the occipital area, then in the frontal area. Patients with an encephalocele may develop hydrocephalus. A posterior encephalocele is found in patients with Meckel syndrome (see *Meckel Syndrome).*

**Etiology** The cause is not known. Failure of the neural tube to close properly during fetal growth probably causes the encephalocele to form. Meckel syndrome, however, is inherited as an autosomal recessive trait.

The anticonvulsant drug valproic acid may cause neural tube defects when taken by pregnant women.

**Epidemiology** Encephalocele occurs in an estimated 1:2,000 live births. Ireland has the highest occurrence of encephalocele; Thailand, a high percentage of frontal encephaloceles. Male and female infants are affected in equal numbers.

**Related Disorders** See *Agenesis of Corpus Callosum; Anencephaly; Hydrocephalus; Meckel Syndrome; Spina Bifida; Walker-Warburg Syndrome.*

**Treatment—Standard** Surgical closure of the encephalocele is generally performed as soon as possible. When the face is involved, repeated plastic surgery may be required over a period of time. When hydrocephaly is also present, the required shunt may have to be lengthened periodically. When bacterial meningitis is present, the addition of dexamethasone to the antibiotic treatment can be helpful in reducing meningeal inflammation.

**Treatment—Investigational** Please contact the agencies listed under Resources, below, for the most current information. Addresses and telephone numbers of these agencies, as well as of individual experts and research centers, may be found in the Master Resources List.

**Resources**

    **For more information on encephalocele:** National Organization for Rare Disorders (NORD); National Hydrocephalus Foundation; Hydrocephalus Parent Support Group; Hydrocephalus Association; Fighters for Encephaly Support Group; National Craniofacial Foundation; FACES—National Association for the Craniofacially Handicapped; Forward Face; Children's Craniofacial Association; AboutFace; Craniofacial Family Association; American Cleft Palate Cranial Facial Association; NIH/National Institute of Child Health and Human Development; NIH/National Institute of Neurological Disorders and Stroke.

    **For genetic information and genetic counseling referrals:** March of Dimes Birth Defects Foundation; Alliance of Genetic Support Groups.

**References**

Interim CDC Recommendations for Folic Acid Supplementation for Women: August 1991, Centers for Disease Control; JAMA, September 4, 1991, vol. 266(9), p. 1191.

Nasal Midline Masses in Infants and Children. Dermoids, Encephaloceles, and Gliomas: A.S. Paller, et al.; Arch. Dermatol., March 1991, vol. 127(3), pp. 362–326.

Birth Defects Encyclopedia: M.L. Buyse, M.D., ed.-in-chief; Blackwell Scientific Publications, 1990, pp. 614–615.

Cephaloceles: Classification, Pathology, and Management: D.J. David, et al.; World J. Surg., July–August 1989, vol. 13(4), pp. 349–357.

Subtorcular Occipital Encephaloceles: Anatomical Considerations Relevant to Operative Management: P.H. Chapman, et al.; J. Neurosurg., September 1989, vol. 71(3), pp. 375–381.

Nasal Encephalocele: Definitive One-Stage Reconstruction: L.A. Sargent, et al.; J. Neurosurg., April 1988, vol. 68(4), pp. 571–575.

# EPILEPSY, MYOCLONIC PROGRESSIVE FAMILIAL

**Description** This central nervous system disorder takes 2 forms: **Lafora disease** and **Unverricht-Lundborg (-Laf) disease.** In both forms, onset is in childhood, and the disorder is progressive, in some cases leading to dementia.

**Synonyms**

    Baltic Myoclonus Epilepsy

    Lafora Body Disease

    Lundborg-Unverricht Disease

    Myoclonic Epilepsy

    Unverricht Syndrome

**Signs and Symptoms** In **Lafora disease,** onset usually is around the age of 15 in the form of grand mal seizures and/or myoclonus. As the disease progresses, mental capacity deteriorates. The presence on biopsy of Lafora bodies in the brain, heart, muscle, and liver is diagnostic.

In **Unverricht-Lundborg disease,** onset may be anywhere between the ages of 6 and 13. The essential and usually earliest symptom is myoclonus. Major seizures are less common. Muscle spasms in the limbs are seen as minor twitching motions; later they may become violent enough to cause the patient to fall to the ground. Mental deterioration develops as the disease progresses.

The course is variable. In advanced cases cerebellar ataxia occurs. Very rarely, deafness may result, especially when there is cerebellar ataxia. Stimulus-sensitive myoclonus may be present. Generalized tonic-clonic seizures may sometimes be combined with petit mal attacks. Emotional instability is common. Electroencephalogram (**EEG**) findings will document the seizures. Unlike Lafora disease, no cell particles are found.

**Etiology** Lafora and Unverricht diseases are inherited through autosomal recessive genes.

**Epidemiology** Males and females are affected in equal numbers in all forms of myoclonic progressive familial epilepsy. The disorder begins in childhood: Lafora disease, at about age 15; and Unverricht-Lundborg disease, at about 6 to 13 years. Unverricht-Lundborg disease is frequently found in persons of Finnish and Swedish heritage.

**Related Disorders** See *Huntington Disease; Kufs Disease; Myoclonus; Tourette Syndrome; Wilson Disease.*

In **juvenile myoclonic epilepsy,** onset is early in life. Characteristic are isolated myoclonic jerks, usually occurring in the morning, which do not necessarily lead to major seizures. A family record of epilepsy may be present. There is some evidence for autosomal recessive inheritance. Diagnosis is by EEG. Occasionally an asymptomatic family member may show similar EEG characteristics. Juvenile myoclonic epilepsy is chronic but not progressive.

**Treatment—Standard** Treatment includes anticonvulsant drugs such as valproic acid and clonazepam. Genetic counseling may be beneficial. Other treatment is symptomatic and supportive.

**Treatment—Investigational** For patients who continue to have seizures despite anticonvulsant medication, zonisamide may be tried.

A study to identify the gene responsible for Lafora disease is under way at The Centre for Research in Neurocience, McGill University. Please contact Guy A. Rouleau, M.D., Iscia Lopes-Cendes, M.D., or Karen Rye, R.N.

Please contact the agencies listed under Resources, below, for the most current information. Addresses and telephone numbers of these agencies, as well as of individual experts and research centers, may be found in the Master Resources List.

**Resources**

**For more information on myoclonic progressive familial epilepsy:** National Organization for Rare Disorders (NORD); NIH/National Institute of Neurological Disorders and Stroke; Epilepsy Foundation of America.

**For genetic information and genetic counseling referrals:** March of Dimes Birth Defects Foundation; Alliance of Genetic Support Groups.

**References**

Diagnosis of Lafora Disease by Skin Biopsy: J.W. White, Jr., et al.; J. Cutan. Pathol., June 1989, vol. 15(3), pp. 171–175.

Juvenile Myoclonic Epilepsy: An Autosomal Recessive Disease: C.P. Panayiotopoulos, et al.; Ann. Neurol., May 1989, vol. 25(5), pp. 440–443.

Juvenile Myoclonic Epilepsy: Characteristics of a Primary Generalized Epilepsy: F.E. Dreifuss; Epilepsia, 1989, vol. 30(4), pp. 1–7, 24–27.

Juvenile Myoclonic Epilepsy: M.J. Clement, et al.; Arch. Dis. Child, September 1988, vol. 63(9), pp. 1049–1053.

Progressive Myoclonus Epilepsy Treated with Zonisamide: T.R. Henry, et al.; Neurology, June 1988, vol. 38(6), pp. 928–931.

Valproate Monotherapy in Children: J.V. Murphy; Am. J. Med., January 25, 1988, vol. 84(1A), pp. 17–22.

# ERB PALSY

**Description** Erb palsy is a disorder, usually seen in newborns or infants, of the peripheral nervous system resulting from an injury to one or more nerves of the upper brachial plexus. Paralysis of the shoulder and upper extremity is characteristic.

**Synonyms**

Erb/Duchenne Palsy

Erb Paralysis

**Signs and Symptoms** Following an injury to the upper brachial plexus, adduction and internal turning of the shoulder occurs, with pronation of the forearm and hand. The shoulder and upper extremity may become paralyzed. There also may be paralysis of the diaphragm on the affected side. Feeling and function in the wrist and hand usually are not affected.

**Etiology** The cause of this disorder is an injury to the nerve roots and surrounding nerves of the upper brachial plexus. The injury may involve abnormal stretching of the shoulder during a difficult labor, breech delivery, or excessive sideways movement of the neck during delivery.

**Epidemiology** Males and females are affected equally. The disorder is most often seen in newborns, but injuries caused by abnormal stretching of the shoulder may cause Erb palsy at any age.

**Related Disorders** See *Parsonnage-Turner Syndrome; Peripheral Neuropathy.*

**Treatment—Standard** Patients usually respond promptly to the standard treatment of physical therapy and splinting of the affected area. Surgery may be necessary to repair damaged nerves when injury has been extensive. Other treatment is symptomatic and supportive.

**Treatment—Investigational** Please contact the agencies listed under Resources, below, for the most current information. Addresses and telephone numbers of these agencies, as well as of individual experts and research centers, may be found in the Master Resources List.

**Resources**

   **For more information on Erb palsy:** National Organization for Rare Disorders (NORD); NIH/National Arthritis and Musculoskeletal and Skin Diseases Information Clearinghouse.

**References**

Brachial Plexus Palsy in the Newborn: S. Jackson, et al.; J. Bone Joint Surg. Am., September 1988, vol. 70(8), pp. 1217–1220.

Duchenne-Erb Palsy: Experience with Direct Surgery: J. Comtet, et al.; Clin. Orthop., December 1988, vol. 237, pp. 17–23.

Preliminary Experience with Brachial Plexus Exploration in Children: Birth Injury and Vehicular Trauma: J. Piatt Jr., et al.; Neurosurgery, April 1988, vol. 22(4), pp. 715–723.

Early Microsurgical Reconstruction in Birth Palsy: H. Kawabata, et al.; Clin. Orthop., February 1987, pp. 233–242.

Erb/Duchenne Palsy: A Consequence of Fetal Macrosomia and Method of Delivery: L. McFarland, et al.; Obstet. Gynecol., December 1986, vol. 68(6), pp. 784–788.

# FAHR DISEASE

**Description** Fahr disease is a rare neurologic condition characterized by abnormal deposition of calcium in certain areas of the brain. The clinical picture is one of progressive deterioration in mental and motor function, mental retardation, spastic paralysis, and athetosis. Parkinson disease may be secondarily associated.

**Synonyms**

> Cerebrovascular Ferrocalcinosis
> Intracranial Calcification
> Nonarteriosclerotic Cerebral Calcification
> Striopallidodentate Calcinosis

**Signs and Symptoms** Abnormal calcium deposits accrue in the basal ganglia, cerebral cortex, dentate nucleus, subthalamus, and red nucleus areas of the brain, attended by loss of brain cells. Calcium may also be deposited in areas of demyelination and in lipid deposits.

The head often appears round and smaller than normal. Dementia and loss of previously attained motor function are characteristic and accompanied by spastic paralysis and occasionally athetosis. Optic atrophy may be present.

Features of Parkinson disease that may be found in Fahr disease include tremors and rigidity, a masklike facies, shuffling walk, and a "pill-rolling" motion of the fingers. Dystonia, chorea, and seizures are occasionally reported. A parkinsonian component is not necessary for the differential diagnosis.

**Etiology** An autosomal recessive inheritance of Fahr disease has been postulated. Some cases occur sporadically, perhaps reflecting fetal infection rather than a genetic origin.

**Epidemiology** Fahr disease is a very rare disorder. Males and females are equally affected.

**Related Disorders** See *Parkinson Disease.*

**Treatment—Standard** Some psychotic symptoms may be ameliorated with lithium carbonate. Other treatment is symptomatic and supportive. Genetic counseling may be beneficial for patients and families with the hereditary form of the disease.

**Treatment—Investigational** A Fahr disease registry has been developed.

Please contact the agencies listed under Resources, below, for the most current information. Addresses and telephone numbers of these agencies, as well as of individual experts and research centers, may be found in the Master Resources List.

**Resources**

   **For more information on Fahr disease:** National Organization for Rare Disorders (NORD); NIH/National Institute of Neurological Disorders and Stroke; Fahr Disease Registry; Parkinson Disease and Movement Disorders Clinic; The Arc (a national organization on mental retardation).

**For genetic information and genetic counseling referrals:** March of Dimes Birth Defects Foundation; Alliance of Genetic Support Groups.

### References

Mendelian Inheritance in Man, 9th ed.: V.A. McKusick; The Johns Hopkins University Press, 1990, pp. 1084–1085.

Idiopathic Nonarteriosclerotic Cerebral Calcification (Fahr's Disease): An Electron Microscopic Study: S. Kobayashi, et al.; Acta Neuropathol. (Berl.), 1987, vol. 73(1), pp. 62–66.

The Treatment of Psychotic Symptoms in Fahr's Disease with Lithium Carbonate: K.M. Munir; J. Clin. Psychopharmacol., February 1986, vol. 6(1), pp. 36–38.

# FAMILIAL DYSAUTONOMIA

**Description** Familial dysautonomia is a rare genetic disorder of the autonomic nervous system (**ANS**) associated with pain, loss of sensation, and unsteadiness.

Two types of the disorder (I and II) are recognized. Type II is better known as congenital sensory neuropathy with anhidrosis. There may be a 3rd type with adult onset of impaired ANS functioning.

### Synonyms

> Congenital Sensory Neuropathy with Anhidrosis (Type II Familial Dysautonomia)
> Hereditary Sensory and Autonomic Neuropathy
> Riley-Day Syndrome

**Signs and Symptoms** Types I and II familial dysautonomia for the most part have similar symptoms. Differential diagnosis can be made by biopsy.

An infant born with this disorder has poor sucking and swallowing reflexes, low ocular fluid pressure, and hypothermia.

There is typically a decreased perception of pain and temperature, which can lead to cutaneous trauma. A lack of tears and insensitivity of the eye to pain from foreign objects can lead to corneal inflammation and ulceration.

Other findings include unstable blood pressure, an absence of sense of taste, impaired speech, drooling, attacks of vomiting, and skin blotching. There may be episodes of pneumonia, absence of tendon reflexes, skeletal defects, and stunted height.

By adolescence, 95 percent of patients have evidence of spinal curvature and may experience increased sweating and an accelerated heart rate. Other adolescent symptoms include weakness, leg cramping, difficulty concentrating, and personality changes characterized by depression, irritability, insomnia, and negativism. Kidney insufficiency develops in 20 percent of patients over 20 years of age. Neurologic deterioration also progresses, and unsteadiness in walking becomes more apparent at this age.

Patients with type II familial dysautonomia also may have anhidrosis and mental retardation.

There may be an adult-onset type of familial dysautonomia, the genetic defect expressed later than in the childhood forms.

Diagnosis is made by subcutaneous injection of histamine. The lack of axon flare response is diagnostic for familial dysautonomia.

**Etiology** Type I familial dysautonomia has a dominant inheritance; type II, a recessive inheritance.

**Epidemiology** Type I familial dysautonomia primarily affects individuals of Ashkenazic Jewish ancestry; the genetic carrier rate is estimated to be 1:30. Both males and females are affected. Type II is not limited to a specific group.

**Related Disorders** Many conditions characterized by the symptom of dysautonomia should not be confused with this specific hereditary disorder. See *Neuropathy, Hereditary Sensory, Type II.*

**Biemond congenital and familial analgesia** symptoms are similar to those of familial dysautonomia, and include insensitivity to pain, a diminished sense of temperature and touch, and absence of tendon reflexes.

**Treatment—Standard** Drugs used to relieve the symptoms of familial dysautonomia are diazepam and metoclopramide. Artificial tears may be needed for the eyes. Physical therapy, chest physiotherapy, occupational therapy, feeding facilitation, and speech therapy may be needed. Patients may also benefit from a variety of orthopedic and ocular aids.

**Treatment—Investigational** Clinical trials are under way to study the taxonomy of familial dysautonomia and treatment of orthostatic hypotension. Italo Biaggioni, M.D., may be contacted at Vanderbilt University.

Please contact the agencies listed under Resources, below, for the most current information. Addresses and telephone numbers of these agencies, as well as of individual experts and research centers, may be found in the Master Resources List.

### Resources

**For more information on familial dysautonomia:** National Organization for Rare Disorders (NORD); Dysautonomia Foundation; National Foundation for Jewish Genetic Diseases; NIH/National Institute of Neurological

Disorders and Stroke.

**For genetic information and genetic counseling referrals:** March of Dimes Birth Defects Foundation; Alliance of Genetic Support Groups.

### References

Cecil Textbook of Medicine, 19th ed.: J.B. Wyngaarden, et al., eds.; W.B. Saunders Company, 1992, p. 2246.

Mendelian Inheritance in Man, 10th ed.: V.A. McKusick; The Johns Hopkins University Press, 1992, pp. 768–769, 1345–1346.

Principles and Practices of Medical Genetics, 2nd ed.: E.H. Allan, et al., eds.; Churchill Livingston Publishers, 1990, pp. 397–441.

Principles of Neurology, 4th ed.: R.D. Adams and M. Victor, eds.; McGraw-Hill, 1989, pp. 453, 1033, 1056.

Neonatal Recognition of Familial Dysautonomia: F.B. Axelrod, et al.; J. Pediatr., June 1987, vol. 110(6), pp. 946–948.

# FIBER TYPE DISPROPORTION, CONGENITAL (CFTD)

**Description** CFTD is a rare hereditary disease affecting the growth of type I muscle fibers. The clinical picture is dominated by hypotonia and weakness, various skeletal deformities, and short stature; however, none of these findings is pathognomonic. The disorder can usually be diagnosed at birth. Function tends to improve as the patient ages.

**Synonyms**
>    Atrophy of Type I Fibers
>    Myopathy of Congenital Fiber Type Disproportion

**Signs and Symptoms** The muscles of a newborn infant with CFTD are unusually weak and hypotonic. The nonprogressive hypotonia may be accompanied by failure to grow and by developmental skeletal anomalies such as scoliosis, dislocated hip joints, foot deformities, and a high-arched palate. Mental retardation may occur in some cases. The clinical findings may occur singly or in combination, but the diagnosis rests on muscle biopsy, which shows type I muscle fibers smaller than type II fibers.

**Etiology** CFTD is inherited as an autosomal recessive trait.

**Epidemiology** CFTD is usually present at birth. Males and females are affected equally.

**Related Disorders** Various neuromuscular disorders, especially the dystrophies, can produce symptoms resembling those of CFTD. See *Muscular Dystrophy, Batten Turner; Muscular Dystrophy, Becker; Muscular Dystrophy, Duchenne; Muscular Dystrophy, Emery-Dreifuss; Muscular Dystrophy, Limb-Girdle; Myotonic Dystrophy.*

   **Gowers muscular dystrophy (late distal hereditary myopathy)** is a hereditary disorder with an early symptom of mild weakness in the small muscles of the hands and feet, spreading proximally to involve neighboring muscles. The disorder is transmitted as an autosomal dominant trait and is rare. Onset usually occurs in middle age or later, and symptoms typically remain mild to moderate.

**Treatment—Standard** Physiotherapy with active and passive exercise is recommended to promote muscle function in CFTD. The effects of the disorder usually diminish as the patient ages. Genetic counseling may be helpful.

**Treatment—Investigational** Please contact the agencies listed under Resources, below, for the most current information. Addresses and telephone numbers of these agencies, as well as of individual experts and research centers, may be found in the Master Resources List.

**Resources**

   **For more information on congenital fiber type disproportion:** National Organization for Rare Disorders (NORD); The Arc (a national organization on mental retardation); NIH/National Institute of Neurological Disorders and Stroke; Muscular Dystrophy Association.

   **For genetic information and genetic counseling referrals:** March of Dimes Birth Defects Foundation; Alliance of Genetic Support Groups.

### References

Congenital Fiber Disproportion. Atrophy of Type I Fibers: Report of 11 Cases: J.A. Levy, et al.; Arq. Neuropsiquiatr., June 1987, vol. 45(2), pp. 153–158.

Mendelian Inheritance in Man, 8th ed.: V.A. McKusick; The Johns Hopkins University Press, 1986, p. 1094.

Muscle Fiber Type Transformation in Nemaline Myopathy and Congenital Fiber Type Disproportion: T. Miike, et al.; Brain Dev., 1986, vol. 8(5), pp. 526–632.

# FREY SYNDROME

**Description** Frey syndrome results from injury to the facial nerve near the parotid glands and is characterized by flushing or sweating on one side of the face when foods are chewed. The symptoms usually are mild and well tolerated by most patients, although symptomatic treatment is necessary in some cases.

**Synonyms**

> Auriculotemporal Syndrome
> Baillarger Syndrome
> Dupuy Syndrome

**Signs and Symptoms** Sweating is the predominant symptom in men; women typically experience flushing symptoms. Chewing food causes sweating and flushing on the cheek and ear on one side of the face.

**Etiology** Frey syndrome usually develops after injury or surgery on the parotid glands, resulting in damage to the facial nerve. The sweating and flushing are due to abnormal regeneration of parasympathetic, rather than sympathetic, nerve fibers following injury. These aberrant parasympathetic nerves are stimulated by eating. It has been suggested that a surgical technique (superficial aponeurotic system preservation technique) may reduce the high risk of Frey syndrome in persons undergoing parotid gland surgery.

**Related Disorders** See *Hyperhidrosis.*

**Treatment—Standard** Treatment is symptomatic and directed toward relieving excessive discomfort. Procaine may be injected into the auriculotemporal nerve. Scopolamine cream, diphemanil methylsulfate, or aluminum chloride hexahydrate antiperspirant may reduce sweating. In severe cases, nerve projections near the ear and cheek may be modified surgically.

**Treatment—Investigational** An orphan drug, glycopurrolate, is being developed by Robins Corporation for treatment of Frey syndrome.

Please contact the agencies listed under Resources, below, for the most current information. Addresses and telephone numbers of these agencies, as well as of individual experts and research centers, may be found in the Master Resources List.

**Resources**

**For more information on Frey syndrome:** National Organization for Rare Disorders (NORD); NIH/National Institute of Neurological Disorders and Stroke.

**References**

Frey's Syndrome: A Preventable Phenomenon: P.C. Bonanno; Plast. Reconstr. Surg., March 1992, vol. 89(3), pp. 452–458.

Facial Flushing in Children: A Variant of the Auriculo-Temporal Syndrome: D.K. Hennon; J. Indiana Dent. Assoc., January–February 1991, vol. 70(1), pp. 25–27.

Birth Defects Encyclopedia: M.L. Buyse, ed.-in-chief; Blackwell Scientific Publications, 1990, pp. 1614–1615.

Dictionary of Medical Syndromes, 3rd ed.: S.I. Magalini, et al., eds.; J.B. Lippincott Company, 1990, pp. 327–328.

The Management of Frey's Syndrome with Aluminium Chloride Hexamydrate Antiperspirant: M.J. Black, et al.; Ann. R. Coll. Surg. Engl., January 1990, vol. 72(1), pp. 49–52.

Treatment of Frey's Syndrome with Topical 2% Diphemanil Methysulfate (Prantal): A Double-Blind Evaluation of 15 Patients: O. Laccourreye, et al.; Laryngoscope, June 1990, vol. 100(6), pp. 651–653.

# GERSTMANN SYNDROME

**Description** The syndrome is characterized by the loss or absence of certain sensory abilities, which occurs as the result of a brain injury or as a developmental disorder.

**Synonyms**

> Gerstmann Tetrad

**Signs and Symptoms** The disorder is defined by 4 specific neurologic deficits: agraphia, acalculia, finger agnosia, and the inability to distinguish between right and left.

**Etiology** In some cases, the syndrome is caused by damage to the focal, sensory centers in the left hemisphere of the brain. Scar tissue, trauma, or brain tumor can be responsible. However, the tetrad can also occur in children of normal intelligence with no sign of brain injury or disease. In these developmental cases, the cause is unknown.

**Epidemiology** The disorder affect males and females of all ages and in equal numbers.

**Treatment—Standard** Treatment in developmental cases involves special education and related rehabilitation and counseling services. When brain injury or tumor is involved, surgery may be used to alleviate the condition. The removal of scar tissue or a tumor along with rehabilitation therapies often restores an individual's normal abilities.

**Treatment—Investigational** Please contact the agencies listed under Resources, below, for the most current information. Addresses and telephone numbers of these agencies, as well as of individual experts and research centers, may be found in the Master Resources List.

**Resources**

**For more information on Gerstmann syndrome:** National Organization for Rare Disorders (NORD); NIH/National Institute of Child Health and Human Development; Learning Disabilities Association of America; American Brain Tumor Association.

**References**

Gerstmann's Syndrome: A.L. Benton; Arch. Neurol., May 1992, vol. 49(5), pp. 445–447.

Right Parietal Stroke with Gerstmann's Syndrome: Appearance on Computed Tomography, Magnetic Resonance Imaging, and Single-Photon Emission Computed Tomography: M.K. Moor, et al.; Arch. Neurol., April 1991, vol. 48(4), pp. 432–435.

Principles of Neurology, 4th ed.: R.D. Adams and M. Victor, eds.; McGraw-Hill, 1989, pp. 4, 116, 132, 388, 365–366.

Developmental Gerstmann's Syndrome: R. PeBenito, et al.; Arch. Neurol., September 1988, vol. 45(9), pp. 977–982.

Developmental Gerstmann Syndrome: Case Report and Review of the Literature: R. PeBenito; J. Dev. Behav. Pediatr., August 1987, vol. 8(4), pp. 229–232.

# GUILLAIN-BARRÉ SYNDROME

**Description** Guillain-Barré syndrome (acute idiopathic polyneuritis) is a rare, rapidly progressive form of ascending polyneuropathy. Although the precise etiology is unknown, a viral enteric or respiratory infection precedes the onset of the syndrome in about half of cases, which has led to postulation of an autoimmune mechanism. Damage to the myelin and nerve axons through immune system mechanisms results in delayed nervous signal transmission, with a corresponding weakness in the muscles innervated by those nerves. With proper treatment, more than half of patients recover completely with no residual neurologic signs. The syndrome is fatal in 2 to 5 percent of cases.

The following subdivisions are recognized: Miller-Fischer syndrome (Fischer syndrome, acute disseminated encephalomyeloradiculopathy); chronic Guillain-Barré syndrome (chronic idiopathic polyneuritis); relapsing Guillain-Barré syndrome; chronic inflammatory demyelinating polyradiculoneuropathy; chronic relapsing polyneuropathy; polyneuropathy; and polyradiculoneuropathy.

**Synonyms**

> Acute Idiopathic Polyneuritis
> Ascending Paralysis
> Kussmaul-Landry Paralysis
> Landry Ascending Paralysis
> Postinfective Polyneuritis

**Signs and Symptoms** In the typical pattern in this ascending polyneuritis, paresthesias begin in the feet, followed by weakness and flaccid paralysis of the legs. Eventually the torso, upper limbs, and face are affected. Symptoms progress over hours to weeks. Deep tendon reflexes may be lost; among the first to go is the ankle jerk. The paralysis may be accompanied by fever, bulbar palsy, and an increase in cerebrospinal fluid protein levels.

Specific symptoms are bilateral and reflect the portion of the nervous system involved. Sensory nerve damage produces numbness and tingling in the feet, hands, gums, and face. The face may appear pouchy and lopsided, and the patient may have difficulty breathing or swallowing food without choking. Involvement of the autonomic nervous system may cause sinus tachycardia or bradycardia, hypertension, postural hypotension, and changes in body temperature, vision, bladder function, and blood chemistries.

**Fischer syndrome** is a rare form of Guillain-Barré syndrome that commonly follows an upper respiratory tract infection. Men are predominantly affected. A generalized weakness occurs that is particularly severe in the ocular muscles, resulting in vision problems. Involvement of facial and neck musculature leads to impaired speech production and a sagging face. Deep tendon reflexes may be lost, and an awkward, unsteady (ataxic) gait is common.

**Chronic idiopathic polyneuritis** produces symptoms indistinguishable from those of Guillain-Barré syndrome except that the eyes and face are involved in only 15 percent of cases. The course is unpredictable; however, symptoms tend to progress over 6 to 12 months, then remit for a variable period before recurring.

**Etiology** An autoimmune mechanism triggered by a preceding viral infection has been postulated as the cause of Guillain-Barré syndrome. The viral infections incriminated have ranged from a common cold to viral hepatitis and mononucleosis. Cases have also occurred following surgery, an insect sting, a swine flu injection, or porphyria.

**Epidemiology** Guillain-Barré syndrome is extremely rare, with a reported incidence of 1 or 2 cases per 100,000 persons.

**Related Disorders** The symptoms of ***Peripheral Neuropathy*** are frequently confused with the early symptoms of Guillain-Barré syndrome. See also under Signs and Symptoms, above.

**Treatment—Standard** The clinical course is highly variable. Paralysis generally peaks in less than 10 days, although it may continue to progress for months. Recovery begins after the condition has stabilized and may take 6 months to 2 years. The prognosis generally correlates with the speed of recovery.

Although no cure for Guillain-Barré syndrome is available, various forms of treatment have proved effective. Physiotherapy is helpful for restoring muscle strength as innervation returns. Strength is usually recovered in the upper body first. Respiratory assistance may be needed by hospitalized patients. Corticosteroids (for chronic Guillain-Barré syndrome) and plasmapheresis may be prescribed. Plasmapheresis appears most beneficial in younger patients with severe locomotor disability at the time of the first plasma exchange. Other therapy is customized to the particular deficit or complication present.

**Treatment—Investigational** Several studies suggest that high-dose intravenous immunoglobulin may be beneficial in severe cases. For information on plasmapheresis, physicians may contact The Johns Hopkins University Hospital.

Please contact the agencies listed under Resources, below, for the most current information. Addresses and telephone numbers of these agencies, as well as of individual experts and research centers, may be found in the Master Resources List.

**Resources**

**For more information on Guillain-Barré syndrome:** National Organization for Rare Disorders (NORD); Guillain-Barré Syndrome Foundation International; NIH/National Institute of Neurological Disorders and Stroke.

**References**

Autoimmune Disease and the Nervous System: Biochemical, Molecular, and Clinical Update: J.E. Graves, et al.; West. J. Med., June 1992, vol. 156(6), pp. 639–646.

Cecil Textbook of Medicine, 19th ed.: J.B. Wyngaarden, et al., eds.; W.B. Saunders Company, 1992, pp. 471, 1855, 2181.

Principles of Neurology, 4th ed.: R.D. Adams and M. Victor, eds.; McGraw-Hill, 1989, pp. 1035–1039.

# HALLERVORDEN-SPATZ DISEASE

**Description** Hallervorden-Spatz disease affects movement. Characteristics are varied, ranging from dystonia to dementia.

**Synonyms**

Progressive Pallid Degeneration Syndrome

**Signs and Symptoms** The most common symptoms are dystonia and choreoathetosis, muscular rigidity, and dementia. Spasticity develops in one-third of cases. Dysarthria, mental retardation, facial grimacing, dysphasia, and visual loss due to optic atrophy are reported less frequently. Symptoms tend to vary among individuals. The clinical syndrome may resemble Parkinson disease in some cases (see ***Parkinson Disease).***

Diagnosis is confirmed by CT scan and MRI, demonstrating the characteristic high-density lesions due to accumulation of large amounts of pigmented material in the globus pallidus and pars reticulata of the substantia nigra. Localized swelling of tissue is also evident. A useful diagnostic test measures the uptake of radioactive ferrous citrate into certain areas of the brain; unusually high uptake is characteristic of the disease.

**Etiology** Hallervorden-Spatz disease is inherited as an autosomal recessive trait. More than one child in a family may be affected. In such cases, siblings are likely to experience similar symptoms.

**Epidemiology** Onset typically occurs during childhood, although occasionally symptoms begin in adulthood. About 70 cases have been reported in the medical literature, most of these in persons of European descent. Males and females are affected in equal numbers. Death usually occurs before the age of 30 years.

**Related Disorders** Other movement disorders such as static encephalopathy, Sandifer syndrome, benign paroxysmal torticollis, and infections and tumors of the spine and soft tissues of the neck may also cause dystonic symptoms or uncontrolled muscle contractions. See ***Huntington Disease; Joseph Disease; Leigh Disease; Olivopontocerebellar Atrophy; Pelizaeus-Merzbacher Brain Sclerosis; Seitelberger Disease; Torsion Dystonia.***

**Treatment—Standard** Treatment is symptomatic and supportive, and may include physical therapy, exercise physiology, occupational therapy, and speech pathology. Genetic counseling may be of benefit.

**Treatment—Investigational** Please contact the agencies listed under Resources, below, for the most current information. Addresses and telephone numbers of these agencies, as well as of individual experts and research centers, may be found in the Master Resources List.

**Resources**

**For more information on Hallervorden-Spatz disease:** National Organization for Rare Disorders (NORD); NIH/National Institute of Neurological Disorders and Stroke; Research Trust for Metabolic Diseases in Children; Dystonia Clinical Research Center; Dystonia Medical Research Foundation.

**For genetic information and genetic counseling referrals:** March of Dimes Birth Defects Foundation; Alliance of Genetic Support Groups.

### References

Clinical Features of Neuroleptic Malignant Syndrome in Basal Ganglia Disease: Spontaneous Presentation on a Patient with Hallervorden-Spatz Disease in the Absence of Neuroleptic Drugs: K. Hayashi, et al.; Anaesthesia, June 1993, vol. 48(6), pp. 499–502.

Hallervorden-Spatz Disease: MR and Pathologic Findings: M. Savoiardo, et al.; Am. J. Neuroradiol., January–February 1993, vol. 14(1), pp. 155–162.

Principles of Neurology, 5th ed.: R.D. Adams and M. Victor, eds.; McGraw-Hill, 1993, pp. 835–836.

Rehabilitation of Patients with Hallervorden-Spatz Syndrome: M.O. Seibel, et al.; Arch. Phys. Med. Rehabil., March 1993, vol. 74(3), pp. 328–329.

Cecil Textbook of Medicine, 19th ed.: J.B. Wyngaarden, et al., eds.; W.B. Saunders Company, 1992, p. 2132.

Mendelian Inheritance in Man, 10th ed.: V.A. McKusick; The Johns Hopkins University Press, 1992, p. 1430.

Nelson Textbook of Pediatrics, 14th ed.: R.E. Behrman, ed.-in-chief; W.B. Saunders Company, 1992, p. 1514.

Hallervorden-Spatz Syndrome and Brain Iron Metabolism: K.F. Swaiman; Arch. Neurol., December 1991, vol. 48(12), pp. 1285–1293.

Harrison's Principles of Internal Medicine, 12th ed.: J.D. Wilson, et al., eds.; McGraw-Hill, 1991, p. 2064

Adult Onset Hallervorden-Spatz Syndrome or Seitelberger's Disease with Late Onset: Variants of the Same Entity? A Clinico-Pathological Study: S. Gaytan-Garcia, et al.; Clin. Neuropathol., May–June 1990, vol. 9(3), pp. 136–142.

Birth Defects Encyclopedia: M.L. Buyse, ed.-in-chief; Blackwell Scientific Publications, 1990, pp. 829–830.

Dictionary of Medical Syndromes, 3rd ed.: S.I. Magalini, et al., eds.; J.B. Lippincott Company, 1990, pp. 383–384.

# HOLOPROSENCEPHALY

**Description** Holoprosencephaly refers to deficiency or failure of cleavage in the fetal prosencephalon, resulting in varying degrees of defects in midline facial development and failure to form 2 symmetric cerebral hemispheres.

**Synonyms**

Arhinencephaly

Lobar Holoprosencephaly

**Signs and Symptoms** The malformation sequence can be mild or severe. Mildly affected children may have hypotelorism, missing incisors, cleft lip and/or cleft palate, delayed development, spastic quadriplegia, seizures, and microcephaly. Mental retardation may also be present. These children may live for months or years.

Many severely affected infants are stillborn or die within a few days. Rarely, severely affected infants are born with cyclopia and cebocephaly.

Other body systems may be affected. The pituitary gland may be absent, and hypoglycemia may occur. Apnea and seizure disorders may be present. Males may have micropenis.

**Etiology** Holoprosencephaly can be inherited, but there is disagreement as to whether transmission is through autosomal dominant or recessive genes. Several reported cases have involved parental consanguinity. In most instances the defect occurs alone (but see Related Disorders, below). A higher incidence of holoprosencephaly has been reported in children of diabetic mothers. Fetal cytomegalovirus (**CMV**) infection has also been associated.

**Epidemiology** Holoprosencephaly is a very rare disorder affecting males and females in equal numbers prenatally. The incidence of holoprosencephalic children with normal chromosomes has been estimated at between 1:16,000 and 1:53,394 live births.

**Related Disorders** See *Trisomy 13 Syndrome; Chromosome 13q- Syndrome; Chromosome 18p- Syndrome; Meckel Syndrome.*

**Treatment—Standard** Ultrasound will detect holoprosencephaly, and a CT scan may determine its severity. Prenatal chromosomal examination of subsequent pregnancies may be indicated.

The child's treatment will involve pediatricians, dentists, special education teachers, surgeons, speech pathologists, psychologists, and others. Plastic reconstructive surgery of the face will be considered in some cases.

Genetic counseling may be beneficial. Family members of affected children should be examined for mild signs, such as hypotelorism or a single incisor instead of 2. Other treatment is symptomatic and supportive.

**Treatment—Investigational** Please contact the agencies listed under Resources, below, for the most current information. Addresses and telephone numbers of these agencies, as well as of individual experts and research centers, may be found in the Master Resources List.

**Resources**

**For more information on holoprosencephaly:** National Organization for Rare Disorders (NORD); NIH/National Institute of Child Health and Human Development; Fighters for Encephaly Defects Support Group; Society for the Rehabilitation of the Facially Disfigured; The Arc (a national organization on mental retardation).

**For genetic information and genetic counseling referrals:** March of Dimes Birth Defects Foundation; Alliance of Genetic Support Groups.

### References

Sonography of Facial Features of Alobar and Semilobar Holoprosencephaly: J.P. McGahan, et al.; AJR Am. J. Roentgenol., January 1990, vol. 154(1), pp. 143–148.

Holoprosencephaly: A Developmental Field Defect: V.P. Johnson; Am. J. Genet., October 1989, vol. 34(2), pp. 258–264.

Smith's Recognizable Patterns of Human Malformation, 4th ed.: K.L. Jones; W.B. Saunders Company, 1988, pp. 546–547.

# HORNER SYNDROME

**Description** The syndrome is characterized by unilateral pupillary constriction, upper eyelid ptosis, and facial anhidrosis related to ipsilateral lesions or damage to the cervical sympathetic chain.

**Synonyms**

      Bernard-Horner Syndrome

      Oculosympathetic Palsy

**Signs and Symptoms** Features include not only miosis, ptosis, and anhidrosis but also enophthalmos, swelling of the lower eyelid, and heterochromia. An increase in vibration occurs when the eye is adjusting to different distances. Cocaine eye drops will dilate the normal pupil more than the affected pupil, thus establishing the diagnosis.

**Etiology** Horner syndrome is caused by a partial interruption of the sympathetic chain due to a lesion or injury. The lesion may be present at birth, inherited as an autosomal dominant trait; may be acquired during infancy; may develop sporadically; or may be caused by trauma.

**Epidemiology** The syndrome affects males and females in equal numbers, and can occur at any age.

**Related Disorders** See *Adie Syndrome.*

**Wallenberg syndrome** is a rare disorder caused by arterial occlusion. Its characteristics include dysarthria, dysphagia, vertigo, nystagmus, ataxia, ipsilateral signs of Horner syndrome, and contralateral loss of thermal and pain senses.

**Treatment—Standard** Treatment depends on the location and cause of the lesion or tumor. In some cases surgical removal of a tumor is appropriate. Malignant tumors may be treated with radiation and chemotherapy.

Genetic counseling is advised for patients with the genetic form of this disorder. Other treatment is symptomatic and supportive.

**Treatment—Investigational** Please contact the agencies listed under Resources, below, for the most current information. Addresses and telephone numbers of these agencies, as well as of individual experts and research centers, may be found in the Master Resources List.

**Resources**

**For more information on Horner syndrome:** National Organization for Rare Disorders (NORD); NIH/National Eye Institute.

**For genetic information and genetic counseling referrals:** March of Dimes Birth Defects Foundation; Alliance of Genetic Support Groups.

**References**

Clinical Ophthalmology, 2nd ed.: J.J. Kanski, ed.; Butterworth-Heinemann, 1990, pp. 474–475.

Principles of Neurology, 4th ed.: R.D. Adams and M. Victor, eds.; McGraw-Hill, 1989, pp. 20–21, 435–436.

Cecil Textbook of Medicine, 18th ed.: J.B. Wyngaarden and L.H. Smith, Jr., eds.: W.B. Saunders Company, 1988, pp. 2113–2114.

Mendelian Inheritance in Man, 8th ed.: V.A. McKusick; The Johns Hopkins University Press, 1986, p. 472.

# HUNTINGTON DISEASE

**Description** Huntington disease (Huntington chorea) is an inherited, progressively degenerative neurologic condition that produces chorea and dementia.

**Synonyms**

      Chronic Progressive Chorea

      Degenerative Chorea

      Hereditary Chorea

      Hereditary Chronic Progressive Chorea

      Huntington Chorea

      Woody Guthrie's Disease

**Signs and Symptoms** Huntington disease runs a 10- to 25-year progressive course. Initial characteristics include mild choreiform movements and personality changes. In time, speech and memory become impaired, and the choreiform movements become severe. With further progression the chorea may subside and akinesia develop, and dementia gradually ensues. Patients with advanced disease are at high risk of pneumonia, the result of being bedridden and emaciated. Death occurs, on the average, about 14 years after onset.

Magnetic resonance imaging and computerized tomography, electroencephalography, neuropsychologic testing, and recently a DNA marker test can be utilized in making the diagnosis.

**Etiology** The mode of inheritance is autosomal dominant. The defective gene responsible for Huntington disease has been located on the short arm of chromosome 4 (4p16.3). There are some indications that the gene produces varying amounts of trinucleotide repeats, which may be the reason for symptom severity as well as age of onset.

**Epidemiology** Huntington disease affects approximately 1:10,000 persons in the United States, with another 150,000 at risk. The disease occurs in both sexes equally, and is most common in whites. Symptoms usually appear between 30 and 50 years of age, although onset may be as late as the 7th or 8th decade. A rarer childhood form of the disease, accounting for 10 percent of cases, can occur in children as young as age 2 years.

Related Disorders See *Hallervorden-Spatz Disease; Olivopontocerebellar Atrophy; Sydenham Chorea; Tourette Syndrome; Wilson Disease.*

**Treatment—Standard** Therapy is symptomatic and supportive. Phenothiazine and other neuroleptics are only marginally effective.

**Treatment—Investigational** Paul F. Consroe, Ph.D., has been awarded a grant from the Office of Orphan Products Development, Food and Drug Administration, for studies involving clinical trials of the orphan drug cannabidiol in the treatment of Huntington disease

Another experimental drug, MK-801, is being tested to determine whether it can block the effects of quinolinic acid, thought to damage brain neurons in persons with Huntington disease. The drug idebenone (AVAN) is being used in Japan to treat patients with cognitive problems resulting from strokes, but it also appears to prevent brain cell degeneration. It is being tested in the United States on a small number of persons with Huntington disease.

Please also contact the agencies listed under Resources, below, for the most current information. Addresses and telephone numbers of these agencies, as well as of individual experts and research centers, may be found in the Master Resources List.

**Resources**

**For more information on Huntington disease:** National Organization for Rare Disorders (NORD); Huntington Disease Society of America; NIH/National Institute of Neurological Disorders and Stroke; Hereditary Disease Foundation; Huntington Society of Canada.

**For genetic information and genetic counseling referrals:** March of Dimes Birth Defects Foundation; Alliance of Genetic Support Groups.

**References**
Cecil Textbook of Medicine, 19th ed.: J.B. Wyngaarden, et al., eds.; W.B. Saunders Company, 1992, pp. 2135–2136.
Mendelian Inheritance in Man, 10th ed.: V.A. McKusick; The Johns Hopkins University Press, 1992, pp. 550–555.
Birth Defects Encyclopedia: M.L. Buyse, ed.-in-chief; Blackwell Scientific Publications, 1990, pp. 882–883.
Proposed Genetic Basis of Huntington Disease: C.D. Laird; Trends Genet., August 1990, vol. 6(8), pp. 242–247.

# HYDRANENCEPHALY

**Description** In hydranencephaly, portions of the cerebral hemispheres may be missing, replaced by fluid within the cranium. The disorder is a very rare form of porencephaly (see Related Disorders, below).

**Synonyms**
  Hydroanencephaly

**Signs and Symptoms** At birth, irritability and spasticity of the arms and legs are common. A neurologic examination may be inconclusive. Other symptoms may include inadequate body temperature regulation, visual impairment, mental retardation, seizures, myoclonus, and respiratory failure. There is usually nothing specific about the neurologic findings.

**Etiology** Genetic inheritance is suspected, although the mode of transmission remains unknown. Prenatal blockage of the carotid artery where it enters the cranium has been postulated as etiologic; however, the reason for the blockage is not known.

**Epidemiology** Hydranencephaly is present at birth. Males and females are affected in equal numbers.

**Related Disorders** See *Hydrocephalus.*

**Porencephaly** is a central nervous system disorder in which cysts develop in cortical brain tissue. Accumulated fluid can be drained by means of a surgical shunt. Some patients may be only mildly affected neurologically and have normal intelligence; for others, the disablement may be severe.

**Treatment—Standard** Treatment is symptomatic and supportive. Increased intracranial pressure often is relieved with a shunt, which must be monitored carefully for potential infection and blockage.

**Treatment—Investigational** Please contact the agencies listed under Resources, below, for the most current information. Addresses and telephone numbers of these agencies, as well as of individual experts and research centers, may be found in the Master Resources List.

**Resources**

**For more information on hydranencephaly:** National Organization for Rare Disorders (NORD); NIH/National Institute of Neurological Disorders and Stroke; The Arc (a national organization on mental retardation); Children's Brain Diseases Foundation for Research.

**For information on shunts:** American Brain Tumor Association.

**For genetic information and genetic counseling referrals:** March of Dimes Birth Defects Foundation; Alliance of Genetic Support Groups.

**References**

Ultrasonographic Prenatal Diagnosis of Hydranencephaly: A Case Report: H.A. Hadi, et al.; J. Reprod. Med., April 1986, vol. 31(4).

Hydranencephaly: Prenatal and Neonatal Ultrasonographic Appearance: D.J. Coady, et al.; Am. J. Perinatol., July 1985, vol. 2(3), pp. 228–230.

# HYDROCEPHALUS

**Description** Hydrocephalus is a condition in which cerebral ventricles dilate because of inhibition of normal flow of cerebrospinal fluid **(CSF).** The CSF accumulates in the skull and puts pressure on the brain tissue. An enlarged head in infants and increased CSF pressure are frequent findings but are not necessary for the diagnosis. The following forms are recognized: communicating hydrocephalus, noncommunicating or obstructive hydrocephalus, internal hydrocephalus, normal-pressure hydrocephalus, and benign hydrocephalus.

**Synonyms**

Hydrocephaly

**Signs and Symptoms** Characteristic features of hydrocephalus in children include cephalomegaly; a thin, transparent scalp; a bulging forehead with prominent fontanelles; and a downward gaze. Other clinical findings include convulsions, abnormal reflexes, a slowed heartbeat and respiratory rate, headache, vomiting, irritability, weakness, and problems with vision. Blindness and continuing mental deterioration from brain atrophy can result if treatment is not instituted.

In adolescent- or adult-onset hydrocephalus, the physiognomic abnormalities are less evident than in children with congenital or early-onset hydrocephalus. Many of the other mental and physiologic manifestations are the same, with the added loss of previously acquired motor coordination. Acquired hydrocephalus in children and adolescents is often associated with symptoms of hypopituitarism, such as delayed growth and obesity, and generalized weakness.

Hydrocephalus is subdivided according to the ventricular defect and the CSF pressure, high or normal. In **communicating hydrocephalus** there is no obstruction in the ventricular system; the CSF flows readily into the subarachnoid space but is insufficiently absorbed, or perhaps produced in too great a quantity to be absorbed. In **noncommunicating (obstructing) hydrocephalus,** a ventricular block to CSF flow causes dilation of the pathways upstream of the block, leading to increased CSF pressure in the skull. **Normal-pressure hydrocephalus,** which affects middle-aged and older persons, is characterized by dilated ventricles but normal lumbar CSF pressure. The hydrocephalus may be detected by pneumoencephalography. Other symptoms of normal-pressure hydrocephalus include dementia, ataxia, and urinary incontinence.

**Etiology** Hydrocephalus can be caused by a birth defect, hemorrhage, viral infection, or meningitis. A genetic predisposition has been proposed, with transmission through autosomal recessive or X-linked genes.

**Epidemiology** Most cases of hydrocephalus are diagnosed in the first 2 years of life, but onset may occur at any age, depending on the etiology. The disorder seems to affect males and females equally, except those inherited as X-linked genetic traits.

**Related Disorders** Among the disorders that can occur in conjunction with hydrocephalus are ***Arnold-Chiari Syndrome; Cardio-Facio-Cutaneous Syndrome;*** epilepsy; meningitis; ***Spina Bifida;*** and ***Walker-Warburg Syndrome.***

**Treatment—Standard** Standard treatment entails placement of a ventriculoperitoneal shunt to drain the excess CSF. Periodic lengthening of the shunt is necessary to accommodate growth in children. A clogged or nonfunctioning shunt may have to be replaced.

**Treatment—Investigational** Please contact the agencies listed under Resources, below, for the most current information. Addresses and telephone numbers of these agencies, as well as of individual experts and research centers, may be found in the Master Resources List.

**Resources**

**For more information on hydrocephalus:** National Organization for Rare Disorders (NORD); Hydrocephalus Parent Support Group; National Hydrocephalus Foundation; Hydrocephalus Association; NIH/National Institute of Neurological Disorders and Stroke; The Arc (a national organization on mental retardation).

**For genetic information and genetic counseling referrals:** March of Dimes Birth Defects Foundation; Alliance of Genetic Support Groups.

**References**

Cecil Textbook of Medicine, 19th ed.: J.B. Wyngaarden, et al., eds.; W.B. Saunders Company, 1992, pp. 2223–2224.
Hydrocephalus in Infancy and Childhood: H.E. James; Am. Fam. Physician, February 1992, vol. 45(2), pp. 733–742.
Mendelian Inheritance in Man, 9th ed.: V.A. McKusick; The Johns Hopkins University Press, 1990, pp. 1248–1250, 1635–1636.
Internal Medicine, 2nd ed.: J.H. Stein, ed.-in-chief; Little, Brown and Company, 1987, p. 2213.

# HYPEROSTOSIS FRONTALIS INTERNA

**Description** Hyperostosis frontalis interna is characterized by excessive growth or thickening of the frontal bone of the skull. The disorder has been found in association with a variety of conditions.

**Synonyms**

Endostosis Crani
Hyperostosis Calvariae Interna
Morgagni-Stewart-Morel Syndrome

**Signs and Symptoms** The excessive growth or thickening of the frontal bone can only be seen on x-ray, and it is suspected that the condition may often go undetected. Many affected persons have no apparent symptoms.

Conditions that may be associated include female virilization, hypertrichosis, other gonadal disturbances, epilepsy, diabetes insipidus, decreased vision, and headaches. Increased serum alkaline phosphatase and elevated serum calcium may be present.

**Etiology** Hyperostosis frontalis interna has been found in multiple generations, suggesting dominant inheritance. It is not known if the disorder is autosomal dominant or X-linked. There are no known cases of male-to-male transmission.

**Epidemiology** Females are affected 9 times more often than males. The disorder usually affects middle-aged or elderly persons, but has been found in adolescents.

It has been suggested that this condition may be a common abnormality found in as many as 12 percent of the female population.

**Related Disorders** See *Acromegaly; Crouzon Disease; Diabetes Insipidus; Myotonic Dystrophy; Paget Disease of Bone.*

In **leontiasis ossea (Virchow disease)** there is an overgrowth of the bones of the face and sometimes of the cranium, resulting in a general enlargement and distortion of all the features.

**Treatment—Standard** There is no present therapy for thickening of the frontal bone. Associated conditions can be treated with standard medications. Genetic counseling may be beneficial for patients and their families. Other treatment is symptomatic and supportive.

**Treatment—Investigational** Please contact the agencies listed under Resources, below, for the most current information. Addresses and telephone numbers of these agencies, as well as of individual experts and research centers, may be found in the Master Resources List.

**Resources**

**For more information on hyperostosis frontalis interna:** National Organization for Rare Disorders (NORD); National Craniofacial Foundation; National Association for the Craniofacially Handicapped; NIH/National Arthritis and Musculoskeletal and Skin Diseases Information Clearinghouse.

**For genetic information and genetic counseling referrals:** March of Dimes Birth Defects Foundation; Alliance of Genetic Support Groups.

**References**

Birth Defects Encyclopedia: M.L. Buyse, M.D., ed.-in-chief; Blackwell Scientific Publications, 1990, pp. 909–910.
Mendelian Inheritance in Man, 9th ed.: V.A. McKusick; The Johns Hopkins University Press, 1990, p. 493.

# ISAACS SYNDROME

**Description** Isaacs syndrome is a peripheral motor neuron disorder that occurs in 3 forms: **generalized-sporadic, generalized-familial,** or **focal**. Muscular stiffness and cramping are present, especially in the limbs.
**Synonyms**
      Continuous Muscle Fiber Activity Syndrome
      Neuromyotonia
      Quantal Squander
**Signs and Symptoms** Myokymia may be present. The involuntary continuous muscle fiber activity results in stiffness and delayed relaxation in affected muscles. When the disorder is focal, muscle relaxation following voluntary movement is delayed; e.g., the patient may be unable to open his or her fist or eyes immediately after closing them tightly for a few seconds. Symptoms can occur whether the patient is awake or asleep. Walking may be difficult. Diagnosis is by electromyography (**EMG**).
**Etiology** The 3 forms of Isaacs syndrome reflect the causes of the abnormal peripheral nerve impulses:
    **Generalized-sporadic:** usually the result of intrathoracic malignancy.
    **Generalized-familial:** inherited as an autosomal dominant trait. Peripheral neuropathy may be linked to this form.
    **Focal:** the result of lesions, often of unknown etiology, on the peripheral nerves.
**Epidemiology** Males and females of all ages are affected in equal numbers.
**Related Disorders** See *Hallervorden-Spatz Disease; Paraplegia, Hereditary Spastic; Stiff Man Syndrome.*
**Treatment—Standard** Anticonvulsant drugs may stop the abnormal impulses and prevent symptom recurrence. Phenytoin especially is helpful with myokymia.
    Genetic counseling may be beneficial in inherited forms of the syndrome. Other treatment is symptomatic and supportive.
**Treatment—Investigational** Oxygen inhalation may help muscle relaxation and hand spasms but does not relieve myokymia.
    Surgery entailing motor nerve block and/or block of the afferent sensitive fibers may help some patients when drug therapies are ineffective.
    Please contact the agencies listed under Resources, below, for the most current information. Addresses and telephone numbers of these agencies, as well as of individual experts and research centers, may be found in the Master Resources List.
**Resources**
    **For more information on Isaacs syndrome:** National Organization for Rare Disorders (NORD); NIH/National Arthritis and Musculoskeletal and Skin Diseases Information Clearinghouse.
    **For genetic information and genetic counseling referrals:** March of Dimes Birth Defects Foundation; Alliance of Genetic Support Groups.
**References**
    Hypoxia-Sensitive Hyperexcitability of the Intramuscular Nerve Axons in Isaacs' Syndrome: K. Oda, et al.; Ann. Neurol., February 1989, vol. 25(2), pp. 140–145.
    Cecil Textbook of Medicine, 18th ed.: J.B. Wyngaarden and L.H. Smith, Jr., eds.; W.B. Saunders Company, 1988, p. 2284.
    Isaacs' Syndrome: T.J. Brown; Arch. Phys. Med. Rehabil., January 1984, vol. 65(1), pp. 27–29.
    Isaacs' Syndrome with Muscle Hypertrophy Reversed by Phenytoin Therapy: J. Zisfein, et al.; Arch. Neurol., April 1983, vol. 40(4), pp. 241–242.

# JOSEPH DISEASE

**Description** Joseph disease is a central nervous system disorder producing a cerebellar deficit and peripheral sensory loss. There are 3 forms: types I, II, III.
**Synonyms**
      Stiatonigral Degeneration
**Signs and Symptoms Type I** Joseph disease is identified by a lurching, unsteady gait that may be accompanied by dysarthria, muscle rigidity, dystonia, athetosis, and irregular eye movements. Mental alertness and intellect usually remain unaffected.
    **Type II** symptoms are similar to those of type I but progress less rapidly. The distinctive characteristic of type II is increased cerebellar dysfunction marked by difficulty in walking and in coordinating movement of the extremities, and by spasticity.

**Type III (Machado disease)** typically presents with ataxia and is distinguished from the other 2 forms by a loss of muscle mass that is due to motor polyneuropathy. Impaired sensation, diminished ability to move the extremities, and diabetes are common.

**Etiology** Joseph disease is inherited as an autosomal dominant trait. The responsible gene has been mapped to chromosome 14q (14q24.3–q31).

**Epidemiology** Individuals of Portuguese ancestry (specifically, the Azores) are most susceptible to Joseph disease. Onset of type I usually occurs around age 20; type II typically begins about age 30; and type III usually is not evident until after age 40.

**Related Disorders** See *Ataxia, Friedreich; Ataxia, Marie; Hallervorden-Spatz Disease; Olivopontocerebellar Atrophy; Parenchymatous Cortical Degeneration of the Cerebellum; Progressive Supranuclear Palsy.*

**Treatment—Standard** Treatment is symptomatic and supportive. Pharmacotherapy with L-dopa and baclofen may help relieve muscle rigidity and spasticity. Genetic testing is recommended for families in which at least one member has been diagnosed with the disease.

**Treatment—Investigational** Please contact the agencies listed under Resources, below, for the most current information. Addresses and telephone numbers of these agencies, as well as of individual experts and research centers, may be found in the Master Resources List.

**Resources**

   **For more information on Joseph disease:** National Organization for Rare Disorders (NORD); International Joseph Diseases Foundation; NIH/National Institute of Neurological Disorders and Stroke; Roger N. Rosenberg, M.D., University of Texas Southwestern Medical School.

   **For genetic information and genetic counseling referrals:** March of Dimes Birth Defects Foundation; Alliance of Genetic Support Groups.

**References**

Machado-Joseph Disease: An Autosomal Dominant Motor System Degeneration: R.N. Rosenberg; Mov. Disord., 1992, vol. 7(3), pp. 193–203.

Machado-Joseph Disease in New England: Clinical Description and Distinction from the Olivopontocerebellar Atrophies: L. Sudarsky, et al.; Mov. Disord., 1992, vol. 7(3), pp. 204–208.

The Machado-Joseph Disease Locus Is Different from the Spinocerebellar Ataxia Locus (SCA1): W.J. Carson, et al.; Genomics, July 1992, vol. 13(3), pp. 852–855.

Mendelian Inheritance in Man, 10th ed.: V.A. McKusick; The Johns Hopkins University Press, 1992, p. 136.

Birth Defects Encyclopedia: M.L. Buyse, ed.-in-chief; Blackwell Scientific Publications, 1990, pp. 1093–1094.

Dictionary of Medical Syndromes, 3rd ed.: S.I. Magalini, et al., eds.; J.B. Lippincott Company, 1990, p. 80.

Waiting for the Family Legacy: The Experience of Being at Risk for Machado-Joseph Disease: M.I. Boutte; Soc. Sci. Med., 1990, vol. 30(8), pp. 839–847.

Principles of Neurology, 4th ed.: R.D. Adams and M. Victor, eds.; McGraw-Hill, 1989, pp. 951–952.

# JOUBERT SYNDROME

**Description** Joubert syndrome is a rare neurologic disorder involving malformation of the area of the brain that controls balance and coordination. Psychomotor retardation, abnormal eye movements, and respiratory irregularities are characteristic.

**Synonyms**

   Cerebellar Hypoplasia
   Cerebellar Vermis Aplasia
   Cerebellarparenchymal Disorder IV
   Familial Cerebellar Vermis Agenesis
   Vermis Cerebellar Agenesis

**Signs and Symptoms** Sleep apnea and periods of deep, abnormal breathing are common in infants and may be triggered by emotional stimulation, e.g., crying. Unusually deep inhalations occasionally may occur. These respiratory irregularities usually decrease with age.

   Abnormal eye movements such as irregular jerking and eye rolling or crossing may be present. Ataxia, dysmetria, hypermetria, and tremors also may be observed. Weakness of the skeletal muscles may be accompanied by clumsy or rapid alternating movements. Mental retardation also may occur.

   CT scans can be diagnostically helpful.

**Etiology** The cause is not known; the disorder may be inherited as an autosomal recessive trait.

**Epidemiology** Onset is usually in infancy. The syndrome is extremely rare; it is estimated that only 10 cases occur each year in the United States. Both males and females can be affected, and the disorder can occur more than once in the same family.

**Related Disorders** See *Dandy-Walker Syndrome; Leber Congenital Amaurosis.*

**Treatment—Standard** Treatment is symptomatic and supportive. Genetic counseling, special education services, and physical therapy may benefit patients and their families.

**Treatment—Investigational** Please contact the agencies listed under Resources, below, for the most current information. Addresses and telephone numbers of these agencies, as well as of individual experts and research centers, may be found in the Master Resources List.

**Resources**

For more information on Joubert syndrome: National Organization for Rare Disorders (NORD); Joubert Syndrome Parents-in-Touch Network; The Arc (a national organization on mental retardation); NIH/National Institute of Neurological Disorders and Stroke; Children's Brain Diseases Foundation for Research; David B. Flannery, M.D., Medical College of Georgia.

For genetic information and genetic counseling referrals: March of Dimes Birth Defects Foundation; Alliance of Genetic Support Groups.

**References**

Mendelian Inheritance in Man, 10th ed.: V.A. McKusick; The Johns Hopkins University Press, 1992, p. 1487.

Dysmorphic Features of Joubert Syndrome: L.A. Squires, et al.; Dysmorphol. Clin. Genet., May 1991, pp. 77–79.

Birth Defects Encyclopedia: M.L. Buyse, ed.-in-chief; Blackwell Scientific Publications, 1990, pp. 995–996.

Joubert's Syndrome Associated with Congenital Fibrosis and Histidinemia: R.E. Appleton, et al.; Arch. Neurol., May 1989, vol. 46(5), pp. 579–582.

# JUMPING FRENCHMEN OF MAINE

**Description** *Jumping Frenchmen* is an appellation for an unusually extreme startle reaction that occurs in selected populations. The symptoms are elicited by sudden, unexpected noise or movement but greatly exceed, in range and severity, the normal startle reaction.

**Synonyms**

Jumping Frenchmen

Latah (observed in Malaysia)

Myriachit (observed in Siberia)

**Signs and Symptoms** The symptoms of jumping Frenchmen of Maine usually become apparent in adolescence and tend to remit with age. The extreme startle reaction response includes jumping, raising the arms, hitting, yelling, echolalia, obeying sudden orders, and echopraxia. The reaction may include violence, and the intensity of the response increases with fatigue and stress. An unexpected event is necessary to elicit the reaction, and affected individuals may become the subjects of practical jokes designed to provoke the reaction.

**Etiology** The cause is unknown.

**Epidemiology** The disorder was originally described in French Canadian lumberjacks in the Moosehead Lake region of Maine in the late 19th and early 20th centuries. Similar behaviors have been observed in specific populations in Southeast Asia, Siberia, India, Somalia, and Yemen. Males appear to be affected more often than females.

**Related Disorders** Several syndromes or reactive behaviors have features in common with jumping Frenchmen of Maine but are unrelated to it. See *Tourette Syndrome,* which is similarly characterized by echolalia or echopraxia. **Hyperexplexia,** thought to be a hereditary disorder, lacks the echolalia, echopraxia, and the forced obedience response characteristic of jumping Frenchmen of Maine. The brief, predominantly unilateral muscle contractions of **startle epilepsy** are not as complex and directed as the startle reaction in jumping Frenchmen of Maine, and affected subjects have other seizure manifestations. Individuals with **Kok disease,** a rare hereditary neurologic disorder, have an excessive startle reaction to sudden, unexpected noise, movement, or touch, but also exhibit specific seizure activity.

**Treatment—Standard** Anticipation of a sudden noise or movement can help the patient avoid the startle response. As the response appears to be reinforced by repetition, elimination of teasing or provocative behavior from others will also help to end episodes.

**Treatment—Investigational** Please contact the agencies listed under Resources, below, for the most current information. Addresses and telephone numbers of these agencies, as well as of individual experts and research centers, may be found in the Master Resources List.

**Resources**

For more information on jumping Frenchmen of Maine: National Organization for Rare Disorders (NORD); NIH/National Institute of Neurological Disorders and Stroke.

**References**

Jumping Frenchmen of Maine: M. Sainte-Hilaire, et al.; Neurology, September 1986, vol. 36(9), pp. 1269–1271.

# KENNEDY DISEASE

**Description** Kennedy disease is an inherited progressive disorder of the muscles.
**Synonyms**
>Bulbospinal Muscular Atrophy, X-Linked
>Calves, Hypertrophy of Spinal Muscular Atrophy
>Kennedy-Type Spinal and Bulbar Muscular Atrophy
>Kennedy-Stefanis Disease
>Spinal and Bulbar Muscular Atrophy
>Spinal Muscular Atrophy, Benign with Hyperatrophy of Calves
>Spinal Muscular Atrophy–Hypertrophy of the Calves
>X-Linked Adult-Onset Spinobulbar Muscular Atrophy
>X-Linked Adult Spinal Muscular Atrophy

**Signs and Symptoms** Onset is between the ages of 15 and 59 and may occur unilaterally. Fasciculations are usually the first symptom. Twitching of the muscles of the face, trunk, arms, and legs slowly progresses to muscle weakness and atrophy. The lips, tongue, mouth, chin, throat, and vocal chords may be affected. Dysphagia and hypertrophy of the calves may occur.

Gynecomastia occurs in most patients. Sexual function is normal until onset, when impotence and infertility may appear. Primary testicular failure with oligospermia and diabetes mellitus can also be present

**Etiology** Kennedy disease is inherited as an X-linked genetic trait and has been mapped to Xq13–q22. Some studies suggest that the defective gene may produce trinucleotide repeats, which determine severity of symptoms and age of onset.

**Epidemiology** Kennedy disease is a rare disorder that affects males only, at a ratio of approximately 1:50,000.

**Related Disorders** See *Adrenoleukodystrophy; Amyotrophic Lateral Sclerosis; Kugelberg-Welander Syndrome.*

**Treatment—Standard** Treatment of Kennedy disease is symptomatic and supportive. Physical therapy may be prescribed.

Genetic counseling may be of benefit for patients and their families.

**Treatment—Investigational** Please contact the agencies listed under Resources, below, for the most current information. Addresses and telephone numbers of these agencies, as well as of individual experts and research centers, may be found in the Master Resources List.

**Resources**
**For more information on Kennedy disease:** National Organization for Rare Disorders (NORD); Families of Spinal Muscular Atrophy; National Ataxia Foundation; NIH/National Institute of Neurological Disorders and Stroke.

**For genetic information and genetic counseling referrals:** March of Dimes Birth Defects Foundation; Alliance of Genetic Support Groups.

**References**
Birth Defects Encyclopedia: M.L. Buyse, ed.-in-chief; Blackwell Scientific Publications, 1990, p. 1177.
Mendelian Inheritance in Man, 9th ed.: V.A. McKusick; The Johns Hopkins University Press, 1990, pp. 1719–1720.
X-Linked Bulbo-Spinal Neuronopathy: A Family Study of Three Patients: J. Wilde, et al.; J. Neurol. Neurosurg. Psychiatry, March 1987, vol. 50(3), pp. 279–284.

# KERNICTERUS

**Description** Kernicterus is a condition in infants characterized by high levels of bilirubin in the blood. The bilirubin accumulates in the brain stem and basal ganglia. The condition is most prevalent in premature or very sick neonates. It is associated with severe neural symptoms in the form of mental retardation and neuromuscular disorders.

**Synonyms**
>Bilirubin Encephalopathy
>Nuclear Jaundice
>Posticteric Encephalopathy

**Signs and Symptoms** Early general symptoms of kernicterus in full-term infants include lethargy, poor feeding, and vomiting; neuromuscular symptoms reflecting degenerative changes include opisthotonos, upward deviation of the eyes, convulsions, and rigidity. Children who survive the initial period may develop the complete neurologic syndrome, with bilateral choreoathetosis, sensorineural hearing loss, extrapyramidal signs, seizures, and loss of upward gaze. In mild cases the dysfunction may be limited to perceptual-motor handicaps and learning disorders.

**Etiology** Historically, kernicterus was a common sequela of severe hemolytic jaundice of the newborn. Today kernicterus commonly results from severe erythroblastosis fetalis, a hemolytic anemia of newborn infants that is caused by transplacental transmission of maternally formed antibody, evoked by maternal-fetal blood group incompatibility. With the availability of specific treatments for jaundice, kernicterus now develops only in premature or very low birth weight infants with hyperbilirubinemia. Factors predisposing to the development of kernicterus include hypoxemia, acidosis, infections, hypoalbuminemia, and hypothermia.

**Epidemiology** Newborn infants of either sex may be affected.

**Related Disorders** Hepatic diseases and hemolytic anemias are among the disorders producing jaundice.

**Treatment—Standard** Various measures can be implemented to avoid or treat kernicterus in neonates. Early frequent feedings increase the frequency of stools, mobilizing the bowel and reducing the levels of bilirubin in the liver and intestines. Infants with high bilirubin levels may be given exchange blood transfusions through a catheter placed in the umbilical vein. Phototherapy is widely used to treat hyperbilirubinemia in infants, although the long-term effects on mental development are unknown.

**Treatment—Investigational** The orphan drug Zixoryn (flumecinol) has been used in the investigational treatment of hyperbilirubinemia in newborns unresponsive to phototherapy.

Please contact the agencies listed under Resources, below, for the most current information. Addresses and telephone numbers of these agencies, as well as of individual experts and research centers, may be found in the Master Resources List.

**Resources**

For more information on kernicterus: National Organization for Rare Disorders (NORD); American Liver Foundation; United Liver Association; Children's Liver Foundation; NIH/National Institute of Child Health and Human Development.

For genetic information and genetic counseling referrals: March of Dimes Birth Defects Foundation; Alliance of Genetic Support Groups.

**References**

Cecil Textbook of Medicine, 18th ed.: J.B. Wyngaarden and L.H. Smith, Jr., eds.; W.B. Saunders Company, 1988, pp. 812, 1076.
Nelson Textbook of Pediatrics, 13th ed.: R.E. Behrman and V.C. Vaughan, III, eds.; W.B. Saunders Company, 1987, pp. 407–409.

# KLÜVER-BUCY SYNDROME

**Description** Damage to the temporal lobes results in the varied characteristics of the syndrome.

**Synonyms**
Bilateral Temporal Lobe Disorder

**Signs and Symptoms** Memory loss, aphasia, dementia, seizures, indiscriminate sexual behavior, an excessive tendency to put all sorts of objects in the mouth, and an almost uncontrollable appetite for food are features of this disorder. Emotional response to stimuli is usually lacking but an easy distractibility by external stimuli (particularly visual) is usually present.

**Etiology** Damage to the temporal lobes may be the result of trauma to the brain itself, the result of degenerative brain disease, or the result of some forms of herpes simplex encephalitis.

**Epidemiology** Males and females are affected equally.

**Related Disorders** See *Alzheimer Disease; Korsakoff Syndrome; Pick Disease.*

**Treatment—Standard** Treatment is symptomatic and supportive.

**Treatment—Investigational** Please contact the agencies listed under Resources, below, for the most current information. Addresses and telephone numbers of these agencies, as well as of individual experts and research centers, may be found in the Master Resources List.

**Resources**

For more information on Klüver-Bucy syndrome: National Organization for Rare Disorders (NORD); NIH/National Institute of Neurological Disorders and Stroke; Alzheimer's Disease and Related Disorders Association.

**References**

Cecil Textbook of Medicine, 19th ed.: J.B. Wyngaarden, et al., eds.; W.B. Saunders Company, 1992, pp. 2080–2087.
Klüver-Bucy Syndrome: A Case Report.: N.A. Fragassi, et al.; Acta Neurol., April 1990, vol. 12(2), pp. 138–142.
Principles of Neurology, 4th ed.; R.D. Adams and M. Victor, eds.; McGraw-Hill, 1989, pp. 360–363, 451–452.
Klüver-Bucy Syndrome with Severe Amnesia Secondary to Herpes Encephalitis: P. Conlon, et al.; Can. J. Psychiatry, November 1988, vol. 33(8), pp. 754–756.

# KORSAKOFF SYNDROME

**Description** Korsakoff syndrome is characterized principally by greatly impaired memory. The disorder is associated with chronic, excessive alcohol ingestion and a deficiency of vitamin B1 (thiamine).

**Synonyms**
> Alcohol Amnestic Disorder Due to Thiamine Deficiency
> Alcoholic Brain Damage
> Korsakoff Psychosis

**Signs and Symptoms** Memory impairment is greatest for new information; past memory is less severely affected. The patient may experience deficits in visual-spatial function and conceptual and abstract reasoning that are much less severe proportionately than the anterograde memory loss.

When **Wernicke encephalopathy** is also present **(Wernicke-Korsakoff syndrome),** signs and symptoms include bilateral 6th nerve palsy, nystagmus, cerebellar ataxia, and mental dysfunction that may include confusion, drowsiness, and disorientation, along with the memory impairment of Korsakoff syndrome.

**Etiology** Korsakoff syndrome results from excessive, prolonged alcohol consumption: malnutrition and thiamine deficiency (affecting the diencephalon), and alcohol neurotoxicity that damages the cerebral cortex. Wernicke encephalopathy usually precedes Korsakoff syndrome.

**Epidemiology** The disease is seen in severe alcoholics.

**Treatment—Standard** Early recognition and treatment of Wernicke encephalopathy may prevent Korsakoff psychosis, and early recognition and treatment of Korsakoff psychosis may permit the patient to return to predisease mental capability; however, only about 25 percent of Korsakoff syndrome patients achieve full recovery.

Treatment consists of abstention from alcohol, and immediate multi-vitamin supplementation to restore the thiamine, B-complex, and other vitamins.

**Treatment—Investigational** Clinical trials are being conducted by Peter R. Martin, M.D., of Vanderbilt University School of Medicine, to study the genetic mechanism of alcoholic organic brain disease.

Please contact the agencies listed under Resources, below, for the most current information. Addresses and telephone numbers of these agencies, as well as of individual experts and research centers, may be found in the Master Resources List.

**Resources**

**For more information on Korsakoff syndrome:** National Organization for Rare Disorders (NORD); NIH/National Digestive Diseases Information Clearinghouse; U.S. Department of Health and Human Services Public Health Service—Alcohol, Drug Abuse, Mental Health Administration; National Institute on Alcohol Abuse and Alcoholism.

**References**

Brain Lesions in Alcoholics: M.E. Charness; Alcohol Clin. Exp. Res., February 1993, vol. 17(1), pp. 2–11.

Neurobehavioral Sequelae of Alcoholism: O.A. Parsons and S.J. Nixon; Neurol. Clin., February 1993, vol. 11(1), pp. 205–218.

Thalamic Amnesia: Korsakoff Syndrome Due to Left Thalamic Infarction: M. Cole, et al.; J. Neurol. Sci., July 1992, vol. 110(1–2), pp. 62–67.

Harrison's Principles of Internal Medicine, 12th ed.: J.D. Wilson, et al.; 1991, pp. 2045–2047, 2147.

Diagnostic and Statistical Manual of Mental Disorders, 3rd ed.: R.L. Spitzer, et al., eds.; American Psychiatric Association, 1984, pp. 326–328.

# KUFS DISEASE

**Description** The cerebral lipofuscinoses are a group of inherited disorders marked by excess accumulation of lipofuscin in the brain. The various diseases in this group are differentiated according to age at onset; Kufs disease is a late adolescent or adult form. Symptoms are predominantly neurologic, resembling those of mental disorders, and dermatologic, resembling ichthyosis. Deposits of lipofuscin are found throughout the central nervous system **(CNS).** The disorder is usually slowly progressive and may be fatal.

**Synonyms**
> Amaurotic Familial Idiocy, Adult
> Ceroid Lipofuscinosis, Adult Form
> Ceroidosis, Adult-Onset
> Lipofuscinosis, Generalized
> Neuronal Ceroid Lipofuscinosis

**Signs and Symptoms** Manifestations of Kufs disease first appear in the late teens or early 20s. The early symptoms of muscle weakness and incoordination increase in severity and may be replaced by seizures and chorea as the disease progresses. Excessive amounts of keratin in the skin lead to ichthyosis vulgaris. Neurologic manifestations begin with confusion and behavioral changes reminiscent of psychosis. Convulsions and more severe mental disturbances resembling mental illness may ensue. The neurologic deficits result from excess accumulation of lipofuscin in the brains of affected individuals.

**Etiology** Kufs disease may be inherited as a dominant or recessive trait. The dominant form produces milder symptoms than the recessive form. An inborn defect in lipid metabolism is responsible for the accumulation of lipofuscin in the CNS.

**Epidemiology** Kufs disease, the adult-onset form of cerebral sphingolipidosis, begins between the ages of 15 and 26 years. It is an extremely rare condition, affecting perhaps a few hundred people in the United States. There is no racial predilection.

**Related Disorders Jansky-Bielschowsky disease** is the late infantile form of cerebral sphingolipidosis, with onset occurring between 3 and 4 years of age; ***Batten Disease*** is the juvenile form, and begins between the ages of 5 and 7 years. Both are inherited as recessive traits and are hereditary disorders of lipid metabolism or storage. The cardinal features of Jansky-Bielschowsky disease are rapid neurologic deterioration, retinal pigment changes, and optic atrophy leading to blindness. It is a rare disease that appears to occur predominantly in persons of Scandinavian ancestry. Batten disease is a rare condition diagnosed from the finding of ceroid lipofuscin pigments and the characteristic "salt-and-pepper" retinal appearance.

Of the 14 known lipid storage diseases, ***Gaucher Disease*** is the most common. Gaucher disease is the comprehensive term for a number of disorders characterized by the defective production or metabolism of glucocerebrosidase and diagnosed from the presence of Gaucher cells in the marrow and other organs. Infantile, juvenile, and adult forms are recognized. See ***Batten Disease; Gaucher Disease; Niemann-Pick Disease; Sandhoff Disease; Tay-Sachs Disease.***

**Treatment—Standard** Treatment of Kufs disease is symptomatic and supportive. Patients and their families may benefit from genetic counseling and services for the mentally disabled.

**Treatment—Investigational** Recent advances in the treatment of Gaucher disease raises hope that other lipid storage disorders may be treatable in the near future.

Please contact the agencies listed under Resources, below, for the most current information. Addresses and telephone numbers of these agencies, as well as of individual experts and research centers, may be found in the Master Resources List.

**Resources**

**For more information on Kufs disease:** National Organization for Rare Disorders (NORD); NIH/National Institute of Neurological Disorders and Stroke; Children's Brain Diseases Foundation for Research; National Tay-Sachs and Allied Diseases Association; The Arc (a national organization on mental retardation).

**For genetic information and genetic counseling referrals:** March of Dimes Birth Defects Foundation; Alliance of Genetic Support Groups.

**References**

Familial Occurrence of Adult-Type Neuronal Ceroid Lipofuscinosis: M. Tobo, et al.; Arch. Neurol., October 1984, vol. 41(10), pp. 1091–1094.

Autofluorescence Emission Spectra of Neuronal Lipopigment in a Case of Adult-Onset Ceroidosis (Kufs Disease): J.H. Dowson, Acta Neuropathol. (Berl.), 1983, vol. 59(4), pp. 241–245.

Adult Ceroid-Lipofuscinosis: Diagnostic Value of Biopsies and of Neurophysiological Investigations: A. Vercruyssen, et al.; J. Neurol. Neurosurg. Psychiatry, November 1982, vol. 45(11), pp. 1056–1059.


# KUGELBERG-WELANDER SYNDROME

**Description** Kugelberg-Welander syndrome is a rare inherited disorder in which degeneration of motor neurons causes progressive weakness and muscle atrophy, notably in the legs, accompanied by loss of reflexes. An early symptom is uncoordinated gait.

**Synonyms**

Juvenile Spinal Muscular Atrophy

Spinal Muscular Atrophy

**Signs and Symptoms** The clinical picture of Kugelberg-Welander syndrome is dominated by muscle atrophy in the limbs and trunk, producing a slumped-forward posture and impaired motor control. Patients with this condition describe difficulty walking, climbing stairs, and getting out of bed. They may lose bowel control, and reflexes may be slowed. Involvement of the ocular muscles leads to profound myopia and impaired vision.

**Etiology** Kugelberg-Welander syndrome is attributed to degeneration of the motor neurons in the spinal cord. It is commonly inherited as an autosomal recessive trait. An autosomal dominant or X-linked recessive transmission has been postulated for some cases.

**Epidemiology** More males than females have Kugelberg-Welander syndrome, and those women who are affected tend to have less severe symptoms. Onset generally occurs between 2 and 17 years of age.

**Related Disorders** See *Werdnig-Hoffmann Disease.*

**Treatment—Standard** Treatment of Kugelberg-Welander syndrome is symptomatic and supportive. The mainstays of treatment are physiotherapy and orthotic supports. Genetic counseling may be offered to patients and their families.

**Treatment—Investigational** Lithium carbonate is being used experimentally in the treatment of Kugelberg-Welander syndrome.

The orphan product, ciliary neurotrophic factor recombinant human, is being investigated for treatment of the spinal muscular atrophies.

Please contact the agencies listed under Resources, below, for the most current information. Addresses and telephone numbers of these agencies, as well as of individual experts and research centers, may be found in the Master Resources List.

**Resources**

**For more information on Kugelberg-Welander syndrome:** National Organization for Rare Disorders (NORD); Families of Spinal Muscular Atrophy; NIH/National Institute of Neurological Disorders and Stroke.

**For genetic information and genetic counseling referrals:** March of Dimes Birth Defects Foundation; Alliance of Genetic Support Groups.

**References**

Mendelian Inheritance in Man, 9th ed.: V.A. McKusick; The Johns Hopkins University Press, 1990, p. 1355.

Chronic Proximal Spinal Muscular Atrophy of Childhood and Adolescence: Sex Influence: I. Hausmanowa-Petrusewicz, et al.; J. Med. Genet., December 1984, vol. 21(6), pp. 447–450.

# LANDAU-KLEFFNER SYNDROME

**Description** Landau-Kleffner syndrome is a neurologic disorder characterized by aphasia and occasionally epileptic seizures and auditory agnosia. The electroencephalogram (**EEG**) is abnormal.

**Synonyms**

Infantile Acquired Aphasia

**Signs and Symptoms** Symptoms develop slowly and include aphasia, paroxysmal abnormalities in the EEG, and occasionally epileptic seizures and auditory agnosia. The aphasia varies among patients and is related to the location and extent of dysfunction in the brain. Some patients improve spontaneously. In general, the prognosis is poorer for those who develop symptoms at an early age. Diagnosis is aided by neuroradiologic examination.

**Etiology** The cause is unknown, but focal encephalitis is a possibility.

**Epidemiology** Only children are affected. The disorder was first identified in 1957; as of 1982 only 80 cases had been reported.

**Related Disorders Epilepsy** is a symptomatic component of Landau-Kleffner syndrome.

**Treatment—Standard** Treatment is generally symptomatic and supportive. Antiepileptic drugs have had varying effectiveness. Some patients may benefit from speech therapy or sign language.

**Treatment—Investigational** A new type of surgery is being investigated for children suffering from Landau-Kleffner syndrome. Subpial transection may restore hearing and speech and eliminate seizures. For more information, contact Rush Presbyterian, St. Luke's Medical Center, in Chicago.

Corticosteroid therapy is being tested. If given early, it can in many cases restore speech and eliminate seizures.

Please contact the agencies listed under Resources, below, for the most current information. Addresses and telephone numbers of these agencies, as well as of individual experts and research centers, may be found in the Master Resources List.

**Resources**

**For more information on Landau-Kleffner syndrome:** National Organization for Rare Disorders (NORD); C.A.N.D.L.E. (Childhood Aphasia, Neurological Disorders, Landau-Kleffner Syndrome, and Epilepsy); NIH/National Institute on Deafness and Other Communication Disorders Information Clearinghouse; American Speech-Language-Hearing Association; Rush Presbyterian, St. Luke's Medical Center.

**References**

Age of Onset and Outcome in "Acquired Aphasia with Convulsive Disorder" (Landau-Kleffner Syndrome): D.V. Bishop; Dev. Med. Child Neurol., December 1985, vol. 27(6), pp. 705–712.

# LENNOX-GASTAUT SYNDROME

**Description** Lennox-Gastaut syndrome is a very rare childhood seizure disorder that is usually apparent in infancy or early childhood.

**Signs and Symptoms** The syndrome may begin in infancy, but onset is most often between 1 and 6 years of age. Seizures generally recalcitrant to usual anticonvulsant medications occur many times a day, with the result that the child's intellectual ability and neurologic system can suffer damage. Pronounced mental retardation is common.

Among the types of seizures seen are "drop attacks," in which a sudden loss of muscle tone causes the child to fall to the ground. Atonic, tonic, and absence seizures and myoclonus also can occur.

Positron emission tomography (**PET**) and electroencephalography (**EEG;** diffuse slow [1- to 2½-Hz] spike-and-wave brain wave pattern on EEG) are abnormal.

**Etiology** The reason or reasons for the brain lesions and irregular brain wave pattern are unknown.

**Epidemiology** Onset is usually between 1 and 6 years of age, but the syndrome may occur earlier than age 1; onset may also be in adulthood. Males and females are affected in equal numbers.

**Related Disorders** See *West Syndrome.*

Symptoms of **epilepsy** and **juvenile myoclonic epilepsy** can be similar to those of Lennox-Gastaut syndrome.

**Treatment—Standard** Anticonvulsant medications often have limited success with this type of epilepsy. A surgical procedure, corpus callosotomy, usually improves the seizures and lessens the need for medication.

Untreated, the syndrome often continues into adulthood.

**Treatment—Investigational** The Food and Drug Administration has approved the anticonvulsant drug felbamate (Felbatol) for use in treating epilepsy in children with Lennox-Gastaut syndrome. Because of serious side effects from this drug, physicians should contact the manufacturer or the Food and Drug Administration before prescribing.

The orphan product topiramate (Topimax) has been approved by the Food and Drug Administration for treatment of Lennox-Gastaut syndrome.

Please contact the agencies listed under Resources, below, for the most current information. Addresses and telephone numbers of these agencies, as well as of individual experts and research centers, may be found in the Master Resources List.

**Resources**

**For more information on Lennox-Gastaut syndrome:** National Organization for Rare Disorders (NORD); Epilepsy Foundation of America; NIH/National Institute of Neurological Disorders and Stroke.

**References**

Cecil Textbook of Medicine, 19th ed.: J.B. Wyngaarden, et al., eds.; W.B. Saunders Company, 1992, p. 2222.

Principles of Neurology, 4th ed.; R.D. Adams and M. Victor, eds.; McGraw-Hill, 1989, p. 252.

Double-Blind, Placebo-Controlled Evaluation of Cinromide in Patients with the Lennox-Gastaut Syndrome: O.W. Renier, et al.; Epilepsia, July–August, 1989, vol. 30(4), pp. 422–429.

# LEUKODYSTROPHY, CANAVAN

**Description** Canavan leukodystrophy is a rare inherited disorder in which spongy degeneration of the central nervous system leads to progressive mental deterioration accompanied by increased muscle tone, poor head control, megalocephaly, and blindness. The disorder is caused by a chemical imbalance in the brain. Symptoms appear in early infancy and progress rapidly, resulting in early death.

**Synonyms**

>   Canavan–Van Bogaert–Bertrand Disease
>   Familial Idiocy with Spongy Degeneration of Neuraxis
>   Spongy Degeneration of the Brain
>   Van Bogaert–Bertrand Syndrome

**Signs and Symptoms** Canavan leukodystrophy is usually noticed by 6 months of age as mental and physical regression occurs. Early symptoms include apathy, floppiness, and loss of previously acquired mental and motor skills. Disease progression is characterized by limb spasticity, atonicity of the neck muscles, and megalocephaly as the brain swells and the bones of the skull fail to fuse normally. Paralysis may ensue. With diminished chest muscle function, the infant is susceptible to respiratory tract disease. Progressive atrophy of the optic muscles results in blindness in many cases; less often, hearing is also impaired. Death typically occurs before the age of 4 years.

Neurologic and radiologic studies aid in the diagnosis. Computed tomography is helpful in distinguishing Canavan leukodystrophy from hydrocephaly; the scans show severe, widespread white matter changes, predominantly demyelination and vacuolation.

**Etiology** Canavan leukodystrophy is transmitted as an autosomal recessive trait. The defective gene has been mapped to chromosome 17 (17pter–p13).

The degenerative brain changes are attributed to insufficient production of aspartoacylase, the enzyme that breaks down N-acetylaspartic acid, which occurs in high levels in the brain. Breakdown of this acid may act to trigger chemical reactions requisite to proper brain function, or the excessively high levels may be damaging per se.

**Epidemiology** Patients with Canavan dystrophy are usually of Eastern European Jewish ancestry. Both sexes are affected. A familial tendency has been recognized.

**Related Disorders** See *Adrenoleukodystrophy; Alexander Disease; Baló Disease; Leukodystrophy, Krabbe; Leukodystrophy, Metachromatic; Tay-Sachs Disease.*

**Treatment—Standard** Treatment is symptomatic and supportive.

**Treatment—Investigational** With the identification of the enzyme defect causing Canavan leukodystrophy, prenatal testing and specific therapies may become available in the future. Basic pathologic (tissue and fluid) research, not intended to provide counseling or devise treatment, is being conducted on various peroxisomal diseases, including Canavan leukodystrophy. For more information: Anne B. Johnson, M.D., Albert Einstein College of Medicine.

Please contact the agencies listed under Resources, below, for the most current information. Addresses and telephone numbers of these agencies, as well as of individual experts and research centers, may be found in the Master Resources List.

**Resources**

**For more information on Canavan leukodystrophy:** National Organization for Rare Disorders (NORD); United Leukodystrophy Foundation; Association Européenne contre les Leucodystrophes; NIH/National Institute of Neurological Disorders and Stroke; National Foundation for Jewish Genetic Diseases; National Tay-Sachs and Allied Diseases Association.

**For genetic information and genetic counseling referrals:** March of Dimes Birth Defects Foundation; Alliance of Genetic Support Groups.

**References**

Human Genetic Disorders: J. NIH Res.; August 1994, vol. 7(8), pp. 115–134.

Protracted Clinical Course for Patient with Canavan Disease: N. Zelnik, et al.; Dev. Med. Child Neurol., April 1993, vol. 35(4), pp. 255–258.

Reliable Prenatal Diagnosis of Canavan Disease (Aspartoacylase Deficiency): Comparison of Enzymatic and Metabolite Analysis: M.J. Bennett, et al.; J. Inherit. Metab. Dis., 1993, vol. 16(5), pp. 831–836.

Biochemical Diagnosis of Canavan Disease: G. Bartalini, et al.; Childs Nerv. Syst., December 1992, vol. 8(8), pp. 468–470.

Cecil Textbook of Medicine, 19th ed.: J.B. Wyngaarden, et al., eds.; W.B. Saunders Company, 1992, pp. 2200–2201,

Mendelian Inheritance in Man, 10th ed.: V.A. McKusick; The Johns Hopkins University Press, 1992, p. 1707.

Nelson Textbook of Pediatrics, 14th ed.: R.E. Behrman, ed.-in-chief; W.B. Saunders Company, 1992, p. 335.

Use of Computerized Tomography, Magnetic Resonance Imaging, and Localized 1H Magnetic Resonance Spectroscopy in Canavan's Disease: A Case Report: H.G. Marks, et al.; Ann. Neurol., July 1991, vol. 30(1), pp. 106–110.

# LEUKODYSTROPHY, KRABBE

**Description** Krabbe leukodystrophy is a rare familial metabolic disorder in which the sphingolipid ceramide galactoside accumulates in the white matter of the brain, owing to a deficiency of the enzyme galactoside β-galactosidase (galactosylceramidase). The resulting demyelination leads to brain degeneration and progressive neurologic dysfunction. The clinical picture includes mental retardation, paralysis, blindness, deafness, and pseudobulbar palsy.

**Synonyms**

Galactocerebrosidase Deficiency
Galactosylceramidase Deficiency
Globoid Leukodystrophy
Leukodystrophy, Globoid Cell
Sphingolipidosis

**Signs and Symptoms** The infantile form of Krabbe leukodystrophy, which accounts for 90 percent of cases, manifests between 3 and 5 months of age. A late-onset form has been identified, with onset at age 6 to 18 months. Apathy, irritability, and fretfulness are among the first symptoms to appear; vomiting and episodes of partial unconsciousness may also occur. These early symptoms are followed by seizures, spastic contractions of the lower extremities, dysphagia, and mental deterioration. With progressive brain degeneration, paraplegia and blindness may occur. Lesions in specific areas of the brain produce decerebrate rigidity. Sensitivity to sounds is a component of the disorder in some cases.

The diagnosis is established by galactocerebrosidase assays performed on fibroblast cells from an infant or fetus. Pathologic examination shows extensive demyelination and characteristic globoid cells filled with unmetabolized cerebroside.

**Etiology** Krabbe leukodystrophy is inherited as a recessive trait. The disorder is caused by a deficiency of galactoside β-galactosidase, an enzyme that aids in the metabolism of galactocerebroside, a component of myelin. The neurologic symptoms are due to demyelination of the brain and brain stem.

**Epidemiology** Krabbe leukodystrophy affects 1:40,000 newborns in the United States. The sex distribution is equal.

**Related Disorders** See *Adrenoleukodystrophy; Alexander Disease; Leukodystrophy, Canavan; Leukodystrophy, Metachromatic.*

**Treatment—Standard** Treatment for Krabbe leukodystrophy is symptomatic and supportive. Prenatal diagnosis is available.

**Treatment—Investigational** Bone marrow transplantation is being studied as possible therapy for mild, early cases of Krabbe leukodystrophy. Other research focuses on defining the gene abnormality that causes leukodystrophy.

Please contact the agencies listed under Resources, below, for the most current information. Addresses and telephone numbers of these agencies, as well as of individual experts and research centers, may be found in the Master Resources List.

**Resources**

**For more information on Krabbe leukodystrophy:** National Organization for Rare Disorders (NORD); United Leukodystrophy Foundation; Adrenoleukodystrophy Project; NIH/National Institute of Neurological Disorders and Stroke; Research Trust for Metabolic Diseases in Children; The Arc (a national organization on mental retardation); Association Européenne contre les Leucodystrophes.

**For genetic information and genetic counseling referrals:** March of Dimes Birth Defects Foundation; Alliance for Genetic Support Groups.

**References**

A Correlative Synopsis of the Leukodystrophies: P. Morell; Neuropediatrics, September 1984, suppl. 15, pp. 62–65.

Prenatal Diagnosis of Krabbe Disease Using a Fluorescent Derivative of Galactosylceramide: M. Zeigler, et al.; Clin. Chim. Acta, October 15, 1984, vol. 142(3), pp. 313–318.

# LEUKODYSTROPHY, METACHROMATIC (MLD)

**Description** MLD is a form of leukoencephalopathy in which sulfatide, a sphingolipid, accumulates in neural and nonneural tissues, producing blindness, convulsions, motor disturbances progressing to paralysis, and dementia. Myelin is lost from the central nervous system **(CNS).** The disorder is inherited as an autosomal recessive trait. Infantile, juvenile, and adult forms are recognized.

**Synonyms**

> Arylsulfatase A Deficiency
> Cerebroside Sulfatase Deficiency
> Diffuse Cerebral Sclerosis
> Greenfield Disease
> Leukoencephalopathy
> Sulfatidosis

**Signs and Symptoms** The early signs and symptoms of MLD may be vague and gradual in onset, and therefore difficult to diagnose correctly. A subtle change in mentation, memory, or posture may be the first symptom observed. In occasional cases the earliest symptom is a disturbance in vision, or numbness somewhere in the body.

Infantile MLD usually is detected in the 2nd year of life, commonly before 30 months of age. Clinical features include blindness, motor disturbances, spasticity, mental deterioration, and occasionally convulsions. A juvenile form has an onset between ages 4 and 10 years. Adult MLD begins after 16 years of age and is characterized by psychiatric disturbances evolving to dementia; truncal ataxia and intention tremor develop later in this form of MLD.

Prenatal diagnosis is possible by measuring arylsulfatase A activity in cultured cells from amniotic fluid.

**Etiology** MLD is caused by a deficiency in arylsulfatase A, an enzyme that acts on the sulfatide of the myelin of nerve cells in the white matter of the CNS. An autosomal recessive inheritance has been identified.

**Epidemiology** Persons of all nationalities and both sexes may be affected by MLD.

**Related Disorders** See *Adrenoleukodystrophy; Alexander Disease; Leukodystrophy, Canavan; Leukodystrophy, Krabbe.*

See also *Pelizaeus-Merzbacher Brain Sclerosis; Sandhoff Disease; Tay-Sachs Disease.*

**Treatment—Standard** Treatment for MLD is symptomatic and supportive.

**Treatment—Investigational** Bone marrow transplantation has been used experimentally for children with mild forms of MLD who have a compatible donor. The safety and efficacy of the procedure in this setting are not known. Laboratory research is directed toward identifying the abnormal gene responsible for MLD.

Please contact the agencies listed under Resources, below, for the most current information. Addresses and telephone numbers of these agencies, as well as of individual experts and research centers, may be found in the Master Resources List.

**Resources**

**For more information on metachromatic leukodystrophy:** National Organization for Rare Disorders (NORD); United Leukodystrophy Foundation; National Tay-Sachs and Allied Diseases Association; NIH/National Institute of Neurological Disorders and Stroke; National Lipid Diseases Foundation; Association Européenne contre les Leucodystrophes.

**For genetic information and genetic counseling referrals:** March of Dimes Birth Defects Foundation; Alliance of Genetic Support Groups.

**References**

Characteristics of the Dementia in Late-Onset Metachromatic Leukodystrophy: E.G. Shapiro, et al.; Neurology, April 1994, vol. 44(4), pp. 662–665.

Principles of Neurology, 5th ed.: R.D. Adams and M. Victor, eds.; McGraw-Hill, 1993, pp. 840–841.

Cecil Textbook of Medicine, 19th ed.: J.B. Wyngaarden, et al., eds.; W.B. Saunders Company, 1992, pp. 2200–2201.

Diagnosis of Arylsulfatase Deficiency: Z.G. Li, et al.; Am. J. Med. Genet., August 1, 1992, vol. 43(6), pp. 976–982.

Nelson Textbook of Pediatrics, 14th ed.: R.E. Behrman, ed.-in-chief; W.B. Saunders Company, 1992, pp. 1526–1527.

Mendelian Inheritance in Man, 10th ed.: V.A. McKusick; The Johns Hopkins University Press, 1992, pp. 1525–1529.

Psychiatric Disturbances in Metachromatic Leukodystrophy: Insights into the Neurobiology of Psychosis: T.M. Hyde, et al.; Arch. Neurol., April 1992, vol. 49(4), pp. 401–406.

# LISSENCEPHALY

**Description** Lissencephaly ("smooth brain"), also called agyria ("without rings"), is a rare brain formation disorder characterized by lack of normal development of convolutions in the cerebral cortex, and by a small brain. Two major subdivisions, including **Miller-Dieker syndrome** and **Norman-Roberts syndrome,** have been identified although as many as 8 variants of the disorder may exist. Persons with this disorder have a small head and characteristic facies; developmental anomalies of the renal, cardiovascular, and gastrointestinal systems may be present as well. The developmental abnormalities begin before birth, perhaps with interruption of normal brain development in the 4th month of gestation.

**Synonyms**

Agyria

**Signs and Symptoms** Lissencephaly can be diagnosed at or soon after birth. In addition to the small head and unusual facies, young infants suffer from failure to thrive, in part due to difficulty in feeding. The newborn is cyanotic and floppy, has a feeble cry, and may have respiratory difficulties, especially while sleeping. Some are jaundiced and have hepatomegaly or splenomegaly. Hair may cover large areas of the body, and the digits may be malformed. As the infant grows, lack of response to stimuli may be noted, with intermittent bouts of hyperactivity. The initial poor muscle tone may be replaced by seizures and pronounced muscle spasms. Psychomotor retardation is prominent. Other developmental anomalies that may be noted early include undescended testicles, hernias, congenital heart disease, solitary kidney, and duodenal atresia.

The facial features of patients with **Miller-Dieker** syndrome include a high, narrow, wrinkled forehead and a wide, flat lip span ("carp mouth"). Skeletal abnormalities show up as a poorly developed jaw and a prominent posterior aspect to the skull. The corneas may be clouded, and the ears may have an unusual shape. By contrast, the physiognomy in **Norman-Roberts syndrome** is characterized by a low sloping forehead and a prominent bridge of the nose.

**Etiology** The gene that causes lissencephaly has been located on the short arm of chromosome 17 (17p13.3). Studies indicate that the majority of cases of this disorder are caused by a de novo mutation. A small number may be inherited as an autosomal recessive trait.

No chromosomal abnormality has been found in Norman-Roberts syndrome.

**Epidemiology** Lissencephaly is a very rare disorder. Males and females seem to be affected in equal numbers.

**Related Disorders** Lissencephaly may occur as part of a suite of disorders, particularly in the triad of hydrocephalus, agyria (lissencephaly), and retinal dysplasia **(HARD).** This triad is known variously as Warburg syndrome, Chemke syndrome, Pagon syndrome, *Walker-Warburg Syndrome,* and cerebro-ocular dysgenesis. When encephalocele is also present, the mnemonic is **HARD + E.**

See *Neu-Laxova Syndrome; Walker-Warburg Syndrome.*

**Treatment—Standard** Treatment of lissencephaly is symptomatic and supportive. Patients and families may benefit from genetic counseling.

**Treatment—Investigational** Please contact the agencies listed under Resources, below, for the most current information. Addresses and telephone numbers of these agencies, as well as of individual experts and research centers, may be found in the Master Resources List.

**Resources**

**For more information on lissencephaly:** National Organization for Rare Disorders (NORD); Lissencephaly Network; NIH/National Institute of Neurological Disorders and Stroke; Children's Brain Diseases Foundation for Research; William B. Dobyns, M.D., Indiana University School of Medicine; David Ledbetter, M.D., NIH/National Institutes of Health, Center for Genome Research.

**For genetic information and genetic counseling referrals:** March of Dimes Birth Defects Foundation; Alliance of Genetic Support Groups.

**References**

Syndromes with Lissencephaly: I. Miller-Dieker and Norman-Roberts Syndromes and Isolated Lissencephaly: W.B. Dobyns, et al.; Am. J. Med. Genet., July 1984, vol. 18(3), pp. 509–526.

Miller-Dieker Syndrome: Lissencephaly and Monosomy 17P: W.B. Dobyns, et al.; J. Pediatr., April 1983, vol. 102(4), pp. 552–558.

# LOCKED-IN SYNDROME

**Description** Locked-in syndrome is a very rare neuromuscular disorder characterized by complete paralysis of voluntary muscles, with the exception of the muscles that control voluntary eye movements. Paralysis can result from lesions in motor nerve centers, or from a blood clot that interferes with oxygen flow to the brain stem, particularly the ventral pons.

**Synonyms**

> Cerebromedullospinal Disconnection
> Deefferented State
> Pseudocoma

**Signs and Symptoms** Complete paralysis of all voluntary muscles occurs. The only muscles that remain unaffected are those that control eye movements. Consciousness is maintained, but individuals are unable to speak. Communication is limited to the use of an eye blink code.

**Etiology** Lesions across the corticospinal and corticobulbar nerve tracts separate all motor nerves except those to the eye muscles. In some cases, the circulation to the brain stem may be blocked by a blood clot. Reduced blood flow and oxygen supply to the internal capsule of the brain can cause tissue death on both sides. If circulation can be restored, the patient's condition may improve.

**Epidemiology** Males and females are affected in equal numbers.

**Related Disorders** See *Reye Syndrome.*

In **akinetic mutism,** patients' eyes are open and they seem to be awake, but they cannot communicate. The disorder is a result of bilateral frontal lobe damage or destruction of the brain's reticular activating system. Muscle response to painful stimuli is poor.

**Treatment—Standard** Functional neuromuscular stimulation may help activate paralyzed muscles. Several devices to facilitate communication are available for people who cannot speak. Other treatment is symptomatic and supportive.

**Treatment—Investigational** Please contact the agencies listed under Resources, below, for the most current information. Addresses and telephone numbers of these agencies, as well as of individual experts and research centers, may be found in the Master Resources List.

**Resources**

**For more information on locked-in syndrome:** National Organization for Rare Disorders (NORD); NIH/National Institute of Neurological Disorders and Stroke.

**References**

Recovery from Locked-in Syndrome After Posttraumatic Bilateral Distal Vertebral Artery Occlusion: J.M. Cabezudo, et al.; Surg. Neurol., February 1986, vol. 25(2), pp. 185–190.

Adaptive Equipment for C6 Quadriplegia: An Approach to Effective, Simple, and Inexpensive Devices: J.R. Basford, et al.; Arch. Phys. Med. Rehabil., December 1985, vol. 66(12), pp. 829–831.

# MARCUS GUNN PHENOMENON

**Description** The primary symptom of this rare genetic disorder is the rapid rising of the upper eyelid of one eye upon movement of the jaw.

**Synonyms**

> Jaw-Winking Syndrome
> Marcus Gunn Ptosis
> Maxillopalpebral Synkinesis

**Signs and Symptoms** In most patients with the disorder, the upper eyelid of one eye droops. Upon movement of the lower jaw, the eyelid of the affected eye involuntarily and rapidly rises, causing the eye to open wider. This first becomes apparent soon after birth when, during feeding, sucking causes the eyelid to move up and down. It usually persists into adult life. Strabismus, anisometropia, or superior rectus muscle palsy may also be present.

**Etiology** Marcus Gunn phenomenon is inherited as an autosomal dominant trait.

**Epidemiology** The disorder is present at birth. Males and females are affected in equal numbers.

**Related Disorders** Marcus Gunn phenomenon may occur in conjunction with certain other eye disorders (see ***Duane Syndrome; Oral-Facial-Digital Syndrome; Retinitis Pigmentosa).***

Certain types of injury to the facial nerve may produce symptoms comparable to Marcus Gunn phenomenon.

**Marin-Amat syndrome** is similar to Marcus Gunn phenomenon except that the eye closes (rather than opens wider) when the jaw moves to open the mouth. This disorder is also referred to as **inverse Marcus Gunn phenomenon.**

**Faciopalpebral synkinesis** occurs when the upper eyelid of one eye rises when an individual smiles.

**Treatment—Standard** Surgery can correct the eyelid abnormalities. Genetic counseling may be helpful for patients and their families.

**Treatment—Investigational** Please contact the agencies listed under Resources, below, for the most current information. Addresses and telephone numbers of these agencies, as well as of individual experts and research centers, may be found in the Master Resources List.

**Resources**

**For more information on Marcus Gunn phenomenon:** National Organization for Rare Disorders (NORD); NIH/National Eye Institute.

**For genetic information and genetic counseling referrals:** March of Dimes Birth Defects Foundation; Alliance of Genetic Support Groups.

**References**

Mendelian Inheritance in Man, 9th ed.: V.A. McKusick; The Johns Hopkins University Press, 1990, p. 599.

Levator Sling for Marcus Gunn Ptosis: S.M. Betharia and S. Kumar; Br. J. Ophthalmol., September 1987, vol. 71(9), pp. 685–689.

Auditory Brain-Stem Responses in Marcus Gunn Ptosis: D.J. Creel, et al.; Electroencephalogr. Clin. Neurophysiol., July 1984, vol. 59(4) pp. 341–344.

The Marcus Gunn Phenomenon: A Review of 71 Cases: S.G. Pratt, et al.; Ophthalmology, January 1984, vol. 91(1), pp. 27–30.

# MEDULLOBLASTOMA

**Description** A medulloblastoma is a cerebellar tumor consisting of undifferentiated glial cells. About half of medulloblastomas invade the pons and medulla, with subsequent extension or metastasis. Headache and vomiting are early symptoms; however, the full spectrum of symptoms varies with the precise location of the tumor.

**Signs and Symptoms** The signs and symptoms of medulloblastoma fall into 2 general categories: those due to increased intracranial pressure **(ICP),** and those due to the tumor's effects on brain tissue. Increased ICP may result from tumor growth in the nonexpansile skull, with subsequent displacement of normal brain tissue. Other tumor mass effects include brain tissue edema and obstruction of cerebrospinal fluid **(CSF)** flow.

The first sign of a medulloblastoma in infants may be cephalomegaly without other apparent symptoms. Older children experience early-morning vomiting, with or without nausea. The vomiting is attributed to increased ICP but may also result from some other disturbance of the brain tissue without ICP changes. Because the child may feel transiently well after vomiting, the diagnosis may be delayed until growth of the tumor produces other symptoms. As the ICP continues to increase, the child may become irritable and lethargic, with personality changes and attention deficit. Vomiting is more frequent as the tumor grows.

Signs of tumor impingement on normal cerebellar tissue include loss of skilled muscle activity controlled by the cerebellum, such as walking and speech. Ataxia and ataxic gait are early manifestations of cerebellar disorder.

The precise location of the tumor determines which of the many other symptoms will occur in a given case. Symptoms commonly observed include muscle weakness, spasticity, hypotonicity, reflex changes, stiff neck muscles, strabismus, and nystagmus.

**Etiology** The cause of medulloblastoma is unknown.

**Epidemiology** Medulloblastomas have been found in persons of all ages, from neonates to people in the 8th decade of life. The greatest prevalence (80 percent) is in children, in whom 3 peaks of onset have been noticed: at 3 years, at 5½ years, and at 7 to 9 years. Twice as many boys as girls are affected, but the sex distinction diminishes with increasing age. In adults, peak onset occurs at 20 to 24 years.

**Treatment—Standard** Treatment of medulloblastoma entails some combination of surgery, radiation therapy, and chemotherapy. Because the tumor frequently obstructs normal CSF flow, a shunt may be inserted to drain the excess fluid and decrease ICP before surgical excision of the tumor is attempted. Posterior fossa craniectomy is the preferred procedure to debulk the tumor and to promote the efficacy of subsequent chemotherapy or radiation therapy.

Medulloblastoma is a highly radiation-sensitive tumor. Radiation therapy is usually begun 7 to 10 days after surgery. Because medulloblastoma may spread extensively throughout the neural axis, the entire central nervous system must be irradiated, with a booster dose to the posterior fossa. Five-year survival rates of 60 to 70 percent have been reported following total excision of the tumor and irradiation.

Treatment is complex in young children, especially those with extensive initial involvement or in whom the tumor cannot be completely excised. Chemotherapy is usually prescribed in these cases to delay recurrence.

**Treatment—Investigational** Please contact the agencies listed under Resources, below, for the most current information. Addresses and telephone numbers of these agencies, as well as of individual experts and research centers, may be found in the Master Resources List.

**Resources**

**For more information on medulloblastoma:** National Organization for Rare Disorders (NORD); American Brain Tumor Association; American Cancer Society; NIH/National Cancer Institute Physician Data Query Phoneline.

**References**

About Medulloblastoma: W. Kretzmer, et al.; Association for Brain Tumor Research, 1985.

# MEIGE SYNDROME

**Description** Meige syndrome is a neurologic movement disorder characterized by blepharospasm, dystonia, and occasionally spasms in the facial musculature. Persons in late middle age and older are affected.

**Synonyms**

> Blepharospasm Oromandibular Dystonic Syndrome
> Bruegel Syndrome

**Signs and Symptoms** The clinical picture of Meige syndrome is dominated by the gradual onset of dyskinesia and dystonia of the facial muscles in middle-aged or older persons. Intermittent involuntary eyelid closure may result from spasms of the muscles around the eye. Spasms of the tongue, throat, and respiratory tract may also occur, leading to breathing difficulties. Occasionally the neuromuscular involvement extends to the trunk and extremities.

**Etiology** The cause is unknown.

**Epidemiology** Meige syndrome typically affects persons of either sex 50 years of age or older, although it can occur at younger ages.

**Related Disorders** See *Benign Essential Blepharospasm.*

**Treatment—Standard** Various drugs may be used to treat the symptoms, particularly the blepharospasm, of Meige syndrome. These drugs include diazepam, levodopa, methyldopa, trihexyphenidyl, lithium, baclofen, and clonazepam.

The orphan drug botulinum A toxin (Oculinum) when injected intramuscularly into eyelid muscles causes temporary paralysis and for this reason has been used to treat the spasms of Meige syndrome. After a few months the spasms return and treatment must be repeated.

**Treatment—Investigational** Please contact the agencies listed under Resources, below, for the most current information. Addresses and telephone numbers of these agencies, as well as of individual experts and research centers, may be found in the Master Resources List.

**Resources**

**For more information on Meige syndrome:** National Organization for Rare Disorders (NORD); NIH/National Institute of Neurological Disorders and Stroke; Dystonia Medical Research Foundation; Benign Essential Blepharospasm Research Foundation.

**References**

The Cecil Textbook of Medicine, 18th ed.: J.B. Wyngaarden and L.H. Smith, Jr., eds.; W.B. Saunders Company, 1988, pp. 2150–2151.

# MELKERSSON-ROSENTHAL SYNDROME

**Description** Melkersson-Rosenthal syndrome is a rare hereditary neurologic condition characterized by chronic noninflammatory facial edema, predominantly of the lips, accompanied by paresis and occasionally lingua plicata (scrotal tongue). Symptoms typically begin before adulthood.

**Synonyms**

> Cheilitis Granulomatosa
> Melkersson Syndrome

**Signs and Symptoms** The chronic facial edema in Melkersson-Rosenthal syndrome is most noticeable in the lips, although sometimes only one lip is involved. Affected tissue sites may permanently increase in size with the buildup of fibrous tissue. Peripheral facial paralysis, unilateral or bilateral, is another diagnostic feature. Lingua plicata occurs in some cases and may be associated with sensory defects on the anterior two-thirds of the tongue. Symptomatic episodes may follow long symptom-free periods.

**Etiology** The cause is not known.

**Epidemiology** Melkersson-Rosenthal syndrome was first identified in European populations. Onset typically is in childhood or adolescence, and more girls than boys have been diagnosed with the syndrome.

**Related Disorders** See *Amyloidosis; Bell's Palsy.*

**Treatment—Standard** Specific treatment of Melkersson-Rosenthal syndrome involves surgery, to decompress the facial nerve and reduce the amount of fibrous tissue in the lips, and triamcinolone injections, for treatment of swelling and fibrosis.

**Treatment—Investigational** Clofazimine, a drug used in the treatment of leprosy, is undergoing trial in the treatment of Melkersson-Rosenthal syndrome.

Please contact the agencies listed under Resources, below, for the most current information. Addresses and telephone numbers of these agencies, as well as of individual experts and research centers, may be found in the Master Resources List.

**Resources**

**For more information on Melkersson-Rosenthal syndrome:** National Organization for Rare Disorders (NORD); NIH/National Institute of Neurological Disorders and Stroke.

**For genetic information and genetic counseling referrals:** March of Dimes Birth Defects Foundation; Alliance of Genetic Support Groups.

**References**

Internal Medicine, 2nd ed.: J.H. Stein, ed.-in-chief; Little, Brown and Company, 1987, p. 486.

Melkersson-Rosenthal Syndrome: M.W. Minor, et al.; J. Allergy Clin. Immunol., July 1987, vol. 80(1), pp. 64–67.

# MENIERE DISEASE

**Description** Meniere disease is associated with endolymphatic hydrops and is characterized by vertigo, fluctuating hearing loss, and tinnitus.

**Synonyms**

> Endolymphatic Hydrops
> Labyrinthine Hydrops
> Labyrinthine Syndrome
> Lermoyez Syndrome

**Signs and Symptoms** The attacks of vertigo usually are sudden in onset, persist for hours, and slowly decrease. Nausea and vomiting may accompany the vertigo. The tinnitus characteristic of Meniere disease may be ever-present or recurrent, and there may be an intermittent hearing loss. Symptoms are unilateral in 85 to 90 percent of cases.

The Lermoyez variant of Meniere disease is distinguished by initial tinnitus and hearing loss and later onset of vertigo, from months to years. In another variant, vertigo is not present and the endolymphatic distention is limited to the cochlea.

**Etiology** The cause of Meniere disease is not known. It is thought that the membrane between the inner and middle ear may become more porous, causing an alteration in the labyrinthine osmotic pressure. Other possible factors include disturbance of the autonomic regulation of the endolymphatic system, local allergy of the inner ear, and vascular disturbance of the stria vascularis. Stress and emotional disturbances can precipitate attacks.

**Epidemiology** A recent study suggests that 0.4 percent of the population in the United States may be affected with Meniere disease. Males are affected more commonly than females, and onset is usually during the 5th decade of life.

**Treatment—Standard** Anticholinergic agents may relieve the tinnitus and gastrointestinal disturbances. Antihistamines and diazepam may also be helpful. Barbiturates such as phenobarbital also are used for general sedation during severe episodes.

**Treatment—Investigational** When recurring attacks of vertigo become more frequent and severe and intensive medical therapy has failed to control them, the patient becomes a candidate for either conservative or destructive surgery.

Conservative approaches are used if residual hearing is good or adequate with a hearing aid. These procedures are the endolymphatic shunt, middle cranial fossa vestibular neurectomy, and retrolabyrinthine vestibular neurectomy.

Destructive approaches are used if residual hearing is poor and cannot be helped with amplification. The 3 such procedures in use today are the oval window labyrinthectomy, postauricular labyrinthectomy, and translabyrinthine vestibular neurectomy.

For further information on experimental surgery, contact Margareta Moller, M.D., Pittsburgh Presbyterian University Hospital; and the Ear Research Foundation, Sarasota, Florida.

Please contact the agencies listed under Resources, below, for the most current information. Addresses and telephone numbers of these agencies, as well as of individual experts and research centers, may be found in the Master Resources List.

**Resources**

**For more information on Meniere disease:** National Organization for Rare Disorders (NORD); E.A.R. Foundation; Meniere Crouzon Syndrome Support Network; Vestibular Disorders Association; American Tinnitus Association; NIH/National Institute on Deafness and Other Communication Disorders Information Clearinghouse.

# MENINGIOMA

**Description** Meningiomas are benign, slow-growing tumors of the meninges that occasionally cause thickening or thinning of adjoining skull bones. Meningiomas are characterized as frontal, temporal, and parietal.

**Synonyms**

> Arachnoidal Fibroblastoma
> Dural Endothelioma
> Leptomeningioma
> Meningeal Fibroblastoma

**Signs and Symptoms** The symptoms of meningioma vary according to the size and location of the tumor. Many, but not all, brain tumors cause headaches.

With **frontal tumors,** progressive weakness develops on one side of the body or in a localized area (e.g., a leg). Focal or generalized seizures and mental changes such as drowsiness, listlessness, dullness, or personality changes may occur. If the tumor is in the dominant hemisphere, aphasia may result. Frontal lobe tumors can also produce anosmia, diplopia, and incontinence.

**Temporal tumors,** particularly in the nondominant hemisphere, usually cause no symptoms other than seizures. Some patients experience anomia if the tumor is in the dominant hemisphere.

**Parietal tumors,** meningiomas over the parietal lobe, may produce either generalized or focal sensory seizures. Astereognosis is also seen.

**Etiology** The cause is unknown. These tumors usually develop from cell clusters associated with arachnoidal villi.

**Epidemiology** Meningiomas most frequently are found in middle-aged persons, and are rare in children. The ratio of affected women to affected men is 3:2. American blacks are seldom affected.

**Treatment—Standard** Many meningiomas can be completely removed surgically. If complete removal is impossible because of the risk of damaging an artery or other local tissue, even partial removal may alleviate symptoms. Because meningiomas grow so slowly, further surgery may not be necessary for many years. Radiation and chemotherapy are usually not used as treatment for meningiomas.

If the patient experiences muscle weakness, coordination problems, or speech impairment, physical, occupational, or speech therapy may be helpful.

**Treatment—Investigational** Please contact the agencies listed under Resources, below, for the most current information. Addresses and telephone numbers of these agencies, as well as of individual experts and research centers, may be found in the Master Resources List.

**Resources**

**For more information on meningioma:** National Organization for Rare Disorders (NORD); American Brain Tumor Association; American Cancer Society; NIH/National Cancer Institute Physician Data Query Phoneline.

**References**

About Meningiomas: B. Fine, et al.; Association for Brain Tumor Research, 1982.

# MOYAMOYA DISEASE

**Description** Moyamoya disease affects the cerebrovascular circulation by gradually narrowing and in some cases eventually occluding the terminal portion of the internal carotid artery.

**Synonyms**

Cerebrovascular Moyamoya Disease

**Signs and Symptoms** The age at onset appears to dictate the manifestations. For example, children may experience seizures or involuntary movements and even exhibit signs of mental retardation. In young patients, moyamoya disease is usually associated with headaches; speech difficulties; paralytic episodes involving the feet, legs, or upper extremities; hemorrhage; and anemia. In adults, disturbance of consciousness or subarachnoid hemorrhage is prominent.

The patient may have syncopal episodes. In addition, these visual abnormalities may occur alone or in combination: hemianopia, diplopia, bilaterally diminished visual acuity, and the inability to recognize objects; papilledema may indicate subarachnoid or cerebral hemorrhage.

Arteriography and magnetic resonance imaging (**MRI**) are diagnostic in moyamoya disease.

**Etiology** Moyamoya disease is idiopathic. In a few patients, it has been attributed to an autosomal recessive trait. Studies have implicated oral contraceptives in a small number of female patients, but this has not been substantiated. Pregnancy also may be a factor.

**Epidemiology** Although onset can be at any age, moyamoya disease often affects females under age 20, especially Japanese girls. In one Japanese study, 7 percent of the cases were familial, and similar cases, including those involving identical twins, have been recognized in Europe.

**Related Disorders** Symptoms of cerebrovascular accidents and malformations can be similar to those of moyamoya disease.

**Treatment—Standard** The disease may plateau in some patients in whom it has been advancing, but it has not responded to therapy in the past. Today, however, both drug therapy and surgical treatment offer hope. Current drug therapy consists of IV verapamil, a calcium-channel blocker. Five surgical procedures are in use: encephalomyosynangiosis (**EMS**); encephaloduroarteriosynangiosis (**EDAS**); encephalomyoarteriosynangiosis (**EMAS**); superficial temporal-to-middle cerebral artery (**STA-MA**) bypass; and indirect non-bypass revascularization. Patient response to these complex procedures varies.

Other treatment is symptomatic and supportive.

**Treatment—Investigational** The potential roles not only of calcium-channel blockers but also of anticoagulants are being investigated.

Please contact the agencies listed under Resources, below, for the most current information. Addresses and telephone numbers of these agencies, as well as of individual experts and research centers, may be found in the Master Resources List.

**Resources**

**For more information on moyamoya disease:** National Organization for Rare Disorders (NORD); NIH/National Institute of Neurological Disorders and Stroke; Children's Brain Diseases Foundation for Research; Families with Moyamoya Support Network; The Arc (a national organization on mental retardation).

**For genetic information and genetic counseling referrals:** March of Dimes Birth Defects Foundation; Alliance of Genetic Support Groups.

**References**

Mendelian Inheritance in Man, 9th ed.: V.A. McKusick; The Johns Hopkins University Press, 1990, p. 1338.

Cerebral Infarction Due to Moyamoya Disease in Young Adults: A. Bruno, et al.; Stroke, July 1988, vol. 19(7), pp. 826–833.

Pitfalls in the Surgical Treatment of Moyamoya Disease: Operative Techniques for Refractory Cases: S. Miyamoto, et al.; J. Neurosurg., April 1988, vol. 68(4), pp. 537–543.

Nelson Textbook of Pediatrics, 13th ed.: R.E. Behrman and V.C. Vaughan, III, eds.; W.B. Saunders Company, 1987, pp. 1324–1325.

Ocular Symptoms of Moyamoya Disease: S. Noda, et al.; Am. J. Ophthalmol., June 15, 1987, vol. 103(6), pp. 812–816.

# MULTIPLE SCLEROSIS (MS)

**Description** The course of MS, a chronic demyelinating central nervous system (**CNS**) disorder, is variable; it may advance, relapse, remit, or stabilize. Demyelinating plaques scattered throughout the CNS interfere with neuro-transmission and cause a range of neurologic symptoms.

**Synonyms**

Disseminated Sclerosis

Insular Sclerosis

**Signs and Symptoms** Symptoms can range from visual impairment, including blind spots, diplopia, and nystagmus, to impairment of speech, paresthesias or numbness, difficult ambulation, and dysfunction of the bladder and bowel. MS is rarely fatal; the average life expectancy is 93 percent that of the general population. One in 5 MS patients experiences but one attack, followed by little or no advance in the disorder. Two-thirds of patients are independently ambulatory 25 years post-diagnosis. Approximately 50 percent of those pursue most of the activities they engaged in prior to onset of the disease. In some, however, paralysis of varying severity necessitates the use of canes, crutches, and other ambulatory aids. In a small minority of patients, the disease accelerates quickly and may result in life-threatening complications.

**Etiology** Multiple sclerosis is idiopathic. An autoimmune association, possibly in a viral or an environmental setting, has been suggested. The human T-lymphotropic virus (**HTLV-I**), a retrovirus that has been associated with other CNS disorders and certain blood malignancies, has been implicated. A hereditary predisposition has been suggested, but a precipitating factor must also be present.

Studies have shown that siblings of a patient with MS are at a 10 to 15 percent higher risk of developing MS than the general population, whose risk is 0.1 percent. A Canadian study indicated that daughters of mothers with MS have a 5 percent risk. Certain histocompatibility antigens may be involved.

A 1989 Australian study implicated a feline virus. Approximately 7 percent of domestic cats have been shown to have a demyelinating disease that closely resembles MS. Both infected cats and patients with MS have yielded a morbillivirus. Confirmatory studies are yet to come.

**Epidemiology** In the United States, MS affects approximately 58:100,000 persons in the United States, numbering approximately 130,000 individuals. The disease may appear at any age, but diagnosis is most often made between the ages of 20 and 40. MS is more common in whites than in American blacks and Orientals. In a few ethnic societies (Eskimos, Bantus, American Indians), MS is rare or absent, which may hint at a genetic link. MS seems to occur more often in temperate regions of the world.

**Related Disorders** See *Amyotrophic Lateral Sclerosis; Ataxia, Friedreich; Charcot-Marie-Tooth Disease; Chronic Inflammatory Demyelinating Polyneuropathy; Dejerine-Sottas Disease; Guillain-Barré Syndrome.*

**Treatment—Standard** Routinely, ACTH, prednisone, or another corticosteroid is given to alleviate attacks, but these drugs have no effect on the progression of the disorder. Several classes of drugs bring symptomatic relief, including muscle relaxants to reduce muscle spasms, and antidepressants, aspirin, or acetaminophen to lessen pain. The orphan drug Betaseron (interferon beta-1b) is being manufactured by Chiron Corporation for use in ambulatory patients with relapsing-remitting MS, to reduce the frequency of clinical exacerbations. Berlex is the distributor in the United States. The Betaseron Patient Information line: (800) 580-3837.

Physical therapy and exercise, particularly aquatic programs, may be beneficial.

**Treatment—Investigational** Research regarding MS is vigorous. Among the drugs and modalities under investigation are the following.

**Amantadine** regimens are being studied in treatment of MS.

**4-Aminopyridine.** Intravenous injections of this drug, which can increase conduction in demyelinated pathways, resulted in varying degrees of improvement of vision, eye movement, coordination, and walking in 10 of the 12 subjects. Investigators at the Rush Medical College in Chicago reported that the improvements lasted about 4 hours, and a current study is evaluating the effects of long-term treatment with 4-aminopyridine.

**Baclofen.** Intrathecal infusion of baclofen through a surgically implanted pump is under study for its effect on spasticity. Infusion into the spinal space, rather than the oral route, seems to afford better reduction in spasticity and improvement of muscle tone for longer periods. Also, a lower dose seems to be required when the drug is infused. Research on baclofen for spasticity is supported by an orphan drug grant from the Food and Drug Administration.

**2-Chlorodeoxyadenosine compound** (Johnson and Johnson's 2-CdA) may slow the progression of chronic-progressive MS.

**Cladribine (Leustatin)** is an orphan product being tested for treating the chronic form of MS. Research is being done by Ernest Beutler, M.D., 10666 N. Torrey Pines Road, La Jolla, CA 92037.

**Colchicine** regimens are being studied in treatment of MS.

**Copolymer 1.** This orphan drug, a synthetic polypeptide developed in Israel and man⸍ Pharmaceuticals, has had a 2-year trial, the results of which have been announced by Dr. Mɪ Einstein College of Medicine. The subjects were 50 patients with relapsing-remitting MS, so. copolymer I and some a placebo. The average number of attacks per patient was markedly lower ⅃. group. Currently an international trial of several hundred patients is ongoing. The drug is currently avaɪ. a "Treatment IND" to patients not in a clinical trial.

**Cyclophosphamide.** Some patients in studies have had temporary improvement. The goal of current treaↆ ment protocols, in which maintenance booster injections are given, is sustaining the effects of the drug.

**EL-970** is being tested in the hope it may improve nerve conduction, increasing visual and motor abilities. Elan Drug Company licensed EL-970 from Rush Presbyterian–St. Luke's Medical Center in Chicago.

**Immunosuppressive drugs.** The immunosuppressive drugs are under investigation for use in MS. Recent research involving one immunosuppressive drug, cyclosporine, however, found that the therapeutic dose required in MS is so high that side effects would be unacceptable.

**α-Interferon.** This antiviral compound has been given experimentally to patients with MS. Early findings indicate that α-interferon may delay attacks, thereby reducing their number.

**β-Interferon.** Intrathecal injections appear to halve the rate of exacerbations in some patients. The injections are given once a week. The drug is expected to be approved in 1995.

**Linomide,** which stimulates the production of natural killer cells, is being tested by Jacob M. Rowe, M.D., University of Rochester Medical Center.

Low-dose **methotrexate** has been shown in clinical trials to have a limiting effect on disease progression. Upper extremity function experienced the best results in the 2-year study at the Mellen MS center in Cleveland.

**Monoclonal antibodies.** Researchers are exploring the potential of monoclonal antibodies in preventing MS progression; these antibodies may interrupt the autoimmune process. Initial trials have shown the treatment to be without adverse effects. Chimeric M-T412 (human murine) IgG monoclonal Anti-CD4 is being tested. The manufacturer is Centocor.

The orphan drug **Myloral** is being tested for treatment of the relapsing-remitting form of MS. Clinical trials exist in the United States and Canada. The manufacturer is Autoimmune.

**T-cell receptor repertoire** clinical trials are under way in an attempt to study their role in MS. David H. Mattson, M.D., University of Rochester, may be contacted.

**Tizanidine HCL (Zanaflex)** , an orphan product being tested for treatment of spasticity associated with MS and spinal cord injuries, is manufactured by Athena Neurosciences, in San Francisco.

**Hyperbaric oxygen.** This method of therapy has been disappointing.

**Irradiation.** This modality is in experimental use to reduce T-cell–producing tissue in patients with MS. Lymphoid irradiation focuses on the spleen and the lymph nodes.

**Photopheresis** as an attempt to stimulate the immune system's defenses against MS is being studied at the University of Pennsylvania.

**Plasmapheresis** is undergoing clinical trials.

Please contact the agencies listed under Resources, below, for the most current information. Addresses and telephone numbers of these agencies, as well as of individual experts and research centers, may be found in the Master Resources List.

## Resources

**For more information on multiple sclerosis:** National Organization for Rare Disorders (NORD); NIH/National Institute of Neurological Disorders and Stroke; National Multiple Sclerosis Society, National Headquarters. (The National Multiple Sclerosis Society maintains over 120 chapters throughout the United States. These chapters provide direct services to people with MS and their families, including occupational and physical therapy, support groups, clinics, and professional and public education. Information about chapters can be obtained from the national office.)

## References

Cecil Textbook of Medicine, 19th ed.: J.B. Wyngaarden, et al., eds.; W.B. Saunders Company, 1992, pp. 2196–2202.

Mendelian Inheritance in Man, 10th ed.: V.A. McKusick; The Johns Hopkins University Press, 1992, pp. 317–318.

High Dose Oral Baclofen: Experience in Patients with Multiple Sclerosis: G.D. Ehrlich, et al.; Neurology, March 1991, vol. 41(3), pp. 335–343.

Treatment of Multiple Sclerosis with Hyperbaric Oxygen: Results of a National Registry: E.P. Kidwell, et al.; Arch. Neurol., February 1991, vol. 48(2), pp. 195–199.

The Supraspinal Anxiolytic Effect of Baclofen for Spasticity: S.R. Hinderer; Am. J. Med. Rehabil., October 1990, vol. 69(5), pp. 254–258.

Intrathecal Baclofen for Severe Spasticity: R.D. Penn, et al.; N. Engl. J. Med., June 8, 1989, vol. 320(23), pp. 1517–1521.

# ꓹUSCULAR DYSTROPHY, BATTEN TURNER

**Description** The disorder is a benign congenital form of muscular dystrophy.

**Synonyms**

Benign Congenital Muscular Dystrophy Syndrome

**Signs and Symptoms** The initial sign in an infant may be floppiness. Later, a mild muscular weakness and hypotonia make the child prone to falling and stumbling. Early motor development and milestone achievements may be minimally retarded. Especially susceptible to weakness and hypotonia are the pelvic girdle, neck, and shoulder girdle. As a rule, walking becomes normal later in life, but physical activities may be hampered. Fractures and paralysis are not part of the symptom complex.

**Etiology** Batten Turner muscular dystrophy is inherited as an autosomal recessive trait.

**Epidemiology** Infants and young children of either sex are affected. The disorder is very rare. Nine cases of Batten Turner muscular dystrophy have been described in the medical literature. Six of these cases were clustered in one family.

**Related Disorders** See *Werdnig-Hoffmann Disease; Leukodystrophy, Canavan.*

**Treatment—Standard** Exercise and avoidance of obesity are important for patients with Batten Turner muscular dystrophy. The outlook for minimal muscular deficiency is excellent. Many patients have no major physical handicaps.

**Treatment—Investigational** Please contact the agencies listed under Resources, below, for the most current information.

**Resources**

**For more information on Batten Turner muscular dystrophy:** National Organization for Rare Disorders (NORD); Muscular Dystrophy Association; Muscular Dystrophy Group of Great Britain and Northern Ireland; Society for Muscular Dystrophy International; NIH/National Institute of Neurological Disorders and Stroke.

**For genetic information and genetic counseling referrals:** March of Dimes Birth Defects Foundation; Alliance of Genetic Support Groups.

**References**

Cecil Textbook of Medicine, 19th ed.: J.B. Wyngaarden, et al., eds.: W.B. Saunders Company, 1992, p. 2256.

Mendelian Inheritance in Man, 10th ed.: V.A. McKusick; The Johns Hopkins University Press, 1992, p. 1578.

Birth Defects Encyclopedia: M.L. Buyse, ed.-in-chief; Blackwell Scientific Publications, 1990, pp. 1190–1191.

Dictionary of Medical Syndromes, 3rd ed.: S.I. Magalini, et al., eds.; J.B. Lippincott Company, 1990, pp. 93–94.

# MUSCULAR DYSTROPHY, BECKER (BMD)

**Description** BMD is a slowly progressive wasting myopathy that affects particularly the hip and shoulder muscles.

**Synonyms**

Benign Juvenile Muscular Dystrophy

Progressive Tardive Muscular Dystrophy

**Signs and Symptoms** Onset of BMD is usually during the patient's 2nd or 3rd decade. On palpation, the muscles have a firm, rubbery feel. Deep tendon reflexes may be absent early in the disorder. Walking is impaired. Eventually, joint contractures and scoliosis may appear. Cardiac complications are rare. Mental retardation also is rare.

It is possible to test for muscular dystrophy in utero and postnatally. The prenatal genetic test identifies the fetus as a carrier of the gene associated with muscular dystrophy. The postnatal test uses antidystrophin antibodies to check for the protein dystrophin in muscle tissue. A deficiency or an abnormality of dystrophin is responsible for the symptoms in BMD.

**Etiology** The disorder is inherited as an X-linked recessive trait. However, approximately 30 percent of patients with any type of muscular dystrophy have no familial history. Diagnosis in these cases is facilitated by the ability to test for dystrophin.

**Epidemiology** BMD is almost exclusively limited to males, with an incidence of about 1:30,000 live births. Females may be carriers; usually they remain asymptomatic, but in most carriers the serum creatine phosphokinase (**CPK**) is high.

**Related Disorders** See *Muscular Dystrophy, Duchenne; Muscular Dystrophy, Limb-Girdle.*

**Gower muscular dystrophy,** usually with onset in adulthood, begins in the hands and feet, slowly progressing to proximal body areas. Only moderate weakness occurs.

**Treatment—Standard** Treatment consists of exercise, physical therapy, and the use of orthoses. Genetic counseling may be helpful.

**Treatment—Investigational** Please contact the agencies listed under Resources, below, for the most current information. Addresses and telephone numbers of these agencies, as well as of individual experts and research centers, may be found in the Master Resources List.

**Resources**

**For more information on Becker muscular dystrophy:** National Organization for Rare Disorders (NORD); Muscular Dystrophy Association; The Arc (a national organization on mental retardation); NIH/National Institute of Neurological Disorders and Stroke; Muscular Dystrophy Group of Great Britain and Northern Ireland; Society for Muscular Dystrophy International.

**For genetic information and genetic counseling referrals:** March of Dimes Birth Defects Foundation; Alliance of Genetic Support Groups.

**References**

Mendelian Inheritance in Man, 9th ed.: V.A. McKusick; The Johns Hopkins University Press, 1990, pp. 1679–1688.

Internal Medicine, 2nd ed.: J.H. Stein, ed.-in-chief; Little, Brown and Company, 1987, pp. 2238–2239.

Preferential Deletion of Exons in Duchenne and Becker Muscular Dystrophies: S.M. Forrest, et al.; Nature, October 15–21, 1987, vol. 329(6140), pp. 638–640.

Evaluation of Carrier Detection Rates for Duchenne and Becker Muscular Dystrophies Using Serum Creatine-Kinase (CK) and Pyruvate-Kinase (PK) Through Discriminant Analysis: M. Zatz, et al.; Am. J. Med. Genet., October 1986, vol. 25(2), pp. 219–230.

# MUSCULAR DYSTROPHY, DUCHENNE (DMD)

**Description** DMD is one of the most frequently encountered types of muscular dystrophy. It is also the fastest in its spread of muscle degeneration. Almost all affected children are boys.

**Synonyms**

Childhood Muscular Dystrophy

Pseudohypertrophic Muscular Dystrophy

**Signs and Symptoms** The weakness associated with DMD usually does not manifest before age 2 to 5 years. Initially, muscle wasting is confined to the pelvic and shoulder girdle muscles. Infiltration of fat and connective tissue produces hypertrophy of the calf muscles. Within several years the disorder affects the musculature of the upper trunk and arms, and finally all major muscles. DMD runs a consistent, predictable course.

The affected child's symptoms include falls, waddling gait, and awkwardness in raising himself from the floor; these are often attributed to clumsiness. By age 3 to 5 years, however, weakness becomes apparent. The parents may be falsely encouraged by a seeming improvement between ages 3 and 7, but it is due to natural growth and development. Weakness progresses rapidly after age 8 or 9, resulting in inability to walk or stand alone. Leg braces may make walking possible for 1 or 2 years, but the patient will need a wheelchair by early adolescence, or before.

As a rule, the next stage produces a marked increase in contractures and scoliosis. Lung capacity may be diminished, increasing susceptibility to respiratory infections. Mental retardation can occur.

Tests are available to detect muscular dystrophy either before or after birth. The prenatal examination determines whether the fetus is carrying the DMD gene. The postnatal test employs antidystrophin antibodies to locate dystrophin in muscle tissue. Individuals with DMD lack dystrophin; those with Becker muscular dystrophy have a normal amount of dystrophin in the tissue, but the molecule is abnormal.

**Etiology** DMD is inherited as an X-linked trait; the responsible gene has been identified on the short arm of the X chromosome (Xp21.2). Approximately 30 percent of patients are without a familial history, however, in which case the disorder is diagnosed by finding a deficiency of dystrophin in the muscles.

**Epidemiology** DMD is almost exclusively limited to boys. The estimated incidence is 1:4,000 male neonates.

**Related Disorders Glycerol kinase deficiency** is a rare inborn error of metabolism that results in adrenal cortical insufficiency and adrenal atrophy. Principal characteristics of the disorder are muscular weakness and developmental delays. The muscle atrophy seen in glycerol kinase deficiency is almost indistinguishable from that in Duchenne muscular dystrophy.

**Treatment—Standard** Treatment consists only of supportive measures. Physical therapy and orthopedic devices can lessen some of the crippling associated with the disease.

**Treatment—Investigational** The gene appears to serve as the blueprint for the manufacture of dystrophin in muscle tissue. Symptoms occur when dystrophin is completely absent from the body. Investigation involving replacement of dystrophin is under way in individuals with DMD. Other studies involve prednisone, which appears to improve muscle strength in affected patients.

Please contact the agencies listed under Resources, below, for the most current information. Addresses and telephone numbers of these agencies, as well as of individual experts and research centers, may be found in the Master Resources List.

### Resources

**For more information on Duchenne muscular dystrophy:** National Organization for Rare Disorders (NORD); Muscular Dystrophy Association; NIH/National Institute of Neurological Disorders and Stroke; Muscular Dystrophy Group of Great Britain and Northern Ireland; Society for Muscular Dystrophy International.

**For genetic information and genetic counseling referrals:** March of Dimes Birth Defects Foundation; Alliance of Genetic Support Groups.

### References

Cecil Textbook of Medicine, 19th ed.: J.B. Wyngaarden, et al., eds.; W.B. Saunders Company, 1992, pp. 2253–2255.

Mendelian Inheritance in Man, 10th ed.: V.A. McKusick; The Johns Hopkins University Press, 1992, pp. 1916–1922.

Principles of Neurology, 4th ed.: R.D. Adams and M. Victor, eds.; McGraw-Hill, 1989, pp. 118–121.

Randomized, Double-Blind Six-Month Trial of Prednisone in Duchenne's Muscular Dystrophy: J.R. Mendell, et al; N. Engl. J. Med., June 15, 1989, vol. 320(24), pp. 1592–1597.

# MUSCULAR DYSTROPHY, EMERY-DREIFUSS

**Description** Emery-Dreifuss muscular dystrophy attacks the musculature of the arms, legs, face, neck, spine, and heart. Encroachment is frequently slow.

**Synonyms**

> Dreifuss-Emery Type Muscular Dystrophy with Contractures
> Rigid Spine Syndrome
> Tardive Muscular Dystrophy

**Signs and Symptoms** As a rule, the first sign of Emery-Dreifuss muscular dystrophy is toe-walking in a child age 4 to 5 years. This initial manifestation of slowly advancing muscle weakness in the legs may later be followed by waddling that is due to pelvic girdle weakness, and significant weakness of the shoulder muscles. Eventually the disorder may affect the nuchal muscles. Flexion contractures of the elbows and ankles may occur. The effect on the heart muscle is of major concern; the potential for severe cardiac complications is high. Mental retardation does not occur.

**Etiology** Emery-Dreifuss is inherited as an X-linked trait. The recent appearance in females of a disorder with symptoms resembling those of Emery-Dreifuss raises the possibility of an additional route of inheritance, however.

**Epidemiology** Emery-Dreifuss is almost exclusively limited to males.

**Related Disorders** See *Muscular Dystrophy, Becker; Muscular Dystrophy, Duchenne; Myotonic Dystrophy.*

**Treatment—Standard** Treatment is supportive, consisting of physical therapy and active and passive exercise. Agencies that provide services to handicapped people and their families may be helpful, as may genetic counseling.

Patients with cardiac complications are usually candidates for a pacemaker; antiarrhythmic drugs may be indicated.

**Treatment—Investigational** Heart transplantation has been attempted in patients with severe cardiac complications.

Please contact the agencies listed under Resources, below, for the most current information. Addresses and telephone numbers of these agencies, as well as of individual experts and research centers, may be found in the Master Resources List.

### Resources

**For more information on Emery-Dreifuss muscular dystrophy:** National Organization for Rare Disorders (NORD); Muscular Dystrophy Association; Muscular Dystrophy Group of Great Britain and Northern Ireland; Society for Muscular Dystrophy International; NIH/National Institute of Neurological Disorders and Stroke.

**For genetic information and genetic counseling referrals:** March of Dimes Birth Defects Foundation; Alliance of Genetic Support Groups.

### References

Mendelian Inheritance in Man, 9th ed.: V.A. McKusick; The Johns Hopkins University Press, 1990, pp. 1688–1690.

Cardiologic Evaluation in a Family with Emery-Dreifuss Muscular Dystrophy: G. Pinelli, et al.; G. Ital. Cardiol., July 1987, vol. 17(7), pp. 589–593.

Lethal Cardiac Conduction Defects in Emery-Dreifuss Muscular Dystrophy: A.H. Oswald, et al.; S. Afr. Med. J., October 1987, vol. 72(8), pp. 567–570.

X-Linked Muscular Dystrophy with Early Contractures and Cardiomyopathy (Emery-Dreifuss Type): A.E. Emery; Clin. Genet., November 1987, vol. 32(5), pp. 360–367.

# Muscular Dystrophy, Fukuyama Type

**Description** The disorder is a rare form of muscular dystrophy, with both muscle and brain pathology.

**Synonyms**
> Cerebromuscular Dystrophy, Fukuyama Type
> Fukuyama Disease
> Micropolygyria with Muscular Dystrophy

**Signs and Symptoms** Affected neonates are floppy and usually have problems sucking and swallowing. Their cries are weak, and there is a loss of muscle tone as well as muscle weakness. Joint contractures in the knees and elbows may be present, and tendon reflexes are decreased or absent. Few children with this form of muscular dystrophy learn to walk. Seizures, mental retardation, and developmental delay also are present. Mild calf hypertrophy may occur.

**Etiology** The condition is inherited as an autosomal recessive trait.

**Epidemiology** This form of muscular dystrophy has been found mainly in Japan but can occur elsewhere. In recent years there have been a few cases in whites reported in the medical literature. Males are affected slightly more often than females.

**Related Disorders** See *Muscular Dystrophy, Batten Turner; Muscular Dystrophy, Duchenne.*

**Treatment—Standard** Physical therapy will help prevent joints from becoming fixed. Anticonvulsant drugs are used to help control seizures. Genetic counseling will benefit patients and their families.

**Treatment—Investigational** For patients who have grand mal status epilepticus, the orphan drug Fosphentoin is being tested.

Please contact the agencies listed under Resources, below, for the most current information. Addresses and telephone numbers of these agencies, as well as of individual experts and research centers, may be found in the Master Resources List.

**Resources**

**For more information on muscular dystrophy, Fukuyama type:** National Organization for Rare Disorders (NORD); Muscular Dystrophy Association; The Arc (a national organization on mental retardation); NIH/National Institute of Neurological Disorders and Stroke; Muscular Dystrophy Group of Great Britain and Northern Ireland; Society For Muscular Dystrophy International.

**For genetic information and genetic counseling referrals:** March of Dimes Birth Defects Foundation; Alliance of Genetic Support Groups.

**References**
Birth Defects Encyclopedia: M.L. Buyse, ed.-in-chief; Blackwell Scientific Publications, 1990, p. 1182.
Mendelian Inheritance in Man, 9th ed.: V.A. McKusick; The Johns Hopkins University Press, 1990, p. 1357.

# Muscular Dystrophy, Landouzy-Dejerine

**Description** Landouzy-Dejerine muscular dystrophy is characterized by muscle weakness of the face and shoulder girdle. The amount of muscle weakness can be slight, slowly progressive, or rapidly progressive.

**Synonyms**
> Dejerine-Landouzy Muscular Dystrophy
> Facioscapulohumeral Muscular Dystrophy
> Muscular Dystrophy, Facioscapulohumeral

**Signs and Symptoms** Weakness of the facial muscles and shoulder girdle typically appears anytime during the first 2 decades of life. Initially the patient has trouble blowing or puckering the lips. As the muscle weakness becomes more severe, a masklike facial expression develops and the individual cannot close the eyes while sleeping.

When the shoulder girdle becomes affected, lifting the arms above the head is difficult. Neck and shoulder blade muscles weaken and become wasted. Some patients may eventually not be able to raise their arms to eye level.

Symptoms manifestation varies even among related family members, and muscle weakness progression can vary widely between patients. Conditions that may be associated include wrist drop, foot drop, forward curvature of the spine, sensorineural hearing loss, and abnormalities of retinal blood vessels.

When Landouzy-Dejerine muscular dystrophy is present during infancy, progression is rapid, causing severe weakness of the muscles and the inability to walk by age 10 years.

**Etiology** The disorder is inherited as an autosomal dominant trait.

**Epidemiology** Landouzy-Dejerine muscular dystrophy is a very rare disorder that affects males and females in equal numbers. The incidence rate varies among different locations and ethnic groups. A high incidence has been found in Utah and southern Germany.

**Related Disorders** See *Central Core Disease; Kugelberg-Welander Syndrome; Nemaline Myopathy; Scapuloperoneal Myopathy.*

**Treatment—Standard** Physical therapy may help prevent contractures in affected persons. Orthopedic devices can be useful, depending on the extent of the disability. Genetic counseling may benefit patients and their families. Other treatment is symptomatic and supportive.

**Treatment—Investigational** Please contact the agencies listed under Resources, below, for the most current information. Addresses and telephone numbers of these agencies, as well as of individual experts and research centers, may be found in the Master Resources List.

**Resources**

**For more information on Landouzy-Dejerine muscular dystrophy:** National Organization for Rare Disorders (NORD); Facioscapulohumeral Society; Muscular Dystrophy Association; NIH/National Institute of Neurological Disorders and Stroke; Muscular Dystrophy Group of Great Britain and Northern Ireland; Society for Muscular Dystrophy International.

**For genetic information and genetic counseling referrals:** March of Dimes Birth Defects Foundation; Alliance of Genetic Support Groups.

**References**

Birth Defects Encyclopedia: M.L. Buyse, ed.-in-chief; Blackwell Scientific Publications, 1990, pp. 1183–1184.

A Clinically Homogeneous Group of Families with Facioscapulohumeral (Landouzy-Dejerine) Muscular Dystrophy: Linkage Analysis of Six Autosomes: S.J. Jacobsen, et al.; Am. J. Hum. Genet., September 1990, vol. 47(3), pp. 376–388.

Mendelian Inheritance in Man, 9th ed.: V.A. McKusick; The Johns Hopkins University Press, 1990, pp. 626–627.

# MUSCULAR DYSTROPHY, LIMB-GIRDLE

**Description** Limb-girdle muscular dystrophy is a rare genetic disorder that is characterized by progressive weakness and wasting of the muscles of the hip and shoulders.

**Synonyms**

Erb Muscular Dystrophy

Leyden-Moebius Muscular Dystrophy

Pelvofemoral Muscular Dystrophy

**Signs and Symptoms** The first sign of the disorder is usually difficulty in walking upstairs or lifting the hands above the head. Weakness of the hip and shoulder muscles may spread from the upper to the lower limbs or vice versa. Winging of the scapulae and difficulty in raising the arms above the head are early signs. Progression typically varies: in many patients it is slow; in others, rapid. However, severe disability in walking is usually seen within 20 to 30 years of onset.

Some affected persons may also develop neck muscle weakness and contractures in later stages of the disorder, muscle pseudohypertrophy; and severe lower back pain. The serum CK activity is elevated, and EMG indicates myopathy. Muscle biopsy is abnormal.

**Etiology** Limb-girdle muscular dystrophy is a rare form of muscular dystrophy that in most cases is inherited as an autosomal recessive trait; very rarely inheritance is autosomal dominant.

**Epidemiology** In general, the disorder is detected between the ages of 10 and 25, although symptoms onset can also occur in middle age. Males and females are affected in equal numbers. A large affected Swiss family has been reported as well as a group of affected patients in Scotland.

**Related Disorders** See *Kugelberg-Welander Syndrome; Muscular Dystrophy, Becker; Scapuloperoneal Myopathy; Polymyositis.*

**Treatment—Standard** Patients may benefit from physical therapy and use of orthoses. Genetic counseling will benefit patients and their families. Other treatment is symptomatic and supportive.

**Treatment—Investigational** Please contact the agencies listed under Resources, below, for the most current information. Addresses and telephone numbers of these agencies, as well as of individual experts and research centers, may be found in the Master Resources List.

**Resources**

**For more information on limb-girdle muscular dystrophy:** National Organization for Rare Disorders (NORD); Muscular Dystrophy Association; NIH/National Institute of Neurological Disorders and Strokes; Muscular Dystrophy Group of Great Britain and Northern Ireland; Society for Muscular Dystrophy International.

**For genetic information and genetic counseling referrals:** March of Dimes Birth Defects Foundation; Alliance of Genetic Support Groups.

### References

Birth Defects Encyclopedia: M.L. Buyse, ed.-in-chief; Blackwell Scientific Publications, 1990, pp. 1184–1185.

Mendelian Inheritance in Man, 9th ed.: V.A. McKusick; The Johns Hopkins University Press, 1990, pp. 627, 1356.

Clinical and Genetic Investigation in Autosomal Dominant Limb-Girdle Muscular Dystrophy: J.M. Gilchrist, et al.; Neurology, January 1988, vol. 38(1), pp. 5–9.

# MUSCULAR DYSTROPHY, OCULO-GASTROINTESTINAL

**Description** Oculo-gastrointestinal muscular dystrophy is a very rare form of muscular dystrophy in which ptosis and external ophthalmoplegia are combined with progressive intestinal pseudo-obstruction.

### Synonyms

Intestinal Pseudo-obstruction with External Ophthalmoplegia

Ophthalmoplegia–Intestinal Pseudo-obstruction

Visceral Myopathy–External Ophthalmoplegia

**Signs and Symptoms** Symptoms onset may occur during childhood or not until late adulthood. Patients with childhood onset tend to have a rapid progression of the disorder; those with adult onset, usually a milder course. Principal characteristics of the disorder are ptosis, external ophthalmoplegia, and progressive intestinal pseudo-obstruction. Abdominal pain, vomiting, diarrhea, constipation, malabsorption leading to an infant's failure to thrive, and enlargement of various parts of the intestine may occur.

**Etiology** Oculo-gastrointestinal muscular dystrophy is thought to be inherited as an autosomal recessive trait.

**Epidemiology** Onset may be at birth or during the 5th decade of life. The ratio of affected females to males is 6:1. About 7 cases of this form of muscular dystrophy have been reported in the medical literature.

**Related Disorders** See *Intestinal Pseudo-obstruction; Kearns-Sayre Syndrome.*

**Oculopharyngeal muscular dystrophy** is a rare disorder that typically presents itself during the 4th to 8th decades and is inherited as an autosomal dominant trait. Characteristics include ptosis, progressive dysphagia, weakness of throat muscles, and, eventually, weakness of the muscles of the shoulder and pelvic girdles. Males and females are affected equally.

**Progressive external ophthalmoplegia** is a rare disorder characterized at first by ptosis of both upper eyelids, followed by ophthalmoplegia. Patients eventually develop a backward tilt of the head in order to compensate for the eye problems. Associated disorders often include diabetes mellitus, hypoparathyroidism, hyperaldosteronism, thyroid disease, ataxia, spasticity, and retinal degeneration. Progressive external ophthalmoplegia can be a symptom of another disorder or it may be inherited.

**Treatment—Standard** In severe cases, patients may require long-term parenteral or enteral nutrition. Genetic counseling may be of benefit for patients and their families. Other treatment is symptomatic and supportive.

**Treatment—Investigational** Cisapride, which induces peristalsis, is being tested for treatment of intestinal pseudo-obstruction.

Please contact the agencies listed under Resources, below, for the most current information. Addresses and telephone numbers of these agencies, as well as of individual experts and research centers, may be found in the Master Resources List.

### Resources

**For more information on oculo-gastrointestinal muscular dystrophy:** National Organization for Rare Disorders (NORD); Muscular Dystrophy Association; Muscular Dystrophy Group of Great Britain and Northern Ireland; Society for Muscular Dystrophy International; NIH/National Institute of Neurological Disorders and Stroke; American Society of Adults with Pseudoobstruction; American Pseudoobstruction and Hirschsprung's Disease Society; Parent Education Network (for information on parenteral or enteral nutrition).

**For genetic information and genetic counseling referrals:** March of Dimes Birth Defects Foundation; Alliance of Genetic Support Groups.

### References

Birth Defects Encyclopedia, M.L. Buyse, ed.-in-chief; Blackwell Scientific Publications, 1990, pp. 1185–1186.

Mendelian Inheritance in Man, 9th ed.: V.A. McKusick; The Johns Hopkins University Press, 1990, p. 1526.

# MUTISM, ELECTIVE

**Description** Elective mutism is a rare pediatric psychiatric disorder in which a child chooses not to speak in a social setting. Comprehension and vocal ability are usually intact.

**Signs and Symptoms** The child may be overly shy, anxious, depressed, and manipulative. Usually mute in school—which he or she may refuse to attend—the child often talks normally at home. Some children, however, remain mute in almost every social setting, substituting gestures, nodding, sound, or words of one syllable for speech. Temper tantrums may occur, and the patient may respond negatively when given a chore. With strangers the child typically is compliant, reticent, and almost rigid. Progress in school and social life may be adversely affected. Usually elective mutism continues for only a few weeks or months, but a few cases on record have endured for several years.

**Etiology** Precipitating factors in elective mutism are recent immigration, hospitalization or trauma at a young age, social isolation, a language or speech disorder, and mental retardation. In addition, the child's family may be innately overly shy and reserved. When immigration is a factor, the diagnosis can only be made after the child has learned the new language.

**Epidemiology** While the onset of elective mutism is usually before age 5 years, it may not be apparent until the child starts school. The disorder occurs slightly more often in females than in males.

**Related Disorders** See *Autism.*

**Delayed speech and language development** may indicate a disorder of the nervous system, a cognitive impairment, or a degree of deafness. Or, delayed development may reflect an emotional, social, family, or behavioral problem. It is important to rule out tracheal and laryngeal dysfunction and an abnormality in oral-motor development.

In **aphasia,** trauma to the area in the brain that controls language adversely affects comprehension or oral expression. The highest incidence of aphasia is in individuals who have had a stroke or head trauma, but in children it may be congenital. The severity of cerebral trauma dictates the severity of the deficit. Severe damage may result in lack of comprehension of information given orally. Minor injuries may result in selective language impairment.

**Pervasive developmental disorders** are a group of uncommon psychiatric disorders with the common denominators of deficient social skills, impaired development of verbal and nonverbal communication, and an inability to participate in activities requiring imagination. The child may be slow in developing intellect, language and speech, and motor activity, including posture. The degree and form of these deficiencies vary widely among afflicted children. The most well-known pervasive developmental disorder is autism.

**Developmental expressive language disorder** is infrequently encountered. The child starts speaking late, and expansion of the words used is slow to evolve. When severe, the disorder is generally apparent before age 3; milder forms may go unnoticed until early adolescence.

**Treatment—Standard** The initial step is a workup, including hearing tests, to confirm elective mutism by exclusion. Upon confirmation, psychotherapy and behavior management constitute treatment. One method used is reinforcement conditioning, in which the patient is rewarded for compliance with an assigned task. A 2nd technique is counterconditioning, which entails substituting new behaviors for the unacceptable previous behaviors. The 3rd approach is shaping, a means of developing complex behaviors through increasing reinforcement of simple behaviors; the goal is that the child in time will adopt the desired complex behavior. Paramount in sustaining the positive changes is resolution of any attendant family problems.

**Treatment—Investigational** Please contact the agencies listed under Resources, below, for the most current information. Addresses and telephone numbers of these agencies, as well as of individual experts and research centers, may be found in the Master Resources List.

**Resources**

**For more information on elective mutism:** National Organization for Rare Disorders (NORD); NIH/National Institute of Mental Health; National Mental Health Association; National Alliance for the Mentally Ill; National Mental Health Consumer Self-Help Clearinghouse.

**References**

Diagnostic and Statistical Manual of Mental Disorders, 3rd ed., revised: R.L. Spitzer, et al., eds.; American Psychiatric Association, 1987, pp. 32–33, 38–39, 45–47, 88–89.

Stranger Reaction and Elective Mutism in Young Children: M. Lesser-Katz; Am. J. Orthopsychiatry, July 1986, vol. 56(3), pp. 458–469.

A Comparison of Elective Mutism and Emotional Disorders in Children: R. Wilkins; Br. J. Psychiatry, February 1985, vol. 146, pp. 198–203.

# Myasthenia Gravis (MG)

**Description** MG is a chronic neuromuscular disease marked by weakness and easy fatigability of the musculature, particularly of the bulbar-innervated muscles. MG is responsive to rest. Any muscle may be involved, but the extraocular muscles and those used in swallowing are most frequently affected.

**Synonyms**

Goldflam Disease

**Signs and Symptoms** The disorder may be so insidious in its initial stage that it is unrecognized. On the other hand, the onset of severe generalized weakness may be sudden. Symptoms correlate with the weakened muscles. Early symptoms reflect fatigue in the muscles employed in speech, swallowing, and chewing. The voice is nasal and tends to fade. Dysphagia poses the threat of food lodging in the trachea. Weakness of the extraocular musculature leads to 2 early signs, ptosis and diplopia, which worsen as the day goes on and improve with rest. Weakness of the limbs is often present and is most intense after exercise and in the evening.

In most patients, intervals of improved strength are interspersed with those of greater weakness. Many events, such as infection, overdoing physical activity, emotional upset, menstruation, and pregnancy can trigger a short-term increase in intensity of symptoms. At its worst, the sudden escalation of MG may lead to **myasthenia gravis crisis**. In that case, the patient experiences sudden, severe muscle weakness, particularly in the muscles used in respiration. The symptoms resemble those of cholinergic crisis, the cause of which is excessive dosage of anticholinesterase agents.

Rarely, patients have become asymptomatic spontaneously.

Maternal MG may result in the infant having a transient form of the disorder. Weakness is apparent at birth and persists for 18 to 50 days, after which function becomes normal.

**Etiology** Evidence indicates that MG is an autoimmune disorder in which antibodies bind to the acetylcholine receptor on muscles, thus interrupting neuromuscular transmission. This interference causes weakening of the muscles upon repeated use.

**Epidemiology** Approximately 100,000 individuals in the United States have MG. Onset is at any age; in females, it is usually at ages 15 to 35 and in males at ages 40 to 70. Younger females tend to have generalized MG, while males are more likely to have localized symptoms in the extraocular muscles. Any type may strike at any age in either sex, however.

**Related Disorders** See *Acoustic Neuroma; Bell's Palsy; Benign Essential Blepharospasm; Eaton-Lambert Syndrome; Schmidt Syndrome.*

**Treatment—Standard** For many years the agents of choice for symptomatic relief have been the anticholinesterase drugs, especially pyridostigmine and neostigmine. Edrophonium is used to diagnose MG. ACTH is indicated for severely ill patients.

Physicians at the National Institute of Neurological and Disorders and Stroke are trying a new drug regimen for MG: a long-term course of alternate-day prednisone in a single high dose. This treatment has been effective over long periods in most of the patients treated, with patients over age 40, especially males, showing the best response.

Thymectomy has been therapeutic in a number of patients, many of whom had advanced disease. Recent studies have led a number of physicians to consider that thymectomy should be done in most patients with MG.

Certain drugs can aggravate symptoms in MG. Contraindicated are curare, quinidine, quinine, and some antibiotics; tonic water is a source of quinine.

**Treatment—Investigational** The National Institute of Neurological Disorders and Stroke has studied plasmapheresis as a treatment for MG. The procedure has been effective in strengthening patients before and after thymectomy. It is also useful in reducing symptoms during treatment with immunosuppressive drugs and in MG crisis.

Cyclosporine, an immunosuppressive drug, is undergoing trials as a treatment for MG. Some patients have shown increased strength after using the drug. Other drugs in this category being tested are azathioprine, cyclophosphamide, and methotrexate.

A new drug, 3,4-DAP, is being studied by Donald B. Sanders, M.D., at Duke University. Preliminary tests indicate that it may restore muscle strength.

Please contact the agencies listed under Resources, below, for the most current information. Addresses and telephone numbers of these agencies, as well as of individual experts and research centers, may be found in the Master Resources List.

**Resources**

**For more information on myasthenia gravis:** National Organization for Rare Disorders (NORD); Myasthenia Gravis Foundation; NIH/National Institute of Neurological Disorders and Stroke; Muscular Dystrophy Association.

## References

Autoimmune Disease and the Nervous System: Biochemical, Molecular, and Clinical Update: J.E. Merrill, et al.; West. J. Med., June 1992, vol. 156(6), pp. 639–646.

Cecil Textbook of Medicine, 19th ed.: J.B. Wyngaarden, et al., eds.; W.B. Saunders Company, 1992, pp. 2265–2267.

Therapeutic Strategies for Myasthenia Gravis: P.A. Keys; DICP, October 1991, vol. 25(1), pp. 1101–1108.

New Treatment Approaches to Myasthenia Gravis: C.W. Havard, et al.; Drugs, January 1990, vol. 39(1), pp. 66–73.

Principles of Neurology, 4th ed.: R.D. Adams and M. Victor, eds.; McGraw-Hill, 1989, pp. 1150–1161.

# MYELITIS

**Description** Myelitis refers to inflammation of segments of the spinal cord. The disease may be acute or chronic and has many subdivisions: acute transverse myelitis; ascending myelitis; Brown-Séquard syndrome; concussion myelitis; Foix-Alajouanine myelitis (subacute necrotizing myelitis); funicular myelitis; systemic myelitis; transverse myelitis.

**Signs and Symptoms** Frequently present are muscle spasms, muscle weakness, malaise, headache, anorexia, and numbness or paresthesias of the legs. Sensorimotor paralysis below the level of the lesion may cause urinary retention, sexual dysfunction, and fecal incontinence. Below the spinal lesion tendon reflexes may be absent. Frequently the thoracic area is affected, resulting in abdominal muscle paralysis. Symptoms may abate minimally in time, but this is cause-dependent.

In **acute transverse myelitis,** there may be congested or obstructed blood vessels, edema, cellular infiltration or loss, and demyelination.

In **ascending myelitis,** loss of sensation becomes more extensive with time.

**Brown-Séquard Syndrome** is a disorder in which spinal cord compression and lesions affect one half of the spinal cord. Inflammation, trauma, foreign bodies, or meningovascular syphilis may be causative. (See **Brown-Séquard Syndrome.**)

In **disseminated myelitis** there is more than one spinal cord segment lesion.

**Etiology** Although myelitis is often idiopathic, a viral infection, trauma to the spinal cord, an immune reaction, or a circulatory deficiency in the cord per se may be the cause. Furthermore, the disorder may be a complication of demyelination, a reaction to rubella or varicella vaccines, or a symptom of neurovascular syphilis or acute encephalomyelitis.

**Epidemiology** Onset may be at any age. Males and females are affected in equal numbers.

**Related Disorders** See **Spinal Stenosis.**

**Cervical spondylitis** is the result of nerve root compression and a narrowed spinal canal. The precipitating factors are collapse of disc spaces, thickening of ligaments, and bony overdevelopment. Pain, initially in the nuchal area, may eventually extend to the shoulders and arms and possibly affect motion.

**Treatment—Standard** Treatment is symptomatic and supportive and depends on etiology.

**Treatment—Investigational** Electrical stimulation is under study as therapy in some cases of myelitis. The multiprogrammable spinal cord stimulator, which is being assessed for its ability to control motor dysfunction, produces epidural spinal electrostimulation (**ESES**). When implanted in the spine, it may improve the range of motion and reduce muscle spasms and pain in some types of myelitis or myelopathy as well as in other neuromuscular disorders that are refractory to more conventional modalities.

Please contact the agencies listed under Resources, below, for the most current information. Addresses and telephone numbers of these agencies, as well as of individual experts and research centers, may be found in the Master Resources List.

**Resources**

**For more information on myelitis:** National Organization for Rare Disorders (NORD); American Paraplegia Society; American Spinal Injury Association; Spinal Cord Society; National Spinal Cord Injury Hotline; NIH/National Institute of Neurological Disorders and Stroke; NIH/National Institute of Allergy and Infectious Diseases.

**References**

Acute Transverse Myelopathy in Childhood: K. Dunne, et al.; Dev. Med. Child Neurol., April 1986, vol. 28(2), pp. 198–204.

Recurrent Transverse Myelitis Associated with Collagen Disease: M. Yamamato; J. Neurol., June 1986, vol. 233(3), pp. 185–187.

Evoked Potentials in Acute Transverse Myelopathy: C.H. Wulff; Dan. Med. Bull., October 1985, vol. 32(5), pp. 282–286.

# MYOCLONUS

**Description** Myoclonus is a movement disorder in which a skeletal muscle undergoes sudden, involuntary contractions. The following are causes of myoclonus.

**Intention myoclonus (action myoclonus):** postanoxic; postencephalitic.

**Arrhythmic myoclonus (stimulus-sensitive myoclonus):** hereditary essential myoclonus (paramyoclonus multiplex); hyperexplexia (essential startle disease); opsoclonus (infantile myoclonic encephalopathy, polymyoclonia familial arrhythmic myoclonus); progressive myoclonic epilepsy; Ramsay Hunt syndrome (dyssynergia cerebellaris myoclonia).

**Rhythmical myoclonus (segmental myoclonus):** nocturnal myoclonus; palatal myoclonus; respiratory myoclonus.

**Signs and Symptoms Intention myoclonus** is marked by episodes triggered by voluntary movements, such as a purposeful action.

In **arrhythmic myoclonus,** muscle jerks are arrhythmic and unforeseeable. The jerking may be confined to a single muscle or involve the whole skeletal musculature. Severity, simultaneity, and symmetry of muscle contractions differ in the individual patient as well as among patients. The stimulus may be visual, auditory, or tactile, or it may be physical fatigue, stress, or anxiety. In women, myoclonus is often more intense premenstrually.

In **hyperexplexia,** the patient's startle reaction is extreme; muscle jerks come and go. **Opsoclonus** is localized; both eyes jerk irregularly. When opsoclonus occurs in infants with generalized myoclonus, the infant is said to have **infantile myoclonic encephalopathy** or **polymyoclonia familial. Progressive myoclonic epilepsy,** which is potentially disabling, combines severe epilepsy with significant stimulus-sensitive myoclonus. In advanced disease, dementia may appear. **Ramsay Hunt syndrome** comprises many disorders: epilepsy, myoclonus, and marked spinocerebellar degeneration as well as other neurologic abnormalities.

**Rhythmical (segmental) myoclonus** has a distinctive hallmark: the muscles jerk at a frequency of 10 to 180 jerks/minute. The affected muscles are generally those innervated by one or more contiguous spinal cord segments. In contrast to arrhythmic myoclonus, this type is not relieved by sleep or coma and is not triggered by sudden stimuli or voluntary movements. In **nocturnal myoclonus** there is frequent jerking of the body or extremities, particularly the legs, 2 to 3 times a minute when falling asleep, sleeping, or during deep relaxation during the day. Insomnia frequently accompanies these attacks. In **palatal myoclonus** there are quick rhythmical contractions of the soft palate and sometimes other muscles, including those of the pharynx, larynx, eyes, face, and diaphragm. **Respiratory myoclonus** causes rapid rhythmic muscular contractions of the diaphragm, sometimes leading to dyspnea.

**Etiology** Several types of arrhythmic myoclonus are hereditary: hereditary essential myoclonus (autosomal dominant), progressive myoclonic epilepsy (usually autosomal recessive, whether alone or in conjunction with a hereditary disease such as Tay-Sachs or Kufs), and Ramsay Hunt syndrome (autosomal dominant).

Myoclonus is believed in the majority of patients to be due to excessive neuronal discharge. Hyperexcitability of foci in the medullary reticular formation or cerebral cortical pathways may be the cause of arrhythmic myoclonus. Some types of intention myoclonus, essential myoclonus, and progressive myoclonus epilepsy may be associated with decreased activity in the brain of the neurotransmitter, serotonin.

Viral, vascular, neoplastic, or traumatic lesions to the central nervous system, and cerebral oxygen deprivation due to cardiac or respiratory failure, can cause myoclonus. Also implicated are certain toxins, including some therapeutic drugs in high doses, and metabolic disorders.

**Epidemiology** Males and females are affected in equal numbers.

**Related Disorders** The differential diagnosis of myoclonus includes fasciculations, tics, chorea, athetosis, dystonia, and hemiballismus. It is important to rule out tremor, particularly that associated with cerebellar disease.

See *Benign Essential Tremor; Huntington Disease; Jumping Frenchmen of Maine; Torsion Dystonia; Tourette Syndrome.*

**Treatment—Standard** Certain drugs are indicated for treating the various types of arrhythmic myoclonus. For example, the benzodiazepine derivatives, especially clonazepam, are given in most forms of arrhythmic myoclonus, including progressive myoclonus epilepsy, Ramsay Hunt syndrome, myoclonus associated with idiopathic epilepsy, infantile spasms, and postencephalitic and postanoxic intention myoclonus. Diazepam is also used in these disorders. The patient may become tolerant to these drugs after a course of several months. Meanwhile, side effects, such as sleepiness, ataxia, lethargy, and aberrant behavior, may appear. Anticonvulsant drugs with antimyoclonic activity may also be useful.

Valproic acid is most therapeutic in the long-term treatment of progressive myoclonus epilepsy; it is less effective in some other forms of the disorder. The drug is not without side effects, however, which may be transient: nausea, vomiting, diarrhea, abdominal pain, and possibly hepatic damage.

ACTH or prednisone is indicated in a few types of myoclonus. These include infantile spasms, infantile myoclonic encephalopathy, and opsoclonus accompanying neuroblastoma.

Rhythmical myoclonus is more refractory. Among the drugs that have recently shown therapeutic potential in the disorder are clonazepam, tetrabenazine, and haloperidol.

**Treatment—Investigational** An antimyoclonic drug, L-5 hydroxytryptophan (L-5HTP), is still undergoing study. This serotonin precursor, in combination with carbidopa, which prevents the conversion of L-5HTP to serotonin outside the central nervous system, is being investigated for its efficacy in postanoxic intention myoclonus, progressive myoclonus epilepsy, essential myoclonus, and palatal myoclonus. The gastrointestinal side effects of diarrhea and nausea are kept to a minimum by correct proportions of carbidopa. Combinations of clonazepam, valproic acid, and L-5HTP with carbidopa may in some patients be the therapy of choice. L-5HTP is being developed by Circa Pharmaceuticals.

Acetazolamide is being studied as treatment for Ramsay Hunt syndrome and severe action myoclonus. The drug may be used in combination with clonazepam, sodium valproate, primidone, and piracetam. The addition of acetazolamide to this combination may reduce the severity of muscle contractions in some patients.

Piracetam (Nootripil) has been approved in England for treatment of cortical myoclonus. The drug is used in combination with other drugs for epilepsy.

Please contact the agencies listed under Resources, below, for the most current information. Addresses and telephone numbers of these agencies, as well as of individual experts and research centers, may be found in the Master Resources List.

**Resources**

**For more information on myoclonus:** National Organization for Rare Disorders (NORD); Myoclonus Research Foundation; National Pediatric Myoclonus Center; Moving Forward; We Move; NIH/National Institute of Neurological Disorders and Stroke; Epilepsy Foundation of America.

**For genetic information and genetic counseling referrals:** March of Dimes Birth Defects Foundation; Alliance of Genetic Support Groups.

**References**

Acetazolamide Improves Action Myoclonus in Ramsay Hunt Syndrome: L. Vaamonde, et al.; Clin. Neuropharmacol., October 1992, vol. 15(5), pp. 392–396.

Cecil Textbook of Medicine, 19th ed.: J.B. Wyngaarden, et al., eds.; W.B. Saunders Company, 1992, pp. 2136–2137.

Mendelian Inheritance in Man, 10th ed.: V.A. McKusick; The Johns Hopkins University Press, 1992, pp. 737, 1574, 1928.

Principles of Neurology, 4th ed.: R.D. Adams and M. Victor, eds.; McGraw-Hill, 1989, pp. 269, 311, 808–811.

Myoclonus: What Causes It, What Controls It: M.H. Van Woert and H.E. Chung; Consultant, April 1982, pp. 263–273.

Treatment of Myoclonus: M.H. Van Woert and H.E. Chung; in Current Status of Modern Therapy, vol. 8: A. Barbeau, ed.; MTP Press, 1980.

Myoclonus: M.H. Van Woert and H.E. Chung; in Handbook of Clinical Neurology, vol. 38: P.J. Vinken and G.W. Bruyn, eds.; North Holland Publishing Co., 1979, pp. 575–593.

# MYOPATHY, CENTRONUCLEAR

**Description** Centronuclear myopathy is a rare muscle-wasting disorder that occurs in 3 different forms based on severity, inheritance, and range of symptoms.

**Synonyms**

Myotubular Myopathy

Myotubular Myopathy, X-Linked

**Signs and Symptoms** Onset of the most severe form of the disorder, **X-linked centronuclear myopathy**, is at birth or during early infancy. Weakness of respiratory muscles causes respiratory distress. Infants are generally weak with poor muscle tone, causing poor sucking and an inability to swallow. Muscles of the jaw, tongue, lips, cheeks, mouth, throat, and neck may be weak. Upper eyelid ptosis and paralysis of the eye may be present.

**Autosomal recessive centronuclear myopathy** is a less severe form of the disorder that presents itself during infancy or childhood. Respiratory distress is present. Progression is slow, with generalized muscle weakness becoming more severe by adolescence or young adulthood. Many patients have a high-arched palate and thin face. Weakness of the upper eyelid, jaw, tongue, lips, mouth, throat, and neck may be present. As the disorder progresses, curvature of the spine becomes apparent in many adolescents. Seizures develop in some patients.

**Autosomal dominant centronuclear myopathy** is the mildest form of the disorder, with onset between the 1st and 3rd decades. Early signs may be a clumsy gait and general weakness of the hips and shoulders. Walking becomes increasingly difficult and eventually leads to use of a wheelchair. Some patients may have facial weakness, but muscles of the throat and eyes usually remain unaffected.

**Etiology** Centronuclear myopathy is inherited as an X-linked, autosomal recessive, or autosomal dominant trait. The X-linked recessive form has been mapped to Xq28.

**Epidemiology** The X-linked form only affects males. About 20 cases have been reported in the medical literature.

The autosomal recessive form affects females slightly more often than males, and has been described in many parts of the world. There appears to be a higher incidence among black persons, but all races can be affected.

The autosomal dominant form affects males twice as often as females. Approximately 20 cases have been reported in the medical literature.

**Related Disorders** See *Dystrophy, Myotonic; Kearns-Sayre Syndrome; Muscular Dystrophy, Emery-Dreifuss; Muscular Dystrophy, Landouzy-Dejerine; Muscular Dystrophy, Limb-Girdle; Muscular Dystrophy, Oculo-Gastrointestinal; Nemaline Myopathy.*

**Treatment—Standard** Patients with the autosomal recessive and X-linked forms of centronuclear myopathy may require the use of mechanical ventilation devices, such as positive end expiratory pressure (**PEEP**) machines.

Patients with the autosomal recessive form who have seizures may benefit from anticonvulsant drugs.

Patients with the autosomal dominant form may require physical therapy and appliances such as walkers and wheelchairs.

Genetic counseling is helpful for patients and their families. Other treatment is symptomatic and supportive.

**Treatment—Investigational** Please contact the agencies listed under Resources, below, for the most current information. Addresses and telephone numbers of these agencies, as well as of individual experts and research centers, may be found in the Master Resources List.

**Resources**

**For more information on centronuclear myopathy:** National Organization for Rare Disorders (NORD); Muscular Dystrophy Association; NIH/National Institute of Neurological Disorders and Stroke.

**For genetic information and genetic counseling referrals:** March of Dimes Birth Defects Foundation; Alliance of Genetic Support Groups; NIH/National Institute of Child Health and Human Development.

**References**

Prenatal Diagnosis of X-Linked Centronuclear Myopathy by Linkage Analysis: S. Liechti-Gallati, et al.; Pediatr. Res., 1993, vol. 33(2), pp. 201–204.

Cecil Textbook of Medicine, 19th ed.: J.B. Wyngaarden, et al., eds.; W.B. Saunders Company, 1992, p. 2275.

Birth Defects Encyclopedia: M.L. Buyse, ed.-in-chief; Blackwell Scientific Publications, 1990, p. 1196.

Mendelian Inheritance in Man, 9th ed.: V.A. McKusick; The Johns Hopkins University Press, 1990, pp. 633, 1367, 1690–1691.

# MYOPATHY, DESMIN STORAGE (DSM)

**Description** DSM is a rare inherited muscle disorder. Three forms have been described, based on age of onset and range of symptoms: **congenital proximal myopathy associated with DSM; cardiomyopathy associated with DSM**; and **autosomal dominant DSM with late onset.**

**Synonyms**

Cardiomyopathy Due to Desmin Defect

Myopathy with Sarcoplasmic Bodies and Intermediate Filaments

**Signs and Symptoms** Major symptoms of the congenital form are usually apparent at birth and include kyphoscoliosis and weakness of face, shoulder, and pelvic muscles. Higher than normal blood pressure in the pulmonary arteries and insufficient heart function may also occur.

The cardiomyopathy associated with DSM may lead to complete atrioventricular block. Ventricular hypertrophy may be present. This form of DSM can occur at any age.

Autosomal dominant DSM with late onset is progressive, with symptoms that usually begin around age 40, with thenar muscle weakness and/or weakness of the muscles used to flex the hand. Muscle weakness and atrophy and decreased tendon reflexes may occur in other muscle groups (e.g., legs and feet) as the disorder progresses.

Desmin storage myopathy is diagnosed by finding desmin on laboratory examination of muscle and heart tissue samples.

**Etiology** The exact biochemical defect that causes desmin storage myopathy is not known. For the form inherited as an autosomal dominant trait, the desmin (**DES**) gene has been localized to the long arm of chromosome 2 (2q35).

**Epidemiology** The disorder is very rare. It may be congenital, or not appear until age 40, depending on which of the 3 forms affects the individual. Approximately 20 cases of DSM have been reported in the medical literature. Males and females are affected in equal numbers.

**Related Disorders** *Muscular Dystrophy, Batten Turner; Fiber Type Disproportion, Congenital; Muscular Dystrophy, Landouzy-Dejerine; Werdnig-Hoffmann Disease.*

**Distal muscular dystrophy** is a rare muscular disorder that may be inherited either as an autosomal recessive or dominant trait. Onset is usually in the adult years. In the autosomal recessive form, weakness and wasting of the muscles on the outside of the leg progress rapidly to the thigh and hand muscles. Major symptoms of the autosomal dominant form of this disorder include clumsiness and weakness starting in the hands, then progressing to the forearm. Leg muscles are affected later or are not affected at all.

**Treatment—Standard** Treatment is symptomatic and supportive. Patients with cardiomyopathy may require a pacemaker. Genetic counseling may benefit the families of those with the inherited form.

**Treatment—Investigational** Please contact the agencies listed under Resources, below, for the most current information. Addresses and telephone numbers of these agencies, as well as of individual experts and research centers, may be found in the Master Resources List.

**Resources**

**For more information on desmin storage myopathy:** National Organization for Rare Disorders (NORD); NIH/National Heart, Lung and Blood Institute Information Center; American Heart Association.

**For genetic information and genetic counseling referrals:** March of Dimes Birth Defects Foundation; Alliance of Genetic Support Groups.

**References**

Familial Desminopathy: Myopathy with Accumulation of Desmin-Type Intermediate Filaments: J. Vajsar, et al.; J. Neurol. Neurosurg. Psychiatry, June 1993, vol. 56(6), pp. 644–648.

Mendelian Inheritance in Man, 10th ed.: V.A. McKusick; The Johns Hopkins University Press, 1992, p. 311.

Congenital Myopathies: H.H. Goebel; Acta Paediatr. Jpn., April 1991, vol. 33(2), pp. 247–255.

Birth Defects Encyclopedia: M.L. Buyse, ed.-in-chief; Blackwell Scientific Publications, 1990, pp. 1191–1192.

Cardiomyopathy and Multicore Myopathy with Accumulation of Intermediate Filaments: E. Bertini, et al.; Eur. J. Pediatr., September 1990, vol. 149(12), pp. 856–858.

Myopathy Associated with Desmin Type Intermediate Filaments: An Immunoelectron Microscopic Study: J.F. Pellissier, et al.; J. Neurol. Sci., January 1989, vol. 89(1), pp. 49–61.

Storage of Phosphorylated Desmin in a Familial Myopathy: L. Rappaport, et al.; FEBS Lett., April 1988, vol. 231(2), pp. 421–425.

# MYOSITIS, INCLUSION BODY (IBM)

**Description** IBM is a slowly progressive inflammatory disease of the skeletal muscles associated with microtubular filament inclusions in muscle cells.

**Signs and Symptoms** The absence of fever, headache, and joint and muscle pain differentiates IBM from polymyositis and dermatomyositis; the histopathology of IBM does, however, include macrophages (also associated with polymyositis). Distal muscle weakness and atrophy are prominent. Facial weakness and dysphagia also have been reported. Serum creatine kinase may be only slightly elevated. Muscle biopsy and electromyography are useful for making a diagnosis. IBM is not usually associated with malignancy, skin changes, or connective tissue disease.

**Etiology** IBM seems to be a distinct type of inflammatory muscle disease. Its cause is unknown.

**Epidemiology** In general, IBM is a disease of the elderly, most often male. On the average, onset occurs at age 53, but it has been reported in patients in their teens.

**Related Disorders** See ***Polymyositis/Dermatomyositis; Mixed Connective Tissue Disease.***

**Distal myopathy** primarily attacks the small muscles of the extremities. As a rule, a patient is over age 40 when he experiences the first symptoms.

Generally, **oculopharyngeal muscular dystrophy** appears in adulthood, with involvement of the extraocular muscles and those muscles employed in swallowing. The characteristic facies, particularly ptosis, is similar to that of myasthenia gravis. The inheritance pattern is frequently autosomal dominant, but at times the disorder may be sporadic or autosomal recessive.

**Treatment—Standard** IBM is unresponsive to corticosteroids and other immunosuppressive drugs. To date, therapy is only symptomatic and supportive.

**Treatment—Investigational** Please contact the agencies listed under Resources, below, for the most current information. Addresses and telephone numbers of these agencies, as well as of individual experts and research centers, may be found in the Master Resources List.

**Resources**

**For more information on inclusion body myositis:** National Organization for Rare Disorders (NORD); Inclusion Body Myositis Association; NIH/National Arthritis and Musculoskeletal and Skin Diseases Information Clearinghouse; Muscular Dystrophy Association.

**References**

Monoclonal Antibody Analysis of Mononuclear Cells in Myopathies. V: Identification and Quantitation of T8+ Cytotoxic and T8+ Suppressor Cells: K. Arahata, et al.; Ann. Neurol., May, 1988, vol. 23(5), pp. 493–499.

Inclusion Body Myositis: A Chronic Persistent Mumps Myositis?: S.M. Chou; Hum. Pathol., August, 1986, vol. 17(8), pp. 765–777.

Mendelian Inheritance in Man, 8th ed.: V.A. McKusick; The Johns Hopkins University Press, 1986, p. 427.

Inclusion Body Myositis and Systemic Lupus Erythematosus: R.A. Yood, et al.; J. Rheumatol., June 1985, vol. 12(3), pp. 568–570.

# MYOSITIS OSSIFICANS

**Description** Myositis ossificans is a progressive disorder characterized by calcifications in the skeletal musculature.

**Synonyms**

> Fibrodysplasia Ossificans Progressiva
> Guy-Patin Syndrome
> Muenchmeyer Syndrome
> Patin Syndrome
> Stone Man

**Signs and Symptoms** The muscles invaded by calcification increasingly weaken and become rigid, thus restricting movement. Related tissue–that linking muscle to muscle and tendon to muscle—and the tendons themselves may be similarly affected. Upon muscular contraction, the patient usually experiences pain and tenderness. Some patients have bruiselike swelling of the skin over the site of the calcifications. In addition, malformations of the big toe and shortened digits may be present. On rare occasions, deafness, baldness, or mental retardation may accompany the disorder. Scoliosis may or may not occur. In the most severely afflicted patients, ambulation may be impaired.

**Etiology** It is thought that myositis ossificans is inherited as an autosomal dominant trait. Muscle injuries that cause calcifications can, however, mimic hereditary myositis ossificans.

**Epidemiology** The medical literature has reported approximately 350 cases of myositis ossificans in this century. The disorder affects males and females in equal numbers; onset is commonly before age 10.

**Related Disorders** In **a variant of myositis ossificans,** calcifications are due to muscle injury. This form is not hereditary.

**Pseudohypoparathyroidism** is hereditary and X-linked. Normal quantities of the parathyroid hormone are present, but response to the hormone is insufficient, adversely affecting bone growth. Headaches, weakness, easy fatigability, lethargy, and blurred vision or photophobia may be present. Paresthesias, stiffness, or cramps in arms or legs; palpitations; and abdominal pain may occur. A round face, thick short stature, shortened digits, and mental deficiencies are also part of the pattern. The prognosis is favorable in most cases. Hormonal and calcium replacement therapy is often beneficial, but the stunting of growth may continue.

**Calcinosis universalis** is a skin disorder in which calcium deposits produce tenderness. Onset of this progressive disorder may be at any age. Calcium deposits around joints or in muscles may cause weakness and edema. Deposits may also settle in the kidneys, stomach, or lungs. The outlook depends on the extent of the disorder and treatment of associated infections.

**Treatment—Standard** Surgery or biopsy of calcifications may sometimes aggravate symptoms; surgery is reserved for the most seriously afflicted patients. Intramuscular injections, muscle trauma, puncture of a vein, or dental surgery may also worsen calcifications.

Corticosteroids and lidocaine may lessen inflammation and muscle stiffness. Prompt treatment of infections is essential. Otherwise, treatment is symptomatic and supportive. Agencies and programs for the handicapped may benefit patients and their families. Genetic counseling can help families with the hereditary form of myositis ossificans.

**Treatment—Investigational** Sonography, x-ray, and scintigraphy are being evaluated for their ability to locate and monitor the growth and size of calcifications in muscles.

Please contact the agencies listed under Resources, below, for the most current information. Addresses and telephone numbers of these agencies, as well as of individual experts and research centers, may be found in the Master Resources List.

**Resources**

**For more information on myositis ossificans:** National Organization for Rare Disorders (NORD); NIH/National Arthritis and Musculoskeletal and Skin Diseases Information Clearinghouse; Muscular Dystrophy Association; International Fibrodysplasia Ossificans Progressiva Association.

**For genetic information and genetic counseling referrals:** March of Dimes Birth Defects Foundation; Alliance of Genetic Support Groups.

**References**

Diagnostic and Therapeutic Aspects of Myositis Ossificans (Author Transl.): P. Jenny, et al.; Z. Kinderchir., March 1982, vol. 35(3), pp. 86–87.

Fibrodysplasia Ossificans Progressiva: The Clinical Features and Natural History of 34 Patients: J.M. Connor, et al.; J. Bone Joint Surg. Br., 1982, vol. 64(1), pp. 76–83.

Treatment of Traumatic Myositis Ossificans Circumscripta: Use of Aspiration and Steroids: J.C. Molloy, et al.; J. Trauma, November 1976, vol. 16(11), pp. 851–857.

# MYOTONIC DYSTROPHY

**Description** Myotonic dystrophy is a rare, slowly progressive, inherited condition in which the relaxing power of the muscles is decreased and muscle atrophy occurs, especially in the muscles of the face and neck. Ocular muscles, the endocrine system, and the cardiovascular system may also be affected. Myotonic dystrophy may be mild or severe. If the latter, mentation may be affected. Onset typically is in late adolescence or young adulthood, but it can be in infancy.

**Synonyms**

> Curschmann-Batten-Steinert Syndrome
> Myotonia Atrophica
> Steinert Disease

**Signs and Symptoms** Early symptoms of myotonic dystrophy are the inability to relax muscles after they have been contracted, and muscle weakness. Depending on the muscles involved, manifestations may include drooping eyelids, a continually furrowed forehead, weakness in lifting, tongue weakness, and inability to relax the hand after shaking hands. The patient may trip or fall easily. Muscles of the face and neck are principally affected, but limb dystrophy is also common. Eventually generalized weakness ensues.

Myotonic dystrophy may be accompanied by mental deterioration or retardation and endocrine abnormalities such as low testosterone levels, amenorrhea, menstrual irregularities, infertility, and glucose intolerance. Death usually occurs in the 5th or 6th decade from cardiac arrythmias, respiratory failure, or intercurrent infection.

**Etiology** Myotonic dystrophy is inherited as a dominant trait with incomplete penetrance. The responsible gene has been localized to chromosome 19. A genetic test is available with a 90 percent predictive accuracy.

**Epidemiology** Equal numbers of males and females are affected. New cases are primarily seen in young adults.

**Related Disorders** See ***Thomsen Disease*** (myotonia congenita), in which there is a similar problem of muscle inability to relax after contraction, but in which the muscles themselves are well-developed and even large.

**Treatment—Standard** Treatment is symptomatic and supportive. Physiotherapy may be helpful in promoting remaining muscle strength. Genetic testing is available.

**Treatment—Investigational** Drugs under investigation for the treatment of myotonic dystrophy include tocainide (Xylotocan) and nifedipine. In addition, it is thought that selenium and vitamin E may increase muscle strength and alleviate some symptoms. Administration of these substances must be supervised to prevent toxic overdose.

Please contact the agencies listed under Resources, below, for the most current information. Addresses and telephone numbers of these agencies, as well as of individual experts and research centers, may be found in the Master Resources List.

**Resources**

**For more information on myotonic dystrophy:** National Organization for Rare Disorders (NORD); Muscular Dystrophy Association; NIH/National Institute of Neurological Disorders and Stroke; NIH/National Arthritis and Musculoskeletal and Skin Diseases Information Clearinghouse.

**For genetic information and genetic counseling referrals:** March of Dimes Birth Defects Foundation; Alliance of Genetic Support Groups.

**References**

Nifedipine in the Treatment of Myotonia in Myotonic Dystrophy: R. Grant, et al.; J. Neurol. Neurosurg. Psychiatry, February 1987, vol. 50(2), pp. 199–206.

Myotonic Dystrophy Treated with Selenium and Vitamin E: G. Orndahl, et al.; Acta Med. Scand., 1986, vol. 219(4), pp. 407–414.

Antimyotonic Therapy with Tocainide Under ECG Control in the Myotonic Dystrophy of Curschmann-Steinert: U. Mielke, et al.; J. Neurol., 1985, vol. 232(5), pp. 271–274.

The Problem of Diagnosis and Therapy of Myotonic Dystrophy: F. Reisecker; Wien Med. Wochenschr., June 30, 1983, vol. 133(12), pp. 319–321.

# NARCOLEPSY

**Description** Narcolepsy is marked by unnatural drowsiness during the day, cataplexy, hallucinations, sleep paralysis, and disrupted sleep during the night.

**Synonyms**

> Gélineau Syndrome
> Paroxysmal Sleep
> Sleep Epilepsy

**Signs and Symptoms** Onset of narcolepsy is generally between ages 10 and 20. The development and the degree of symptoms vary greatly among patients. The various symptoms usually appear singly. Each onset may be separated by years from another, and there is variability in symptoms sequence. Initial manifestations are mild. These intensify over the years, sometimes without change for months or years; at other times, changes can be rapid.

**Exaggerated daytime drowsiness** is usually the initial symptom, and may be described by the patient as sleepiness, tiredness, lack of energy, a sleep attack, or an inability to resist sleep. This unending susceptibility to drowsiness or falling asleep occurs daily, but the severity varies throughout each day. Total sleep time in each 24 hours is generally normal.

**Cataplexy** is a sudden loss of voluntary muscle tone. The usual background of an attack is anger, elation, or surprise. The episode may be a short period of partial muscle weakness, or almost complete loss of muscle control that persists for several minutes and climaxes in postural collapse. During the attack, the cataplectic patient cannot move or speak despite consciousness and at least partial awareness of surrounding activities.

**Hypnagogic hallucinations** are startling occurrences during the beginning or end of a sleep period. The hallucinations may pertain to any or all of the senses and be almost indistinguishable from reality.

In **sleep paralysis,** the patient wants to move but cannot do so and feels panic. The timing of this symptom coincides with falling asleep or waking up.

Many awakenings are typical in **disrupted nighttime sleep.** Nightmares, the urge to urinate, or sleep apnea (common in narcolepsy) may awaken the patient. At times there is no apparent reason for awakening, and frequently this type of awakening is associated with a craving for food, especially something sweet.

**Etiology** The cause is unknown. The disorder is known to be familial, and HLA associations have been reported.

**Epidemiology** The American Narcolepsy Association estimates the incidence of narcolepsy to be approximately 200,000 individuals in the United States. Approximately 5 percent of patients are symptomatic by age 10; 25 percent after age 20; and 18 percent after age 30. Onset after age 40 is unlikely. Narcolepsy tends to remain a lifelong condition.

**Related Disorders** Symptoms resembling those of narcolepsy may occur secondary to intracranial tumors, head trauma, cerebral arteriosclerosis, psychosis, and uremia. Cataplexy can be differentiated from familial periodic paralysis; in the latter, episodes are longer lasting and the metabolism of potassium is faulty.

**Treatment—Standard** Specific treatment for narcolepsy is lacking, but there are several drugs that may bring symptomatic relief. The treatment selected relates to the symptoms and prior response to therapy. In some patients, the disorder has more of an element of cataplexy, and in others, sleep attacks predominate. Those who are not seriously hampered by sleep attacks, sleepiness, or cataplexy may not require drug therapy.

Drugs indicated include methamphetamines and amphetamines, although their side effects are potentially harmful. The most frequently encountered side effects are personality changes (particularly tenseness and irritability) and depression. These manifest during the late afternoon and evening as the drugs wear off, or on weekends if the patient has a tendency to reduce the dose during that period. Methylphenidate is the analeptic drug of choice in sleep attacks and drowsiness.

Treatment of cataplexy includes imipramine, desimipramine, and chlorimipramine. Two recognized side effects are sleepiness and impotence. Chlorimipramine is currently the most effective of these compounds.

Tolerance and the need for excessively high doses or the necessity to assess the symptom status may make withdrawal of drug therapy necessary. Sudden cessation of analeptic medications may result in exaggerated drowsiness and often a severe depression. Sudden withdrawal from imipraminic compounds may result in a marked acceleration of the cataplectic symptoms.

Sleep habits are an essential part of therapy. Assuring regular bedtimes and prevention of interruptions are important. Intervals of naps during the day may avert the hard-to-control continual need for daytime sleep. A physician-directed program can set the most beneficial sleep pattern.

**Treatment—Investigational** Two of the National Institutes of Health–the National Institute of Mental Health and the National Institute of Neurological Disorders and Stroke–support research in sleep disorders, including narcolepsy. γ-Hydroxybutyrate **(GHB),** an orphan drug, is on trial for cataplexy in sleep disorder centers and is currently regarded favorably in the treatment of narcolepsy and cataplexy. Fewer episodes of sleep paralysis and hypnagogic hallucinations have also been recorded, and some patients have been able to stop or reduce their use of stimulants while taking GHB. Controlled studies of this drug, sponsored by a Food and Drug Administration Orphan Drug research grant, began in 1985. GHB is produced by Biocraft Laboratories.

Vitoxazine hydrochloride is also under study, especially in the control of cataplectic symptoms. For further information contact Stuart Pharmaceuticals, Division of ICI Americas.

Studies have begun in regard to human brain tissue in narcolepsy. Preliminary supposition is that narcoleptic patients may have an excess of dopamine receptors in the amygdala, the area that controls emotions.

The orphan drug modafinil is being studied for treatment of narcolepsy. It is manufactured by Cephalon.

Please contact the agencies listed under Resources, below, for the most current information. Addresses and telephone numbers of these agencies, as well as of individual experts and research centers, may be found in the Master Resources List.

## Resources

**For more information on narcolepsy:** National Organization for Rare Disorders (NORD); Narcolepsy and Cataplexy Foundation of America; Narcolepsy Network; NIH/National Institute of Neurological Disorders and Stroke.

## References

Cecil Textbook of Medicine, 19th ed.: J.B. Wyngaarden, et al., eds.; W.B. Saunders Company, 1992, pp. 2065–2066.
Mendelian Inheritance in Man, 10th ed.: V.A. McKusick; The Johns Hopkins University Press, 1992, pp. 752–753.
Narcolepsy: M.S. Aldrich; Neurology, July 1992, vol. 42(7 suppl. 6), pp. 34–43.
Birth Defects Encyclopedia: M.L. Buyse, ed.-in-chief; Blackwell Scientific Publications, 1990, pp. 1214–1215.
Narcolepsy Update: J.W. Richardson, et al.; Mayo Clin. Proc., July 1990, vol. 65(7), pp. 991–998.
Principles of Neurology, 4th ed.: R.D. Adams and M. Victor, eds.; McGraw-Hill, 1989, pp. 314–317.

# NEMALINE MYOPATHY

**Description** Nemaline myopathy is a congenital disease of the skeletal muscles. Under the microscope, nemaline rods—fine threads—are seen in the muscle fibers.

## Synonyms

Congenital Rod Disease

Rod Myopathy

**Signs and Symptoms** Skeletal muscle floppiness may be apparent in the newborn. The musculature of the thin thighs and upper arms is very weak, as are the trunk muscles; posture may be affected. Neurologic examination of the infant may reveal absence of the deep tendon reflexes, impaired muscle tone, and soft muscles. Involvement of the muscles used in respiration or swallowing may be life-threatening. This condition may be fatal before the age of 2 years. The disease may progress during childhood, but increase in muscle mass during the growing years may offset the progression and the child may show general improvement. The facial muscles can be markedly affected. A high-arched palate, thin face, prominent jaw, and pectus carinatum are sometimes seen. In the adult-onset cases, varying degrees of weakness of shoulder, pelvic girdle, or facial muscles are seen. Cardiomyopathy may also occur.

**Etiology** Nemaline myopathy is inherited as an autosomal dominant trait; a recessive inheritance has also been reported. The biochemical defect involved is not known.

**Epidemiology** The age of onset varies from early childhood to middle life. More females are affected than males.

**Related Disorders** See *Central Core Disease; Congenital Fiber Type Disproportion; Leukodystrophy, Canavan; Muscular Dystrophy, Limb-Girdle; Myopathy, Centronuclear; Werdnig-Hoffmann Disease.*

**Treatment—Standard** Treatment is symptomatic and supportive.

**Treatment—Investigational** Please contact the agencies listed under Resources, below, for the most current information. Addresses and telephone numbers of these agencies, as well as of individual experts and research centers, may be found in the Master Resources List.

## Resources

**For more information on nemaline myopathy:** National Organization for Rare Disorders (NORD); NIH/National Institute of Neurological Disorders and Stroke.

**For genetic information and genetic counseling referrals:** March of Dimes Birth Defects Foundation; Alliance of Genetic Support Groups.

## References

Intranuclear Rods in Severe Congenital Nemaline Myopathy: Z. Rifai, et al.; Neurology, November 1993, vol. 43(11), pp. 2372–2377.
Anaesthesia for Cardiac Surgery in Children with Nemaline Myopathy: T. Asai, et al.; Anaesthesia, May 1992, vol. 47(5), pp. 576–583.

Assignment of a Gene (NEMI) for Autosomal Dominant Nemaline Myopathy to Chromosome I: N.G. Laing, et al.; Am. J. Hum. Genet., March 1992, vol. 50(3), pp. 576–583.

Cecil Textbook of Medicine, 19th ed.: J.B. Wyngaarden, et al., eds.; W.B. Saunders Company, 1992, pp. 2256.

Mendelian Inheritance in Man, 10th ed.: V.A. McKusick; The Johns Hopkins University Press, 1992, pp. 754–755, 1582.

Familial Nemaline Myopathy: Case Reports: K. Antoniades, et al.; Oral Surg. Oral Med. Oral Pathol., July 1991, vol. 72(1), pp. 51–54.

Birth Defects Encyclopedia: M.L. Buyse, ed.-in-chief; Blackwell Scientific Publications, 1990, pp. 1196–1197.

Dictionary of Medical Syndromes, 3rd ed.: S.I. Magalini, et al., eds.; J.B. Lippincott Company, 1990, p. 625.

Principles of Neurology, 4th ed.: R.D. Adams and M. Victor, eds.; McGraw-Hill, 1989, p. 1143.

# NEU-LAXOVA SYNDROME

**Description** Major characteristics of this disorder are generalized edema, unusual facies, fetal growth retardation, joint contractures, scaly skin, and central nervous system abnormalities.

**Signs and Symptoms** Fetal growth retardation as well as generalized edema, especially of the scalp, hands, and feet, are typically present. The skin may be thin and scaly (ichthyotic) or tight and shiny.

Microcephaly with distinct facial features is always present. A short neck, micrognathia, microphthalmia, exophthalmos, hypertelorism, absent eyelids, a broad nasal bridge, and a sloping forehead may also be present.

Limb abnormalities include contractures, syndactyly, and rocker-bottom feet. Less frequent features are underdeveloped skeletal muscle, abnormal external genitalia, cataracts, polymicrogyria, aplasia of the corpus callosum, incomplete development of the cerebellum, and lissencephaly.

**Etiology** The syndrome is thought to be inherited as an autosomal recessive trait. One reported case seems to have occurred sporadically.

**Epidemiology** The disorder is very rare; approximately 20 cases have been reported in the medical literature. Males and females are affected in equal numbers.

**Related Disorders** See *Cerebro-Oculo-Facio-Skeletal Syndrome; Lissencephaly; Pterygium Syndrome, Multiple.*

**Treatment—Standard** Genetic counseling may be of benefit for families of affected patients. Other treatment is symptomatic and supportive.

**Treatment—Investigational** Please contact the agencies listed under Resources, below, for the most current information. Addresses and telephone numbers of these agencies, as well as of individual experts and research centers, may be found in the Master Resources List.

**Resources**

**For more information on Neu-Laxova syndrome:** National Organization for Rare Disorders (NORD); NIH/National Institute of Neurological Disorders and Stroke.

**For genetic information and genetic counseling referrals:** March of Dimes Birth Defects Foundation; Alliance of Genetic Support Groups.

**References**

Mendelian Inheritance in Man, 10th ed.: V.A. McKusick; The Johns Hopkins University Press, 1992, p. 1586.

Neu-Laxova Syndrome: Prenatal Ultrasonographic Diagnosis, Clinical and Pathological Studies, and New Manifestations: I. Shapiro, et al.; Am. J. Med. Gen., June 1, 1992, vol. 43(3), pp. 602–605.

Neu Laxova Syndrome in Two Egyptian Families: N.A. Meguid, et al.; Am. J. Med. Gen., October 1, 1991, vol. 41(1), pp. 30–31.

Birth Defects Encyclopedia: M.L. Buyse, ed.-in-chief; Blackwell Scientific Publications, 1990, pp. 1226–1227.

Neu-Laxova Syndrome: A Case Report: K. Broderick, et al.; Am. J. Obstet. Gynecol., March 1988, vol. 158(3 pt 1), pp. 574–575.

Smith's Recognizable Patterns of Human Malformation, 4th ed.: K.L. Jones, ed.; W.B. Saunders Company, 1988, p. 150.

# NEURASTHENIA

**Description** Neurasthenia is a mental disorder triggered by stress or anxiety. Symptoms include weakness, chest pain, tachycardia, hyperventilation.

**Synonyms**

Cardiac Neurosis

Chronic Asthenia

Da Costa Syndrome

Irritable Heart

Neurocirculatory Asthenia

Soldier's Heart

Subacute Asthenia

**Signs and Symptoms** Major characteristics include a feeling of weakness or fatigue, which may be accompanied by chest pain, palpitations, tachycardia, and cold, clammy hands and feet. The individual often sighs a lot. Hyperventilation and hyperhidrosis may be present. Neurasthenia may accompany depression or other psychological disorders.

**Angiopathic neurasthenia (angioparalytic neurasthenia; pulsating neurasthenia)** is a mild form of the disorder in which the patient feels a pulsing or throbbing sensation throughout the entire body. **Gastric neurasthenia,** also a mild form, is accompanied by dyspepsia and distention. **Neurasthenia gravis** refers to an extreme and persistent form. **Neurasthenia precox (primary neurasthenia)** occurs most often in adolescents and is characterized by nervous exhaustion.

Tests should be done to rule out any underlying organic cause that might lead to the symptoms of neurasthenia.

**Etiology** Neurasthenia is a mental disorder caused by emotional stress or anxiety.

**Epidemiology** The disorder is fairly common and may occur at any time in the life cycle. Males and females are affected in equal numbers.

**Related Disorders** See *Encephalomyelitis, Myalgic; Myasthenia Gravis; Panic-Anxiety Syndrome.*

The symptoms and signs of **hyperthyroidism** include sweating, nervousness, emotional instability, fatigue, insomnia, increased appetite, weight loss, or diarrhea. Tachycardia or atrial fibrillation may occur. Patients may experience heat intolerance, trembling of the hands, or muscle weakness. In older persons depression or heart failure may occur. Thyroid gland enlargement, warm smooth skin, or exophthalmos may be present.

**Treatment—Standard** Treatment includes reassurance that the symptoms are not due to organic causes. Counseling will help the patient learn how to control feelings of stress and anxiety. Biofeedback, sedatives, or tranquilizers may be required.

**Treatment—Investigational** Please contact the agencies listed under Resources, below, for the most current information. Addresses and telephone numbers of these agencies, as well as of individual experts and research centers, may be found in the Master Resources List.

**Resources**

**For more information on neurasthenia:** National Organization for Rare Disorders (NORD); National Mental Health Association; National Alliance for the Mentally Ill; National Mental Health Consumer Self-Help Clearinghouse; NIH/National Institute of Mental Health.

**References**

Feelings of Fatigue and Psychopathology: A Conceptual History: G.E. Berrios; Compr. Psychiatry, March–April 1990, vol. 31(2), pp. 140–151.

Neurasthenia in the 1980s: Chronic Mononucleosis, Chronic Fatigue Syndrome, and Anxiety and Depressive Disorders: D.B. Greenberg; Psychosomatics, Spring 1990, vol. 31(2), pp. 129–137.

Old Wine in New Bottles: Neurasthenia and Me: S. Wessely; Psychol. Med., February 1990, vol. 20(1), pp. 35–53.

Cecil Textbook of Medicine, 18th ed.: J.B. Wyngaarden and L.H. Smith, Jr., eds.; W.B. Saunders Company, 1988, pp. 1322, 1324, 2124–2125, 2286.

Internal Medicine, 2nd ed.: J.H. Stein, ed.-in-chief; Little, Brown and Company, 1987, pp. 374–375.

# NEUROACANTHOCYTOSIS

**Description** The primary characteristics of this disorder are acanthocytosis with normal lipoproteins, and chorea.

**Synonyms**

Choreoacanthocytosis

Levine-Critchley Syndrome

**Signs and Symptoms** Onset of neuroacanthocytosis is usually during adolescence or early adult life. The disorder begins with tics of the face, mouth, and tongue, and slowly progresses to chorea of the trunk and limbs. Dyskinesia of the mouth, tongue, and face become apparent, along with tongue, cheek, and lip biting. Tendon reflexes are absent. Personality changes as well as comprehension, judgment, memory, and cognitive deficits are seen in over half of the cases. Muscle weakness and atrophy eventually affect the arms, legs, and trunk. Approximately half of affected patients have seizures. Parkinson disease has been associated with neuroacanthocytosis in some patients.

**Etiology** The disorder usually is inherited as an autosomal recessive trait. However, there has been one documented family that is thought to have autosomal dominant inheritance.

**Epidemiology** Males and females are affected in equal numbers. Neuroacanthocytosis has been found in the United States, Japan, Great Britain, and Finland.

**Related Disorders** See *Acanthocytosis; Huntington Disease; Parkinson Disease; Sydenham Chorea; Tourette Syndrome; Wilson Disease.*

**Treatment—Standard** Some patients with chorea benefit from dopamine-blocking drugs such as haloperidol. Anticonvulsant drugs are used to help control seizures. Genetic counseling may be of benefit for patients and their families. Other treatment is symptomatic and supportive.

**Treatment—Investigational** Please contact the agencies listed under Resources, below, for the most current information. Addresses and telephone numbers of these agencies, as well as of individual experts and research centers, may be found in the Master Resources List.

**Resources**

For more information on **neuroacanthocytosis:** National Organization for Rare Disorders (NORD); NIH/National Institute of Neurological Disorders and Stroke.

For **genetic information and genetic counseling referrals:** March of Dimes Birth Defects Foundation; Alliance of Genetic Support Groups.

**References**

Birth Defects Encyclopedia: M.L. Buyse, ed.-in-chief; Blackwell Scientific Publications, 1990, pp. 4–5.

Hematology, 4th ed.: W.J. Williams, et al, eds.; McGraw-Hill, 1990, pp. 584–585.

Mendelian Inheritance in Man, 9th ed.: V.A. McKusick; The Johns Hopkins University Press, 1990, p. 5.

Regional Brain Glucose Metabolism in Neuroacanthocytosis: R.M. Dubinsky, et al.; Neurology, September 1989, vol. 39(9), pp. 1253–1255.


# NEUROLEPTIC MALIGNANT SYNDROME (NMS)

**Description** NMS is an idiosyncratic reaction to neuroleptics. Haloperidol, chlorpromazine, fluphenazine, thioridazine, trifluoperazine, and perphenazine are among the drugs most commonly involved.

**Signs and Symptoms** Manifestations include irregular pulse, tachycardia, tachypnea, hyperpyrexia (102° to 104° F; 39° to 40° C), diaphoresis, hyper- or hypotension, incontinence, seizures, tremors, muscle rigidity, and altered mental status. Liver or kidney failure, hyperkalemia, rhabdomyolysis, or arterial and venous blood clots may also occur.

**Etiology** NMS may be due to a neuroleptic-induced blockade of dopamine neurotransmission. Hyperthermia may be due to the resultant muscle rigidity produced by striatal dopamine blockade and/or direct hypothalamic thermoregulatory injury.

**Epidemiology** Any individual taking neuroleptics may be affected. Men appear to be at higher risk than women.

**Related Disorders** See ***Malignant Hyperthermia; Tardive Dyskinesia.***

**Treatment– Standard** Neuroleptic medications should be withdrawn, and measures instituted to provide adequate hydration and nutrition as well as the lowering of body temperature. Medications may include dantrolene, bromocriptine, and levodopa. Secondary complications such as acidosis, hypoxia, and renal insufficiency must be treated independently.

Most patients recover completely, but fatalities have occurred.

**Treatment—Investigational** Please contact the agencies listed under Resources, below, for the most current information. Addresses and telephone numbers of these agencies, as well as of individual experts and research centers, may be found in the Master Resources List.

**Resources**

For more information on **neuroleptic malignant syndrome:** National Organization for Rare Disorders (NORD); National Mental Health Association; National Alliance for the Mentally Ill; National Mental Health Consumer Self-Help Clearinghouse; NIH/National Institute of Mental Health; Malignant Hyperthermia Association of the United States.

**References**

Clinical Differentiation Between Lethal Catatonia and Neuroleptic Malignant Syndrome: E. Castillo, et al.; Am. J. Psychiatry, March 1989, vol. 146(3), pp. 324–328.

Patients with Neuroleptic Malignant Syndrome Histories: What Happens When They Are Hospitalized?: A.J. Gelenberg, et al.; J. Clin. Psychiatry, May 1989, vol. 50(5), pp. 18–25.

Recurrence of Neuroleptic Malignant Syndrome: V.L. Susman, et al.; J. Nerv. Ment. Dis., April 1988, vol. 176(4), pp. 234–241.


# NEUROPATHY, CONGENITAL HYPOMYELINATION

**Description** Congenital hypomyelination neuropathy is a neurologic disorder present at birth. Symptoms include respiratory difficulty and delayed motor development.

**Synonyms**

Congenital Dysmyelinating Neuropathy

Congenital Hypomyelination (Onion Bulb) Polyneuropathy
Hypomyelination Neuropathy

**Signs and Symptoms** Symptoms and signs and their severity vary from patient to patient: delayed motor development, muscle weakness, hypotonia, impaired muscle coordination, areflexia, difficulty in walking or crawling, and mild distal palsy. In some infants, respiratory problems or dysphagia may occur. Abnormal microscopic changes in certain nerves (e.g., sural nerves) can occur.

**Etiology** A recurrent loss and repair of myelin results in congenital hypomyelination neuropathy, but the underlying cause is unknown. It has been hypothesized, but not established, that the disorder is a subtype of Dejerine-Sottas disease, which is inherited as an autosomal dominant trait. Other disorders characterized by the loss and repair of the myelin sheath may be immune-mediated.

**Epidemiology** Congenital hypomyelination neuropathy is present at birth. Males and females are affected in equal numbers.

**Related Disorders** See *Dejerine-Sottas Disease; Guillain-Barré Syndrome.*

**Treatment—Standard** Treatment is symptomatic and supportive. Diagnostic procedures include electromyography as well as nerve and muscle biopsies.

**Treatment—Investigational** Please contact the agencies listed under Resources, below, for the most current information. Addresses and telephone numbers of these agencies, as well as of individual experts and research centers, may be found in the Master Resources List.

**Resources**

**For more information on congenital hypomyelination neuropathy:** National Organization for Rare Disorders (NORD); NIH/National Institute of Neurological Disorders and Stroke.

**For genetic information and genetic counseling referrals:** March of Dimes Birth Defects Foundation; Alliance of Genetic Support Groups.

**References**

Two Cases of Congenital Hypomyelination Neuropathy: N. Tachi, et al.; Brain Dev., 1984, vol. 6(6), pp. 560–565.

Congenital Hypomyelination Neuropathy in a Newborn: S. Hakamada, et al.; Neuropediatrics, August 1983, vol. 14(3), pp. 182–183.

Congenital Hypomyelination Polyneuropathy: Pathological Findings Compared with Polyneuropathies Starting Later in Life: F. Guzzetta, et al.; Brain, June 1982, vol. 105(pt. 2), pp. 395–416.

# NEUROPATHY, GIANT AXONAL

**Description** Giant axonal neuropathy is a genetic disorder that first appears between infancy and 8 years, and is slowly progressive. Both central and peripheral nervous systems are involved.

**Synonyms**

Congenital Giant Axonal Neuropathy

**Signs and Symptoms** Features include loss of sensation in the legs and feet, ataxia, weakness, hyporeflexia, and poor vision. Hearing may be affected. Tightly curled, kinky hair, often very pale in color, is characteristic of the disorder but is not present in all patients. Other symptoms and signs include nystagmus, dysarthria, unusual leg posture, fasciculations, diminished tendon reflexes, and epilepsy. Progressive intellectual deterioration can occur.

Diagnosis can be made by sural nerve biopsy.

**Etiology** Giant axonal neuropathy is inherited as an autosomal recessive trait.

**Epidemiology** The disorder is present at birth. Males and females are affected in equal numbers.

**Related Disorders** See *Seitelberger Disease; Incontinentia Pigmenti.*

**Treatment—Standard** Treatment is symptomatic and supportive. Genetic counseling will benefit patients and their families.

**Treatment—Investigational** Please contact the agencies listed under Resources, below, for the most current information. Addresses and telephone numbers of these agencies, as well as of individual experts and research centers, may be found in the Master Resources List.

**Resources**

**For more information on giant axonal neuropathy:** National Organization for Rare Disorders (NORD); Children's Brain Diseases Foundation for Research; The Arc (a national organization on mental retardation); NIH/National Institute of Neurological Disorders and Stroke.

**For genetic information and genetic counseling referrals:** March of Dimes Birth Defects Foundation; Alliance of Genetic Support Groups.

**References**

Giant Axonal Neuropathy with Inherited Multisystem Degeneration in a Tunisian Kindred: M.B. Hamida, et al.; Neurology, February 1990, vol. 40(2), pp. 245–250.

A Giant Axonal Neuropathy: Review: R.A. Ouvrier; Brain Dev., 1989, vol. 11(4), pp. 207–214.

Giant Axonal Neuropathy: Observations on a Further Patient: M. Donaghy, et al.; J. Neurol. Neurosurg., Psychiatry, July 1988, vol. 51(7), pp. 991–994.

Childhood Giant Axonal Neuropathy: Case Report and Review of the Literature: R. Tandan, et al.; J. Neurol. Sci., December 1987, vol. 82(1–3), pp. 205–228.

Giant Axonal Neuropathy: Correlation of Clinical Findings with Postmortem Neuropathology: C. Thomas, et al.; Ann. Neurol., July 1987, vol. 22(1), pp. 79–84.

Giant Axonal Neuropathy: Central Abnormalities Demonstrated by Evoked Potentials: A. Majnemer, et al.; Ann. Neurol., April 1986, vol. 19(4), pp. 394–396.

Mendelian Inheritance in Man, 8th ed.: V.A. McKusick; The Johns Hopkins University Press, 1986, pp. 506, 893, 1090–1091.

Congenital Giant Axonal Neuropathy: R.B. Kinney, et al.; Arch. Pathol. Lab. Med., July 1985, vol. 109(7), pp. 639–641.

Giant Axonal Neuropathy: A Conditional Mutation Affecting Cytoskeletal Organization: M.W. Klymkowsky, et al.; J. Cell Biol., January 1985, vol. 100(1), pp. 245–250.

# NEUROPATHY, HEREDITARY SENSORY, TYPE I

**Description** Hereditary sensory neuropathy type I is a rare autosomal dominant disorder accompanied by slowly progressive loss of sensation primarily in the feet and legs, and by ulcers on the feet.

**Synonyms**

> Acrodystrophic Neuropathy
> Hereditary Sensory and Autonomic Neuropathy Type I
> Hereditary Sensory Radicular Neuropathy
> Mutilating Acropathy

**Signs and Symptoms** Primary characteristics are loss of sensation, usually affecting the feet and legs more severely than the hands and forearms. Pain and temperature sensations are affected more than touch-pressure. Some patients experience lancinating pains. As the disorder progresses, perforating ulcers may develop on the feet. Reflexes in the legs are decreased or absent. Deafness occasionally occurs.

**Etiology** Inheritance is autosomal dominant. Symptoms are caused by degeneration of nerve fibers. Diagnosis is by biopsy.

**Epidemiology** The disorder is present at birth, but symptom development is usually in adulthood, occasionally during childhood (generally between 10 and 30 years of age).

**Related Disorders** See *Charcot-Marie-Tooth Disease; Neuropathy, Hereditary Sensory, Type II; Peripheral Neuropathy; Syringomyelia; Roussy-Lévy Syndrome.*

**Treatment—Standard** Treatment is symptomatic and supportive. Genetic counseling may be beneficial.

**Treatment—Investigational** Please contact the agencies listed under Resources, below, for the most current information. Addresses and telephone numbers of these agencies, as well as of individual experts and research centers, may be found in the Master Resources List.

**Resources**

**For more information on hereditary sensory neuropathy type I:** National Organization for Rare Disorders (NORD); NIH/National Institute of Neurological Disorders and Stroke.

**For genetic information and genetic counseling referrals:** March of Dimes Birth Defects Foundation; Alliance of Genetic Support Groups.

**References**

Persistent Skin Ulcers, Mutilations, and Acro-Osteolysis in Hereditary Sensory and Autonomic Neuropathy with Phospholipid Excretion: Report of a Family: M. Bockers, et al.; J. Am. Acad. Dermatol., October 1989, vol. 21(4 pt. 1), pp. 736–739.

Cecil Textbook of Medicine, 18th ed.: J.B. Wyngaarden and L.H. Smith, Jr., eds.; W.B. Saunders Company, 1988, p. 2284.

Mendelian Inheritance in Man, 8th ed.: V.A. McKusick; The Johns Hopkins University Press, 1986, pp. 506, 893, 1090–1091.

# NEUROPATHY, HEREDITARY SENSORY, TYPE II

**Description** Hereditary sensory neuropathy type II is a rare autosomal recessive disorder with symptoms presenting in childhood. Paronychial infection and kinesthetic loss in arms and legs are characteristic.

**Synonyms**

> Congenital Sensory Neuropathy
> Hereditary Sensory and Autonomic Neuropathy Type II
> Hereditary Sensory Radicular Neuropathy, Recessive Form

**Signs and Symptoms** Slowly progressive abnormalities of sensation occur diffusely, involving hands, feet, face, and trunk. Usually touch and pressure sensations are more affected than pain and temperature sensations. Characteristics include paronychia and whitlow, generally accompanied by pus and infection, and by ulcers on the fingers and soles, in some cases leading to osteomyelitis or osteolysis. There may be kinesthetic loss affecting the skin and sometimes the muscles, tendons, or joints, resulting in unsteady movement. Fractures of the limbs may occur without the patient's awareness. Tendon reflexes may be absent. Sweating may be impaired.

**Etiology** The disorder is inherited as an autosomal recessive trait.

**Epidemiology** Although the condition is present at birth, symptoms usually develop during infancy or childhood. Males and females are affected in equal numbers.

**Related Disorders** See *Charcot-Marie-Tooth Disease; Neuropathy, Hereditary Sensory, Type I; Peripheral Neuropathy; Roussy-Lévy Syndrome; Syringomyelia.*

**Treatment—Standard** Treatment is symptomatic and supportive. Genetic counseling may be of benefit.

**Treatment—Investigational** Please contact the agencies listed under Resources, below, for the most current information. Addresses and telephone numbers of these agencies, as well as of individual experts and research centers, may be found in the Master Resources List.

**Resources**

For more information on hereditary sensory neuropathy type II: National Organization for Rare Disorders (NORD); NIH/National Institute of Neurological Disorders and Stroke.

For genetic information and genetic counseling referrals: March of Dimes Birth Defects Foundation; Alliance of Genetic Support Groups.

**References**

Persistent Skin Ulcers, Mutilations, and Acro-Osteolysis in Hereditary Sensory and Autonomic Neuropathy with Phospholipid Excretion: Report of a Family: M. Bockers, et al.; J. Am. Acad. Dermatol., October 1989, vol. 21(4 pt. 1), pp. 736–739.

Cecil Textbook of Medicine, 18th ed.: J.B. Wyngaarden and L.H. Smith, Jr., eds.; W.B. Saunders Company, 1988, pp. 2264–2265.

Paucifascicular Congenital Sensory Neuropathy in Identical Twins: G.B. Croall, et al.; Am. J. Dis. Child, June 1986, vol. 140(6), pp. 589–595.

# OBSESSIVE-COMPULSIVE DISORDER

**Description** Obsessive-compulsive disorder is a psychiatric condition in which persistently recurrent ideas and fantasies and specific repetitive actions and impulses cause marked distress and interfere with the person's normal routine. Inner conflict, anxiety, and depression are common associated characteristics.

**Synonyms**

Obsessive-Compulsive Neurosis

**Signs and Symptoms** Common obsessions range from worrying over whether one has locked a door or been contaminated by contact with another person or thing, to repeated impulses toward violence. The individual usually recognizes that these ideas, images, or impulses are intrinsic to himself and attempts to suppress them. Compulsive behaviors include repetitive hand-washing, verifying, and touching. The individual may resist such impulses, but acting on them relieves tension. The course of the disorder is variable and chronic, with mild, moderate, or severe symptomatic episodes followed by intermittent periods of remission.

**Etiology** The cause of obsessive-compulsive disorder is not known.

**Epidemiology** Symptoms are commonly first seen in the teen and early adult years, although childhood onset is possible. Males and females are affected in equal numbers. The mild form of this disorder may be quite common; only a small percentage of affected persons are impaired significantly enough to warrant treatment.

**Related Disorders** The disorder may be differentiated from **obsessive-compulsive personality disorder,** whose characteristics are perfectionism and inflexibility, exemplified by such behaviors as avoidance of decision-making; preoccupation with details, rules, and efficiency; and inability to express affection.

**Treatment—Standard** Appropriate treatment options for obsessive-compulsive disorder include insight psychotherapy, supportive therapy, behavioral techniques, or pharmacologic therapy. Fluoxetine (Prozac), clomipramine (Anafranil), and fluvoxamine (Luvox) are effective for treatment of this condition.

**Treatment—Investigational** Intravenous use of clomipramine is under study for treatment of persons who have side effects to the oral form of the drug.

Please contact the agencies listed under Resources, below, for the most current information. Addresses and telephone numbers of these agencies, as well as of individual experts and research centers, may be found in the Master Resources List.

**Resources**

**For more information on obsessive-compulsive disorder:** National Organization for Rare Disorders (NORD); Obsessive-Compulsive Foundation; NIH/National Institute of Mental Health; National Mental Health Association; National Alliance for the Mentally Ill; National Mental Health Consumer Self-Help Clearinghouse.

**References**

Diagnostic and Statistical Manual of Mental Disorders, 3rd ed., revised: R.L. Spitzer, et al., eds.; American Psychiatric Association, 1987, pp. 245–247, 354–356.

Biological Factors in Obsessive-Compulsive Disorders: S.M. Turner, et al.; Psychol. Bull., 1985, vol. 97(3), pp. 430–450.

Intravenous Chlorimipramine in the Treatment of Obsessional Disorder in Adolescence: Case Report: L.B. Warneke; J. Clin. Psychiatry, March 1985, vol. 46(3), pp. 100–103.

Psychotherapeutic Management of Obsessive-Compulsive Patients: L. Salzman; Am. J. Psychother., July 1985, vol. 39(3), pp. 323–330.

Evidence for a Biological Hypothesis of Obsessive-Compulsive Disorder: J.Lieberman; Neuropsychobiology, 1984, vol. 11, pp. 14–21.

Successful Treatment of Obsessive-Compulsive Disorder with ECT: L.A. Melman, et al.; Am. J. Psychiatry, April 1984, vol. 141(4), pp. 596–597.

# OLIVOPONTOCEREBELLAR ATROPHY

**Description** Olivopontocerebellar atrophy describes 5 inherited forms of ataxia characterized by degeneration of the cerebellar cortex, the middle peduncles, and the inferior olivary bodies: type I (Menzel type); type II (Fickler-Winkler type; Dejerine-Thomas type); type III (with retinal degeneration); type IV (Schut-Haymaker type); and type V (with dementia and extrapyramidal signs).

**Synonyms**

Multiple Systems Atrophy

**Signs and Symptoms** Manifestations vary and include ataxia, spasticity, and chorea. Retinitis pigmentosa, ophthalmoplegia, dysphagia, and dementia may also be present. As discussed above, 5 clinical types of olivopontocerebellar atrophy have been described.

**Olivopontocerebellar atrophy type I (Menzel type)** is characterized by cerebellar degeneration, speech disturbances, and chorea. Average age at onset of symptoms is 30 years.

**Olivopontocerebellar atrophy type II (Fickler-Winkler or Dejerine-Thomas type)** is not well understood; the disorder appears to manifest at around age 50 years.

**Olivopontocerebellar atrophy type III (with retinal degeneration)** is characterized by blindness, tremor, weakness, and ataxia.

**Olivopontocerebellar atrophy type IV (Schut-Haymaker type)** is accompanied by abnormalities of the spinal cord and cranial nerves. Spastic paraplegia and other symptoms manifest during the middle 20s.

**Olivopontocerebellar atrophy type V (with dementia and extrapyramidal signs)** manifests as cerebellar atrophy, tremor, ataxia, rigidity, and mental deterioration in affected adults.

**Etiology** Types I and III through V are inherited as autosomal dominant traits. Olivopontocerebellar atrophy type II is inherited as an autosomal recessive trait.

**Epidemiology** The 5 forms of the disorder appear to affect males and females in equal numbers.

**Related Disorders** See *Ataxia, Friedreich; Ataxia, Marie; Ataxia Telangiectasia; Charcot-Marie-Tooth Disease.*

**Treatment—Standard** Treatment of olivopontocerebellar atrophy is symptomatic and supportive. Pharmacologic therapy with propranolol or dantrolene sodium may be beneficial in the management of static tremors and muscle spasms, respectively. Physical therapy may be helpful; genetic counseling is recommended.

**Treatment—Investigational** Please contact the agencies listed under Resources, below, for the most current information. Addresses and telephone numbers of these agencies, as well as of individual experts and research centers, may be found in the Master Resources List.

**Resources**

**For more information on olivopontocerebellar atrophy:** National Organization for Rare Disorders (NORD); National Ataxia Foundation; NIH/National Institute of Neurological Disorders and Stroke.

**For genetic information and genetic counseling referrals:** March of Dimes Birth Defects Foundation; Alliance of Genetic Support Groups.

**References**

Mendelian Inheritance in Man, 9th ed.: V.A. McKusick; The Johns Hopkins University Press, 1990, pp. 671–674, 1392.

Olivopontocerebellar Atrophy with Dementia, Blindness, and Chorea. Response to Baclofen: D.A. Trauner; Arch. Neurol., August 1985, vol. 42(8), pp. 757–758.

An Apology and an Introduction to the Olivopontocerebellar Atrophies: R.C. Duvoisin; Adv. Neurol., 1984, vol. 41, pp. 5–12.

# ONDINE'S CURSE

**Description** Ondine's curse is characterized by dysfunction of the central regulation of respiration. The disorder typically affects infants. Insufficient aeration of the lungs due to shallow breathing may cause brain damage and death.

**Synonyms**

>Congenital Central Hypoventilation Syndrome
>Primary Central Hypoventilation Syndrome

**Signs and Symptoms** The clinical picture is dominated by nocturnal hypoventilation, resulting in hypoxemia, hypercapnia, and acidosis. Other symptoms and signs include restlessness, hypertension, hypotonia, tachycardia, apnea, stupor, and coma. Approximately 70 percent of infants also have epileptic seizures. Severity of the symptoms in infants may decrease with age.

**Etiology** Although the genetic defect is not known, it is thought that most cases are inherited as an autosomal recessive trait.

**Epidemiology** Congenital central hypoventilation syndrome begins in infancy. Rarely, trauma (surgical or accidental) may precipitate the syndrome in adolescents and adults. Males and females are affected in equal numbers. Approximately 65 cases have been reported in the medical literature.

**Related Disorders** Congenital central hypoventilation syndrome must be distinguished from infantile apnea, characterized by intermittent cessation of breathing, and from chronic obstructive lung disease, characterized by dyspnea, coughing, and an onset coinciding with bronchiolitis. See ***Apnea, Infantile.***

**Treatment—Standard** Monitoring of sleep patterns is recommended.

Respiratory stimulants such as almitrine and dimefline may be prescribed to deepen nocturnal respiration and improve blood gas values. Tracheostomy and cribral cannulation have been used for surgical correction. Assisted breathing techniques include diaphragmatic pacing (electrophrenic or radio frequency respiration).

**Treatment—Investigational** An MK8-Bird respirator and compressor have been used in treatment. For more information, contact William Tamborlane, Jr., M.D., Yale University School of Medicine.

For information on clinical trials to study diaphragm pacing, contact John Elefteriades, M.D., Yale University School of Medicine.

Please contact the agencies listed under Resources, below, for the most current information. Addresses and telephone numbers of these agencies, as well as of individual experts and research centers, may be found in the Master Resources List.

**Resources**

**For more information on Ondine's curse:** National Organization for Rare Disorders (NORD); NIH/National Institute of Neurological Disorders and Stroke; NIH/National Institute of Child Health and Human Development; Congenital Central Hypoventilation Syndrome Family Support Network.

**References**

Ventilatory Response to Exercise in Children with Congenital Central Hypoventilation Syndrome: J.Y. Paton,, et al.; Am. Rev. Respir. Dis., May 1993, vol. 147(5), pp. 1185–1191.

Cecil Textbook of Medicine, 19th ed.: J.B. Wyngaarden, et al., eds.; W.B. Saunders Company, 1992, pp. 378–380.

Congenital Central Hypoventilation Syndrome: Diagnosis, Management, and Long-Term Outcome in Thirty-Two Children: D.E. Weese-Mayer, et al.; J. Pediatr., March 1992, vol. 120(3), pp. 381–387.

Mendelian Inheritance in Man, 10th ed.: V.A. McKusick; The Johns Hopkins University Press, 1992, p. 1246.

Nelson Textbook of Pediatrics, 14th ed.: R.E. Behrman, ed.-in-chief; W.B. Saunders Company, 1992, p. 465.

Neuropsychologic Abnormalities in Children with Congenital Central Hypoventilation Syndrome: J.M. Silvestri, et al.; J. Pediatr., March 1992, vol. 120(3), pp. 388–393.

Medical and Psychosocial Outcome of Children with Congenital Central Hypoventilation Syndrome: C.L. Marcus, et al.; J. Pediatr., December 1991, vol. 119(6), pp. 888–895.

Birth Defects Encyclopedia: M.L. Buyse, ed.-in-chief; Blackwell Scientific Publications, 1990, p. 934.

Dictionary of Medical Syndromes, 3rd ed.: S.I. Magalini, et al., eds.; J.B. Lippincott Company, 1990, p. 648.

# PANIC-ANXIETY SYNDROME

**Description** Panic-anxiety syndrome is a psychiatric disorder characterized by acute attacks of anxiety or panic with no apparent cause. These attacks tend to be unpredictable and recurrent.

**Synonyms**

>Anxiety Neurosis
>Anxiety State
>Panic Disorder

**Signs and Symptoms** The primary feature is acute anxiety, or panic, that initially develops abruptly for no evident reason and interferes temporarily with rational thoughts and behavior. Later, the patient may relate certain events with his feelings of anxiety or panic. Psychological symptoms may include intense apprehension; unreasonable fear of impending doom, such as fear of dying or becoming insane; or dread of losing self-control. Cardiorespiratory symptoms are the most common physical manifestations, such as dyspnea, tachycardia, palpitations, sweating, trembling, and dizziness or faintness. Patients also may experience chest pain, feelings of unreality, unusual sensations (burning or pricking), or hot and cold flashes. Attacks occur suddenly, typically last only a few minutes to an hour, and follow a chronic course.

Secondary complications may develop. Fear of losing control may result in **agoraphobia,** the fear of being in places or situations that are difficult to escape from or in which help might not be available. Fear of future attacks may cause patients to experience nervousness, muscle tension, and increased blood pressure and heart rate between attacks. Attempts to alleviate the constant nervousness can lead to abuse of alcohol or antianxiety medications. Depressive disorders also can develop as an associated complication.

**Etiology** Although the specific cause of panic-anxiety disorder is unknown, disruption of important interpersonal relationships may predispose to the development of the condition. Excessive secretion of the hormone norepinephrine, which stimulates the autonomic nervous system, is one possible effect of panic-anxiety disorders which may produce some of the symptoms, such as tachycardia. Hypersensitivity to lactates, which usually accumulate during physical exertion, also may be a contributing factor. Studies with caffeine suggest a potential relationship between panic-anxiety syndrome and abnormalities in the neural systems involving adenosine.

Researchers have been able to trigger panic attacks by exposing patients to carbon dioxide or some other substances. Cholecystokinin has been found to provoke panic attacks 20 seconds after injection. The significance of this finding is unclear.

**Epidemiology** Females tend to be affected more frequently than males in panic disorder with agoraphobia, but panic disorder without agoraphobia is equally common in males and females. The average age of onset is usually in the late 20s.

**Related Disorders Phobias** can cause physical symptoms that resemble panic-anxiety syndrome; however, these symptoms occur only in response to specific stimuli. Panic-anxiety syndrome may be differentiated by the unpredictability of the anxiety attacks.

**Withdrawal from barbiturates and substance intoxications** (caffeine, alcohol, or amphetamines) also may produce symptoms of panic attacks.

The chronic anxiety characteristic of **generalized anxiety disorder** often resembles the anxiety that can develop between attacks in panic-anxiety syndrome. However, the typical recurrent fits of panic associated with the latter are not evident in generalized anxiety disorder.

Panic attacks can occur with such other psychiatric disorders as **major depression** or **somatization disorder.**

**Treatment—Standard** Alprazolam and imipramine hydrochloride are the main therapeutic agents used to treat panic-anxiety syndrome.

**Treatment—Investigational** Please contact the agencies listed under Resources, below, for the most current information. Addresses and telephone numbers of these agencies, as well as of individual experts and research centers, may be found in the Master Resources List.

**Resources**

For more information on **panic-anxiety syndrome:** National Organization for Rare Disorders (NORD); Anxiety Disorders Association of America; Mental Health Association; NIH/National Institute of Mental Health; National Mental Health Consumer Self-Help Clearinghouse.

**References**

Diagnostic and Statistical Manual of Psychiatric Illness, 3rd ed., revised: R.L. Spitzer, et al., eds.; American Psychiatric Association, 1987, pp. 235–241.

Neuroendocrine Correlates of Lactate-Induced Anxiety and Their Response to Chronic Alprazolam Therapy: D.B. Carr, et al.; Am. J. Psychiatry, April 1986, vol. 4(143), pp. 483–494.

Increased Anxiogenic Effects of Caffeine in Panic Disorders: D.S. Charney, et al.; Arch. Gen. Psychiatry, March 1985, vol. 3(42), pp. 233–243.

Noradrenergic Function and the Mechanism of Action of Antianxiety Treatment: D.S. Charney and G.R. Heninger; Arch. Gen. Psychiatry, May 1985, vol. 5(42), pp. 473–481.

# PARAMYOTONIA CONGENITA

**Description** A nonprogressive myotonia characterizes this disorder, which is usually apparent during infancy.

**Synonyms**

Eulenburg Disease

Myotonia Congenita Intermittens

Paralysis Periodica Paramyotonica
Von Eulenburg Paramyotonia Congenita

**Signs and Symptoms** The muscles of the face, tongue, and hands are most often affected. The myotonia may be provoked and worsened with exposure to cold temperatures, and weakness may occur. Rewarming may relieve these symptoms. Cold exposure often leads to stiffness or to passive resistance to stretch, followed by weakness or paralysis. Muscle soreness occurs during attacks. Calf hypertrophy can occur. Paradoxical myotonia may be present.

**Etiology** Paramyotonia congenita is inherited as an autosomal dominant trait.

**Epidemiology** The disorder is very rare. Three large families with multiple generations of affected members have accounted for at least 60 cases. Males and females are affected in equal numbers.

**Related Disorders** See *Myotonic Dystrophy; Thomsen Disease.*

**Hyperkalemic periodic paralysis** is inherited as an autosomal dominant trait and typically detected during infancy. The disorder is characterized by periodic muscle weakness (with or without myotonia) in the calves, thighs, lower back, arms, neck, and/or eyelids. Attacks may occur once a week or several times a day, and typically last from 30 minutes to 1 hour. Periods of muscle weakness usually follow rest after exercise, hunger, infection, exposure to cold temperatures, or emotional stress.

**Treatment—Standard** Acetazolamide or thiazide diuretic drugs may reduce the number of paralytic attacks in some patients. Tocainide may help reduce the cold-induced symptoms. Verapamil and mexiletine may be useful in some cases. Genetic counseling may be of benefit for patients and their families. Other treatment is symptomatic and supportive.

**Treatment—Investigational** Please contact the agencies listed under Resources, below, for the most current information. Addresses and telephone numbers of these agencies, as well as of individual experts and research centers, may be found in the Master Resources List.

**Resources**

**For more information on paramyotonia congenita:** National Organization for Rare Disorders (NORD); NIH/National Arthritis and Musculoskeletal and Skin Diseases.

**For genetic information and genetic counseling referrals:** March of Dimes Birth Defects Foundation; Alliance of Genetic Support Groups.

**References**

Cecil Textbook of Medicine, 19th ed.: J.B. Wyngaarden, et al., eds.; W.B. Saunders Company, 1992, p. 2284.

Birth Defects Encyclopedia: M.L. Buyse, ed.-in-chief; Blackwell Scientific Publications, 1990, pp. 1365–1366.

Mendelian Inheritance in Man, 9th ed.: V.A. McKusick; The Johns Hopkins University Press, 1990, p. 708.

Paramyotonia Congenita or Hyperkalemic Periodic Paralysis? Clinical and Electrophysiological Features of Each Entity in One Family: S.M. de Silva, et al.; Muscle Nerve, January 1990, vol. 13(1), pp. 21–26.

Principles of Neurology, 4th ed.: R.D. Adams and M. Victor, eds.; McGraw-Hill, 1989, p. 1163.

# PARAPLEGIA, HEREDITARY SPASTIC

**Description** Hereditary spastic paraplegia is characterized by slow, progressive degeneration of the corticospinal tract. Manifestations of the disorder vary in accordance with the extent of neurologic damage and the mode of genetic inheritance, but they generally include muscle spasticity, weakness, and paralysis.

**Synonyms**

Spasmodic Infantile Paraplegia
Spastic Congenital Paraplegia
Strümpell-Lorrain Familial Spasmodic Paraplegia

**Signs and Symptoms** Symptoms may first appear in early childhood or later in life. Weakness, stiffness, delay in walking, and spasticity of leg muscles may progress to muscle groups in other parts of the body. Increased tendon reflexes, generalized weakness, and urinary disturbances develop as the disorder progresses.

**Etiology** The disorder may be inherited as an autosomal dominant or recessive trait.

**Related Disorders** See *Arteriovenous Malformation; Werdnig-Hoffmann Disease.*

**Treatment—Standard** Treatment of hereditary spastic paraplegia is symptomatic and supportive. Foot bracing and physical therapy may be beneficial. Genetic counseling is recommended.

**Treatment—Investigational** The Food and Drug Administration has awarded an orphan drug research grant to John H. Growdon, M.D., Massachusetts General Hospital, Boston, for studies on the experimental drug L-threonine for hereditary spastic paraplegia.

Infusion of the drug baclofen by a surgically implanted pump is being studied for spasticity, under a Food and Drug Administration orphan drug grant. Infusion of the drug directly into the spinal space, rather than oral administration, seems to provide patients with better relief of spasticity and improve muscle tone for longer periods of time. Less baclofen is needed when administered in this way.

Please contact the agencies listed under Resources, below, for the most current information. Addresses and telephone numbers of these agencies, as well as of individual experts and research centers, may be found in the Master Resources List.

### Resources
**For more information on hereditary spastic paraplegia:** National Organization for Rare Disorders (NORD); NIH/National Institute of Neurological Disorders and Stroke; International Tremor Foundation.

**For genetic information and genetic counseling referrals:** March of Dimes Birth Defects Foundation; Alliance of Genetic Support Groups.

### References
Familial Spastic Paraparesis Syndrome Association with HTLV-1 Infection: E.F. Solazar-Grueso, et al.; N. Engl. J. Med., September 13, 1990, vol. 323(11), pp. 732–737.

Intrathecal Baclofen for Severe Spasticity: R.D. Penn, et al.; N. Engl. J. Med., June 8, 1989, vol. 320(23), pp. 1517–1521.

Familial Spastic Paraplegia, Mental Retardation, and Precocious Puberty: M.I. Raphaelson, et al.; Arch. Neurol., December 1983, vol. 40(13), pp. 809–810.

# PARENCHYMATOUS CORTICAL DEGENERATION OF THE CEREBELLUM

**Description** Deterioration of the superficial layer of the cerebellum occurs in parenchymatous cortical degeneration of the cerebellum. Disability increases as the disease progresses.

### Synonyms
Parenchymatous Cerebellar Disease

**Signs and Symptoms** Deterioration of the cerebellum gradually leads to slurring of speech, tremor of the lower extremities, and incoordination of the upper extremities.

Microscopic examination reveals the loss of certain cells and fibers of the cerebellar cortex, such as Purkinje cells, granular cells, and olivocerebellar fibers.

**Etiology** Parenchymatous cortical degeneration of the cerebellum may be inherited, or may be associated with underlying disease, especially cancer or alcoholism.

**Epidemiology** Symptom onset is usually during adulthood, although it may occur at any time.

**Treatment—Standard** Treatment is symptomatic and supportive.

**Treatment—Investigational** Please contact the agencies listed under Resources, below, for the most current information. Addresses and telephone numbers of these agencies, as well as of individual experts and research centers, may be found in the Master Resources List.

### Resources
**For more information on parenchymatous cortical degeneration of the cerebellum:** National Organization for Rare Disorders (NORD); NIH/National Institute of Neurological Disorders and Stroke; NIH/National Institute on Aging; International Tremor Foundation.

**For genetic information and genetic counseling referrals:** March of Dimes Birth Defects Foundation; Alliance of Genetic Support Groups.

# PARKINSON DISEASE

**Description** Parkinson disease is a slowly progressive neurologic condition marked by tremor, muscular rigidity, slowness of movement, and difficulty initiating voluntary movements. Degenerative changes occur in the substantia nigra and other pigmented regions of the brain, accompanied by a decrease in dopamine levels in the brain. Parkinsonian symptoms occasionally develop secondary to cerebral trauma or encephalitis, or exposure to certain drugs and toxins. The disease may not become incapacitating for many years.

### Synonyms
Hunt Corpus Striatum Syndrome
Juvenile Parkinsonism of Hunt
Pallidopyramidal Syndrome
Paralysis Agitans
Parkinsonism
Shaking Palsy

**Signs and Symptoms** Onset is insidious and often marked by a slight tremor, especially in the hands. Initially, the tremor occurs at rest, then becomes more pronounced with fatigue and emotional stress, diminishing during voluntary movements. The tremor may be limited to the arms or extend to the neck, jaw, and legs. Voluntary movements such as walking become increasingly difficult, and gait becomes slow, stiff, and shuffling. Cognition and sensation generally remain normal, although some patients experience mild to severe dementia. The depression that commonly develops may be part of the disease or a reactive response.

As the disease advances, a stooped posture and an immobile, unblinking facial expression with frequent drooling develops. Seborrhea may arise on the face and scalp.

**Etiology** In most cases, the cause of Parkinson disease is unknown. A few cases result from carbon monoxide or manganese poisoning. Drug-induced parkinsonian symptoms can develop from dopamine-receptor antagonistic drugs used to treat psychiatric disorders. These symptoms usually disappear when the drugs are withdrawn or the dosage is decreased, or with time during treatment.

**Epidemiology** Although 10 to 20 percent of all cases are diagnosed in individuals under age 40 years, Parkinson disease occurs primarily in the middle-aged and elderly populations. Between 300,000 and 500,000 cases of classic Parkinson disease are found in the United States. The National Institute of Neurological Disorders and Stroke reported recently that from a study of the prevalence of major neurologic disorders in a biracial population, the incidence of Parkinson disease demonstrates no gender or racial differences.

**Juvenile parkinsonism of Hunt** is an extremely rare hereditary syndrome with onset in teens, 20s, or early 30s.

**Parkinsonism dementia complex** is associated with motor neuron disease or amyotrophic lateral sclerosis. Consumption of a locally grown **toxic bean** causes a rare form of parkinsonism in western Pacific islands.

A **drug-induced parkinsonism** was identified in young heroin addicts who abused a "designer drug," originally in a fairly localized community in California. Primates given the same toxic substance are considered a model for this disorder.

**Treatment—Standard** Some patients can enjoy a normal life span with drug treatment that provides varying degrees of symptomatic relief. A combination of levodopa and carbidopa is the treatment of choice, although this drug combination tends to become less effective over time.

Other useful drugs include anticholinergics and amantadine, a dopamine-releasing agent. Anticholinergic agents, such as trihexyphenidyl, benztropine mesylate, biperiden, and diphenhydramine, help control tremors and rigidity. Amantadine hydrochloride also helps reduce tremors and rigidity. Bromocriptine and pergolide, which are dopamine agonists, may be useful in some cases, particularly in conjunction with the levodopa/carbidopa combination.

An orphan drug, deprenyl, is a monoamine-oxidase inhibitor that was approved by the Food and Drug Administration for use in the United States in 1989. This drug has been used in late-stage Parkinson disease to enhance the levodopa/carbidopa combination. Recent research suggests that the progression of more advanced symptoms may be delayed significantly by using deprenyl in the early stages of Parkinson disease.

Physical therapy involves exercises that may improve walking and speaking. Exercise does not stop the progression of the disease, but tends to reduce disability and improve emotional well-being.

**Treatment—Investigational** Dopamine agonists are a class of drugs being investigated for the treatment of Parkinson disease. A surgical treatment procedure in the very early stages of experimentation involves implanting cells from the patient's adrenal gland or from fetal tissue into the brain to increase the amount of dopamine available to the affected structures.

Development of new drugs continues worldwide. In Italy, Farmitlalia Carlo Erba is investigating the drug cabergoline. In Japan, Thomai is studying the dopamine D-2 agonist talipexole. In Israel, Teva Pharmaceuticals is developing TVP101. Merrell-Dow is testing MDL72974A. Hoffmann–La Roche is studying RO196327 and N-(2 aminoethyl)-5-chloro-2-pyridine carboxamide. SmithKline Beecham is developing ropinerole. Britannia Pharmaceuticals in Surrey, UK, is testing apomorphine HCL injection for treatment of the on-off fluctuations associated with late-stage Parkinson disease.

Also being studied are catechol-O-methyltransferase **(COMT)** inhibitors for use with or in place of carbidopa/levodopa in early-stage Parkinson disease.

Surgical procedures such as pallidotomy and high-frequency thalamic stimulation are being investigated.

Please contact the agencies listed under Resources, below, for the most current information. Addresses and telephone numbers of these agencies, as well as of individual experts and research centers, may be found in the Master Resources List.

**Resources**

**For more information on Parkinson disease:** National Organization for Rare Disorders (NORD); Parkinson's Disease Foundation; United Parkinson Foundation; NIH/National Institute of Neurological Disorders and Stroke.

**References**

Bilateral Fetal Mesencephalic Grafting in Two Patients with Parkinsonism Induced by 1-Methyl-4 Phenyl-1,2,3,6-Tetrahydropyridine: H. Widner, et al.; N. Engl. J. Med., November 26, 1992, vol. 327(22).

Survival of Implanted Fetal Dopamine Cells and Neurologic Improvement 12 to 42 Months After Transplantation for Parkinson's Disease: C.R. Freed, et al.; N. Engl. J. Med., November 26, 1992, vol. 327(22), pp. 1549–1555.

Unilateral Transplantation of Human Fetal Mesencephalic Tissue into the Caudate Nucleus of Patients with Parkinson's Disease: D.D. Spencer, et al.; N. Engl. J. Med., November 26, 1992, vol. 327(22), pp. 1541–1547.

Mendelian Inheritance in Man, 9th ed.: V.A. McKusick; The Johns Hopkins University Press, 1990, pp. 707, 710–711, 1409, 1703.

Cecil Textbook of Medicine, 18th ed.: J.B. Wyngaarden and L.H. Smith, Jr., eds.; W.B. Saunders Company, 1988, pp. 2143–2147.

# PARSONNAGE-TURNER SYNDROME

**Description** Parsonnage-Turner syndrome is characterized by neuritis of the brachial plexus.

**Synonyms**

Brachial Plexus Neuritis

Idiopathic Brachial Plexus Neuropathy

Neuralgic Amyotrophy

**Signs and Symptoms** The chief symptom is severe, sharp, lancinating pain in the shoulder, scapular region, and upper arm. The pain may be accompanied by unilateral or bilateral muscle weakness, atrophy, and hyperesthesia. Persons with this disorder generally recover within a few months, although symptoms may persist for several years.

**Etiology** The etiology is unknown. The syndrome may develop after immunization, viral infection, surgery, or Lyme disease. An autoimmune association is suspected.

**Epidemiology** Parsonnage-Turner syndrome occurs most often in young males, but anyone can be affected.

**Related Disorders** See *Peripheral Neuropathy.*

**Rheumatoid arthritis** is distinguished by morning stiffness, pain or tenderness, and swelling of one or more joints, chiefly in the hands, knees, feet, jaw, and spine. It is thought to be an autoimmune disorder.

**Treatment—Standard** Most patients with Parsonnage-Turner syndrome recover without treatment. Physical therapy may be helpful. Other measures are symptomatic and supportive.

**Treatment—Investigational** Please contact the agencies listed under Resources, below, for the most current information. Addresses and telephone numbers of these agencies, as well as of individual experts and research centers, may be found in the Master Resources List.

**Resources**

**For more information on Parsonnage-Turner syndrome:** National Organization for Rare Disorders (NORD); NIH/National Arthritis and Musculoskeletal and Skin Diseases Information Clearinghouse.

**References**

Postpartum Idiopathic Brachial Neuritis: D. Dimitru, et al.; Obstet. Gynecol., March 1989, vol. 73(3), pp. 473–475.

Hypertrophic Brachial Plexus Neuritis: A Pathological Study of Two Cases: M. Cusiamano, et al.; Ann. Neurol., November 1988, vol. 24(5), pp. 615–622.

Brachial Neuritis Involving the Bilateral Phrenic Nerves: N. Walsh, et al.; Arch. Phys. Med. Rehabil., January 1987, vol. 68(1), pp. 46–48.

Injury to the Brachial Plexus During Putti-Platt and Bristow Procedures: A Report of Eight Cases: R. Richards, et al.; Am. J. Sports Med., July–August 1987, vol. 15(4), pp. 374–380.

Surgery for Lesions of the Brachial Plexus: D. Kline, et al.; Arch. Neurol., February 1986, vol. 43(2), pp. 170–181.

Brachial Neuritis: L. Dillin, et al.; J. Bone Joint Surg. Am., July 1985, vol. 67(6), pp. 878–883.

# PELIZAEUS-MERZBACHER BRAIN SCLEROSIS

**Description** Pelizaeus-Merzbacher brain sclerosis is a progressive disease of the central nervous system associated with deterioration of the white matter of the brain. The pathologic changes in the brain consist of destruction of the myelin sheath surrounding nerve cell axons, with accumulation of the breakdown products of myelin. Affected areas include the subcortical cerebrum, cerebellum, and brain stem.

The disease exists in 3 forms: classic X-linked; acute infantile; and autosomal dominant or late onset.

**Synonyms**

Aplasia Axialis Extracorticalis Congenita

Diffuse Familial Brain Sclerosis

Sudanophilic Leukodystrophy

**Signs and Symptoms** The manifestations of **classical X-linked Pelizaeus-Merzbacher brain sclerosis** appear in early infancy. The child grows slowly and fails to develop normal control of the head and eyes. Tremor, spasticity, head tremors, grimacing, unsteadiness, muscle contractures, weakness, dementia, choreoathetosis, optic atrophy, and ocular nystagmus eventually develop. Skeletal deformations and convulsions also are sometimes seen.

Onset of the **acute infantile form** is during the first few weeks of life. Symptoms include muscle weakness and spasticity.

In the **autosomal dominant adult-onset form,** the symptoms and signs are frequently confused with those of multiple sclerosis. They are slowly progressive and may include ataxia, spasticity, hyperreflexia, weakness of the arms and legs, and the loss of previously acquired motor skills.

Chorionic villus sampling will detect if the fetus has the defective gene for classic Pelizaeus-Merzbacher brain sclerosis.

**Etiology** The classic form of Pelizaeus-Merzbacher brain sclerosis is X-linked. The associated gene, known as proteolipid protein **(PLP),** has been located on the long arm of the X chromosome (Xq21.3–q22). The acute infantile form is autosomal recessive, and the adult-onset form, autosomal dominant. Some cases may be sporadic.

The reasons for the degeneration of the white matter of the brain are not understood. The problem may be defective function of the PLP gene; the proteolipid proteins are a major structural component of myelin.

**Epidemiology** The classic and infantile forms begin during the first few weeks of life; symptoms of the adult-onset form generally begin during the 3rd or 4th decade of life. The classic form affects males; the other 2 affect both sexes in equal numbers.

**Related Disorders** Pelizaeus-Merzbacher brain sclerosis belongs to a group of degenerative brain diseases known as leukodystrophies, which are characterized by destruction of the white matter of the brain. See ***Adrenoleukodystrophy; Alexander Disease; Leukodystrophy, Canavan; Leukodystrophy, Krabbe; Leukodystrophy, Metachromatic; Refsum Syndrome.***

**Treatment—Standard** Treatment for Pelizaeus-Merzbacher brain sclerosis is symptomatic. Supportive care, including emotional support for family members, is recommended as needed. Genetic counseling may be beneficial.

**Treatment—Investigational** Please contact the agencies listed under Resources, below, for the most current information. Addresses and telephone numbers of these agencies, as well as of individual experts and research centers, may be found in the Master Resources List.

**Resources**

**For more information on Pelizaeus-Merzbacher brain sclerosis:** National Organization for Rare Disorders (NORD); United Leukodystrophy Foundation; NIH/National Institute of Neurological Disorders and Stroke; Research Trust for Metabolic Diseases in Children; Association Européenne contre les Leucodystrophes.

**For genetic information and genetic counseling referrals:** March of Dimes Birth Defects Foundation; Alliance of Genetic Support Groups.

**References**

Visual Evoked Potential Characteristics and Early Diagnosis of Pelizaeus-Merzbacher Disease: P. Apkarian, et al.; Arch. Neurol., September 1993, vol. 50(9), pp. 981–985.

Cecil Textbook of Medicine, 19th ed.: J.B. Wyngaarden, et al., eds.; W.B. Saunders Company, 1992, p. 2201.

Mendelian Inheritance in Man, 10th ed.: V.A. McKusick; The Johns Hopkins University Press, 1992, pp. 835, 1624, 1943.

Nelson Textbook of Pediatrics, 14th ed.: R.E. Behrman, ed.-in-chief; W.B. Saunders Company, 1992, p. 1528.

Pelizaeus-Merzbacher Disease: Detection Mutations THR181–PRO and LEU223–PRO in the Proteolipid Protein Gene, and Prenatal Diagnosis: S. Strautnieks, et al.; Am. J. Hum. Genet., October 1992, vol. 51(4), pp. 871–878.

Complete Deletion of the Proteolipid Protein Gene (PLP) in a Family with X-Linked Pelizaeus-Merzbacher Disease: W.H. Raskind, et al.; Am. J. Hum. Genet., December 1991, vol. 49(6), pp. 1355–1360.

Birth Defects Encyclopedia: M.L. Buyse, ed.-in-chief; Blackwell Scientific Publications, 1990, p. 1373.

Dictionary of Medical Syndromes, 3rd ed.: S.I. Magalini, et al., eds.; J.B. Lippincott Company, 1990, pp. 677–678.

Pelizaeus-Merzbacher Disease: An X-Linked Neurologic Disorder of Myelin Metabolism with a Novel Mutation in the Gene Encoding Proteolipid Protein: S. Gencic, et al.; Am. J. Hum. Genet., September 1989, vol. 45(3), pp. 435–442.

Principles of Neurology, 4th ed.: R.D. Adams and M. Victor, eds.; McGraw-Hill, 1989, pp. 786–788.

# PERIPHERAL NEUROPATHY

**Description** Peripheral neuropathy produces sensory, motor, and autonomic symptoms. These can appear alone or in combination.

**Synonyms**

Mononeuritis Multiplex

Mononeuropathy

Polyneuropathy

**Signs and Symptoms** Symptoms reflect disease of a single nerve (mononeuropathy, mononeuritis), several nerves in asymmetric areas of the body (mononeuritis multiplex), or symmetric involvement (polyneuropathy, polyneuritis, multiple peripheral neuritis). As a rule, lesions are degenerative; their sites are the nerve roots or the peripheral nerves. Tinel sign is helpful in locating the site of damage in some neuropathies, but electrical nerve conduction studies are the sine qua non.

Involvement of a single nerve produces mononeuropathy (mononeuritis), as in the compression and entrapment syndromes. Symptoms include weakness, pain, and paresthesias. In mononeuritis multiplex the nerves destined to be ultimately affected may all be diseased at onset or they may become involved as the disorder advances. The symptoms of multineural disease frequently mimic those of polyneuropathy.

Polyneuropathy is usually bilaterally symmetric, with a diverse spectrum of symptoms due to the variability of nerve involvement and the range of etiologies, including malnutrition, poisoning, diseases such as diabetes mellitus, and metabolic disorders. Development may take months or years, commonly starting with sensory disorders in the legs such as peripheral tingling, numbness, or burning pain. When the sensory loss is major, nontender ulcers on the digits or Charcot joints may be evident. A neurologic examination will show absence or weakening of the Achilles and other deep tendon reflexes. Weakness and atrophy of distal limb muscles and flaccid tone signal that the motor nerve fibers are affected.

**Etiology** Peripheral neuropathy has many different causes:

**Mechanical pressure** (e.g., compression, direct trauma, penetrating injuries, contusions, fracture, or dislocated bones), which can result in mononeuritis and sometimes mononeuritis multiplex.

Another type of mechanically induced neuritis may be due to heavy muscular activity and forced overextension of a nerve, as in certain construction or craft activities.

**Neuropathy due to pressure,** which commonly involves the superficial nerves (ulnar, radial, or peroneal) and may result from prolonged use of crutches, or staying in one position for too long. A tumor may exert such pressure, and nerves in narrow canals such as in the entrapment syndromes may be similarly affected.

**Intraneural hemorrhage** or **exposure to cold temperatures or to radiation.**

**Vascular or collagen disorders,** such as polyarteritis nodosa, atherosclerosis, systemic lupus erythematosus, scleroderma, sarcoidosis, and rheumatoid arthritis, which can result in mononeuritis multiplex.

**Related Disorders** See *Guillain-Barré Syndrome.*

**Treatment—Standard** Depending upon the type of peripheral neuropathy, the patient may recover without residual effects or partially recover and have sensory, motor, or vasomotor deficits and, if severely afflicted, chronic muscular atrophy.

Therapy is cause-oriented, e.g., control of diabetes, nutritional needs, changing recreational or work habits, or surgery to remove a tumor or a ruptured intervertebral disc. In entrapment or compression neuropathy, splinting or surgical decompression of the ulnar or median nerves is frequently curative. Peroneal and radial compression neuropathies require avoidance of pressure. Recovery is frequently slow; physical therapy and/or splints may be useful in preventing contractures.

**Treatment—Investigational** Please contact the agencies listed under Resources, below, for the most current information. Addresses and telephone numbers of these agencies, as well as of individual experts and research centers, may be found in the Master Resources List.

**Resources**

**For more information on peripheral neuropathy:** National Organization for Rare Disorders (NORD); NIH/National Institute of Neurological Disorders and Stroke.

**References**

Cecil Textbook of Medicine, 18th ed.: J.B. Wyngaarden and L.H. Smith, Jr., eds.; W.B. Saunders Company, 1988, p. 507.

# PICK DISEASE

**Description** Pick disease is a degenerative neurologic condition affecting the frontal and temporal lobes of the brain. It is characterized by progressive dementia.

**Synonyms**

Diffuse Degenerative Cerebral Disease

Lobar Atrophy

**Signs and Symptoms** Clinically, Pick disease closely resembles Alzheimer disease. In the early stages, memory is usually intact, and disorientation may be less pronounced than in Alzheimer disease. It is characterized by early dysphasia, apathy, and personality change. In later stages, however, there is loss of motor control and language functions, and severe dementia.

The disease is characterized by uneven atrophy of the brain, with marked changes in the frontal and temporal lobes, and other areas apparently intact. Brain tissue from persons with Pick disease does not exhibit the neurofibrillary tangles and senile plaques characteristic of Alzheimer disease. Pick argentophilic inclusion bodies are found in certain nerve cells of the brain.

Diagnosis of Pick disease is usually made after a careful history and physical examination, including thorough neurologic evaluation, psychometric studies, magnetic resonance imaging and computed tomography, and electroencephalographic testing.

**Etiology** The cause is unknown, although some cases have been reported with dominant inheritance.

**Epidemiology** Females are affected more often than males. The disease usually begins in the 5th or 6th decade, but onset may be as early as age 30. The reported incidence in the United States is much lower than that of Alzheimer disease. Investigators in Michigan have reported 12 cases of Pick disease in 35 years; in Minnesota, however, Pick disease accounts for about 4 percent of dementias.

**Related Disorders** See *Alzheimer Disease; Huntington Disease.*

Dementia can be a symptom of many disorders, mimicking Alzheimer and Pick diseases.

**Treatment—Standard** Treatment is symptomatic and supportive. Patients with progressive dementia often experience frustration, anxiety, and depression resulting from their inability to function at their previous level. These problems can be minimized by maintaining a stable home environment and a structured routine that does not place excessive demands on the patient. Sedatives should generally be avoided.

**Treatment—Investigational** The National Institute of Neurological Disorders and Stroke is seeking patients with Pick disease and other types of frontal lobe atrophy to participate in a neurobehavioral study. For more information, contact Jordan Grafman, Ph.D.

Please contact the agencies listed under Resources, below, for the most current information. Addresses and telephone numbers of these agencies, as well as of individual experts and research centers, may be found in the Master Resources List.

**Resources**

**For more information on Pick disease:** National Organization for Rare Disorders (NORD); NIH/National Institute of Neurological Disorders and Stroke; NIH/National Institute on Aging; Alzheimer's Disease and Related Disorders Association.

**References**

Harrison's Principles of Internal Medicine, 12th ed.: J.D. Wilson, et al., eds.; McGraw-Hill, 1991, p. 2062.

Mendelian Inheritance in Man, 9th ed.: V.A. McKusick; The Johns Hopkins University Press, 1990, p. 748.

# POST-POLIO SYNDROME

**Description** Post-polio syndrome is characterized by progressive muscle weakness and deterioration of function in the previously affected muscles of an individual who had poliomyelitis at least 10 years earlier. Partial or complete recovery from the initial episode of polio is common, followed years later by a gradual recurrence of muscle weakness for which there is no other apparent cause.

**Synonyms**

Polio Sequelae

**Signs and Symptoms** Muscle function gradually decreases and muscle weakness develops, usually in the limbs that previously had been most affected by the polio virus. Occasionally muscles are affected that are fully recovered or never had been involved in the initial polio episode. This latent polio syndrome may involve the muscles necessary for respiration, and cause other symptoms such as fatigue, muscle pain, and fasciculations.

**Etiology** The exact cause of post-polio syndrome remains unknown. Research has failed to prove early theories of reactivation of the dormant polio virus and a more rapid aging in certain parts of the nervous system of post-polio patients than their unaffected peers. Scientists recently determined that post-polio syndrome is not a form of amyotropic lateral sclerosis.

In a 1987 study of patients with post-polio syndrome, it was found that nerve cells in affected muscles may grow many small sprouts from the axons of healthy nerve cells during the recovery phase. These sprouts acquire the function of the polio-damaged neurons. After years of functioning beyond capacity, the healthy nerve cells can weaken and lose the ability to maintain the sprouts. The muscle becomes weaker as the sprouts begin to shrink. This discovery may be helpful in the development of an experimental treatment to improve the sprouting of axons.

Other research being conducted to determine the cause of post-polio syndrome includes investigating the presence of abnormal proteins in cerebrospinal fluid, and examining the effect of the polio virus on nerve cells in muscle fibers of post-polio patients.

**Epidemiology** Approximately 20 percent of persons who recovered from poliomyelitis more than 10 years earlier may be affected by post-polio syndrome. Symptoms of this syndrome can appear 30 or more years after the initial polio episode.

**Related Disorders** Symptoms of poliomyelitis (infantile paralysis) are similar to those of post-polio syndrome.

**Treatment—Standard** Persons who had polio before the vaccine was developed should be evaluated for post-polio syndrome, including a complete physical examination and comprehensive muscle testing and gait analysis. Rehabilitation in the form of physical and occupational therapy may be helpful. Exercise, not exceeding 5 to 20 minutes' duration, and regular rest periods may be advised. Swimming is a particularly good form of exercise for post-polio patients. Changes in braces and medication and diet modification may be recommended. Excess weight is very disabling for weakened muscles. Occasionally a respirator is prescribed, such as an intermittent positive pressure ventilation system, if breathing has been affected.

**Treatment—Investigational** Please contact the agencies listed under Resources, below, for the most current information. Addresses and telephone numbers of these agencies, as well as of individual experts and research centers, may be found in the Master Resources List.

**Resources**

   **For more information on post-polio syndrome:** National Organization for Rare Disorders (NORD); Post-Polio National (Post-Polio League for Information and Outreach); Polio Information Center; British Polio Fellowship; Centers for Disease Control; International Polio Network.

   **For rehabilitation services:** National Easter Seal Society.

**References**

   Mouth Intermittent Positive Pressure Ventilation in the Management of Post-Polio Respiratory Insufficiency: J.R. Bach, et al.; Chest, June 1987, vol. 91(6), pp. 859–864.

   Handbook of the Late Effects of Poliomyelitis for Physicians and Survivors: G. Laurie, et al., eds.; G.I.N.I., 1984.

   Late Effects of Poliomyelitis: L. Halstead, et al., eds.; Symposia Foundation, 1984.

# PRIMARY LATERAL SCLEROSIS

**Description** Primary lateral sclerosis is an adult neurologic disease that affects the central motor neurons (corticospinal tract). It is characterized by progressive muscle weakness in the facial area and the extremities, associated with spasticity and hyperactive deep tendon reflexes.

**Synonyms**

   Central Motor Neuron Disease

   Motor Neuron Disease

**Signs and Symptoms** Initially there are few symptoms, and neurologic dysfunction progresses slowly. Spasticity in the hands, feet, or legs produces slowness and stiffness of movement. Dragging of the feet is followed by inability to walk. Facial involvement may result in dysarthria. Sensory function and intellectual function remain intact. The disease may progress gradually over a number of years, with wasting and weakening of the affected muscles.

**Etiology** The etiology is unknown.

**Epidemiology** Males and females are affected equally.

**Related Disorders** See *Amyotrophic Lateral Sclerosis; Werdnig-Hoffmann Disease.*

   **Multifocal motor neuropathy** is clinically similar to amyotrophic lateral sclerosis. However, lower motor neurons are mainly affected. The disease is characterized by slowly progressive muscle wasting and weakness without spasticity and stiffness. Immunosuppressive drugs have produced improvement in some cases.

**Treatment—Standard** Symptomatic treatment includes the use of baclofen and diazepam for spasticity and quinine to control cramps. Other measures may include physical therapy to prevent joint immobility and speech therapy for patients with dysarthria.

**Treatment—Investigational** Current research on motor neuron diseases involves nerve growth factors, axonal transport, androgen receptor in motor neurons, and DNA/RNA changes.

   Syntex-Synergen Neuroscience of Boulder, Colorado, is sponsoring an orphan product (ciliary neurotrophic factor, recombinant human) for treatment of motor neuron diseases, including primary lateral sclerosis.

   Please contact the agencies listed under Resources, below, for the most current information. Addresses and telephone numbers of these agencies, as well as of individual experts and research centers, may be found in the Master Resources List.

**Resources**

   **For more information on primary lateral sclerosis:** National Organization for Rare Disorders (NORD); NIH/National Institute of Neurological and Disorders and Stroke; Amyotrophic Lateral Sclerosis Association.

**References**

   Harrison's Principles of Internal Medicine, 12th ed.: J.D. Wilson, et al., eds.; McGraw-Hill, 1991, p. 2074.

   Chronic Progressive Spinobulbar Spasticity: A Rare Form of Primary Lateral Sclerosis: J.L. Gastaut, et al.; Arch. Neurol., May 1988, vol. 45(5), pp. 509–513.

# PROGRESSIVE SUPRANUCLEAR PALSY (PSP)

**Description** PSP is characterized by impaired motor control, abnormal eye movements, and dementia.

**Synonyms**

    Nuchal Dystonia Dementia Syndrome

    Steele-Richardson-Olszewski Syndrome

**Signs and Symptoms** Onset of symptoms is between ages 50 and 70 years. Characteristic features include bradykinesia, visual impairment, and falling. Loss of voluntary (but preservation of reflexive) eye movements, particularly of vertical gaze, is accompanied by spastic weakness of the pharyngeal musculature, and signs of Parkinson disease. The face is expressionless, and speech is forced and slurred. Apathy and dementia develop late in the course of the disorder, which progresses over a 6- to 8-year period. Degenerative changes occur in the basal ganglia, brain stem, and cerebellum.

**Etiology** The cause of PSP is unknown.

**Epidemiology** Males are affected twice as often as females.

**Related Disorders** See *Parkinson Disease.*

    **Lacunar state** is characterized by a progression of neurologic symptoms similar to that found in cases of stroke.

    **Pseudobulbar palsy** is characterized by symptoms similar to those of PSP; however, eye movements in affected individuals are normal.

**Treatment—Standard** Medical treatment of PSP is generally disappointing. Tricyclic antidepressant drugs such as amitryptiline and imipramine may bring symptomatic relief in some cases. Agents such as carbidopa/levodopa, bromocriptine, trihexyphenidyl, amantadine, and benztropine may relieve extrapyramidal symptoms early in the course. Pergolide has been helpful in some cases.

    Walking aids, such as a walker weighted in front, and wearing shoes with built-up heels, may help prevent patients from falling backwards.

**Treatment—Investigational** The National Institute of Neurological Disorders and Stroke is seeking individuals affected by progressive supranuclear palsy for participation in a clinical research study. For more information, contact Irene Litvan, M.D., at the Experimental Therapeutics Branch.

    Idazoxan, a British drug developed as an antidepressant, is being studied as treatment for PSP, with some promising results, by John H. Growdon, M.D., Harvard Medical School. The drug was not effective as an antidepressant and is no longer being manufactured in Britain.

    Please contact the agencies listed under Resources, below, for the most current information. Addresses and telephone numbers of these agencies, as well as of individual experts and research centers, may be found in the Master Resources List.

**Resources**

    **For more information on progressive supranuclear palsy:** National Organization for Rare Disorders (NORD); NIH/National Institute of Neurological Disorders and Stroke; International Tremor Foundation; Society for Progressive Supranuclear Palsy; Progressive Supranuclear Palsy Research Fund; We Move.

**References**

    Scientific American MEDICINE: E. Rubinstein and D. Federman, eds.; Scientific American, 1978–1991, pp. 11:IV:8–9.

    Progressive Supranuclear Palsy: H.L. Klawans; United Parkinson Foundation, 1981.

# PSEUDOTUMOR CEREBRI

**Description** Pseudotumor cerebri is a syndrome of increased intracranial pressure. Although symptoms can mimic those of a brain tumor, no tumor is present.

**Synonyms**

    Benign Intracranial Hypertension

**Signs and Symptoms** Symptoms include headache that typically is mild and resistant to analgesics. Features seen occasionally include papilledema with progressive visual loss, memory impairment, dizziness, and asthenia.

    Spinal fluid pressure is elevated. Electroencephalogram findings usually are normal.

**Etiology** In most cases no specific cause can be identified. Possible causes include increased intracranial pressure secondary to chronic carbon dioxide retention and hypoxia, a parathyroid or adrenal gland disorder, iron deficiency anemia, and venous sinus thrombosis. Agents that have been implicated include corticosteroids, sex hormones, tetracycline, nalidixic acid, and vitamin A in excessive amounts.

**Epidemiology** The female-to-male ratio is 8:1, and prevalence is highest among overweight females between the ages of 15 and 50. The general public appears to be affected at a rate of 0.9:100,000 persons, but this incidence increases to 13 to 15:100,000 persons among those who are 10 percent overweight, and to 19.3:100,000 persons among those who are 20 percent or more over their ideal weight.

**Related Disorders** See *Arachnoiditis.*

**Epiduritis** is characterized by inflammation of the dura mater. Symptoms can be similar to those of pseudotumor cerebri.

**Treatment—Standard** The cause determines treatment. Implicated medications should be discontinued. Lumbar punctures, performed daily at first, may lower pressure and relieve some of the symptoms. Occasionally a lumbar-peritoneal shunt may be required. Diuretics may be used.

**Treatment—Investigational** Please contact the agencies listed under Resources, below, for the most current information. Addresses and telephone numbers of these agencies, as well as of individual experts and research centers, may be found in the Master Resources List.

**Resources**

**For more information on pseudotumor cerebri:** National Organization for Rare Disorders (NORD); NIH/National Institute of Neurological Disorders and Stroke.

**References**

Internal Medicine, 3rd ed.: J.H. Stein, ed.-in-chief; Little, Brown and Company, 1990, p. 2023.

Clinical Course and Prognosis of Pseudotumor Cerebri: A Prospective Study of 24 Patients: P.S. Sorenson, et al.; Acta Neurol. Scand., February 1988, vol. 77(2), pp. 164–172.

The Incidence of Pseudotumor Cerebri: Population Studies in Iowa and Louisiana: F.J. Durcan, et al.; Arch. Neurol., August 1988, vol. 45(1), pp. 875–877.

Optic Nerve Head Drusen and Pseudotumor Cerebri: B. Katz, et al.; Arch. Neurol., January 1988, vol. 45(1), pp. 45–47.

Pseudotumor Cerebri in Men: K.B. Digre, et al.; Arch. Neurol., August 1988, vol. 45(8), pp. 866–872.

# REFLEX SYMPATHETIC DYSTROPHY SYNDROME (RSDS)

**Description** The wide variety of disorders encompassed in this syndrome are all characterized by chronic, severe pain that occurs with posttraumatic vasomotor changes. RSDS is easily misdiagnosed as just a painful nerve injury.

**Synonyms**

> Algoneurodystrophy
> Causalgia Syndrome
> Posttraumatic Dystrophy
> Reflex Neurovascular Dystrophy
> Shoulder-Hand Syndrome
> Steinbrocker Syndrome

**Signs and Symptoms** The usual presenting symptom is burning pain and stiffness in an arm or leg (although any area of the body may be affected) at the site of a previous injury but extending beyond the area of the earlier injury. Pain severity may be worse than the original injury. In the early stages, there may also be erythema, tenderness, and swelling. Hyperhidrosis may be present, and heat may intensify the discomfort. Range of motion may be decreased.

In some patients the condition progresses. Pain worsens, and range of motion is further restricted. The skin may appear pale, pitted, or cyanotic.

A further stage may be associated with a decrease in pain, although more commonly pain becomes intractable and only mild relief can be obtained with treatment. Severe tendon contractures and muscle atrophy may accompany loss of strength. At this late stage, changes may become permanent. Osteoporosis and grooved nails may be present.

**Etiology** The cause is unclear, but a number of factors may contribute, particularly changes in autonomic nervous system function.

RSDS may be associated with infections, burns, radiation therapy, and hemiparesis. Spinal disorders such as cervical osteoarthritis also may be associated with the syndrome. No cause is found, however, in approximately 30 percent of cases.

**Epidemiology** RSDS appears to be more common among women than men, and among individuals over 50 years of age. It has also been seen among children and young adults.

**Related Disorders** See *Erythromelalgia.*

**Treatment—Standard** Although no standard treatment for RSDS has been developed, prevention and early treatment of symptoms are recommended. Daily physical therapy should begin as soon as the diagnosis is confirmed. Whirlpool and paraffin wax baths are sometimes beneficial. Ice or heat applications should be avoided in most cases because they seem to cause overstimulation of nerve endings, resulting in increased discomfort.

Transcutaneous electrical nerve stimulation **(TENS)** may be used in the early stages of RSDS or added to an existing therapy program. Local or systemic glucocorticosteroids can be effective but must be used cautiously. Side effects are rarely seen with the lower doses recommended for RSDS, but weight gain, moon facies, and digestive upsets have been reported. Nonsteroidal anti-inflammatory medications, other analgesics, and muscle relaxants are sometimes helpful. Other agents that have been used include guanethidine, propranolol, nifedipine, phenytoin, and tricyclic antidepressants.

Sympathetic blockade can be helpful for the intractable pain of the later stage of the disorder. A stellate ganglion block is used for upper extremity pain, and a lumbar sympathetic block is performed for lower extremity pain. Surgical or chemical sympathectomy may be undertaken if blockade is inadequate.

**Treatment—Investigational** Preliminary investigation of dorsal column stimulation, which involves a spinal implant device, shows promise. A similar device, the implanted morphine pump, is being used to deliver morphine directly to the spinal fluid.

Guanethidine monosulfate is being used experimentally as a treatment. Ciba-Geigy Corporation may be contacted.

Please contact the agencies listed under Resources, below, for the most current information. Addresses and telephone numbers of these agencies, as well as of individual experts and research centers, may be found in the Master Resources List.

**Resources**

**For more information on reflex sympathetic dystrophy syndrome:** National Organization for Rare Disorders (NORD); Reflex Sympathetic Dystrophy Syndrome Association; Arthritis Foundation; NIH/National Arthritis and Musculoskeletal and Skin Diseases Information Clearinghouse.

**References**

Signs and Symptoms of Reflex Sympathetic Dystrophy: A Prospective Study of 829 Patients: P.H.J.M. Veldman, et al.; Lancet, October 1993, vol. 342(8878), pp. 1012–1016.

Reflex Sympathetic Dystrophy Syndrome: Diagnosis and Treatment: R.W. Rothrock and D. Weiss; Osteopathic Medical News, February 1987, pp. 20–25.

# RESTLESS LEGS SYNDROME

**Description** Restless legs syndrome is a neurologic disorder in which aching and crawling sensations occur in the legs, usually at night. Patients attempt to relieve these irritating sensations by constantly moving their feet and legs. This syndrome can be hereditary, or it can develop as a complication of alcoholism, iron deficiency anemia, pregnancy, or diabetes.

**Synonyms**

Anxietas Tibialis
Ekbom Syndrome
Hereditary Acromelalgia

**Signs and Symptoms** Attacks commonly begin at times when the legs are resting, such as when going to bed or sitting still. Intense discomfort involving aching sensations and paresthesias occurs between the knee and ankle. These often intolerable sensations precipitate movement of the legs and feet, and interfere with the ability to fall asleep and maintain sleep. Myoclonic leg jerks just prior to the onset of sleep are reported more frequently in persons with restless legs syndrome, even when awake, than in the normal adult population. Psychological stress typically exacerbates symptoms.

**Etiology** Restless legs syndrome is inherited as an autosomal dominant trait in about one-third of all cases. Some research suggests that restless legs syndrome may be related to a defect in the way sleep is organized in the brain.

**Epidemiology** Onset usually occurs in adolescence, and the course is chronic. Alcoholism, anemia, diabetes, and pregnancy increase the risk of developing this disorder. Males and females are equally affected.

**Related Disorders** See *Myoclonus.*

**Treatment—Standard** Treatment is symptomatic. The application of cold compresses sometimes helps relieve aching sensations in the legs. Drug therapy with clonazepam, carbamazepine, and low doses of a combination of L-dopa and carbidopa has been reported to be effective. Patients with an inherited form of this disorder may benefit from genetic counseling.

**Treatment—Investigational** Arthur Walters, M.D., and Wayne Hening, M.D., at Robert Wood Johnson Medical School are conducting research on the disorder.

Please contact the agencies listed under Resources, below, for the most current information. Addresses and telephone numbers of these agencies, as well as of individual experts and research centers, may be found in the Master Resources List.

**Resources**

**For more information on restless legs syndrome:** National Organization for Rare Disorders (NORD); Restless Legs Syndrome Foundation; NIH/National Institute of Neurological Disorders and Stroke.

**For genetic information and genetic counseling referrals:** March of Dimes Birth Defects Foundation; Alliance of Genetic Support Groups.

### References

Mendelian Inheritance in Man, 9th ed.: V.A. McKusick; The Johns Hopkins University Press, 1990, p. 16.

Restless Legs Syndrome: Harvard Medical School Health Letter; August 1987, vol. 10(12), pp. 2–3.

# RETT SYNDROME

**Description** Rett syndrome, a degenerative disease with progressive encephalopathy, is behaviorally similar to autism and characterized by developmental regression or loss of previously acquired skills. It is found exclusively in girls.

**Synonyms**

Cerebroatrophic Hyperammonemia

**Signs and Symptoms** Rett syndrome manifests after the first 7 to 18 months of the female infant's life. Rapid deterioration occurs for the next 18 months and leads to mental and physical retardation. Patients develop severe dementia, lose purposeful movements of the hands, and appear autistic. A repetitive hand-wringing movement is characteristic. Walking, if acquired at all, is characterized by a broad-based gait. Microcephaly develops with increasing age. Later, seizures, gait apraxia, and truncal ataxia are prominent. There is continued deterioration often resulting in death before 40 years of age.

**Etiology** Rett syndrome is an X-linked dominant genetic disorder.

**Epidemiology** Approximately 1,200 cases in females have been reported worldwide in the medical literature. The Texas Rett Syndrome Registry at Baylor College of Medicine in Houston, the largest Rett syndrome registry in the world, estimates the disorder may affect about 1:22,800 females between 2 and 18 years of age.

**Related Disorders** See *Autism; Cerebral Palsy.*

**Treatment—Standard** Physical therapy may help prevent stiffening and encourage mobility. Braces and splints are sometimes used to treat toe-walking, scoliosis, and clenched hands. Hydrotherapy or underwater jet massage may also be helpful. Seizures associated with Rett syndrome are treated with anticonvulsive medications. Music therapy has been helpful in achieving communication with some patients. Special education and related services in school are recommended.

**Treatment—Investigational** Research on the syndrome is being conducted by Alan Percy, M.D., and Diane Donley, M.D., at the University of Alabama School of Medicine; Daniel Glaze, M.D., at Baylor College of Medicine; and Sakkubai Naidu, M.D., at the John F. Kennedy Institute for Handicapped Children in Baltimore.

Please contact the agencies listed under Resources, below, for the most current information. Addresses and telephone numbers of these agencies, as well as of individual experts and research centers, may be found in the Master Resources List.

### Resources

**For more information on Rett syndrome:** National Organization for Rare Disorders (NORD); International Rett Syndrome Association; The Arc (a national organization on mental retardation); NIH/National Institute of Neurological Disorders and Stroke.

**For genetic information and genetic counseling referrals:** March of Dimes Birth Defects Foundation; Alliance of Genetic Support Groups.

### References

Epidemiology of Rett Syndrome: A Population-Based Registry: C.A. Kozinetz, et al.; Pediatrics, February 1993, vol. 91(2), pp. 445–450.

Neuroanatomy of Rett Syndrome: A Volumetric Imaging Study: A.L. Reiss, et al.; Ann. Neurol., August 1993, vol. 34(2), pp. 227–234.

The Pattern of Growth Failure in Rett Syndrome: R.J. Schultz, et al.; Am. J. Dis. Child, June 1993, vol. 147(6), pp. 633–637,

Principles of Neurology, 5th ed.: R.D. Adams and M. Victor, eds.; McGraw-Hill, 1993, pp. 827–828.

The Rett Syndrome: An Introductory Overview 1990: B. Hagberg; Brain Dev., May 1993, (14 suppl.), pp. S5–8.

Rett Syndrome: An Update and Review for the Primary Pediatrician: S.R. Braddock, et al.; Clin. Pediatr., October 1993, vol. 32(10), pp. 613–626.

Mendelian Inheritance in Man, 10th ed.: V.A. McKusick; The Johns Hopkins University Press, 1992, pp. 1957–1958.

Nelson Textbook of Pediatrics, 14th ed.: R.E. Behrman, ed.-in-chief; W.B. Saunders Company, 1992, pp. 1528–1529.

Rett Syndrome: A Search for Gene Sources: H.O. Akesson, et al.; Am. J. Med. Genet., January 1992, vol. 42(1), pp. 104–108.

# ROSENBERG-CHUTORIAN SYNDROME

**Description** Rosenberg-Chutorian syndrome is a very rare disorder whose major characteristics are sensorineural hearing loss, optic atrophy resulting in loss of vision, and noninflammatory degenerative polyneuropathy of the upper and/or lower limbs.

**Synonyms**

> Optic Atrophy, Polyneuropathy, and Deafness
> Polyneuropathy–Deafness–Optic Atrophy

**Signs and Symptoms** Symptoms of Rosenberg-Chutorian syndrome become apparent during infancy or puberty. Optic atrophy causes loss of visual clearness beginning with night blindness and/or poor vision in dim light. A defect in the inner ear resulting in sensorineural deafness causes hearing loss. Dysarthria as well as rhinolalia may also be found in some affected individuals. It is felt that the hearing loss is a contributing factor to the speech impairments.

Polyneuropathy is another major symptom of Rosenberg-Chutorian syndrome. Weakness and wasting of the muscles in the arms and legs is found in most affected individuals. Demyelination has been present in a few affected individuals. The tarsal bone as well as the bones of the chest and spine may also be affected.

**Etiology** Rosenberg-Chutorian syndrome is thought to be inherited as an X-linked semidominant trait.

**Epidemiology** Rosenberg-Chutorian syndrome affects males more often than females. Males tend to have more severe symptoms.

**Related Disorders** See *Charcot-Marie-Tooth Disease; Neuropathy, Hereditary Sensory, Type I; Refsum Syndrome; Wolfram Syndrome.*

**Treatment—Standard** Treatment of Rosenberg-Chutorian syndrome is symptomatic and supportive. Physical and occupational therapy may be useful to maintain function. A hearing aid may be of help to individuals with milder hearing loss. Orthopedic devices may also be of benefit. Genetic counseling is beneficial for patients and their families.

**Treatment—Investigational** Please contact the agencies listed under Resources, below, for the most current information. Addresses and telephone numbers of these agencies, as well as of individual experts and research centers, may be found in the Master Resources List.

**Resources**

**For more information on Rosenberg-Chutorian syndrome:** National Organization for Rare Disorders (NORD); NIH/National Institute of Neurological Disorders and Stroke.

**For genetic information and genetic counseling referrals:** March of Dimes Birth Defects Foundation; Alliance of Genetic Support Groups.

**References**

Wolfram Syndrome: A Mitochondrial-Mediated Disorder?: J.I. Rotter, et al.; Lancet, 1993, vol. 342, pp. 598–600.

Mendelian Inheritance in Man, 10th ed.: V.A. McKusick; The Johns Hopkins University Press, 1992, pp. 1935.

Birth Defects Encyclopedia: M.L Buyse, ed.-in-chief; Blackwell Scientific Publications, 1990, p. 510.

Principles of Neurology, 4th ed.; R.D. Adams and M. Victor, eds.; McGraw-Hill, 1989, p. 1935.

# ROUSSY-LÉVY SYNDROME

**Description** Roussy-Lévy syndrome is a rare genetic motor sensory disorder. Major symptoms include clawfoot, muscle weakness, atrophy of the leg muscles, and tremor in the hands.

**Synonyms**

> Charcot-Marie-Tooth Disease (Variant)
> Charcot-Marie-Tooth–Roussy-Lévy Disease
> Hereditary Areflexic Dystasia
> Hereditary Motor Sensory Neuropathy

**Signs and Symptoms** Although the disorder begins in early childhood and has a slowly progressive course, disability is not inevitable. Affected persons have symptoms and signs similar to other hereditary motor sensory neuropathies, i.e., weakness and atrophy of the leg muscles with some loss of feeling and areflexia. Pes cavus, difficulty walking, and a slight hand tremor may be present.

**Etiology** Roussy-Lévy is inherited as an autosomal dominant trait.

**Epidemiology** Onset is in early childhood, unlike other hereditary motor sensory neuropathies. Males and females are affected in equal numbers.

**Related Disorders** See *Ataxia, Friedreich; Charcot-Marie-Tooth Disease; Dejerine-Sottas Disease; Refsum Syndrome; Neuropathy, Hereditary Sensory, Type I.*

**Treatment—Standard** Treatment may include use of braces for the foot deformity, or orthopedic surgery on the feet to correct the imbalance of the affected muscles. Genetic counseling may be beneficial. Other treatment is symptomatic and supportive.

**Treatment—Investigational** Please contact the agencies listed under Resources, below, for the most current information. Addresses and telephone numbers of these agencies, as well as of individual experts and research centers, may be found in the Master Resources List.

**Resources**

    **For more information on Roussy-Lévy syndrome:** National Organization for Rare Disorders (NORD); NIH/National Institute of Neurological Disorders and Stroke; Charcot-Marie-Tooth Association; Charcot-Marie-Tooth Disease/Peroneal Muscular Atrophy Association; International Tremor Foundation.

    **For genetic information and genetic counseling referrals:** March of Dimes Birth Defects Foundation; Alliance of Genetic Support Groups.

**References**

Progressive Ataxia and Distal Muscular Atrophy—Differential Diagnostic Considerations on Roussy-Lévy Syndrome: F. Aksu, et al.; Klin. Pediatr., March–April 1986, vol. 198(2), pp. 114–118.

Treatment of Severe Concave Clubfoot in Neural Muscular Atrophy: G. Imhauser; Z. Orthop., November–December 1984, vol. 122(6), pp. 827–834.

Roussy-Lévy Hereditary Areflexic Dystasia: Its Historical Relation to Friedreich's Disease, Charcot-Marie-Tooth Atrophy and Dejerine-Sottas Hypertrophic Neuritis; The Present Status of the Original Family; The Nosologic Role of this Entity: J. Lapresle; Rev. Neurol. (Paris), 1982, vol. 138(12), pp. 967–978.

# SCAPULOPERONEAL MYOPATHY

**Description** Scapuloperoneal myopathy is a hereditary condition in which muscle wasting and consequent weakness of the scapular and peroneal musculature are hallmarks. It can be a single entity, but it may accompany several other disorders.

**Synonyms**

    Myogenic (Facio)-Scapulo-Peroneal Syndrome

    Scapuloperoneal Muscular Dystrophy

**Signs and Symptoms** Onset of muscle wasting and weakness may occur during the childhood years, but these features may have their onset in adulthood as well. The patient's initial complaint is likely to be one of weakness in the proximal muscles of the arms or legs. A few patients have wasting of the facial muscles. Both the rate of progression and the degree of weakness vary among patients. Cardiac arrythmias and sudden death have been reported. Serum CK activity is moderately elevated.

**Etiology** Scapuloperoneal myopathy is hereditary; the trait is autosomal dominant.

**Epidemiology** Males and females are affected in equal numbers.

**Related Disorders Davidenkov syndrome (Kaeser syndrome; neurogenic scapuloperoneal amyotrophy)** is marked by peroneal muscle weakness and atrophy, with pedal abnormalities and an unusual gait. These signs and symptoms precede involvement of the shoulder muscles. Unlike scapuloperoneal myopathy, in this syndrome the nerve impulses may become significantly delayed. Pain, paresthesias in the legs, and muscle contractures may also occur.

**Treatment—Standard** Treatment of scapuloperoneal myopathy consists of programmed therapeutic exercise and physical therapy interspersed with rest. Genetic counseling is advisable for patients and their families. Other treatment is symptomatic and supportive.

**Treatment—Investigational** Please contact the agencies listed under Resources, below, for the most current information. Addresses and telephone numbers of these agencies, as well as of individual experts and research centers, may be found in the Master Resources List.

**Resources**

    **For more information on scapuloperoneal myopathy:** National Organization for Rare Disorders (NORD); NIH/National Arthritis and Musculoskeletal and Skin Diseases Information Clearinghouse.

    **For genetic information and genetic counseling referrals:** March of Dimes Birth Defects Foundation; Alliance of Genetic Support Groups.

**References**

Scapuloperoneal Myopathy: D.H. Todman, et al.; Clin. Exp. Neurol., 1984, vol. 20, pp. 169–174.

Scapuloperoneal Syndrome with Cardiomyopathy: Report of a Family with Autosomal Dominant Inheritance and Unusual Features: A. Chakrabarti, et al.; J. Neurol. Neurosurg. Psychiatry, December 1981, vol. 44(12), pp. 1146–1152.

# SEITELBERGER DISEASE

**Description** Seitelberger disease is an inherited central nervous system condition in which progressive muscular and coordination difficulties, speech and vision deficits, and impaired cerebral function develop.

**Synonyms**
Infantile Neuroaxonal Dystrophy

**Signs and Symptoms** Onset is usually before age 2 years, often at birth. The disease is characterized by involuntary jerking of the head, eyes, or limbs; hypotonia; impaired ability to speak or walk; loss of coordination; spasticity; and loss of reflexes. In later stages, there may be progressively impaired vision, nystagmus, dementia, and seizures. Most affected children die before age 6 years.

**Etiology** The disease is inherited as an autosomal recessive trait. There is some indication that it is the infantile form of Hallervorden-Spatz syndrome.

**Epidemiology** There is a slight predilection for females, with onset usually before the age of 2 years.

**Related Disorders** See *Hallervorden-Spatz Disease; Leukodystrophy, Metachromatic.*

**Primary optic atrophy,** which causes diminished visual acuity and decreased ability to see light, can be a symptom of Seitelberger disease. Symptoms may be caused by degeneration, shrinkage, or disappearance of nerve fibers.

**Treatment—Standard** Treatment is symptomatic and supportive, and services for visually and physically impaired persons can provide assistance. Genetic counseling may benefit families of affected patients.

**Treatment—Investigational** Please contact the agencies listed under Resources, below, for the most current information. Addresses and telephone numbers of these agencies, as well as of individual experts and research centers, may be found in the Master Resources List.

**Resources**

**For more information on Seitelberger disease:** National Organization for Rare Disorders (NORD); Children's Brain Diseases Foundation for Research; NIH/National Institute of Neurological Disorders and Stroke; United Leukodystrophy Foundation; National Ataxia Foundation; Association Européenne contre les Leucodystrophes.

**For genetic information and genetic counseling referrals:** March of Dimes Birth Defects Foundation; Alliance of Genetic Support Groups.

**References**

Histological and Ultrastructural Features of Dystrophic Isocortical Axons in Infantile Neuroaxonal Dystrophy (Seitelberger Disease): M.H. Mitchell, et al.; Acta Neuropathol. (Berl.), 1985, vol. 66(2), pp. 89–97.

Neuroaxonal Dystrophy in Childhood: Report of Two Second Cousins with Hallervorden-Spatz Disease, and a Case of Seitelberger Disease: K. Kristensson, et al.; Acta Paediatr. Scand., November 1982, vol. 71(6), pp. 1045–1049.

# SHY-DRAGER SYNDROME

**Description** Shy-Drager syndrome is a progressive disorder of unknown cause marked by autonomic insufficiency associated with degeneration of cell bodies of preganglionic sympathetic nerves in the intermediolateral column of the spinal cord. Degeneration in other parts of the central nervous system can produce olivopontocerebellar and parkinsonian syndromes.

**Synonyms**
Orthostatic Hypotension in Neurologic Disease
Postural Hypotension
Progressive Autonomic Failure

**Signs and Symptoms** Onset of symptoms occurs at ages 40 to 75 years. The hallmark of the disorder is orthostatic hypotension. Urinary and bowel dysfunction, sexual impotence, and anhidrosis occur, followed by parkinsonian neurologic disturbances, cerebellar incoordination, muscle wasting and fasciculations, and coarse tremors of the legs. Late in the course, affected persons may develop stridor and sleep apnea. Chewing, swallowing and speaking may become more difficult. The disease progresses over many years, with potentially serious neurologic complications.

**Etiology** The cause is not known, although environmental or genetic factors have been suggested. Symptoms result from an impairment of the autonomic nervous system.

**Epidemiology** Males are more commonly afflicted than females. Incidence in the United States is believed to be 25,000 to 100,000 persons. Most cases are probably undiagnosed or misdiagnosed as Parkinson disease.

**Related Disorders** See *Parkinson Disease.* See also *Corticobasal Degeneration; Creutzfeldt-Jakob Disease; Joseph Disease; Olivopontocerebellar Atrophy.*

The very rare **Bradbury-Eggleston syndrome (idiopathic orthostatic hypotension)** differs from Shy-Drager syndrome in that there is no evidence of symptoms related to neurologic impairment (e.g., tremor). The cause is unknown.

**Dopamine-β-hydroxylase deficiency** is a very rare inherited neurometabolic disorder characterized by orthostatic hypotension. Symptoms develop because of the enzyme deficiency. They are similar to those of Bradbury-Eggleston syndrome. No other neurologic symptoms are noted in persons with this disorder.

**Treatment—Standard** Therapy should include counterpressure, as in the use of elastic stockings. Antiparkinsonian medication must be used cautiously because it may lower blood pressure. Dietary increases of salt used with fludrohydrocortisone to increase intravascular pressure also should be used with care.

**Treatment—Investigational** The orphan drug midodrine is being investigated as a treatment for Shy-Drager syndrome. For more information, contact Roberts Pharmaceuticals.

The National Institute of Neurological Disorders and Stroke is seeking certain individuals affected by Shy-Drager syndrome for participation in a clinical research project. For more information, contact David Goldstein, M.D.

For information on a clinical trial to study the cause and possible treatment of Shy-Drager syndrome, Italo Biaggioni, M.D., or David Robertson, M.D., may be contacted at Vanderbilt University.

Several studies are investigating the use of the drug xamoterol for treatment of orthostatic hypotension associated with Shy-Drager syndrome.

Please contact the agencies listed under Resources, below, for the most current information. Addresses and telephone numbers of these agencies, as well as of individual experts and research centers, may be found in the Master Resources List.

### Resources

**For more information on Shy-Drager syndrome:** National Organization for Rare Disorders (NORD); Shy-Drager Syndrome Support Group; International Tremor Foundation; We Move; NIH/National Institute of Neurological Disorders and Stroke.

### References

Genitourinary Dysfunction in Multiple System Atrophy: Clinical Features and Treatment in 62 Cases: R.O. Beck, et al.; J. Urol., May 1994, vol. 151(5), pp. 1336–1341.

Online Mendelian Inheritance in Man (OMIM): V.A. McKusick; The Johns Hopkins University, last edit 5/24/94, entry number 146500.

Cognitive and Motor Performance in Multiple System Atrophy and Parkinson Disease Compared: D. Testa, et al.; Neuropsychologia, February 1993, vol. 31(2), pp. 207–210.

Principles of Neurology, 5th ed.: R.D. Adams and M. Victor, eds.; McGraw-Hill, 1993, p. 322.

Cecil Textbook of Medicine, 19th ed.: J.B. Wyngaarden, et al., eds.; W.B. Saunders Company, 1992, pp. 2092–2093, 2138.

Effect of Xamoterol in Shy-Drager Syndrome: A. Obara, et al.; Circulation, February 1992, vol. 85(2), pp. 606–611.

Mendelian Inheritance in Man, 10th ed.: V.A. McKusick; The Johns Hopkins University Press, 1992, pp. 486–487.

Harrison's Principles of Internal Medicine, 12th ed.: J.D. Wilson, et al., eds.; McGraw-Hill, 1991, p. 2071–2072.

# SPASMODIC TORTICOLLIS

**Description** Spasmodic torticollis is characterized by repetitive or continuous spasm of the cervical muscles, resulting in twisting of the neck and an unusual head posture.

### Synonyms

Spasmodic Wryneck

**Signs and Symptoms** The onset may be gradual, with the head tending to rotate to one side when the patient attempts to hold it straight or is experiencing stress. One shoulder may be higher than the other. The symptoms may slowly progress, often reaching a plateau after 2 to 5 years.

In some cases pain is present, usually unilateral and in one site, often at the side of the neck, the back, or the shoulder. The severity of pain varies from person to person. After a night's sleep, for a period of 10 minutes to 4 hours, spasmodic torticollis may be relieved or subside completely. Lying supine also may relieve the spasms.

Approximately 5 percent of patients recover spontaneously, most often within 5 years. Recovery seems to be more common in milder cases and in those with onset before age 40. The disorder may recur after apparent remission.

**Etiology** In most cases, etiology is unknown. Occasionally, basal ganglia disease, central nervous system infection, or tumors in the neck have been thought to be the underlying cause.

**Epidemiology** Onset is generally in the 4th or 5th decade of life but may occur at any age. Females are affected slightly more often than males.

**Related Disorders** See *Torsion Dystonia.*

**Treatment—Standard** Treatment is not always effective. Medications reported to be useful for some patients include clonazepam and diazepam; trihexyphenidyl and procyclidine; baclofen; carbamazepine; amitriptyline; amantadine; reserpine; bromocriptine; perphenazine/amitriptyline; and lithium.

Physical therapy may reduce pain associated with spasms. Cervical collars or orthopedic devices are generally not effective. Although surgery is not usually beneficial, it may be helpful in severe cases. Transcutaneous electrical nerve stimulation (**TENS**), biofeedback, nerve blocks, and relaxation techniques may also relieve pain. Supportive counseling is often of benefit. An occupational therapist may be able to help patients increase their comfort and improve mobility.

**Treatment—Investigational** The use of electronic spinal implants to improve motor function is being studied. A double-blind controlled study involving 300 patients using an electronic orphan device is being conducted by Neuromed, Fort Lauderdale, Florida.

Clinical trials of the orphan drug botulinum toxin for treating spasmodic torticollis are in progress. The NIH is giving botulinum injections to persons who qualify for the program. For additional information, contact Mark Hallet, M.D., National Institutes of Health.

Porton Products Limited has received orphan product designation from the Food and Drug Administration for clostridium botulinum type F neurotoxin.

Please contact the agencies listed under Resources, below, for the most current information. Addresses and telephone numbers of these agencies, as well as of individual experts and research centers, may be found in the Master Resources List.

**Resources**

**For more information on spasmodic torticollis:** National Organization for Rare Disorders (NORD); National Spasmodic Torticollis Association; Dystonia Medical Research Foundation; NIH/National Institute of Neurological Disorders and Stroke; International Tremor Foundation; We Move.

**References**

Cecil Textbook of Medicine, 18th ed.: J.B. Wyngaarden and L.H. Smith, Jr., eds.; W.B. Saunders Company, 1988, p. 2150.

# SPINA BIFIDA

**Description** A closure defect of the posterior portion of the neural tube produces spina bifida; part of the contents of the spinal canal protrude through this opening. In the most severe form, **rachischisis,** the opening is extensive.

**Synonyms**

Rachischisis Posterior

**Signs and Symptoms** Physical findings in spina bifida can range from mild to severe. The mildest form of the condition, spina bifida occulta, causes few, if any, symptoms and may go undetected. The lack of closure affects only a small area of the spine. Spina bifida occulta is sometimes found on x-ray, and is occasionally suspected because of a dimple or tuft of hair overlying the affected area. Impaired bladder control is a common finding, even with relatively mild forms of the condition.

In the more severe forms of spina bifida, a meningocele or meningomyelocele protrudes from the lower back. This sac, which may be as large as a grapefruit, may be covered with skin, or the nerve tissue may be exposed, and it may contain spinal fluid.

The malformation of the lower spinal cord causes abnormalities of the lower trunk and extremities of varying severity. If the condition is mild, the person may only experience muscle weakness and impaired skin sensations. In more severe cases, the legs may be paralyzed and without sensation.

Although spina bifida is usually present at birth, it occasionally is first seen during adolescence, when rapid growth stretches shortened nerves and causes progressive weakness.

**Etiology** The cause of spina bifida is not known. Hereditary and other prenatal factors may contribute.

**Epidemiology** In the United States, it is estimated that spina bifida occurs in approximately 1:2,000 live births. The condition is more frequent in Ireland and Wales and less common in Israel and among Jews in general. Spina bifida is also 3 to 4 times more common among lower socioeconomic groups of all cultures.

**Related Disorders** See *Caudal Regression Syndrome.*

**Treatment—Standard** The mildest forms of spina bifida generally require no treatment, but in moderate-to-severe conditions, surgery may be considered, as early as a few hours after birth. Special surgical considerations include imminent breakage of the sac, and placement of a shunt to drain the fluid. A coiled catheter may be implanted, which will expand as the child grows.

Cases of anaphylactic shock have occurred in children with spina bifida who have undergone surgery. These children seem to have an extreme hypersensitivity to latex. It has been suggested that any elective surgeries be postponed until the reason for the increased risk of anaphylaxis in these children can be determined.

Leg paralysis may lead to contractures, and physical therapy, further surgery, orthopedic devices, and range of motion exercises may help the patient minimize the disability.

The U.S. Public Health Service advises women of childbearing age to take 0.4 mg of folic acid daily (but not more than 1.0 mg), since it has been shown to prevent neural tube defects, including spina bifida.

**Treatment—Investigational** Various aspects of the causes of spina bifida, hydrocephalus, and related defects are being investigated, including the effects of drugs, chemicals, viruses, and other agents on nervous system development.

The National Institute of Neurological Disorders and Stroke is sponsoring a nationwide project involving 55,000 affected individuals, to collect and analyze information about spina bifida and related conditions.

Please contact the agencies listed under Resources, below, for the most current information. Addresses and telephone numbers of these agencies, as well as of individual experts and research centers, may be found in the Master Resources List.

**Resources**

**For more information on spina bifida:** National Organization for Rare Disorders (NORD); Spina Bifida Association of America; National Easter Seal Society; NIH/National Institute of Neurological Disorders and Stroke; Spina Bifida Association of Canada; International Federation for Hydrocephalus and Spina Bifida.

**For genetic information and genetic counseling referrals:** March of Dimes Birth Defects Foundation; Alliance of Genetic Support Groups.

**References**

Cecil Textbook of Medicine, 19th ed.: J.B. Wyngaarden, et al., eds.; W.B. Saunders Company, 1992, pp. 2239–2240.

Mendelian Inheritance in Man, 10th ed.: V.A. McKusick; The Johns Hopkins University Press, 1992, pp. 1028–1029.

Morbidity Mortality Weekly: September 11, 1992, vol. 41(suppl. 44 14), pp. 1–7.

Birth Defects Encyclopedia: M.L. Buyse, ed.-in-chief; Blackwell Scientific Publications, 1990, pp. 1120–1121.

Principles of Neurology, 4th ed.: R.D. Adams and M. Victor, eds.; McGraw-Hill, 1989, pp. 976–977.

Spina Bifida Today: D.G. McLone; Semin. Neurol., September 1989, vol. 9(3), pp. 169–175.

# SPINAL STENOSIS

**Description** Spinal stenosis is characterized by measurable constriction or compression of the space within the spinal canal, nerve root canals, or vertebrae.

**Synonyms**

>Cervical Spinal Stenosis
>Degenerative Lumbar Spinal Stenosis
>Lumbosacral Spinal Stenosis
>Stenosis of the Lumbar Vertebral Canal

**Signs and Symptoms** The nerve and blood vessel compression associated with spinal stenosis can lead to intermittent limping and other difficulties with walking, urinary incontinence, temporary paralysis of the legs, and pain or burning sensations in the lower back and legs.

Diagnosis relies on imaging procedures, such as magnetic resonance imaging, computed tomography, myelography, and intraoperative spinal sonography.

**Etiology** Symptoms may be associated with spinal injury or surgery, or with abnormal bone growth or deterioration, as in osteoarthritis or Paget disease of bone. The constriction is sometimes progressive. Spinal stenosis may be inherited, at least in some cases, as an autosomal dominant trait.

**Epidemiology** Spinal stenosis tends to affect males more often than females, and is usually found among middle-aged or elderly persons, although it can be present at birth. Persons engaging in extremely rough contact sports may have a greater incidence of the condition than the general population.

**Related Disorders** See *Achondroplasia,* which may precede the development of spinal stenosis; and *Paget Disease of Bone.*

**Sciatica** is characterized by pain that travels along the route of the sciatic nerve. The cause can be peripheral nerve root compression from spinal disc abnormalities, tumors, or, rarely, from infection.

**Cauda equina syndrome** is characterized by dull pain in the upper sacral region with loss of sensation in the buttocks, genitalia, or thighs, and disturbance of bowel and bladder function. The condition is caused by compression of the cauda equina below the first lumbar vertebra. Symptoms are sometimes successfully managed with surgical decompression.

A **herniated intervertebral lumbar disc** (or "slipped" disc) refers to an abnormal protrusion of the fibrous disc tissue into the spinal canal, causing local compression and nerve injury. This painful condition is common, and may require surgical intervention.

**Treatment—Standard** Surgery to decompress the affected areas of the spinal canal may be helpful; other treatment is symptomatic and supportive.

**Treatment—Investigational** Internal spinal fixation devices are being evaluated to alleviate pressure on nerves or blood vessels in the spinal canal, by mechanically altering the position of the bony vertebrae.

Please contact the agencies listed under Resources, below, for the most current information. Addresses and telephone numbers of these agencies, as well as of individual experts and research centers, may be found in the Master Resources List.

### Resources

**For more information on spinal stenosis:** National Organization for Rare Disorders (NORD); National Scoliosis Foundation; NIH/National Arthritis and Musculoskeletal and Skin Diseases Information Clearinghouse.

**For genetic information and genetic counseling referrals:** March of Dimes Birth Defects Foundation; Alliance of Genetic Support Groups.

### References

Decompressive Lumbar Laminectmy for Spinal Stenosis: H.R. Silvers; J. Neurosurg., May 1993, vol. 78(5), pp. 695–701.
Lumbar Spinal Stenosis: S.F. Ciricillo; West. J. Med., February 1993, vol. 158(2), pp. 171–177.
Mendelian Inheritance in Man, 10th ed.: V.A. McKusick; The Johns Hopkins University Press, 1992, p. 675.
Principles of Neurology, 4th ed.: R.D. Adams and M. Victor, eds.; McGraw-Hill, 1989, pp. 162–168.

# STIFF-MAN SYNDROME

**Description** Stiff-man syndrome is a very rare neurologic disorder characterized by diffuse hypertonia that includes the voluntary muscles of the neck, trunk, shoulders, and proximal extremities, and by painful muscle spasms.

### Synonyms

Moersch-Woltmann Syndrome

**Signs and Symptoms** Onset is gradual. Initial symptoms include aching and tightness of the involved muscles, possibly bilaterally. As muscular rigidity progresses, pain may increase, and patients may have difficulty making sudden movements. In severe cases, bone fractures may result from the extreme twisting and contracting of the muscles. Hyperhidrosis and tachycardia may accompany muscle spasms. Contractions usually are relieved by sleep.

The course of this disorder is progressive, with eventual involvement of the muscles of the back and abdomen. As stiffness increases, patients may develop kyphosis or lordosis.

**Etiology** The cause of stiff-man syndrome is unknown. Genetic factors have not been established clearly, although the disorder appears to be familial.

An autoimmune association has been postulated. External factors such as sudden noise and emotional stimuli can precipitate muscle spasms.

**Epidemiology** About 70 percent of affected persons are male.

**Related Disorders** See *Torsion Dystonia.*

**Treatment—Standard** Diazepam may provide dramatic relief of muscle rigidity and spasms.

**Treatment—Investigational** Pietro DeCamilli, M.D., and Michele Solemana, M.D., at Yale University theorize that stiff-man syndrome may be an autoimmune disorder and are studying the use of plasma exchange combined with steroid drugs as a potential treatment. The effectiveness and side effects of this therapy currently are being investigated.

Please contact the agencies listed under Resources, below, for the most current information. Addresses and telephone numbers of these agencies, as well as of individual experts and research centers, may be found in the Master Resources List.

### Resources

**For more information on stiff-man syndrome:** National Organization for Rare Disorders (NORD); Mark Hallet, M.D., NIH/National Institute of Neurological Disorders and Stroke.

### References

Autoantibodies to GABA-ergic Neurons and Pancreatic Beta Cells in Stiff Man Syndrome: M. Solimena, et al.; N. Engl. J. Med., May 31, 1990, vol. 322(2), pp. 1555–1560.
Mendelian Inheritance in Man, 9th ed.: V.A. McKusick; The Johns Hopkins University Press, 1990, pp. 553, 880.

# SYDENHAM CHOREA

**Description** Sydenham chorea is an acute, usually self-limited, disorder of early life that occurs in about 5 to 10 percent of cases of rheumatic fever, beginning several months after the polyarthritis has subsided.

### Synonyms

Chorea Minor
Infectious Chorea

Rheumatic Chorea

St. Vitus Dance

**Signs and Symptoms** Affected individuals develop rapid, involuntary, nonrepetitive movements that gradually become severe, affecting gait, arm movements, and speech. Fatigue and restlessness may precede the onset of chorea. Clumsiness and facial grimacing are common. The disorder is bilateral in 75 percent of cases. Choreic movements disappear with sleep. Occasionally the patient may require sedation to avoid self-injury. The disorder subsides in 3 to 6 months with no neurologic residua.

**Etiology** Sydenham chorea is a complication of streptococcal infection.

**Epidemiology** Onset of choreic symptoms may occur up to 6 months after the streptococcal infection has been cleared. Girls are affected more often than boys, usually between the ages of 5 and 15 years.

**Related Disorders** See *Cerebral Palsy; Huntington Disease; Tourette Syndrome; Wilson Disease.*

Scarlet fever and rheumatic fever may precede the development of Sydenham chorea. See *Rheumatic Fever.*

**Treatment—Standard** No medication is consistently effective in the treatment of Sydenham chorea. Tranquilizers, barbiturates, salicylates, or corticosteroids may be helpful in some patients. Symptoms disappear even without treatment after 6 to 8 months.

**Treatment—Investigational** Please contact the agencies listed under Resources, below, for the most current information. Addresses and telephone numbers of these agencies, as well as of individual experts and research centers, may be found in the Master Resources List.

**Resources**

For more information on Sydenham chorea: National Organization for Rare Disorders (NORD); NIH/National Institute of Neurological Disorders and Stroke; Centers for Disease Control.

**References**

Harrison's Principles of Internal Medicine, 12th ed.: J.D. Wilson, et al., eds.; McGraw-Hill, 1991, p. 935.

Scientific American MEDICINE: E. Rubinstein and D. Federman, eds.; Scientific American, 1978–1991, p. 15:VII:2.

Carbamazepine: An Alternative Drug for the Treatment of Nonhereditary Chorea: M. Roig, et al.; Pediatrics, September 1988, vol. 82(pt. 2), pp. 492–495.

Tetrabenazine Therapy of Dystonia, Chorea, Tics and Other Dyskinesias: J. Jankovic, et al.; Neurology, March 1988, vol. 38(3), pp. 391–394.

# SYRINGOBULBIA

**Description** Syringobulbia is a slowly progressive neurologic disorder in which cavitation occurs in the brain stem. The cavity (syrinx) in *Syringomyelia* is usually in the central portion of the spinal cord, but may extend from the cervical to the lumbar regions. In syringobulbia, the syrinx is in the lower brain stem.

Syringobulbia is often associated with craniovertebral anomalies, including *Arnold-Chiari Syndrome.*

**Signs and Symptoms** Features of syringobulbia may include vocal cord paralysis, atrophy and fibrillation of the tongue muscle, dysarthria, vertigo, and nystagmus. There also may be anhidrosis and flushing on the affected side of the face (see *Horner Syndrome).*

**Etiology** The defect may be congenital but does not increase in size and cause symptoms until later in life (e.g., early adulthood). Brain stem injury from trauma, tumors, or compression may also cause syringobulbia.

**Epidemiology** Syringobulbia can affect persons of either sex. Onset usually is before 30 years of age.

**Related Disorders** See *Syringomyelia; Arnold-Chiari Syndrome.*

The symptoms in some forms of amyloid neuropathy are similar to those of syringobulbia (see *Amyloidosis).*

Neoplasms and vascular malformations in the brain stem may cause neurologic symptoms similar to those of syringobulbia.

**Treatment—Standard** Surgical drainage may be indicated in some cases. Nonsurgical treatment of syringobulbia is symptomatic and supportive. Radiation therapy has not been beneficial.

**Treatment—Investigational** Please contact the agencies listed under Resources, below, for the most current information. Addresses and telephone numbers of these agencies, as well as of individual experts and research centers, may be found in the Master Resources List.

**Resources**

For more information on syringobulbia: National Organization for Rare Disorders (NORD); American Syringomyelia Alliance Project; NIH/National Institute of Neurological Disorders and Stroke; National Spinal Cord Injury Hotline; American Spinal Injury Association; National Spinal Cord Injury Association.

**References**

Harrison's Principles of Internal Medicine, 12th ed.: J.D. Wilson, et al., eds.; McGraw-Hill, 1991, p. 2086.

Infantile Hypoventilation Syndrome, Neurenteric Cyst, and Syringobulbia: H.D. Chung, et al.; Neurology (NY), April 1982, vol. 32(4), pp. 441–444.

# SYRINGOMYELIA

**Description** Syringomyelia is a slowly progressive neurologic disorder in which cavitation occurs in the spinal cord. The cavity (syrinx) is usually paramedian and may extend up into the medulla oblongata (see **Syringobulbia)** or down as far as the lumbar region.

Syringomyelia is often associated with craniovertebral anomalies, including **Arnold-Chiari Syndrome.**

**Synonyms**

Morvan Disease

Myelosyringosis

**Signs and Symptoms** If the syrinx is located in the cervical or thoracic areas of the spine, the initial symptoms may include loss of pain and temperature perception in the upper extremities and chest, spreading to the shoulders and back. Reflexes may be absent. The sense of touch is not affected, however.

When the lumbar and sacral segments of the spine are affected, typical findings include spasticity, muscle weakness, and ataxia in the lower extremities as well as paralysis of the bladder.

Syringomyelia is a slowly progressive disorder. Erosion of the bony spinal canal, osteoporosis, joint contractures, and progressive scoliosis may occur.

Diagnosis relies on imaging techniques such as delayed computed tomographic metrizamide myelography or magnetic resonance imaging.

**Morvan disease** is a severe form of syringomyelia accompanied by ulceration of fingers and toes.

**Etiology** Autosomal dominant inheritance for some cases has been suggested. Syringomyelia may also be caused by injury of the spinal cord from trauma, tumors, or compression.

**Epidemiology** Usually, males and females under age 30 years are affected. About 1,000 cases are identified in the United States each year.

**Related Disorders** See **Syringobulbia; Arnold-Chiari Syndrome.**

The symptoms in some forms of amyloid neuropathy are similar to those of syringomyelia (see **Amyloidosis).**

Neoplasms and vascular malformations in the spinal cord may also cause neurologic symptoms similar to those of syringomyelia.

**Treatment—Standard** Syringoperitoneal shunting to drain the fluid has been effective in reversing or arresting neurologic deterioration in some patients. Radiation therapy has not been beneficial.

Intraoperative sonography (**IOS**) has been used during surgery to evaluate the effectiveness of the procedure as it is being performed.

**Treatment—Investigational** Please contact the agencies listed under Resources, below, for the most current information. Addresses and telephone numbers of these agencies, as well as of individual experts and research centers, may be found in the Master Resources List.

**Resources**

**For more information on syringomyelia:** National Organization for Rare Disorders (NORD); American Syringomyelia Alliance Project; NIH/National Institute of Neurological Disorders and Stroke.

**References**

Harrison's Principles of Internal Medicine, 12th ed.: J.D. Wilson, et al., eds.; McGraw-Hill, 1991, p. 2086.

Mendelian Inheritance in Man, 9th ed.: V.A. McKusick; The Johns Hopkins University Press, 1990, pp. 890–891, 1490.

# TARDIVE DYSKINESIA

**Description** Tardive dyskinesia is a neurologic syndrome associated with the long-term use of neuroleptic drugs, producing symptoms that mimic certain neurologic diseases but are neurotoxic side effects of the drugs. The syndrome usually appears late in the course of drug therapy and may persist indefinitely after discontinuation of the medication.

**Synonyms**

Oral-Facial Dyskinesia

Tardive Dystonia

**Signs and Symptoms** Typical involuntary and abnormal facial movements include grimacing, sticking out the tongue, and sucking and smacking of the lips. Involuntary, rapid movements of the arms and legs (chorea and athetosis) also may occur. These symptoms often remain long after the neuroleptic drugs have been discontinued, although some may disappear with time.

**Etiology** Tardive dyskinesia results from long-term use (3 months to years) of neuroleptic drugs, prescribed not only for the treatment of psychoses but also for certain gastrointestinal and neurologic disorders.

**Epidemiology** Prevalence in patients being treated with neuroleptics depends on the specific drug, dosage, and duration of treatment. The risk is higher for women and with advancing age.

**Related Disorders** The following disorders all have symptoms that may mimic those of tardive dyskinesia. See ***Cerebral Palsy; Huntington Disease; Tourette Syndrome.***

**Treatment—Standard** Prevention is important because most symptomatic treatment is unsatisfactory and potentially dangerous. The neuroleptic drug must be discontinued as soon as any involuntary facial movements are observed. Psychiatric disorders treated with neuroleptic drugs may go into remissions, at which time the drugs should be reduced and discontinued when possible to prevent tardive dyskinesia.

**Treatment—Investigational** The use of vitamin E is being evaluated for the possible treatment of tardive dyskinesia. Patients involved in this study have persistent, moderate-to-severe symptoms of tardive dyskinesia, and are between the ages of 18 and 70 years. Information about this research project can be obtained from Denise Juliano, Neuropsychiatric Research Hospital, Washington, DC.

Please contact the agencies listed under Resources, below, for the most current information. Addresses and telephone numbers of these agencies, as well as of individual experts and research centers, may be found in the Master Resources List.

**Resources**

**For more information on tardive dyskinesia:** National Organization for Rare Disorders (NORD); Tardive Dyskinesia/Tardive Dystonia National Association; NIH/National Institute of Mental Health; National Mental Health Association; Dystonia Medical Research Foundation.

**References**

Internal Medicine, 3rd ed.: J.H. Stein, ed.-in-chief; Little, Brown and Company, 1990, pp. 1955, 2003.

Facial Dyskinesia: J. Janovic, et al.; Adv. Neurol., 1988, p. 49.

Suppression of Tardive Dyskinesia with Amoxapine: Case Report: D.A. D'Mello, et al.; J. Clin. Psychiatry, March 1986, vol. 47(3), p. 148.

Diagnostic and Statistical Manual of Mental Disorders, 3rd ed.: American Psychiatric Association, 1984, pp. 76–77.

# TARSAL TUNNEL SYNDROME

**Description** Tarsal tunnel syndrome is a compression neuropathy of the posterior tibial nerve at the ankle.

**Synonyms**

Posterior Tibial Nerve Neuralgia

**Signs and Symptoms** Symptoms typically are painful burning, tingling, or numbness in the foot. Pain is often more intense at night, and is relieved by moving the foot.

**Etiology** The posterior tibial nerve may become compressed where it enters a confined compartment or tunnel inferior to the medial malleolus of the tibia at the ankle. An old fracture, hypertrophied adjacent muscles, or vascular compression may be responsible for the compression; but in some cases no abnormality can be demonstrated.

**Epidemiology** Onset can be at any age. Males and females appear to be affected in equal numbers. The disorder is most common among individuals who stand for long periods.

**Related Disorders** See ***Erythromelalgia; Peripheral Neuropathy.***

**Burning feet syndrome (Gopalan syndrome)** is thought to be caused by deficiency of a B vitamin. Symptoms include severe burning, aching, cramping, and pins-and-needles sensations in the soles of the feet. In some cases the palms of the hands are affected.

**Treatment—Standard** Tension on the affected nerve should be alleviated by immobilization of the foot or adaptation of the shoe. Anti-inflammatory drugs and local corticosteroid injection are the usual treatment. Surgery should be reserved for cases that do not respond to conservative treatment.

**Treatment—Investigational** Please contact the agencies listed under Resources, below, for the most current information. Addresses and telephone numbers of these agencies, as well as of individual experts and research centers, may be found in the Master Resources List.

**Resources**

**For more information on tarsal tunnel syndrome:** National Organization for Rare Disorders (NORD); NIH/National Arthritis and Musculoskeletal and Skin Diseases Information Clearinghouse.

**References**

Tarsal Tunnel Syndrome: A Case Report and Review of the Literature: G.M. O'Malley, et al.; Orthopedics, June 1985, vol. 8(6), pp. 758–760.

Tarsal Tunnel Syndrome: E.L. Radin; Clin. Orthop., December 1983, vol. 181, pp. 167–170.

# TETHERED SPINAL CORD SYNDROME

**Description** The syndrome is characterized by progressive neurologic deterioration, the result of unnatural stretching of the spinal cord due to vertebral adhesions. Tethered spinal cord syndrome is usually the result of spina bifida.

**Synonyms**

> Congenital Tethered Cervical Spinal Cord Syndrome
> Occult Spinal Dysraphism Sequence
> Tethered Cervical Spinal Cord Syndrome
> Tethered Cord Malformation Sequence

**Signs and Symptoms** Affected children at birth commonly have a characteristic lesion on the skin of the lower back, which may consist of tufts of hair, skin tags, dimples, or fatty tumors. Initial symptoms are usually urologic and may include incontinence and repeated urinary tract infections. Progressive foot and spinal deformities are characteristic. Other symptoms may include weakness of the lower extremities, fecal incontinence, low back pain, or a combination of these.

Adult onset is very rare. The most common symptom is diffuse leg pain, which may reach as high as the rectum. Progressive sensory and motor deficits may occur in the lower extremities, as well as bladder and bowel dysfunction.

It is believed that the amount of traction exerted on the spinal cord, rather than the type or distribution of lesions, probably determines the age of onset of symptoms. Less severe traction usually produces no symptoms in childhood, but may result in neurologic dysfunction in later life because of repeated tugging at the base of the cord during natural head and neck flexion, or when the condition is aggravated by trauma or disease.

**Etiology** Vertebral adhesions are believed to cause the tethering or compression of nerve roots, and to be the result of structural defects arising from improper closure of the neural tube at approximately 28 days of embryonic development.

Children with cutaneous hemangiomas on the lower back may also have tethered spinal cords. (See also **diastematomyelia**, below.)

**Epidemiology** First-degree relatives of those with the malformation appear to be at slightly higher risk of developing it. Individuals with previously repaired defects of the neural tube are also particularly susceptible. Males and females are affected equally.

**Related Disorders** See *Spina Bifida.*

**Diastematomyelia** is believed to be caused by genetic or environmental factors during embryonic development that cause a longitudinal division in half of the spinal cord. In some cases, abnormalities of the vertebrae occur because of the adjustment necessary for encasing the 2 halves of the cord. Diastematomyelia is often associated with spina bifida, clubfoot, or tethered spinal cord syndrome. Symptoms may include pain, weakness of legs, and urinary and fecal incontinence. Surgery during infancy is often recommended. Later in life, surgery is performed only if neurologic symptoms develop.

**Treatment—Standard** The appearance of surface lesions on the lower back at birth should lead to further testing for tethered spinal cord syndrome. Magnetic resonance imaging **(MRI)** is usually the technique of choice for identifying the tethered cord. Preoperative evaluation of potential sites of tethering, based on MRI findings, is vital for planning surgery. Removal of adhesions at the lower base of the spine through surgery is often recommended, and results are usually successful. Early management usually prevents neuromuscular, lower limb, or urologic problems. It is best to treat the tethered cord before serious complications become apparent, as neurologic damage may not be reversible.

In cases where surgical release of the tethered spinal cord is ineffective, a posterior rhizotomy may relieve pain.

**Treatment—Investigational** Please contact the agencies listed under Resources, below, for the most current information. Addresses and telephone numbers of these agencies, as well as of individual experts and research centers, may be found in the Master Resources List.

**Resources**

**For more information on tethered spinal cord syndrome:** National Organization for Rare Disorders (NORD); NIH/National Institute of Neurological Disorders and Stroke; Spina Bifida Association of America; Spina Bifida Association of Canada; International Federation for Hydrocephalus and Spina Bifida.

**References**

Lumbar Cutaneous Hemangiomas As Indicators of Tethered Spinal Cords: A.L. Albright, et al.; Pediatrics, June 1989, vol. 83(6), pp. 977–980.

Tethered Cord Syndrome: A Pediatric Case Study: L. Greif, et al.; J. Neurosci. Nurs, April 1989, vol. 21(2), pp. 86–91.

Urologic Aspects of Tethered Cord: R.C. Flanigan, et al.; Urology, January 1989, vol. 33(1), pp. 80–82.

Diagnosis of Tethered Cords by Magnetic Resonance Imaging: W.A. Hall, et al.; Surg. Neurol., July 1988, vol. 30(1), pp. 60–64.

Smith's Recognizable Patterns of Human Malformation, 4th ed.: K.L. Jones; W.B. Saunders Company, 1988, p. 550.

# THALAMIC SYNDROME

**Description** Thalamic syndrome is a rare neurologic disorder characterized by pain and loss of sensation, usually in the face, arm, or leg.

**Synonyms**
> Dejerine-Roussy Syndrome
> Retrolenticular Syndrome
> Thalamic Hyperesthetic Anesthesia
> Thalamic Pain Syndrome

**Signs and Symptoms** All types of sensations can be involved, including touch, taste, and temperature awareness as well as pain. Half of the body is usually affected (e.g., hemihypoesthesia, transient hemiparesis). The pain may increase with stimulation, e.g., on touch or exposure to cold temperatures. Responses to touch vary from hyperpathia to dysesthesia and then hyperresponsiveness. Mild muscular weakness or hemiparesis may be present.

**Etiology** The cause is damage to the thalamus, producing nerve cell loss that may be due, for example, to a blood clot, air embolus, lesion, or tumor.

**Epidemiology** Males and females are affected in equal numbers.

**Related Disorders** See *Reflex Sympathetic Dystrophy Syndrome; Guillain-Barré Syndrome.*

Major symptoms of the very prevalent **carpal tunnel syndrome** include a sensation of numbness, tingling, burning, and a slight pain in the hand and wrist. The sensation is often temporary at first, but can become chronic; left untreated, muscles in the hand may become atrophied.

**Treatment—Standard** Surgical lesions can interrupt the sensory pathway of the brain and may help decrease the pain without affecting sensory ability.

**Treatment—Investigational** Please contact the agencies listed under Resources, below, for the most current information. Addresses and telephone numbers of these agencies, as well as of individual experts and research centers, may be found in the Master Resources List.

**Resources**

For more information on thalamic syndrome: National Organization for Rare Disorders (NORD); NIH/National Institute of Neurological Disorders and Stroke; International Tremor Foundation.

**References**

Brain Glucose Metabolism in Thalamic Syndrome: E.C. Laterre, et al.; J. Neurol. Neurosurg. Psychiatry, March 1988, vol. 51(3), pp. 427–428.

Cecil Textbook of Medicine, 18th ed.: J.B. Wyngaarden and L.H. Smith, Jr., eds.; W.B. Saunders Company, 1988, pp. 2128–2129.

Thalamic Pain Syndrome of Dejerine-Roussy: F. Mauguiere and J.E Desmedt; Arch. Neurol., December 1988, vol. 45(12), pp. 1312–1320.

# THOMSEN DISEASE

**Description** Thomsen disease is a rare, nonprogressive, inherited neuromuscular condition, usually beginning in infancy, that is characterized by muscle stiffness on first attempting movement and also by muscle inability to relax following movement. If all the body muscles are involved, the entire body may become stiff.

**Synonyms**
> Myotonia Congenita
> Thomsen-Becker Myotonia

**Signs and Symptoms** When movement is attempted after rest, muscles become rigid. Contraction may continue for 30 seconds or more after mechanical stimulation, but the stiffness subsides as the same movement is repeated a few times. Slowness in chewing, swallowing, talking, and walking are typical, and muscles are often large and well-developed for the child's age. The symptoms may improve as the child grows older, and life span is normal.

**Etiology** Thomsen disease is inherited as an autosomal dominant trait.

**Epidemiology** Thomsen disease usually begins at birth or shortly after, although, rarely, it appears at puberty. Males seem to be affected more often than females.

**Related Disorders** See *Myotonic Dystrophy,* in which there is a similar problem of muscle inability to relax after contraction. Differentiation can be made, however, by the muscular weakness and atrophy seen in myotonic dystrophy.

**Schwartz-Jampel syndrome (chondrodystrophic myotonia)** is characterized by failure of muscle development to keep pace with overall growth. The condition begins in early infancy.

**Treatment—Standard** The antiarrhythmic drug tocainide is used as a treatment for Thomsen disease. Careful monitoring of dosage and heart function is important. Procainamide, phenytoin, and quinine also have been effective.

There is usually a poor response to physical therapy in Thomsen disease, but active and passive exercises may be helpful in some instances. Agencies that provide services to handicapped persons and their families may be of benefit. Genetic counseling also may be useful.

**Treatment—Investigational** The experimental antimyotonic drug mexiletine may improve muscle weakness in some patients, but this treatment is still under investigation.

Please contact the agencies listed under Resources, below, for the most current information. Addresses and telephone numbers of these agencies, as well as of individual experts and research centers, may be found in the Master Resources List.

**Resources**

**For more information on Thomsen disease:** National Organization for Rare Disorders (NORD); NIH/National Institute of Neurological Disorders and Stroke; NIH/National Arthritis and Musculoskeletal and Skin Diseases Information Clearinghouse; Muscular Dystrophy Association.

**For genetic information and genetic counseling referrals:** March of Dimes Birth Defects Foundation; Alliance of Genetic Support Groups.

**References**

Mendelian Inheritance in Man, 9th ed.: V.A. McKusick; The Johns Hopkins University Press, 1990, p. 638.

Nelson Textbook of Pediatrics, 13th ed.: R.E. Behrman and V.C. Vaughan, III, eds.; W.B. Saunders Company, 1987, p. 1339.

Successful Treatment with Tocainide of Recessive Generalized Congenital Myotonia: E.W. Streib; Ann. Neurol., May 1986, vol. 19(5), pp. 501–504.

Value of Mexiletine in the Treatment of Thomsen-Becker Myotonia: F. Himon, et al.; Arch. Fr. Pediatr., January 1986, vol. 43(1), pp. 49–50.

# TINNITUS

**Description** Tinnitus is a person's subjective experience of sound that does not exist in the environment.

**Signs and Symptoms** The sounds of tinnitus have variously been described as clicking, buzzing, whistling, ringing, roaring, etc. They may be continuously present, or intermittent. There frequently is an associated hearing loss.

**Etiology** Many ear disorders are associated with tinnitus, including infection, obstruction, tumors, and Meniere syndrome. Certain medications and environmental toxins may be implicated, as may head injuries and alcohol abuse.

**Epidemiology** More than 37 million persons in the United States have tinnitus. Males and females are affected in equal numbers.

**Related Disorders Bruits,** heard in auscultation by the examiner, can sometimes be heard by the patient and may be mistaken for tinnitus.

Internal (though imaginary) sounds are a feature of some mental illnesses such as schizophrenia.

**Treatment—Standard** Treatment of any underlying disease may cure the tinnitus. Otherwise, relief may be obtained through the use of pleasant background noise, e.g., music or other sounds attractive to the patient, such as ocean surf.

**Treatment—Investigational** A surgical procedure using microsurgical techniques is sometimes suggested in the most severe cases of tinnitus. The surgery seeks to relieve pressure on the portion of the 8th cranial nerve associated with hearing. Margareta Moller, M.D., Allegheny General Hospital, may be contacted.

In another procedure being studied, lidocaine is delivered inside the eardrum through a grommet (intratympanic instillation). Treatment with lidocaine is continued for 5 weeks. Some patients experience temporary improvement.

A synthetic form of prostaglandin E1 (misoprostol) is being investigated.

Research indicates that alprazolam may be useful in reducing symptoms. The dosage required to achieve satisfactory results can vary greatly, however, and some patients experience side effects at even low doses.

In other studies, the following drugs have been investigated for treatment of tinnitus: oxazepam, clonazepam, sodium amylobarbitone, flunarizine, and eperisone hydrochloride.

Please contact the agencies listed under Resources, below, for the most current information. Addresses and telephone numbers of these agencies, as well as of individual experts and research centers, may be found in the Master Resources List.

**Resources**

**For more information on tinnitus:** National Organization for Rare Disorders (NORD); American Tinnitus Association; NIH/National Institute on Deafness and Other Communication Disorders.

### References

Principles of Neurology, 5th ed.: R.D. Adams and M. Victor, eds.; McGraw-Hill, 1993, pp. 252–253.

Synthetic Prostaglandin E1 Misoprostol As a Treatment for Tinnitus: W. Briner, et al.; Arch. Otolaryngol. Head Neck Surg., June 1993, vol. 119(6), pp. 652–654.

Cecil Textbook of Medicine, 19th ed.: J.B. Wyngaarden, et al., eds.; W.B. Saunders Company, 1992, pp. 2108–2109.

Erythromycin Ototoxicity: Prospective Assessment with Serum Concentrations and Audiograms in a Study of Patients with Pneumonia: D.J. Swanson, et al.; Am. J. Med., January 1992, vol. 92(1), pp. 61–68.

Tinnitus and Vertigo in Patients with Temporomandibular Disorder: R.A. Chole, et al.; Arch. Otolaryngol. Head Neck Surg., August 1992, vol. 118(8), pp. 817–821.

Tinnitus: Imaging Algorithms: R.A. Willinsky; Can. Assoc. Radio. J., April 1992, vol. 43(2), pp. 93–99.

Tinnitus Suppression Following Cochlear Implantation: A Multifactorial Investigation: C.R. Souliere, et al.; Arch. Otolaryngol. Head Neck Surg., December 1992, vol. 118(12), pp. 1291–1297.

Diseases of the Nose, Throat, Ear, Head and Neck, 14th ed.: J.J. Ballenger; Lea and Febiger, 1991, pp. 1194–1195.

Harrison's Principles of Internal Medicine, 12th ed.: J.D. Wilson, et al., eds.; McGraw-Hill, 1991, p. 156.

# TORSION DYSTONIA

**Description** Torsion dystonia is a neurologic disorder characterized by involuntary contortions of muscles in the neck, torso, and extremities. Occasionally only one or a few muscles are involved. The disorder is most noticeable on walking, when involvement of several muscle groups may produce a sideways gait, with the body twisting as if writhing.

**Synonyms**

Dystonia Lenticularis

Ziehen-Oppenheim Disease

**Signs and Symptoms** In the early stages, the symptoms may be mild and sporadic, occurring only after prolonged activity or stress. As the disease progresses, the contortions begin to occur during any physical activity, particularly walking; in advanced disease they also occur during rest. Not all cases are progressive, however, and the dystonia may plateau at a mild level.

Secondary symptoms include foot drag, cramps in the hands and feet, difficulty in grasping objects, and unclear speech. The contractured tendons and buildup of connective tissue in muscle may cause permanent physical deformities.

**Etiology** Torsion dystonia may be inherited as a recessive, dominant, or X-linked trait, or may be acquired. A chromosome marker for hereditary forms of dystonia, identified in 1989, indicates that the gene is located on the long arm of chromosome 9.

In the autosomal recessive form, muscle contractions of the feet and hands typically appear in childhood or adolescence. Symptoms spread quickly to involve the trunk and extremities, but progression slows after adolescence. This form is more severe than the autosomal dominant form.

In the autosomal dominant form, muscles in the torso and neck are affected first. Symptoms progress slowly, but new muscle groups may be initially involved well beyond adolescence.

An X-linked form of torsion dystonia has been described in which the initial symptom is spasmodic eye blinking.

Torsion dystonia acquired as a result of brain injury due to infection, trauma, birth injury, or stroke is frequently unilateral and nonprogressive.

**Epidemiology** The autosomal recessive form usually becomes apparent by puberty and primarily affects Ashkenazic Jews. The defective gene is carried by 1:100 Ashkenazic Jews in the United States. Males and females are affected in equal numbers.

Onset of the rarer autosomal dominant form is in late adolescence or early adulthood.

The average age at onset for the X-linked form seems to be about the late 30s.

**Related Disorders** Torsion dystonia must be differentiated from other conditions associated with involuntary contortions. See **Ataxia, Marie; Cerebral Palsy; Glutaricaciduria I; Spasmodic Torticollis; Tardive Dyskinesia.**

**Segawa dystonia** is extremely rare. A chemical imbalance in the central nervous system causes lack of muscle control. Movement in the morning is almost normal but by the afternoon is disabling. Onset is in early childhood; symptoms worsen for a few years and then become static. Segawa dystonia is often misdiagnosed as cerebral palsy. The disorder is inherited as an autosomal dominant trait.

**Treatment—Standard** Drugs used to treat dystonia include trihexyphenidyl, benztropine, diazepam, clonazepam, baclofen, carbamazepine, levodopa, bromocriptine, chlorpromazine, thiopropazate, haloperidol, pimozide, tetrabenazine, and amantadine.

**Treatment—Investigational** Surgical techniques in development for the treatment of torsion dystonia include the implantation of electrical devices to stimulate nerve impulse transmission. Other surgical procedures are ablative. A high-risk procedure involves destruction of the cells of the basal ganglia that are transmitting incorrect instructions. In severe cases, the nerves connecting with the contracting muscles may be severed.

Botulinum toxin, an orphan drug approved by the Food and Drug Administration in 1989, is being tested in connection with certain forms of dystonia. The drug is manufactured by Oculinum.

Sinemet, being tested at the National Institute of Neurological Disorders and Stroke in Bethesda, Maryland, for treatment of Segawa dystonia, has dramatically alleviated symptoms in patients with this inherited disorder. Sinemet's property of stimulating the production of dopamine is useful in this case, since children with Segawa dystonia are deficient in dopamine. For more information, contact John K. Fink, M.D.

Please contact the agencies listed under Resources, below, for the most current information. Addresses and telephone numbers of these agencies, as well as of individual experts and research centers, may be found in the Master Resources List.

### Resources

**For more information on torsion dystonia:** National Organization for Rare Disorders (NORD); NIH/National Institute of Neurological Disorders and Stroke; Dystonia Medical Research Foundation; National Foundation for Jewish Genetic Diseases; We Move.

**For genetic information and genetic counseling referrals:** March of Dimes Birth Defects Foundation; Alliance of Genetic Support Groups.

### References

Cecil Textbook of Medicine, 19th ed.: J.B. Wyngaarden, et al., eds.; W.B. Saunders Company, 1992, pp. 2134–2135.
The Dystonias: C.H. Markham; Curr. Opin. Neurol. Neurosurg., June 1992, vol. 5(3), pp. 301–307.
Mendelian Inheritance in Man, 10th ed.: V.A. McKusick; The Johns Hopkins University Press, 1992, pp. 328–329, 1349, 1974.
The Genetics of Primary Torsion Dystonia: U. Miller; Hum. Genet., January 1990, vol. 84(4), pp. 107–115.
Autosomal Dominant Torsion Dystonia in a Swedish Family: L. Forsgren, et al.; Adv. Neurol., 1988, vol. 50, pp. 83–92.
Clinical Course of Idiopathic Torsion Dystonia Among Jews in Israel: R. Inzelberg, et al.; Adv. Neurol., 1988, vol. 50, pp. 93–100.

# TOURETTE SYNDROME

**Description** Tourette syndrome is a neurologic disorder characterized by motor and vocal tics, manifested as involuntary muscle movements of the extremities, shoulder, and face, and uncontrollable noises, sounds, and sometimes inappropriate words. Tourette syndrome is not a progressive or degenerative disorder; rather, symptoms tend to be variable and follow a chronic waxing and waning course throughout an otherwise normal life span.

### Synonyms

> Brissaud II
> Chronic Multiple Tics
> Coprolalia–Generalized Tic Disorder
> Tics

**Signs and Symptoms** Onset usually occurs in childhood with a tic in a facial muscle, causing excessive blinking, nose twitching, or grimacing. Other gestures include involuntary head shaking, shoulder jerking, arm flapping, foot stamping, and the uncontrollable imitation of another person's movements. Some patients may have self-mutilating symptoms.

The sounds produced can be inarticulate and incoherent, such as grunts, barks, screams, or sniffing, or they can include words. **Coprolalia** occurs in approximately 30 percent of all patients. Involuntary repetition of a word or sentence spoken by the patient or another person (**palilalia** or **echolalia**) also is common.

Tics may subside when the patient is concentrating on a particular task, but intensify during stress. Over periods of months to years, some symptoms may disappear and be replaced by new tics; or new symptoms may be added to old ones.

**Etiology** Seventy percent of all cases appear to be genetic, inherited as an autosomal dominant trait, although an X-linked Tourette modifier gene has been described. Research suggests that there may be a biochemical dysfunction that affects neurotransmitter systems in the brain.

The effect of gene penetrance is suggested by the high prevalence of first-degree relatives with mild tic conditions in families with Tourette syndrome. Some relatives may have chronic tics, while others may not display any tics but exhibit obsessive-compulsive behaviors, which recent research indicates are frequently associated with Tourette syndrome. Attention deficit disorder also occurs more frequently in patients with Tourette syndrome.

Genetic studies suggest that only about 10 percent of affected relatives have symptoms severe enough to interfere with normal, daily living. The chance of an affected parent having a child with Tourette symptoms has been estimated to be approximately 40 to 50 percent. In many cases, however, the child will have a mild form of the syndrome, although severity of symptoms currently cannot be predicted.

**Epidemiology** A childhood onset between the ages of 2 and 16 years is most typical, although there are rare cases with later onset as well as symptoms appearing at 1 year of age. The male-to-female ratio is 4:1. Tourette syndrome occurs in all nationalities and across all economic groups.

**Related Disorders Transient tics of childhood** are common among children. These motor or vocal tics usually disappear within 1 year.

**Chronic tics** begin in childhood, or after age 40. Usually either motor or vocal tics are present, not both, and are more limited than in Tourette syndrome.

**Treatment—Standard** Haloperidol in low doses helps suppress symptoms in many patients, but side effects often limit its use.

Clonidine appears to improve motor, vocal, and behavioral symptoms in approximately 50 percent of patients, according to some reports.

Pimozide, an approved orphan drug with dopaminergic blocking action, appears to be as effective as haloperidol with fewer side effects for some Tourette patients. Other dopamine-blocking drugs (e.g., fluphenazine) also are useful for reducing Tourette symptoms.

Supportive psychotherapy can help patients adjust to this chronic, often socially crippling disorder.

**Treatment—Investigational** Please contact the agencies listed under Resources, below, for the most current information. Addresses and telephone numbers of these agencies, as well as of individual experts and research centers, may be found in the Master Resources List.

**Resources**

**For more information on Tourette syndrome:** National Organization for Rare Disorders (NORD); Tourette Syndrome Association; NIH/National Institute of Neurological Disorders and Stroke.

**For genetic information and genetic counseling referrals:** March of Dimes Birth Defects Foundation; Alliance of Genetic Support Groups.

**References**

Antineuronal Antibodies in Movement Disorders: L.S. Kiessling, et al.; Pediatrics, July 1993, vol. 92(1), pp. 39–43.

Cecil Textbook of Medicine, 19th ed.: J.B. Wyngaarden, et al., eds.; W.B. Saunders Company, 1992, p. 2137.

Mendelian Inheritance in Man, 10th ed.: V.A. McKusick; The Johns Hopkins University Press, 1992, p. 270.

Diagnostic and Statistical Manual of Mental Disorders, 3rd ed., revised: R.L. Spitzer, et al., eds.; American Psychiatric Association, 1987, pp. 79–82.

# TRICHOTILLOMANIA

**Description** Trichotillomania is characterized by an overwhelming and irresistible impulse to pull out one's hair. Patches of baldness result, usually on the most easily accessible areas, such as the scalp, eyebrows, eyelashes, or beard. Trichotillomania is classified as a disorder of impulse control.

**Synonyms**

Hair Pulling

**Signs and Symptoms** The principal feature is the recurrent failure to resist impulses to pull out, or break off, one's hair. Extreme tension usually precedes the act, with a feeling of release following. Patches of baldness generally result, but the scalp surface is not scarred. Short, broken strands of hair appear together with long, normal hairs. The affected areas may itch or tingle but are not routinely painful. Other areas often involved are the eyebrows, eyelashes, and beard; less commonly involved is hair from the truncal, axillary, and pubic areas.

Trichophagy commonly follows the hair pulling. Other acts of self-mutilation may accompany trichotillomania, e.g., head-banging, nail-biting, and excoriation. Children with the disorder often suck their fingers. Affected individuals usually deny that the hair-pulling behavior exists, and often take pains to conceal or camouflage the resultant baldness, e.g., with wigs or false eyelashes.

Duration of the disorder varies from 1 year, in about one-third of cases, to 2 decades in others. Frequent periods of worsening symptoms and remissions are common.

Scalp biopsy will usually show trichomalacia and plugs of fibrous keratin along with an absence of inflammation or scarring.

**Etiology** The cause is not known. The disorder may be a subcategory of ***Obsessive-Compulsive Disorder.*** Psychoactive substance abuse may contribute to development of trichotillomania.

In children, approximately one-fourth of reported cases have been linked to stressful situations, such as disturbances in mother-child relationships, fear of being left alone, and recent loss of a loved one. In adults, trichotillomania commonly accompanies a psychotic disorder.

**Epidemiology** Females are more frequently affected than males. The disorder usually occurs in childhood, but cases have been reported with onset as late as 62 years. Eldest and only children are most often afflicted. The disorder is more common in individuals with mental retardation, schizophrenia, obsessive-compulsive disorder, or borderline personality disorder.

**Related Disorders** See *Obsessive-Compulsive Disorder.*

**Treatment—Standard** Medications used in treating trichotillomania include chlorpromazine, isocarboxazid, amitriptyline, and imipramine. Psychoanalysis, intensive psychotherapy, and behavior-modification therapy may be helpful in some cases.

**Treatment—Investigational** Clomipramine, a treatment approved by the Food and Drug Administration for obsessive-compulsive disorder, is being investigated as a treatment for trichotillomania.

The National Institute of Mental Health is looking for males from ages 6 to 60 years for a study on trichotillomania. Please contact Marge Lenane.

Please contact the agencies listed under Resources, below, for the most current information. Addresses and telephone numbers of these agencies, as well as of individual experts and research centers, may be found in the Master Resources List.

**Resources**

**For more information on trichotillomania:** National Organization for Rare Disorders (NORD); Obsessive-Compulsive Foundation; National Mental Health Association; National Alliance for the Mentally Ill; National Mental Health Consumer Self-Help Clearinghouse; NIH/National Institute of Mental Health; Wayne Goodman, M.D., Yale University School of Medicine.

**References**

Return of Symptoms After Discontinuation of Clomipramine in Patients with Obsessive-Compulsive Disorder: M.T. Pato, et al.; Am. J. Psychiatry, December 1988, vol. 145(12), pp. 1521–1525.

Tricotillomania: S.A. Muller; Dermatol. Clin., July 1987, vol. 5(3), pp. 595–601.

Trichotillomania in Childhood: A.P. Oranje, et al.; J. Am. Acad. Dermatol., October 1986, vol. 15(4 pt. 1), pp. 614–619.

Diagnostic and Statistical Manual of Mental Disorders, 3d. ed.: R.L. Spitzer, et al., eds.; American Psychiatric Association, 1984, pp. 326–328.

# TRIGEMINAL NEURALGIA

**Description** Trigeminal neuralgia is characterized by excruciating episodic pain in the areas supplied by the trigeminal nerve.

**Synonyms**

> Fothergill Disease
> Tic Douloureux

**Signs and Symptoms** Brief (seconds to minutes) but intense bursts of pain occur along the maxillary and mandibular nerves, usually in adults over age 50 years. Pain may be triggered by talking, brushing teeth, touching the face, chewing, or swallowing. No other clinical or pathologic signs are present. During an attack, the pain is usually limited to one side of the face.

**Etiology** The cause is unknown. Vascular compression of the root entry zone of the trigeminal nerve, as well as toxic, nutritional, and infectious factors have been discussed.

**Epidemiology** Trigeminal neuralgia usually affects older adults of both sexes. It is more common in women than in men.

**Related Disorders Glossopharyngeal neuralgia** is characterized by severe paroxysmal pain originating on the side of the throat and radiating to the ear. The petrosal and jugular ganglia of the glossopharyngeal nerve are involved.

**Sphenopalatine ganglion neuralgia (Sluder neuralgia)** is characterized by burning and boring pain in the area of the superior maxilla. Pain radiates to the neck and shoulder.

**Postherpetic pain** may also occur in the face.

**Treatment—Standard** Carbamazepine, phenytoin, and baclofen have been reported to be effective in treating trigeminal neuralgia. Surgical therapy includes radiofrequency coagulation of the gasserian ganglion and the Jannetta procedure, involving removal of vascular structures pressing on the trigeminal ganglion.

**Treatment—Investigational** Tinzanidine, used experimentally as a treatment in trigeminal neuralgia, has been approved for study in the United States by the Food and Drug Administration. Although this orphan drug is available experimentally in the United States, conclusive results have not yet been reported.

Please contact the agencies listed under Resources, below, for the most current information. Addresses and telephone numbers of these agencies, as well as of individual experts and research centers, may be found in the Master Resources List.

**Resources**

**For more information on trigeminal neuralgia:** National Organization for Rare Disorders (NORD); Trigeminal Neuralgia Association; NIH/National Institute of Dental Research, Clinical Pain Division; NIH/National Institute of Neurological Disorders and Stroke.

**References**

Scientific American MEDICINE: E. Rubinstein and D. Federman, eds.; Scientific American, 1978–1991, p. 11:II:7.

Trigeminal Neuralgia: Treatment by Microvascular Decompression: P.J. Jannetta; *in* Neurosurgery: Wilkins, et al., eds.; McGraw-Hill, 1984.

# TUBEROUS SCLEROSIS (TS)

**Description** TS is characterized by seizures, mental retardation, developmental delay, and skin and ocular lesions. The disorder's manifestations and severity vary.

**Synonyms**

Bourneville Pringle Syndrome

Epiloia

Phakomatosis

**Signs and Symptoms** The first signs occur during infancy or early childhood, but in some cases onset is not till the 2nd or 3rd decade. Seizures are the first indications in about 80 percent of patients. Myoclonic jerks may be present, as well as hypsarrhythmia, which can be detected by electroencephalogram. Forty to 50 percent of affected persons are severely mentally retarded.

Prenatal benign brain tumors may be detected with a CT scan; they may calcify within the first years after birth.

Between 60 and 90 percent of infants have hypomelanotic macules at birth. Adenoma sebaceum appears between the ages of 3 and 5 years and proliferates during puberty. Collagen accumulates in the skin of the lower back and nape of the neck and appears as slightly elevated, yellowish-brown patches with an orange-peel (peau d'orange) texture. Periungual or subungual fibromas may develop, and café au lait spots and nodules appear on the skin. About 50 percent of patients develop retinal hamartomas.

Delayed speech, slow motor development, and learning disabilities may be associated. Typical behavior patterns include manifestations resembling childhood autism; episodes of screaming, crying, and rage; and catatonic rigidity.

**Etiology** TS is believed to be inherited as an autosomal dominant trait. It is thought that 2 genes are involved: TSC 1, not precisely located but known to be on the long arm of chromosome 9; and TSC 2, recently discovered on the short arm of chromosome 16 (16p13.3). Fifty to 80 percent of cases occur as a new mutation.

**Epidemiology** Some estimates indicate that 1:5,000 to 1:6,000 newborns are affected. Approximately 40,000 to 80,000 persons in the United States have tuberous sclerosis. Males and females are affected equally, and the disorder occurs in all races.

**Related Disorders** See *Epidermal Nevus Syndrome; Hypomelanosis of Ito.*

**Treatment—Standard** Although mental impairment does not always occur, its severity has a direct correlation with early onset and duration or severity of the seizures. Early diagnosis and seizure control are important. Treatment is limited to abolishing or minimizing symptoms and includes anticonvulsants. Conventional anticonvulsants include closely monitored use of phenobarbital, phenytoin, clonazepam, valproic acid, carbamazepine, ethosuximide, or acetazolamide. Some "infantile spasms" can be treated with prednisone or adrenocorticotropic hormone **(ACTH).** Immunizations, such as DPT and rubella, can prompt seizures in children.

Dermabrasion or laser therapy is used to eliminate facial angiofibromas. Surgery may be required for rapidly growing tumors.

Intracranial hypertension caused by a benign tumor may require a shunting procedure or surgical removal of the tumor. Some rhabdomyomas require surgery. Large cystic lesions of the kidneys may require surgical decompression or excision, possibly leading to removal of a kidney.

**Treatment—Investigational** Investigators are trying to locate and study the 2 TS genes. Blood and skin cells from TS individuals have been banked at the Camden Cell Repository, New Jersey; at Massachusetts General Hospital; and at the newly established Neonatal Brain Bank at the University of Miami School of Medicine. These specimens are available for worldwide research.

A new drug, Vigabatrin, is being studied for use in treating infantile spasms associated with tuberous sclerosis.

Please contact the agencies listed under Resources, below, for the most current information. Addresses and telephone numbers of these agencies, as well as of individual experts and research centers, may be found in the Master Resources List.

**Resources**

**For more information on tuberous sclerosis:** National Organization for Rare Disorders (NORD); National Tuberous Sclerosis Association; NIH/National Institute of Neurological Disorders and Stroke; The Arc (a national organization on mental retardation).

**For information about seizures:** The Epilepsy Foundation of America.

**For genetic information and genetic counseling referrals:** March of Dimes Birth Defects Foundation; Alliance of Genetic Support Groups.

**References**

Cecil Textbook of Medicine, 19th ed.: J.B. Wyngaarden, et al., eds.; W.B. Saunders Company, 1992, p. 2144.

Mendelian Inheritance in Man, 10th ed.: V.A. McKusick; The Johns Hopkins University Press, 1992, pp. 1116–1118.

Neurocutaneous Syndromes: E.S. Roach; Pediatr. Clin. North Am., August 1992, vol. 39(4), pp. 591–602.

Disorders of Hypopigmentation in Children: F.J. Pinto; Pediatr. Clin. North Am., August 1991, vol. 38(3), pp. 991–1017.

Tuberous Sclerosis and Allied Disorders, Clinical, Cellular, and Molecular Studies: W.G. Johnson and M.R. Gomez, eds.; Ann. N. Y. Acad. Sci., 1991, p. 615.

Clinical Dermatology, 2nd ed.: T.P. Habif, ed.; C.V. Mosby Company, 1990, pp. 654–655.

# VASCULAR MALFORMATIONS OF THE BRAIN

**Description** Vascular malformations of the brain include arteriovenous malformations, cavernous angiomas (or hemangiomas), venous malformations, and telangiectasia.

**Synonyms**

Intracranial Vascular Malformations

Occult Intracranial Vascular Malformations

**Signs and Symptoms** Manifestations of cerebrovascular malformations vary according to the type and severity of the disorder.

**Arteriovenous malformations (AVMs)** are congenital. These anomalous shunts can produce neurologic symptoms as they enlarge and compress neural tissue, or in response to hemorrhage. Parenchymal (or subarachnoid) hemorrhage, focal epilepsy, and progressive focal sensory-motor deficits may occur.

**Cavernous angiomas (or hemangiomas)** may be congenital or appear shortly after birth. These raised red or purplish lesions may contain mature vasculature and lymphatics. They rarely involute spontaneously.

**Venous malformations** vary in size and may cause headaches, seizures, strokes, or hemorrhage.

**Telangiectasia** can occur on the face, eyes, meninges, and mucous membranes.

**Etiology** Vascular malformations of the brain may be congenital (inherited as an autosomal dominant trait with variable expression and incomplete penetrance) or acquired, the result of an injury or trauma.

**Epidemiology** Vascular malformations of the brain generally affect males and females in equal numbers, although AVMs occur more frequently in males. A hereditary form of cavernous malformations may be found more frequently in Mexican-Americans.

**Related Disorders** See *Moyamoya Disease.*

**Embolic, hemorrhagic, and thrombotic strokes** should be considered in the differential diagnosis of cerebrovascular malformations.

**Treatment—Standard** Surgical excision may be indicated. Intravascular thrombosing via intra-arterial catheters and coagulation with focused proton beams may also be effective.

Cavernous angiomas may resolve in response to systemic administration of prednisone, but electrocoagulation or surgical excision may be required. Anticonvulsants are used to control seizures when present.

**Treatment—Investigational** Several types of surgery are being investigated for treatment of vascular malformations of the brain: charged-particle radiosurgery, interventriculostomy, and catheter placement.

Please contact the agencies listed under Resources, below, for the most current information. Addresses and telephone numbers of these agencies, as well as of individual experts and research centers, may be found in the Master Resources List.

**Resources**

**For more information on vascular malformations of the brain:** National Organization for Rare Disorders (NORD); NIH/National Institute of Neurological Disorders and Stroke; National Vascular Malformation Foundation.

**For genetic information and genetic counseling referrals:** March of Dimes Birth Defects Foundation; Alliance of Genetic Support Groups.

**References**

Cerebral Cavernous Malformations: Incidence and Familial Occurrence: D. Rigamonti, et al.; N. Engl. J. Med., August 11, 1988, vol. 319(6), pp. 343–347.

Clinical, Radiological, and Pathological Spectrum of Angiographically Occult Intracranial Vascular Malformations. Analysis of 21 Cases and Review of the Literature: R.D. Lobato, et al.; J. Neurosurg., April 1988, vol. 68(4), pp. 518–531.

Vascular Malformations of the Brain: B.M. Stein and J.P. Mohr; N. Engl. J. Med., August 11, 1988, vol. 319(6), pp. 368–370.

# WALKER-WARBURG SYNDROME

**Description** Walker-Warburg syndrome is also known as **HARD +/- E syndrome** ([**H**]ydrocephalus, [**A**]gyria, [**R**]etinal [**D**]ysplasia and, if present, [**E**]ncephalocele).

**Synonyms**
> Cerebroocular Dysgenesis
> Chemke Syndrome
> HARD +/- E Syndrome
> Pagon Syndrome

**Signs and Symptoms** Lissencephaly, malformations of the cerebellum, hydrocephalus, and retinal abnormalities are typically present and are accompanied by mental impairment, seizures, hypotonia, and, eventually, spastic quadriplegia. Anterior chamber dysgenesis has been found in some affected individuals.

Additional conditions that may be found in some patients with Walker-Warburg syndrome are Dandy-Walker syndrome, encephalocele, cleft palate and cleft lip, microcephaly, and microphthalmia.

**Etiology** The disorder is inherited as an autosomal recessive trait.

**Epidemiology** The syndrome is very rare; approximately 60 patients have been reported in the medical literature. Females are affected slightly more often than males.

**Related Disorders** See *Dandy-Walker Syndrome; Encephalocele; Hydrocephalus; Lissencephaly; Muscular Dystrophy, Fukuyama Type.*

**Treatment—Standard** When hydrocephalus is present, a shunt procedure may be necessary. Genetic counseling may be of benefit for patients and their families. Other treatment is symptomatic and supportive.

**Treatment—Investigational** Please contact the agencies listed under Resources, below, for the most current information. Addresses and telephone numbers of these agencies, as well as of individual experts and research centers, may be found in the Master Resources List.

**Resources**

**For more information on Walker-Warburg syndrome:** National Organization for Rare Disorders (NORD); Muscular Dystrophy Association; Lissencephaly Network; Hydrocephalus Parent Support Group; National Hydrocephalus Foundation; Hydrocephalus Association; NIH/National Institute of Neurological Disorders and Stroke.

**For genetic information and genetic counseling referrals:** March of Dimes Birth Defects Foundation; Alliance of Genetic Support Groups.

**References**

Birth Defects Encyclopedia: M.L. Buyse, ed.-in-chief; Blackwell Scientific Publications, 1990, p. 1774.

Mendelian Inheritance in Man, 10th ed.: V.A. McKusick, ed.; The Johns Hopkins University Press, 1990, pp. 1449–1450.

Smith's Recognizable Patterns of Human Malformation, 4th ed.: K.L. Jones, ed.; W.B. Saunders Company, 1988, p. 158.

# WERDNIG-HOFFMANN DISEASE

**Description** Werdnig-Hoffmann disease is an inherited neuromuscular condition of infants. It is characterized by degenerative changes in the ventral horn cells of the spinal cord, resulting in progressive atrophy and weakness of the muscles of the trunk and extremities.

**Synonyms**
> Infantile Spinal Muscular Atrophy
> Werdnig-Hoffmann Paralysis

**Signs and Symptoms** Onset occurs before age 2 years and may even develop in utero. The earlier the onset, the graver the prognosis. Initial signs include hypotonia and weakness of the skeletal musculature, with hypermobility of joints; absent tendon reflexes; fasciculations of the tongue; and a froglike position, with hips abducted and knees flexed. Mental development is normal. Typically, the child never gains head control, does not turn over, and never sits or stands.

The rate of progression varies. In the form that begins in utero, generalized muscle atrophy and weakness progress rapidly. Within a few months, respiratory and excretory difficulties develop, and the infant is unable to swallow. Death occurs because of respiratory failure or aspiration of food. The form that begins during the first few months of life may have a more slowly progressive course, even extending into adult life. Very infrequently the disease may become arrested.

**Etiology** Werdnig-Hoffmann disease is an autosomal recessive disorder. In rare instances there appears to be autosomal dominant inheritance.

**Epidemiology** Males and females are affected equally. There may be no known family history of the disease, since the genetic defect is recessive. The estimated incidence is 1:1,000,000 live births per year.

**Treatment—Standard** Medical management is symptomatic. Physical therapy, respiratory care, and aggressive treatment of respiratory infections are used. Orthopedic devices may be helpful when the condition is relatively static.

**Treatment—Investigational** Please contact the agencies listed under Resources, below, for the most current information. Addresses and telephone numbers of these agencies, as well as of individual experts and research centers, may be found in the Master Resources List.

**Resources**

**For more information on Werdnig-Hoffmann disease:** National Organization for Rare Disorders (NORD); Muscular Dystrophy Association; NIH/National Institute of Neurological Disorders and Stroke; Families of Spinal Muscular Atrophy; Muscular Dystrophy Group of Great Britain and Northern Ireland.

**For genetic information and genetic counseling referrals:** March of Dimes Birth Defects Foundation; Alliance of Genetic Support Groups.

**References**

Cecil Textbook of Medicine, 19th ed.: J.B. Wyngaarden, et al., eds.; W.B. Saunders Company, 1992, p. 2140.

Mendelian Inheritance in Man, 10th ed.: V.A. McKusick; The Johns Hopkins University Press, 1992, pp. 1563–1564.

Birth Defects Encyclopedia: M.L. Buyse, ed.-in-chief; Blackwell Scientific Publications, 1990, pp. 1576–1577.

EMG Evaluation of the Floppy Infant: Differential Diagnosis and Technical Aspects: H.R. Jones, Jr.; Muscle Nerve, April 1990, vol. 13(4), pp. 338–347.

Principles of Neurology, 4th ed.: R.D. Adams and M. Victor, eds.; McGraw-Hill, 1989, pp. 1146–1147.

# WEST SYNDROME

**Description** West syndrome is a rare form of infantile spasm often accompanied by an EEG hypsarrhythmic pattern.

**Synonyms**

Infantile Myoclonic Seizures
Jackknife Convulsion
Massive Myoclonia

**Signs and Symptoms** Symptoms most often appear in the first few weeks or months after birth, although onset has been reported up to 2 years. The spasms that occur may be violent jackknife or "salaam" movements, or no more than a mild twitching of the nose or mouth. The spasms are most common upon awakening. Other forms of seizures accompany the infantile spasms in about one-third of cases. Mental retardation has been reported in over 75 percent of affected children.

Normal pregnancy, birth, and development may precede symptoms onset in some infants, but for others there are precipitating factors such as birth hypoxia, injury, and infection.

Hypsarrhythmia will be seen on EEG initially in 65 percent of cases, and will be evident in almost all cases within a few weeks. Positron emission tomography is useful in showing sites of injury.

**Etiology** Some cases of West syndrome may be inherited as an X-linked genetic trait.

Other causes include developmental or brain defects, perinatal injury, cerebral anoxia, metabolic problems, meningitis, and brain tumors.

**Epidemiology** The syndrome is rare, affecting both males and females, although males predominate in the X-linked form.

**Related Disorders** See *Lennox-Gastaut Syndrome; Myoclonus.*

**Treatment—Standard** Drug treatment includes high-dose adrenocorticotropic hormone (**ACTH**), and vigabatrin in combination with other anticonvulsant drug treatment.

Surgical procedures may be necessary to treat forms of the syndrome caused by the presence of cysts, tumors, or malformations of the brain.

Genetic counseling may be helpful in connection with the hereditary form of West syndrome. Other treatment is symptomatic and supportive.

**Treatment—Investigational** Please contact the agencies listed under Resources, below, for the most current information. Addresses and telephone numbers of these agencies, as well as of individual experts and research centers, may be found in the Master Resources List.

**Resources**

**For more information on West syndrome:** National Organization for Rare Disorders (NORD); Epilepsy Foundation of America; The Arc (a national organization on mental retardation); NIH/National Institute of Neurological Disorders and Stroke.

**For genetic information and genetic counseling referrals:** March of Dimes Birth Defects Foundation; Alliance of Genetic Support Groups.

**References**

Brain-Adrenal Axis Hormones Are Altered in the CSF of Infants with Massive Infantile Spasms: T.Z. Baram, et al.; Neurology, June 1992, vol. 42(6), pp. 1171–1175.

Mendelian Inheritance in Man, 10th ed.: V.A. McKusick; The Johns Hopkins University Press, 1992, p. 1890.

Nelson Textbook of Pediatrics, 14th ed.: R.E. Behrman, ed.-in-chief; W.B. Saunders Company, 1992, p. 1495.

Treatment of Infantile Spasms: Medical or Surgical?: W.D. Shields, et al.; Epilepsia, 1992, vol. 33(suppl. 5), pp. 26–29.

The Use of Positron Emission Tomography in the Clinical Assessment of Epilepsy: H.T. Chugani; Semin. Nucl. Med., October 1992, vol. 22(4), pp. 247–253.

Outcome for West Syndrome Following Surgical Treatment: B.M. Uthman, et al.; Epilepsia, September–October 1991, vol. 32(5), pp. 668–671.

Seizures in Series: Similarities Between Seizures of the West and Lennox-Gastaut Syndromes: J.F. Donat, et al.; Epilepsia, July–August 1991, vol. 32(4), pp. 504–509.

# WIEACKER SYNDROME

**Description** Wieacker syndrome is a rare genetic disorder affecting males and characterized by congenital contractures of the feet.

**Synonyms**

Wieacker-Wolff Syndrome

**Signs and Symptoms** Contractures of the feet at birth, slowly progressive atrophy of certain muscles, and mild mental retardation are present. Affected persons are unable to move their eyes despite the wish to do so, and have impaired use of face and tongue muscles.

**Etiology** The syndrome is inherited as an X-linked recessive trait.

**Epidemiology** The disorder is rare, present at birth, and affects only males.

**Related Disorders** See *Apraxia.*

**Treatment—Standard** Physical and speech therapy, special education, and surgery may be beneficial, especially if started early. Genetic counseling is useful.

**Treatment—Investigational** Detection of the female carrier condition may be possible in some instances.

Please contact the agencies listed under Resources, below, for the most current information. Addresses and telephone numbers of these agencies, as well as of individual experts and research centers, may be found in the Master Resources List.

**Resources**

**For more information on Wieacker syndrome:** National Organization for Rare Disorders (NORD); The Arc (a national organization on mental retardation); NIH/National Arthritis and Musculoskeletal and Skin Diseases Information Clearinghouse; NIH/National Institute of Neurological Disorders and Stroke.

**For genetic information and genetic counseling referrals:** March of Dimes Birth Defects Foundation; Alliance of Genetic Support Groups.

**References**

Mendelian Inheritance in Man, 9th ed.: V.A. McKusick; The Johns Hopkins University Press, 1990, p. 1732.

Close Linkage of the Wieacker-Wolff Syndrome to the DNA Segment DXYS in Proximal Xq: P. Wieacker, et al.; Am. J. Med. Genet., September 1987, vol. 28(1), pp. 245–253.

A New X-Linked Syndrome with Muscle Atrophy, Congenital Contractures, and Oculomotor Apraxia: P. Wieacker, et al.; Am. J. Med. Genet., April 1985, vol. 20(4), pp. 597–606.

# 4 | CARDIOVASCULAR AND RESPIRATORY DISEASES
### By Amnon Rosenthal, M.D.

In this brief introduction, I have outlined an approach to the recognition and detection of rare cardiovascular and respiratory diseases in the infant, child, and young adult. Only a broad classification and generalizations are provided. In general, cardiovascular diseases in childhood are congenital, acquired, or associated with other hereditary conditions. The rarity of any of these is related to the population examined, methods used in detection, and the training and subspecialty expertise of the physician. For example, ventricular septal defect, which is a congenital cardiac malformation, is seen frequently by the pediatric cardiologist, less often by the pediatrician or general practitioner, and rarely by an internist. Since many of these defects close spontaneously with advancing age, they occur more frequently in the infant than in the child and are truly rare in adults. Many of the rare diseases described are specific to infancy, with few survivors into adulthood (e.g., hypoplastic left heart syndrome), while others may be silent in childhood and are more frequently observed in adults (e.g., mitral valve prolapse syndrome). Some diseases are rare at any age (e.g., primary pulmonary artery hypertension or Romano-Ward syndrome).

In more than 90 percent of infants and children with cardiovascular disease, the condition is congenital and not acquired. The prevalence of congenital heart disease is approximately 8:1,000 to 10:1,000 live births. The diagnosis of significant congenital cardiac defects can usually be made reliably in the fetus as early as the eighteenth week of gestation by fetal echocardiography. In the postnatal period, the clinician should have a high index of suspicion for the possible presence of congenital heart disease in the following circumstances.

(1) A history of prematurity or being small for gestational age.

(2) An identifiable syndrome with or without associated chromosomal abnormality. For example, heart disease is very common in children with Down syndrome. Nearly 50 percent have an atrioventricular septal defect, ventricular septal defect, or patent ductus arteriosus. Turner syndrome is frequently associated with left heart lesions, especially coarctation of the aorta; and Noonan syndrome with right heart lesions, such as pulmonary stenosis or atrial septal defect.

(3) The presence of other noncardiac congenital malformations. Nearly a quarter of all children with congenital cardiac disease have associated noncardiac anomalies. The presence of congenital heart disease should be especially suspected in those infants and children with anomalies in the musculoskeletal system, central nervous system, and gastrointestinal system.

(4) Delayed height and weight maturation during infancy.

(5) Recurrent respiratory infections or episodes of bronchospasm.

The history and physical examination are particularly useful in eliciting symptoms and signs that may clearly point to involvement of the cardiovascular system. The assessment should include evaluation of growth and development, blood pressure measurement, and auscultation for abnormal heart sounds and murmurs. The possible presence of congestive heart failure or a chronic shunt hypoxemia (cyanosis) is almost invariably indicative of cardiac disease. Other symptoms and signs that point to the possible presence of cardiac disease include syncope (e.g., orthostatic hypotension, congenital complete heart block); dyspnea (e.g., fibrosing alveolitis) or wheezing (e.g., cor triatriatum); easy fatigability (e.g., pulmonary artery hypertension); chest pain (e.g., mitral valve prolapse); palpitations (e.g., Wolff-Parkinson-White syndrome); a cerebrovascular accident (e.g., arteriovenous malformation); and seizures or abortive sudden death (e.g., Romano-Ward syndrome). If pulmonary disease is present, evidence of cor pulmonale should be sought.

Primary physicians should employ commonly used studies that they themselves can interpret. The most useful are the chest x-ray, electrocardiogram, and performance of systemic arterial oxygen saturation by pulse volume oximeter. These, in addition to the history and physical examination, will usually lead to the strong suspicion or identification of cardiac disease. Performance of more extensive studies, such as echocardiograms, radionuclide imaging, exercise testing, or Holter monitoring, should be at the discretion of the cardiologist. Adequate performance of an echocardiogram requires great skill, knowledge of the pediatric cardiac disease searched for, and, in infants and young children, adequate sedation. It is also rather expensive.

In addition to referral to a cardiologist, multiple consultations are often necessary in the management of patients with hereditary, metabolic, or acquired diseases. These consultations may include the geneticist (e.g., for Marfan syndrome); pulmonologist (e.g., fibrosing alveolitis); endocrinologist (e.g., Turner syndrome); rheumatologist (e.g., collagen diseases); or an expert in metabolic diseases (e.g., Pompe disease).

A pediatric cardiologist should be consulted when an infant exhibits one or more of the following: (a) central cyanosis; (b) persistent tachypnea; (c) congestive heart failure; (d) absent or weak femoral pulses; (e) loud murmur; (f) a heart rate greater than 200 or slower than 80 beats per minute; (g) chest x-ray with cardiomegaly, increased or decreased pulmonary vascularity; and (h) an abnormal electrocardiogram. In children and adolescents, consultation should be obtained when the following are present: (a) loud systolic murmur (grade 3/6 or greater); (b) any diastolic murmur; (c) cyanosis or clubbing; (d) chest pain suggestive of angina; (e) systemic hypertension with or without decreased femoral pulses; (f) palpitations, syncope, or exercise intolerance; (g) an abnormal rhythm; (h) an ECG with ventricular hypertrophy; and (i) cardiomegaly or pulmonary congestion on chest x-ray.

General principles in the management of children with any cardiac disease include appropriate dietary and nutritional recommendations, activity recommendations, the need for antimicrobial prophylaxis in the prevention of infective endocarditis at times of predictable risk, and appropriate therapy of intercurrent infections. Also important is attention to the psychosocial aspects of the cardiac disease; genetic counseling; advice with respect to travel, insurance, or employability; and sometimes the need for home therapy, including oxygen, intravenous administration, or other devices. Special considerations may be required for both cardiac and noncardiac surgery, as well as the anesthetic used.

## References

Moss and Adams Heart Disease in Infants, Children, and Adolescents, Including the Fetus and Young Adult, 5th ed.: G.C. Emmanouilides, et al., eds.; Williams and Wilkins, 1995.

Developmental Cardiology: Morphogenesis and Function: E.B. Clark and A. Takao, eds.; Futura Publishing Company, 1990.

The Science and Practice of Pediatric Cardiology, vols. 1–2: A. Garson, et al., eds.; Lea and Febiger, 1990.

Fetal, Neonatal, and Infant Cardiac Disease: J.H. Moller and W.A. Neal, eds.; Appleton and Lange, 1989.

Smith's Recognizable Patterns of Human Malformations, 4th ed.: K.L. Jones; W.B. Saunders Company, 1988.

# CARDIOVASCULAR AND RESPIRATORY DISEASES
*Listings in This Section*

# α-1-ANTITRYPSIN (AAT) DEFICIENCY

**Description** A deficiency of AAT allows proteolytic enzymes to attack various tissues of the body, causing emphysema and also affecting the liver, joints, and blood.

α-1-Antitrypsin is a nonspecific serum protease inhibitor (antiprotease) of proteolytic enzymes released by neutrophils in response to infection, or in the inflammatory process. A relative deficiency of AAT results in uncontrolled protease activity, especially in the basilar regions of the lung.

**Synonyms**

Homozygous α-1-Antitrypsin Deficiency

Serum Protease Inhibitor Deficiency

**Signs and Symptoms** The most common manifestation of AAT deficiency is progressive panacinar emphysema. In persons who are homozygous for the condition, the initial symptoms may be seen as early as the 2nd decade, with clinical disease developing by the time the individual reaches the 30s or early 40s. In patients with intermediate levels of antitrypsin, symptoms onset occurs during the 40s. The earliest symptom is most often progressive shortness of breath, but chronic cough or frequent respiratory infections may also be present. Full clinical disease develops by the mid to late 50s.

Other early signs, also frequently seen in asymptomatic AAT-deficient persons, suggest hyperinflation and loss of elastic recoil in the lungs: low forced expiratory volume, low diffusing capacity, and abnormalities seen on lung scan. Arterial hypoxemia without carbon dioxide retention is also present. The perfusion defects are most often seen in the basilar areas of the lung, particularly early in the disease course. Also helpful for diagnosis are a missing or greatly reduced α-1-globulin peak, and low serum AAT levels.

Hepatic symptoms of AAT deficiency may appear during the neonatal period, childhood, or adolescence. Infants may have jaundice and ascites and feed poorly. Affected children and adolescents experience fatigue, decreased appetite, swelling of the legs or abdomen, and hepatomegaly. About 25 percent of infants with hepatic symptoms experience no further complications, and liver involvement seems to end after infancy. In the rest (estimated at a small percentage of all cases), cirrhosis eventually develops. The resulting increased intrahepatic venous pressure is associated with nosebleeds, bruising, ascites, gastric and esophageal varices, and occasional internal bleeding. All tests of hepatic function will probably have abnormal results. Later in the course of the cirrhosis, drowsiness may occur after protein-rich meals, as the liver is unable to synthesize urea. Susceptibility to infection may also complicate later stages of the disease.

Hepatic cellular pathology findings in adults with AAT deficiency emphysema are similar to those of infants with symptomatic hepatic involvement, but no hepatic symptoms seem to result in these cases.

Other less common manifestations of AAT deficiency include erosive joint destruction and hematologic abnormalities involving clotting mechanisms.

**Etiology** α-1-Antitrypsin phenotypes result from a number of different alleles at the α-1-antitrypsin locus on chromosome 14. For this reason there is great variability of the enzyme, with about 70 different genetic variants recorded so far. Serum deficiencies result from impaired release of AAT from the liver cells after synthesis. Normally levels of AAT are low, rising quickly in response to physiologic stress. AAT-deficient patients appear to have close-to-normal antiprotease levels until infection, surgery, pregnancy, or other stressful conditions occur; then they are unable to release enough of the protein to meet their needs. Liver involvement seems to result from impairment in storage or release of antiprotease in the hepatocyte. It is not known why only some persons with AAT deficiency have liver involvement.

**Epidemiology** Deficiencies of AAT are most common in persons of northern and central European descent. The condition may be suspected when emphysema occurs in a woman, a relatively young man, a nonsmoker, or someone with a family history of emphysema.

**Related Disorders** Other disorders of protease-antiprotease imbalance include adult respiratory distress syndrome, chronic bronchitis, certain pneumonias, and pancreatitis (see **Respiratory Distress Syndrome, Adult).**

**Treatment—Standard** Symptomatic treatment for AAT-associated emphysema includes oxygen therapy and antibiotics for the frequent respiratory infections. Exercise programs help increase the person's overall functioning.

Treatment of hepatic disease is also symptomatic. Phenobarbital or cholestyramine are directed against jaundice and itching, and diuretics and potassium are used to maintain electrolyte balance. Proper nutrition is essential. Surgically created shunts to lower intrahepatic venous pressure may become necessary. Liver transplantations have been attempted, but with limited success.

The orphan biological product, α-1-proteinase inhibitor (Prolastin—Cutter Biological, Miles), inhibits the action of α-1-proteinase and thus replaces the deficient α-1-antitrypsin.

**Treatment—Investigational** Research is under way to determine if hepatic release of AAT can be induced with danazol, a modified synthetic testosterone. This approach has increased serum levels to 50 percent of normal, which is low but may be sufficient to prevent tissue damage in otherwise healthy nonsmoking individuals.

Other agents being investigated include synthetic neutrophil elastase inhibitors, certain acylating agents, sulfonyl fluorides, short-chain fatty acids, and chloromethyl ketone peptides. An aerosolized synthetic form of Prolastin is also being developed to deliver the drug directly to the lungs.

Lung transplants for patients with AAT have been performed at the Minnesota Heart and Lung Institute in Minneapolis, the University of California at San Diego, and Barnes Hospital in St. Louis.

Another new drug being tested, in collaboration with the manufacturer, Syndergen, and the NIH/National Heart, Lung and Blood Institute, is secretory leukocyte protease inhibitor **(SLPI).**

An AAT deficiency registry has been established by the NIH/National Heart, Lung and Blood Institute at 22 clinical centers throughout the country. Patients who participate in the registry are seen every 6 months during a 5-year period.

Please contact the agencies listed under Resources, below, for the most current information. Addresses and telephone numbers of these agencies, as well as of individual experts and research centers, may be found in the Master Resources List.

### Resources

**For more information on α-1-antitrypsin deficiency:** National Organization for Rare Disorders (NORD); Alpha-1-Antitrypsin Deficiency National Association; American Lung Association; American Liver Foundation; NIH/National Heart, Lung and Blood Institute; Children's Liver Foundation.

**To locate α-1-antitrypsin deficiency registry clinics:** Alpha-1-Antitrypsin Deficiency Registry.

**For genetic information and genetic counseling referrals:** March of Dimes Birth Defects Foundation; Alliance of Genetic Support Groups.

### References

The Metabolic Basis of Inherited Disease, 7th ed.: C.R. Scriver, et al., eds.; McGraw-Hill, 1995, p. 4125.

Alpha-1-Antitrypsin Deficiency: Noninfectious Disorders of the Respiratory Tract: R.H. Schwartz; in Pediatric Respiratory Disease Diagnosis and Treatment: B.C. Hillman, ed.; W.B. Saunders Company, 1993.

Mendelian Inheritance in Man, 10th ed.: V.A. McKusick; The Johns Hopkins University Press, 1992, pp. 92–94.

Alpha-1-Antitrypsin Deficiency and Liver Disease: P. Birrer; J. Inherit. Metab. Dis., 1991, vol. 14(4), pp. 512–525.

Alpha-1-Antitrypsin Deficiency: Pathogenesis and Treatment: R.G. Crystal; Hosp. Pract., February 15, 1991, vol. 26(2), pp. 81–84, 88–89, 93–94.

Birth Defects Encyclopedia: M.L Buyse, ed.-in-chief; Blackwell Scientific Publications, 1990, p. 91.

Rare Deficiency Types of α-1-Antitrypsin: Electrophoretic Variation and DNA Haplotypes: D.W. Cox and G.D. Billingsley; Am. J. Hum. Genet., 1989, vol. 44, p. 844.

Liver Disease in α-1-Antitrypsin Deficiency: S.G. Eriksson; Scand. J. Gastroenterol., 1985, vol. 20, p. 907.

Pulmonary Diseases and Disorders, 2nd ed.: A.P. Fishman, ed.; McGraw-Hill, 1980, vol. 2, pp. 1204–1269, 1544.

# ALVEOLITIS, EXTRINSIC ALLERGIC

**Description** Extrinsic allergic alveolitis is a lung disease usually associated with certain occupations that provide the possibility of recurrent organic dust inhalation. Acute respiratory symptoms and fever may begin several hours after exposure. Chronic disease, marked by gradual changes in lung tissue, is associated with repeated episodes or long-term exposure (over years) to a specific organic dust.

Associated forms of the disease include bird breeder disease, bathtub refinisher's lung, mushroom picker disease, mushroom worker's lung, laboratory technician's lung, pituitary snuff-taker's lung, plastic worker's lung, epoxy resin lung, malt worker's lung, maple bark stripper disease, sequoiosis, suberosis, bagassosis, wheat weevil disease, farmer's lung, ventilation pneumonitis, and cheese worker's lung.

### Synonyms

Allergic Interstitial Pneumonitis

Extrinsic Allergic Pneumonia

Hypersensitivity Pneumonitis

**Signs and Symptoms** Symptoms generally include dyspnea, wheezing, and dry coughs that seem to shake the entire body. Additional symptoms may include chills, sweating, aching, and fatigue. Most cases involve typical episodes that are mild and short and may be misdiagnosed. The chronic disease that develops with prolonged exposure to the irritant may be characterized by fever, rales, cyanosis, and, possibly, expectoration of blood.

**Etiology** Repeated exposure to organic substances, often associated with a specific occupation, is linked to the disorder. The irritants may include avian dust, a paint catalyst used in bathtub refinishing, mushroom compost, rat or gerbil urine residue, snuff, plastic residue, heated epoxy residue, and a variety of molds, including moldy barley, maple bark dust, redwood bark dust (sequoiosis), cork dust (suberosis), sugar cane dust (bagasse), moldy wheat and hay dust, moldy water from heating and cooling systems, and cheese mold.

**Epidemiology** Males and females are both affected, depending on their occupations and individual allergic reactions.

**Related Disorders** See *Alveolitis, Fibrosing.*

**Asthma** is often associated with allergies.

**Desquamative interstitial pneumonia** is a chronic pneumonia of unknown etiology characterized by dyspnea and a harsh cough that does not seem to clear the obstruction. Symptoms are caused by desquamation in the lungs and thickening of the air passage walls.

**Treatment—Standard** Identification and, if possible, avoidance of the irritant are the initial concerns of treatment. In an occupational setting, improved ventilation and air filtering masks are recommended for mild symptoms. If permanent lung changes have not occurred, corticosteroids and avoidance measures often reduce severity and may resolve acute symptoms. Corticosteroids may also be tried in persistent cases. Change of occupation may be necessary.

**Treatment—Investigational** Please contact the agencies listed under Resources, below, for the most current information. Addresses and telephone numbers of these agencies, as well as of individual experts and research centers, may be found in the Master Resources List.

**Resources**

**For more information on extrinsic allergic alveolitis:** National Organization for Rare Disorders (NORD); American Lung Association; NIH/National Institute of Allergy and Infectious Diseases; National Institute of Environmental Health Sciences.

**References**

Extrinsic Allergic Alveolitis in Children: Apropos of 4 Cases: M. Bost, et al.; Pediatrie, June 1984, vol. 39(4), pp. 253–260.

Diagnostic Approach to New or Unrecognized Risks in Hypersensitivity Pneumopathies: C. Molina; Rev. Fr. Mal. Respir., 1983, vol. 11(4), pp. 427–438.

Allergic Alveolitis: Pathogenesis and Diagnosis: K.C. Bergman; A. Gesamte Inn. Med., January 1980, vol. 35(2), pp. 77–80.

# ALVEOLITIS, FIBROSING

**Description** Fibrosing alveolitis is an inflammatory lung disorder characterized by abnormal formation of fibrous tissue between alveoli.

**Synonyms**

> Alveolocapillary Block
> Cryptogenic Fibrosing Alveolitis
> Diffuse Fibrosing Alveolitis
> Hamman-Rich Syndrome
> Interstitial Diffuse Pulmonary Fibrosis
> Pulmonary Fibrosis, Idiopathic

**Signs and Symptoms** Manifestations include progressive dyspnea and coughing that may not ease bronchial irritation. Rapid, shallow breathing and coughing occur with moderate exercise. The skin may appear cyanotic, and fingers or toes may become clubbed. Loss of appetite and weight, fatigue, fever, weakness, and vague chest pains are common. Infections occur easily, and untreated individuals develop complications that include emphysema, pulmonary infections, or cardiac disease. Imaging techniques monitor progressive lung changes.

**Etiology** The cause is unknown. Scleroderma, a blood factor associated with rheumatoid arthritis, or an autoimmune factor may be involved.

**Epidemiology** The disease affects males and females equally, primarily during middle age.

**Related Disorders** See *Alveolitis, Extrinsic Allergic.*

**Treatment—Standard** Early treatment with systemic corticosteroids (high doses followed by a lower maintenance dosage) may prevent widespread or permanent lung morbidity. Azathioprine may be effective in cases resistant to steroids. Other treatments include oxygen administered in high concentrations if blood oxygen is diminished, antibiotics for bacterial infections, and digitalis or diuretics for heart problems. Other treatment is symptomatic and supportive.

**Treatment—Investigational** Lung transplantation is under investigation as a possible treatment.

Please contact the agencies listed under Resources, below, for the most current information. Addresses and telephone numbers of these agencies, as well as of individual experts and research centers, may be found in the Master Resources List.

**Resources**

**For more information on fibrosing alveolitis:** National Organization for Rare Disorders (NORD); American Lung Association; NIH/National Heart, Lung and Blood Institute.

**References**

Bronchoalveolar Lavage Fluid Neutrophils Increase After Corticosteroid Therapy in Smokers with Idiopathic Pulmonary Fibrosis: K.L. Christopher, et al.; Am. Rev. Respir. Dis., January 1986, vol. 133(1), pp. 104–109.

Concentration, Biosynthesis and Degradation of Collagen in Idiopathic Pulmonary Fibrosis: M. Selman, et al.; Thorax, May 1986, vol. 41(5), pp. 355–359.

Effect of Intermittent High Dose Parenteral Corticosteroids on the Alveolitis of Idiopathic Pulmonary Fibrosis: B.A. Keogh, et al.; Am. Rev. Respir. Dis., January 1983, vol. 127(1), pp. 18–22.

# ARTERIOVENOUS MALFORMATION (AVM)

**Description** AVM is a congenital disorder involving abnormal vascular communication between arteries and veins. AVM may occur in the central nervous system, spine, liver, or limbs.

**Signs and Symptoms Spinal AVM** is characterized by back pain associated with sensory loss and leg weakness, and, infrequently, acute hemorrhage. Urination is impaired early. Rarely, a murmur at auscultation can be heard over the spine, or a skin angioma may be seen. An x-ray of the spine may reveal the distinctive wormlike impression of tangled vessels.

There are 3 types of lesions. **Type I,** the most common, occurs in adults. It is a single coiled feeding vessel, usually with a single feeding artery arising from another artery between the ribs or a lumbar segmental artery. Located dorsally, Type I AVM is often surgically accessible.

**Type II** is less common, occurs in adults, and also has a single feeding vessel. A glomus-type anomaly, Type II presents delayed opacification after contrast medium injection prior to x-ray.

**Type III** typically occurs in the neck area in children and has the poorest overall prognosis. There are multiple feeding vessels with a large malformation that often appears to fill the entire spinal canal, demonstrating rapid flow with marked arteriovenous shunting. The multiple arterial feeders and the location inside the spinal canal usually prohibit surgery, and bleeding occurs more frequently.

Large **cranial AVM** in infants result in congestive heart failure within 24 hours of delivery. Forty percent of older patients with cranial AVM initially have focal or generalized seizures. Headaches may occur with or without bleeding. A ruptured AVM causes bleeding in the subarachnoid space under the inner membrane of the brain or inside the brain itself. Clinical symptoms are similar to those of ruptured cerebral aneurysms. A steal syndrome occurs as blood is shunted away from normal brain tissue toward the AVM, causing focal neurologic deficits secondary to ischemia. Bleeding to the affected brain area, AVM size, and individual response to treatment affect outcome.

A CT scan or MRI of spinal cord AVM may be useful for both screening and follow-up. Digital intravenous computerized angiography may eventually replace common angiography as a diagnostic tool.

**Etiology** AVMs are congenital defects of unknown etiology.

**Epidemiology** Onset of symptoms ranges from early childhood to the 9th decade, affecting males slightly more often than females.

**Treatment—Standard** If spinal cord function is threatened, spinal AVM surgery using specialized microtechniques is indicated.

Treatment of cranial AVM includes anticonvulsants. Embolization or surgical removal may be attempted. If all the arterial feeders can be identified and embolized or ligated, the condition may be successfully treated (see below). In most instances, however, the location and size of the lesions preclude satisfactory therapy.

**Treatment—Investigational** Occlusion of feeder arteries by embolization (collapsing of the veins by shooting plastic pellets into them through a catheter) is being evaluated as a treatment for spinal AVM.

Cranial AVM patients are being treated experimentally with stereotactic Bragg-peak proton-beam therapy. This therapy is designed to induce subendothelial deposits of a collagen and hyaline substance that will narrow small vessel lumens and thicken the malformation's walls during the first 12 to 24 months following this procedure.

Please contact the agencies listed under Resources, below, for the most current information. Addresses and telephone numbers of these agencies, as well as of individual experts and research centers, may be found in the Master Resources List.

**Resources**

**For more information on arteriovenous malformations:** National Organization for Rare Disorders (NORD); National Vascular Malformation Foundation; NIH/National Institute of Neurological Disorders and Stroke.

## References

Moss and Adams Heart Disease in Infants, Children, and Adolescents, Including the Fetus and Young Adult, 5th ed.: G.C. Emmanouilides, et al., eds.; Williams and Wilkins, 1995, pp. 791–810.

Harrison's Principles of Internal Medicine, 12th ed.: J.D. Wilson, et al., eds.; McGraw-Hill, 1991, pp. 2000–2001.

Cecil Textbook of Medicine, 18th ed.: J.B. Wyngaarden and L.H. Smith, Jr., eds.; W.B. Saunders Company, 1988, p. 2060.

# ATRIAL SEPTAL DEFECTS

**Description** A small opening (foramen ovale) is present in all normal infants at birth, but closes in the majority with advancing age. If the septum separating the 2 atria is incompletely and abnormally formed before birth, a large opening may persist. The defect leads to an increased workload on the right heart, and excessive blood flow to the lung. Symptoms tend to be absent or mild at first, so that the defect is often not recognized until school age or adulthood. In adults, various cardiorespiratory problems and heart failure begin to develop. Atrial defects can take several forms, including the most common, ostium secundum defect, the less frequent ostium primum defect, and sinus venosus defect, or coronary sinus defect.

**Signs and Symptoms** In **ostium secundum defect,** the middle portion of the atrial septum, in the region of the foramen ovale, fails to close during fetal development. Although superficially similar to patent foramen ovale, the ostium secundum defect develops differently and has a different course.

In **ostium primum defect,** which may be associated with Down syndrome, the lower part of the atrial septum fails to develop normally. Often, the valves separating the atrium from the ventricle on each side (tricuspid valve—right side; mitral valve—left side) are also malformed, and the ventricular septum may be deficient.

**Sinus venosus defect** occurs high in the atrial septum and is often associated with anomalous entry of the right pulmonary veins into the right atrium or superior vena cava.

Many children are asymptomatic. A few have mild growth retardation and an unusual susceptibility to respiratory infections. At approximately 40 years of age (and earlier at high altitudes where there is more constriction of the pulmonary arteries), patients may begin to have difficulties because of gradually developing hypertension in pulmonary circulation, changing the direction in which the blood is shunted through the defect.

Clinical consequences of right-to-left shunts include cyanosis, clubbing of the fingertips, and polycythemia. Patients are predisposed to brain abscesses. Severe cases may result in heart failure, with edema and breathlessness. Arrhythmias, including atrial fibrillation, may occur in the disease's later stages. Patients are also predisposed to paradoxical embolism, especially during pregnancy. Death may result without surgical repair of the defect.

**Etiology** The causes of the arrest in embryonic development resulting in atrial septal defects are poorly understood. The defects may occur in association with a variety of other congenital cardiac defects, or in infants small for gestational age. Ostium primum defects often occur in individuals with Down syndrome or Ellis–van Creveld syndrome. There appears to be familial inheritance in some cases. In rare instances, ostium primum defects may be inherited as an autosomal recessive genetic trait. Some ostium secundum defects may be inherited as an autosomal dominant genetic trait.

**Epidemiology** Approximately 1 percent of live births have some type of congenital heart defect; of these, about 10 percent are atrial septal defects. Females are affected more often than males (2–3:1).

**Related Disorders** See *Cor Triatriatum.*

**Atrioventricular septal defect** is a congenital heart defect characterized by improperly developed atrial and ventricular septa and atrioventricular valves. Symptoms and prognosis depend on the severity of the malformation. There is an incomplete form (atrial septal defect primum), transitional form (atrial septal defect and small ventricular septal defect), or complete form (large atrial and ventricular defects). In addition, the extent of leakage of the valves between the atria and ventricles and size of the ventricles influence symptoms and prognosis.

Other related disorders include **cor triloculare biatriatum,** in which there are 3 heart chambers (2 atria and 1 ventricle), and **cor triloculare biventricularis** (2 ventricles and 1 large atrium).

**Treatment—Standard** The definitive treatment is surgery, suturing shut the hole in the septum, or patching it with a graft. The success rate is high for this procedure. For ostium primum (endocardial cushion) defects, which may require repairing or replacing of the atrioventricular valves, the success rate is considerably lower. Surgery is optimally performed between the ages of 3 and 6.

Digitalis can be used as a preoperative, palliative treatment for arrhythmias, tachycardias, and heart failure. Sodium restriction, diuretics, and rest are also effective in treating congestive heart failure. Respiratory infections are treated vigorously and early. Because of the risk of bacterial endocarditis, patients should be given antibiotics prophylactically with surgery and procedures such as tooth extractions.

Genetic counseling may be of benefit for some patients and their families. Other treatment is symptomatic and supportive.

**Treatment—Investigational** Clinical trials utilizing a variety of devices delivered by catheters have been very promising. Children undergo cardiac catheterization, during which a prosthetic device (self-centering double disk, double-umbrella disk, or button device), which covers and closes the opening in the septum, is implanted.

Please contact the agencies listed under Resources, below, for the most current information. Addresses and telephone numbers of these agencies, as well as of individual experts and research centers, may be found in the Master Resources List.

**Resources**

**For more information on atrial septal defects:** National Organization for Rare Disorders (NORD); American Heart Association; American Lung Association; NIH/National Heart, Lung and Blood Institute.

**For genetic information and genetic counseling referrals:** March of Dimes Birth Defects Foundation; Alliance of Genetic Support Groups.

**References**

International Experience with Secundum Atrial Defect Occlusion by the Buttoned Device: Rao, P.S., et al.; Am. Heart J., 1994, vol. 128, pp. 1022–1035.

Acyanotic Congenital Heart Disease: Atrial and Ventricular Septal Defects, Atrioventricular Canal, Patent Ductus Arteriosus, Pulmonic Stenosis: L.T. Mahoney; Cardiol. Clin., November 1993, vol. 11(4), pp. 603–616.

Echocardiographic Follow-up of Atrial Septal Defect After Catheter Closure by Double-Umbrella Device: C. Boutin, et al.; Circulation, August 1993, vol. 88(2), pp. 621–627.

Experimental Atrial Septal Closure with a New, Transcatheter, Self-Centering Defice: G.S. Das, et al.; Circulation, October 1993, vol. 88(4 pt. 1), pp. 1754–1764.

Long-Term Follow-up (9 to 20 Years) After Surgical Closure of Atrial Septal Defect at a Young Age: F. Meijboom, et al.; Am. J. Cardiol., December 15, 1993, vol. 72(18), pp. 1431–1434.

Secundum Atrial Septal Defect Repair: Long-Term Surgical Outcome and the Problem of Late Mitral Regurgitation: M.E. Speechly-Dick, et al.; Postgrad. Med. J., December 1993, vol. 69(818), pp. 912–915.

Transcatheter Closure of Atrial Septal Defect and Patent Ductus Arteriosus: T.R. Hoyd and R.H. Beekman; in Textbook of International Cardiology, 2nd ed.: E.J. Topol, ed.; W.B. Saunders, 1993, pp. 1298–1311.

Cecil Textbook of Medicine, 19th ed.: J.B. Wyngaarden, et al., eds.; W.B. Saunders Company, 1992, pp. 280–283.

Mendelian Inheritance in Man, 10th ed.: V.A. McKusick; The Johns Hopkins University Press, 1992, pp. 132–133, 1244.

Nelson Textbook of Pediatrics, 14th ed.: R.E. Behrman, ed.-in-chief; W.B. Saunders Company, 1992, pp. 1169–1172.

Birth Defects Encyclopedia: M.L Buyse, ed.-in-chief; Blackwell Scientific Publications, 1990, pp. 209–210.

Dictionary of Medical Syndromes, 3rd ed.: S.I. Magalini, et al., eds.; J.B. Lippincott Company, 1990, pp. 76–77.

# BROAD BETA DISEASE

**Description** This hereditary lipid transport disorder is marked by the presence of xanthomas under certain skin areas. The patient is predisposed to obesity, atherosclerosis, and occlusion of blood vessels.

**Synonyms**

> Familial Broad Beta Disease
> Familial Dysbetalipoproteinemia
> Hyperlipoproteinemia, Type III
> Xanthoma Tuberosum

**Signs and Symptoms** Xanthomas appear in adults on the palms of the hands, fingers (occasionally), knees, elbows, arms, legs, and buttocks, and within the Achilles tendon. The cornea may also be affected (arcus lipidus corneae).

The primary complications are cardiovascular. An imbalance of cholesterol-transporting protein-lipid molecules and other fats leads to elevated cholesterol and triglyceride blood levels. The patient's obesity resulting from this disorder increases the risk of cardiovascular disease.

**Etiology** Broad beta disease is believed to be an inherited autosomal dominant trait. It has been associated rarely with diabetes or hypothyroidism.

**Epidemiology** Slightly more males than females are affected. In males, symptoms begin during early adulthood; in females, they begin approximately 15 years later. It is estimated that 1:500 people in the United States are affected.

**Related Disorders** See *Hyperchylomicronemia.*

Broad beta disease is one of several forms of **hyperlipoproteinemia.**

**Treatment—Standard** Reducing the amounts of cholesterol and fats in the patient's diet may prevent xanthomas and hyperlipidemia. Xanthomas can sometimes be removed surgically. The blood levels of total cholesterol and low density lipoproteins may be lowered in some patients by the administration of niacin, gemfibrozil, clofibrate, and/or lovastatin. Other drugs, such as cholestyramine and colestipol, are not effective and may actually raise blood levels of β-lipoproteins. Treatment of cardiovascular disease is symptomatic.

**Treatment—Investigational** The drug simvastatin may be effective in lowering the serum level of β-lipoproteins. Studies are under way to determine the long-term safety and effectiveness of this treatment.

Please contact the agencies listed under Resources, below, for the most current information. Addresses and telephone numbers of these agencies, as well as of individual experts and research centers, may be found in the Master Resources List.

**Resources**

**For more information on broad beta disease:** National Organization for Rare Disorders (NORD); National Lipid Diseases Foundation; American Heart Association; NIH/National Heart, Lung and Blood Institute.

**For genetic information and genetic counseling referrals:** March of Dimes Birth Defects Foundation; Alliance of Genetic Support Groups.

**References**

Clinical Features of Type III Hyperlipoproteinemia: Analysis of 64 Patients: G. Feussner, et al.; Clin. Investig., May 1993, vol. 71(5), pp. 362–366.

Cecil Textbook of Medicine, 19th ed.: J.B. Wyngaarden, et al., eds.; W.B. Saunders Company, 1992, pp. 1082–1090.

Mendelian Inheritance in Man, 10th ed.: V.A. McKusick; The Johns Hopkins University Press, 1992, pp. 569–570.

The Role of Apolipoprotein E Genetic Variant in Lipoprotein Disorders: S.C. Rall, et al.; J. Intern. Med., June 1992, vol. 231(6), pp. 653–659.

Long-Term Effects of Sinvastatin in Familial Dysbetalipoproteinemia: P.M. Stuyt, et al.; J. Intern. Med., August 1991, vol. 230(2), pp. 151–155.

Birth Defects Encyclopedia: M.L Buyse, ed.-in-chief; Blackwell Scientific Publications, 1990, pp. 906–907.

Dictionary of Medical Syndromes, 3rd ed.: S.I. Magalini, et al., eds.; J.B. Lippincott Company, 1990, pp. 437–439.

The Effective Reduction of Plasma Lipoprotein Levels in Familial Dysbetalipoproteinemia (Type III Hyperlipoproteinemia): P.M. Stuyt, et al.; Am. J. Med., January 1990, vol. 88(1N), pp. 42N–45N.

Drug Therapy of Hypercholesterolemia: D.R. Illingworth; Clin. Chem., 1988, vol. 34(8B), pp. 123–132.

Hyperlipoproteinemia with Genfibrozil to Retard Progression of Coronary Artery Disease: P.T. Kuo, et al.; Am. Heart J., July 1988, vol. 116(1 pt. 1), pp. 85–90.

# BRONCHOPULMONARY DYSPLASIA (BPD)

**Description** Bronchopulmonary dysplasia is a chronic bronchial tube and lung disease that affects infants who have been on a ventilator for a prolonged period of time. This disorder usually becomes manifest in the late neonatal period, has certain blood gas and radiographic abnormalities, and has an apparent lung injury causing a respiratory disorder. Pulmonary distress syndrome may also be present.

**Signs and Symptoms** The symptoms of bronchopulmonary dysplasia may be inflammation, difficulty breathing, collapsed lungs, flat chest, low birth weight, air flow obstruction, lung air leaks, abnormal blood gas, and scarring in the alveolar walls of the lungs. On chest x-ray, the lungs may appear hazy. Infection can be found in or near the trachea, and the alveolar epithelium begins to separate, forming necrotic tissue. In more severe and chronic cases, cor pulmonale develops, with pulmonary artery hypertension and congestive heart failure.

**Etiology** Bronchopulmonary dysplasia is associated with the prolonged use of ventilators with newborns. It is more common among premature infants and often follows infantile respiratory distress syndrome. In many cases the infant does not wean from the ventilator in the 5- to 6-day period when respiratory distress syndrome should clear up. Undernutrition may also be a factor in the development of bronchopulmonary dysplasia. Because infants with a low birth weight have a very small reserve of calories and nutrients, their capability of fighting this disease is greatly diminished.

**Epidemiology** Bronchopulmonary dysplasia affects males and females in equal numbers. Between one-fourth and two-thirds of infants with respiratory distress syndrome end up developing bronchopulmonary dysplasia. Most infants who develop this disorder are about 28 days old, have a low birth weight, have received supplemental oxygen, and have been on a ventilator. In the United States, bronchopulmonary dysplasia has become the most common form of chronic lung disease in infants.

**Related Disorders** See *Respiratory Distress Syndrome, Infant.*

**Pulmonary interstitial emphysema** is a disorder in which the normal lung air spaces have air leaks. This disorder usually occurs when infants have trouble breathing, are on a ventilator, and have serious lung disease. It may also occur sporadically. One or both lungs may be involved. The disorder may be concentrated in one area of one lung, or it may be widespread in both lungs.

**Treatment—Standard** Bronchopulmonary dysplasia requires constant monitoring of arterial oxygenation. Further ventilation and oxygen support may be required. This support should be reduced as tolerated. When chronic lung disease is present, the blood gas level should be allowed to rise above normal while weaning from the ventilator. This procedure may be used as long as the infant is not having too much difficulty breathing and acid balance remains normal. Nutrition plays an important part in the treatment of infants with bronchopulmonary dysplasia. Because of the extra work required for breathing, the infant may need an increase in calories. Increased nutrition can be provided by using intravenous or tube feedings. Diuretic therapy may be instituted to help prevent lung congestion. Furosemide or a combination of chlorothiazide and spironolactone may be needed for several weeks after the infant has been weaned off the ventilator or in those patients with cor pulmonale and congestive heart failure. The vaporized drug terbutaline may be used to help lung mechanics in infants using ventilators.

**Treatment—Investigational** Please contact the agencies listed under Resources, below, for the most current information. Addresses and telephone numbers of these agencies, as well as of individual experts and research centers, may be found in the Master Resources List.

**Resources**

**For more information on bronchopulmonary dysplasia:** National Organization for Rare Diseases (NORD); National Heart, Lung and Blood Institute Information Center; American Lung Association.

**References**

Late Pulmonary Sequelae of Bronchopulmonary Dysplasia: W.H. Northway, Jr., et al.; N. Engl. J. Med., December 1990, vol. 323(26), pp. 1793–1799.

Response of Pulmonary Mechanics to Terbutaline in Patients with Bronchopulmonary Dysplasia: D.S. Brudno, et al.; Am. J. Med. Sci., March 1989, vol. 297(3), pp. 166–168.

Pulmonary Disease and Disorders, 2nd ed.: A.P. Fishman, et al., eds.; McGraw-Hill, 1988, pp. 2261–2262.

Antireflux Surgery in Infants with Bronchopulmonary Dysplasia: R.M. Giuffre, et al.; Am. J. Dis. Child., June 1987, vol. 141(6), pp. 648–651.

# CHURG-STRAUSS SYNDROME

**Description** Churg-Strauss syndrome is a lung disorder that often occurs as a complication of other conditions. Angiitis or vasculitis is accompanied by granulomas.

**Synonyms**

Allergic Angiitis and Granulomatosis
Allergic Granulomatosis and Angiitis
Allergic Granulomatous Angiitis
System Vasculitis with Asthma and Eosinophilia

**Signs and Symptoms** An allergic reaction or asthma may precede the syndrome's development by several years. Asthma tends to subside as vasculitis occurs. Lung tissue infiltrations (short-term or persistent), fever, and weight loss are often initial signs. Interstitial lung disease, ophthalmic lesions, and seizures may develop.

Granulomas may infiltrate tissue and cause deterioration; they may be accompanied by eosinophils, which can unite with the granulomas to form larger lesions. Histiocytes and a variable number of giant cells may invade tissues, especially in the lungs. Vascular growths can bring about both deterioration and infiltrating inflammation. Lesions can heal with or without scar formation.

Malaise, skin rash, kidney inflammation, peripheral neuropathy, asymmetric polyarthralgia, or arthritis may occur.

**Etiology** Although the exact etiology is unknown, the disease may be associated with an autoimmune disorder, possibly involving antibodies to thyroglobulin, parietal cells, adrenal cells, or thyroid.

**Epidemiology** Onset may occur from 15 to 70 years of age. The disease affects both males and females.

**Related Disorders** See *Polyarteritis Nodosa; Wegener Granulomatosis.*

**Treatment—Standard** Corticosteroids and/or cyclophosphamide are used for inflammation and kidney problems. Intravenous methylprednisolone may be effective in severe cases. Other treatment is symptomatic and supportive.

**Treatment—Investigational** Plasma exchange in conjunction with corticosteroids and cyclophosphamide is being evaluated. Studies are also being conducted in the use of sandoglobulin as a treatment for Churg-Strauss syndrome.

Please contact the agencies listed under Resources, below, for the most current information. Addresses and telephone numbers of these agencies, as well as of individual experts and research centers, may be found in the Master Resources List.

**Resources**

**For more information on Churg-Strauss syndrome:** National Organization for Rare Disorders (NORD); American Lung Association; NIH/National Heart, Lung and Blood Institute.

**References**

Complications of Plasma Exchange in the Treatment of Polyarteritis Nodosa and Churg-Strauss Angiitis and the Contribution of Adjuvant Immunosuppressive Therapy: A Randomized Trial in 72 Patients: F. Lhote, et al.; Artif. Organs, February 1988, vol. 12(1), pp. 27–33.

Internal Medicine, 2nd ed.: J.H. Stein, ed.-in-chief; Little, Brown and Company, 1987, pp. 1285–1286.

Allergic Angiitis of Churg-Strauss Syndrome: Response to Pulse Methylprednisolone: R. MacFadyen, et al.; Chest, April 1987, 91(4), pp. 629–631.

Systemic Vasculitis with Asthma and Eosinophilia: A Clinical Approach to the Churg-Strauss Syndrome: J.G. Lanham, et al.; Medicine (Baltimore), March 1984, 63(2), pp. 65–81.

Conjunctival Involvement in Churg-Strauss Syndrome: C.L. Shields, et al.; Am. J. Ophthalmol., November 1986, 102(5), pp. 601–605.

# COR TRIATRIATUM

**Description** Cor triatriatum is a rare congenital heart defect characterized by a small extra chamber above the left atrium into which the pulmonary veins drain. As a result, the passage of blood to the left atrium and ventricle is slowed, simulating obstruction of the mitral valve.

**Synonyms**

Triatrial Heart

**Signs and Symptoms** Depending on the size of the opening between the extra chamber and the left atrium proper, symptoms develop early in infancy when the opening is small. Symptoms include tachypnea, wheezing, coughing, and pulmonary congestion. Progressive enlargement of the heart occurs, often resulting in the development of high pulmonary artery pressure and right heart congestive failure. Heart murmurs may be present. In older patients, generalized edema, extreme dyspnea, poor oxygenation of the tissues, and tachycardia occur. Frequent pneumonias and bronchitis are likely, in turn precipitating heart failure. Patients are also at risk for bacterial endocarditis. Diagnosis can be made through echocardiography, magnetic resonance imaging, or heart catheterization and angiography.

**Etiology** The cause of cor triatriatum is unknown.

**Epidemiology** Infants of both sexes may be affected.

**Related Disorders** The condition simulates **mitral valve stenosis.**

**Treatment—Standard** Most patients will require surgery, which should be performed at a young age. Prior to surgery, congestive heart failure should be managed by diuretics and, if necessary, fluid and salt restriction. Digitalis should also be administered to increase the strength and decrease the rate of heart contractions. Oxygen therapy may also prove beneficial. Respiratory infections are treated vigorously and early.

**Treatment—Investigational** Please contact the agencies listed under Resources, below, for the most current information. Addresses and telephone numbers of these agencies, as well as of individual experts and research centers, may be found in the Master Resources List.

**Resources**

**For more information on cor triatriatum:** National Organization for Rare Disorders (NORD); American Heart Association; American Lung Association; NIH/National Heart, Lung and Blood Institute.

**References**

Moss and Adams Heart Disease in Infants, Children, and Adolescents, Including the Fetus and Young Adult, 5th ed.: G.C. Emmanouilides, et al., eds.; Williams and Wilkins, 1995, pp. 863–868.

Cor Triatriatum: Diagnosis, Operative Approach, and Late Results: J.A. Van Son, et al.; Mayo Clin. Proc., September 1993, vol. 68(9), pp. 854–859.

Cor Triatriatum Sinister, Not Mitral Stenosis, in an Adult with Previous Sydenham's Chorea: Diagnosis and Preoperative Assessment by Cross Sectional Echocardiography: M.A. De Belder, et al.; Br. Heart J., July 1992, vol. 68(1), pp. 9–11.

Asymptomatic Cor Triatriatum Incidentally Revealed by Computed Tomography: F. Tanaka; Chest, July 1991, vol. 199(1), pp. 272–274.

Birth Defects Encyclopedia: M.L Buyse, ed.-in-chief; Blackwell Scientific Publications, 1990, pp. 839–840.

Dictionary of Medical Syndromes, 3rd ed.: S.I. Magalini, et al., eds.; J.B. Lippincott Company, 1990, p. 601.

# CYSTIC FIBROSIS (CF)

**Description** Cystic fibrosis is an inherited disorder that affects the exocrine glands. The main consequences are related to the mucus-producing glands. The secreted mucus is thick and sticky, clogging and obstructing air passages in the lungs and pancreatic bile ducts. Cystic fibrosis also causes dysfunction of the salivary and sweat glands.

**Synonyms**

Fibrocystic Disease of the Pancreas

Mucosis

Mucoviscidosis

Pancreatic Fibrosis

**Signs and Symptoms** Ten to 15 percent of those affected manifest symptoms at birth in the form of an intestinal blockage known as **meconim ileus.** In other patients, symptoms appear during the first few months of life.

**Pulmonary problems:** Most cystic fibrosis patients develop lung disease. Thick mucus obstructs the airways of the lungs, interfering with the patient's breathing and causing damage to the lung tissue. Cystic fibrosis patients are susceptible to lung infections, especially those caused by *Staphylococcus aureus* and *Pseudomonas aeruginosa*. Early symptoms include a dry, hacking, nonproductive cough; increased respiratory rate, often with wheezing; prolonged expiratory phases of respiration; and decreased activity. Later signs include increased cough with sputum production, rales, musical rhonchi, and scattered or localized wheezes; repeated episodes of respiratory infection; and signs of obstructive lung disease. Other symptoms include increased front-to-back measurement of the chest, a depressed diaphragm, and palpable liver border. There may also be decreased appetite, weight loss, failure to gain weight or grow, decreased exercise tolerance, and digital clubbing.

Advanced signs of the disease include chronic, paroxysmal, productive cough, often associated with vomiting; marked increase in respiratory rate; exertional dyspnea; orthopnea; diffuse and localized rales and rhonchi; signs of marked obstructive lung disease; marked increase in front-to-back measurement (barrel chest, pigeon breast); depressed diaphragm; decreased air exchange; noisy respiration (wheezing, bubbling, audible rales); marked decrease in appetite associated with weight loss; growth failure and stunting; muscular weakness and flabbiness; cyanosis; fever; tachycardia; hemoptysis; atelectasis; pneumothorax; lung abscess; signs of cardiac failure associated with cor pulmonale (edema; enlarged, tender liver; venous distention); visual impairment; bone pain; and osteoarthropathy. Upper respiratory symptoms include nasal polyps and chronic sinusitis.

**Gastrointestinal problems:** In cystic fibrosis, thick mucus blocks the pancreatic duct that carries digestive enzymes to the intestines, causing incomplete digestion of food. Pancreatic and nutritional symptoms may include intestinal obstruction, intussusception, fecal masses, poor weight gain despite voracious appetite, easy bruising secondary to vitamin K deficiency, malnutrition, poor muscle tone, small flabby muscles, lack of subcutaneous fat, and vitamin deficiencies. There may also be a distended abdomen; greasy, floating, foul-smelling stools; chronic diarrhea in infancy; rectal prolapse; cramps and excessive foul gas; hypoproteinemia with generalized edema; pancreatitis; and diabetes.

**Biliary problems:** Biliary cirrhosis and portal hypertension symptoms include jaundice; firm, nodular liver, often palpable in midline; splenomegaly; hypersplenism; anemia; hematemesis and melena from esophageal varices; and ascites.

**Problems of the sweat glands:** Hyponatremia and hypochloremia also occur. Because of the high concentration of sodium and chloride secreted by the sweat glands, those suffering from cystic fibrosis experience extreme heat exhaustion and dehydration during periods of exercise, hot weather, or febrile states. In addition, severe muscle cramps, weakness, and shock may occur. The child's forehead often tastes salty.

**Genital tract/reproductive problems:** Symptoms may include aspermia, blockage or absence of the vas deferens, cervical polyps, and increased viscosity of mucus. Approximately 95 percent of males are sterile. Women usually have reproductive problems as well. Menstrual cycles may become irregular, and vaginal infections may occur as side effects of antibiotic treatment. Although conception may be difficult for women with cystic fibrosis, they are not sterile and can give birth to normal children.

Patients should be suspected of having cystic fibrosis when the following conditions are encountered: chronic cough, recurrent bronchitis or pneumonia, allergy (e.g., rhinitis, postnasal drip), asthma, nasal polyposis, chronic sinusitis, tuberculosis, pulmonary lesions, intestinal obstruction in the newborn, failure to thrive/malnutrition, celiac disease, malabsorption, rectal prolapse, dysautonomia, agammaglobulinemia, cirrhosis of the liver, heat stroke, diagnosis of cystic fibrosis in a sibling, or a chest x-ray that reveals irregularity of aeration with patchy areas of atelectasis and generalized overinflation.

**Etiology** Cystic fibrosis is inherited as an autosomal recessive disorder. The gene that causes cystic fibrosis was identified in 1989. Recent investigations indicate that a malformed protein located in the cell membrane may be linked to the disease, causing an abnormal flow of chloride in and out of the cell. The thick mucus that characterizes the disease may be caused by limited secretion of chloride. The same defect in cells lining the sweat glands is thought to alter the salt concentration in the sweat of cystic fibrosis patients. Another theory asserts that this defect is a byproduct of the disease rather than the primary defect. According to this theory, the gene produces an enzyme that changes the chemical structure of the mucus. This overactive enzyme may also alter the chloride channels in sweat cell membranes, leading to production of abnormally salty sweat.

**Epidemiology** There are about 33,000 cases of cystic fibrosis in the United States. It mostly affects white children and young adults, although there is a small but significant number of blacks and Orientals affected.

**Treatment—Standard** There is presently no cure for cystic fibrosis. Various treatments can help patients lead normal, active lives. Genetic tests are available to determine if parents are carriers of the cystic fibrosis gene. Scientists are also developing a neonatal screening test for cystic fibrosis. Since early treatment may lead to better quality of life for cystic fibrosis patients, early diagnosis will be of great help to children with the disease.

In the area of physical therapy, postural drainage, specifically bronchial drainage, carried out twice a day is the most important form of preventive therapy and is often used in conjunction with aerosol inhalation. Breathing exercises help improve the patient's respiration, ventilation, and posture. Aerosol therapy entails the inhalation of particulate water and medication via nebulizers and is effective in wetting and thinning the mucus secretions in the airways. Pancreatic deficiency is treated by replacement therapy and diet. Prophylaxis against respiratory infections helps maintain clear airways. A diet high in protein, calories, and vitamins is recommended. Patients should be given extra salt with their food and occasionally take salt tablets in order to be protected from acute salt loss. The steroid prednisone has been used to control severe reactive airway disease in cystic fibrosis patients.

Up until the end of 1991, 312 people with cystic fibrosis had undergone lung transplants. The 3-year survival rate was 52 percent.

**Treatment—Investigational** Clinical trials of the orphan drug DNase were begun in June of 1990. DNase is an enzyme that affects the thickness of mucus secretions. One study of DNase is being conducted at the National Heart, Lung and Blood Institute; the other study is under way at the University of Washington in Seattle. DNase is manufactured by Genentech.

Scientists are studying an aerosol antihypertensive drug, amiloride, which may delay, but not prevent, lung damage in people with cystic fibrosis. More research is needed to determine the safety and effectiveness of this treatment.

A new treatment, secretory leukocyte protease inhibitor (**SLPI**) is to be used in clinical trials with human patients in collaboration with the National Heart, Lung and Blood Institute and the manufacturer, Synergen. Information on the trials can be obtained from the Cystic Fibrosis Foundation.

Univax Biologics has received orphan drug designation for mucoid expolysacchride *Pseudomonas* hyperimmune globulin (**MEPIG**) for the prevention of lung infections due to *Pseudomonas aeruginosa*.

The orphan product tobramycin for inhalation is being tested for the treatment of bronchopulmonary infections of *Pseudomonas aeruginosa*. The product is manufactured by Pathogensis Corporation.

Drs. T. Kennedy and J. Hoidal are working on an inhaled, aerosolized orphan drug, dextran sulfate (Unedex), as an adjunct to the treatment of cystic fibrosis. They are also studying the orphan product 2-0-desulfated heparin (Aeropin).

The Food and Drug Administration has approved the orphan drug amibride HCL solution for inhalation for testing as a treatment for cystic fibrosis patients. The drug is manufactured by Glaxo. Other drugs being tested include adenosine triphosphate and uridine triphosphate. These 2 drugs work on a chloride in the nasal passages to thin sputum. Recombinant human deoxyribonuclease also works as a mucolytic agent.

Research on the use of ibuprofen to reduce the effects of chronic bronchitis that often afflicts cystic fibrosis patients is also very promising.

For additional information on the treatment of cystic fibrosis, see "Cystic Fibrosis: New Treatments Give Victims Precious Time" in the Prevalent Health Conditions/Concerns area of NORD Services.

Clinical trials are under way to study the use of 1-antitrypsin (ProlastinR) in cystic fibrosis. Interested persons may wish to contact Melvin Berger, M.D., Ph.D.

The orphan product cystic fibrosis transmembrane conductance regulator, sponsored by Genzyme Corp., is being tested as a protein replacement therapy in patients with cystic fibrosis.

The orphan product recombinant human gelsolin is being tested for the treatment of respiratory symptoms of cystic fibrosis. The product is manufactured by Biogen.

Several researchers are studying gene therapy for cystic fibrosis by inserting the normal CFTR gene into an adenovirus and delivering the virus directly into the lung. When the virus is modified with the normal CFTR gene, its ability to reproduce itself is destroyed so that it cannot cause a cold. This research is being conducted by Dr. Ronald Crystal of The National Heart, Lung and Blood Institute, Dr. Michael J. Welsh of Howard Hughes Medical Institute, and Dr. James Wilson of the University of Pennsylvania.

Please contact the agencies listed under Resources, below, for the most current information. Addresses and telephone numbers of these agencies, as well as of individual experts and research centers, may be found in the Master Resources List.

**Resources**

**For more information on cystic fibrosis:** National Organization for Rare Disorders (NORD); Cystic Fibrosis Foundation; NIH/National Digestive Diseases Information Clearinghouse; Cystic Fibrosis Research Trust; Canadian Cystic Fibrosis Foundation.

**For genetic information and genetic counseling referrals:** March of Dimes Birth Defects Foundation; Alliance of Genetic Support Groups.

**References**

Cecil Textbook of Medicine, 18th ed.: J.B. Wyngaarden and L.H. Smith, Jr., eds.: W.B. Saunders Company, 1988, p. 1534.
Cystic Fibrosis: T.F. Boat; *in* Textbook of Respiratory Medicine: J.F. Murray and J.A. Nodel, eds.; W.B. Saunders Company, 1988.
Heart-Lung Transplantation for Cystic Fibrosis: J. Scott, et al.; Lancet, July 23, 1988, vol. II(8604), pp. 192–194.
Cystic Fibrosis: L.M. Taussig, ed.; Thieme-Stratton, 1984.

# DEGOS DISEASE

**Description** Degos disease is a systemic disorder that affects small and medium-sized arteries, causing occlusive arteriopathy. The disorder usually progresses through 2 stages, affecting first the skin and later other organs.

**Synonyms**
> Degos-Kohlmeier Disease
> Kohlmeier-Degos Disease
> Malignant Atrophic Papulosis

**Signs and Symptoms** Major symptoms of Degos disease appear in 2 stages: skin lesions, and lesions that affect other organs. Skin lesions begin as circular reddish papules on the skin that heal and leave scars with a flat white center and a raised red edge. This stage of the disease may last for a period of time ranging from weeks to years. A few cases have been reported with no involvement beyond the skin lesion stage.

The occlusive arteriopathy that is characteristic of Degos disease restricts blood flow and leads to severe tissue necrosis. Multiple areas of necrosis may occur in connective tissue near skin lesions and in other organs.

The gastrointestinal tract is usually involved in the 2nd stage of Degos disease. Lesions frequently develop on the walls of the small intestine. Gastrointestinal symptoms include abdominal pain, diarrhea, and weight loss. The intestinal lesions frequently ulcerate and perforate the intestinal wall, resulting in peritonitis.

In approximately 20 percent of cases, Degos disease affects the central nervous system. Small areas of the brain may be damaged as a result of infarcts. Major neurologic symptoms may include mental dysfunction, paresthesia, weakness of the limbs on one side, and/or other motor abnormalities. Other neurologic symptoms may include ptosis, ophthalmoplegia, and/or obtundation.

In a few cases of Degos disease, plaques have appeared on the bulbar conjunctiva. Chorioretinal lesions have also occurred.

**Etiology** The cause of Degos disease is not known. The disease process causes the cells lining the arteries to multiply, which contributes to arterial occlusion. Areas of necrosis may appear as a result of occlusive arteriopathy. The effects of Degos disease depend upon the location of the occluded arteries and necrotic lesions.

**Epidemiology** Degos disease affects more males than females. In most cases, primary symptoms (skin lesions) first appear in adulthood. However, there have been a few reported cases in which infants and children are affected.

**Related Disorders** See *Buerger Disease; Lichen Sclerosus et Atrophicus; Lymphomatoid Granulomatosis; Scleroderma.*

**Vasculitis,** a vascular inflammatory disorder, may occur alone or in conjunction with allergic and rheumatic diseases. Inflammation of the vascular walls constricts the blood vessels and may cause ischemia, necrosis, thrombosis, and, rarely, an aneurysm. Any size vessel and any part of the vascular system may be affected, with symptoms being localized or striking larger areas of the body. Vasculitis may be the primary disorder, or secondary to other disease processes. Because of the varied situations in which vasculitis can arise, symptoms and signs are relative to the system involved. Degos disease is a systemic form of vasculitis that primarily affects the skin and small intestine.

**Cutaneous (dermal) necrotizing vasculitis,** a vascular inflammatory disease that also affects the skin, may occur alone or in conjunction with infectious, allergic, or rheumatic illnesses. Males and females are affected equally. Inflamed vessel walls and skin lesions appear primarily on the back, buttocks, interior forearms, hands, and lower extremities. The lesions may be nodular, macular, or purpural, and may persist for several weeks and leave darkened spots and scarring. Some lesions are annular. Ulcers, vesicles, or bullae are signs of greater severity. The lesions characteristic of cutaneous necrotizing vasculitis usually affect only the skin, while in Degos disease lesions may affect other organs (e.g., small intestine) and cause associated complications.

**Treatment—Standard** Treatment is supportive and symptomatic. Examination of the gastrointestinal tract on a regular basis may detect intestinal perforation before symptoms of acute complications (e.g., peritonitis) appear.

**Treatment—Investigational** Please contact the agencies listed under Resources, below, for the most current information. Addresses and telephone numbers of these agencies, as well as of individual experts and research centers, may be found in the Master Resources List.

**Resources**

**For more information on Degos disease:** National Organization for Rare Disorders (NORD); NIH/National Digestive Diseases Information Clearinghouse.

**References**

Degos Disease and Spastic Paraplegia: T.A. Leslie, et al.; Clin. Exp. Dermatol., July 1993, vol. 18(4), pp. 344–346.

Endoscopic and Histopathologic Features of Degos Disease: M.K. Casparis, et al.; Endoscopy, July 1991, vol. 23(4), pp. 231–233.

Dictionary of Medical Syndromes, 3rd ed.: S.I. Magalini, et al., eds.; J.B. Lippincott Company, 1990, p. 504.

Malignant Atrophic Papulosis (Degos Syndrome): A. Stejskalova, et al.; Sb. Lek., January 1990, vol. 92(1), pp. 1–5.

Gastrointestinal Disease, 4th ed.: M.H. Sleisenger, et. al.; W.B. Saunders Company, 1989, pp. 1918, 1949.

The Pathology and Pathogenesis of Malignant Atrophic Papulosis (Degos Disease): A Case Study with Reference to Other Vascular Disorders: W.M. Molenaar, et al.; Pathol. Res. Pract., February 1987, vol. 182(1), pp. 98–106.

CNS Involvement in Malignant Atrophic Papulosis (Kohlmeier-Degos Disease): Vasculopathy and Coagulopathy: D.K. Dastur, et al.; J. Neurol. Neurosurg. Psychiatry, February 1981, vol. 44(2), pp. 156–160.

# DEXTROCARDIA WITH SITUS INVERSUS

**Description** The condition is characterized by a right-sided positioning of the heart, with reversal of its chambers and the abdominal viscera.

**Synonyms**

> Heterotaxy Syndrome
> Mirror-Image Dextrocardia
> Situs Inversus Totalis

**Signs and Symptoms** The cardiac silhouette is positioned on the right side of the chest, with the apex pointing to the right; the position of the chambers and of the abdominal organs is reversed. Heart sounds emanating more clearly from the right chest provide physical evidence of the condition. Chest roentgenography reveals malpositioning of the heart. The electrocardiogram shows inversion of electrical waves. Most patients live a normal life without associated symptoms or disability. However, about 20 percent of patients have Kartagener syndrome, or the triad of situs inversus, sinusitis, and bronchiectasis. While situs inversus totalis is rarely associated with congenital heart disease, situs inversus of the abdominal organs and a normally positioned heart are commonly associated with heart defects. Similarly, a heart in the right chest with normal or ambiguous abdominal situs is often associated with severe heart defects.

**Etiology** The disorder, present at birth, is transmitted by autosomal recessive genes.

**Epidemiology** The incidence of dextrocardia with complete situs inversus is about 2:10,000 live births. Males and females are affected in equal numbers.

**Related Disorders** See *Kartagener Syndrome.*

**Treatment—Standard** Treatment is symptomatic and supportive. If the condition is associated with other more serious heart malformations, the prognosis and treatment will vary. Genetic counseling may be helpful.

**Treatment—Investigational** Please contact the agencies listed under Resources, below, for the most current information. Addresses and telephone numbers of these agencies, as well as of individual experts and research centers, may be found in the Master Resources List.

**Resources**

**For more information on dextrocardia with situs inversus:** National Organization for Rare Disorders (NORD); American Heart Association; NIH/National Heart, Lung and Blood Institute.

**For genetic information and genetic counseling referrals:** March of Dimes Birth Defects Foundation; Alliance of Genetic Support Groups.

**References**

Moss and Adams Heart Disease in Infants, Children, and Adolescents, Including the Fetus and Young Adult, 5th ed.: G.C. Emmanouilides, et al., eds.; Williams and Wilkins, 1995, pp. 1307–1317.

The Heart, Arteries and Veins, 7th ed.: J.W. Hurst, et al., eds.; McGraw-Hill, 1990, pp. 255, 757–758.

Internal Medicine, 2nd ed.: J.H. Stein, ed.-in-chief; Little, Brown and Company, 1987, pp. 525.

A Possible Increase in the Incidence of Congenital Heart Defects Among the Offspring of Affected Parents: V. Rose, et al.; J. Am. Coll. Cardiol., August 1985, vol. 6(2), pp. 376–382.

# DILATATION OF THE PULMONARY ARTERY, IDIOPATHIC (IDPA)

**Description** IDPA is a rare congenital defect in which the main pulmonary artery is dilated in the absence of any apparent anatomic or physiologic cause.

**Signs and Symptoms** IDPA generally produces no symptoms because there is no circulation abnormality. The minimal clinical signs consist of a pulmonary ejection sound that disappears on inhalation, a soft pulmonary ejection systolic murmur, and splitting of the 2nd sound on inhalation. The disorder does not cause pulmonary valve disease, nor does bacterial endocarditis occur. The electrocardiogram is normal, and diagnosis is made when chest x-ray films reveal a dilated main pulmonary artery without cardiac chamber enlargement. An echocardiogram confirms the diagnosis.

**Etiology** The cause is unknown; however, a defect in the normal development of pulmonary artery elastic tissue before or after birth has been postulated. The dilatation also may be a consequence of a generalized connective tissue disease, because it is occasionally found in Marfan syndrome or Ehlers-Danlos syndrome (see **Marfan Syndrome; Ehlers-Danlos Syndrome**).

**Treatment—Standard** Treatment is not required. Affected persons have a normal life expectancy, provided there are no cardiac lesions.

**Treatment—Investigational** Please contact the agencies listed under Resources, below, for the most current information. Addresses and telephone numbers of these agencies, as well as of individual experts and research centers, may be found in the Master Resources List.

**Resources**

**For more information on idiopathic dilatation of the pulmonary artery:** National Organization for Rare Disorders (NORD); NIH/National Heart, Lung and Blood Institute; American Lung Association.

# EISENMENGER SYNDROME

**Description** The syndrome is characterized by a congenital ventricular septal defect. Pulmonary vascular resistance (**PVR**) increases as the child matures, resulting in high pulmonary artery pressure. The term *Eisenmenger syndrome* has also been applied to the association of other congenital heart defects with advanced pulmonary vascular disease.

The patient has dyspnea, cyanosis, and polycythemia. In some cases, the patient's condition does not deteriorate until age 40 or 50.

**Signs and Symptoms** Onset of noticeable symptoms usually occurs between ages 5 and 15. Cyanosis develops, especially during exertion, and a heart murmur may be detected. In persistent ductus arteriosus (without a ventricular septal defect), the feet will appear more bluish than the hands. Swelling due to soft-tissue proliferation at the fingertips and toes (clubbing) may also occur. Dyspnea and easy fatigability are common, and angina and syncope may occur.

Older patients have an abnormally high blood pressure, and atrial fibrillation may be present in the later stages.

An enlarged right ventricle and loud pulmonary valve closure may be evident on medical examination. Signs of pulmonary hypertension may be identified by a heaving parasternal cardiac impulse; a loud pulmonary second sound transmitted to the apex of the heart, by high diastolic pressure closing the valve forcibly; a pulmonary ejection click; a high-frequency decrescendo murmur during diastole down the left edge of the sternum; and a pansystolic murmur caused by incomplete closure of the tricuspid valve.

Failure of the right cardiac ventricle is characterized by dyspnea and fluid retention, often resulting in edema.

Hemoptysis may occur in advanced stages. Chest x-rays may show enlarged pulmonary arteries close to the lungs and ischemia in the periphery of the lungs. An enlarged atrium and tissue death due to pulmonary infarction may occur during late stages.

**Etiology** The cause of the defective development of the fetal heart and pulmonary vasculature are not known.

**Epidemiology** Male and female infants are affected in equal numbers.

**Related Disorders** See **Pulmonary Hypertension, Primary; Ventricular Septal Defects.**

**Treatment—Standard** Treatment is symptomatic and supportive. Anticoagulants should be avoided because of the risk of hemorrhaging in the lungs.

**Treatment—Investigational** Repair of the cardiac defect with lung transplantation or combined heart and lung transplantation has been performed with a reasonable success rate.

Please contact the agencies listed under Resources, below, for the most current information. Addresses and telephone numbers of these agencies, as well as of individual experts and research centers, may be found in the Master Resources List.

**Resources**

**For more information on Eisenmenger syndrome:** National Organization for Rare Disorders (NORD); NIH/National Heart, Lung and Blood Institute.

**For genetic information and genetic counseling referrals:** March of Dimes Birth Defects Foundation; Alliance of Genetic Support Groups.

**References**

Experience with Pediatric Lung Transplantation: B.E. Noyes, et al.; J. Pediatr., 1994, vol. 124, pp. 261–268.

Abnormal Architecture of the Ventricles in Hearts with an Overriding Aortic Valve and a Perimembranous Ventricular Septal Defect ("Eisenmenger VSD"): A. Oppenheimer-Dekker, et al.; Int. J. Cardiol., November 1985, vol. 9(3), pp. 341–355.

Eisenmenger's Syndrome and Pregnancy: S. Lieber, et al.; Acta Cardiol. (Brux.), 1985, vol. 40(4), pp. 421–424.

Combined Heart and Lung Transplantation: S.W. Jamieson, et al.; Lancet, May 1983, vol. 1(8334), pp. 1130–1132.

# EMPHYSEMA, CONGENITAL LOBAR

**Description** Congenital lobar emphysema is a respiratory disorder of varying degrees of severity in which air enters the lungs but cannot escape. In some cases, it is apparent at birth or shortly after birth. In others, it does not become manifest until adulthood. It may be so severe as to cause associated heart problems. Or it may be so mild that it does not cause any breathing difficulties and never becomes apparent.

**Synonyms**

> Congenital Pulmonary Emphysema
> Emphysema, Localized Congenital
> Lobar Emphysema, Infantile
> Lobar Tension Emphysema in Infancy

**Signs and Symptoms** Congenital lobar emphysema is characterized by dyspnea, an enlarged chest area over the affected lobe of the lung, and displacement of the space in the lung section nearest to the diseased lobe. The infant may experience severe difficulty in breathing when a cold or respiratory infection occurs, when trying to eat, or when crying. The disorder most often affects the left side of the lung in the upper lobe. The second most often affected section of the lung is the middle right lobe. There may be an absence of bronchial cartilage, or too much connective tissue within the lung. The lung tissue may be very fragile and may collapse easily.

**Etiology** In many cases, the cause is unknown. In some cases, the disorder is inherited as an autosomal recessive gene. In at least one case, the disorder was inherited as an autosomal dominant gene.

**Epidemiology** Congenital lobar emphysema is a very rare disorder that affects males and females in equal numbers. It is usually apparent at birth or shortly after. However, in some cases it may not become apparent until later in life, if at all.

**Related Disorders** See ***Respiratory Distress Syndrome, Infant; α-1-Antitrypsin Deficiency; Pulmonary Hypertension, Secondary.***

**Cor pulmonale** is associated with enlargement of the right ventricle of the heart, occurring as a result of severe pulmonary disease. Symptoms usually include dyspnea, exertional syncope, and substernal angina.

**Interstitial pneumonia** is characterized by exertional dyspnea, coughing, and anorexia; the symptoms may range from mild to severe, depending on the extent of involvement. Fever usually is not present, nor is there an overproduction of mucus.

**Treatment—Standard** Treatment of congenital lobar emphysema depends on the condition of the patient at the time of diagnosis. The extent of disease is usually determined by CT and radionuclide V/Q scans. Lung function tests help determine exactly which part of the lung is affected and if surgery is necessary. When the condition seriously affects the patient's ability to breathe, the usual treatment is surgical removal of the affected area in the lungs.

**Treatment—Investigational** Treatment of congenital lobar emphysema with the orphan drug alpha-1-proteinase inhibitor 2,3 (Prolastin) is being studied. The product is manufactured by Cutter Biological, a division of Miles Labs. Further studies are necessary to determine the long-term safety and effectiveness of this therapy.

Please contact the agencies listed under Resources, below, for the most current information. Addresses and telephone numbers of these agencies, as well as of individual experts and research centers, may be found in the Master Resources List.

**Resources**

**For more information on congenital lobar emphysema:** National Organization for Rare Disorders (NORD); National Heart, Lung and Blood Institute Information Center; American Lung Association.

**For genetic information and genetic counseling referrals:** March of Dimes Birth Defects Foundation; Alliance of Genetic Support Groups.

**References**

Birth Defects Encyclopedia: M.L Buyse, ed.-in-chief; Blackwell Scientific Publications, 1990, pp. 1083–1084.

Mendelian Inheritance in Man, 9th ed.: V.A. McKusick; The Johns Hopkins University Press, 1990, pp. 294, 1238.

Congenital Lobar Emphysema: The Roles of CA and V/Q Scan: R.I. Markowitz, et al.; Clin. Pediatr., January 1989, vol. 28(1), pp. 19–23.

Pulmonary Disease and Disorders, 2nd ed.: A.P. Fishman, et al., eds.; McGraw-Hill, 1988, pp. 1259–1269.

Congenital Lobar Emphysema: L.K. Lacquet, et al.; Prog. Pediatr. Surg., 1977, vol. 10, pp. 307–320.

# ENDOCARDIAL FIBROELASTOSIS (EFE)

**Description** EFE, a serious and rare heart disorder affecting infants and children, is characterized by a thickened endocardium that shows an increase in collagenous and elastic tissue. These lesions cause cardiac hypertrophy and congestive heart failure. Two forms are recognized: the rare restrictive cardiomyopathy and the more common congestive cardiomyopathy.

**Synonyms**

> Endocardial Dysplasia
> Endocardial Sclerosis
> Fetal Endomyocardial Fibrosis
> Subendocardial Sclerosis

**Signs and Symptoms** Elastic tissue proliferates in the subendocardium, causing a diffuse, milky-white thickening of the endocardium and subendocardium. The onset of symptoms, which generally occurs between 4 and 12 months of age, is rapid and most commonly features dyspnea, grunting respirations, cough, irritability, weakness, and pallor. The physical examination may reveal respiratory distress; intercostal retractions; fine, moist rales; and a gallop rhythm of the heart. The chest film shows an enlarged heart.

Left ventricular hypertrophy suggests the diagnosis. The earliest signs of myocardial damage are shown in subtle S-T segment and T-wave changes on the electrocardiogram **(ECG).** Serial ECGs reveal progression or regression of the disorder. Ventricular failure may also be encountered, with tachycardia and atrial and ventricular arrhythmias. Severe mitral regurgitation is common.

**Etiology** The cause is not known. EFE may be hereditary.

**Epidemiology** EFE affects less than 1 percent of infants and children with congenital heart disease. Infants and children of both sexes between the ages of 4 months and 2 years are affected. A few adult cases have been reported.

**Related Disorders Idiopathic cardiomyopathy,** a disorder of unknown origin, is characterized by cardiac hypertrophy and dilatation. **Viral myocarditis** is marked by severe dyspnea, an enlarged heart, tachycardia, arrhythmias, and generalized edema.

**Treatment—Standard** Response to treatment is most favorable when the damage is noted early. Bed rest may facilitate healing of the myocardial lesions while the myocardium is working at a reduced load. Further therapy is directed at control of congestive heart failure, with agents such as afterload reduction digitalis and diuretics. Associated arrhythmias require appropriate antiarrhythmic therapy. Anticoagulation may be necessary. Prognosis is guarded despite therapy. Cardiac transplantation is effective surgical treatment.

**Treatment—Investigational** Please contact the agencies listed under Resources, below, for the most current information. Addresses and telephone numbers of these agencies, as well as of individual experts and research centers, may be found in the Master Resources List.

**Resources**

   **For more information on endocardial fibroelastosis:** National Organization for Rare Disorders (NORD); American Heart Association; NIH/National Heart, Lung and Blood Institute.

**References**

Moss and Adams Heart Disease in Infants, Children, and Adolescents, Including the Fetus and Young Adult, 5th ed.: G.C. Emmanouilides, et al., eds.; Williams and Wilkins, 1995, pp. 495–510, 1354–1358.

Cecil Textbook of Medicine, 18th ed.: J.B. Wyngaarden and L.H. Smith, Jr., eds.; W.B. Saunders Company, 1988, p. 351.

The Heart, Arteries and Veins, 17th ed.: J.S. Hurst, et al., eds.; McGraw-Hill, 1990, pp. 725–726, 1312–1313.

# ENDOMYOCARDIAL FIBROSIS (EMF)

**Description** A heart disease of unknown etiology, EMF is commonly characterized by a gross fibrosis of the endocardium lining of one or both ventricles, which progresses toward ventricular cavities constriction and involvement of the chordae tendineae and atrioventricular valves. EMF may be progressive **Loeffler disease,** a heart and small-arteries disease of unknown origin characterized by eosinophilia, gross fibrosis of the endocardium, small-vessel arteritis, and infiltration of other organs.

**Synonyms**

> Davies Disease
> Fibroelastic Endocarditis

**Pathophysiology, Signs, and Symptoms** Fibrotic lesions may be over 1 cm thick, project into the myocardium, and frequently affect the heart asymmetrically. The left ventricle may be involved at its base, or on its posterior left wall, including the chordae tendineae. The right ventricle may be involved at its apex and along the inflow tract, encasing the tricuspid valve's papillary muscles and chordae tendineae. Thrombosis often develops on the surface of the fibrotic lesions, and calcification may occur.

**Left ventricular fibrosis** is characterized by restricted left ventricle filling with diminished diastolic compliance. Mitral valve incompetence is frequent, resulting in mitral regurgitation, left atrial dilatation, pulmonary venous hypertension, left ventricular enlargement, and first-degree arteriovenous block. Atrial fibrillation is common. A chest x-ray may reveal a normal or mildly enlarged heart except for left atrial enlargement and signs of pulmonary venous hypertension. The electrocardiogram (**ECG**) shows a low QRS voltage and a nonspecific S-T segment with T-wave changes.

**Right ventricular fibrosis** is characterized by restricted filling of the right ventricle and poor ventricular compliance. It is often associated with tricuspid valve incompetence. Tricuspid regurgitation, right atrial dilatation, and systemic venous hypertension result. Ascites, hepatosplenomegaly, and jugular vein distention with facial edema may be present. Findings similar to left ventricular fibrosis are seen on ECG. Chest x-rays show an enlarged right atrium.

**Biventricular fibrosis** is a combination of right and left ventricular fibrosis.

The extracardiac manifestations of **Loeffler disease** include stroke, petechial hemorrhages, and hepatomegaly.

**Etiology** Suggested causes have included filariasis and diet. An immunologic mechanism is currently suspected.

**Epidemiology** EMF is endemic in the tropics but rare in Europe and North America. All races can be affected, mostly children and young adults. The disease has occurred in a few patients over age 60.

**Treatment—Standard** Open-heart surgery is the only effective treatment. The procedure involves endomyocardiectomy to allow normal diastolic ventricular filling; repair or replacement of the mitral or tricuspid valve (or both) to ensure valvular competence; and leaving a portion of fibrous endocardium on the left ventricular septum to prevent postoperative heart block. Cardiac transplantation may also be an option.

**Treatment—Investigational** Please contact the agencies listed under Resources, below, for the most current information. Addresses and telephone numbers of these agencies, as well as of individual experts and research centers, may be found in the Master Resources List.

**Resources**

**For more information on endomyocardial fibrosis:** National Organization for Rare Disorders (NORD); American Heart Association; NIH/National Heart, Lung and Blood Institute; Centers for Disease Control.

**References**

Cecil Textbook of Medicine, 18th ed.: J.B. Wyngaarden and L.H. Smith, Jr., eds.; W.B. Saunders Company, 1988, pp. 361–362.

# GOODPASTURE SYNDROME

**Description** Goodpasture syndrome is a rare disease that causes inflammation of pulmonary and renal membranes. It is classified into 3 groups according to its etiology: autoimmune or antibody-induced disease, systemic vasculitis, and idiopathic Goodpasture. When the disease is antibody-induced, the antibodies that cause inflammation appear to be deposited in the capillary membranes of the lungs and kidneys.

**Synonyms**

Pneumorenal Syndrome

**Signs and Symptoms** Lung hemorrhage and renal dysfunction are the major features of Goodpasture syndrome. Symptoms include hemoptysis, rhonchi, and dyspnea, and, less commonly, coughing, chills, hypertension, fatigue, and weakness. Fibrous tissue may form in the lungs.

Glomerulonephritis may progress rapidly to renal failure. Anemia and pallor give evidence of renal dysfunction, and hematuria and proteinuria may be present.

Although symptoms may recur during therapy, continued treatment is effective for many patients.

**Etiology** The known causes of Goodpasture syndrome are toxins, such as hydrocarbon chemical exposure, and infections, such as influenza. Even simple infections can cause Goodpasture syndrome in some patients. Antiglomerular basement membrane (**anti-GBM**) antibodies appear to circulate throughout the blood and damage pneumorenal membranes.

**Epidemiology** Goodpasture syndrome occurs worldwide and at any age, and seems to be more frequent in males.

**Related Disorders** See *Wegener Granulomatosis.*

A lung disorder similar to Goodpasture syndrome that occurs mostly in young children is **idiopathic pulmonary hemosiderosis.** This disorder is marked by chronic secondary anemia; however, it does not produce the antibody reaction found in Goodpasture syndrome.

A lung and kidney disorder that also has some clinical similarities to Goodpasture syndrome is **bacterial endocarditis.** This disease also affects the heart and can cause heart murmurs and embolism. Other symptoms are skin lesions, splenomegaly, and intermittent high fever.

**Treatment—Standard** The use of plasmapheresis combined with immunosuppressive drugs to treat Goodpasture syndrome has been successful in most patients. Corticosteroids alone or in combination with azathioprine or mercaptopurine may be of benefit in some cases. In some patients hemodialysis and/or renal transplantation seem to be the best treatment options; transplantation must await decrease in levels of circulating anti-GBM antibody.

Goodpasture syndrome has been considered a highly fatal disease, but the mortality rate for the syndrome dropped from 86 percent in 1955 to 13 percent in 1982 as a result of improved therapy. These studies have also shown that as many as 51 percent of patients no longer require renal dialysis.

**Treatment—Investigational** Researchers are investigating the benefits of selective methods of plasmapheresis over nonspecific methods in the treatment of Goodpasture syndrome as well as many other autoimmune disorders. Cascade filtration, cryofiltration, immunoabsorption, enzymatic degradation, and continuous electrophoresis are among the procedures under investigation.

Please contact the agencies listed under Resources, below, for the most current information. Addresses and telephone numbers of these agencies, as well as of individual experts and research centers, may be found in the Master Resources List.

**Resources**

**For more information on Goodpasture syndrome:** National Organization for Rare Disorders (NORD); Immune Deficiency Foundation; National Kidney Foundation; American Lung Association; NIH/National Kidney and Urologic Diseases Information Clearinghouse.

**References**

Immunomodulation with Apheresis Technics: A. Liebert, et al.; Allerg. Immunol. (Leipz.), 1986, vol. 32(1), pp. 5–18.

The Clinical Spectrum of Acute Glomerulonephritis and Lung Haemorrhage (Goodpasture's Syndrome): S. Holdsworth, et al.; Q. J. Med., April 1985, vol. 55(216), pp. 75–86.

Goodpasture's Syndrome: Development of Its Prognosis from 1955 to 1982: J. Marcandoro, et al.; Presse Med., May 28, 1985, vol. 12(23), pp. 1483–1487.

# HEART BLOCK, CONGENITAL

**Description** This rare congenital heart disease involves the conduction system of the heart, and results in a slow heart rate. There are 3 forms of congenital heart block: first, second, and third degree.

**Synonyms**

Atrioventricular (AV) Block

**Signs and Symptoms First-degree atrioventricular (AV) block** is characterized by slowed conduction of electrical impulses within the AV node and is detectable only by electrocardiogram. The condition is benign and not associated with symptoms. **Second-degree AV block** may be associated with symptoms. In **third-degree (complete) AV block,** no atrial impulses are conducted to the ventricles. There is independent beating of the atria and ventricles. Some patients may be asymptomatic, but others develop fatigue with exertion, lightheadedness, syncope, or sudden death.

**Etiology** The etiology is unknown. Some cases may be caused during pregnancy by an intrauterine infection or by the presence of an autoimmune disorder, such as systemic lupus erythematosus, in the mother.

**Epidemiology** Males and females are affected equally.

**Related Disorders Mobitz type I (Wenkebach) AV block** is characterized by progressive slowing of AV conduction of atrial impulses. It is usually transient. **Mobitz type II AV block** has an acute onset and generally indicates organic heart disease.

**Bundle branch block** is due to a lesion in a bundle branch. It is occasionally congenital and usually indicates prior cardiac surgery or cardiovascular disease. Right bundle branch block, characterized by a slowing of conduction in the bundle branches, may occur in patients with no clinical evidence of cardiovascular disease.

**Treatment—Standard** Atropine increases AV conduction. Complete heart block often requires a pacemaker.

**Treatment—Investigational** For pregnant women affected with connective tissue disease, especially systemic lupus erythematosus, plasmapheresis may be useful. Dexamethasone is under investigation for this situation.

Please contact the agencies listed under Resources, below, for the most current information. Addresses and telephone numbers of these agencies, as well as of individual experts and research centers, may be found in the Master Resources List.

**Resources**

**For more information on congenital heart block:** National Organization for Rare Disorders (NORD); American Heart Association; NIH/National Heart, Lung and Blood Institute; International Bundle Branch Block Association; Coalition of Heritable Disorders of Connective Tissue.

**For genetic information and genetic counseling referrals:** March of Dimes Birth Defects Foundation; Alliance of Genetic Support Groups.

## References

Permanent Pacing in Children: Acute Lead Implantation and Long-Term Followup: G.A. Jerwer; Pediatr. Cardiol., 1995, vol. 4, pp. 31–41.

Complete Heart Block in Children: M. Dick; Curr. Opin. Pediatr., 1990, vol. 2, p. 957–962.

Internal Medicine, 2nd ed.: J.H. Stein, ed.-in-chief; Little, Brown and Company, 1987, pp. 301–570.

Maternal Antibodies Against Fetal Cardiac Antigens in Congenital Complete Heart Block: P.V. Taylor, et al.; N. Engl. J. Med., September 1986, vol. 315(11), pp. 667–672.

Connective Tissue Disease, Antibodies to Ribonucleoprotein, and Congenital Heart Block: J.S. Scott, et al.; N. Engl. J. Med., July 1983, vol. 28(309), pp. 209–212.

Delayed Maternal Lupus After Delivery of Offspring with Congenital Heart Block: B.S. Kasinath, et al.; Arch. Intern. Med., December 1982, vol. 142(13), p. 2317.

# HYPOPLASTIC LEFT HEART SYNDROME

**Description** Hypoplastic left heart syndrome is a congenital heart defect characterized by an underdeveloped left atrium and ventricle and narrowed valves connecting the chambers to each other (mitral valve) and to an abnormally formed aorta (aortic valve).

**Synonyms**

Aortic Atresia, Mitral Atresia, Univentricular Heart

**Signs and Symptoms** Diagnosis is usually confirmed in newborns by echocardiography. Underdevelopment of the left side of the heart impairs blood flow from the lungs to the systemic circulation. There is poor systemic perfusion, metabolic acidosis, and shock. Blood also accumulates in the lungs, and congestive heart failure develops. Symptoms may include tachypnea, dyspnea, rales, cyanosis, and hepatomegaly. Without surgical intervention, death usually occurs in the newborn period, with very few patients surviving infancy.

**Etiology** The causes of the arrest in embryonic development of the left heart are poorly understood. Less than 10 percent of the cases appear to be familial. Diagnosis can be made in the fetus as early as 18 weeks of gestation.

**Epidemiology** Hypoplastic left heart syndrome may affect infants of both sexes.

**Treatment—Standard** Emergency medical treatment is directed to maintenance of adequate systemic perfusion by infusion of prostaglandin E-1 (**PGE-1**), which keeps the ductus arteriosus patent. Digoxin and diuretics are also useful. More definitive surgical therapy is available and includes the Norwood procedure followed by a bidirectional Glenn and Fontan procedure. Another surgical option is cardiac transplantation.

**Treatment—Investigational** Please contact the agencies listed under Resources, below, for the most current information. Addresses and telephone numbers of these agencies, as well as of individual experts and research centers, may be found in the Master Resources List.

**Resources**

**For more information on hypoplastic left heart syndrome:** National Organization for Rare Disorders (NORD); Congenital Heart Anomalies Support, Education, and Resources; American Heart Association; NIH/National Heart, Lung and Blood Institute.

**For genetic information and genetic counseling referrals:** March of Dimes Birth Defects Foundation; Alliance of Genetic Support Groups.

## References

Improving Results with First Stage Palliation for Hypoplastic Left Heart Syndrome: M.D. Iannetoni, et al.; J. Thorac. Cardiovasc. Surg., 1994, vol. 107, pp. 934–940.

Current Approach to Hypoplastic Left Heart Syndrome: Palliation, Transplantation, or Both?: V.A. Starnes, et al.; J. Thorac. Cardiovasc. Surg., July 1992, vol. 104(1), pp. 189–194, discussion pp. 194–195.

Fontan Procedure for Hypoplastic Left Heart Syndrome: W.I. Norwood, et al.; Ann. Thorac. Surg., December 1992, vol. 54(6), pp. 1025–1029, discussion pp. 1029–1030.

Mendelian Inheritance in Man, 10th ed.: V.A. McKusick; The Johns Hopkins University Press, 1992, p. 1473.

Nelson Textbook of Pediatrics, 14th ed.: R.E. Behrman, ed.-in-chief; W.B. Saunders Company, 1992, pp. 1163–1164.

Outcome and Assessment After the Modified Fontan Procedure for Hypoplastic Left Heart Syndrome: P.E. Farrell, Jr., et al.: Circulation, January 1992, vol. 85(1), pp. 116–122.

Hypoplastic Left Heart Syndrome: W.I. Norwood, Jr.; Ann. Thorac. Surg., September 1991, vol. 52(3), pp. 688–695.

Hypoplastic Left Heart Syndrome: Prenatal Diagnosis, Clinical Profile, and Management: D.M. Blake, et al.; Am. J. Obstet. Gynecol., September 1991, vol. 165(3), pp. 529–534.

Intrapartum Course of Fetuses with Isolated Hypoplastic Left Heart Syndrome: G.M. Jackson, et al.; Am. J. Obstet. Gynecol., October 1991, vol. 165(4 pt. 1), pp. 1068–1972.

Transplantation After First-Stage Reconstruction for Hypoplastic Left Heart Syndrome: E.L. Bove; Ann. Thorac. Surg., September 1991, vol. 52(3), pp. 701–704, discussion pp. 704–707.

Birth Defects Encyclopedia: M.L Buyse, ed.-in-chief; Blackwell Scientific Publications, 1990, pp. 166–169.

Dictionary of Medical Syndromes, 3rd ed.: S.I. Magalini, et al., eds.; J.B. Lippincott Company, 1990, p. 451.

Hypoplastic Left Heart Syndrome: L.L. Bailey, et al.; Pediatr. Clin. North Am., February 1990, vol. 37(1), pp. 137–150.

Cardiac Malformations in Relatives of Infants with Hypoplastic Left-Heart Syndrome: J.I. Brenner, et al.; Am. J. Dis. Child., December 1989, vol. 143(12), pp. 1492–1494.

Fetal, Neonatal and Infant Cardiac Disease: J.H. Moller and W.A. Neal, eds.; Appleton and Lange, 1989.

# JERVELL AND LANGE-NIELSEN SYNDROME

**Description** Jervell and Lange-Nielsen syndrome is characterized by congenital deafness, syncope, and prolonged Q-T interval, causing seizures and ventricular fibrillation. Physical activity, excitement, or stress may trigger the onset of these symptoms.

**Synonyms**

> Cardioauditory Syndrome of Jervell and Lange-Nielsen
> Deafness, Congenital, and Functional Heart Disease
> Prolonged Q-T Interval with Congenital Deafness
> Surdicardiac Syndrome

**Signs and Symptoms** Symptoms of Jervell and Lange-Nielsen syndrome are usually apparent during early childhood. There is bilateral sensorineural hearing loss. Some patients may have slight hearing in the low tones but usually not enough for them to learn to speak without special education.

Syncope or periods of unconsciousness may occur as a result of Stokes-Adams attacks. Ventricular fibrillation may also occur, resulting in syncope, loss of consciousness, seizures, and even death. Physical activity, excitement, or stress may trigger the onset of these attacks. Severity and frequency of these spells vary greatly from patient to patient, usually decreasing as the patient grows older. The inability to control urination may be present during seizures. The presence of seizures has led to the misdiagnosis of epilepsy in some cases.

**Etiology** Jervell and Lange-Nielsen syndrome is inherited as an autosomal recessive trait.

**Epidemiology** Jervell and Lange-Nielsen syndrome affects males and females in equal numbers. Approximately 1:300,000 people are afflicted with this disorder. The incidence among deaf children is 1:100.

**Related Disorders** See *Romano-Ward Syndrome.*

**Epilepsy,** a disorder of the central nervous system, is characterized by recurrent paroxysmal electrical disturbances in the brain. Manifestations include loss of consciousness, convulsions, spasms, sensory confusion, and disturbances in the autonomic nervous system. Attacks are frequently preceded by an "aura," a feeling of unease or sensory discomfort; the aura marks the beginning of the seizure in the brain. If the electrical disturbances or symptoms respond to medication, the patient can expect an otherwise normal life.

**Treatment—Standard** The cardiac disturbances in Jervell and Lange-Nielsen syndrome are treated with the drug propranolol in most cases. Electrophysiologic studies and autonomic nervous system surgical intervention, or a combination of surgical and drug therapy, may help control arrhythmias. Genetic counseling may be of benefit for patients and their families. Other treatment is symptomatic and supportive.

**Treatment—Investigational** Treatment of Jervell and Lange-Nielsen syndrome with an implantable automatic defibrillator is being investigated in conjunction with antiarrythmic drug therapy. Another implantable device, the Q-T–sensitive cybernetic pacemaker, is also being tested. Effectiveness and side effects of these implanted devices have not been fully documented and more extensive research is needed before their therapeutic value is known.

Please contact the agencies listed under Resources, below, for the most current information. Addresses and telephone numbers of these agencies, as well as of individual experts and research centers, may be found in the Master Resources List.

**Resources**

**For more information on Jervell and Lange-Nielsen syndrome:** National Organization for Rare Disorders (NORD); American Heart Association; International Long QT Syndrome Registry; NIH/National Heart, Lung and Blood Institute Information Center.

**For genetic information and genetic counseling referrals:** March of Dimes Birth Defects Foundation; Alliance of Genetic Support Groups.

**References**

Birth Defects Encyclopedia: M.L Buyse, ed.-in-chief; Blackwell Scientific Publications, 1990, pp. 281–282.

The Congenital Long QT Syndrome: R.G. Weintraub, et al.; J. Am. Coll. Cardiol., September 1990, vol. 16(3), pp. 674–680.

Mendelian Inheritance in Man, 9th ed.: V.A. McKusick; The Johns Hopkins University Press, 1990, p. 1132.

Hereditary Long Q-T Syndrome Presenting As Epilepsy: Electroenceph Laboratory Diagnosis: S.M. Gospe, et al.; Ann. Neurol., May 1989, vol. 25(5), pp. 514–516.

The Long Q-T Interval and Syndromes: C.E. Kossmann; Adv. Intern. Med., 1987, vol. 32, pp. 87–110.

Heart Disease: A Textbook of Cardiovascular Medicine, 3rd ed.: E. Braunwald, ed.; W.B. Saunders Company, pp. 749, 1635.

# LYMPHOMATOID GRANULOMATOSIS

**Description** Lymphomatoid granulomatosis is a vascular disease that is rare and progressive and characterized by nodular lesions that infiltrate and destroy veins and arteries, especially in the lungs. The condition can be benign or malignant.

**Synonyms**

>Benign Lymphangiitis and Granulomatosis
>Malignant Lymphangiitis and Granulomatosis
>Pulmonary Angiitis
>Pulmonary Wegener Granulomatosis

**Signs and Symptoms** The destructive lesions can occur in the lungs, kidneys, central nervous system, or skin. The patient may have a cough with or without hemoptysis, dyspnea, chest pain, malaise, fever, weight loss, diarrhea, arthralgia, and myalgia. Macules, nodules, and sometimes ulcerations appear when the skin is affected.

Respiratory distress and eventually failure of the respiratory system can result. In severe cases, the lesions sometimes take on the characteristics of **malignant lymphoma.** Lung biopsy may be necessary for diagnosis.

**Etiology** While the exact cause is unknown, some cases are thought to result from an allergic reaction to an unknown antigen. Others appear to be autoimmune-related.

**Epidemiology** Although lymphomatoid granulomatosis can affect individuals of any age, it occurs more often in persons over 40 years, and it is slightly more common in males than females.

**Related Disorders** See *Wegener Granulomatosis; Churg-Strauss Syndrome.*

**Treatment—Standard** The administration of corticosteroid drugs or cyclophosphamide or both in combination is standard treatment. Other therapy depends on symptoms.

**Treatment—Investigational** The orphan drug prednimustine is being tested as a treatment for malignant lymphomatoid granulomatosis. For more information, please contact Smith Kline and French Laboratories.

Please contact the agencies listed under Resources, below, for the most current information. Addresses and telephone numbers of these agencies, as well as of individual experts and research centers, may be found in the Master Resources List.

**Resources**

**For more information on lymphomatoid granulomatosis:** National Organization for Rare Disorders (NORD); American Lung Association; American Cancer Society; NIH/National Cancer Institute Physicians Data Query Phoneline; NIH/National Heart, Lung and Blood Institute.

**References**

Benign Lymphocytic Angiitis and Granulomatosis: H. Tukianen, et al.; Thorax, August 1988, vol. 43(8), pp. 649–650.

Lymphomatoid Granulomatosis: A Review of 12 Cases: J. Prenovault, et al.; Can. Assoc. Radiol. J., December 1988, vol. 39(4), pp. 263–266.

Necrotizing Vasculitis with Granulomatosis: I. Yevich; Int. J. Dermatol., October 1988, vol. 27(8), pp. 540–546.

Internal Medicine, 2nd ed.: J.H. Stein, ed.-in-chief; Little, Brown and Company, 1987, p. 665.

Pulmonary Diseases and Disorders, 2nd ed.: A.P. Fishman, ed.; McGraw-Hill, 1980, vol. 2, p. 1127.

# MADELUNG DISEASE

**Description** Madelung disease is a disorder of lipid storage that results in an unusual accumulation of fat deposits around the neck and shoulder areas.

**Synonyms**

>Benign Symmetrical Lipomatosis
>Launois-Bensaude Syndrome
>Multiple Symmetric Lipomatosis

**Signs and Symptoms** Madelung disease is characterized by massive deposits of fat predominantly around the head and neck and sometimes in the upper trunk. It is often associated with excessive use of alcohol. There may also be glucose intolerance, liver disease, and malignant tumors of the lungs.

**Etiology** The exact cause of Madelung disease is not known. The body's inability to properly metabolize fat indicates that it may be an endocrine disorder. A predisposition to the disorder may be inherited. However, the mode of transmission has not been determined.

**Epidemiology** Madelung disease most frequently affects middle-aged alcoholic males. However, this disease is also found in women and in persons who do not consume alcohol. It is seen more often in Europe than in the United States.

**Treatment—Standard** Treatment consists of surgical removal of the fatty deposits from the areas around the head, neck, shoulders, and trunk. Liposuction has been used successfully to remove single fatty tumors. Ultrasound is a helpful diagnostic tool.

**Treatment—Investigational** Please contact the agencies listed under Resources, below, for the most current information. Addresses and telephone numbers of these agencies, as well as of individual experts and research centers, may be found in the Master Resources List.

**Resources**

   **For more information on Madelung disease:** National Organization for Rare Disorders (NORD); NIH/National Digestive Diseases Information Clearinghouse.

**References**

Madelung's Lipomatosis of The Neck: A Sonographic Diagnosis: M. Drockur, et al.; HNO, March 1989, vol. 37(3), pp. 117–119.

The Metabolic Basis of Inherited Disease, 6th ed.: C.R. Scriver, et al., eds.; McGraw-Hill, 1989, pp. 1129–1266.

Madelung's Disease (Benign Symmetric Lipomatosis): N.A. Plotnicov, et al.; Oral Surg. Oral Med. Oral Pathol., August 1988, vol. 66(2), pp. 171–175.

Multiple Familial Angiolipomatosis: Treatment of Liposuction: W.R. Kanter, et al.; Ann. Plast. Surg., March 1988, vol. 20(3), pp. 277–279.

Madelung's Lipomatosis of the Neck: Expression of an Alcohol-Induced Endocrine Disorder: D. Knovver, et al.; HNO, November 1986, vol. 34(11), pp. 474–476.

# MITRAL VALVE PROLAPSE SYNDROME (MVPS)

**Description** MVPS is a cardiac disorder that may occur alone or be associated with other disorders, such as connective tissue disease or congential heart disease. Mitral regurgitation may cause other complications.

**Synonyms**

   Ballooning Posterior Leaflet Syndrome
   Barlow Syndrome
   Billowing Posterior Mitral Leaflet Syndrome
   Click-Murmur Syndrome
   Mitral Click-Murmur Syndrome
   Mitral Leaflet Syndrome

**Signs and Symptoms** Most patients have no noticeable symptoms. When these occur, they may initially include fatigue, weakness, palpitations, and dizzy spells. Other persons experience atypical chest pain or have a history of heart murmur. In some severe cases, patients demonstrate an inability to breathe except when sitting upright. Arrhythmia may develop. Examination may reveal a single or multiple midsystolic click. Mitral regurgitation does not occur in all cases and may be minor, slowly progressive, or sudden and severe. Rare cases may result in endocarditis, transient ischemic episodes, stroke, congestive heart failure, or sudden death.

Diagnostic tests include stationary and ambulatory electrocardiogram recordings and echocardiography, and, less often, cardiac catheterization and angiography, radionuclide studies, and exercise testing. The diagnosis is usually established by physical examination and is confirmed by echocardiography.

**Etiology** The syndrome can be inherited as an autosomal dominant trait. Some cases result from neuroendocrine or autonomic nerve dysfunction. Mitral valve leaflets may be myxomatous or redundant; and chordae tendineae may become elongated, causing prolapse of the mitral valve into the left atrium. Abnormally contracting left ventricular wall segments may also be a cause, as may rheumatic fever.

**Epidemiology** The syndrome affects both males and females and often appears in women of childbearing age.

**Related Disorders** See *Marfan Syndrome; Rheumatic Fever.*

**Treatment—Standard** Patients should receive antibiotics prior to surgery or dental procedures. Oral contraceptives for women with mitral valve prolapse are contraindicated, since serious complications may occur. Surgical replacement of the affected valve is indicated with severe mitral regurgitation.

**Treatment—Investigational** β-Blockers and moricizine may alleviate arrhythmias and tachycardia, as well as palpitations, dizziness, and syncope.

Please contact the agencies listed under Resources, below, for the most current information. Addresses and telephone numbers of these agencies, as well as of individual experts and research centers, may be found in the Master Resources List.

**Resources**

   **For more information on mitral valve prolapse:** National Organization for Rare Disorders (NORD); American Heart Association; NIH/National Heart, Lung and Blood Institute.

   **For genetic information and genetic counseling referrals:** March of Dimes Birth Defects Foundation; Alliance of Genetic Support Groups.

**References**

The Floppy, Myxomatous Mitral Valve, Mitral Valve Prolapse and Mitral Regurgitation: C.F. Wolley, et al.; Prog. Cardiovasc. Dis., 1991, vol. 33, pp. 397–433.

Mitral Valve Prolapse Syndrome: Evidence of Hyperadrenergic State: H. Boudoulas, et al.; Postgrad. Med., February 1988, pp. 152–162.

Internal Medicine, 2nd ed.: J.H. Stein, ed.-in-chief; Little, Brown and Company, 1987, pp. 475–482.

Complex Ventricular Arrhythmias Associated with the Mitral Valve Prolapse Syndrome: Effectiveness of Moricizine (Ethmozine) in Patients Resistant to Conventional Antiarrhythmics: C.M. Pratt, et al.; Am. J. Med., April 1986, vol. 80(4), pp. 626–632.

Mitral Valve Prolapse in Women with Oral Contraceptive-Related Cerebrovascular Insufficiency: Associated Persistent Hypercoagulable State: M.B. Elam, et al.; Arch. Intern. Med., January 1986, vol. 146(1), pp. 73–77.

# ORTHOSTATIC HYPOTENSION

**Description** Orthostatic hypotension is an extreme and rapid drop in blood pressure occurring when a person suddenly stands. A defect in the baroreceptors is often involved.

**Synonyms**

Low Blood Pressure

Postural Hypotension

**Signs and Symptoms** Symptoms, which usually appear after sudden standing, may include dizziness, lightheadedness, blurred vision, and syncope.

**Etiology** Hypovolemia, resulting from excessive use of diuretics or vasodilators or from prolonged bed rest, is a common cause. Other types of drugs that can cause orthostatic hypotension include phenothiazines, tricyclic antidepressants, the monoamine oxidase inhibitors, and α-adrenergic blocking agents. Specific drugs include alcohol, vincristine, barbiturates, L-dopa, and quinidine.

Conditions associated with orthostatic hypotension include the prolonged bed rest mentioned above, Addison disease, arteriosclerosis, diabetes, and certain neurologic disorders. Tilt table study may be helpful in establishing the diagnosis.

**Epidemiology** The disorder affects both men and women and is more common in the elderly.

**Related Disorders** See ***Shy-Drager Syndrome.***

In **vasovagal syncope,** blood circulation in the brain is temporarily impaired, possibly from emotional stress, pain, mild shock, fasting, fever, anemia, mild heart disease, and prolonged bed rest. Symptoms, which include orthostatic hypotension, fainting, and pale, cold extremities, may occur at irregular intervals and last from minutes to hours.

Symptoms of **idiopathic orthostatic hypotension** include lowered blood pressure, hypohidrosis, decreased salivation, and impotence. Idiopathic damage to the autonomic nervous system is implicated.

**Treatment—Standard** When due to hypovolemia because of medications, the condition is easily and rapidly reversed by correcting dosage or discontinuing the medication. When due to extended bed rest, the condition may be improved by allowing the patient to sit up each day with increasing frequency. Oral ephedrine may be given. In some cases, sodium intake is increased or sodium-retaining drugs prescribed. β-Blockers may also be useful. In some extreme cases, physical counterpressure is required; e.g., the use of elastic hose, or whole-body inflatable suits.

**Treatment—Investigational** Drugs under investigation for treating this disorder are DL-*threo*-3,4-dihydroxyphenylserine, phenylpropanolamine, midodrine, oral ergotamine tartrate or subcutaneous dihydroergotamine, and caffeine. Subcutaneous somatostatin appears to help certain individuals with postprandial hypotension.

Please contact the agencies listed under Resources, below, for the most current information. Addresses and telephone numbers of these agencies, as well as of individual experts and research centers, may be found in the Master Resources List.

**Resources**

**For more information on orthostatic hypotension:** National Organization for Rare Disorders (NORD); NIH/National Institute of Neurological Disorders and Stroke; David Robertson, M.D., Director of Clinical Research Center, Vanderbilt University.

**References**

Orthostatic Hypotension: J. Susman; Am. Fam. Physician, June 1988, vol. 37(6), pp. 115–118.

Postural Hypotension: Its Meaning and Management in the Elderly: M.J. Rosenthal, et al.; Geriatrics, December 1988, vol. 43(12), pp. 31–34, 39–42.

Treatment of Orthostatic Hypotension: Interaction of Pressor Drugs and Tilt Table Conditioning: R.D. Hoeldtke, et al.; Arch. Phys. Med. Rehabil., October 1988, vol. 69(10), pp. 895–898.

# PERNIOSIS

**Description** Perniosis, a vascular disorder caused by prolonged exposure to cold damp weather, is characterized by skin lesions on the lower legs, hands, toes, feet, ears, and face.

**Synonyms**

> Chilblains
> Cold-Induced Vascular Disease
> Erythema, Pernio
> Pernio

**Signs and Symptoms** The disorder usually occurs in cold weather with high humidity and generally lasts several weeks, with some cases persisting into warmer weather. It is characterized by a bluish-red skin discoloration that can cause pain, intense itching, burning, and swelling of the skin, especially as the body becomes warmer. Lesions usually occur on the fingers, toes, lower legs, heels, ears, or nose, and acrocyanosis may be seen on fingertips or extremities. Bullae that ulcerate if rubbed or irritated may appear in severe cases.

Thigh perniosis commonly affects individuals who wear tight-fitting slacks. It is characterized by red or bluish plaques on the outside thighs that cause swelling, burning, itching, and occasionally ulceration. Symptoms can be relieved or avoided by exposure to a warm temperature and looser-fitting thermal insulated clothing.

**Etiology** The cause is not known. The disease may result from an allergic reaction or hypersensitivity to the cold. Prolonged exposure, insufficient protective clothing, and circulatory or cardiovascular disease may be causative factors.

**Epidemiology** Females are affected more often than males; children, adults with poor circulation, and smokers are affected most often. The disorder is rarely seen in the United States.

**Related Disorders** See *Raynaud Disease; Urticaria, Cold.*

**Vasculitis,** a vascular inflammatory disorder, may occur alone or in conjunction with allergic and rheumatic diseases. Inflammation of the vascular walls constricts the blood vessels and may cause ischemia, necrosis, thrombosis, and, rarely, an aneurysm. Any size vessel and any part of the vascular system may be affected, with symptoms being localized or striking larger areas of the body. Vasculitis may be the primary disorder, or secondary to other disease processes. Because of the varied situations in which vasculitis can arise, symptoms and signs are relative to the system involved.

**Treatment—Standard** Affected areas should be warmed slowly, and patients should refrain from scratching or rubbing affected skin. Symptoms may be relieved with nifedipine, and corticosteroid creams may relieve itching. Other treatment is symptomatic and supportive.

**Treatment—Investigational** Please contact the agencies listed under Resources, below, for the most current information. Addresses and telephone numbers of these agencies, as well as of individual experts and research centers, may be found in the Master Resources List.

**Resources**

**For more information on perniosis:** National Organization for Rare Disorders (NORD); NIH/National Heart, Lung and Blood Institute.

**References**

The Treatment of Chilblains with Nifedipine: The Results of a Pilot Study, a Double-Blind Placebo-Controlled Randomized Study and a Long-Term Open Trial: M. Rustin, et al.; Br. J. Dermatol., February 1989, vol. 120(2), p. 267.

Chronic Pernio: A Historical Perspective of Cold-Induced Vascular Disease: J. Jacob, et al.; Arch. Intern. Med., August 1986, vol. 146(8), pp. 1589–1592.

# PULMONARY ALVEOLAR PROTEINOSIS

**Description** Pulmonary alveolar proteinosis is a rare chronic lung disorder in which the alveoli fill with a protein/phospholipid material that interferes with ventilation. Individual cases vary from mild to severe.

**Synonyms**

> Phospholipidosis

**Signs and Symptoms** Although some patients are asymptomatic, most cases are characterized by progressively severe dyspnea, especially following exertion. The disorder may remain stable and confined, spread throughout the lungs, or spontaneously clear. Commonly affected regions include the lower and posterior lung; occasionally the disease is restricted to the anterior segments.

**Etiology** Although the exact etiology is unknown, exposure to aluminum dust or an impaired immune system has been associated with rare cases.

**Epidemiology** The disease affects males more often than females, usually between ages 20 and 50.

**Related Disorders** Symptoms of **pneumonia** may be similar.

**Treatment—Standard** Mild cases may go into spontaneous remission. Lavage (performed once or several times as needed) under general anesthesia is indicated in more severe cases. The clinician should promptly identify and treat secondary lung infections.

**Treatment—Investigational** Please contact the agencies listed under Resources, below, for the most current information. Addresses and telephone numbers of these agencies, as well as of individual experts and research centers, may be found in the Master Resources List.

**Resources**

**For more information on pulmonary alveolar proteinosis:** National Organization for Rare Disorders (NORD); American Lung Association; NIH/National Heart, Lung and Blood Institute.

**References**

Morphologic Diagnosis of Idiopathic Pulmonary Alveolar Lipoproteinosis Revisited: I. Rubinstein, et al.; Arch. Int. Med., April 1988, vol. 148(4), pp. 813–816.

Bronchopulmonary Lavage in Pulmonary Alveolar Proteinosis: Chest Radiograph Observations: M.E. Gale, et al.; AJR, May 1986, vol. 146(5), pp. 981–985.

Total Lung Lavage for Pulmonary Alveolar Proteinosis in an Infant Without the Use of Cardiopulmonary Bypass: F. Moazam, et al.; J. Pediatr. Surg., August 1985, vol. 20(4), pp. 398–401.

# PULMONARY HYPERTENSION, PRIMARY (PPH)

**Description** PPH is a rare and progressive vascular disease characterized by pulmonary artery hypertension and widespread multiple lesions that affect the pulmonary arterioles leading to the capillaries. The pumping ability of the right ventricle eventually diminishes.

**Synonyms**

Primary Obliterative Pulmonary Vascular Disease

**Signs and Symptoms** Symptoms include dyspnea (with or without exertion), excessive fatigue, weakness, angina, and syncope. Facial puffiness and eyelid swelling may be present. Cyanosis, coughing, hemoptysis, hypotension, and cardio- and hepatomegaly also may occur. Heart failure may ensue. Cardiac catheterization and pulmonary angiography may be necessary for diagnosis if routine laboratory tests prove inconclusive.

PPH can occur in full-term newborns with no underlying structural heart disease, or in association with meconium aspiration. Infants will have severe hypoxemia and acidosis because of diminished pulmonary blood flow and large right-to-left shunt at a persistent patent ductus arteriosus and/or patent foramen ovale.

**Etiology** The etiology is unknown, but a genetic predisposition to the disorder may exist through autosomal dominant or recessive genes. In infants, the disorder is believed to be caused by perinatal hypoxemia immediately before, during, or after birth.

**Epidemiology** Although it can occur in the newborn, the condition appears more frequently in females between age 20 and 50. In males, it usually occurs later in life. The disorder also occurs more frequently at higher altitudes.

**Related Disorders** See *Pulmonary Hypertension, Secondary.*

**Cor pulmonale** is associated with enlargement of the right ventricle of the heart, occurring as a result of severe pulmonary disease. Symptoms usually include dyspnea, exertional syncope, and substernal angina.

**Interstitial pneumonia** is characterized by exertional dyspnea, coughing, and anorexia; the symptoms may range from mild to severe, depending on the extent of involvement. Fever usually is not present, nor is there an overproduction of mucus.

**Pulmonary veno-occlusive disease** is characterized by obstruction in the pulmonary venules leading to pulmonary hypertension and a radiographic picture of pulmonary edema.

**Treatment—Standard** Treatment is supportive. Physical activity and exercise should be limited. The disorder has been treated with nifedipine, isoproterenol, phentolamine, phenoxybenzamine, and prazosin. Prostacyclin may be used to dilate the pulmonary blood vessels. Vasodilator drugs, α-adrenergic blocking agents, β-agonists, and prostaglandins may also be used. However, drugs cannot cure or halt the progression of the disease. Genetic counseling may be beneficial. Lung or heart/lung transplantation is used in severe cases unresponsive to other therapies.

**Treatment—Investigational** Epoprostenol is under investigation; for more information contact Burroughs Wellcome. Clinical trials are under way to study family members of patients with PPH; for more information contact John H. Newman, M.D., at Vanderbilt University.

Please contact the agencies listed under Resources, below, for the most current information. Addresses and telephone numbers of these agencies, as well as of individual experts and research centers, may be found in the Master Resources List.

## Resources

**For more information on primary pulmonary hypertension:** National Organization for Rare Disorders (NORD); United Patients' Association for Pulmonary Hypertension; Foundation for Pulmonary Hypertension; American Heart Association; American Lung Association; NIH/National Heart, Lung and Blood Institute.

**For genetic information and genetic counseling referrals:** March of Dimes Birth Defects Foundation; Alliance of Genetic Support Groups.

## References

Current Approach to Treatment of Primary Pulmonary Hypertension: B.M. Groves, et al.; Chest, March 1988, vol. 93(suppl.), pp. 175S–178S.

Familial Pulmonary Capillary Hemangiomatosis Resulting in Primary Pulmonary Hypertension: D. Langleben, et al.; Ann. Intern. Med., July 1988, vol. 109(2), pp. 106–109.

Pulmonary Diseases and Disorders, 2nd ed.: A.P. Fishman; McGraw-Hill, 1988, pp. 999–1025.

Internal Medicine, 2nd Ed.: J.H. Stein, ed.-in-chief; Little, Brown and Company, 1987, pp. 527, 675.

Mendelian Inheritance in Man, 8th ed.: V.A. McKusick; The Johns Hopkins University Press, 1986, pp. 647, 1158.

# PULMONARY HYPERTENSION, SECONDARY (SPH)

**Description** SPH affects the blood vessels in the lungs and is usually associated with other lung diseases, such as interstitial pneumonia, or related diseases in other organs.

## Synonyms

Pulmonary Arterial Hypertension

**Signs and Symptoms** Dyspnea (especially after exertion), anxiety, tachypnea, angina, and, in extreme cases, heart failure can occur. Echocardiography or right-sided cardiac catheterization are used in diagnosis. In 98 percent of patients, a presumptive diagnosis can be made by diameter measurements of the right and left descending pulmonary arteries. A right pulmonary artery diameter greater than 16.7 mm and a left pulmonary artery diameter greater than 16.9 mm indicate excessively high pulmonary hypertension.

**Etiology** There are a number of causes, including lung disease, congenital heart disease, pulmonary artery embolism or thrombosis, pulmonary vasoconstriction, and the CREST syndrome. High altitudes, thickening of the blood, and portal hypertension may be implicated. SPH may also occur for unknown reasons.

**Epidemiology** The disease affects both males and females.

**Related Disorders** See *Pulmonary Hypertension, Primary.*

**Treatment—Standard** Physical activity should be restricted and underlying causes treated. Oxygen inhalation and vasodilators, such as epoprostenol, hydralazine, and nifedipine, may be used.

**Treatment—Investigational** Heart/lung transplantation is performed in severe cases.

Please contact the agencies listed under Resources, below, for the most current information. Addresses and telephone numbers of these agencies, as well as of individual experts and research centers, may be found in the Master Resources List.

## Resources

**For more information on secondary pulmonary hypertension:** National Organization for Rare Disorders (NORD); United Patients' Association for Pulmonary Hypertension; Foundation for Pulmonary Hypertension; American Heart Association; American Lung Association; NIH/National Heart, Lung and Blood Institute.

## References

Current Approach to Treatment of Primary Pulmonary Hypertension: B.M. Groves, et al.; Chest, March 1988, vol. 93(3), pp. 175S–178S.

Functional Tricuspid Regurgitation and Right Ventricular Dysfunction in Pulmonary Hypertension: D.A. Morrison, et al.; Am. J. Cardiol., July 1988, vol. 62(1), pp. 108–112.

Prediction of Favourable Responses to Long-Term Vasodilator Treatment of Pulmonary Hypertension by Short-Term Administration of Epoprostenol CC (Prostacyclin) or Nifedipine: A. Rozkovec, et al.; Br. Heart J., June 1988, vol. 59(6), pp. 696–705.

Pulmonary Diseases and Disorders, 2nd ed.: A.P. Fishman; McGraw-Hill, 1988, pp. 999–1025.

# RESPIRATORY DISTRESS SYNDROME, ADULT (ARDS)

**Description** ARDS, a life-threatening pulmonary disorder, is precipitated by a variety of direct lung injuries or acute illnesses that damage the microvasculature of the lungs. Major symptoms include dyspnea, tachypnea, hyperventilation, and hypoxemia.

## Synonyms

Acute Respiratory Distress Syndrome
Pump Lung

Shock Lung

Wet Lung

**Signs and Symptoms** The onset of ARDS is often within 24 to 48 hours after the pulmonary insult. Dyspnea with intercostal retractions and use of the accessory muscles of respiration are often the first signs. A few fine inspiratory crackles also may be evident in the physical examination. The chest film usually reveals diffuse, bilateral infiltrates. Early analysis of arterial blood gases shows a reduced arterial oxygen tension despite an increased inspired oxygen fraction and an increased carbon dioxide tension.

Complications include pulmonary emboli and barotrauma, secondary infection, stress ulceration and hemorrhage, renal insufficiency, arrhythmias, and anemia. Chronic lung disease, multiple-organ failure, and irreversible respiratory dysfunction may also develop. Death is most often the result of multiple organ failure.

**Etiology** ARDS is caused by injuries and illnesses such as shock, sepsis or pneumonia, trauma, aspiration of gastric contents, inhalation injury, drug overdose, metabolic disorders (including pancreatitis and uremia), and hematologic disorders (including intravascular coagulation and massive blood transfusion). The major cause of ARDS appears to be the sepsis syndrome.

**Epidemiology** The syndrome affects males and females of any age who suffer acute injury or illness to the lungs.

**Related Disorders** See *Respiratory Distress Syndrome, Infant.*

Symptoms of bronchial asthma, pneumonia, and emphysema can be similar to ARDS.

**Treatment—Standard** Supportive therapies include mechanical ventilation, fluid management, and pharmacologic agents. Mechanical ventilation usually necessitates nasal or endotracheal intubation and the use of positive end-expiratory pressure. Packed red blood cells can correct anemia, and crystalloids can correct hypovolemia. Treatment of secondary infections includes use of antibiotics and surgical drainage of closed space infections. Infection is the most serious complication because it frequently leads to sepsis. Infection control measures are recommended. Other agents that have been suggested include dopamine to augment cardiac output and diuretics to reduce preload and hydrostatic forces. Treatment is considered to be successful when the patient no longer needs mechanical assistance to breathe. Extracorporeal membrane oxygenator **(ECMO)** has been utilized successfully in treating ARDS.

**Treatment—Investigational** Ketoconazole (antifungal) and prostaglandin E-1 are being investigated for preventing secondary infections. The ability of monoclonal antibodies to endotoxin to decrease the progression of sepsis syndrome to ARDS is being studied. Replacing surfactant, which becomes depleted in ARDS, is also under investigation. The synthetic lung surfactant colfosceril palmitate/cetyl alcohol/tyloxapol (Exosurf—Burroughs Wellcome Co.) is being tested in the treatment of ARDS.

Please contact the agencies listed under Resources, below, for the most current information. Addresses and telephone numbers of these agencies, as well as of individual experts and research centers, may be found in the Master Resources List.

**Resources**

**For more information on adult respiratory distress syndrome:** National Organization for Rare Disorders (NORD); American Lung Association; NIH/National Heart, Lung and Blood Institute.

**References**

Trends in Respiratory Medicine: Adult Pulmonary Diseases (roundtable discussion): J. Respir. Dis., October 1989, vol. 10, pp. 39–51.

Adult Respiratory Distress Syndrome in Pediatric Patients: II. Management: J. Royall, et al.; J. Pediatr., March 1988, vol. 112(3), pp. 335–347.

Ketoconazole Prevents Acute Respiratory Failure in Critically Ill Surgical Patients: G.J. Slotman, et al.; J. Trauma, May 1988, vol. 28(5), pp. 648–654.

Pulmonary Extraction and Pharmacokinetics of Prostaglandin E1 During Continuous Intravenous Infusion in Patients with Adult Respiratory Distress Syndrome: J.W. Cox, et al., Am. Rev. Respir. Dis., January 1988, vol. 137(1), pp. 5–12.

Internal Medicine, 2nd Ed.: J.H. Stein, ed.-in-chief; Little, Brown and Company, 1987, pp. 612, 614, 618, 1537.

Adult Respiratory Distress Syndrome: Update for 1984: M. Iannuzzi and T.L. Petty; J. Respir. Dis., February 1984, vol. 2, pp. 118–125.

# RESPIRATORY DISTRESS SYNDROME, INFANT (IRDS)

**Description** IRDS is an acute respiratory disorder that affects premature infants who have a deficiency of alveolar surfactant. Clinical manifestations include breathing difficulty and atelectasis.

**Synonyms**

Infantile Respiratory Distress Syndrome

Hyaline Membrane Disease

**Signs and Symptoms** IRDS is characterized by rapid respirations with an expiratory grunt, cyanosis, and chest retractions, which generally develop within the first hours of life. Chest film findings include diffuse reticulogranular densities, air bronchograms, and underinflation. Arterial blood gas analysis often shows hypoxemia and hypercapnia.

**Etiology** IRDS is caused by the absence of surfactant in the lungs of premature infants. The type II alveolar cells that synthesize surfactant are not completely differentiated until 32 weeks of gestation, explaining why IRDS is seen in premature infants. Because surfactant acts to decrease surface tension in the alveoli, surfactant-deficient infants have progressive alveolar collapse.

**Epidemiology** Male and female premature infants of less than 37 weeks' gestation are affected in equal numbers. The risk of IRDS is higher in infants of diabetic mothers.

**Related Disorders** See *Bronchopulmonary Dysplasia; Respiratory Distress Syndrome, Adult; Pulmonary Alveolar Proteinosis.*

**Transient tachypnea of the newborn** often resembles mild IRDS and is caused by delayed absorption of fetal pulmonary fluid. Predisposing conditions include premature birth (but close to term), cesarean section, precipitous delivery, breech delivery, and maternal diabetes. Mechanical ventilation is rarely needed, and recovery is usually within 2 to 3 days.

Symptoms of **bronchial asthma, pneumonia,** and **emphysema** can be similar to IRDS.

**Treatment—Standard** Conventional treatment in IRDS involves mechanical ventilation using positive end-expiratory pressure and fluid and nutritional support. The synthetic lung surfactant colfosceril palmitate/cetyl alcohol/tyloxapol (Exosurf Pediatric, Burroughs Wellcome Co.) is being used in IRDS. The treatment is administered 30 minutes after birth to high-risk infants through the ventilator tube.

Survanta (developed by Abbott Laboratories), Human Surf, and Surfactant TA are other surfactants now approved for treating IRDS.

**Treatment—Investigational** Recombinant human super-oxid dismutase (Bio-Technology General Corporation) is being tested as a treatment to prevent bronchopulmonary dysplasia in premature infants weighing less than 1,500 grams.

The orphan drug protirelin (UCB Pharmaceuticals) is being tested for the treatment of IRDS.

The orphan drug pulmonary surfactant replacement, procine (Curosurf, manufactured by Chiesi Pharmaceuticals) is being tested for the treatment and prevention of IRDS.

Please contact the agencies listed under Resources, below, for the most current information. Addresses and telephone numbers of these agencies, as well as of individual experts and research centers, may be found in the Master Resources List.

**Resources**

**For more information on infant respiratory distress syndrome:** National Organization for Rare Disorders (NORD); American Lung Association; NIH/National Heart, Lung and Blood Institute.

**References**

Changes in Pulmonary Mechanics After the Administration of Surfactant to Infants with Respiratory Distress Syndrome: J.M. Davis, et al.; N. Engl. J. Med., August 1988, vol. 319(8), pp. 476–479.

Internal Medicine, 2nd ed.: J.H. Stein, ed.-in-chief; Little, Brown and Company, 1987, p. 576.

Pulmonary Surfactant Replacement in Respiratory Distress Syndrome: D. Vidyasagar, et al.; Clin. Perinatol., December 1987, vol. 14(4), pp. 991–1015.

Randomized Controlled Trial of Exogenous Surfactant for the Treatment of Hyaline Membrane Disease: J.D. Gitlin, et al.; Pediatrics, January 1987, vol. 79(1), pp. 31–37.

# ROMANO-WARD SYNDROME

**Description** This genetic heart disorder is characterized primarily by symptoms occurring during infancy or early childhood, with adult onset possible. Recurrent symptoms include syncope, convulsive seizures, and/or arrhythmias with angina.

**Synonyms**

Q-T Prolongation with Extracellular Hypokalemia

Q-T Prolongation Without Congenital Deafness

**Signs and Symptoms** Initial symptoms include recurring, unexpected partial or total loss of consciousness accompanied by arrhythmias with long Q-T intervals. Overexertion, excitement, or stress may trigger recurrent symptoms, which can also appear without any precipitating factors. The severity of attacks and types of symptoms may vary: e.g., a prolonged Q-T interval may occur with mild angina and without loss of consciousness; or loss of consciousness or grand mal seizures may occur followed by temporary disorientation. Lowered blood potassium levels may be symptomatic and linked to arrhythmias.

**Etiology** The syndrome is thought to be an inherited autosomal dominant trait with variable penetrance.

**Epidemiology** Approximately 155 cases, affecting both sexes equally, have been reported in the 20th century.

**Related Disorders** See *Jervell and Lange-Nielsen Syndrome.*

**Treatment—Standard** Propranolol is the suggested treatment. Therapies for arrhythmias include surgical removal of certain afferent cardiac nerves or a combination of surgical and pharmaceutical intervention. Raising potassium levels may improve some symptoms, and genetic counseling may be beneficial. First-degree relatives should be investigated. Other treatment is symptomatic and supportive.

**Treatment—Investigational** Treatment with an implantable automatic cardioverter-defibrillator is being investigated in conjunction with antiarrhythmic drug therapy. The implantable Q-T–sensitive cybernetic pacemaker is also under investigation.

Please contact the agencies listed under Resources, below, for the most current information. Addresses and telephone numbers of these agencies, as well as of individual experts and research centers, may be found in the Master Resources List.

**Resources**

**For more information on Romano-Ward syndrome:** National Organization for Rare Disorders (NORD); American Heart Association; International Long QT Syndrome Registry; NIH/National Heart, Lung and Blood Institute.

**For genetic information and genetic counseling referrals:** March of Dimes Birth Defects Foundation; Alliance of Genetic Support Groups.

**References**

The Q-T–Sensitive Cybernetic Pacemaker: A New Role for an Old Parameter?: P.E. Puddu, et al.; Pace, January 1986, vol. 9(1 pt. 1), pp. 108–123.

Management of the Prolonged Q-T Syndrome and Recurrent Ventricular Fibrillation with an Implantable Automatic Cardioverter-defibrillator: E.V. Platia, et al.; Clin. Cardiol., September 1985, vol. 8(9), pp. 490–493.

Prolonged Q-T Syndrome (Romano-Ward Syndrome): Description of a Case Diagnosed in Infancy: V. Meschi, et al.: Pediatr. Med. Chir., January–February 1985, vol. 7(1), pp. 131–136.

# TETRALOGY OF FALLOT

**Description** Tetralogy of Fallot is the most prevalent form of cyanotic congenital heart disease. It consists of 4 defects: a ventricular septal defect; subpulmonary stenosis; overriding aorta; and right ventricular hypertrophy. Untreated cases become progressively more severe. There is further diminution in pulmonary blood flow and increasing cyanosis with its associated complications.

**Synonyms**

Pink Tetralogy of Fallot (Acyanotic Tetralogy of Fallot)

Pseudotruncus Arteriosus

**Signs and Symptoms** Symptoms can appear at birth or within the first year. The most common symptom is cyanosis at rest or with crying. Excessive fatigue may adversely affect the infant's appetite, resulting in slow weight gain and impeded growth. Exertion can bring about severe, life-threatening attacks of hyperpnea and hypoxia. A characteristic squatting posture is sometimes assumed to aid with difficult breathing. Other symptoms of inadequate tissue oxygenation are cyanosis, clubbing of the fingertips, and polycythemia.

Various complications can occur, such as relative anemia in infancy, polycythemia in children and adults, coagulation defects, infective endocarditis, embolisms in the systemic circulation, cerebral infarctions, infectious sinusitis, and brain abscesses. Congestive heart failure is rare except with endocarditis or arrhythmias. Severe right ventricle obstructions with pulmonary atresia are known as **pseudotruncus arteriosus** (or **pulmonary atresia with ventricular septal defect).**

The physical examination, electrocardiography, echocardiography, and cardiac catheterization data aid in diagnosis and therapy. X-rays usually reveal a characteristic shape of the heart. Periodic measurements of systemic blood oxygen saturation and hemoglobin are advisable.

**Etiology** No specific etiologic agent has been identified. Approximately 25 percent of patients have an associated extracardiac congenital abnormality.

**Epidemiology** About 1 percent of newborns have congenital heart defects. Of these, about 10 percent have tetralogy of Fallot, which occurs more often in males than females.

**Related Disorders** Other congenital heart defects include atrial defects, abnormal distribution of the coronary arteries, pulmonary valve stenosis, malformations of the aorta and pulmonary artery, and anomalous positions of the heart. See *Atrial Septal Defects; Ventricular Septal Defects.*

**Treatment—Standard** Surgical correction of the malformation is best accomplished during infancy. When repair is not feasible, palliative measures taken in infancy or early childhood include construction of a shunt between the aorta and the pulmonary artery. Presurgical, palliative medical treatment includes maintenance of adequate hydration and appropriate hemoglobin, and avoidance of strenuous exercise. Medications may also be needed to treat arrhythmias. Because they are susceptible to bacterial endocarditis, patients should be given antibiotics at times of predictable risk (e.g., tooth extractions and surgery). Similarly, respiratory infections are treated vigorously and early. Severe hypoxic spells may require the administration of oxygen, morphine, sodium bicarbonate, and other drugs to improve oxygen concentration.

**Treatment—Investigational** Please contact the agencies listed under Resources, below, for the most current information. Addresses and telephone numbers of these agencies, as well as of individual experts and research centers, may be found in the Master Resources List.

**Resources**

**For more information on tetralogy of Fallot:** National Organization for Rare Disorders (NORD); American Heart Association; NIH/National Heart, Lung and Blood Institute; Congenital Heart Anomalies Support, Education, and Resources.

**For genetic information and genetic counseling referrals:** March of Dimes Birth Defects Foundation; Alliance of Genetic Support Groups.

**References**

Moss and Adams Heart Disease in Infants, Children, and Adolescents, Including the Fetus and Young Adult, 5th ed.: G.C. Emmanouilides, et al., eds.; Williams and Wilkins, 1995, pp. 998–1017.

Echocardiographically Guided Repair of Tetralogy of Fallot: G. Santoro, et al.; Am. J. Cardiol., April 15, 1994, vol. 73(11), pp. 808–811.

Surgery for Tetralogy of Fallot at Less Than Six Months of Age: M. Sousa Uva, et al.; J. Thorac. Cardiovasc. Surg., May 1994, vol. 107(5), pp. 1291–1300.

Long-Term Outcome in Patients Undergoing Surgical Repair of Tetralogy of Fallot: J.G. Murphy, et al.; N. Engl. J. Med., August 26, 1993, vol. 329(9), pp. 593–599.

Preoperative Management of Neonatal Tetralogy of Fallot with Absent Pulmonary Valve Syndrome: M.K. Heinemann, et al.; Ann. Thorac. Surg., January 1993, vol. 55(1), pp. 172–174.

Tetralogy of Fallot and Pulmonary Atresia/Ventricular Septal Defect: C.A. Warnes; Cardiol. Clin., November 1993, vol. 11(4), pp. 643–650.

Cecil Textbook of Medicine, 19th ed.: J.B. Wyngaarden, et al.,eds.; W.B. Saunders Company, 1992, pp. 285–287.

Mendelian Inheritance in Man, 10th ed.: V.A. McKusick; The Johns Hopkins University Press, 1992, pp. 1068–1069.

Nelson Textbook of Pediatrics, 14th ed.: R.E. Behrman, ed.-in-chief; W.B. Saunders Company, 1992, pp. 1147–1153.

Birth Defects Encyclopedia: M.L Buyse, ed.-in-chief; Blackwell Scientific Publications, 1990, pp. 846–847.

Dictionary of Medical Syndromes, 3rd ed.: S.I. Magalini, et al., eds.; J.B. Lippincott Company, 1990, pp. 300–301.

# TRUNCUS ARTERIOSUS, PERSISTENT

**Description** Persistent truncus arteriosus is a serious congenital heart defect with a high mortality rate. The truncus arteriosus is a fetal structure that later is divided into the aorta and pulmonary artery by the development of the bulbar septum. The disorder is nearly always accompanied by a ventricular septal defect. Persistence beyond the fetal stage causes blood from both ventricles to mix, affecting the pulmonary and systemic circulation. If the infant survives congestive heart failure in infancy, extreme hypertension in the lungs eventually causes pulmonary vascular obstructive disease.

**Synonyms**

Buchanan Syndrome

**Signs and Symptoms** Similar to those of a severe ventricular septal defect, the symptoms and signs are those related to unrelenting congestive heart failure, an enlarged heart, pulmonary plethora, and gradual development of pulmonary vascular obstructive disease. There may be associated truncal valve stenosis or regurgitation. The infant's appetite is adversely affected, resulting in slow weight gain and impeded growth. Diagnosis is established by echocardiography or heart catheterization. In the absence of surgical correction, nearly 90 percent of infants die by 6 months of age.

**Etiology** The causes of the arrest in embryonic development resulting in congenital heart disease are poorly understood. About 35 percent of patients with truncus arteriosus have *DiGeorge Syndrome.*

**Epidemiology** Persistent truncus arteriosus may affect infants of both sexes. It is usually fatal during early infancy.

**Related Disorders** See *Tetralogy of Fallot; Ventricular Septal Defects.* Other related disorders are **interrupted aortic arch** and **pseudotruncus arteriosus.**

**Treatment—Standard** Surgical repair in the neonatal period has dramatically increased survival. In addition to surgical intervention, standard medical therapeutic measures for heart failure are used.

**Treatment—Investigational** Please contact the agencies listed under Resources, below, for the most current information. Addresses and telephone numbers of these agencies, as well as of individual experts and research centers, may be found in the Master Resources List.

**Resources**

**For more information on persistent truncus arteriosus:** National Organization for Rare Disorders (NORD); American Heart Association; NIH/National Heart, Lung and Blood Institute.

**For genetic information and genetic counseling referrals:** March of Dimes Birth Defects Foundation; Alliance of Genetic Support Groups.

## References

Moss and Adams Heart Disease in Infants, Children, and Adolescents, Including the Fetus and Young Adult, 5th ed.: G.C. Emmanouilides, et al., eds.; Williams and Wilkins, 1995, pp. 1026–1041.

Fate of Small Homograft Conduits After Early Repair of Truncus Arteriosus: M.K. Heinemann, et al.; Ann. Thorac. Surg., June 1993, vol. 55(6), pp. 1409–1411, discussion pp. 1411–1412.

Repair of Truncus Arteriosus in the Neonate: F.L. Hanley, et al.; J. Thorac. Cardiovasc. Surg., June 1993, vol. 105(6), pp. 1047–1056.

Results of a Policy of Primary Repair of Truncus Arteriosus in the Neonate: E.L. Bove, et al.; J. Thorac. Cardiovasc. Surg., June 1993, vol. 105(6), pp. 1057–1065, discussion pp. 1065–1066.

Current Method of Repair of Truncus Arteriosus: K. Turley; J. Card. Surg., March 1992, vol. 7(1), pp. 1–4.

Nelson Textbook of Pediatrics, 14th ed.: R.E. Behrman, ed.-in-chief; W.B. Saunders Company, 1992, pp. 1161–1162.

The Role of Coronary Artery Abnormalities in the Prognosis of Truncus Arteriosus: C.C. Lenox, et al.; J. Thorac. Cardiovasc. Surg., December 1992, vol. 104(6), pp. 1728–1742.

Harrison's Principles of Internal Medicine, 12th ed.: J.D. Wilson, et al., eds.; McGraw-Hill, 1991, p. 928.

Repair of Truncus Arteriosus in Infancy: J.M. Pearl, et al.; Ann. Thorac. Surg., October 1991, vol. 52(4), pp. 780–786.

Birth Defects Encyclopedia: M.L. Buyse, ed.-in-chief; Blackwell Scientific Publications, 1990, pp. 849–850.

Dictionary of Medical Syndromes, 3rd ed.: S.I. Magalini, et al., eds.; J.B. Lippincott Company, 1990, p. 142.

# VENTRICULAR SEPTAL DEFECTS

**Description** Ventricular septal defects, a relatively common form of congenital heart disease, may occur at any part of the interventricular septum but are generally paramembranous. The size of the defect determines clinical severity; large defects can result in infant mortality. Ventricular septal defects may close spontaneously (more common with small defects) or become relatively less significant as the heart matures and grows. The disease can result in congestive heart failure, characterized by tachypnea, wheezing, tachycardia, hepatomegaly, and failure to thrive. In addition, persistent high pulmonary artery blood pressure can permanently damage the lungs.

**Synonyms**

Common Ventricle (Cor Triloculare Biatriatum)

Roger Disease (Maladie de Roger)

**Signs and Symptoms** Small defects may be asymptomatic, as may be the case in patients with **Roger disease.** With moderate defects, signs of congestive heart failure may appear, such as fatigue or breathing difficulty during activity or feeding. In infants, poor feeding due to fatigue, cold grayish extremities, and rapid shallow breathing may indicate heart disease. Ventricular septal defects of moderate size are also characterized by cardiomegaly, characteristic heart murmurs, and an abnormal electrocardiogram.

A very large opening causes severe symptoms. If the septum is entirely absent, the 2 ventricles constitute a single chamber, a condition known as **common ventricle** or **cor triloculare biatriatum.** In infants and children, large defects generally cause growth retardation, heart failure, and pulmonary artery hypertension. In older children and adults, dyspnea after physical exertion, chest pain, episodes of fainting, hemoptysis, and hypoxia (including cyanosis, clubbing of the fingers, and polycythemia) may occur as a result of pulmonary vascular obstructive disease (see *Eisenmenger Syndrome).*

Infective endocarditis is associated more with small- or moderate-sized septal defects.

The patterns and quality of the heart sounds, electrocardiography, echocardiography, and cardiac catheterization data help determine the exact anatomic defect and differentiate ventricular septal defects from other similar conditions.

**Etiology** The causes of the arrest in embryonic development resulting in congenital heart disease are poorly understood. In most infants, ventricular septal defects occur as the only malformation. However, many malformation syndromes are associated with ventricular septal defects, including maternal alcoholism, trisomy syndromes, maternal ingestion of phenylhydantoin, postrubella infection, and maternal phenylketonuria.

**Epidemiology** Approximately 1 percent of newborns have a congenital heart defect; 25 to 30 percent of these are ventricular septal defects. Females are affected more often than males.

**Related Disorders** Other associated or related congenital heart defects include atrioventricular septal defects, atrial septal defects, valve defects of various kinds, malformation of the aorta and pulmonary artery, and anomalous positions of the heart in the chest. See *Tetralogy of Fallot; Atrial Septal Defects; Eisenmenger Syndrome.*

**Treatment—Standard** Surgery is not indicated for small ventricular septal defects. Medical management includes treatment of congestive heart failure with digoxin, diuretics, and rest. Nutritional considerations are paramount in infants. Because they are susceptible to bacterial endocarditis, patients should be given appropriate antibiotics at times of predictable risk (e.g., dental work and surgery). Similarly, respiratory infections are treated vigorously and early.

Indications for surgical repair in infancy are intractable congestive heart failure, poor weight gain, and significant pulmonary artery hypertension. The development of pulmonary vascular obstructive disease may be prevented if surgical closure of the defect is undertaken in the first 2 years of life. In older children, persistent large left-to-right shunt and cardiomegaly are also treated surgically.

If symptoms persist after conservative treatment, surgery is recommended, especially since it is successful even in infants, and because pulmonary vascular disease may be prevented in the first 2 years of life.

**Treatment—Investigational** Studies are under way to devise nonsurgical techniques that may be utilized to close ventricular septal defects. A self-centering double disk or double-umbrella disk, which covers and closes the opening in the septum, is implanted during cardiac catheterization.

The use of special surgical glue (fibrin seal) is also being studied for use in the treatment of ventricular septal defects. The glue has been used to close mild to moderate septal defects.

Please contact the agencies listed under Resources, below, for the most current information. Addresses and telephone numbers of these agencies, as well as of individual experts and research centers, may be found in the Master Resources List.

**Resources**

**For more information on ventricular septal defects:** National Organization for Rare Disorders (NORD); Congenital Heart Anomalies Support, Education, and Resources; American Heart Association; NIH/National Heart, Lung and Blood Institute.

**For genetic information and genetic counseling referrals:** March of Dimes Birth Defects Foundation; Alliance of Genetic Support Groups.

**References**

Moss and Adams Heart Disease in Infants, Children, and Adolescents, Including the Fetus and Young Adult, 5th ed.: G.C. Emmanouilides, et al., eds.; Williams and Wilkins, 1995, pp. 724–745.

Novel Technique for Extending the Use of Allografts in Cardiac Operations: R.E. Michler, et al.; Ann. Thorac. Surg., January 1994, vol. 57(1), pp. 83–87.

Intraoperative Device Closure of Ventricular Septal Defects: S.B. Fishberger, et al.; Circulation, November 1993, vol. 88(5 pt. 2), pp. II 205–209.

Second Natural History Study of Congenital Heart Defects: Ventricular Septal Defect: D.R. Pieroni, et al.; Circulation, February 1993, vol. 87(2 suppl.), pp. I 80–88.

Cecil Textbook of Medicine, 19th ed.: J.B. Wyngaarden, et al., eds.; W.B. Saunders Company, 1992, pp. 283–284.

Natural and Modified History of Isolated Ventricular Septal Defect: A 17-Year Study: P. Frontera-Izquierdo, et al.; Pediatr. Cardiol., October 1992, vol. 13(4), pp. 193–197.

Nelson Textbook of Pediatrics, 14th ed.: R.E. Behrman, ed.-in-chief; W.B. Saunders Company, 1992, pp. 1167–1168.

Primary Surgical Closure of Large Ventricular Septal Defects in Small Infants: J.T. Hardin, et al.; Ann. Thorac. Surg., March 1992, vol. 53(3), pp. 397–401.

Restrictive Ventricular Septal Defect: How Small Is Too Small to Close?: C.L. Backer, et al.; Ann. Thorac. Surg., November 1993, vol. 56(5), pp. 1014–1019.

Surgical Management of Isolated Multiple Ventricular Septal Defects: Logical Approach in 130 Cases: A. Serraf, et al.; J. Thorac. Cardiovasc. Surg., March 1992, vol. 103(3), pp. 437–442, discussion p. 443.

Harrison's Principles of Internal Medicine, 12th ed.: J.D. Wilson, et al., eds.; McGraw-Hill, 1991, pp. 283–284.

Birth Defects Encyclopedia: M.L Buyse, ed.-in-chief; Blackwell Scientific Publications, 1990, pp. 1763–1764.

Fetal, Neonatal and Infant Cardiac Disease: J.H. Moller and W.A. Neal, eds.; Appleton and Lange, 1989.

# WOLFF-PARKINSON-WHITE (WPW) SYNDROME

**Description** WPW syndrome is a genetic disorder resulting in cardiac arrhythmias. An extra conduction pathway in the heart (bundle of Kent) pre-excites the ventricles. Palpitations, weakness, and dyspnea may occur.

**Synonyms**

Accessory Atrioventricular Pathways

Preexcitation Syndrome

**Signs and Symptoms** Symptoms include arrhythmias, such as atrial flutter, atrial fibrillation, or supraventricular tachycardia **(SVT).** In atrial flutter, the atria of the heart contract very fast, faster than the ventricles; atrial fibrillation is a "twitching" of the atria instead of regular contractions, which causes the ventricles to respond irregularly. Symptoms associated with atrial flutter may include irregular pulse, tachycardia, pallor, nausea, weakness, dyspnea, syncope, and fatigue. SVT is a condition in which the heart rate suddenly increases to 100 to 200 beats per minute. A sudden, rapid, regular fluttering sensation and tightness in the chest may occur. These patients may also experience weakness, syncope, palpitations, and dyspnea. Angina may occur in older patients. Diagnosis may be made with electrocardiogram and electrophysiologic study.

**Etiology** WPW syndrome is inherited as an autosomal dominant trait characterized by an additional conduction pathway, the bundle of Kent, which sends extra electrical impulses from the atria to the ventricles.

**Epidemiology** This rare congenital disorder affects males and females equally, and symptoms can occur at any age.

**Related Disorders Lown-Ganong-Levine (LGL) syndrome** is a genetic disorder involving cardiac arrhythmias that are slightly different from WPW syndrome. The ventricles receive part or all of their electrical impulses from an irregular conduction pathway instead of from the bundle of His. If LGL patients have atrial flutter, atrial fibrillation, or paroxysmal atrial arrhythmias, then palpitations, faintness, weakness, and nausea may occur as they do in WPW syndrome.

**Sinus tachycardia** is a cardiac arrhythmia that causes the heartbeat to gradually increase to more than 100 beats per minute. The disorder may be caused by emotional stress, exercise, infection, and certain drugs.

**Sick sinus syndrome** is characterized by irregular atrial activity. Bradycardia and tachycardia usually occur. Gradual supraventricular tachycardia, atrial flutter, and atrial fibrillation may also develop. Palpitations, weakness, faintness, and nausea are common symptoms.

**Atrial ectopic tachycardia** usually occurs gradually. It is the result of premature electrical impulses located within the atrial myocardium. Rapid, regular fluttering sensations and tightness in the chest may occur, as may palpitations, weakness, faintness, shortness of breath, and polyuria.

**Treatment—Standard** Initial SVT treatment may involve lying down, stimulation of gagging or vomiting, the Valsalva maneuver, or carotid sinus massage. Intravenous Adenosive administration is effective and rapid-acting in termination SVT. Quinidine and procainamide may help control atrial flutter, fibrillation, and PSVT. Flecainide is used in preventing SVT in the absence of underlying heart disease. Localization and ablation of the accessory connection can usually be achieved by catheter radiofrequency energy. Ablation of the accessory pathway by catheter has largely replaced pharmacologic therapy, operative surgical division, or cryoablation. Implantation of a pacemaker may control tachycardia. Affected individuals should avoid excessive ingestion of caffeinated beverages and foods. Genetic counseling may be beneficial. Other treatment is symptomatic and supportive.

**Treatment—Investigational** Edrophonium may be helpful for SVT in WPW patients, but it has not yet been approved by the Food and Drug Administration.

Please contact the agencies listed under Resources, below, for the most current information. Addresses and telephone numbers of these agencies, as well as of individual experts and research centers, may be found in the Master Resources List.

**Resources**

**For more information on Wolff-Parkinson-White syndrome:** National Organization for Rare Disorders (NORD); American Heart Association; NIH/National Heart, Blood and Lung Institute.

**For genetic information and genetic counseling referrals:** March of Dimes Birth Defects Foundation; Alliance of Genetic Support Groups.

**References**

Supraventricular Tachycardia Study Group: Flecainide Acetate Prevents Recurrence of Paroxysmal Supraventricular Tachycardia: R. Henthorn, et al.; Circulation, 1991, vol. 83, pp. 119–125.

Use of Radiofrequency Energy to Ablate Accessory Connections in Children: M. Dick, et al.; Circulation, 1991, vol. 84, pp. 2318–2324.

Internal Medicine, 3rd ed.: J.H. Stein, ed.-in-chief; Little, Brown and Company, 1990, pp. 77–78.

Mendelian Inheritance in Man, 9th ed.: V.A. McKusick; The Johns Hopkins University Press, 1990, p. 985.

Comparative Quantitative Electrophysiologic Effects of Adenosine Triphosphate on the Sinus Node and Atrioventricular Node: A.D. Sharma and G.J. Klein; Am. J. Cardiol., February 1, 1988, vol. 61(4), pp. 330–335.

# YELLOW NAIL SYNDROME

**Description** Yellow nail syndrome is characterized by yellow, thickened, and curved nails with almost complete cessation of nail growth. Cuticle loss may also be associated with this syndrome. Onycholysis may cause loss of some of the nails.

**Signs and Symptoms** Yellow nail syndrome is characterized by slow-growing, yellow, thickened nails with an associated loss of cuticles. The nails may become convex and loose. This condition is usually associated with pleural effusion or lymphedema of the extremities. Edema of the legs as well as the face may also be present. Respiratory diseases such as bronchiectasis, bronchitis, and sinusitis may also occur with yellow nail syndrome.

**Etiology** The cause of yellow nail syndrome is not known. Because the disease is often associated with respiratory infections, the immune system may be involved.

**Epidemiology** Women may be afflicted with this syndrome more often than men. Onset varies from birth to old age.

**Treatment—Standard** There is no known treatment for yellow nail syndrome. The nails may improve when the related disorder is treated.

**Treatment—Investigational** Please contact the agencies listed under Resources, below, for the most current information. Addresses and telephone numbers of these agencies, as well as of individual experts and research centers, may be found in the Master Resources List.

## Resources

**For more information on yellow nail syndrome:** National Organization for Rare Disorders (NORD); American Lung Association; NIH/National Heart, Lung and Blood Institute Information Center.

## References

Clinical Dermatology, 2nd ed.: T.P. Habif; C.V. Mosby Company, 1990, pp. 632.

Cecil Textbook of Medicine, 18th ed.: J.B. Wyngaarden and L.H. Smith, Jr., eds.: W.B. Saunders Company, 1988, p. 2347.

Pulmonary Diseases and Disorders, 2nd ed.: A.P. Fishman; McGraw-Hill, 1988, vol. 1, p. 374.

Yellow Nail Syndrome: G.P. Pavvlidakey, et al.; J. Am. Acad. Dermatol., September 1984, vol. 11(3), pp. 509–512.

Pleural Effusion Associated with Primary Lymphedema: A Perspective on the Yellow Nail Syndrome: D.J. Beer, et al.; Am. Rev. Respir. Dis., March 1978, vol. 117(3), pp. 595–599.

# 5 | HEMATOLOGIC/ONCOLOGIC DISORDERS
## By Laurence A. Boxer, M.D.

## Clinical Disorders of Anemia and Erythrocytosis

The classification of anemia can be based on physiologic, morphologic, or etiologic factors. The prospective approach to any individual patient requires integration of history, physical findings, blood counts, red cell indices, reticulocyte count, red blood cell morphology, specific tests such as hemoglobin electrophoresis and Coombs test, and, finally, a search to determine the underlying disease or process. The approach to the diagnosis of anemia in patients takes into consideration the following broad categories: 1) decreased production of red blood cells or blood loss; 2) red blood cell size: normocytic, macrocytic, or microcytic; 3) knowledge of the relative frequency of the causes of anemia at various ages; and 4) appreciation that the diagnosis of anemia depends on normal values corresponding to the patient's age, sex, and cardiopulmonary status (see Figure 5.1).

The history can help focus on a diagnosis, but physical examination is more often nonspecific. In children, signs of anemia include pallor, color of mucous membranes, jaundice, tachycardia, palpitation, fatigue, dyspnea, poor feeding, and weight gain or other evidence of cardiac decompensation. Bruising, petechial and overt bleeding, splenomegaly, and other abdominal organomegaly or lymphadenopathy might suggest an underlying process causing the anemia. In children it is important to be alert to the specific dysmorphic features of Diamond-Blackfan and Fanconi anemias, the vascular and skin changes of sickle cell anemia and sickle C disease, and the facies of β-thalassemia trait, which can be established by hemoglobin electrophoresis. Careful examination of the peripheral smear often reveals abnormalities pointing to a specific diagnosis or underlying abnormalities. Perhaps the most difficult group of patients are those with hemolytic anemia and red cell aplasia. Under these circumstances, as well as in hemoglobinopathies, critical information is obtainable by examining the hemogram and peripheral blood smears. For these patients the reticulocyte count corrected as the reticulocyte index (reticulocyte count × hematocrit ÷ by age-appropriate hematocrit) × ½ is an important guide to further evaluation.

The hemolytic anemias are a complex group of disorders associated with an elevated reticulocyte index. The correct diagnosis for an individual patient may be apparent after a history, physical examination, and routine blood study. The smear may allow the crucial distinction to be made between immune and nonimmune hemolysis; this determination will then guide further evaluation. Spherocytes and microspherocytes are classic markers of immune hemolytic anemia; fragmented red blood cells are markers of intravascular nonimmune myelocytic anemia. Since extravascular hemolysis within the spleen does not result in hemoglobinemia, hemoglobinuria, or hemosiderinuria, detection of any of these implies an intravascular hemolytic process. Acute severe intravascular hemo-

**Figure 5.1    A diagnostic approach to anemia**

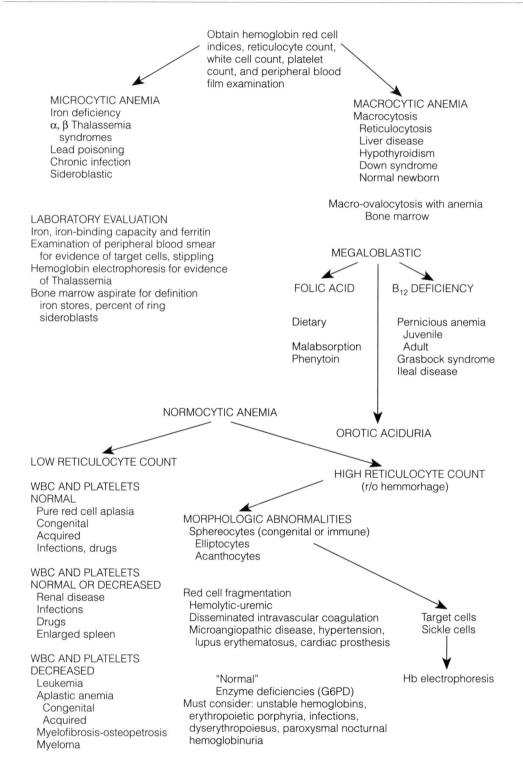

lysis may cause detectable hemoglobinemia, which can be seen on visual inspection of the patient's plasma. Hemoglobinuria may be detected with recent intravascular hemolysis. Chronic intravascular hemolysis can be detected by assays for urinary hemosiderin. Frequently, however, additional tests including hemoglobin electrophoresis, haptoglobin determination, red cells' osmotic fragility, specific assays of red blood cell enzymes, acid hemolysis tests, sugar water test, and tests for unstable hemoglobin must be performed to identify the basis for the anemia.

Examination of the bone marrow is important in the diagnosis in relatively few cases of anemia. These include megaloblastic, sideroblastic, aplastic, and dyserythropoietic anemias; acute leukemia; neuroblastoma; lipid storage diseases; and myeloma.

Similarly, when erythrocytosis has been identified, the physician has two goals in dealing with the patient: identification of the correctable cause and reduction of the red cell mass. Polycythemia vera is a form of myeloproliferative syndrome in which the granulocyte, monocyte, and platelet counts as well as the red cell count are usually elevated. This disorder appears to represent occupancy of the bone marrow by the progeny of a neoplastic clone of stem cells, which proliferate with an appropriate exuberance for any given level of external stimulants. Elevation of the counts in all three major cell lineages—red blood cells, white blood cells, and platelets—and the presence of splenomegaly should lead one to suspect this diagnosis strongly as a cause of erythrocytosis. Erythropoietin levels are normal in polycythemia vera, which distinguishes it from the secondary causes of red cell elevation.

## Clinical Disorders of Granulopoiesis

Neutropenia is defined as an absolute decrease in the number of circulating, terminally differentiated neutrophils. For whites over 1 year of age, the lower limit of the normal range for the peripheral blood neutrophil count is 1,500 cells/mm³ of blood. For white infants under 1 year, the lower limit of normal is generally considered to be 1,000 cells/mm³ of blood. Blacks have slightly lower values on average.

Neutropenia appears secondary to or in association with a number of pathophysiologic conditions, including viral and severe bacterial infections; exposure to drugs, such as certain antibiotics and anticonvulsants; autoimmune processes, such as those seen with systemic lupus erythematosus; marrow infiltrative processes, such as leukemia, metastatic tumor, and myelofibrosis; and inborn errors of metabolism, such as propionic acidemia and isovaleric acidemia. Finally, some chronic primary neutropenic disorders occur with a well-defined genetic basis (e.g., cyclic neutropenia); and some occur in association with disorders of immune function. Neutropenia can also occur as a consequence of extramedullary physiologic processes.

To establish a diagnosis of cyclic neutropenia, serial blood counts with white blood cell differential counts are essential (see Table 5.1). Usually these should be obtained twice weekly for 6 to 8 weeks in order to confirm the neutrophil cycling at 21-day intervals. Bone marrow aspirate or biopsy or both are particularly important for ruling out the possibility of malignant marrow disorders, such as leukemia or metastatic tumor. Other tests that may be useful in ruling out alternative diagnoses include an antineutrophil antibody assay, antinuclear antibody assay, and antimicrobial serologic assays when specific infections such as hepatitis or cytomegalic disease or the infections caused by Epstein-Barr or human immunodeficiency virus are suspected. Blood cultures and cultures of other apparent sites of infection may document the presence of an organism causing neutropenia. A bone marrow test with corticosteroids may prove useful in assessing marrow reserve, which is normal in patients with chronic benign neutropenia. Other conditions that may be associated with chronic idiopathic neutropenia include Shwachman syndrome, X-linked agammaglobulinemia, dysgammaglobulinemia, and depressed cellular immunity. Other rare dis-

**Table 5.1    Laboratory evaluation of neutropenia**

Complete blood count, including platelet count

Serial absolute neutrophil counts: 2×/week for 6 weeks
Bone marrow aspirate
Serologic studies
    Antineutrophil antibody assay
    Antinuclear antibody assay
    Immunoglobulins (IgG, IgA, IgM)
    Antiviral antibody studies

Cultures to screen for infections

Radiography of long bones (for Shwachman syndrome and Fanconi anemia)

Screening for nutritional deficiency states
    Serum copper, folate, and vitamin B12 levels

Lymphocyte quantitation and function
    T- and B-cell numbers
    Skin test reactivity

Colony-forming unit (CFU) and colony-stimulating activity (CSA) assays

Hydrocortisone stimulation test

Special studies
    Bone marrow chromosome analysis (for preleukemia states and Fanconi anemia)
    Plasma and urinary amino acid screening (for metabolic acidemias)
    Sucrose hemolysis/Ham tests (for paroxysmal nocturnal hemoglobinuria)
    Pancreatic enzyme determination in duodenal fluid (for Shwachman syndrome)
    Electron microscopic evaluation of neutrophils

orders associated with neutropenia but with distinctive features permitting separation from idiopathic neutropenia include cartilage-hair hypoplasia, dyskeratosis congenita, and Fanconi anemia.

## Recurrent Infections

The differential diagnosis for a patient who presents with recurrent infection is formidable, given the complexity of the immune response. The similarities in the clinical presentation of many of the phagocyte disorders can further complicate attempts to establish the diagnosis. Even when appropriate phagocyte function tests are performed, the results can be difficult to interpret in light of the intrinsic variability of these tests from day to day and from laboratory to laboratory. With these caveats in mind, however, the clinician can approach the patient with recurrent infection in an orderly manner and often establish a diagnosis if in fact a phagocytic defect is responsible. A useful algorithm for approaching these patients is presented in Figure 5.2.

## Phagocyte Disorders

When considering the history, one must take into account the frequency of infections, the patient's age, and the associated medical conditions. For example, recurrent otitis media in a 2-year-old boy is far less worrisome than a similar history in a 40-year-old. Another consideration is that the more unusual or severe the infection, the less frequently it has to occur before a phagocyte evaluation is indicated. Infections in unexpected anatomical locations should also alert the physician to a possible underlying immune disorder. Hepatic, pulmonary, and rectal abscesses as well as disseminated systemic infections may be indicative of an underlying phagocytic defect. Finally, the identification of certain pathogens such as the catalase-positive organisms including *Serratia marcescens, Aspergillus, Nocardia,* and *Pseudomonas cepacia* in children and young adults should suggest an evaluation for chronic granulomatous disease. Certain unusual findings can be help-

**Figure 5.2    Algorithm for the workup of a patient with recurrent infection**

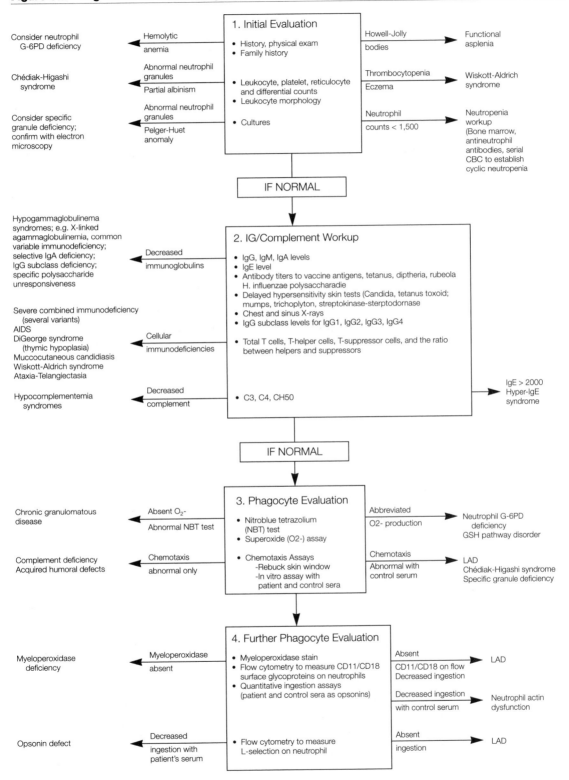

Modified from J.T. Curnutte and L.A. Boxer; Disorders of granulopoiesis and granulocyte function *in* Hematology of Infancy and Childhood, 3rd ed.: D.G. Nathan and F.A. Oski, eds.; W.B. Saunders Company, 1987, p. 835. Used with permission.

ful in determining which patients warrant further testing. For example, an infant with a history of delayed separation of the umbilical cord who has had several bouts of pneumonia and is noted to have neutrophilia should be evaluated for leukocyte adhesion deficiency; and the child with nystagmus, fair skin, and recurrent staphylococccal infections should be evaluated for Chédiak-Higashi syndrome.

## Primary Immune Deficiencies

A number of physical findings may be present in the patient with cellular immune deficiency. These include absent or diminished tonsils or lymph nodes, indicative of cellular immune deficiency; skin abnormalities such as alopecia, eczema, pyoderma, or telangiectasia; evidence of hematologic disease, such as pallor, petechiae, jaundice, mouth ulcerations; and generalized lymphadenopathy and splenomegaly, which may suggest HIV disease, a phagocyte disorder, or possible associated hematologic disorder.

Since 80 percent of patients with primary immune disease also have an antibody deficiency, tests for antibody function as well as immunoglobin levels are appropriate. Patients with an unusually convincing history of recurrent infections should be given other tests for immune deficiency even if the initial screening tests are normal. Subsequent testing must be individualized for each patient based on the results indicated in Figure 5.2. A very low neutrophil count, for example, may indicate severe congenital neutropenia, cyclic neutropenia, idiopathic neutropenia, marrow failure, or replacement of marrow via tumor if other hematopoietic cell lines are affected. Once initial antibody screening is completed, other tests may include antibody responses to pneumovax vac-

**Table 5.2   Characteristic clinical patterns in some primary immunodeficiencies**

| Features | Diagnosis |
|---|---|
| **Newborns and infants to 6 months** | |
| Hypocalcemia, heart disease, unusual facies | DiGeorge syndrome |
| Cyanosis, heart disease, midline liver | Congenital asplenia |
| Delayed umbilical cord attachment, leukocytosis, recurrent infections | Leukocyte adhesion deficiency syndrome |
| Diarrhea, pneumonia, thrush, failure to thrive | Severe combined immunodeficiency |
| Maculopapular rash, alopecia, lymphadenopathy, hepatosplenomegaly | Severe combined immunodeficiency |
| Melena, draining ears, eczema | Wiskott-Aldrich syndrome |
| Oculocutaneous albinism, recurrent infections, neutropenia | Chédiak-Higashi syndrome |
| Recurrent pyogenic infections, sepsis | C3 deficiency |
| Chronic gingivitis, recurrent aphthous ulcers and skin infections, severe neutropenia | Severe congenital neutropenia |
| **Newborns and children from 6 months to 5 years** | |
| Severe progressive infectious mononucleosis | X-linked lymphoproliferative syndrome |
| Paralytic disease following oral polio immunization | X-linked agammaglobulinemia |
| Recurrent cutaneous and systemic staphyloccocal infections, coarse facial features | Hyperimmunoglobulin E syndrome |
| Persistent thrush, nail dystrophy, endocrinopathies | Chronic mucocutaneous candidiasis |
| Recurrent deep-seated skin abscesses | Specific granule deficiency |
| **Children over 5 years and adults** | |
| Progressive dermatomyositis with chronic echovirus encephalitis | X-linked agammaglobulinemia |
| Sinopulmonary infections, neurologic deterioration, telangiectasia | Ataxia-telangiectasia |
| Lymphadenopathy, dermatitis, antral obstruction, pneumonias, small bone osteomylelitis | Chronic granulomatous disease |
| Recurrent meningococcal meningitis | C5, C6, C7, or C8 deficiency |
| Sinopulmonary infections, malabsorption, splenomegaly, autoimmunity | Common variable immunodeficiency |

Adapted from L.A. Boxer and R.A. Blackwood: Recurrent Infections in Practical Strategies in Pediatric Diagnosis and Therapy: R.M. Kliegman, M.L. Nieder, D.M. Super, (eds.): W.B. Saunders Company. In Press. Used with permission.

cine; IgG subclass levels for IgG1, IgG2, IgG3, IgG4; and delayed hypersensitivity skin test. Table 5.2 presents the characteristic clinical features of some of the primary immunodeficiencies as they appear in newborn and infants to 6 months of age; in children between the ages of 6 months and 5 years; and in older children and adults. Awareness of the clinical features of the immunodeficiencies will lead to a more rational interpretation of the findings from the diagnostic tests.

## Lymphocyte Disorders

There is a heterogeneous group of primary disorders involving both the cell-mediated and humoral arms of the immune system. These disorders affecting T-cell function (cell-mediated immunity) tend to be more severe than primary B-cell disorders, while combined defects carry the worst prognosis.

It is important to bear in mind with the B-cell disorders that circulating mature B lymphocytes differentiate into plasma cells that produce specific antibodies required for the phagocytosis of encapsulated pathogens and the neutralization of viruses. In order for B lymphocytes to differentiate into plasma cells, T lymphocyte–derived cytokines are required for the terminal differentiation of immature B lymphocytes into mature B lymphocytes and ultimately plasma cells. The antibody immunodeficiency states can be divided into those that are due to genetic defects and B-lymphocyte maturation occurring primarily at the pre-B-cell or immature B-lymphocyte stage, and those that are due to defective interaction between T and B lymphocytes occurring at the mature B-lymphocyte stage.

Children with altered lymphocyte function suffer from recurrent infections. They often have unusual responses to usually benign infectious agents, or they develop infections with unusual organisms. *Pneumocystic carinii*, cytomegalic virus, rubeola, and varicella often cause fatal pneumonia in these patients. In fact, pneumonitis with any of these agents should suggest a potential immunodeficiency. These children often have higher incidence of malignancy and autoimmune disorders. A partial list of primary disorders of lymphocyte function is shown in Table 5.3, and their evaluation is described in Figure 5.2.

## Bleeding Tendency

The history and physical findings are important in classifying a patient with a bleeding tendency. A carefully constructed family pedigree may indicate the hereditary nature of the bleeding manifestation (X-linked inheritance with factor VIII and IX deficiencies; autosomal dominant inheritance [although not solely] with von Willebrand disease; recessive inheritance with factor V and factor VII deficiencies). Characteristic of the hemophilias are bleeding at circumcision (but not invariably), and deep hematoma and hemarthrosis if the disorder is severe. In contrast, thrombocytopenia and abnormalities of platelet function and of von Willebrand factor are frequently manifested by epistaxis, bruising, and petechiae. Neonates with factor XIII deficiency characteristically have umbilical cord bleeding. Prolonged hemorrhage after a tooth extraction or after nasopharyngeal surgery, such as tonsillectomy, is a reliable symptom of an abnormal bleeding tendency. Negative personal and family histories are rare in a child with hereditary hemorrhagic disease unless the child is very young or the disease is quite mild. Nevertheless, mild hemophilia may result in bleeding with only severe trauma or major surgery. Hemorrhagic disorders are classified in Table 5.4.

Patients with a positive family history of bleeding or significant hemorrhagic episodes in the past or those who are scheduled for major surgery should have certain laboratory tests performed to determine and classify a potential bleeding diathesis (see Table 5.5). These include platelet count or estimation of the platelet number on blood smear; bleeding time by the template method, which

**Table 5.3  Disorders of lymphocyte function**

| Disorder | Genetics | Onset | Manifestations | Pathogenesis | Associated features |
|---|---|---|---|---|---|
| Brutons agammaglobulinemia | X-linked (Xq21.3–q22) | infancy 6–9 months | recurrent high-grade infections, sinusitis, pneumonia, meningitis | arrest in B-cell differentiation (pre B-B level) | lymphoid hypoplasia |
| Common variable immunodeficiency | AR; AD | 2nd–3rd decade | sinusitis, bronchitis, pneumonia, chronic diarrhea | arrest in B to plasma cell differentiation | autoimmune disease, RA, SLE, Graves disease, ITP, malignancy |
| Transient hypogamma-globulinemia of infancy | ? | 4th–9th month | recurrent viral and pyrogenic infections | delayed development of plasma cell maturation | frequently in families with immunodeficiences |
| IgA deficiency | X-linked, AR, ? 6p21.3 | variable | sinopulmonary infections gastrointestinal infections may be normal | failure of IgA expressing B-cell differentiation | IgG subclass deficiency, common variable immunodeficiency, autoimmune diseases |
| IgG subclass deficiency | AR 2p11; 14q32.3 | variable | variable (normal to recurrent sinopulmonary infections and gastrointestinal infections) | defect in isotype IgG production | IgA deficiency |
| IgM deficiency | AR | 1st year | recurrent septicemia | defective helper T cell–B cell interaction | Whipple disease, regional enteritis, lymphoid hyperplasia |
| Immunodeficiency with increased IgM | X-linked, AR, ? (Xq24–q26) | 2–3 years old | recurrent pyrogenic infections (otitis media, sinusitis, tonsilitis, pneumonia) | defect in IgG and IgA synthesis | hematologic autoimmune disease |
| DiGeorge anomaly | ? (22) | early infancy | variable | hypoplasia of 3rd and 4th pharyngeal pouch | hypoparathyroidism, aortic arch anomalies, micrognathia, hypertelorism |
| Wiskott-Aldrich syndrome | X-linked (Xp11–p11.3) | early infancy | recurrent otitis media, pneumonia, meningitis with encapsulated organisms | unknown | recurrent infections, atopic dermatitis, platelet dysfunction |

**Table 5.3 Disorders of lymphocyte function (continued)**

| Disorder | Genetics | Onset | Manifestations | Pathogenesis | Associated features |
|---|---|---|---|---|---|
| Ataxia telangiectasia | AR (11q22.3) | 2–5 years old | sinopulmonary infections | unknown (defect in DNA repair) | neurologic and endocrine dysfunction, malignancy, telangiectasias |
| Cartilage-hair hypoplasia (short-limbed dwarf) | AR | birth | variable | unknown | metaphyseal dysplasia, short extremities |
| Severe combined immunodeficiency | X-linked (Xq13.1–q21.1) AR | 1–3 months | candidiasis, all types of infections (bacterial, viral, fungal, protozoal) | IL-2R γ depletion severe T-cell depletion | severe graft-versus-host disease from maternal-fetal transfusions |
| Severe combined immunodeficiency (ADA deficiency) | AR (20q13–ter) | 1–3 months | candidiasis, all types of infections (bacterial, viral, fungal, protozoal) | enzyme deficiency results in dATP-induced lymphocyte toxicity | multiple skeletal abormalities, chrondo-osseous dysplasia |
| Severe combined immunodeficiency (PNP deficiency) | AR 14q13.1 | 1–3 months | candidiasis, all types of infections (bacterial, viral, fungal, protozoal) | enzyme deficiency results in dGTP induced T-cell toxicity | neurologic disorders, severe graft-versus-host disease from transfusions |
| Severe combined immunodeficiency (reticular dysgenesis) | AR | 1–3 months | candidiasis, all types of infections (bacterial, viral, fungal, protozoal) | defective maturation of common stem cell affecting myeloid and lymphoid cells | agammaglobulinemia, alymphocytosis, agranulocytosis |

AR = autosomal recessive, RA = rheumatoid arthritis, SLE = systemic lupus erythematosis, ITP = idiopathic thrombocytopenia purpura, IL-2R γ = interleukin-2 receptorgamma chain, d = deoxy

Adapted from L.A. Boxer and R.A. Blackwood: Recurrent Infections in Practical Strategies in Pediatric Diagnosis and Therapy: R.M. Kliegman, M.L. Nieder, D.M. Super, (eds.): W.B. Saunders Company. In Press. Used with permission.

**Table 5.4    Classification of hemorrhagic disorders**

Disorders due to abnormalities of platelet-vessel interaction
    Hereditary hemorrhagic telangiectasia
    Secondary vasculitis
        Systematic lupus erythematosus
        Sepsis
    Scurvy
    Henoch-Schoenlein syndrome (anaphylactoid purpura)

Thrombocytopenias
    Increased destruction of trapping
        Idiopathic thrombocytopenic purpura
        Immunologic drug purpura
        Splenomegaly
        Acute infection and inflammatory disorders
        Hemolytic-uremic syndrome
        Thrombotic thrombocytopenic purpura
        Giant hemangioma
        Cyanotic congenital heart disease
        Intravascular coagulation
        Isoimmune thrombocytopenias
        Wiskott-Aldrich syndrome
    Decreased production
        Leukemia and other malignancies
        Aplastic anemias
        Drugs and toxins
        Hereditary thrombocytopenias
        Thrombopoietin deficiency

Disorders of platelet function
    Thromboasthenia or Glanzmann disease
    Bernard-Soulier giant platelet syndrome
    Platelet release abnormality
        Storage pool disease
        Abnormal release mechanism
    von Willebrand disease
    Acquired disorders

Disorders of coagulation system
    Congenital deficiencies
        Factor VIII (classic hemophilia A) and von Willebrand disease
        Factor IX (Christmas disease)
        Factor XI
        Factor XIII (fibrin-stabilizing factor deficiency)
        Factor I (afibrinogenemia, dysfibrinogenemia)
        Factor II (hypoprothrombinemia, dysprothrombinemias)
        Factor V
        Factor VII
        Factor X
        $\alpha$-2-antiplasmin deficiency
    Acquired deficiencies due to decreased production
        Vitamin K–dependent coagulation factors
        Liver disease
        Altered bowel flora
        Malabsorption
        Coumadin treatment
    Hypothyroidism
    Acquired deficiencies due to increased destruction
        Disseminated intravascular coagulation
        Purpura fulminans
        Necrotizing enterocolitis
        Localized venous and arterial thrombosis
    Pathologic anticoagulants

**Table 5.5    Use of screening tests for classifying hemorrhagic disorders**

| Disorder | Platelet Count | BT | PTT | PT | TT |
|---|---|---|---|---|---|
| Afribrinogenemia | N | Mild Abn | No clot | No clot | No clot |
| Dysfibrinogenemia | N | N | N | Mild Abn | Abn |
| II, V, X deficiencies | N | N | Abn | Abn | N |
| VII deficiency | N | N | N | Abn | N |
| VIII, IX, XI, XII deficiencies | N | N | Abn | N | N |
| XIII deficiency | N | N | N | N | N |
| von Willebrand disease | N | Abn | Abn | N | N |
| Platelet function defects | N or low | Abn | N | N | Abn |

BT=bleeding time; PTT=partial thromboplastin time; PT=prothrombin time; TT=thrombin time; N=normal for age; Abn=abnormal prolongation of clotting test time.

is a measure of platelet-vessel interaction; partial thromboplastin time, which measures thrombin generation in the intrinsic pathway and is a function of all the coagulation factors except factor VII; the prothrombin time, which measures thrombin generation in the extrinsic pathway and is a function of factors II, V, VII, and X activity and the fibrinogen level; and thrombin time, which estimates the amount and function of fibrinogen as particular sensitivity to the presence of fibrin degradation products or heparin.

## Oncology

Adequate tissue must be obtained from the tumor to establish the specific diagnosis and subtype of cancer. Rare exceptions are those incidences in which a biopsy might be life-threatening and the location is virtually pathognomonic of a specific histology. Brain tumors and anterior mediastinal tumors that compress the trachea and blood vessels are two notable examples. In the latter situation, which usually involves a lymphoma, steroids may reduce the tumor size and relieve symptoms before biopsy is attempted. More often, an adequate sample must be obtained before definitive therapy unless complete surgical excision is definitively diagnostic and therapeutic. The specific diagnosis is seldom a problem in the leukemias, since bone marrow aspiration usually affords a ready answer. The solid tumors present the greatest difficulty.

A second diagnostic principle is to establish the extent of the disease. In the leukemias this can be readily accomplished by physical examination, routine laboratory tests, chest x-ray, and examination of the cerebral spinal fluid.

With solid tumors, determining the extent of the disease often involves major surgery and an extensive examination using diagnostic imaging techniques. A coordinated approach involving the surgeon and pathologist is crucial for planning treatment and for judging its success. In addition, modern oncology demands an extensive biological classification of leukemias and solid tumors, often requiring sophisticated scientific approaches using cytogenetics, molecular biology, and immunophenotyping as well as light and electron microscopy with special stains to determine the presence of glycogen, enzymes, or other substances that help classify a variety of tumors.

# HEMATOLOGIC / ONCOLOGIC DISORDERS
*Listings in This Section*

# ACANTHOCYTOSIS

**Description** Acanthocytosis is an inherited blood disorder characterized by the presence of malformed erythrocytes (acanthocytes) in the circulating blood and the absence of chylomicrons and very low density lipoproteins (**VLDL**) in plasma. The disorder leads to ataxia, retinitis pigmentosa, and malabsorption of fat in the alimentary tract that results in steatorrhea.

**Synonyms**

A-β-Lipoproteinemia

Bassen-Kornzweig Syndrome

Low-Density β-Lipoprotein Deficiency

**Signs and Symptoms** With onset usually beginning in the first year of life, symptoms of this disorder can occur in the alimentary, neuromuscular, skeletal, and ocular systems.

Some of the symptoms related to the alimentary tract are loss of appetite, copious loose stools, vomiting, and reduced ability to absorb nutrients from food. Although patients tend to have very high levels of fat in the mucous membrane cells of the intestine, they do not metabolize fats well and excrete only 15 to 20 percent of the fat they ingest. They also have trouble absorbing fat-soluble vitamins A, E, and K; vitamin K deficiency then causes reduced levels of coagulation factor in the blood.

During the first 10 years of life, fully one-third of patients have neuromuscular problems. Slow growth is a common symptom, as is loss of stretch reflexes. Patients generally have ataxia before they turn 20 and are usually unable to stand without assistance by the time they reach 40 because of spinocerebellar degeneration resulting in loss of position and vibration sense. Patients may also have retrospinal demyelination and some loss of sensation to touch, pain, and temperature. Muscle weakness and atrophy sometimes occur and, rarely, cardiac problems. Approximately one-third of patients become mentally retarded.

The symptoms related to the skeletal system, which include kyphoscoliosis, lordosis, pes cavus, and clubfoot, are probably due to muscle imbalances that develop at key stages of bone growth.

Retinitis pigmentosa, loss of clear vision, nystagmus, and ophthalmoplegia are some of the common symptoms related to the eyes. Retinitis pigmentosa usually begins about the time the patient reaches age 10. Loss of clear vision, which can lead to blindness, begins between the ages of 7 and 30.

Laboratory studies reveal the characteristic spiny cytoplasmic projections of acanthocytes, low levels of plasma cholesterol, and an absence or deficiency of VLDLs or **LDLs** (low density lipoproteins). The patient is unable to form chylomicrons in the lymph vessels. Diagnosis of this disorder is based on the demonstration of large intracellular fat particles in biopsy specimens of the jejunum, on the patient's failure to form chylomicrons following a meal, and on the absence of apolipoprotein B in plasma as determined by immunochemical means.

**Etiology** A genetically transmitted autosomal recessive disorder, acanthocytosis often occurs in patients with consanguineous parentage.

**Epidemiology** This extremely rare disorder affects equal numbers of males and females.

**Related Disorders** See *Tangier Disease.*

**Treatment—Standard** Restriction of triglycerides in the patient's diet has been successful in helping to relieve symptoms in the gastrointestinal tract. Vitamin E administered in large doses has been shown to improve neuromuscular symptoms and prevent retinopathy in some patients, but it cannot stop the disease from progressing.

Other treatments depend on symptoms. A mentally retarded or blind child may benefit from programs offered by social service agencies. The patient's family should receive genetic counseling.

**Treatment—Investigational** Please contact the agencies listed under Resources, below, for the most current information. Addresses and telephone numbers of these agencies, as well as of individual experts and research centers, may be found in the Master Resources List.

**Resources**

**For more information on acanthocytosis:** National Organization for Rare Disorders (NORD); National Lipid Diseases Foundation; NIH/National Diabetes, Digestive and Kidney Diseases Information Clearinghouse; National Tay-Sachs and Allied Diseases Association; Foundation Fighting Blindness; Research Trust for Metabolic Diseases in Children.

**For genetic information and genetic counseling referrals:** March of Dimes Birth Defects Foundation; Alliance of Genetic Support Groups.

**References**

The Metabolic Basis of Inherited Disease, 6th ed.: C.R. Scriver, et al., eds.; McGraw-Hill, 1989, pp. 1145–1151.

# AFIBRINOGENEMIA, CONGENITAL

**Description** Congenital afibrinogenemia is a blood disorder in which the protein necessary for coagulation is absent, causing severe to mild hemorrhaging.

**Signs and Symptoms** Two-thirds of infants with congenital afibrinogenemia experience bleeding problems. The severity and frequency of bleeding from surgery or trauma varies from mild to severe. Hemorrhaging is noticeable from the umbilical cord, in the stools, when vomiting, after circumcision, from the use of forceps during delivery, and in hematomas.

Other symptoms include severe bleeding after minor trauma, with the loss of baby teeth, or during the extraction of teeth. Patients may bruise easily and hemorrhage from the gums. Hemarthrosis, nosebleeds, a ruptured spleen, menorrhagia, and bleeding in the chest cavity and gastrointestinal area are common.

**Etiology** Congenital afibrinogenemia is thought to be inherited as an autosomal recessive trait.

**Epidemiology** Males and females are affected in equal numbers. Approximately 130 cases have been reported.

**Related Disorders** See *Factor IX Deficiency; Factor XIII Deficiency; Hageman Factor Deficiency; Hemophilia; von Willebrand Disease.*

**Treatment—Standard** Infusions of cryoprecipitate concentrate are the treatment of choice in order to raise the fibrogen level in the blood so clots can form. Fibrogen concentrates may be given, but there is a risk of contracting an infection.

Genetic counseling may be of benefit for patients and their families. Other treatment is symptomatic and supportive.

**Treatment—Investigational** Please contact the agencies listed under Resources, below, for the most current information. Addresses and telephone numbers of these agencies, as well as of individual experts and research centers, may be found in the Master Resources List.

**Resources**

**For more information on congenital afibrinogenemia:** National Organization for Rare Disorders (NORD); National Hemophilia Foundation; NIH/National Heart, Lung and Blood Institute Information Center.

**For genetic information and genetic counseling referrals:** March of Dimes Birth Defects Foundation; Alliance of Genetic Support Groups.

**References**

Cecil Textbook of Medicine, 19th ed.: J.B. Wyngaarden, et al., eds.; W.B. Saunders Company, 1992, p. 1073.

Birth Defects Encyclopedia: M.L. Buyse, ed.-in-chief; Blackwell Scientific Publications, 1990, pp. 62–63.

Hematology, 4th ed.: W.J. Williams, et al., eds.; McGraw-Hill, 1990, pp. 1474–1475.

Mendelian Inheritance in Man, 9th ed.: V.A. McKusick; The Johns Hopkins University Press, 1990, pp. 1199–1200.

Prophylactic Cryoprecipitate in Congenital Afibrinogenemia: R.C. Rodriguez, et al.; Clin. Pediatr., November 1988, vol. 27(11), pp. 543–545.

# AGAMMAGLOBULINEMIAS, PRIMARY

**Description** Primary agammaglobulinemias are genetic antibody deficiency disorders characterized by abnormal B-lymphocyte development and function in the presence of basically normal T lymphocytes, although T cell–mediated immune deficits may occur secondary to the disorder. Primary agammaglobulinemias are categorized into 3 types: X-linked agammaglobulinemia **(XLA)**, X-linked agammaglobulinemia with growth hormone deficiency, and autosomal recessive agammaglobulinemia.

**Synonyms**

Antibody Deficiency

Gammaglobulin Deficiency

Immunoglobulin Deficiency

**Signs and Symptoms** Bacterial infections, the most frequent symptoms of these antibody deficiencies, result from failures in specific immune responses that are triggered by defects in T and B lymphocytes, which make antibodies. Autoimmune disorders also occur more frequently than normal in patients with some of these diseases. *Giardia lamblia* is a frequent cause of chronic intestinal inflammation and diarrhea in patients with all forms of agammaglobulinemia. Infections begin to occur in boys with X-linked agammaglobulinemia (also known as Bruton agammaglobulinemia) late in the first year of life, only after maternal IgG antibodies have been catabolized. Subsequently these patients suffer recurrent pyogenic infections in the skin, middle ear, and upper and lower respiratory tracts. Most of the infections in XLA patients are bacterial, but persistent viral and parasitic infections can occur as well. Infection by enteroviruses and the poliomyelitis virus results in unusually severe illness. Echovirus infections can cause a syndrome that resembles dermatomyositis. Infections caused by mycoplasma bacteria can lead to severe arthritis. *Hemophilus influenzae* is the most common pyogen found in XLA patients, but they also have recurrent infections with pneumococci, streptococci, and staphylococci, and to a lesser degree with pseudomonas.

XLA patients have abnormally low levels of IgA, IgG, and IgM antibodies in their blood. Their neutrophils are compromised in terms of their ability to engulf microbes that require antibodies for opsonization. Transient, persistent, or cyclical neutropenia may occur. The number of B cells and their plasma cell progeny are reduced consistently by 100-fold or more. XLA patients are virtually devoid of tonsils, which are made up mostly of B lymphocytes.

A single family has been described to have X-linked agammaglobulinemia with growth hormone deficiency. The boys in the family have reduced or undetectable numbers of B cells and may also have panhypogammaglobulinemia and substantial amounts of IgA and IgM. Researchers are unable to explain why growth hormone coexists with XLA. The patients' T cells appear normal.

Familial agammaglobulinemia also occurs in girls, suggesting that one form of the disorder is inherited as an autosomal trait. Because autosomal recessive agammaglobulinemia is rare, researchers have not yet been able to document the exact mode of transmission or the B-cell defect.

**Etiology** XLA is inherited as an X-linked trait that is believed to be intrinsic to the B-lymphocyte lineage. The gene for XLA has been mapped to Xq21.3–22. Obligate heterozygous carriers have normal immune systems. As noted above, one very rare form is autosomal recessive. The disease has been shown to occur in brothers and in males whose sisters later had male children with XLA.

**Epidemiology** These rare inherited disorders occur almost exclusively in males.

**Related Disorders** See *Acquired Immune Deficiency Syndrome; Ataxia Telangiectasia; DiGeorge Syndrome; Nezelof Syndrome; Severe Combined Immunodeficiency; Wiskott-Aldrich Syndrome.*

**IgA deficiency** is a related antibody deficiency disorder characterized by low levels of IgA in the blood in the presence of normal or increased levels of IgG and IgM. It is the most common primary immunodeficiency. Other deficiencies of immunoglobulin isotypes are **IgM deficiency** and **IgG subclass deficiencies**.

**Selective IgG subclass deficiency:** Patients with recurrent pyogenic infections may have selected deficiency of IgG$_1$, IgG$_2$, IgG$_3$, and IgG$_4$, or a combination of these subclasses. The basis of IgG subclass deficiency is not understood.

**Common variable immunodeficiency:** Most patients with immunodeficiency do not fall precisely into defined syndromes. Some patients are said to have "acquired" or "late-onset" agammaglobulinemia. Deterioration of T-cell function also may be observed in some instances. Undue susceptibility to pyogenic infections, particularly with recurrent sinusitis and pneumonia, is the prominent clinical feature of acquired agammaglobulinemia. A prominent complication of acquired agammaglobulinemia that is rarely seen in the X-linked disease is a spruelike syndrome.

**Hyper-IgM immunodeficiency** is due to a genetic defect in the CD40 ligand, a type II membrane glycoprotein expressed on activated T cells. In order for B lymphocytes to undergo isotype switching from IgM to IgG synthesis, the B lymphocytes must receive 2 signals. The 1st signal is a cytokine, such as interleukin-2, required for IgG synthesis. The 2nd signal involves the physical engagement of CD40 on the B cell with CD40 ligand expressed on activated T cells. The gene for the CD40 ligand maps to Xq26. Several mutations in the CD40 ligand have been found in males affected with the X-linked form of hyper-IgM syndrome.

**Treatment—Standard** Intravenous administration of gammaglobulin therapy is the standard treatment. The optimal dose for each XLA patient should be determined empirically but is at least 300 mg/kg every month. Bacterial infections can be controlled with antibiotics. Patients should avoid exposure to infectious diseases, immunizations, corticosteroids, and immunosuppressive drugs.

Selective IgA deficiency is more difficult to treat. Gammaglobulins and fresh or frozen plasma can result in anaphylaxis. Only blood transfusions with multiple washed red blood cells or blood products from other IgA deficient individuals should be use.

Genetic counseling may be of benefit for those with primary agammaglobulinemias and their families. Other treatment is symptomatic and supportive.

**Treatment—Investigational** Prenatal testing is being developed for mothers who already have one child with X-linked primary agammaglobulinemia.

Please contact the agencies listed under Resources, below, for the most current information. Addresses and telephone numbers of these agencies, as well as of individual experts and research centers, may be found in the Master Resources List.

**Resources**

**For more information on primary agammaglobulinemias:** National Organization for Rare Disorders (NORD); NIH/National Institute of Allergy and Infectious Diseases; Immune Deficiency Foundation; Centers for Disease Control.

**For genetic information and genetic counseling referrals:** March of Dimes Birth Defects Foundation; Alliance of Genetic Support Groups.

### References

Carrier Detection and Prenatal Diagnosis of X-Linked Agammaglobulinemia: O. Journet; Am. J. Med. Genet., July 1992, vol. 15(43), pp. 885–887.

Cecil Textbook of Medicine, 19th ed.: J.B. Wyngaarden, et al., eds.; W.B. Saunders Company, 1992, pp. 1446–1453.

Clinical Use of Immune Serum Globulin As Replacement Therapy in Patients with Primary Immunodeficiency Syndromes: S.A. Schwartz; Clin. Rev. Allergy, Spring–Summer 1992, vol. 10(1–2), pp. 1–12.

Mendelian Inheritance in Man, 10th ed.: V.A. McKusick; The Johns Hopkins University Press, 1992, pp. 1200, 1773–1777.

Home Treatment of Hypogammaglobulinaemia with Subcutaneous Gammaglobulin by Rapid Infusion: A. Gardulf; Lancet, July 1991, vol. 338(8760), pp. 162–166.

Molecular Analysis of X-Linked Agammaglobulinemia with Growth Hormone Deficiency: M.E. Conley; J. Pediatr., September 1991, vol. 119(3), pp. 392–397.

X-Linked Agammaglobulinemia: E. Timmers; Clin. Immunol. Immunopathol., November 1991, vol. 61(2 pt. 2), pp. S83–93.

Birth Defects Encyclopedia: M.L. Buyse, ed.-in-chief; Blackwell Scientific Publications, 1990, pp. 947–962.

Genetic Deficiencies in Specific Immune Responses: F.S. Rosen; Seminars in Hematology, October 1990, vol. 27(4), pp. 333–341.

Hematology, 4th ed.: W.J. Williams, et al., eds.; McGraw-Hill, 1990, pp. 970–971.

Fundamental Immunology, 2nd ed.: W.E. Paul, ed.; Raven Press, 1989, pp. 1039–1057.

The Metabolic Basis of Inherited Disease, 6th ed.: C.R. Scriver et al., eds.; McGraw-Hill, 1989, pp. 2689–2690.

Primary Hypogammaglobulinemia: A Survey of Clinical Manifestations and Complications: R.A. Hermaszewshi; Q. J. Med., January 1986, vol. 86(1), pp. 31–42.

Immunodeficiency: R.H. Buckley; J. Allergy Clin. Immunol., December 1983, vol. 72(6), pp. 627–641.

# AGRANULOCYTOSIS, ACQUIRED

**Description** Acquired agranulocytosis is a blood disorder characterized by a pronounced reduction in the number of granular leukocytes in the circulating blood (often fewer than 500 granulocytes/mm³) due to an impairment in granulocyte production in bone marrow. Patients are susceptible to bacterial infections that cause ulcers in mucous membranes.

**Synonyms**

> Agranulocytic Angina
> Malignant Neutropenia
> Primary Granulocytopenia

**Signs and Symptoms** The first symptoms of bacterial infection may be weakness, chills, fever, or extreme exhaustion. The onset of acute granulocytopenia is marked by infected ulcers in the mucous membranes of the cheek, throat, and intestinal tract. The patient may have difficulty swallowing. Resulting granulocytopenia causes a decrease in the number of neutrophils. If left untreated, the patient may quickly progress into bacterial shock.

Chronic granulocytopenia generally progresses slowly, beginning with many different infections in the patient's bronchopulmonary system, skin, and perirectal region. Canker sores and chronic gingivitis may be a recurrent feature in the mouth, and other infections may recur regularly.

**Etiology** This disorder is usually drug-induced and dose-related. The most common causes of granulocyte destruction or impairment are chemotherapeutic antineoplastic agents. Other chemical or pathogenic agents that are less commonly involved include chemotherapeutic antimetabolites, alkylating agents, antithyroid drugs, dibenzepin compounds, phenothiazine derivatives, anticonvulsants, antihistamines, sulfonamides, synthetic penicillins, benzene, arsenic, chloramphenicol, and nitrous oxide.

Granulocyte production can also be impaired by drugs regardless of the dosage. The drugs implicated in acute idiosyncratic forms of this disorder include indomethacin, cinchona alkaloids, phenylbutazone, thiazides, procainamide, and nitrofurantoin. The drugs implicated in chronic forms include gold salts, chloramphenicol, and phenylbutazone.

A number of drugs destroy granulocyte precursors in bone marrow and produce granulocytopenia. They include phenytoin, pyrimethamine, methotrexate, and cytarabine. In rare instances, acute agranulocytosis results from the destructive action of leukocyte antibodies that are induced by such drugs as phenylbutazone, gold salts, sulfapyridine, aminopyrine, meralluride, and dipyrine.

Granulocytopenia associated with this disease most often results from stepped-up destruction of neutrophils caused by macrophage destruction of leukocytes, whole-body infections, some form of hypersplenism such as Felty syndrome, an intrinsic granulocyte defect such as in Chédiak-Higashi syndrome, congestive splenomegaly associated with collagen disease, and, in rare instances, leukocyte isoantibodies. Acute reversible neutropenia mediated by complement can occasionally occur in hemodialysis.

Aside from antineoplastic chemotherapeutic agents, the drugs that induce granulocytopenia most frequently are phenylbutazone, which carries the highest relative risk, sulfonamides, antithyroid compounds, and phenothiazines.

**Treatment—Standard** The drugs or other agents that induce this disorder must be identified and eliminated from the patient's regimen. Broad-spectrum antibacterial therapy can be beneficial if the patient has a fever over 38.3° C (100.94° F), is in shock, or has a positive blood culture or significant local infection. In adults initially, the antimicrobial therapy should be combined with gentamicin or tobramycin plus cephalothin, oxacillin, or carbenicillin. The antibiotics should be administered for 7 to 10 days after the fever abates, but no longer, or the patient will be exposed to superinfections and renal complications. When granulocyte levels return to 500 mm³, fever and infections will generally abate.

Corticosteroids are sometimes used to treat shock induced by bacteria, but they should not be used for acute granulocytopenia because they can impede the movement of granulocytes into tissue by masking bacterial infections. Patients with hypogammaglobulinemia should be given human gammaglobulin. Patients with severe neutropenia and sepsis that is resistant to antibiotics have been shown to benefit from massive infusions of leukocytes from matched donors, but the procedure is risky and costly and should not be used routinely.

Mouth and throat ulcers can be soothed with gargles of salt or hydrogen peroxide or with anesthetic lozenges. Mouth washes containing nystatin are used for oral thrush. Patients may have to go on a semisolid or liquid diet when mucous membranes are acutely inflamed.

Patients with chronic granulocytopenia need to be hospitalized during acute episodes and so should be instructed to recognize symptoms early. Chronic patients must be monitored for bacteria resistant to antibiotics and for opportunistic infections.

**Treatment—Investigational** In recent years, recombinant DNA technology has been able to clone molecularly the genes of granulocyte-colony stimulating factor (**G-CSF**) and granulocyte macrophage-CSF (**GM-CSF**) from various species to produce recombinant human (**rh**) factors. These rhG-CSF and rhGM-CSF glycoproteins stimulate the proliferation and differentiation of hematopoietic progenitors and ultimately increase the number of granulocytes and macrophages and improve their function. This technology has proved to be effective in the treatment of agranulocytosis and granulocytopenia.

Please contact the agencies listed under Resources, below, for the most current information. Addresses and telephone numbers of these agencies, as well as of individual experts and research centers, may be found in the Master Resources List.

**Resources**

**For more information on acquired agranulocytosis:** National Organization for Rare Disorders (NORD); NIH/National Heart, Lung and Blood Institute.

**References**

Approach to the Patient with Prolonged Granulocytopenia: P.A. Pizzo; Recent Results Cancer Res., 1993, vol. 132, pp. 57–65.

Instant Therapy of Acquired Agranulocytosis and Sepsis by Recombinant Granulocyte-Macrophage Colony-Stimulating Factor in a Polytrauma Patient: W. Gross-Weege, et al.; Clin. Investig., October 1993, vol. 71(10), pp. 791–794.

Invasive Candidiasis During Granulocytopenia: E. Anaissie, et al.; Recent Results Cancer Res., 1993, vol. 132, pp. 137–145.

Case Report: Role of Granulocyte Colony Stimulating Factor in Radiotherapy: B. Zachariah; Am. J. Med. Sci., October 1992, vol. 304(4), pp. 252–253.

Cecil Textbook of Medicine, 19th ed.: J.B. Wyngaarden, et al., eds.; W.B. Saunders Company, 1992, pp. 2082, 2211.

Harrison's Principles of Internal Medicine, 12th ed.: J.D. Wilson, et al., eds.; McGraw-Hill, 1991, p. 376.

Hematology, 4th ed.: W.J. Williams, et al., eds.; McGraw-Hill, 1990, pp. 812–815.

GM-CSF Treatment in Aplasia After Cytotoxic Therapy: C. Gattringer, et al.; Onkologie, February 1989, vol. 12(1), pp. 16–18.

Various Human Hematopoietic Growth Factors (Interleukin-3, GM-CSF, G-CSF) Stimulate Clonal Growth of Nonhematopoietic Tumor Cells: W.E. Berdel, et al.; Blood, January 1989, vol. 73(1), pp. 80–83.

# AMELOBLASTOMA

**Description** Ameloblastoma is a neoplastic disorder of the jaw and sinuses.

**Synonyms**

   Adamantinoma
   Mandibular Ameloblastoma
   Maxillary Ameloblastoma
   Odontogenic Tumor

**Signs and Symptoms** The primary symptom is neoplasm in the jaw or sinus area, often at the site of the 3rd molar, which may spread to the nose, eye socket, and skull. Early diagnosis and treatment are required to arrest progression of the cancer. Metastasis is usually to the lymphatic system and then to the lungs.

**Etiology** The cause of ameloblastoma is not understood. Irritation from dental growth, extraction, or caries has been suggested. Other causes include injury to the mouth or jaw and infection or inflammation of the teeth or gums. Viral infections and inadequate diet are also suspected causes.

**Epidemiology** Males and females of all ethnic backgrounds and ages are affected in equal numbers.

**Related Disorders Hard odontoma** differs from ameloblastoma in that it spreads directly, whereas the ameloblastoma infiltrates other spaces.

**Globulomaxillary cysts** grow between the teeth, causing them to spread. The cysts are either oval or heart shaped and may be removed or drained. Treatment may cause loss of teeth.

**Treatment—Standard** Diagnosis is by x-ray or magnetic resonance imaging. Surgical removal of cysts or tumors should include a wide margin of healthy tissue to prevent recurrence. If the tumor does recur, surgery is repeated. Radiation is the treatment of choice for metastasized tumors. Chemotherapy is usually not as effective in these cases.

**Treatment—Investigational** Please contact the agencies listed under Resources, below, for the most current information.

**Resources**

**For more information on ameloblastoma:** National Organization for Rare Disorders (NORD); NIH/National Institute of Dental Research; NIH/National Cancer Institute; American Cancer Society.

**References**

Ameloblastic Carcinoma: Report of an Aggressive Case and Review of the Literature: R.A. Bruce, et al.; J. Craniomaxillofac. Surg., August 1991, vol. 19(6), pp. 267–271.

Diseases of the Nose, Throat, Ear, Head, and Neck, 14th ed.: J.J. Ballenger; Lea and Febiger, 1991, pp. 213, 328.

Maxillary Ameloblastoma: Case Report: F.J. Sacaccia, et al.; Am. J. Otolaryngol., January–February, 1991, vol. 12(1), pp. 20–25.

Metastasizing Ameloblastoma: E.H. Laughlin, Cancer, August 1991, vol. 64(3), pp. 776–780.

Ameloblastoma Metastatic to the Lung: R.P. Clay, et al.; Ann. Plast. Surg., February 1989, vol. 22(2), pp. 160–162.

Ameloblastoma in Young Persons: A Clinicopathologic Analysis and Etiologic Investigation: M.A. Kahn; Oral Surg. Oral Med. Oral. Pathol., June 1989, vol. 67(6), pp. 706–715.

Diagnosis and Treatment of Metastatic Ameloblastoma: A.H. Eliasson, et al.; South. Med. J., September 1989, vol. 82(9), pp. 1165–1168.

# ANEMIA, APLASTIC

**Description** In aplastic anemia, suppression of the bone marrow can cause pancytopenia. In some cases, however, the disorder may be discriminatory and affect only the red blood cells, the white cells, or the platelets.

**Synonyms**

Aregenerative Anemia

Erythroblastophthisis

Hypoplastic Anemia

Panmyelopathy

Panmyelophthisis

Progressive Hypoerythemia

Refractory Anemia

Toxic Paralytic Anemia

**Signs and Symptoms** Onset of aplastic anemia may be sudden, but as a rule it is gradual. Weeks or months may pass before the effect of the causative toxin becomes apparent.

The initial symptoms may be increasing weakness, fatigue, and lethargy. Exertion may be followed by headache and respiratory problems. The patient may have bacterial infections more often and be sicker than is usual. While the manifestations depend upon the extent of the pancytopenia, the usual symptoms of anemia are exaggerated.

The typical patient's skin is pale and waxy, but that of a patient with the chronic form of the disorder may show significant brown pigmentation. If marked thrombocytopenia is present, bleeding into the epidermis and the mucous membranes may become apparent. Petechiae also may be noted, and trauma may produce purpura. Other signs may be mucosal ulceration, tachycardia, and systolic murmur.

**Etiology** Aplastic anemia results from failure of the bone marrow cells to mature. About 50 percent of cases are idiopathic; in most of these, the patients are in their teens and 20s.

Acquired aplastic anemia may be due to exposure to chemicals such as benzene, urethane, and those in some solvents and insecticides. Other causative agents are inorganic arsenic and radiation, and drugs such as phenylbutazone, chloramphenicol, antibiotics, anti-inflammatory agents, and anticonvulsants.

The exact mechanism involved in the adverse reaction is not known. An inborn hypersensitivity may be the explanation.

**Epidemiology** Approximately 1.5:1,000,000 to 2:1,000,000 people in the United States have been affected by aplastic anemia. It is diagnosed with greater frequency in Asian populations for unknown reasons.

**Related Disorders** Bone marrow failure may also occur in renal failure, hepatic disease, endocrine abnormalities, late-stage malignancies (particularly with metastasis to the bone marrow), chronic infections, and certain hereditary diseases.

**Treatment—Standard** In chemical-, radiation-, or drug-related aplastic anemia, the offender must be removed.

A bone marrow transplant offers maximum effectiveness; the marrow of a sibling is compatible in about 30 percent of cases. Repeated blood transfusions lower the chances of a successful transplant and should be avoided if at all possible. Antilymphocyte globulin is the treatment of choice for patients who do not have an HLA-compatible sibling. Androgenic steroids (e.g., oxymetholone) may also trigger bone marrow production in less severe aplastic anemia.

When an immunologic cause has been identified, immunosuppressive drugs such as prednisone, cyclosporine-A, and cyclophosphamide may be effective.

The outcome is poor in severe aplastic anemia, with only 20 percent of patients surviving 2 years with supportive therapy alone. Marrow production may resume once removal of the causative toxin is accomplished. The idiopathic form of the disorder may have a longer course with a less optimistic prognosis, but remission may occur. Transfusions may lead to an overall increase in tissue iron stores without trauma to the tissue. Infections (e.g., septicemia) may also intervene.

**Treatment—Investigational** A new biotechnology product is undergoing study. Recombinant human granulocyte–colony stimulating factor (**rhG-CSF**) is being given in extremely severe refractory cases. It leads to transient but not sustained rises of the neutrophils.

The drugs E(rGM-CSF) (Schering Corp.) and interleukin-1 alpha human recombinant (Immunex Corp.) are under investigation as treatment for aplastic anemia.

To help induce remission in patients with moderate or severe aplastic anemia and for those who are not good candidates for bone marrow transplantation, researchers are studying lymphocyte immune globulin (antithymocyte globulin).

Please contact the agencies listed under Resources, below, for the most current information. Addresses and telephone numbers of these agencies, as well as of individual experts and research centers, may be found in the Master Resources List.

**Resources**

**For more information on aplastic anemia:** National Organization for Rare Disorders (NORD); Aplastic Anemia Foundation of America; NIH/National Heart, Lung and Blood Institute Information Center.

**References**

Cecil Textbook of Medicine, 19th ed.: J.B. Wyngaarden, et al., eds.; W.B. Saunders Company, 1992, pp. 831–836.

Nelson Textbook of Pediatrics, 14th ed.: R.E. Behrman, ed.-in-chief; W.B. Saunders Company, 1992, pp. 1258–1269.

The Use of Colony-Stimulating Factors in Primary Hematologic Disorders: S.D. Naser; Cancer, August 1992, vol. 70(4 suppl.), pp. 921–927.

Treatment of Aplastic Anaemia with Antilymphocyte Globulin and High-Dose Methylprednisolone: N. Novitzky; Am. J. Hematol., April 1991, vol. 36(4), pp. 227–234.

Hematology, 4th ed.: W.J. Williams, et al., eds.; McGraw-Hill, 1990, pp. 158–174.

Current Considerations of the Etiology of Aplastic Anemia: A.M. Gewirtz; Crit. Rev. Oncol. Hematol., 1985, vol. 4(1), pp. 1–30.

# ANEMIA, DIAMOND-BLACKFAN

**Description** Diamond-Blackfan anemia is a hereditary congenital autoimmune blood disorder.

**Synonyms**

Blackfan-Diamond Anemia

Constitutional Erythroid Hypoplasia

**Signs and Symptoms** The infant with Diamond-Blackfan anemia has a moderate to severe deficiency of red blood cells. At approximately 1 month of age, the infant may appear unusually weak, pale, and sluggish. Normal growth may not occur, and facial characteristics such as a snub nose, widely spaced eyes, and a prominent upper lip may be apparent. Vertebral fusion may produce a webbed or shortened and rigid neck. The shoulder blades may protrude, and the hands may be deformed. Spontaneous remissions are possible, but usually drug therapy is responsible for improvement.

**Etiology** Diamond-Blackfan anemia may be either autosomal dominant or recessive, and is autoimmune-related. Patients have an erythroid-precursor antibody.

**Epidemiology** Males and females are affected in equal numbers. Since its discovery in 1938, about 150 verified cases of Diamond-Blackfan anemia have been reported in the United States.

**Related Disorders** See *Anemia, Aplastic; Anemia, Fanconi.*

**Treatment—Standard** Corticosteroid therapy is begun as soon as possible. Blood transfusions may also be necessary, but when multiple they carry the risk of complications: cardiac and hepatic disorders and iron overload. Prevention of infections is essential since they can aggravate the blood disorder. When treatment is effective, the patient's future health is usually unaffected. Genetic counseling may be helpful. Other treatment is symptomatic and supportive.

**Treatment—Investigational** Experimental bone marrow transplants are reserved for the gravest cases. Interleukin-3 shows promise in raising the red cell count in some patients refractory to corticosteroids.

Please contact the agencies listed under Resources, below, for the most current information. Addresses and telephone numbers of these agencies, as well as of individual experts and research centers, may be found in the Master Resources List.

**Resources**

**For more information on Diamond-Blackfan anemia:** National Organization for Rare Disorders (NORD); Diamond-Blackfan Anemia Support Group; NIH/National Heart, Lung and Blood Institute; Aplastic Anemia Foundation of America.

**For genetic information and genetic counseling referrals:** March of Dimes Birth Defects Foundation; Alliance of Genetic Support Groups.

**References**

Defective Erythroid Progenitor Differentiation System in Congenital Hypoplastic (Diamond-Blackfan) Anemia: J.M. Lipton, et al.; Blood, April 1986, vol. 67(4), pp. 962–968.

Diamond-Blackfan Syndrome in Adult Patients: E.P. Balaban, et al.; Am. J. Med., March 1985, vol. 78(3), pp. 533–538.

# ANEMIA, FANCONI

**Description** Fanconi anemia is a hereditary aplastic anemia encountered mainly in children and associated with cardiac, renal, and skeletal congenital anomalies as well as changes in skin pigmentation.

**Synonyms**

>  Aplastic Anemia with Congenital Anomalies
>  Congenital Pancytopenia
>  Constitutional Aplastic Anemia
>  Fanconi Panmyelopathy

**Signs and Symptoms** The first signs may be easy bruising and unprovoked epistaxis. Tests reveal inadequate production of red blood cells, white blood cells, and platelets. Diagnosis is generally made before age 9, usually between ages 2 and 6, by which time aplastic anemia per se is present.

The child's growth may be retarded or may stop. Microcephaly, hypogenitalism, hyperreflexia, and patchy hyperpigmentation may be evident. The upper extremities are likely to reflect the impact of the disorder on the skeleton, such as aplasia of the thumbs and radii. Examination usually reveals a spleen too small for the child's age. Renal abnormalities, as well as strabismus and microphthalmia, may also be present.

Monitoring is essential because patients with Fanconi anemia are cancer-prone, especially to leukemia.

**Etiology** Fanconi anemia is inherited as an autosomal recessive trait, perhaps precipitated by an environmental factor. Cell hypersensitivity to environmental carcinogens has been implicated.

**Epidemiology** Males are affected more often than females. Incidence is approximately 1:120,000 individuals.

**Treatment—Standard** Treatment usually includes methyltestosterone, methyltestosterone plus prednisone, and blood transfusions. Another therapeutic approach is to give cyclophosphamide, alone or in combination with procarbazine and antithymocyte globulin, followed by thoracoabdominal irradiation to prepare the patient for allogeneic bone marrow transplantation.

**Treatment—Investigational** An experimental method of lessening the likelihood of rejection of a bone marrow transplant is the use of cyclosporin A to remove donor T lymphocytes. The long-term outcome is not yet known.

Under a grant from the National Organization for Rare Disorders, Blanche Alter, M.D., is studying several possible treatments. For tissue donation contact Dr. Alter at Mount Sinai School of Medicine.

Dr. Arleen Auerbach is conducting clinical trials in the genetic, developmental, endocrine, hematologic, neurologic, gastrointestinal, metabolic, and orthopedic aspects of Fanconi anemia.

Drs. Johnson M. Liu and Neal S. Young at the National Heart, Lung and Blood Institute are developing alternative clinical protocols for the eventual treatment of pancytopenia of Fanconi anemia. Their focus is on correction of the defect by gene therapy.

Another study is being conducted on blood cells taken from the umbilical cord of a compatible donor.

Please contact the agencies listed under Resources, below, for the most current information. Addresses and telephone numbers of these agencies, as well as of individual experts and research centers, may be found in the Master Resources List.

## Resources

**For more information on Fanconi anemia:** National Organization for Rare Disorders (NORD); Fanconi Anemia Research Fund; International Fanconi Registry; Aplastic Anemia Foundation of America; NIH/National Heart, Lung and Blood Institute.

**For genetic information and genetic counseling referrals:** March of Dimes Birth Defects Foundation; Alliance of Genetic Support Groups.

## References

Cecil Textbook of Medicine, 19th ed.: J.B. Wyngaarden, et al., eds.; W.B. Saunders Company, 1992, pp. 831, 944.

Fanconi's Anemia: Current Concepts: B.P. Alter; Am. J. Pediatr. Hematol. Oncol., May 1992, vol. 14(2), pp. 170–176.

Mendelian Inheritance in Man, 10th ed.: V.A. McKusick; The Johns Hopkins University Press, 1992, pp. 1368–1372.

Nelson Textbook of Pediatrics, 14th ed.: R.E. Behrman, ed.-in-chief; W.B. Saunders Company, 1992, p. 1719.

Birth Defects Encyclopedia: M.L. Buyse, ed.-in-chief; Blackwell Scientific Publications, 1990, pp. 1359–1361, 1784.

Hematology, 4th ed.: W.J. Williams, et al., eds.; McGraw-Hill, 1990, pp. 159, 163.

Human Umbilical Cord Blood: A Clinically Useful Source of Transplantable Hematopoietic Stem/Progenitor Cells: H.E. Broxmeyer, et al.; Int. J. Cell Cloning, January 1990, vol. 8(suppl. 1), pp. 76–91.

Fanconi Anemia, Dyskeratosis Congenita, and WT Syndrome: N.T. Shahidi; Am. J. Med. Genet. Suppl., 1987, vol. 3, pp. 263–278.

Fanconi Anemia Study May Give Cancer Insight: Dermatology News, July–August, 1986.

# ANEMIA, HEMOLYTIC, ACQUIRED AUTOIMMUNE

**Description** Acquired autoimmune hemolytic anemia is characterized by the destruction of red blood cells before the completion of their usual 120-day life span and by the accompanying failure of the bone marrow to compensate for their loss. The severity of this type of anemia is determined by the life span of the red blood cell and by the capacity of the bone marrow to continue red cell production. The disorder commonly occurs as the result of, or in conjunction with, another medical condition.

**Synonyms**

Immune Hemolytic Anemia

**Signs and Symptoms** General symptoms of acquired autoimmune hemolytic anemia include fatigue, chills, backache, difficulty in breathing upon exertion, and palpitations. Symptoms may become specific to a subcategory of this anemia, namely warm antibody hemolytic anemia, cold antibody hemolytic anemia, or paroxysmal cold hemoglobinuria (see Related Disorders below).

**Etiology** Injury to the immune system by such disorders as chronic lymphatic leukemia, lymphoma, lupus erythematosus, or by such viral infections as chickenpox or mumps may be responsible. Exogenous causes of hemolytic anemia include such medications as sulfonamides, phenothiazines, quinine, quinidine, and methyldopa. Other cases of acquired autoimmune hemolytic anemia have no known cause.

**Epidemiology** Idiopathic cases of acquired autoimmune hemolytic anemia affect twice as many women as men, specifically women under 50 years old.

**Related Disorders** See *Hemoglobinuria, Paroxysmal Nocturnal.*

The following disorders may precede the development of acquired autoimmune hemolytic anemia and may prove useful in identifying an underlying cause of some forms of this disorder. See *Leukemia, Chronic Lymphatic; Lymphoma; Lupus Erythematosus.*

**Treatment—Standard** When acquired autoimmune hemolytic anemia is caused by other diseases, diagnosis and treatment of the underlying disorder usually bring marked improvement of the anemia. Mild cases may require no treatment. Hemolytic anemia caused by medication usually subsides after discontinuance of the medication. Idiopathic cases usually require therapy with prednisone and/or splenectomy.

**Treatment—Investigational** Sandoglobulin is being investigated as a potential therapy.

Please contact the agencies listed under Resources, below, for the most current information. Addresses and telephone numbers of these agencies, as well as of individual experts and research centers, may be found in the Master Resources List.

## Resources

**For more information on acquired autoimmune hemolytic anemia:** National Organization for Rare Disorders (NORD); NIH/National Heart, Lung and Blood Institute Information Center.

## References

Elucidation of Alloantibodies in Autoimmune Haemolytic Anemia: P. James, et al.; Vox. Sang., 1988, vol. 54(3), pp. 167–171.

Isolation of Peptide Associated with Autoimmune Haemolytic Anemia from Red Cell Membranes: E. Kajii, et al.; Clin. Exp. Immunol., September 1988, vol. 73(3), pp. 406–409.

Rapid Transient Reversal of Anemia and Long-Term Effects of Maintenance Intravenous Immunoglobulin for Autoimmune Hemolytic Anemia in Patients with Lymphoproliferative Disorders: E.C. Besa; Am. J. Med., April 1988, vol. 84(4), pp. 691–698.

Internal Medicine, 2nd ed.: J.H. Stein, ed.-in-chief; Little, Brown and Company, 1987, pp. 918–923.

# ANEMIA, HEMOLYTIC, COLD-ANTIBODY

**Description** Cold-antibody hemolytic anemia develops when a temperature of 30° C (86° F) or below causes agglutination and consequent complement fixation when IgM antibodies and erythrocytes bind. As a result, changes in the surface membranes of the red blood cells lead to their removal from the circulating macrophages.

**Synonyms**

> Anemia, Autoimmune Hemolytic
> Cold Agglutinin Disease
> Cold-Antibody Disease

**Signs and Symptoms** It is thought that IgM antibody–erythrocyte binding occurs distally. Temperatures can drop to as low as 32° C to 28° C (89.6° F to 82.4° F) in the ear lobes, fingertips, the tip of the nose, and the cheeks for lengthy periods.

Patients with cold-antibody hemolytic anemia may have weakness, dizziness, headache, tinnitus, spots before the eyes, fatigue, or sleepiness; they may behave oddly or be irritable. Gastrointestinal upsets and amenorrhea may occur, as may jaundice and splenomegaly, and, less often, hemoglobinuria. Cardiac failure or shock may develop.

**Etiology** Cold-antibody hemolytic anemia is idiopathic.

**Epidemiology** Usually the elderly are involved, particularly those whom infectious mononucleosis, lymphoproliferative disease, or mycoplasma pneumonia has rendered susceptible.

**Related Disorders** See *Hemoglobinuria, Paroxysmal Cold.*

**Treatment—Standard** Avoidance of cold may be beneficial. Immunosuppressive drugs such as chlorambucil or cyclophosphamide may sometimes lower the cold agglutinin concentration in severely afflicted patients.

When blood transfusions are necessary, certain precautions are essential. Cross-matching to ensure compatibility should be carried out at 37° C (98.6° F), and the blood should be heated by an on-line warmer to prevent binding of the new erythrocytes with antibodies.

**Treatment—Investigational** Plasmapheresis may be effective in some patients, but the side effects and efficacy are still being studied. It is currently reserved for the gravest cases.

Sandoglobulin is also undergoing investigation as a treatment for cold-antibody hemolytic anemia.

Please contact the agencies listed under Resources, below, for the most current information. Addresses and telephone numbers of these agencies, as well as of individual experts and research centers, may be found in the Master Resources List.

**Resources**

**For more information on cold-antibody hemolytic anemia:** National Organization for Rare Disorders (NORD); NIH/National Heart, Lung and Blood Institute.

**References**

Benefit of a 37 Degree Extracorporeal Circuit in Plasma Exchange Therapy for Selected Cases with Cold Agglutinin Disease: C. Andrzejewski, Jr., et al.; J. Clin. Apheresis, 1988, vol. 4(1), pp. 13–17.

Isolation of a Peptide Associated with Autoimmune Haemolytic Anaemia from Red Cell Membranes: E. Kajii, et al.; Clin. Exp. Immunol., September 1988, vol. 73(3), pp. 406–409.

Patients with Red Cell Autoantibodies: Selection of Blood for Transfusion: R.J. Sokol, et al.; Clin. Lab. Haematol., 1988, vol. 10(3), pp. 257–264.

Internal Medicine, 2nd ed.: J.H. Stein, ed.-in-chief; Little, Brown and Company, 1987, pp. 1058–1059.

# ANEMIA, HEMOLYTIC, HEREDITARY NONSPHEROCYTIC

**Description** Hereditary nonspherocytic hemolytic anemia is a term used to describe a heterogeneous group of genetic blood disorders characterized by defective erythrocytes that are not spherocytes. The disorders are thought to be caused by deficiencies in hereditary enzymes, such as glucose-6-phosphate dehydrogenase **(G6PD),** which will be discussed here.

G6PD deficiency is recognized as the most common inherited enzyme abnormality in humans. There are close to 300 distinct variants that have been classified into 5 main groups according to their erythrocyte enzymatic activity and the presence of hemolysis. In general terms, patients with hereditary nonspherocytic hemolytic anemia who have a G6PD deficiency have inherited an uncommon variant that has severely decreased enzyme activity, extremely abnormal kinetics, and reduced heat stability, factors that could account for its defective function.

**Signs and Symptoms** The signs and symptoms of moderate anemia, recurrent jaundice, and splenomegaly or hepatomegaly usually occur in childhood, but some newborns are jaundiced at birth. If the newborn's erythrocytes contain Heinz bodies, a diagnosis of nonspherocytic hemolytic anemia can be made. In some instances a marked decrease in hemoglobin level may be present.

**Etiology** G6PD deficiency is inherited as a partially dominant X-linked trait. The hemolysis characteristic of these disorders may result from oxidant stress and in turn leads to the symptoms described above. Fava beans and certain drugs, such as some sulfonamides, antimalarial drugs, and phenacetin, can precipitate hemolytic crises.

**Epidemiology** Males, as hemizygotes with respect to the enzyme, are more likely to be seen clinically.

**Treatment—Standard** Any precipitating agent for the hemolysis should be discontinued. Patients with this disease may occasionally need blood transfusions. If the need for transfusions becomes chronic, then iron chelation therapy (deferoxamine) is given when indicated. Splenectomy is not beneficial for nonspherocytic hemolytic anemia.

**Treatment—Investigational** Please contact the agencies listed under Resources, below, for the most current information. Addresses and telephone numbers of these agencies, as well as of individual experts and research centers, may be found in the Master Resources List.

**Resources**

For more information on hereditary nonspherocytic hemolytic anemia: National Organization for Rare Disorders (NORD); NIH/National Heart, Lung and Blood Institute.

For genetic information and genetic counseling referrals: March of Dimes Birth Defects Foundation; Alliance of Genetic Support Groups.

**References**

Chronic Nonspherocytic Hemolytic Anemia (CNSHA) and Glucose 6 Phosphate Dehydrogenase (G6PD) Deficiency in a Patient with Familial Amyloidotic Polyneuropathy (FAP): L. Vives-Corrons, et al.; Human Genetics, January 1989, vol. 81(2), pp. 161–164.

The Metabolic Basis of Inherited Disease, 6th ed.: C.R. Scriver et al., eds.; McGraw-Hill, 1989, pp. 2247–2249.

Cecil Textbook of Medicine, 18th ed.: J.B. Wyngaarden and L.H. Smith, Jr., eds.; W.B. Saunders Company, 1988, p. 880.

# Anemia, Hemolytic, Hereditary Spherocytic

**Description** Hereditary spherocytic hemolytic anemia is an intracorpuscular abnormality in which defects within the red blood cell shorten its survival. The membrane of the cell is abnormal in lipid content and surface area, both of which are smaller than normal. The red blood cells are sphere shaped; it is difficult for them to course through the splenic circulation, and when they cannot do so they are lost. The spheroid shape is the hallmark of hereditary spherocytic hemolytic anemia, and it is the result of the inherent metabolic defect.

**Synonyms**

Acholuric Jaundice (Chronic Acholuric Jaundice)
Chronic Familial Icterus
Congenital Hemolytic Anemia
Congenital Hemolytic Jaundice
Hereditary Spherocytosis

**Signs and Symptoms** Hereditary spherocytic hemolytic anemia may be present at birth or may not be apparent for years. The nature of the disorder varies significantly among patients. In many patients, the symptoms are mild enough to go unrecognized. Tiredness and moderate persistent jaundice may be present. Onset of puberty may be late. Splenomegaly is commonly found, and it may sometimes manifest in abdominal discomfort.

An infection is the most common trigger of an aplastic crisis, which signals temporary deficiency of red blood cell production. Trauma or pregnancy may intensify the crisis. The patient may complain of fever, headache, abdominal pain, anorexia, vomiting, and lethargy. Children may have epistaxis.

Occasionally hepatomegaly, cholelithiasis, or leg ulcers may develop. Congenital deformities, perhaps polydactylism or a tower-shaped skull, may be present.

**Etiology** Hemolytic anemias have 2 distinct findings: (1) a reduction in the life span of the erythrocytes, and (2) the retention of iron within the body, mainly in the reticuloendothelial system. In all hemolytic anemias, there is overdestruction of red blood cells.

The abnormality of the red blood cell membrane in spherocytic hemolytic anemia is usually inherited as an autosomal dominant metabolic trait, but severe forms are inherited in an autosomal recessive manner. Usually there is a familial history of anemia, jaundice, or splenomegaly. At times, the disorder may skip one or more generations. No familial history can be traced in some cases.

**Epidemiology** The greatest incidence of hereditary spherocytic hemolytic anemia is in northern Europeans.

**Related Disorders** Spherocytes may be present in hemoglobin C disease, autoimmune hemolytic anemia, drug-induced hemolytic anemia, alcoholism, and individuals with burns.

**Treatment—Standard** Hereditary spherocytosis usually has a lengthy chronic course. The only currently recognized specific treatment is splenectomy, which is carried out in patients under age 45 who have had jaundice and biliary colic or aplastic crises. Splenectomy should be avoided in children under age 5 years because of the risk of overwhelming bacterial infection. Following the surgery the patient becomes asymptomatic.

During an aplastic crisis, transfusions may be indicated to avert cardiovascular collapse. If the crisis is triggered by an intercurrent infection, antibiotic treatment may be warranted.

Genetic counseling may be of benefit for patients and their families. Other treatment is symptomatic and supportive.

**Treatment—Investigational** Please contact the agencies listed under Resources, below, for the most current information. Addresses and telephone numbers of these agencies, as well as of individual experts and research centers, may be found in the Master Resources List.

**Resources**

**For more information on hereditary spherocytic hemolytic anemia:** National Organization for Rare Disorders (NORD); NIH/National Heart, Lung and Blood Institute; NIH/National Cancer Institute Physicians Data Query Phoneline; American Cancer Society.

**For genetic information and genetic counseling referrals:** March of Dimes Birth Defects Foundation; Alliance of Genetic Support Groups.

**References**

Cecil Textbook of Medicine, 19th ed.: J.B. Wyngaarden, et al., eds.; W.B. Saunders Company, 1992, p. 858–860.

Homozygosity for Dominant Form of Hereditary Spherocytosis: F. Duru; Br. J. Heamotol., November 1992, vol. 82(3), pp. 596–600.

Mendelian Inheritance in Man, 10th ed.: V.A. McKusick; The Johns Hopkins University Press, 1992, pp. 1025–1028, 1702.

Splenic Sequestration Associated with Sickle Cell Trait and Hereditary Spherocytosis: Y.M. Yang; Am. J. Hematol., June 1992, vol. 40(2), pp. 110–116.

Current Problems in Haematology, II: Hereditary Spherocytosis: J.C. Smiley; J. Clin. Pathol., June 1991, vol. 44(6), pp. 441–444.

Birth Defects Encyclopedia: M.L. Buyse, ed.-in-chief; Blackwell Scientific Publications, 1990, pp. 1573–1575.

Hematology, 4th ed.: W.J. Williams, et al., eds.; McGraw-Hill, 1990, pp. 558–569.

The Metabolic Basis of Inherited Disease, 6th ed.: C.R. Scriver, et al., eds.; McGraw-Hill, 1989, p. 362.

# ANEMIA, HEMOLYTIC, WARM-ANTIBODY

**Description** Warm-antibody hemolytic anemia is an autoimmune disorder in which IgM antibodies bind with erythrocytes, removing them from circulation and aborting their normal life span of 120 days. Bone marrow production of new cells cannot replace their numbers. The extent of the anemia depends on the duration of the survival of the coated red cells and the ability of the marrow to maintain manufacture of red cells.

Immune hemolytic anemias are classified by the temperature at which erythrocyte removal occurs. Warm-antibody hemolytic anemia is associated with temperatures of 37° C (98.6° F) or higher, while cold-antibody hemolytic anemia generally has its onset at lower temperatures.

**Synonyms**

Autoimmune Hemolytic Anemias

Warm-Reacting Antibody Disease

**Signs and Symptoms** The severity of symptoms depends upon the speed of onset, the rate of annihilation of red blood cells, and whether an underlying disorder is present; symptoms vary from patient to patient. The manifestations of sudden onset are often paleness, tiredness, exertion-produced breathing problems, dizziness, and palpitations. The slower the onset, the less marked the anemia, and a patient may be asymptomatic. Jaundice and splenomegaly are usually part of the complex.

**Etiology** Approximately 25 percent of reported cases of this disorder are idiopathic; an estimated 65 percent have a precipitating disorder, such as chronic lymphocytic leukemia or another disease of the lymph system. Other associated disorders are systemic lupus erythematosus (**SLE**), rheumatoid arthritis, and ulcerative colitis. Another 10 to 15 percent of cases are considered to be reactions to drugs, e.g., methyldopa.

**Epidemiology** Warm-antibody hemolytic anemia may affect anyone. Individuals with diseases that alter the immune system are at higher risk. Chronic lymphatic leukemia, lymphoma, and SLE may precede the development of warm-antibody hemolytic anemia.

**Related Disorders** See *Hodgkin Disease; Systemic Lupus Erythematosus.*

**Chronic lymphatic leukemia** is marked by an oversupply of white blood cells in the bone marrow, spleen, liver, and blood. As the disease advances, the leukemic cells invade other areas, including the intestinal tract, kidneys, lungs, gonads, and lymph nodes. The patient may experience tiredness, weakness, itchiness, night sweats, abdominal discomfort, or weight loss. Splenomegaly is generally present.

**Treatment—Standard** Corticosteroids are the drugs of choice in warm-antibody hemolytic anemia. For the few patients who are refractory, immunosuppressive drugs are indicated. Advanced disease may require splenectomy. In those with an underlying disorder, treatment of that disorder usually significantly improves the anemia. In drug-induced anemia, symptoms generally abate when the medication is discontinued.

**Treatment—Investigational** Sandoglobulin is being investigated as a potential therapy.

Please contact the agencies listed under Resources, below, for the most current information. Addresses and telephone numbers of these agencies, as well as of individual experts and research centers, may be found in the Master Resources List.

**Resources**

**For more information on warm-antibody hemolytic anemia:** National Organization for Rare Disorders (NORD); NIH/National Heart, Lung and Blood Institute.

**References**

Incomplete Warm Hemolysins, II: Corresponding Antigens and Pathogenic Mechanisms in Autoimmune Hemolytic Anemias Induced by Incomplete Warm Hemolysins: M.W. Wolf, et al.; Clin. Immunopathol., April 1989, vol. 51(1), pp. 68–76.

Production of Human Warm-Reacting Red Cell Monoclonal Antoantibodies by Epstein-Barr Virus Transformation: C. Andrzejewski, et al.; Transfusion, March–April 1989, vol. 29(3), pp. 196–200.

Cecil Textbook of Medicine, 18th ed.: J.B. Wyngaarden and L.H. Smith, Jr., eds.; W.B. Saunders Company, 1988, pp. 917–920.

Internal Medicine, 2nd ed.: J.H. Stein, ed.-in-chief; Little, Brown and Company, 1987, pp. 1057–1059.

# ANEMIA, MEGALOBLASTIC

**Description** Megaloblasts in the marrow and hypersegmented polymorphonuclear leukocytes are hallmarks of megaloblastic anemia. Leukopenia and thrombocytopenia may also be present.

**Synonyms**

Megaloblastic Anemia of Pregnancy

**Signs and Symptoms** As a rule, onset is slow. The initial symptoms may be diarrhea, vomiting, anorexia, and weight loss. Malabsorption may result. Hepatomegaly and splenomegaly may occur. The patient may be jaundiced or pale, and weakness, palpitations, breathing problems, aching limbs, and feeling inappropriately hot or cold may be complaints. Oral infection, neurologic lesions, and irritability also may occur.

**Etiology** Megaloblastic anemia is due to a deficiency of either vitamin B12 or folic acid. Any of a number of factors may cause these deficiencies: inadequate diet, malabsorption, certain diseases or parasites, or immunosuppressive drugs. In addition, during pregnancy the fetal blood requirement may result in maternal megaloblastic anemia.

**Related Disorders Folic acid deficiency** causes megaloblastic anemia and other blood findings. Folic acid is available from many plants and from animal tissues, but long cooking destroys it. Infertility, gastrointestinal problems, certain skin diseases, obstetric disorders, neuropathy, and, perhaps, psychiatric disorders may be associated with the deficiency.

See also *Anemia, Pernicious.*

**Treatment—Standard** Treatment includes intramuscular injections of vitamin B12 or oral iron supplements. A lifetime maintenance dose of vitamin B12 is essential. Folic acid deficiency is treated by oral administration of folate.

**Treatment—Investigational** Please contact the agencies listed under Resources, below, for the most current information. Addresses and telephone numbers of these agencies, as well as of individual experts and research centers, may be found in the Master Resources List.

**Resources**

**For more information on megaloblastic anemia:** National Organization for Rare Disorders (NORD); NIH/National Heart, Lung and Blood Institute.

**References**

Megaloblastic Anemia Due to Vitamin B12 Deficiency Caused by Small Intestinal Bacterial Overgrowth: Possible Role of Vitamin B12 Analogues: M.F. Murphy, et al.; Brit. J. Haematol., January 1986, vol. 62(1), pp. 7–12.

Bone Marrow Status of Anaemic Pregnant Women on Supplemental Iron and Folic Acid in a Nigerian Community: L.A. Okafor, et al.; Angiology, August 1985, vol. 36(8), pp. 500–503.

Homocystinuria and Megaloblastic Anemia Responsive to Vitamin B-12 Therapy: S. Schuh, et al.; N. Engl. J. Med., March 15, 1984, vol. 310(11), pp. 686–690.

# ANEMIA, PERNICIOUS

**Description** Pernicious anemia is characterized by a deficiency of vitamin B12 that is generally due to a failure of the gastric mucosa to secrete intrinsic factor, which is needed to absorb vitamin B12 from the diet. In some cases, intestinal abnormalities prevent absorption of the vitamin.

**Synonyms**

Addison-Biermer Anemia

Addisonian Pernicious Anemia (Addison Anemia)
Biermer Anemia
Cytogenic Anemia
Malignant Anemia
Primary Anemia

**Signs and Symptoms** Because the human liver stores enough vitamin B12 to last 3 to 5 years, pernicious anemia progresses slowly as the hepatic reserves of vitamin B12 are used. Once symptoms appear, however, they must be treated or the disease can be fatal. Symptoms and signs include weakness, easy fatigability, dyspnea, tachycardia, and angina. Patients may also have gastrointestinal problems, such as anorexia, abdominal pain, indigestion, belching, and possibly intermittent constipation and diarrhea. Weight loss is common. In some cases there is genitourinary involvement as well as hepato- or splenomegaly. Diagnosis is confirmed through the Schilling test.

Neurologic involvement can occur, most often in the peripheral nerves but also in the spinal cord. Early neurologic symptoms and signs include paresthesias and loss in the extremities of vibration and position awareness. Ataxia, a positive Babinski sign, and hyperactive reflexes are among the characteristics that may develop. Patients may be depressed and irritable and may experience the paranoia known as megaloblastic madness.

**Etiology** Pernicious anemia is known to be familial, and a predisposition to the disease may be inherited as an autosomal dominant trait. The most common cause of vitamin B12 deficiency is the failure of the gastric mucosa to secrete intrinsic factor, but other causes may be involved, including gastrectomy, malabsorption syndromes, congenital absence of absorptive sites for vitamin B12 in the ileum, absence of absorptive sites due to regional enteritis or surgical resection of the small intestine, chronic atrophic gastritis, chronic pancreatitis, myxedema, blind loop syndrome, and fish tapeworm infestation.

**Epidemiology** Pernicious anemia primarily affects adults and rarely occurs before the age of 35. It is most common in the moderate climates of North America and Europe among people of Scandinavian, English, and Irish extraction. It is extremely rare in Orientals. A juvenile version of pernicious anemia afflicts infants, children, and adolescents and resembles the adult version in all respects except for certain biochemical reactions.

**Related Disorders** See *Anemia, Megaloblastic.*

**Treatment—Standard** Intramuscular injection of vitamin B12 is the standard therapy. A physician must closely monitor the amount given. Patients generally continue to receive maintenance doses of vitamin B12 for life.

**Treatment—Investigational** Please contact the agencies listed under Resources, below, for the most current information. Addresses and telephone numbers of these agencies, as well as of individual experts and research centers, may be found in the Master Resources List.

**Resources**

**For more information on pernicious anemia:** National Organization for Rare Disorders (NORD); NIH/National Heart, Lung and Blood Institute.

**For genetic information and genetic counseling referrals:** March of Dimes Birth Defects Foundation; Alliance of Genetic Support Groups.

**References**

Cecil Textbook of Medicine, 19th ed.: J.B. Wyngaarden, et al., eds.; W.B. Saunders Company, 1992, pp. 693, 847.

Long-Term Neurologic Consequences of Nutritional Vitamin B12 Deficiency in Infants: S.M. Graham, et al.; J. Pediatr., November 1992, vol. 121(5 pt. 1), pp. 710–714.

Mendelian Inheritance in Man, 10th ed.: V.A. McKusick; The Johns Hopkins University Press, 1992, p. 844.

Pernicious Anemia: Early Identification to Prevent Permanent Sequelae: A.B. Karnad, et al.; Postgrad. Med., February 1992, vol. 91(2), pp. 231–237.

Human Gastric Intrinsic Factor: Characterization of cDNA and Genomic Clones and Localization to Human Chromosome 11: J.E. Hewitt, et al.; Genomics, June 1991, vol. 10(2), pp. 432–440.

Birth Defects Encyclopedia: M.L. Buyse, ed.-in-chief; Blackwell Scientific Publications, 1990, p. 135.

Hematology, 4th ed.: W.J. Williams, et al., eds.; McGraw-Hill, 1990, pp. 459–461.

# ANEMIA, SIDEROBLASTIC

**Description** Sideroblastic anemias are disorders in which synthesis of hemoglobin is abnormal because of insufficient or ineffective use of intracellular iron, which may be in abundant supply.

**Synonyms**

Idiopathic Refractory Sideroblastic Anemia
Iron Overload Anemia
Sideroblastosis

**Signs and Symptoms** The patient experiences general weakness, fatigue, and difficulty in breathing. Exertion may cause chest pains resembling angina.

In contrast to most other forms of anemia, the blood serum has unusually high levels of iron and iron-containing substances; it also contains sideroblasts. The mucous membranes and the skin of hands and arms may be pale, often with a lemon-yellow cast. Upon occasion, subcutaneous bleeding may produce a brownish-red effect. Splenomegaly or hepatomegaly may be present. A complication in a late stage of sideroblastic anemia is acute leukemia, which occurs in approximately 10 percent of cases.

**Etiology** Hereditary sideroblastic anemia is generally inherited as an X-linked trait, but may in rare cases be autosomal recessive. Autosomal dominant inheritance of sideroblastic anemia with erythrocyte dimorphism has been reported.

Acquired forms are most often idiopathic, but in some cases can be attributed to such factors as alcohol abuse and certain drugs (e.g., antituberculosis agents or chloramphenicol). The disorder also may be a symptom of a granulomatous disease, a tumor, rheumatoid arthritis, or myelodysplasia.

**Epidemiology** Inherited forms usually develop in childhood. The idiopathic acquired disease occurs most often in the elderly. Incidence of other acquired forms depends on the precipitating condition.

**Related Disorders Idiopathic hemochromatosis** is a hereditary disorder of iron metabolism marked by an overload of iron in the tissues, particularly in the liver, pancreas, and heart, and by a bronze cast to the skin. Cirrhosis of the liver, diabetes mellitus, and associated bone and joint changes may also be present.

See *Thalassemia Major; Thalassemia Minor.*

**Treatment—Standard** Hereditary sideroblastic anemia often improves with the use of pyridoxine. There is presently no specific therapy for idiopathic sideroblastic anemia. When a precipitating agent has been determined, its use should be discontinued. Pyridoxine has not proved generally effective in cases of acquired sideroblastic anemia. Supportive treatment, including transfusion, may be beneficial in all cases of sideroblastic anemia.

To remove an overload of iron in sideroblastic anemia, deferoxamine is infused subcutaneously or intramuscularly and has frequently been effective; however, a combination of deferoxamine with ascorbate has been even more effective in many cases.

**Treatment—Investigational** Please contact the agencies listed under Resources, below, for the most current information. Addresses and telephone numbers of these agencies, as well as of individual experts and research centers, may be found in the Master Resources List.

**Resources**

**For more information on sideroblastic anemia:** National Organization for Rare Disorders (NORD); NIH/National Heart, Lung and Blood Institute; Leukemia Society of America.

**For genetic information and genetic counseling referrals:** March of Dimes Birth Defects Foundation; Alliance of Genetic Support Groups.

**References**

Harrison's Principles of Internal Medicine, 12th ed.: J.D. Wilson, et al., eds.; McGraw-Hill, 1991, p. 1522.

Mendelian Inheritance in Man, 9th ed.: V.A. McKusick; The Johns Hopkins University Press, 1990, pp. 858, 1476, 1563–1564.

Idiopathic Refractory Sideroblastic Anemia, Incidence and Risk Factors for Leukemia Transformation: D.S. Chang, et al.; Cancer, August 1979, vol. 44(2), pp. 724–731.

# ANGIOEDEMA, HEREDITARY

**Description** In hereditary angioedema, circumscribed obstruction of lymphatic vessels or the veins causes temporary edema in areas of the skin, mucous membranes, and, sometimes, the internal organs.

**Synonyms**

Complement-Mediated Urticaria Angioedema

Hereditary Angioneurotic Edema

**Signs and Symptoms** Most commonly, edema affects the backs of the hands or feet, the eyelids, lips, and genitalia. Edema in the mucous membrane lining of the respiratory and gastrointestinal tracts is more usual in hereditary angiodema than in other forms of angioedema. Also, the patient with the hereditary type complains of firm and painful rather than pruritic swellings. Urticaria rarely is present.

Transient attacks recur, becoming more severe. Injury or severe pain, surgery, dental procedures, viral illness, and stress can trigger or worsen the episodes.

Clues to edema in the gastrointestinal tract include nausea, vomiting, acute abdominal pain, and perhaps signs of obstruction. An edematous pharynx or larynx can be life-threatening.

**Etiology** Hereditary angioedema is autosomal dominant. Either 1 of 2 defects is present: more commonly, a deficiency of complement component C1 esterase inhibitor; less commonly, synthesis of an abnormal form of this protein.

**Epidemiology** Males and females are affected equally.

**Related Disorders Acute, nonhereditary angioedema** affects the skin and mucous membranes and commonly clears spontaneously in 1 to 2 days. Any number of allergens may be responsible, including drugs, insect stings and bites, and certain foods, especially eggs, shellfish, nuts, and fruits.

**Chronic nonhereditary angioedema** may be due to constant exposure to an allergen, or to stress. Angioedema may also appear during certain illnesses, including systemic lupus erythematosus and chronic sinus or dental infection.

**Treatment—Standard** Hereditary angioedema is refractory to the routine therapies for acute or chronic angioedema, but several drugs can be preventive. Prophylactic drugs that yield long-term protection include androgens, such as danazol, and oxymetholone. For women, androgens with few masculinizing effects should be prescribed, and the minimal effective dosage should be used.

To avert episodes associated with surgery, dental work, and similar stresses, short-term treatment prior to the expected period of stress is indicated. Fresh frozen plasma, or preparations of the missing enzyme partially purified from whole blood, are effective in these situations.

In acute attacks that threaten airway obstruction, it is essential to maintain or create an airway. A tracheotomy may be indicated and oxygen needed. Epinephrine and antihistamine may be given, but their value is uncertain in this setting.

Genetic counseling may be of benefit for patients with hereditary angioedema and their families.

**Treatment—Investigational** An effective drug that is still only in experimental use is epsilon-aminocaproic acid.

The orphan drug tranexamic acid is used prophylactically in patients with hereditary angioneurotic edema and those with other congenital coagulopathies who are undergoing surgical procedures, such as dental extractions. This drug has been approved for marketing for these procedures only. For additional information contact Kabivitrum.

Other agents under investigation include the orphan drug C1-esterase-inhibitor (human, pasteurized) (Behringwerke Aktiegesellschaft) for prevention and treatment of acute attacks; the orphan drug C1-inhibitor (human) vapor heated immuno (Immuno Clinical Research Corp.) for the treatment of short-term protection for those who require dental or other surgical procedures; and the drug cinnarizine (Searle Pharmaceuticals). The safety and efficacy of these drugs have yet to be proved.

Please contact the agencies listed under Resources, below, for the most current information. Addresses and telephone numbers of these agencies, as well as of individual experts and research centers, may be found in the Master Resources List.

**Resources**

**For more information on hereditary angioedema:** National Organization for Rare Disorders (NORD); NIH/National Heart, Lung and Blood Institute.

**For genetic information and genetic counseling referrals:** March of Dimes Birth Defects Foundation; Alliance of Genetic Support Groups.

**References**

Hereditary Angioedema: Uncomplicated Maxillofacial Surgery Using Short-Term C1 Inhibitor Replacement Therapy: A. Leimgruber; Int. Arch. Allergy Immunol., 1993, vol. 101(1), pp. 107–112.

Cecil Textbook of Medicine, 19th ed.: J.B. Wyngaarden, et al., eds.; W.B. Saunders Company, 1992, p. 1457.

Hereditary Angioedema: D.M. Elnicki; South. Med. J., November 1992, vol. 85(11), pp. 1084–1090.

Mendelian Inheritance in Man, 10th ed.: V.A. McKusick; The Johns Hopkins University Press, 1992, pp. 75–78.

Long-Term Treatment of Hereditary Angioedema with Attenuated Androgens: A Survey of a 13-Year Experience: C. Cicardi; J. Allergy Clin. Immunol., April 1991, vol. 87(4), pp. 768–773.

Oral Manifestations and Dental Management of Patients with Hereditary Angioedema: J.C. Atkinson; J. Oral. Pathol. Med., March 1991, vol. 20(3), pp. 139–142.

Birth Defects Encyclopedia: M.L. Buyse, ed.-in-chief; Blackwell Scientific Publications, 1990, pp. 143–144.

Dictionary of Medical Syndromes, 3rd ed.: S.I. Magalini, et al., eds.; J.B. Lippincott Company, 1990, p. 52.

The Metabolic Basis of Inherited Disease, 6th ed.: C.R. Scriver, et al., eds.; McGraw-Hill, 1989, pp. 2728–2730.

# ANTITHROMBIN III (AT III) DEFICIENCY, CONGENITAL

**Description** Since antithrombin III limits blood coagulation, congenital antithrombin III deficiency is characterized by a marked tendency toward venous or arterial thrombosis. There are 3 recognized forms of the disorder: classical AT III deficiency and 2 variants, AT III-Ia and AT III-Ib.

**Signs and Symptoms** Patients usually suffer the first episode of thrombosis between the ages of 10 and 35. Precipitating events include surgery, pregnancy, childbirth, trauma, or use of oral contraceptives. Because pregnancy and estrogen use are significant risk factors, women tend to develop thrombosis at an earlier age than men.

About 40 percent of patients with congenital AT III deficiency develop pulmonary embolisms. Embolisms also commonly occur in the veins deep in the legs and pelvic region, the more superficial veins in the legs, and the mesenteric veins. Edema is common in affected legs and pelvic areas. Clots that form in the heart may result in thromboembolism to other organs, such as the brain or kidneys.

Diagnosis of AT III is confirmed by the blood antithrombin III assay. Any individual with a history of venous thromboembolism before the age of 40 should be evaluated for ATIII deficiency even if the blood level is normal. Studies suggest that early diagnosis and treatment may reduce the incidence of thrombosis. Anticoagulants may prevent recurrences.

**Etiology** Congenital AT III deficiency is inherited as an autosomal dominant gene. In the classical form of the disorder, an insufficient amount of antithrombin is produced in the liver. In the variant forms, AT III-Ia and AT III-Ib, both normal and abnormal AT III are produced but interact so that the result is inhibition of normal antithrombin.

**Epidemiology** The disease is thought to occur in about 1:3,000 to 1:5,000 individuals.

**Related Disorders Acquired antithrombin III deficiency** occurs when AT III levels fall below 75 percent of normal, increasing the risk of thromboembolism. This condition develops after major trauma calling for sustained or large-scale blood coagulation; if there is urinary loss of antithrombin III during failure of renal filtration; or if AT III is destroyed when proteins are broken down, as in starvation. Other causal conditions include liver failure, severe blood loss, late pregnancy, and estrogen use. Acquired antithrombin III deficiency can usually be reversed.

**Treatment—Standard** The goal of treatment is to prevent thrombosis, primarily through the use of oral anticoagulants, such as coumadin drugs, heparin, and intravenous concentrated AT III. The orphan drug thrombate III (Miles Labs) is now a standard therapy. When the risk of thrombosis is high, as during pregnancy or with surgery, AT III replacement therapy is particularly important. Antithrombin III should also be replaced to help dissolve blood clots after thrombosis has occurred.

Heparin and AT III replacement can cause bleeding, so the amount of therapy must be carefully monitored. AT III can also increase the patient's risk of developing hepatitis.

Women who are prone to this disorder should refrain from taking estrogen. Patients who have any of the following characteristics should be screened for AT III deficiency: a family history of thrombosis, a thrombosis before age 35, recurrence of thrombosis even with heparin therapy, deep vein thrombosis early in pregnancy, or loss of large amounts of protein in the urine.

A drug known as AT nativ has received Food and Drug Administration approval as a treatment for congenital antithrombin III deficiency. It is manufactured by Kabivitrum.

**Treatment—Investigational** AT III replacement is under development by the following pharmaceutical companies: Miles; Kabivitrum; Hoechst-Roussel Pharmaceuticals; and Cutter Laboratories.

Human antithrombin III is under clinical investigation in preventing or arresting episodes of thrombosis in patients with congenital antithrombin III deficiency, especially those who have suffered trauma or are about to undergo surgery or childbirth. For additional information on human antithrombin III: The American Red Cross.

Please contact the agencies listed under Resources, below, for the most current information. Addresses and telephone numbers of these agencies, as well as of individual experts and research centers, may be found in the Master Resources List.

**Resources**

**For more information on congenital antithrombin III deficiency:** National Organization for Rare Disorders (NORD); NIH/National Heart, Lung and Blood Institute; American Liver Foundation; United Liver Association; Children's Liver Foundation.

**References**

Pregnancy and Thrombophilia in Women with Congenital Deficit of Antithrombin III, Protein C, Protein S or Plasminogen: Analysis of 39 Cases: M. Montague; Med. Clin., February 1993, vol. 100(6), pp. 201–204.

Cecil Textbook of Medicine, 19th ed.: J.B. Wyngaarden, et al., eds.; W.B. Saunders Company, 1992, pp. 1011–1012.

Congenital Antithrombin III Deficiency Causing Mesenteric Venous Infarction: A Lesson to Remember: A Case History: H.P. Grewal; Angiology, July 1992, vol. 43(7), pp. 618–620.

Hypercoagulability and Thrombosis: R.L. Bick; Hematol. Oncol. Clin. North Am., December 1992, vol. 6(6), pp. 1421–1431.

Mendelian Inheritance in Man, 10th ed.: V.A. McKusick; The Johns Hopkins University Press, 1992, pp. 87–92.

Incidence and Clinical Characteristics of Hereditary Disorder Associated with Venous Thrombosis: M.D. Tabernero, et al.; Am. J. Hematol., April 1991, vol. 36(4), pp. 249–254.

Recurrent Venous Thrombosis and Hypercoagulable States: C.D. Bolan; Am. Fam. Physician, November 1991, vol. 44(5), pp. 1741–1751.

Birth Defects Encyclopedia: M.L. Buyse, ed.-in-chief; Blackwell Scientific Publications, 1990, pp. 152–153.

Dictionary of Medical Syndromes, 3rd ed.: S.I. Magalini, et al., eds.; J.B. Lippincott Company, 1990, p. 57.

Hematology, 4th ed.: W.J. Williams, et al., eds.; McGraw-Hill, 1990, pp. 1545, 1626.

Substitution of AT III: H.K. Breddin, et al.; Wien. Klin. Wochenschr., December 21, 1984 (in English), vol. 96(24), pp. 875–878.

Antithrombin III Deficiency and Thromboembolism: E. Thaler, et al.; Clin. Haematol., June 1981, vol. 10(2), pp. 369–390.

# BANTI SYNDROME

**Description** Banti syndrome is a chronic splenic disease characterized by splenomegaly that results from thrombosis of the splenic or portal veins, cirrhosis of the liver, narrowing of splenic or portal veins, or birth abnormalities.

**Synonyms**
Hypersplenism

**Signs and Symptoms** In the early stages of the disease, patients have splenomegaly, anemia, fatigue, and weakness. In later stages the anemia worsens and esophageal hemorrhaging may occur, which causes bloody vomitus and dark stools. Hepatomegaly may eventually develop. The course of the disease is similar to that of cirrhosis of the liver, except that splenomegaly is the major symptom.

**Etiology** Banti syndrome is the result of chronic hypertension in the vein that transports blood from the spleen; the hypertension is caused by liver cirrhosis, thrombosis or constriction of the splenic or portal veins, or birth abnormalities. The accumulation of trapped blood then causes splenomegaly.

**Related Disorders** See *Primary Biliary Cirrhosis; Gaucher Disease; Felty Syndrome.*

**Treatment—Standard** Treatment varies with the cause of the syndrome. If thrombosis or narrowing of a vein is the cause, a surgical shunt can be used to reroute the blood and bypass the obstruction. If cirrhosis is the cause, treatment is appropriate to the type and underlying cause of cirrhosis. Ethamolin, an orphan drug, has been approved by the Food and Drug Administration for use in the treatment of bleeding esophageal varices; its manufacturer is Glaxo Pharmaceuticals.

**Treatment—Investigational** Please contact the agencies listed under Resources, below, for the most current information. Addresses and telephone numbers of these agencies, as well as of individual experts and research centers, may be found in the Master Resources List.

**Resources**
**For more information on Banti syndrome:** National Organization for Rare Disorders (NORD); NIH/National Institute of Diabetes, Digestive and Kidney Diseases Information Clearinghouse.

**References**
Evaluation of Splenic Embolization in Patients with Portal Hypertension and Hypersplenism: A. Alwmark, et al.; Ann. Surg., November 1982, vol. 196(5), pp. 518–245.

# BERNARD-SOULIER SYNDROME

**Description** Bernard-Soulier syndrome is an inherited coagulation disorder characterized by abnormalities of blood platelets. Patients have a tendency to bleed excessively and bruise easily. There are 2 forms of the disease, which differ according to the way they are inherited: autosomal recessive (thrombasthenia–thrombocytopenia) and autosomal dominant (thrombopathic thrombocytopenia).

**Synonyms**
Hereditary Giant Platelet Syndrome

**Signs and Symptoms** From the time of birth and throughout life, patients tend to bleed excessively from cuts and other injuries and commonly have nosebleeds and unusually heavy menstrual flow. They also bruise easily and the bruises tend to linger. Subcutaneous bleeding causes purpura in both small spots and large areas. Thrombopathic thrombocytopenia, the autosomal dominant form of this disorder, has been linked with monoclonal gammopathy, hereditary kidney disease, and deafness.

Laboratory studies show that platelets are reduced in number, are larger than normal, and are abnormally shaped; they also exhibit unusual biochemical reactions and have a shortened life span.

**Etiology** Bernard-Soulier syndrome is inherited either through an autosomal recessive or an autosomal dominant gene. Thrombocytopenia, the autosomal recessive form, is thought to be caused by a defects in platelet membrane glycoproteins.

**Related Disorders** See *Thrombasthenia; May-Hegglin Anomaly; Chédiak-Higashi Syndrome*.

**Treatment—Standard** The standard therapy for this disorder consists of transfusion of normal blood or platelets when the patient's bleeding poses a danger. The patient should not be given aspirin and related drugs for arthritis because of their effect on platelet aggregation.

**Treatment—Investigational** Please contact the agencies listed under Resources, below, for the most current information. Addresses and telephone numbers of these agencies, as well as of individual experts and research centers, may be found in the Master Resources List.

**Resources**

**For more information on Bernard-Soulier syndrome:** National Organization for Rare Disorders (NORD); NIH/National Heart, Lung and Blood Institute.

**For genetic information and genetic counseling referrals:** March of Dimes Birth Defects Foundation; Alliance of Genetic Support Groups.

**References**

Defective Adhesion of Blood Platelets to Vascular Microfibrils in the Bernard-Soulier Syndrome: F. Fauvel-Lafeve, et al.; Blood, October 1993, vol. 82(7), pp. 1985–1988.

Cecil Textbook of Medicine, 19th ed.: J.B. Wyngaarden, et al., eds.; W.B. Saunders Company, 1992, p. 997.

Mendelian Inheritance in Man, 10th ed.: V.A. McKusick; The Johns Hopkins University Press, 1992, pp. 1404–1405.

Nelson Textbook of Pediatrics, 14th ed.: R.E. Behrman, ed.-in-chief; W.B. Saunders Company, 1992, p. 1281.

Dictionary of Medical Syndromes, 3rd ed.: S.I. Magalini, et al., eds.: J.B. Lippincott Company, 1990, pp. 105–106.

Hematology, 4th ed.: W.J. Williams, et al., eds.; McGraw-Hill, 1990, pp. 1407–1409.

Hereditary Types of Thrombocytopenia with Giant Platelets and Inclusion Bodies: A. Greinacher, et al.; Blutalkohol, February 1990, vol. 60(2), pp. 53–60.

Bernard-Soulier Syndrome: Whole Blood Diagnostic Assays of Platelets: W.L. Nichols, et al.; Mayo Clin. Proc., May 1989, vol. 64(5), pp. 522–530.

Bernard-Soulier Syndrome: M.C. Berndt, et al.; Baillieres Cl. Haematol., July 1988, vol. 2(3), pp. 585–607.

# CARCINOMA, RENAL CELL

**Description** Renal cell carcinoma, the most common form of kidney cancer in adults, is a malignant disease that occurs in 4 stages. Hematuria is often the first sign.

**Synonyms**

Grawitz Tumor

Hypernephroma

Nephrocarcinoma

Renal Adenocarcinoma

**Signs and Symptoms** Onset is commonly marked by hematuria. Other signs include flank pain, a palpable abdominal mass, hypertension, hypercalcemia, anemia, hepatosis, weight loss, fever, blood clots, and congestive heart failure. Symptoms may not appear until the cancer has spread to the lymph nodes, the lungs, or the long bones. Early diagnosis is important so that prompt treatment can begin. CT scans and sonography are common diagnostic tools.

Staging determines if and where the cancer has spread. In Stage 1 the tumor is confined to kidney tissue; in Stage 2 the tumor involves the fat or adrenal tissues of the kidney; in Stage 3 the tumor moves into the vena cava, the regional kidney nodes, or the lymph nodes and vena cava; in Stage 4 the tumor spreads to other organs (liver, colon, pancreas, or stomach) or to distant corporeal sites.

**Etiology** The exact cause of renal cell carcinoma is unknown. It appears to be more common among pipe and cigar smokers. Patients with von Hippel–Lindau disease, horseshoe kidneys, adult polycystic kidney disease, and kidney failure are also more prone to develop renal cell carcinoma.

Members of the same family may have a genetic predisposition toward developing renal cell carcinoma. Recent research suggests the short arm of chromosome 3 may be responsible. However, the method of inheritance is still unknown.

**Epidemiology** Two to 3 times more males than females are affected, and the disease is more common among those who smoke pipes or cigars. Individuals with other types of kidney disorders or with a family history of renal malignancy are more likely to contract the disease. Renal cell carcinoma accounts for 6 percent, or approximately 18,000 new cases, of kidney malignancies per year in the United States.

**Related Disorders** See *Benign Familial Hematuria; IgA Nephropathy; Polycystic Kidney Diseases.*

**Treatment—Standard** Treatment depends on the stage of the tumor. Surgery is the treatment of choice for primary tumors. CT scan, magnetic resonance imaging (**MRI**) scan, venacavogram, bone scan, and chest x-ray can determine the extent of metastases. Treatment may include radiation, chemotherapy, immunotherapy, hormonal therapy, and the drug vinblastine. Proleukin (interleukin-2) was approved in 1992 for postnephrectomy treatment of metastatic neoplasms. The Cetus Corporation is the manufacturer.

**Treatment—Investigational** Several orphan products are being tested for the treatment of renal cell carcinoma. Roferon-A (interferon α-2a2,6) and intron A (interferon α-2b2,6); poly I: C12u (Ampligen), developed by HEM Research; r-IFN-beta (interferon-β [recombinant]) for treatment of systemic metastatic renal cell carcinoma, manufactured by Biogen; and autolymphocyte therapy, manufactured by Cellcor. More research is needed to determine the long-term safety and effectiveness of all the above.

Please contact the agencies listed under Resources, below, for the most current information. Addresses and tele-

phone numbers of these agencies, as well as of individual experts and research centers, may be found in the Master Resources List.

## Resources

**For more information on renal cell carcinoma:** National Organization for Rare Disorders (NORD); American Cancer Society; National Kidney Foundation; NIH/National Kidney and Urologic Diseases Information Clearinghouse; NIH/National Cancer Institute Physician Data Query Phoneline.

## References

Renal Cell Carcinoma: A Clinicopathologic and DNA Flow Cytometric Analysis of 103 Cases: D. McLemore, et al.; Cancer, November 1989, vol. 64(10), pp. 2133–2140.

Role of Interferons in the Therapy of Metastatic Renal Cell Carcinoma: J.R. Quesada; Urology, October 1989, vol. 34(4), pp. 80–83, discussion pp. 87–96.

Small Renal Neoplasms: Clinical, Pathologic, and Imaging Features: E. Levine, et al.; AJR Am. J. Roentgenol., July 1989, vol. 153(1), pp. 69–73.

Therapeutic Options in Renal Cell Carcinoma: A.C. Buzaid, et al.; Semin. Oncol., February 1989, vol. 16(1), pp. 12–19.

Cecil Textbook of Medicine, 18th ed.: J.B. Wyngaarden and L.H. Smith, Jr., eds.; W.B. Saunders Company, 1988, pp. 652–653.

# CASTLEMAN DISEASE

**Description** Castleman disease is a rare lymph system disorder marked by benign neoplasms in lymph node tissue throughout the body but especially in the neck, base of the head, chest, or stomach.

## Synonyms

Angiofollicular Lymph Node Hyperplasia
Angiomatous Lymphoid
Castleman Tumor
Giant Benign Lymphoma
Hamartoma

**Signs and Symptoms** The neoplasms are single, solid, and contained, and are usually surrounded by normal nodes. Occasionally, neoplasms grow in the veins and mimic an aneurysm. The major symptoms are tumors, respiratory tract infections, dyspnea, coughing, bloody sputum, pain or pressure in the chest or back, fever, and lethargy. Other features include microcyte anemia, hypergammaglobulinemia, and growth retardation.

**Etiology** Although the exact cause is unknown, the disease is thought to reflect the effect of increased IL-6 production.

**Epidemiology** Castleman disease affects equal numbers of males and females of any age.

**Related Disorders** See *Hodgkin Disease.*

Another related disease, **malignant lymphoma,** is marked by circumscribed solid tumors made up of cells that most often appear in lymphatic sites, such as lymph nodes and the spleen. Symptoms may mimic Hodgkin disease or leukemia.

**Treatment—Standard** Surgical excision of the neoplasm is the usual treatment.

**Treatment—Investigational** Please contact the agencies listed under Resources, below, for the most current information. Addresses and telephone numbers of these agencies, as well as of individual experts and research centers, may be found in the Master Resources List.

## Resources

**For more information on Castleman disease:** National Organization for Rare Disorders (NORD); American Cancer Society; NIH/National Cancer Institute Physician Data Query Phoneline.

## References

Castleman Disease: An Unusual Retroperitoneal Mass: D.P. Bartkowski, et al.; J. Urol., January 1988, vol. 139(1), pp. 118–120.

Computerized Tomography of Castleman Disease Simulating a False Renal Artery Aneurysm: A Case Report: L. Friedman, et al.; J. Urol., July 1987, vol. 138(1), pp. 123–124.

Castleman Disease in Children: R.W. Powell, et al.; J. Pediatr. Surg., August 1986, vol. 21(8), pp. 678–682.

# CHÉDIAK-HIGASHI SYNDROME

**Description** A form of albinism, Chédiak-Higashi syndrome is a hereditary disorder characterized by decreased pigmentation, ocular problems, leukocyte anomalies, and increased susceptibility to infections and certain cancers.

## Synonyms

Begnez-Cesar Syndrome

Chédiak-Steinbrinck-Higashi Syndrome
Leukocytic Anomaly Albinism
Oculocutaneous Albinism

**Signs and Symptoms** Because patients have partial albinism, Chédiak-Higashi syndrome can be diagnosed in early infancy when strong light causes ocular discomfort and nystagmus. The number of the patient's leukocytes and platelets is reduced, and neutrophils and lymphocytes contain characteristic inclusions. The patient suffers frequent infections accompanied by high fever and has a tendency to bleed excessively on injury and to bruise easily. The patient's defective blood cells can infiltrate other organs, including the lungs, brain, kidneys, adrenal glands, and liver.

Prenatal diagnosis is based on amniocentesis and chorionic villus sampling. Children who have Chédiak-Higashi syndrome are weak; grow poorly; have splenomegaly, hepatomegaly, and enlarged lymph nodes; and are highly susceptible to leukemias and lymphomas.

**Etiology** Chédiak-Higashi syndrome is transmitted as an autosomal recessive trait. The patient's defective cells are unable to release enzymes into intracellular compartments to destroy foreign material, such as bacteria; they are also unable to produce normal amounts of melanin.

**Related Disorders** See *May-Hegglin Anomaly.*

**Treatment—Standard** The disorder is difficult to treat, and treatment varies according to symptoms. Infections must be kept in check with vigorous antibiotic therapy. Transfusions of leukocytes may also be useful in treating infections. Whole-blood transfusions may be necessary if bleeding becomes excessive after injury or surgery. Any cancers must be treated with accepted cancer therapy. The patient should avoid exposure to sunlight as much as possible and use sunscreens and sunglasses.

**Treatment—Investigational** In patients refractory to standard drug therapy, splenectomy may be beneficial. Severe cases may indicate bone marrow transplantation from allogenic or nonallogenic donors. However, the safety and efficacy of both procedures have yet to be determined.

Please contact the agencies listed under Resources, below, for the most current information. Addresses and telephone numbers of these agencies, as well as of individual experts and research centers, may be found in the Master Resources List.

**Resources**

**For more information on Chédiak-Higashi syndrome:** National Organization for Rare Disorders (NORD); National Organization for Albinism and Hypopigmentation; NIH/National Institute of Allergy and Infectious Diseases.

**For genetic information and genetic counseling referrals:** March of Dimes Birth Defects Foundation; Alliance of Genetic Support Groups.

**References**

Cecil Textbook of Medicine, 19th ed.: J.B. Wyngaarden, et al., eds.; W.B. Saunders Company, 1992, pp. 2322–2323.

Chédiak-Higashi Syndrome: Clinical, Hematologic, and Immunologic Improvement after Splenectomy: H.A. Harfi, et al.; Ann. Allergy, August 1992, vol. 69(2), pp. 147–150.

Mendelian Inheritance in Man, 10th ed.: V.A. McKusick; The Johns Hopkins University Press, 1992, pp. 1279–1281.

Nelson Textbook of Pediatrics, 14th ed.: R.E. Behrman, ed.-in-chief; W.B. Saunders Company, 1992, pp. 566–567.

Prenatal Diagnosis of Chédiak-Higashi Syndrome: R. Diukman, et al.; Prenat. Diagn., November 1992, vol. 12(11), pp. 877–885.

Unrelated Donor Bone Marrow Transplantation for Correction of Lethal Congenital Immunodeficiencies: A.H. Filopovich, et al.; Blood, July 1992, vol. 80(1), pp. 270–276.

Peripheral Neuropathy in the Chédiak-Higashi Syndrome: V.P. Misra, et al.; Acta Neuropathol., 1991, vol. 81(3), pp. 354–358.

Birth Defects Encyclopedia: M.L. Buyse, ed.-in-chief; Blackwell Scientific Publications, 1990, pp. 310–311.

Dictionary of Medical Syndromes, 3rd ed.: S.I. Magalini, et al., eds.: J.B. Lippincott Company, 1990, pp. 175–176.

Hematology, 4th ed.: W.J. Williams, et al., eds.; McGraw-Hill, 1990, pp. 822–824.

Smith's Recognizable Patterns of Human Malformation, 4th ed.: K.L. Jones; W.B. Saunders Company, 1988, p. 542.

# CYCLIC NEUTROPENIA

**Description** A rare blood disorder, cyclic neutropenia is marked by an abnormally severe decrease in the number of circulating neutrophils and other blood components. The decrease occurs at regular intervals, with resulting infections and fever.

**Synonyms**

Cyclic Hematopoiesis
Periodic Neutropenia

**Signs and Symptoms** Patients have a dramatic drop in neutrophil levels below 500/mm³ for 6 to 8 days every 21 days in a constant and consistent cycle that may also affect reticulocytes and platelets. At the same time, levels of eosinophils and monocytes may rise abnormally.

The change in neutrophil levels is usually accompanied by infections and sometimes by aphthous stomatitis. Patients commonly have fatigue, weakness, and fever, and sometimes skin infections, dental problems, and cervical adenopathy. Over the long term, cyclic neutropenia may cause the parotid gland to become inflamed. If the disorder occurs in infancy or childhood, patients tend to improve as they grow older.

**Etiology** When the disease occurs in infants and children, it may be inherited as an autosomal dominant trait. When it occurs in adults, it is believed to be an acquired disease of unknown etiology. Studies suggest that the cyclic nature of the disorder is caused by leukocytes not properly maturing in the patient's bone marrow.

**Epidemiology** Cyclic neutropenia occurs worldwide in equal numbers of males and females. Approximately one-quarter of patients have a family history of the disease.

**Treatment—Standard** Antibiotics are given to treat infections. Granulocyte-colony stimulating factor has been used to increase neutrophil production. Patients require careful oral and dental care. Persons with inherited forms of the disease should receive genetic counseling. Other treatments depend on symptoms.

**Treatment—Investigational** Recombinant growth factor granulocyte stimulating factor (**G-CSF**) appears to alleviate symptoms in cyclic neutropenia by shortening the duration of severe nutropenia.

Please contact the agencies listed under Resources, below, for the most current information. Addresses and telephone numbers of these agencies, as well as of individual experts and research centers, may be found in the Master Resources List.

**Resources**

**For more information on cyclic neutropenia:** National Organization for Rare Disorders (NORD); NIH/National Heart, Lung and Blood Institute.

**For genetic information and genetic counseling referrals:** March of Dimes Birth Defects Foundation; Alliance of Genetic Support Groups.

**References**

A Randomized Controlled Phase III Trial of Recombinant Human G-CSF for Treatment of Severe Chronic Neutropenia: D.C. Dale, et al.; Blood, May 15, 1993, vol. 81, pp. 2496–2502.

Mendelian Inheritance in Man, 9th ed.: V.A. McKusick; The Johns Hopkins University Press, 1990, pp. 660–661.

Treatment of Cyclic Neutropenia with Granulocyte-Colony Stimulating Factor: W.B. Hammond, et al.; N. Engl. J. Med., May 18, 1989, vol. 320, pp. 1306–1311.

Adult-Onset Cyclic Neutropenia Is a Benign Neoplasm Associated with Clonal Proliferation of Large Granular Lymphocytes: T.P. Loughran, Jr., and W.P. Hammond, 4th; J. Exp. Med., December 1, 1986, vol. 164(6), pp. 2089–2094.

Cyclic Hematopoiesis: Human Cyclic Neutropenia: R.D. Lange; Exp. Hematol., July 1983, vol. 11(6), pp. 435–451.

Human Cyclic Neutropenia: Clinical Review and Long-Term Follow-up of Patients: D.G. Wright, et al.; Medicine (Baltimore), January 1981, vol. 60(1), pp. 1–13.

# EWING SARCOMA

**Description** Ewing sarcoma is an inherited malignant neoplastic disease characterized by round-cell tumors that usually occur in the extremities. It occurs most frequently in young persons aged 10 to 20.

**Synonyms**

Endothelioma, Diffuse, of Bones

Myeloma, Endothelial

**Signs and Symptoms** Tumors that are painful to touch (but not always visible) develop, usually in the bones of the arms and legs; however, they can occur in any bone. The tumor tends to involve wide areas of the long bones, sometimes as much as the entire shaft. The femur and humerus are most commonly affected; however, tumors sometimes occur in the pelvis as well. The pain of the tumor worsens with time, and intermittent pain often gets worse at night. Tenderness and swelling are usually present in the area around the tumor; the skin over the tumor may be warm; and blood vessels may be evident on the surface of the skin. The patient may develop anemia and fever. The tumor can spread to lymph nodes, lungs, or the skull if the disease is left untreated.

**Etiology** Ewing sarcoma is not transmitted with a known hereditary pattern. Cytogenetic analysis of fresh Ewing sarcoma tissue has demonstrated consistent rearrangement of chromosome 22, most commonly t(11;22)(q24;q12).

**Epidemiology** Ewing sarcoma occurs most frequently in young men 10 to 20 years of age.

**Related Disorders** The most common primary bone tumor is **osteosarcoma,** which is a painful and highly malignant neoplasm that usually occurs in the knee area, although it can occur in any bone, and commonly metastasizes to the lungs. Patients are usually between 10 and 20 years of age, but osteosarcoma can occur in persons of any age.

**Malignant lymphoma of the bone** is characterized by a small round-cell tumor that may occur in any bone and can spread to soft tissue or other bones. It most commonly affects individuals in their 40s and 50s. Pain and swelling are common. The standard treatment is a combination of radiation therapy and chemotherapy.

Another malignant bone tumor is **chondrosarcoma,** which affects cartilage. If the disease is severe, the tumors grow rapidly and metastasize. Chondrosarcomas can also seed themselves in surrounding soft tissue. Surgery is the usual treatment.

The most commonly occurring benign bone tumor is **osteochondroma,** which may be a single or multiple neoplasm that occurs most frequently in young persons between 10 and 20 years of age. Researchers have discovered a strong tendency among family members to develop these tumors.

**Treatment—Standard** Combinations of surgery, radiation therapy, and chemotherapy are used to treat Ewing sarcoma. The 5-year survival rate is approximately 50 percent.

**Treatment—Investigational** Please contact the agencies listed under Resources, below, for the most current information. Addresses and telephone numbers of these agencies, as well as of individual experts and research centers, may be found in the Master Resources List.

**Resources**

**For more information on Ewing sarcoma:** National Organization for Rare Disorders (NORD); American Cancer Society; NIH/National Cancer Institute Physician Data Query Phoneline.

**For genetic information and genetic counseling referrals:** March of Dimes Birth Defects Foundation; Alliance of Genetic Support Groups.

**References**

Mendelian Inheritance in Man, 9th ed.: V.A. McKusick; The Johns Hopkins University Press, 1990, p. 315.

Long-Term Results in 144 Localized Ewing's Sarcoma Patients Treated with Combined Therapy: G. Bacci, et al.; Cancer, April 15, 1989, vol. 63(8), pp. 1477–1486.

Immunohistological Characterization of a Ewing's Sarcoma Case: S. Lizard-Nacol, et al.; Cancer Detect. Prev., 1988, vol. 12(1–6), pp. 297–302.

# Factor IX Deficiency

**Description** Factor IX deficiency is an inherited coagulation disorder characterized by severe and prolonged hemorrhaging and, in extreme cases, articular pain and bone deformities. The disorder mimics classic hemophilia A but occurs only 20 percent as often. The mostly male patients have a deficiency of factor IX, which is a component of thromboplastin, at birth; however, the severity of the deficiency varies from family to family. Rarely, a mild form of the disorder is found in female carriers.

**Synonyms**

Christmas Disease

Hemophilia B

Plasma Thromboplastin Component Deficiency

**Signs and Symptoms** Patients have prolonged episodes of hemorrhaging that are either spontaneous or related to injury and that occur at or near the surface of the skin or internally. In mild cases, patients hemorrhage only after surgery or tooth extractions. In more severe cases, hemorrhage can occur in any part of the body, including the central nervous system and the gastrointestinal tract. In extreme cases, internal hemorrhaging in muscle, joints, and bone builds up and can cause pain and deformity. Ultimately, the tips of long bones are eroded and chronic problems develop, such as cell necrosis, periosteal pain, and the formation of pseudocysts. Patients who receive transfusions over a long period sometimes develop substances in their blood that inhibit factor IX activity.

**Etiology** Factor IX deficiency is an X-linked recessive genetic trait whose penetrance is incomplete. Patients have diminished amounts of thromboplastin in their blood as a result of the deficient factor IX.

**Epidemiology** While factor IX deficiency most commonly affects males, researchers have documented some occurrence in female carriers of the genetic trait.

**Related Disorders** See *Hemophilia; von Willebrand Disease.*

**Treatment—Standard** Patients are transfused with fresh-frozen plasma for minor hemorrhaging, or prothrombin complex concentrates rich in factor IX for severe episodes. Patients risk getting hepatitis or AIDS if they receive infected prothrombin concentrates that have not been properly screened. An increased load of factor IX might result in coagulation in the veins.

Pseudocysts in bones, muscles, or joints that result in pain and disability can be surgically removed, but patients need to be carefully monitored during any type of surgery, including dental surgery. Patients and their families should receive genetic counseling. Other therapies depend on symptoms.

**Treatment—Investigational** Monoclonal factor IX has been developed for use in factor IX replacement therapy and to treat complications of hemorrhaging. The manufacturer is Armour Pharmaceutical Company.

Please contact the agencies listed under Resources, below, for the most current information. Addresses and telephone numbers of these agencies, as well as of individual experts and research centers, may be found in the Master Resources List.

**Resources**

**For more information on factor IX deficiency:** National Organization for Rare Disorders (NORD); National Hemophilia Foundation; Canadian Hemophilia Society; World Federation of Hemophilia; Haemophilia Society; NIH/National Heart, Lung and Blood Institute.

**For genetic information and genetic counseling referrals:** March of Dimes Birth Defects Foundation; Alliance of Genetic Support Groups.

**References**

The Metabolic Basis of Inherited Disease, 6th ed.: C.R. Scriver, et al., eds.; McGraw-Hill, 1989, pp. 2116–2119.

Internal Medicine, 2nd ed.: J.H. Stein, ed.-in-chief; Little, Brown and Company, 1987, p. 1014.

Introduction of Split Tolerance and Clinical Cure in High-Responding Hemophiliacs with Factor IX Antibodies: I.M. Nilsson, et al.; Proc. Natl. Acad. Sci., December 1986, vol. 83(23), pp. 9169–9173.

Repair of Ventricular Septal Defect and Aortic Regurgitation Associated with Severe Hemophilia B: A. Mazzucco, et al.; Ann. Thorac. Surg., July 1986, vol. 42(1), pp. 97–99.

# FACTOR XIII DEFICIENCY

**Description** Factor XIII deficiency is an extremely rare inherited disorder that prevents the patient's blood from clotting normally and can result in slow internal bleeding. Two forms of the disease are acquired factor XIII deficiency and congenital factor XIII deficiency.

**Synonyms**

>
> Fibrin Stabilizing Factor Deficiency
>
> Fibrinase Deficiency
>
> Fibrinoligase Deficiency
>
> Laki-Lorand Factor Deficiency
>
> Plasma Transglutaminase Deficiency

**Signs and Symptoms** Internal bleeding may seep into surrounding soft tissue several days after trauma, even mild trauma such as a bump or bruise. Pain and swelling may precede the bleeding. If the bleeding persists, large cysts can form in the surrounding tissue spaces, destroy surrounding bone, and cause peripheral nerve damage, usually in the thigh and buttocks areas. At birth, the patient may bleed from the umbilical cord, a phenomenon that rarely occurs in other blood disorders. The most serious hemorrhaging occurs in the central nervous system following mild head trauma. Hemorrhaging may stop spontaneously without treatment.

Women with this condition who become pregnant usually have miscarriages. Men may be sterile or have extremely low sperm counts. Replacing factor XIII does not correct sterility. Some of the less frequently seen signs of this disorder are poor wound healing, excessive bleeding from wounds, retroperitoneal hematomas, and blood in the urine.

The following symptoms are seldom or never seen, helping to differentiate factor XIII deficiency from other bleeding disorders: excessive blood loss during menstruation, ocular hemorrhage, gastrointestinal bleeding, arthritis caused by an accumulation of blood in the joints, postoperative hemorrhage, mucous membrane bleeding, and petechiae.

The condition is not generally a threat to patients who need surgery because even small amounts of factor XIII present in blood transfusions will prevent postoperative hemorrhaging. Excessive bleeding from wounds, abrasions, or even spontaneous abortions is not common unless the patient uses aspirin or similar medications.

**Etiology** Although the exact cause of this disorder is unknown, it may be acquired in conjunction with other disorders or inherited as an autosomal dominant or autosomal recessive gene. Congenital factor XIII deficiency is inherited as a dominant trait. Those who acquire it through autosomal recessive genes have reduced levels of factor XIII in their blood but are usually symptomless.

**Epidemiology** Factor XIII deficiency occurs equally in men and women. The disorder has been seen in pregnant women at term, in newborns, in persons who have undergone major surgery, in those who have sickle cell disease, and in many children with Schoenlein-Henoch purpura.

The disorder sometimes occurs secondary to hepatic carcinoma and cirrhosis. In such cases, levels of factor XIII can be returned to normal when the underlying liver disease is treated. Patients previously treated with isoniazid or who have chronic kidney failure may develop anticoagulation antibodies.

**Related Disorders** See *von Willebrand Disease; Factor IX Deficiency; Hemophilia; Purpura, Schoenlein-Henoch.*

**Treatment—Standard** Since normal plasma contains just 10 percent of factor XIII, patients who receive small infusions of fresh or frozen plasma, cryoprecipitate, or factor XIII concentrates every 3 to 4 weeks can have a normal response to trauma. Because some patients have a high incidence of intracranial bleeding, preventive treatment is necessary. Pregnant women can be given exogenous factor XIII to help prevent spontaneous abortion. Patients and their families may need genetic counseling. Other treatments depend on symptoms.

**Treatment—Investigational** Isolated factor XIII preparations are under development as a potential treatment, as is the orphan drug fibrogammin. For more information on fibrogammin, please contact Hoechst-Roussel Pharmaceuticals.

Please contact the agencies listed under Resources, below, for the most current information. Addresses and telephone numbers of these agencies, as well as of individual experts and research centers, may be found in the Master Resources List.

**Resources**

**For more information on factor XIII deficiency:** National Organization for Rare Disorders (NORD); National Hemophilia Foundation; World Federation of Hemophilia; NIH/National Heart, Lung and Blood Institute.

**For genetic information and genetic counseling referrals:** March of Dimes Birth Defects Foundation; Alliance of Genetic Support Groups.

**References**

Cecil Textbook of Medicine, 19th ed.: J.B. Wyngaarden, et al., eds.; W.B. Saunders Company, 1992, pp. 1010–1011.
Mendelian Inheritance in Man, 10th ed.: V.A. McKusick; The Johns Hopkins University Press, 1992, pp. 379–381.
Birth Defects Encyclopedia: M.L. Buyse, ed.-in-chief; Blackwell Scientific Publications, 1990, pp. 680–681.
Hematology, 4th ed.: W.J. Williams, et al., eds.; McGraw-Hill, 1990, pp. 1491–1492.
Internal Medicine, 2nd ed.: J.H. Stein, ed.; Little, Brown and Company, 1987, p. 1017.

# GASTRIC LYMPHOMA, NON-HODGKIN TYPE

**Description** Non-Hodgkin gastric lymphoma is an extremely rare malignant stomach neoplasm that is characterized by a bulky mass, abdominal pain, and anemia.

**Synonyms**

Stomach Lymphoma, Non-Hodgkin Type

**Signs and Symptoms** X-rays reveal a bulky mass in the stomach that is often associated with hemorrhagic gastritis, stress ulcer, or monilial gastritis. Endoscopic biopsy and brushing cytology are also used to diagnose this disease.

**Etiology** The cause is not known.

**Epidemiology** Only about 5 percent of the total of all primary malignant stomach neoplasms are non-Hodgkin gastric lymphoma. The disease occurs about 10 years earlier than stomach carcinoma and is most common in persons of Japanese, Thai, and Finnish heritage and in those who live in the mountain regions of Colombia. Males are affected more often than females.

**Related Disorders** See *Zollinger-Ellison Syndrome; Familial Polyposis; Peutz-Jeghers Syndrome.*

**Gastric carcinoma,** the 3rd most commonly occurring gastrointestinal cancer in the United States, is characterized by a distended stomach, enlarged gastric folds, obstructing lesions, and an ulcerated mass in the stomach. It generally affects men older than 50 years of age and persons who consume foods high in salt and nitrates rather than a diet high in vegetables and fresh fruits.

**Treatment—Standard** Stomach surgery, multiagent chemotherapy, radiation therapy, or combined radiation therapy and chemotherapy are used to treat this cancer. A chemotherapeutic regimen of cyclophosphamide, nitrogen mustard, Oncovin (vincristine), procarbazine, and prednisone (C-MOPP) is currently being used with success. Also in use is a combination of cyclophosphamide, Oncovin (vincristine), doxorubicin, and prednisone (CHOP) administered along with radiation and other chemicals.

The Food and Drug Administration has recently given approval for Leukine (Immunex Corp.) to be used in the treatment of non-Hodgkin lymphoma.

**Treatment—Investigational** The drug 2-chlorodeoxyadenosine (2CdA) is being tested in the treatment of leukemias and malignant lymphomas such as gastric lymphoma. The orphan product technetium Tx-99 murine monoclonal antibody (IgG2a) to BCE (Immuraid-LL-2 [99mTc]) is being studied for its use in evaluating the extent of non-Hodgkin B-cell lymphoma and of some forms of leukemia. The product is sponsored by Immunomedics. Another orphan product, Cladribine (leustatin injection), is being investigated for the treatment of this disorder. The sponsor is R.W. Johnson Research Institute.

Please contact the agencies listed under Resources, below, for the most current information. Addresses and telephone numbers of these agencies, as well as of individual experts and research centers, may be found in the Master Resources List.

**Resources**

**For more information on non-Hodgkin gastric lymphoma:** National Organization for Rare Disorders (NORD);

American Cancer Society; NIH/National Cancer Institute Physician Data Query Phoneline; Cancer Information Service.

**References**

Internal Medicine, 3rd ed.: J.H. Stein, ed.-in-chief; Little, Brown and Company, 1990, p. 347.

Recent Results of Multimodal Therapy of Gastric Lymphoma: M.H. Shiu, et al.; Cancer, October 1, 1986, vol. 54(10), pp. 594–597.

The Role of Brushing Cytology in the Diagnosis of Gastric Malignancy: I. Cook, et al.; Acta Cytol., July–August, 1988, vol. 32(4), pp. 461–464.

# GLIOBLASTOMA MULTIFORME

**Description** Glioblastoma multiforme is a highly malignant primary brain tumor that grows rapidly and has the ability to invade surrounding tissue by spreading in a butterfly pattern through the white matter of the cerebral hemispheres. The tumor may invade the dura mater or spread to the ventricles of the brain via cerebrospinal fluid. It rarely metastasizes outside the brain and spinal cord.

**Synonyms**

> Giant Cell Glioblastoma
>
> Spongioblastoma Multiforme

**Signs and Symptoms** Due to the tumor's rapid growth pattern, an increase in cranial pressure is usually the first symptom of glioblastoma multiforme. Pressure builds because the cranium is unable to expand to accommodate the growing tumor. The patient may complain of a generalized headache that is more painful in the morning, accompanied by vomiting but rarely nausea. These symptoms may be preceded by subtle personality changes.

Glioblastoma multiforme most commonly occurs in the frontal, temporal, and parietal lobes of the cerebral hemispheres, although it may occur in other areas of the hemispheres as well.

Glioblastomas in the frontal lobe usually cause memory impairment or other intellectual disabilities. Patients may show little or no emotions and may suffer convulsions and hemiplegia of the side of the body opposite the tumor.

Tumors in the temporal lobe can cause seizures, poor coordination of body parts or other motor disturbances, and interference with the ability to interpret language.

The symptoms of parietal lobe tumors are agraphia, paresthesia or similar sensory changes, spatial disorientation or loss of position awareness of body parts, and seizures.

**Etiology** While the cause of glioblastoma multiforme, like most brain tumors, is unknown, tumors have been reported in family members. However, researchers have not proved heredity as a means of transmission.

Certain chemicals in the workplace have been associated with some tumors, including vinyl chloride, chemicals used in rubber manufacturing, and chemical sprays used by farmers. Some studies suggest that children exposed to lead or barbiturates may be at a slightly higher risk of developing this tumor. Other studies indicate that a rare virus may cause glioblastomas, but the research is inconclusive.

**Epidemiology** Men are twice as likely as women to be afflicted by glioblastoma multiforme, and the tumor occurs more frequently in whites than in nonwhites and most often in people between the ages of 48 and 60, although it has been seen in preteens as well. Men with blood type A appear to be at a higher risk.

**Related Disorders** See *Astrocytoma, Malignant.*

**Treatment—Standard** Surgery with or without radiation therapy and chemotherapy is the standard treatment for accessible glioblastomas. If the tumor is not accessible, a biopsy may be performed to determine if the tumor is amenable to other treatments, and steroid medications may be given to control swelling. To ameliorate symptoms and increase the effectiveness of other therapies, subtotal decompressive resection may be performed. If the tumor has invaded the brain extensively, either biopsy or partial resection may be performed, primarily to relieve symptoms.

Aggressive surgery or total resection, often done with the use of an operating microscope, attempts to remove all identifiable tumor. A laser or ultrasonic aspirator can be used in some cases. Surgeons use lasers to vaporize tissue beyond the tumor's border and try to remove tumor infiltrates with a minimal amount of damage to normal tissue. Because glioblastomas infiltrate so extensively, even aggressive resection cannot totally remove the tumor, and follow-up radiation therapy and chemotherapy are needed. If the tumor recurs, a 2nd or even 3rd operation may be performed. External irradiation to both the tumor and the entire brain usually follows surgery almost immediately.

Either during or after radiation therapy, cytotoxic drugs are given in an attempt to destroy any remaining tumor cells. However, since cytotoxins are not completely cell-specific, they may also cause damage to normal tissue. Carmustine (**BCNU**) and lomustine (**CCNU**) are the most commonly used drugs.

**Treatment—Investigational** Brachytherapy is an experimental treatment for glioblastoma multiforme that surgically implants radioactive pellets, such as iodine, iridium, or gold isotopes, directly into the tumor. It is used primarily when a recurrent tumor is confined to one side of the brain and measures less than 2½ inches.

Other therapies under investigation are the use of cell radiosensitizers to increase the effectiveness of radiation; the use of different types of radiation, such as neutrons, hyperthermia, and photoradiation; intraoperative radiation; and hyperfractionation.

Immunotherapy with such drugs as interferon, levamisole, interleukin-2, thymosine, and BCG (bacille Calmette-Guérin), is also being tried. Clinical trials are under way of the orphan drug sodium monomercaptoundecahydro-closo-dodecaborate (Boralife), used as an alternative to conventional photon therapy.

Please contact the agencies listed under Resources, below, for the most current information. Addresses and telephone numbers of these agencies, as well as of individual experts and research centers, may be found in the Master Resources List.

**Resources**

**For more information on glioblastoma multiforme:** National Organization for Rare Disorders (NORD); NIH/National Institute of Neurological Disorders and Stroke; American Brain Tumor Association; American Cancer Society; NIH/National Cancer Institute Physician Data Query Phoneline.

**References**

About Glioblastoma Multiforme and Malignant Astrocytoma: D.P. Hesser et al., eds.; Association for Brain Tumor Research, 1985.

# GLUCOSE-6-PHOSPHATE DEHYDROGENASE (G6PD) DEFICIENCY

**Description** G6PD deficiency is a genetically determined enzyme abnormality that usually has no symptoms but can lead to serious medical consequences, such as hemolytic anemia or favism. G6PD is an enzyme present in all cells that is essential to glucose metabolism and provides erythrocytes with a defense against the destructive effects of certain drugs.

**Signs and Symptoms** Most patients are asymptomatic; however, the symptoms that do occur range in intensity from mild and chronic to life-threatening, and they usually mimic those of acute hemolytic anemia, i.e., shock, fever, chills, pain in the abdomen and back, and sometimes hemoglobinuria and renal failure. Drugs implicated in causing hemolytic anemia include acetanilid, methylene blue, nalidixic acid, naphthalene, niridazole, nitrofurantoin, pamaquine, pentaquine, phenylhydrazine, primaquine, sulfacetamide, sulfamethoxazole, sulfanilamide, sulfapyridine, thiacolesulfone, toluidine blue, and trinitrotoluene. Aspirin, certain derivatives of vitamin K, fava beans, diabetes acidosis, and acute viral or bacterial infections can also cause acute hemolytic anemia in G6PD-deficient patients.

**Etiology** G6PD deficiency is an X-linked genetically transmitted trait.

**Epidemiology** G6PD deficiency is the most common genetically determined enzyme deficiency in humans, affecting an estimated 400 million people in the world. It occurs most frequently in tropical and subtropical Asia, tropical Africa, areas of the Mediterranean, the Middle East, and New Guinea. Scientists have identified more than 300 different varieties of this deficiency, all of which result from G6PD gene mutations. Some variations are more common among black American males. The condition is difficult to diagnose because serious symptoms do not occur until the patient is exposed to certain drugs.

**Related Disorders Favism** occurs when individuals with G6PD deficiency consume fava beans or inhale fava pollen. Researchers believe that 2 chemicals present in high concentrations in fava beans, divicine and isouramil, are responsible for the reactions, which include jaundice, severe anemia, possible coma, fever, pallor, tachycardia, weakness, pain in the abdomen or back, and dark red urine. Onset is sudden, occurring within 5 to 24 hours after the person ingests fava beans or only minutes after he or she inhales the pollen.

**Treatment—Standard** Preventive measures should be taken, such as screening patients for G6PD deficiency before they are given antimalarial drugs or any of the drugs listed in the Signs and Symptoms section above. If hemolysis occurs after any of these drugs are administered, the drug should be discontinued and hydration should be maintained. People found to have G6PD deficiency should avoid fava beans and areas where they are grown. Patients and their families should receive genetic counseling. Other treatments depend on symptoms.

**Treatment—Investigational** Please contact the agencies listed under Resources, below, for the most current information. Addresses and telephone numbers of these agencies, as well as of individual experts and research centers, may be found in the Master Resources List.

**Resources**

**For more information on glucose-6-phosphate dehydrogenase deficiency:** National Organization for Rare Disorders (NORD); NIH/National Diabetes, Digestive and Kidney Diseases Information Clearinghouse; Research Trust for Metabolic Diseases in Children.

**For genetic information and genetic counseling referrals:** March of Dimes Birth Defects Foundation; Alliance of Genetic Support Groups.

### References

Mendelian Inheritance in Man, 9th ed.: V.A. McKusick; The Johns Hopkins University Press, 1990, pp. 357–358, 1213–1215, 1595–1611.

Chronic Nonspherocytic Hemolytic Anemia (CNSHA) and Glucose-6-Phosphate Dehydrogenase (G6PD) Deficiency in a Patient with Familial Amyloidotic Polyneuropathy (FAP): Molecular Study of a New Variant (G6PD Clinic) with Markedly Acidic PH Optimum: J.L. Vives-Corrons, et al.; Hum. Genet., January 1989, vol. 81(2), pp. 161–164.

Diverse Point Mutations in the Human Glucose-6-Phosphate Dehydrogenase Gene Cause Enzyme Deficiency and Mild or Severe Hemolytic Anemia: T.J. Vulliamy, et al.; Proc. Natl. Acad. Sci. USA, July 1988, vol. 85(14), pp. 5171–5175.

The Suitability of Saliva for Detection of Glucose-6-Phosphate Dehydrogenase Deficiency: A.H. Beaumont, et al.; Mol. Biol. Rep., 1988, vol. 13(2), pp. 73–78.

Tolerability of Tiaprofenic Acid in Patients with Glucose-6-Phosphate Dehydrogenase (G6PD) Deficiency: Q. Mela, et al.; Drugs, 1988, vol. 35 (suppl. 1), pp. 107–110.

Internal Medicine, 2nd ed.: J.H. Stein, ed.-in-chief; Little, Brown and Company, 1987, pp. 1052–1054.

# GRANULOMATOUS DISEASE, CHRONIC (CGD)

**Description** CGD is a very rare blood disorder that affects neutrophils and is characterized by widespread granulomatous lesions. The affected patient is unable to resist infections.

**Synonyms**

Chronic Dysphagocytosis

Granulomatosis, Chronic, Familial

Granulomatosis, Septic, Progressive

**Signs and Symptoms** Patients suffer repeated infections that include suppurative lymphadenitis, liver abscesses, pneumonia, and osteomyelitis. Chronic infections may be evident in the liver, gastrointestinal tract, eyes, and brain. Hypergammaglobulinemia, anemia, leukocytosis, and hepatomegaly are characteristic. Dermatitis, diarrhea, perianal abscesses, and rhinitis may also be present. The widespread granulomatous lesions may occur in any organ and commonly cause obstruction of the gastrointestinal tract.

**Etiology** The cause of the X-linked form of CGD is a lack of cytochrome b, a component of the NADPH oxidase enzyme responsible for making $H_2O_2$. The gene for the X-linked form of CGD has been located in the middle of the short arm of the X chromosome, but autosomal variants of the disorder may involve other genes in females and males coding for other protein components that are necessary for NADPH oxidase activity.

**Epidemiology** The disorder affects only 1:1,000,000 persons, males more often than females. Symptoms usually occur during childhood but may be delayed to early teens and rarely into adulthood.

**Related Disorders** See *Wegener Granulomatosis; Churg-Strauss Syndrome; Polyarteritis Nodosa.*

**Treatment—Standard** The standard treatment is antibiotic therapy with such agents as trimethoprim and sulfamethoxazole; corticosteroid drugs are also beneficial. Patients and their families may require genetic counseling. Any other therapy should be based on symptoms and designed to help the patient's body resist infection. The orphan drug interferon-γ attenuates the number of infections.

**Treatment—Investigational** Bone marrow transplants can be successful when the procedure is performed on a young patient.

Clinical trials are under way at Johns Hopkins Hospital to study compassionate treatment of recombinant human interferon-γ therapy in patients with CGD and active infection. Intraconazole is being studied at the National Institutes of Health for treatment of aspergillosis in patients with CGD. In an effort to prevent onset of CGD, researchers at Stanford University are investigating the transfusion of bone marrow stem cells into fetuses.

Please contact the agencies listed under Resources, below, for the most current information. Addresses and telephone numbers of these agencies, as well as of individual experts and research centers, may be found in the Master Resources List.

**Resources**

**For more information on chronic granulomatous disease:** National Organization for Rare Disorders (NORD); NIH/National Institute of Allergy and Infectious Diseases.

**For genetic information and genetic counseling referrals:** March of Dimes Birth Defects Foundation; Alliance of Genetic Support Groups.

**References**

Research Highlights: J.E. Smith, Ph.D.; NIH Research Resources Reporter, March 1989.

Clinical Features and Current Management of Chronic Granulomatous Disease: C.B. Forrest, et al.; Hematol. Oncol. Clin. North Am., June 1988, vol. 2(2), pp. 253–266.

Detection of Carriers of the Autosomal Form of Chronic Granulomatous Disease: A.J. Verhoeven, et al.; Blood, February 1988, vol. 71(2), pp. 505–507.

Recombinant Human Interferon-Gamma Reconstitutes Defective Phagocyte Function in Patients with Chronic Granulomatous Disease in Childhood: J.M. Sechler, et al.; Proc. Natl. Acad. Sci. USA, July 1988, vol. 85(13), pp. 4874–4878.

Corticosteroids in Treatment of Obstructive Lesions of Chronic Granulomatous Disease: T.W. Chin, et al.; J. Pediatrics, September 1987, vol. 111(3), pp. 512–518.

Internal Medicine, 2nd ed.: J.H. Stein, ed.-in-chief; Little, Brown and Company, 1987, pp. 1286–1288.

Mendelian Inheritance in Man, 8th ed.: V.A. McKusick; The Johns Hopkins University Press, 1986, p. 973.

# HAGEMAN FACTOR DEFICIENCY

**Description** Hageman factor deficiency is a genetic blood disorder caused by a lack of blood factor XII (the Hageman factor), a single-chain glycoprotein necessary for blood clotting. Because other blood-clotting factors tend to compensate for factor XII, there are usually no symptoms and the disorder is only accidentally discovered through preoperative blood tests.

**Signs and Symptoms** Although it happens rarely, Hageman factor deficiency can lead to blood clots at an early age that inhibit circulation and might cause myocardial infarction or thrombophlebitis.

Patients are not prone to unusual bleeding, and petechiae and ecchymoses are absent. However, the blood of affected patients takes an abnormally long time to clot, and serum prothrombin and thromboplastin time are usually abnormal. The blood level of Hageman factor tends to vary greatly in affected patients.

Diagnosis is made if blood from a person suspected to have the disorder does not correct the deficiency in blood from a person known to have the disorder.

**Etiology** Although the exact mechanism is not well understood, Hageman factor deficiency is genetically transmitted through autosomal recessive genes believed to be defective on chromosome 5.

**Epidemiology** Men and women are affected in equal numbers. Orientals inherit Hageman factor deficiency more often than people of European descent. The parents of affected patients are closely related in about 10 percent of cases.

**Related Disorders** See *Factor IX Deficiency; Factor XIII Deficiency.*

**Treatment—Standard** Because bleeding caused by this disorder is usually mild, Hageman factor deficiency is generally not treated.

**Treatment—Investigational** Please contact the agencies listed under Resources, below, for the most current information. Addresses and telephone numbers of these agencies, as well as of individual experts and research centers, may be found in the Master Resources List.

**Resources**

**For more information on Hageman factor deficiency:** National Organization for Rare Disorders (NORD); National Hemophilia Foundation; NIH/National Heart, Lung and Blood Institute.

**References**

Immunoblotting Studies of Coagulation Factor XII, Plasma Prekallikrein, and High Molecular Weight Kininogen: B. Lammle, et al.; Semin. Thromb. Hemost., January 1987, vol. 13(1), pp. 106–114.

The Contact Activation System: Biochemistry and Interactions of These Surface-Mediated Defense Reactions: R.W. Colman, et al.; Crc. Crit. Rev. Oncol. Hematol., 1986, vol. 5(1), pp. 57–85.

Mendelian Inheritance in Man, 7th ed.: V.A. McKusick; The Johns Hopkins University Press, 1986, pp. 1015–1016.

The Metabolic Basis of Inherited Disease, 5th ed.: J.B. Stanbury, et al., eds.; McGraw-Hill, 1983, pp. 1548–1549.

# HEMANGIOMA-THROMBOCYTOPENIA SYNDROME

**Description** In hemangioma-thrombocytopenia syndrome, the low number of blood platelets causes bleeding in association with a cavernous hemangioma.

**Synonyms**

Kasabach-Merritt Syndrome

**Signs and Symptoms** Hemangioma-thrombocytopenia syndrome is marked by a benign cavernous hemangioma that occurs along with an abnormally low number of blood platelets. The resultant purpura typically develops within the first 6 weeks of life but may appear later in childhood as the hemangioma grows. Usually only one hemangioma is found on the neck, arm, leg, or trunk of the body. Less common are internal tumors of the tongue, thorax, spleen, liver, gastrointestinal tract, or bones. Hemangiomas are rarely found both internally and externally. Hemangiomas may become engorged before a bleeding spell occurs. The cause is idiopathic, but it can be triggered by trauma.

Thrombocytopenia may occur within the first month of life in association with a placental chorioangioma or large hemangiomas of the skin. A decrease in hemoglobin, erythrocytes, or proteins such as prothrombin and fibrinogen may also occur. However, fibrinogen deficiency usually affects older children and adults.

**Etiology** The exact cause is not known. It is thought that the thrombocytopenia may be a result of platelet destruction in association with growth of the hemangioma. There is no evidence that the syndrome is hereditary.

**Epidemiology** Males and females are affected in equal numbers. Approximately 1:500 cases of hemangiomas have associated thrombocytopenia.

**Related Disorders** See *Blue Rubber Bleb Nevus; Cavernous Hemangioma; Essential Thrombocytopenia.*

**Treatment—Standard** Diagnosis is confirmed with magnetic resonance imaging, CT scans, and x-rays. Some hemangiomas resolve spontaneously, but large surface tumors can be excised followed by immediate correction of the blood abnormalities. Laser surgery is beneficial in some cases. If the hemangioma is inoperable, or if multiple hemangiomas are present, radiation may be indicated. Platelet transfusion is beneficial to counteract hemorrhaging.

**Treatment—Investigational** Please contact the agencies listed under Resources, below, for the most current information. Addresses and telephone numbers of these agencies, as well as of individual experts and research centers, may be found in the Master Resources List.

**Resources**

For more information on hemangioma-thrombocytopenia syndrome: National Organization for Rare Disorders (NORD); NIH/National Heart, Lung and Blood Institute Information Center.

For genetic information and genetic counseling referrals: March of Dimes Birth Defects Foundation; Alliance of Genetic Support Groups.

**References**

Mendelian Inheritance in Man, 10th ed.: V.A. McKusick; The Johns Hopkins University Press, 1992, p. 460.

Nelson Textbook of Pediatrics, 14th ed.: R.E. Behrman, ed.-in-chief; W.B. Saunders Company, 1992, pp. 1280–1281.

Birth Defects Encyclopedia: M.L. Buyse, ed.-in-chief; Blackwell Scientific Publications, 1990, pp. 852–853.

Clinical Dermatology, 2nd ed.: T.P. Habif, M.D., ed.; C.V. Mosby Company, 1990, p. 583.

Hemangioma Thrombocytopenia Syndrome: A Case Masquerading As an Encephalocele: D.M. Orenstein, et al.; Am. J. Dis. Child., June 1977, vol. 131(6), pp. 680–681.

# HEMOCHROMATOSIS, HEREDITARY

**Description** Hereditary hemochromatosis is a metabolic disorder characterized by excessive absorption of iron in the gastrointestinal tract. The accumulation of iron eventually damages numerous organs. Involvement of the liver, pancreas, or heart may lead to serious consequences, particularly in elderly patients. Joints and skin may also become diseased.

**Synonyms**

Bronze Diabetes
Familial Hemochromatosis
Iron Overload Disease
Primary Hemochromatosis
Troisier-Hanot-Chauffard Syndrome

**Signs and Symptoms** Symptoms develop usually in men between ages 40 and 60 years, and later in women. The symptoms vary according to the organs involved. Early symptoms are nonspecific and include weakness, weight loss, apathy, loss of libido, and pain in the extremities. Muscle tenderness and cramps in the legs may develop.

Later stages of the disease are characterized by cirrhosis of the liver, diabetes, gradual darkening of the skin, and congestive heart failure. Enlargement of the liver may begin years before it becomes impaired. Eventually, this organ becomes firm and smooth, with iron deposits in the parenchymal cells. Cancer of the liver is more prevalent in patients with hemochromatosis than in unaffected individuals.

When the heart muscle is involved, cardiac enlargement, arrhythmias, and congestive heart failure may result. Involvement of the pituitary gland can cause secondary dysfunction of the various endocrine glands it regulates: thyroid dysfunction may lead to increased sensitivity to cold; secondary adrenocortical insufficiency, to weakness and lack of resistance to stress; and secondary gonadal dysfunction, to testicular atrophy, loss of libido, and amenorrhea.

**Etiology** Hemochromatosis is inherited as an autosomal recessive trait. The defective gene is on the short arm of chromosome 6 close to HLA-A (6p21.3). Carriers can be identified through testing. The exact enzymatic deficiency is unknown. Relatives of an individual who is homozygous for the mutant gene can be identified by tissue typing; however, the test is expensive and impractical for mass screening. Researchers have measured the degree of saturation of transferrin in the serum to screen for the disease. This test is inexpensive and can detect the disorder before organs become damaged.

**Epidemiology** Hemochromatosis affects an estimated 600,000 to 1.6 million Americans, with carriers ranging from 24 million to 32 million. The disorder is diagnosed rarely, however; fewer than 250,000 cases have been identified in the United States.

Hemochromatosis is expressed fully in homozygotes only. Heterozygotes may develop it if they have diabetes or are alcoholic. Symptoms occur more often in men than in women because women lose blood during menstruation and pregnancy.

**Treatment—Standard** After hemochromatosis has been diagnosed, damage to organs can be prevented by repeated phlebotomies to remove iron. Beginning this treatment early in the course will improve the prognosis. In those cases where multiple phlebotomies cause anemia, injections of deferoxamine may reduce levels of iron without producing anemia. Secondary disorders are treated symptomatically.

**Treatment—Investigational** Gary M. Brittenham, M.D., has been awarded a grant from the Office of Orphan Products Development, Food and Drug Administration, for his research work on chelation therapy with oral iron chelators.

Please contact the agencies listed under Resources, below, for the most current information. Addresses and telephone numbers of these agencies, as well as of individual experts and research centers, may be found in the Master Resources List.

**Resources**

**For more information on hereditary hemochromatosis:** National Organization for Rare Disorders (NORD); Hereditary Hemochromatosis Research Foundation; NIH/National Diabetes, Digestive and Kidney Diseases Information Clearinghouse; Iron Overload Diseases Association.

**For genetic information and genetic counseling referrals:** March of Dimes Birth Defects Foundation; Alliance of Genetic Support Groups.

**References**

Cecil Textbook of Medicine, 19th ed.: J.B. Wyngaarden, et al., eds.; W.B. Saunders Company, 1992, pp. 1133–1136.
Idiopathic Hemochromatosis: T.B. Kinney, et al.; Am. Fam. Physician, September 1991, vol. 44(3), pp. 873–875.
Immunogenetics of Hereditary Hemochromatosis: C.F. Bryan; Am. J. Med. Sci., January 1991, vol. 301(1), pp. 47–49.
Birth Defects Encyclopedia: M.L. Buyse, ed.-in-chief; Blackwell Scientific Publications, 1990, pp. 856–858.
Mendelian Inheritance in Man, 9th ed.: V.A. McKusick; The Johns Hopkins University Press, 1990, pp. 1235–1238.
Overview of Hemochromatosis: L.H. Smith, Jr.; West. J. Medicine, September 1990, vol. 153(3), pp. 296–308.

# HEMOGLOBINURIA, PAROXYSMAL COLD (PCH)

**Description** PCH is an extremely rare autoimmune hemolytic disorder. Healthy erythrocytes are destroyed prematurely and suddenly after exposure to temperatures of 15°C (59°F) or lower.

**Synonyms**

> Donath-Landsteiner Hemolytic Anemia
> Donath-Landsteiner Syndrome

**Signs and Symptoms** Attacks of PCH can occur within minutes or up to 8 hours after exposure to cold. Symptoms and signs may include fever, malaise, anorexia, pain in the flanks and in the back and legs, headache, vomiting, diarrhea, mild anemia, and hemoglobinuria. Jaundice may follow attacks. The liver and spleen may be enlarged.

**Etiology** Most cases occur after a viral infection, such as chickenpox or mumps, or in conjunction with congenital or acquired syphilis. Hemolysis is mediated by a complement-fixing IgG antibody. The disease may also affect individuals with no histories of other disorders. Localized exposure to cold water, by hand washing or drinking, may also trigger an attack in some severe cases.

**Epidemiology** Anyone may acquire PCH. An individual with a viral infection, such as chickenpox or mumps, or with syphilis is at higher risk of contracting the disorder.

**Related Disorders** See *Anemia, Hemolytic, Cold-Antibody; Hemoglobinuria, Paroxysmal Nocturnal.*

**Treatment—Standard** Treatment of the accompanying viral infection by supportive therapy, bed rest, and protection of the affected individual from cold temperatures is usually effective. If the disorder is chronic, it may respond to treatment with glucocorticoids or immunosuppressive drugs, such as cyclophosphamide. The following guidelines must be met when blood transfusions are needed: blood should be cross-matched at 37° C to find compatible units, and the blood should be warmed by an on-line warmer to prevent new erythrocytes from being coated with antibodies and destroyed.

**Treatment—Investigational** Please contact the agencies listed under Resources, below, for the most current information. Addresses and telephone numbers of these agencies, as well as of individual experts and research centers, may be found in the Master Resources List.

**Resources**

**For more information on paroxysmal cold hemoglobinuria:** National Organization for Rare Disorders (NORD); NIH/National Heart, Lung and Blood Institute.

**References**

Cecil Textbook of Medicine, 18th ed.: J.B. Wyngaarden and L.H. Smith, Jr., eds.; W.B. Saunders Company, 1988, p. 921.

Internal Medicine, 2nd ed.: J.H. Stein, ed.-in-chief; Little, Brown and Company, 1987, p. 1059.

Donath-Landsteiner Hemolytic Anemia Due to an Anti-Pr-Like Biphasic Hemolysin: W.J. Judd, et al.; Transfusion, September–October, 1986, vol. 26(5), pp. 423–425.

An Unusual Donath-Landsteiner Antibody Detectable at 37 Degrees C by the Antiglobulin Test: S. Lindgren, et al.; March–April, 1985: vol. 25(2), pp. 142–144.

# HEMOGLOBINURIA, PAROXYSMAL NOCTURNAL (PNH)

**Description** PNH is an anemia caused by a defect in the membrane of erythrocytes. The breakdown of red blood cells causes hemoglobinuria and hemoglobinemia, which occur at night in classical PNH but in fact may occur more often throughout the day or intermittently.

**Synonyms**

Marchiafava-Micheli Syndrome

**Signs and Symptoms** Severe abdominal or back pain may occur during hemolysis. Hemoglobinuria, paleness, and jaundice may be present. Venous thrombosis may occur, usually in the spleen, liver, and inferior vena cava. The spleen and the liver may be enlarged. Patients usually experience mild anemia for several years before the major symptoms of hemoglobinuria become apparent.

**Etiology** PNH results from a defect in the membrane of erythrocytes that leads to complement-mediated intravascular hemolysis. The molecular defect appears to be an acquired somatic mutation of the X-linked PIG-A (phosphatidylinositol glycan class A) gene, which participates in an early step of glycosylphosphatidylinositol anchor synthesis. Aplastic anemia may develop in 20 to 30 percent of cases. An infection, the administration of iron or of a vaccine, or menstruation may precipitate hemolysis, which results in hemoglobinemia and hemoglobinuria.

**Epidemiology** PNH may occur at any age but is most common between 20 and 45 years of age. No racial predominance has been noted.

**Related Disorders** See *Hemoglobinuria, Paroxysmal Cold.*

**Treatment—Standard** Androgens may be administered in some cases. Packed red blood cells may be transfused during crises. Used cautiously, anticoagulants such as heparin appear useful in treating thrombi. Iron supplements may be prescribed. Normal bone marrow has been transplanted in some patients. Other treatment may be symptomatic.

**Treatment—Investigational** Please contact the agencies listed under Resources, below, for the most current information. Addresses and telephone numbers of these agencies, as well as of individual experts and research centers, may be found in the Master Resources List.

**Resources**

**For more information on paroxysmal nocturnal hemoglobinuria:** National Organization for Rare Disorders (NORD); NIH/National Heart, Lung and Blood Institute.

**References**

Abnormalities of PIG-A Transcripts in Granulocytes from Patients with Paroxysmal Nocturnal Hemoglobinuria: T. Miyata, et al.; N. Engl. J. Med., January 1994, vol. 330(4), pp. 249–255.

PIG-A the Target Gene in Paroxysmal Nocturnal Hemoglobinuria: R.S. Schwartz; N. Engl. J. Med., January 1994, vol. 330, (4), pp. 283–284.

Internal Medicine, 3rd ed.: J.H. Stein, ed.-in-chief; Little, Brown and Company, 1990, pp. 1113–1114.

Thrombolytic Therapy for Inferior Vena Cava Thrombosis in Paroxysmal Nocturnal Hemoglobinuria: P.W. Sholar, et al.; Ann. Intern. Med., October 1985, vol. 103(4), pp. 539–541.

# HEMOPHILIA

**Description** Hemophilia is an inherited blood-coagulation disorder caused by inactive or deficient blood proteins, usually factor VIII. It is found in males almost exclusively and can be classified as mild, moderate, or severe. The level of severity is determined by the percentage of active clotting factor in the blood (normal percentage ranges from 50 to 150 percent). People who have severe hemophilia have less than 1 percent in their blood.

There are 3 major types of hemophilia: hemophilia A (also known as classical hemophilia or factor VIII deficiency or antihemophilic globulin [**AHG**] deficiency); hemophilia B (Christmas disease or factor IX deficiency); and hemophilia C (factor XI deficiency). Von Willebrand disease and other rare clotting disorders have similar symptoms but are not usually called hemophilia.

**Synonyms**

    Antihemophilic Globulin (AHG) Deficiency
    Christmas Disease
    Classical Hemophilia
    Factor VIII Deficiency
    Factor IX Deficiency
    Factor XI Deficiency
    von Willebrand Disease (Vascular Hemophilia)

**Signs and Symptoms** The most serious symptom of hemophilia is uncontrolled internal bleeding that begins spontaneously without an apparent cause and, over time, can cause permanent damage to joints and muscles. A hemophiliac bleeds for a longer period of time than normal. External bleeding can usually be controlled, and minor cuts can be treated as normal.

**Etiology** Hemophilia is a recessive genetic condition linked to the X chromosome. Although most patients have a family history of the disease, as many as one-third of new cases are found in persons without a family history. A hemophiliac male cannot pass the disease on to his sons, but all of his daughters will be genetic carriers capable of passing the disease on to succeeding generations.

**Epidemiology** An estimated 20,000 males in the United States have hemophilia, not including the many mild cases that remain undiagnosed until they are discovered following major trauma or surgery. Hemophilia occurs in 1:4,000 male newborns. Medical advances have enabled hemophiliacs to reach a near-normal life expectancy.

**Related Disorders** See *von Willebrand Disease.*

**Treatment—Standard** While there is no cure for hemophilia, the disorder can be controlled through infusions of a blood-clotting factor, generally factor VIII. The clotting factor remains active in the hemophiliac's blood for only a short time; new infusions are required each time internal bleeding occurs to avoid permanent damage. This therapy is necessary for the life of the patient.

The Food and Drug Administration has approved the drug desmopressin (Stimate) for treatment of moderately severe cases of hemophilia. Desmopressin acetate nasal spray (Rorer Pharmaceutical Corp.) has been approved for treatment of mild hemophilia A. Genetically engineered factor VIII became available for the treatment of hemophilia after factor VIII derived from human blood was found to contain the AIDS and hepatitis viruses.

Three biological products have been approved for treatment of hemophilia B: bebulin VH (a factor IX complex containing other clotting proteins) (Osterreichisches Institute fur Haemoderivate, Vienna, Austria); mononine (a factor IX product) (Armour Pharmaceuticals); and alpha nine (a coagulation factor IX [human]) (Alpha Therapeutic Corp.).

Monoclonal factor IX (Green Cross and Armour Pharmaceutical) is a treatment for hemophilia B. Recombinant antihemophilic factor (Cutter Biological) is a treatment for hemorrhage in hemophilia A.

The Food and Drug Administration has approved the orphan drug tranexamic acid (Cyclokapron) for short-term use (2 to 8 days) in hemophiliacs before and after minor surgery, such as a tooth extraction. This drug reduces the need for blood transfusions after surgery. Approval was also received for antihemophilic factor recombinant (Kogenate) to prevent bleeding or prophylactically to prepare patients for surgery.

Genetic counseling may be of benefit for patients and their families.

**Treatment—Investigational** The National Hemophilia Foundation has funded AIDS-related research in collaboration with the Centers for Disease Control and commercial research into the preparation of factor VIII by recombinant gene technology.

Researchers at the National Institute of Diabetes, Digestive and Kidney Diseases have developed a method for culturing endothelial cells and a cell line that produces factor VIII:C, the clotting factor missing from the blood of persons with hemophilia A.

Dr. Harvey Pollard, Chief of the Laboratory of Cell Biology and Genetics, and his colleagues have cultured endothelial cells from the adrenal glands of cows that produce large amounts of factor VIII:C. Hemophiliacs frequently develop antibodies against factor VIII:C obtained from blood donors and therefore must use factor VIII:C from animal or other nonhuman sources. Factor VIII:C obtained from human sources might also expose hemophiliacs to hepatitis and AIDS. Large-scale production of endothelial-produced factor VIII:C may provide a viable alternative to current therapies.

Shirley I. Miekka, Ph.D., at the American Red Cross in Washington, D.C., is studying coagulation factor X as a treatment for hemophilia under a Food and Drug Administration grant.

E(rGM-CSF) is another drug being tested for hemophilia. The drug is manufactured by Schering Corp.

Clinical trials are under way at Brigham and Women's Hospital to study radiation synovectomy using 165-dysprosium ferric hydroxide macroaggregate (165DY-FHMA) in order to treat inflammation of the knee in hemophiliac patients.

The orphan product coagulation factor IX (recombinant) is being tested for the treatment of hemophilia B. The manufacturer is Genetics Institute.

Please contact the agencies listed under Resources, below, for the most current information. Addresses and telephone numbers of these agencies, as well as of individual experts and research centers, may be found in the Master Resources List.

**Resources**

**For more information on hemophilia:** National Organization for Rare Disorders (NORD); National Hemophilia Foundation; World Federation of Hemophilia; Canadian Hemophilia Society; Haemophilia Society; NIH/National Heart, Lung and Blood Institute.

**For genetic information and genetic counseling referrals:** March of Dimes Birth Defects Foundation; Alliance of Genetic Support Groups.

**References**

Mendelian Inheritance in Man, 10th ed.: V.A. McKusick; The Johns Hopkins University Press, 1992, pp. 1848–1865.

Cecil Textbook of Medicine, 19th ed.: J.B. Wyngaarden, et al., eds.; W.B. Saunders Company, 1992, pp. 1004–1007.

Nasal Spray Desmopressin (DDAVP) for Mild Hemophilia A and von Willebrand Disease: E.H. Rose, et al.; Ann. Intern. Med., April 1991, vol. 114, pp. 563–568.

Birth Defects Encyclopedia: M.L. Buyse, ed.-in-chief; Blackwell Scientific Publications, 1990, pp. 859–861.

# HEMORRHAGIC TELANGIECTASIA, HEREDITARY

**Description** Hereditary hemorrhagic telangiectasia is an inherited disorder characterized by capillary lesions on the skin, mucous membranes, and many internal organs. Patients often suffer anemia caused by hemorrhaging telangiectases.

**Synonyms**

Osler-Weber-Rendu Syndrome

Rendu-Osler-Weber Syndrome

**Signs and Symptoms** Lesions that are red to violet in color develop chiefly on the patient's cheeks, ears, lips, and tongue and in the nasal mucosa. The lesions may also occur in the gastrointestinal tract, lungs, brain, spinal cord, and liver. Hemorrhaging occurs either spontaneously or as a result of injury. Epistaxis and gastrointestinal hemorrhaging become more severe with age and can cause chronic anemia. Arteriovenous fistulae are formed that can cause cyanosis, polycythemia, clubbed fingers, and possibly stroke. The mortality from hereditary hemorrhagic telangiectasia is less than 10 percent, but this disorder can lead to many complications because it is often misdiagnosed or undiagnosed.

**Etiology** Hereditary hemorrhagic telangiectasia is transmitted as an autosomal dominant characteristic. Telangiectases in the lungs, brain, and liver are thought to be caused by arteriovenous fistulae that form to replace the capillaries that normally connect venules and arterioles. When the capillaries are missing, the lesions bleed profusely.

**Epidemiology** Hereditary hemorrhagic telangiectasia affects both sexes and all ages. In Europe, the incidence of the disease has been reported to be 1:50,000. However, because the disorder is often misdiagnosed, this estimate may be inaccurate.

**Related Disorders** See *von Willebrand Disease; Scleroderma; Raynaud Disease and Phenomenon.*

Other related disorders are **Calcinosis-Raynaud-Sclerodactyly-Telangiectasia (CRST); multiple phlebectasia; spider nevi;** and **cherry angiomas (senile hemangiomas; DeMorgan** or **ruby spots).** CRST is characterized by calcium salt deposits in focal nodules in various body tissues other than the parenchymatous viscera. Multiple phlebectasias are enlarged veins. Spider nevi are small, visible, abnormally enlarged arteries that have radiating branches resembling spider legs. Cherry angiomas are red papules caused by a weakening of the capillary wall.

**Treatment—Standard** Treatment is designed to stop the hemorrhaging and remove or block exceptionally large lesions or arteriovenous fistulae. Cauterization of telangiectases in the nasal mucosa stops the growth of new lesions and thus offers temporary benefit. Surgical excision of arteriovenous fistulae has been accomplished, and balloon embolotherapy has been found effective in occluding pulmonary arteriovenous fistulae. Application of a compress saturated with vasoconstrictors, such as phenylephrine, has been used to control epistaxis. Anemia can be treated by blood transfusions or iron replacement therapy using iron dextran administered either orally or intravenously. Surgery may be necessary for gastrointestinal lesions that produce severe hemorrhaging.

**Treatment—Investigational** Estrogen and progesterone therapy to prevent hemorrhaging has been investigated. Estrogen has not been effective, but progesterone holds some promise.

Small oral doses of aminocaproic acid are being tested for the treatment of recurrent gastrointestinal and nasal bleeding and moderate anemia associated with hereditary hemorrhagic telangiectasia. Side effects of hypotension and rhabdomyolysis occur rarely. Contact Martin D. Phillips, M.D., at the University of Texas for more information. Additional studies are needed to determine the safety and efficacy of this treatment.

Please contact the agencies listed under Resources, below, for the most current information. Addresses and telephone numbers of these agencies, as well as of individual experts and research centers, may be found in the Master Resources List.

**Resources**

**For more information on hereditary hemorrhagic telangiectasia:** National Organization for Rare Disorders (NORD); Hereditary Hemorrhagic Telangiectasis Registry; NIH/National Heart, Lung and Blood Institute; NIH/National Institute of Child Health and Human Development; Dr. Robert I. White, Jr., Yale University.

**For genetic information and genetic counseling referrals:** March of Dimes Birth Defects Foundation; Alliance of Genetic Support Groups.

**References**

Brief Report: Treatment of Bleeding in Hereditary Hemorrhagic Telangiectasia with Aminocaproic Acid: H. I. Saba, et al.; N. Engl. J. Med., June 1994, vol. 330(25), pp. 1789–1790.

Stopping Bleeding in Hereditary Telangiectasia: M.D. Phillips; N. Engl. J. Med., June 1994, vol. 330(25), pp. 1822–1823.

Harrison's Principles of Internal Medicine, 12th ed.: J.D. Wilson, et al., eds.; McGraw-Hill, 1991, p. 326.

# HERMANSKY-PUDLAK SYNDROME

**Description** Hermansky-Pudlak syndrome is a hereditary disorder composed of 3 characteristics: albinism, red blood cells that lack dense bodies, and abnormal storage of a ceroid or fatlike material in various body systems.

**Synonyms**

Albinism with Hemorrhagic Diathesis and Pigmented Reticuloendothelial Cells

Delta Storage Pool Disease

**Signs and Symptoms** Childhood onset often begins with easy bruising, bleeding gums, nosebleeds, and excessive bleeding after surgery or accidents. Other symptoms include oculocutaneous albinism, storage pool–deficient platelets, and ceroid deposits. The skin, hair, and eyes may vary from very pale to almost normal coloring. Legal blindness and visual acuities of 20/200 or worse are common. The blood storage abnormality may cause excessive bleeding, especially in women during menstruation. Bleeding may become life-threatening, especially after taking aspirin. Ceroid deposits may cause restrictive lung disease, inflammatory bowel disease, kidney failure, and heart disease.

**Etiology** Research suggests that an abnormality of lysosomal function may be responsible for Hermansky-Pudlak syndrome, but the exact cause is unknown. The disorder is inherited as an autosomal recessive genetic trait.

**Epidemiology** The incidence rate is 1:2,000 in persons of Puerto Rican descent. The syndrome occurs most often in those whose ancestry can be traced specifically to northwest Puerto Rico and to Spain. It is the 3rd most prevalent form of albinism. Males and females are affected in equal numbers.

**Related Disorders** See *Albinism; Chédiak-Higashi Syndrome.*

**Treatment—Standard** Treatment is designed to stop hemorrhaging or replace lost blood. Transfusions of normal blood platelets or administration of cyroprecipitate may prove beneficial. Menorrhagia is treated with oral contraceptives. Desmopressin acetate (**DDAVP**) has proved very effective.

Genetic counseling may be of benefit for patients and their families. Other treatment is symptomatic and supportive.

**Treatment—Investigational** Please contact the agencies listed under Resources, below, for the most current information. Addresses and telephone numbers of these agencies, as well as of individual experts and research centers, may be found in the Master Resources List.

**Resources**

**For more information on Hermansky-Pudlak syndrome:** National Organization for Rare Disorders (NORD); Hermansky-Pudlak Syndrome Network; NIH/National Arthritis and Musculoskeletal and Skin Diseases Information Clearinghouse.

**For genetic information and genetic counseling referrals:** March of Dimes Birth Defects Foundation; Alliance of Genetic Support Groups.

**References**

Hematology, 4th ed.: W.J. Williams, et al., eds.; McGraw-Hill, 1990, p. 1177.

Hermansky-Pudlak Syndrome: Case Report and Clinicopathologic Review: J.P. Schachne, et al.; J. Am. Acad. Dermatol., May 1990, vol. 22(5 pt. 2), pp. 926–932.

Mendelian Inheritance in Man, 9th ed.: V.A. McKusick; The Johns Hopkins University Press, 1990, p. 1206.

The Metabolic Basis of Inherited Disease, 6th ed.: C.R. Scriver, et al., eds.; McGraw-Hill, 1989, pp. 2905, 2916, 2929–2930.

Elevated Urinary Dolichol Excretion in the Hermansky-Pudlak Syndrome: Indicator of Lysosomal Dysfunction: C.J. Witkop, et al.; Am. J. Med., March 1987, vol. 82(3), pp. 463–670.

# HISTIOCYTOSIS X

**Description** Histiocytosis X is an older term for Langerhans cell histiocytosis **(LCH),** a name given to a group of childhood blood disorders characterized by an abnormal proliferation of histiocytes throughout the body but especially in the skin, bones, brain, lungs, spleen, and liver. The child develops nonmalignant growths that represent accumulations of histiocytes. The clinical course of these disorders is aggressive, and treatment depends on the extent of damage to the affected organ, which varies according to the extent and location of the growths.

**Synonyms**

> Eosinophilic Granuloma
> Hand-Schüller-Christian Syndrome
> Langerhans Cell Granulomatosis
> Langerhans Cell Histiocytosis
> Letterer-Siwe Disease

**Signs and Symptoms** Symptoms vary widely from child to child and according to the organ affected. Patients with acute forms of this disease have splenomegaly, bone marrow damage, and abnormal blood counts due to blood cell deficiencies. Platelet deficiencies may cause excessive hemorrhaging; erythrocyte loss can cause anemia; and leukocyte deficiencies may cause infection.

Secondary lung infection or histiocytic infiltration may result in breathing difficulties. When bone is affected, the patient will have pain at the site. The patient's skin may have lesions containing small sacs of pus, scaly or greasy rashes, purplish-red spots, hemorrhaging beneath the skin, knots visible under the skin, and small, hard, red elevations on the surface of the skin.

Diabetes insipidus occurs if the hypothalamus and pituitary are affected. Pituitary damage can cause growth problems, thyroid deficiencies, and sex hormone abnormalities. In chronic cases, healing and scarring may be difficult to differentiate from histiocyte growth, particularly in the lungs and liver. Effects in the mouth include gingival swelling, tooth loss, and premature tooth eruption. The patient's eyeballs may protrude, and clear vision may be lost.

Rarely, in patients who have had no signs of the disease for many years, neurologic damage leads to difficulty in walking and controlling the body. Some limited short-term symptoms may heal spontaneously and permanently, but more widespread symptoms may continue for years.

**Etiology** Researchers are unable to explain what causes histiocytes to grow and spread abnormally. Some theories suggest that infections or immune system deficiencies are involved, since Langerhans cells respond to immune system stimuli.

**Epidemiology** While a few cases of this disease have occurred in family members, most are nonfamilial. The disease occurs most frequently in children, although onset can begin in adulthood as well. Children under 2 years of age are the most severely affected.

**Related Disorders Hemophagocytic lymphohistiocytosis (hemophagocytic reticulosis),** a genetic blood disorder with onset in infancy, is characterized by blood cell abnormalities, splenomegaly, hepatomegaly, fever, liver damage, neurologic damage, easy hemorrhaging, and fever.

**Infection-associated hemophagocytic syndrome** is characterized by hepatic lesions and lesions in the central nervous system that are associated with infectious agents or a family history of the disease.

**Treatment—Standard** Although the histiocytic growths resulting from this disorder are not malignant, some therapies are similar to those used in cancer patients. Chemotherapy is routinely used to treat chronic and aggressive forms of histiocytosis X that are widespread. Radiotherapy and steroid injections are used to treat local lesions, depending on where they are, whether or not pain is severe, and if function might be diminished. Long-term therapy with corticosteroids or radiation may be used for adults with lung involvement only. Other therapies depend on symptoms. Some forms of this disorder may require no treatment at all once a confirmed diagnosis has been made.

**Treatment—Investigational** Experimental research is under way in the United States, Germany, Austria, and Italy into the use of bone marrow transplants, immune system modulators, and other procedures to treat this disorder. Definitive results have not yet been achieved.

Researchers at the Histiocytosis Center, Yale University, are investigating treatments for histiocytosis.

Please contact the agencies listed under Resources, below, for the most current information. Addresses and telephone numbers of these agencies, as well as of individual experts and research centers, may be found in the Master Resources List.

**Resources**

**For more information on histiocytosis X:** National Organization for Rare Disorders (NORD); American Lung Association; Histiocytosis-X Association; NIH/National Heart, Lung and Blood Institute; Diane Komp, M.D., Yale University School of Medicine; Izaak Walton Killam Hospital for Children, Halifax, Nova Scotia.

**References**
Point of View: Histiocytosis Syndromes in Children: B. Favara, et al.; Lancet, January 24, 1987, pp. 208–209.
Editorial: Langerhans Cell Histiocytosis: D. Komp; N. Engl. J. Med., 1987, vol. 316(12), pp. 747–748.

# HODGKIN DISEASE

**Description** Hodgkin disease is a form of malignant lymphoma. Its characteristics include lymph node, lymphoid tissue, and spleen enlargement and the presence of Reed-Sternberg cells.

**Synonyms**
Hodgkin Lymphoma

**Signs and Symptoms** Initially, lymph nodes begin to swell, most frequently in the neck (two-thirds of the time) but also in the chest, armpits, abdomen, and groin. Eventually, the tissue around the nodes may be affected, as well as the patient's lungs, liver, spleen, and bone marrow. Patients may or may not have night sweats, weight loss, and fever. In rare cases bone pain is present. Reed-Sternberg cells are found in the affected lymph nodes. Since enlarged lymph nodes are symptoms of other cancers and infectious diseases, diagnosis can be difficult.

**Etiology** The cause is unknown. A viral agent may be involved.

**Epidemiology** Symptoms usually occur in patients between the ages of 15 and 40 years, although in rare instances Hodgkin disease affects persons over 50; it also may occur in children. Four distinct types of malignant cells have been recognized. The most common type affects young women primarily. Two other less common types affect male teenagers and older men predominantly, and the rarest form affects older men and women. Clusters of this disease have appeared in certain geographic areas and occasionally in families, but these are rare.

**Related Disorders** A group of cancers known as **non-Hodgkin lymphomas** is also characterized by enlarged lymph nodes that begin in the neck or groin and usually spread. Patients can be affected at any age and may have leukemia, anemia, and night sweats.

**Burkitt lymphoma** is another lymphatic cancer that is possibly infectious and affects not only the lymph nodes but also bone marrow, the central nervous system, kidneys, and gonads. It occurs in Central Africa but less commonly in the United States.

**Treatment—Standard** The stage of the disease determines the appropriate treatment, which depends on the number of tumors and their location and whether or not the patient has fever, night sweats, and weight loss. Staging is generally done according to the Ann Arbor classification system.

Radiation therapy is used to shrink affected lymph nodes and destroy diseased lymphocytes. Chemotherapeutic regimens are also used, including such combinations as MOPP (nitrogen mustard, Oncovin [vincristine], prednisone, and procarbazine); ABVD (Adriamycin [doxorubicin], bleomycin, vinblastine, and dacarbazine); MOP-BAP (nitrogen mustard, Oncovin, procarbazine, bleomycin, Adriamycin, and prednisone); and ChlVPP (chlorambucil, vinblastine, prednisone, and procarbazine). MOPP and ABVD can be used together but alternated every month. Other treatments depend on symptoms.

**Treatment—Investigational** Fournier, a French pharmaceutical company, has developed an experimental drug, LF1695, for use in children with immune system damage due to Hodgkin disease, Chagas disease, and Shwachman syndrome. For information, contact Fournier Laboratories, BP90, Daix, 21121 Fontaine, Les Dijon, France.

Please contact the agencies listed under Resources, below, for the most current information. Addresses and telephone numbers of these agencies, as well as of individual experts and research centers, may be found in the Master Resources List.

**Resources**
**For more information on Hodgkin disease:** National Organization for Rare Disorders (NORD); American Cancer Society; NIH/National Cancer Institute Physician Data Query Phoneline.

**References**
Treatment Strategies for Hodgkin's Disease: G. Bonadonna; Semin. Hematol., April 1988, vol. 25(2 suppl. 2), pp. 51–57.
Internal Medicine, 3rd Ed.: J.H. Stein, ed.-in-chief; Little, Brown and Company, 1987, pp. 1136–1141.
Winning the Battle Against Hodgkin's Disease: K. Consalvo and M. Gallagher; RN, December 1986, pp. 20–25.

# IDIOPATHIC EDEMA

**Description** Idiopathic edema is a common disorder characterized by episodic or persistent swelling due to salt and water retention that is not caused by cardiac, hepatic, or splenic disease. It occurs in women almost exclusively and usually affects the face, abdomen, and extremities.

**Synonyms**

>Cyclic Edema
>Distress Edema
>Periodic Edema
>Periodic Swelling
>Stress Edema

**Signs and Symptoms** Swelling occurs either occasionally or chronically and develops rapidly, especially in the feet, hands, and face. Significant pitting edema in the lower extremities occurs after standing for a long time. Patients may also have a bloated abdomen and gain weight, sometimes as much as 10 to 12 lb in a 24-hour period. Other signs and symptoms are a drop in urine output, irritability, depression, fatigue, headache, and tension. Idiopathic edema is often associated with the menstrual cycle.

**Etiology** The cause is unknown; an imbalance of estrogens or progesterone is suspected. The patients' abnormal aldosterone response to standing upright apparently plays a role in their retention of sodium and water.

**Epidemiology** Almost all patients are women who are middle-aged or younger.

**Related Disorders** See *Angioedema, Hereditary.*

**Treatment—Standard** The drugs captopril and spironolactone have been found to be successful in restoring normal aldosterone response and reversing the edema.

**Treatment—Investigational** Please contact the agencies listed under Resources, below, for the most current information. Addresses and telephone numbers of these agencies, as well as of individual experts and research centers, may be found in the Master Resources List.

**Resources**

  **For more information on idiopathic edema:** National Organization for Rare Disorders (NORD); NIH/National Digestive Diseases Information Clearinghouse.

**References**

Idiopathic Edema in a Male: I. Weinberger, et al.; American J. Med. Sci., July–August 1984, vol. 288(1), pp. 27–31.

Long-Term Furosemide Treatment in Idiopathic Edema: M. Shichiri, et al.; Arch. Intern. Med., November 1984, vol. 144(11), pp. 2161–2164.

Therapeutic Response of Idiopathic Edema to Captopril: D. Docci, et al.; Nephron, 1983, vol. 34(3), pp. 198–200.

# KIKUCHI DISEASE

**Description** Kikuchi disease is a noncancerous disorder of the lymph nodes whose symptoms often mimic those of malignant lymphoma.

**Synonyms**

>Histiocytic Necrotizing Lymphadenitis
>Kikuchi-Fujimoto Disease
>Kikuchi Histiocytic Necrotizing Lymphadenitis
>Necrotizing Lymphadenitis

**Signs and Symptoms** The patient may have a fever and present with swollen, hard, painful, and tender lymph nodes. Inflammation and abnormal tissue usually resolve spontaneously within weeks or months without treatment. Since this disorder can only be determined by a biopsy of the affected tissue, it may be overlooked by unsuspecting patients.

**Etiology** The exact cause of Kikuchi disease is unknown. Many researchers suspect that a virus may be responsible.

**Epidemiology** Originally identified in Japan in 1972, Kikuchi disease primarily affects young adults. Fewer than 50 cases have been reported.

**Related Disorders** See *Hodgkin Disease.*

  **Burkitt lymphoma** is a cancer of the lymphatic system that may involve the kidneys, sex glands, jaw, bone marrow, or central nervous system. It can be infectious and is associated with the Epstein-Barr virus. Central African children are often affected.

  Pancytopenia, splenomegaly, and Still disease (juvenile rheumatoid arthritis) have been associated with Kikuchi disease in some patients. They are not necessary for a differential diagnosis.

**Treatment—Standard** Treatment is symptomatic and supportive. The disorder usually resolves spontaneously within a few weeks or months.

**Treatment—Investigational** Please contact the agencies listed under Resources, below, for the most current information. Addresses and telephone numbers of these agencies, as well as of individual experts and research centers, may be found in the Master Resources List.

**Resources**

**For more information on Kikuchi disease:** National Organization for Rare Disorders (NORD); NIH/National Institute of Allergy and Infectious Diseases.

**References**

Cutaneous Manifestations of Kikuchi's Histiocytic Necrotizing Lymphadenitis: T.T. Kuo; Am. J. Surg. Pathol., September 1990, vol. 14(9), pp. 872–876.

Kikuchi-Fujimoto Disease Mimicking Malignant Lymphoma: G.A. Chamulak, et al.; Am. J. Surg. Pathol., June 1990, vol. 14(6), pp. 514–523.

Necrotizing Lymphadenitis (Kikuchi's Disease): Report of Four Cases of an Unusual Pseudolymphomatous Lesion and Immunologic Marker Studies: P.D. Unger, et al.; Arch. Pathol. Lab. Med., November 1987, vol. 111(11), pp. 1031–1034.

Necrotising Lymphadenitis Without Granulocytic Infiltration (Kikuchi's Disease): M.H. Ali, et al.; J. Clin. Pathol., November 1985, vol. 38(11), pp. 1252–1257.

# LEUKEMIA, CHRONIC MYELOGENOUS

**Description** Chronic myelogenous leukemia is characterized by excessive numbers of leukocytes in the blood, bone marrow, liver, and spleen that infiltrate the lungs, kidneys, intestinal tract, lymph nodes, and gonads. In the first or chronic phase of the disease, leukocytes are overproduced in the bone marrow. In the advanced or acute phase, known as the blast crisis, immature blast cells or promelocytes make up more than 50 percent of the cells in the bone marrow, and the disease becomes extremely aggressive and unresponsive to therapy. The majority of patients (approximately 85 percent) enter the advanced phase.

**Synonyms**

Chronic Granulocytic Leukemia

Chronic Myelocytic Leukemia

Chronic Myeloid Leukemia

**Signs and Symptoms** Patients usually present with nonspecific symptoms, such as weakness, fatigue, night sweats, splenomegaly, weight loss, abdominal discomfort, or itchiness. Routine blood tests may reveal the underlying problem. In the acute phase, patients have hepatosplenomegaly, pain in bones, extreme weight loss, high fever, excessive calcium in the blood, arthralgia, and hemorrhagic purplish patches in the epidermis and mucous membranes.

**Etiology** While the precise cause is unknown, researchers have implicated excessive radiation exposure as a high-risk factor. Patients have a proliferation of abnormal and useless neoplastic cells in their blood, 90 percent of which have a consistent rearrangement of chromosomes that results from the transfer of genetic material from chromosome 9 to chromosome 22, or vice versa. Known as the Philadelphia chromosome, chromosome 22 becomes shorter than normal and is suspected of playing a role in the onset or development of the disease.

In some cases chronic myelogenous leukemia may be associated with translocation (t[5;12][q33;p13]). The genes directly affected are known as platelet-derived growth factor receptor B gene on chromosome 5 and the TEL (translocation, Ets, leukemia) gene on chromosome 12.

**Epidemiology** Chronic myelogenous leukemia occurs slightly more often in men than in women, and patients are usually in their 40s or 50s, although the disease can occur at any age.

**Related Disorders** See *Polycythemia Vera.*

**Treatment—Standard** Chemotherapy and radiation therapy are used to reduce the number of leukocytes and the size of the spleen in an attempt to induce remission. Busulfan and hydroxyurea are commonly prescribed. Other chemotherapeutic agents, splenectomy, and bone marrow transplantation are sometimes tried to keep patients from entering the acute phase. Marrow transplants are the most successful, and the best results are achieved in patients under 40 who have not entered the acute phase. Once the acute phase begins, transplants are not very successful.

Some patients in the acute phase appear to improve temporarily with prednisone and vincristine therapy, but because the acute phase of this disease proceeds aggressively and rapidly, a second remission is less likely.

The Food and Drug Administration recently approved the orphan drug idarubicin hydrochloride (Idamycin) (Adria Laboratories) for the treatment of chronic myelogenous leukemia.

**Treatment—Investigational** The orphan drug recombinant interferon α-2a (Roferon-A) (Hoffmann–La Roche) is under investigation as a treatment for chronic myelogenous leukemia.

Amgen is developing the drug recombinant methionyl granulocyte colony stimulating factor (Neupogen) to treat myelodysplastic syndromes.

Walter A. Blatter, M.D., was awarded a grant by the Office of Orphan Products Development for his work with immunotherapy of myelcid leukemia using anti-o-blocked ricin immunoconjugate.

For acute attacks of chronic myelogenous leukemia, Medarex has developed the biologic monoclonal antibody PM81.

Please contact the agencies listed under Resources, below, for the most current information. Addresses and telephone numbers of these agencies, as well as of individual experts and research centers, may be found in the Master Resources List.

### Resources

**For more information on chronic myelogenous leukemia:** National Organization for Rare Disorders (NORD); Leukemia Society of America; American Cancer Society; NIH/National Cancer Institute Physician Data Query Phoneline.

### References

Interferon-Alpha Produces Sustained Cytogenic Responses in Chronic Myelogenous Leukemia: M. Talpaz, et al.; Ann. Intern. Med., April 1991, vol. 114, pp. 532–538.

Internal Medicine, 3rd ed.: J.H. Stein, ed.-in-chief; Little, Brown and Company, 1990, pp. 1561–1563.

Blast Crisis of Philadelphia Chromosome-Positive Chronic Myelocytic Leukemia (CML): B. Anger, et al.; Blut, September 1988, vol. 57(3), pp. 131–137.

Bone Marrow Transplantation for Chronic Myelogenous Leukemia in Chronic Phase: J.M. Goldman, et al.; Ann. Intern. Med., June 1988, vol. 108(6), pp. 806–814.

# LEUKEMIA, HAIRY CELL

**Description** Hairy cell leukemia is a neoplastic disease characterized by the presence in the blood of abnormal mononuclear cells (hairy cells) and pancytopenia.

### Synonyms

Leukemic Reticuloendotheliosis

**Signs and Symptoms** Symptoms usually occur gradually and include vague abdominal pain, a feeling of fullness in the stomach, weakness, malaise, fatigue, weight loss, and easy bruising. Hairy cells heavily infiltrate the splenic pulp and sinuses, bone marrow, lymph nodes, and the liver. In chronic cases, splenectomy provides long-term survival. However, in acute cases, the prognosis is not as good.

**Etiology** The cause is not known.

**Epidemiology** Approximately 2,000 to 3,000 people in the United States are affected every year.

**Related Disorders Letterer-Siwe disease (Abt-Letterer-Siwe disease; systemic aleukemic reticuloendotheliosis)** is an inherited autosomal recessive hereditary disorder characterized by swollen lymph nodes, hepatomegaly, splenomegaly, and a persistent, spiking, low-grade fever. Other symptoms are pallor and discrete yellowish-brown maculopapular lesions that are sometimes ulcerated.

**Treatment—Standard** Until recently, splenectomy was the standard treatment. Methotrexate was also used, along with leucovorin as an antidote against its toxic effects, as were glucocorticoids for vasculitic symptoms, and alkylation agents.

Within recent years, the Food and Drug Administration has approved the orphan drug α-interferon, manufactured by Hoffmann–La Roche and Schering Corporation, as a treatment for hairy cell leukemia. Clinical trials of this drug showed that 92 to 94 percent of treated patients were alive 2 years after treatment was begun, compared with fewer than 50 percent of patients who were treated by conventional therapies. In 75 to 90 percent of treated patients, the disease went into remission. α-Interferon may be injected daily for up to 6 months, followed by maintenance injections 3 times a week. Flulike side effects diminish over time.

Leustatin (cladribine or 2CDA) has been approved for treatment of HCL, and the orphan drug Nipent (Warner-Lambert) has been approved for patients refractory to ordinary therapy.

**Treatment—Investigational** Under investigation is the use of interleukin-2 to restore the patient's natural killer cell activity.

Clinical trials are also being conducted on the drug deoxycoformycin. For information, contact The Comprehensive Cancer Center (Dr. Eric Kraut), Ohio State University, Columbus, Ohio, or the Investigational Drug Branch of the National Cancer Institute in Bethesda, Maryland.

Please contact the agencies listed under Resources, below, for the most current information. Addresses and telephone numbers of these agencies, as well as of individual experts and research centers, may be found in the Master Resources List.

### Resources

**For more information on hairy cell leukemia:** National Organization for Rare Disorders (NORD); Hairy Cell Leukemia Foundation; Leukemia Society of America; American Cancer Society; NIH/National Cancer Institute Physician Data Query Phoneline.

### References

Lasting Remissions in Hairy-Cell Leukemia Induced by a Single Infusion of 2-Chlorodeoxyadenosine: L. Piro, et al.; N. Engl. J. Med., April 1990, vol. 322(16), pp. 1117–1121.

Splenectomy for Hairy Cell Leukemia: A Clinical Review of 63 Patients: A.S. Van Norman, et al.; Cancer, February 1, 1986, vol. 57(3), pp. 644–648.

Recombinant Alpha-2 Interferon in the Treatment of Hairy Cell Leukemia: J.A. Thompson, et al.; Cancer Treat. Rep., July–August 1985, vol. 69(7–8), pp. 791–793.

Therapeutic Options in Hairy Cell Leukemia: J.E. Groopman; Semin. Oncol., December 1985, vol. 12(4 suppl. 5), pp. 30–34.

# LYMPHADENOPATHY, ANGIOIMMUNOBLASTIC, WITH DYSPROTEINEMIA (AILD)

**Description** A progressive immune disorder that affects people over 50, AILD is characterized by an abnormal proliferation of immunoblasts, capillaries, and plasma cells in lymph nodes that leaves the patient vulnerable to life-threatening infections. It is believed to be caused by chronic stimulation of the immune system resulting from drug therapy given for another condition, by viral infections, or by other stimuli.

**Synonyms**

Immunoblastic Lymphadenopathy

**Signs and Symptoms** The major symptoms of AILD are enlarged lymph nodes, acute infections, anemia, hypergammaglobulinemia, hepatosplenomegaly, chills, acute fever, sweating, weight loss, general discomfort, and sometimes a skin rash. In some cases, acute lymphoma develops.

**Etiology** AILD is believed to be an overreaction to immune system stimuli, such as drug therapy, viral infections, insect bites, or immunizations; or it could be an early form of a lymphoproliferative disorder.

**Epidemiology** AILD usually affects men and women over 50 in equal numbers.

**Related Disorders** See *Acquired Immune Deficiency Syndrome.*

**Dermatopathic lymphadenopathy (lipomelanic reticulosis)** is a skin condition marked by enlarged lymph nodes and abnormal proliferation of histiocytes and macrophages that contain fat and melanin. Other skin conditions that involve exfoliation or pruritus are thought to be the cause.

**Treatment—Standard** Corticosteroids and cyclophosphamides, which reduce swollen lymph nodes and diminish blood cell deficiencies, are the standard treatment for this disorder. The patient must be carefully shielded against infections. Other therapies depend upon symptoms.

**Treatment—Investigational** Please contact the agencies listed under Resources, below, for the most current information. Addresses and telephone numbers of these agencies, as well as of individual experts and research centers, may be found in the Master Resources List.

**Resources**

**For more information on angioimmunoblastic lymphadenopathy with dysproteinemia:** National Organization for Rare Disorders (NORD); Immune Deficiency Foundation; NIH/National Cancer Institute Physician Data Query Phoneline; NIH/National Institute of Allergy and Infectious Diseases.

**References**

Effect of Cyclophosphamide Therapy on Oncogene Expression in Angioimmunoblastic Lymphadenopathy: D.M. Klinman, et al.; Lancet, November 8, 1986, vol. 2(8515), pp. 1055–1058.

Angioimmunoblastic Lymphadenopathy: W.P. Su; Dermatol. Clin., October 1985, vol. 3(4), pp. 759–768.

Modulation of C-MYB Transcription in Autoimmune Disease by Cyclophosphamide: J.D. Mountz, et al.; J. Immunol., October 1985, vol. 135(4), pp. 2417–2422.

# LYMPHANGIOMA, CAVERNOUS

**Description** Cavernous lymphangioma is a congenital lymphatic disorder characterized by dilated lymph vessels and benign lesions under the skin that are made up of lymphoid tissue. Usually present at birth, lymphangioma may also develop later in life.

**Synonyms**

Chylangioma

**Signs and Symptoms** Deep-seated, benign lesions that are gray, pink, or yellow in color appear around the patient's neck and on the upper extremities, as well as in the mouth, on the tongue, around the eyes and eyelids, and on the lower extremities. These soft tumors of the lymph vessels vary in shape and size. If the lymphangiomas are punctured or cut, prolonged draining of lymph fluid results.

**Etiology** The cause is unknown.

**Epidemiology** Cavernous lymphangioma affects males and females in equal numbers, usually at birth.

**Related Disorders** See *Lymphedema, Hereditary.*

**Treatment—Standard** Surgery is used to remove the involved tissue. Other treatment depends on symptoms.

**Treatment—Investigational** Please contact the agencies listed under Resources, below, for the most current information. Addresses and telephone numbers of these agencies, as well as of individual experts and research centers, may be found in the Master Resources List.

**Resources**

**For more information on cavernous lymphangioma:** National Organization for Rare Disorders (NORD); American Cancer Society; NIH/National Cancer Institute Physician Data Query Phoneline.

**References**

Cavernous Lymphangioma of the Duodenum: Case Report and Review of the Literature: M. Davis, et al.; Gastrointest. Radiol., 1987, vol. 12(1), pp. 10–12.

Cavernous Lymphangioma of the Lip: Report of a Case: B.L. Eppley, et al.; J. Am. Dent. Assoc., April 1985, vol. 110(4), pp. 503–504.

# LYMPHANGIOMYOMATOSIS

**Description** A progressive disorder that primarily affects the lungs of women of childbearing age, lymphangiomyomatosis is characterized by abnormal growth of smooth muscle cells into spindle shapes. The irregularly shaped cells block airways over time and cause breathing difficulties. The disorder may also affect the smooth muscle tissue of the thoracic duct, lymph nodes, and the liver, and can lead to weight loss despite a proper diet. Injections of chorionic gonadotropin and other hormones have been shown to trigger this disorder in some rare cases.

**Synonyms**

> Lymphangioleiomatosis
> Pulmonary Lymphangiomyomatosis

**Signs and Symptoms** The patient usually develops shortness of breath first and then excess fluid or air in the pleurae. Hemorrhaging may eventually occur in the lungs, followed by bloody expectorations. When lymphangiomyomatosis occurs in the lymphatic vessels of the intestines and liver, causing vessel rupture or blockage, chyle and other fluids collect in the walls of the abdominal or thoracic cavity. Excessive urinary fat cell loss turns the urine milky and may cause weight loss. Symptoms and signs become more severe with hormone injections or a pregnancy. In very rare cases, manifestations are confined to lymphatic vessels in the patient's legs.

**Etiology** While the exact cause of this disorder is not known, the fact that it occurs only in women leads researchers to believe that it may be transmitted as a sex-linked trait or genetic disposition. Hormone therapy given to the patient to combat some other malady has also been implicated.

**Epidemiology** Lymphangiomyomatosis occurs only in women and usually in their childbearing years.

**Treatment—Standard** Treatment depends on symptoms. Shunts or tubes are used to drain pleural fluid, and bronchodilators can relieve breathing problems. Oophorectomy has been beneficial for some patients. Tamoxifen has been shown to be successful in arresting the progression of the disease. Pleurodesis of tetracycline diminishes accumulations of fluid. A fat replacement diet may or may not be beneficial. In extreme cases, excision of abnormal lung tissue may benefit the patient.

**Treatment—Investigational** Scientists are investigating the role of hormone therapy in the development of lymphangiomyomatosis and whether or not a genetic disposition is a prerequisite to the disorder. Also under investigation is the therapeutic value of progestin for lymphangiomyomatosis; however, more research is needed.

Please contact the agencies listed under Resources, below, for the most current information. Addresses and telephone numbers of these agencies, as well as of individual experts and research centers, may be found in the Master Resources List.

**Resources**

**For more information on lymphangiomyomatosis:** National Organization for Rare Disorders (NORD); American Lung Association; NIH/National Heart, Lung and Blood Institute.

**For genetic information and genetic counseling referrals:** March of Dimes Birth Defects Foundation; Alliance of Genetic Support Groups.

**References**

Successful Treatment of Pulmonary Lymphangiomyomatosis with Oophorectomy and Progesterone: D. Adamson, et al.; Am. Rev. Respir. Dis., October 1985, vol. 132(4), pp. 916–921.

Pulmonary Lymphangiomyomatosis Associated with Tuberous Sclerosis: Treatment with Tamoxifen and Tetracycline-Pleurodesis: C.M. Luna, et al.; Chest, September 1985, vol. 88(3), pp. 473–475.

# LYMPHEDEMA, HEREDITARY

**Description** Hereditary lymphedema is an inherited lymph-system disorder characterized by swelling of subcutaneous tissue caused by obstruction of lymphatic vessels and resulting edema of lymph fluid.

There are 3 forms of hereditary lymphedema: congenital (Milroy disease; Nonne-Milroy-Meige syndrome); lymphedema praecox (Meige disease); and lymphedema tarda.

**Signs and Symptoms** The edema generally occurs below the waist, but may also be present in the face, larynx, and upper extremities. Patients with an edematous leg may feel uncomfortable but there is usually no pain. The swelling may begin in the foot and move upwards. Radioisotope lymphangiogram and scintilymphangiography may prove helpful in confirming the diagnosis.

Patients with **Milroy disease** have nonulcerating lymphedema from birth. **Meige disease** usually occurs in the 1st or 2nd decade of the patient's life and can cause severe lymphedema in areas below the waist. Initially the patient presents with redness, swelling, pain, and inflammation. Related abnormalities can also occur, such as distichiasis, extradural cysts, vertebral abnormalities, cerebrovascular malformation, pleural effusion, cleft palate, hearing loss, and yellowing of nails.

Onset of **lymphedema tarda** usually occurs after age 35.

**Etiology** Hereditary lymphedema is transmitted as an autosomal dominant trait; less commonly, autosomal or sex-linked recessive. It occurs rarely as a spontaneous change in genetic material of the fetus.

**Epidemiology** Women are affected more often than men.

**Related Disorders** See *Angioedema, Hereditary.*

**Traumatic lymphedema** results from an injury to the lymphatic system, such as a bruise, that blocks the lymph vessels.

**Treatment—Standard** The leg should be elevated to reduce swelling. Other measures include use of support hose and, in some instances, pneumatic compression. Foot and skin hygiene is necessary to prevent lymphangitis and drying of the skin. Microsurgical anastomosis procedures have recently been used with some success.

Treatment of other symptoms and signs is symptomatic and supportive. Genetic counseling may benefit patients and their families.

**Treatment—Investigational** Please contact the agencies listed under Resources, below, for the most current information. Addresses and telephone numbers of these agencies, as well as of individual experts and research centers, may be found in the Master Resources List.

**Resources**

For more information on hereditary lymphedema: National Organization for Rare Disorders (NORD); National Lymphedema Network; National Lymphatic and Venous Diseases Foundation; NIH/National Heart, Lung and Blood Institute.

For genetic information and genetic counseling referrals: March of Dimes Birth Defects Foundation; Alliance of Genetic Support Groups.

**References**
Mendelian Inheritance in Man, 11th ed.: V.A. McKusick; The Johns Hopkins University Press, 1994, pp. 893–895, 897.

Cecil Textbook of Medicine, 19th ed.: J.B. Wyngaarden, et al., eds.; W.B. Saunders Company, 1992, p. 368.

Nelson Textbook of Pediatrics, 14th ed.: R.E. Behrman, ed.-in-chief; W.B. Saunders Company, 1992, p. 1290.

Textbook of Dermatology, 5th ed.: R.H. Champion, et al., eds.: Blackwell Scientific Publications, 1992, pp. 2018–2023.

Harrison's Principles of Internal Medicine, 12th ed.: J.D. Wilson, et al., eds.; McGraw-Hill, 1991, pp. 1025–1026.

Hereditary Lymphedema and Distichiasis: T. Kolin, et al.; Arch. Ophthalmol., July 1991, vol. 109(7), pp. 980–981.

Birth Defects Encyclopedia: M.L. Buyse, ed.-in-chief; Blackwell Scientific Publications, 1990, pp. 1087–1089.

Dictionary of Medical Syndromes, 3rd ed.: S.I. Magalini, et al., eds.: J.B. Lippincott Company, 1990, pp. 637–638.

Congenital Hereditary Lymphedema (Nonne/Milroy): D.D. Farhud, et al.; Pediatr. Padol, 1989, vol. 24(4), pp. 305–307.

Lymphangiosarcoma in Chronic Hereditary Oedema (Milroy's Disease): L.A. Brostrom, et al.; Ann. Chir. Gynaecol., 1989, vol. 78(4), pp. 320–323.

Pulmonary Diseases and Disorders, 2nd ed.: A.P. Fishman; McGraw-Hill, 1988, p. 2134.

Hereditary Late-Onset Lymphedema with Pleural Effusion and Laryngeal Edema: F.A. Herbert, et al.; Arch. Intern. Med., May 1983, vol. 143(5), pp. 913–915.

Familial Lymphedema Praecox: Meige's Disease: E.S. Wheeler, et al; Plast. Reconstr. Surg., May 1981, vol. 67(3), pp. 362–364.

# LYMPHOCYTIC INFILTRATE OF JESSNER

**Description** In lymphocytic infiltrate of Jessner, benign solid lesions composed of accumulated lymphocytes appear on the epidermis of the neck, face, or back. They may disappear spontaneously without leaving scars after remaining unchanged for several years.

**Synonyms**

Benign Lymphocytic Infiltrate of the Skin

Jessner-Kanof Lymphocytic Infiltration of the Skin

**Signs and Symptoms** The lesions typically are smooth and pink or red, have no hair follicles, and are sometimes clear in the center. They most commonly appear on the cheeks, eyelids, and upper face but may also occur on the back and neck. The surrounding skin is usually pruritic and erythematous. Rarely, lesions are sensitive to sunlight. After several years, the lesions generally disappear.

**Etiology** The exact reason for the abnormal lymphocytic accumulation in the skin is not known.

**Epidemiology** Males and females are affected in equal numbers.

**Related Disorders** See *Leprosy; Systemic Lupus Erythematosus; Mycosis Fungoides.*

**Lymphocytoma cutis** is a related disorder marked by skin nodules composed of accumulated lymphocytes and histiocytes. These lesions may be widespread or limited to a small area, are purple to yellow-brown in color, often form glistening spherical masses, and have a narrow noninfiltrating layer that separates them from the epidermis.

**Treatment—Standard** Chloroquine or other antimalarial drugs are usually administered for periods ranging from 6 weeks to 3 months. Superficial radiation may also be given in small doses to eliminate the lesions. Other therapy depends on symptoms.

**Treatment—Investigational** Thalidomide has been used experimentally when the lesions caused by lymphocytic infiltrate of Jessner resist other treatment; however, this drug has been shown to result in birth defects when taken by pregnant women, and it has been disapproved for use in the United States.

Please contact the agencies listed under Resources, below, for the most current information. Addresses and telephone numbers of these agencies, as well as of individual experts and research centers, may be found in the Master Resources List.

**Resources**

**For more information on lymphocytic infiltrate of Jessner:** National Organization for Rare Disorders (NORD); NIH/National Arthritis and Musculoskeletal and Skin Diseases Information Clearinghouse.

**References**

Lymphocytic Infiltration of the Skin (Jessner): A T-Cell Lymphoproliferative Disease: R. Willemze, et al.; Br. J. Dermatol., May 1984, vol. 110(5), pp. 523–529.

Treatment of Jessner-Kanof Disease with Thalidomide: G. Moulin, et al.; Ann. Dermatol. Venereol., 1983, vol. 110(8), pp. 611–614.

Lymphocytic Infiltration of the Skin (Jessner and Kanof): W. Kenneth Blaylock; *in* Clinical Dermatology: J. Demis, et al.; Harper and Row, 1982.


# LYNCH SYNDROMES

**Description** The Lynch syndromes are hereditary disorders that cause colorectal cancers usually prior to age 60. **Lynch syndrome I** is a hereditary site-specific cancer; **Lynch syndrome II** is a cancer family syndrome.

**Synonyms**

Hereditary Nonpolyposis Colorectal Carcinoma

**Signs and Symptoms** Onset is marked by colorectal polyps that may be accompanied by pain or bleeding, diarrhea, abdominal pain, and weight loss. These polyps need to be differentiated from those associated with familial polyposis. Small bowel polyps may be present upon examination. Primary cancers can also develop in the urologic system, brain, stomach, breasts, or female genital tract. The polyp is often the precursor of subsequent neoplasmic growth, especially if other family members have developed colon or rectal cancer.

**Lynch syndrome I** is characterized by hereditary cancers that usually develop in the rectum or colon or in closely related areas such as the small bowel.

**Lynch syndrome II** is characterized by carcinoma of the colorectal or other corporeal site.

**Etiology** The Lynch syndromes are believed to be inherited as an autosomal dominant genetic trait. The gene responsible is reputed to be on the long arm (q) of the 18th chromosome.

**Epidemiology** The Lynch syndromes comprise 5 to 6 percent of the 160,000 new cases of colorectal cancers annually in the United States. The average age of the patient is 40 to 50, whereas the average age of most colorectal cancer patients is 60. Other forms of cancer associated with the Lynch syndromes can occur at any age.

**Related Disorders** See *Familial Polyposis; Peutz-Jeghers Syndrome; Carcinoid Syndrome.*

**Crohn disease** is a bowel disease characterized by severe chronic inflammation of the wall or any part of the gastrointestinal tract. Pain, bloating, and diarrhea are often present. A solid abdominal mass may be palpated. Fissures, abscesses, scarring, obstruction to varying degrees, and fistulae develop as a result of the chronic inflammation.

**Treatment—Standard** The standard treatment is colectomy. At age 25, family members should undergo a colonoscopy and fecal occult blood test every 2 to 3 years (or earlier if malignant polyps have been found).

Genetic counseling is important for patients and their families. Other treatment is symptomatic and supportive.

**Treatment—Investigational** Fluorouracil with interferon α-2a is being developed by Hoffmann–La Roche for the treatment of colorectal cancers.

For metastasized colorectal cancers, anti-TAP immunotoxin is being developed by Xoma Corporation; disaccharide tripeptide glycerol dipalmitoyl, by Immuno Therapeutics; Leucovorin adjunct with fluorouracil 2,3, by Burroughs Wellcome; levoleucovorin with fluorouracil, by Lederle Laboratories; and trimetrexate glucuronate 2,5, by U.S. Bioscience.

Research to determine the exact location of the gene responsible for colorectal cancers is ongoing. It is hoped that a genetic test to identify those susceptible to the Lynch syndromes as well as preventive measures will be developed.

Please contact the agencies listed under Resources, below, for the most current information. Addresses and telephone numbers of these agencies, as well as of individual experts and research centers, may be found in the Master Resources List.

### Resources

**For more information on Lynch syndromes:** National Organization for Rare Disorders (NORD); American Cancer Society; NIH/National Cancer Institute Physician Data Query Phoneline.

**For genetic information and genetic counseling referrals:** March of Dimes Birth Defects Foundation; Alliance of Genetic Support Groups.

### References

Mendelian Inheritance in Man, 10th ed.: V.A. McKusick; The Johns Hopkins University Press, 1992, pp. 180–181, 183–184.

The Molecular Basis of Colon Cancer: A.K. Rustgi, et al.; Annu. Rev. Med., 1992, vol. 43, pp. 61–68.

Genetics of Colon Cancer: D.J. Ahne; West. J. Med., June 1991, vol. 154(4), pp. 700–705.

Hereditary Nonpolyposis Colorectal Cancer (Lynch Syndromes I and II): Genetics, Pathology, Natural History, and Cancer Control (Pt. I): H.T. Lynch, et al.; Cancer Genet. Cytogenet., June 1991, vol. 53(2), pp. 143–160.

The Lynch Syndrome II and Urological Malignancies: H.T. Lynch, et al.; J. Urol., January 1990, vol. 143(1), pp. 24–28.

Adenocarcinoma of the Small Bowel in Lynch Syndrome II.: H.T. Lynch, et al.; Cancer, November 1989, vol. 64(10), pp. 2178–2183.

Gastrointestinal Disease, Pathophysiology Diagnosis Management, 4th ed.: M.H. Sleisenger; W.B. Saunders Company, 1989, pp. 1525–1528.

# MALIGNANT MELANOMA

**Description** Malignant melanoma is a skin neoplasm derived from epidermal or nevose melanin cells. The neoplastic cells eventually invade the dermis and adjacent tissue and frequently metastasize widely. Subtypes of this neoplasm are known as juvenile melanoma, malignant lentigo melanoma, and acral lentiginous melanoma.

**Signs and Symptoms** The early stages of this disease are usually asymptomatic, but later, a lesion appears that does not heal, or a mole begins to change in color or size.

**Juvenile melanoma** is marked by a benign pink to purplish-red papule on the face (usually the cheeks) that has a slightly scaly surface. It usually occurs before the juvenile reaches puberty and is often mistaken for the malignant form of the disease.

A **malignant lentigo melanoma** is a brown or black precancerous spot on the epidermis (usually of the face) that is irregular in shape and resembles a freckle. It most often occurs in older persons.

An **acral lentiginous melanoma** is a malignant neoplasm that occurs on areas of the epidermis that have no hair follicles and have not been overly exposed to the sun.

**Etiology** While the exact cause of this disease is unknown, research indicates that individuals who allow their skin to be exposed to the sun excessively, particularly before puberty, and who live in sunny climates are at greater risk of developing malignant melanoma. Studies have also found that some persons may have a genetic predisposition to the disease that is inherited as an autosomal dominant trait.

**Epidemiology** In recent years, malignant melanoma has increased in incidence at a much greater rate than any other malignant neoplastic disease. It affects equal numbers of males and females, although blue-eyed and fair-complected whites are at greater risk than other populations.

**Related Disorders Squamous cell carcinoma** is a common epithelial neoplasm that often occurs in sun-exposed skin. The carcinoma may also develop in mucous membranes and elsewhere on the body. Cutaneous squamous cell carcinoma is a red, scaly, sharply outlined keratosis that may develop on normal tissue or on precancerous leukoplakia. There may be satellite nodules. The tumor can reach to the lower reticular dermis. The most common cause of cutaneous squamous cell carcinoma is exposure to the sun. The cancer may also arise on the site of preexisting lesions such as a scar from a burn or from trauma, or a lesion of systemic lupus erythematosus.

**Basal cell carcinoma** is a common skin cancer characterized by hard and shiny nodules, hardened scarlike patches that hemorrhage, or ulcerated and encrusted lesions. A biopsy is necessary to distinguish it from localized dermatitis or psoriasis.

**Kaposi sarcoma** is a malignant neoplasm associated with acquired immunodeficiency syndrome (**AIDS**) and characterized by small tumors, plaques, papules, nodules, or ulcers that are tan to purple in color. The neoplasms occur in the oropharyngeal and gastrointestinal tracts and infiltrate the lungs, liver, and bone. Before AIDS was first recognized, Kaposi sarcoma was usually found only in elderly Jewish or Mediterranean men and in persons with compromised immune systems. Today about 30 percent of AIDS patients have Kaposi sarcoma.

The lesions of **seborrheic keratosis** can resemble those of the early stages of malignant melanoma.

**Treatment—Standard** Treatment varies with the stage of disease and the location of the lesion. In stage 1, the lesion is surgically excised along with a 5-cm margin around the lesion. Smaller margins are excised in certain areas, such as the face. In stage 2, which involves the lymph nodes, a lymphadenectomy is performed. Once the disease has metastasized, chemotherapy is administered. Dacarbazine has been shown to be effective in some patients. High-dose combinations of cisplatin, cyclophosphamide, and carmustine have also been beneficial for some patients.

**Treatment—Investigational** Interferon is under investigation as a treatment for this disease, either alone or in combination with other agents. Autologous bone marrow transplantation is also being used on an experimental basis.

Several new products are under investigation. Clinical trials of a polyvalent antigen vaccine for treatment of melanoma are being conducted by Jean Claude Bystryn, M.D., of New York University Medical Center. Interleukin-2 and tumor-infiltrating lymphocytes are being studied in patients with melanoma at Brigham and Women's Hospital, Boston. Researchers at the Food and Drug Administration are testing the orphan product malphalan (Alkeran) for injection as a treatment for metastatic melanoma.

Please contact the agencies listed under Resources, below, for the most current information. Addresses and telephone numbers of these agencies, as well as of individual experts and research centers, may be found in the Master Resources List.

**Resources**

**For more information on malignant melanoma:** National Organization for Rare Disorders (NORD); Skin Cancer Foundation; American Cancer Society; NIH/National Cancer Institute Physician Data Query Phoneline.

**References**

Internal Medicine, 3rd ed.: J.H. Stein, ed.-in-chief; Little, Brown and Company, 1990, pp. 1154–1156.

Malignant Melanoma: Treatment with High Dose Combination Alkylating Agent Chemotherapy and Autologous Bone Marrow Support: T.C. Shea; Arch. Dermatol., June 1988, vol. 124(6), pp. 878–884.

Changing Trends in Melanoma: C.M. Balch, ed.-in-chief; Mel. Let., 1987, vol. 5(1).

Immunotherapy for Malignant Melanoma: Vaccines: J.C. Bystryn; Mel. Let., 1986, vol. 4(2).

# MASTOCYTOSIS

**Description** Mastocytosis is an inherited blood disorder marked by abnormal mast cell infiltration of skin, bone, bone marrow, lungs, liver, spleen, and occasionally the meninges. In adults the solid organs are affected more than the skin, whereas in children the reverse is true (see ***Urticaria Pigmentosa***). **Mast cell leukemia** is one form of mastocytosis.

**Synonyms**

> Cutaneous Mastocytosis
> Systemic Mast Cell Disease

**Signs and Symptoms** Patients with mastocytosis initially feel a vague sense of discomfort or poor health, accompanied by weight loss, diarrhea, nausea, vomiting, weakness, and irregular heartbeat. In children, the skin is primarily affected. The skin is marked with dilated blood vessels, thick and discolored spots that run together, patches resulting from a proliferation of leukocytes, and chronic skin growths that are flat and patterned. The affected skin may show minimal discoloration, but gentle rubbing or stroking can produce swelling and redness.

Adults tend to have greater involvement of internal organs, including mucous membranes in the nose, mouth, and rectum. Lymph nodes, spleen, and liver become swollen, and bone softens and deteriorates, although new bone may grow as the hard outer layer or the spongy inner substance of bone thickens. Patients rarely may have duodenal ulcers that are associated with hemorrhaging or pain in the upper abdomen.

**Etiology** The precise method of genetic transmission of this disorder is not known. The gene responsible for mast cell leukemia has been mapped to chromosome 4 (4q12). Histamine seems to be overproduced and released from mast cells that infiltrate various organs.

**Epidemiology** Mastocytosis most commonly affects adult men and women in equal numbers, although it can also begin in childhood.

**Related Disorders** See ***Urticaria Pigmentosa***.

**Treatment—Standard** A combination of the antihistamines chlorpheniramine and cimetidine is used to control the growth of mast cells and block the effects of histamine release. More recently, oral cromolyn sodium (Gastrocrom R) has been developed; it not only relieves symptoms but prevents recurrence. The drug's manufacturer has established a patient assistance program to provide free Gastrocrom R for needy patients. Contact Fisons Corporation.

Surgical excision of mast cells may be necessary to improve organ function in advanced stages of the disorder.

**Treatment—Investigational** L. Jackson Roberts, II, M.D., at Vanderbilt University Hospital is conducting clinical trials to study systemic mast cell stimulation.

Please contact the agencies listed under Resources, below, for the most current information. Addresses and telephone numbers of these agencies, as well as of individual experts and research centers, may be found in the Master Resources List.

**Resources**

**For more information on mastocytosis:** National Organization for Rare Disorders (NORD); Mastocytosis Chronicles; NIH/National Arthritis and Musculoskeletal and Skin Diseases Information Clearinghouse; NIH/National Cancer Institute Physician Data Query Phoneline.

**References**

Human Genetics Disorders: Journal of NIH Research, August 1994, vol. 6(8), pp. 115–134.

Mastocytosis: A Review: D.H. Stein; Pediatr. Dermatol., November 1986, vol. 3(5), pp. 365–375.

# MAY-HEGGLIN ANOMALY

**Description** May-Hegglin anomaly is a sometimes symptomless hereditary condition characterized by abnormalities of blood platelets and certain leukocytes. Treatment is usually not necessary; prognosis is good.

**Synonyms**

Döhle Bodies Myelopathy

Hegglin Disease

Leukocytic Inclusions with Platelet Abnormality

**Signs and Symptoms** Some patients with May-Hegglin anomaly may show symptoms from birth but others remain asymptomatic for life. The symptoms that do occur include purpura, epistaxis, excessive bleeding from the mouth during dental work, headaches, and muscular weakness on one side of the body due to intracranial bleeding. Excessive bleeding may be brought about when steroid therapy used to treat some other disorder is discontinued.

Laboratory results show giant, oddly shaped platelets and characteristic inclusions in the polymorphonuclear leukocytes. There also might be slightly fewer platelets than normal.

**Etiology** May-Hegglin anomaly is an inherited blood disorder transmitted by an autosomal dominant gene.

**Epidemiology** This anomaly occurs primarily in persons of Greek or Italian descent.

**Related Disorders** Related disorders of abnormal platelet function are Bernard-Soulier syndrome, thrombasthenia, Chédiak-Higashi syndrome, the gray platelet syndrome, and various defects related to collagen-induced platelet aggregation. See *Bernard-Soulier Syndrome; Thrombasthenia; Chédiak-Higashi Syndrome.*

Platelet disorders have also been linked with such congenital conditions as Wiskott-Aldrich syndrome, Down syndrome, thrombocytopenia with absent radius syndrome, and von Willebrand disease.

**Treatment—Standard** May-Hegglin anomaly generally does not require therapy. In severe, rare cases, patients may require transfusions of platelets.

**Treatment—Investigational** Please contact the agencies listed under Resources, below, for the most current information. Addresses and telephone numbers of these agencies, as well as of individual experts and research centers, may be found in the Master Resources List.

**Resources**

**For more information on May-Hegglin anomaly:** National Organization for Rare Disorders (NORD); NIH/National Heart, Lung and Blood Institute.

**For genetic information and genetic counseling referrals:** March of Dimes Birth Defects Foundation; Alliance of Genetic Support Groups.

**References**

Cecil Textbook of Medicine, 19th ed.: J.B. Wyngaarden, et al., eds.; W.B. Saunders Company, 1992, pp. 990–992.

May-Hegglin Anomaly: A Rare Cause of Thrombocytopenia: A. Greinacher, et al.; Eur. J. Pediatr., September 1992, vol. 151(9), pp. 668–671.

Mendelian Inheritance in Man, 10th ed.: V.A. McKusick; The Johns Hopkins University Press, 1992, p. 701.

Coronary Thrombosis in a Patient with May-Hegglin Anomaly: S. McDunn, et al.; Am. J. Clin. Pathol., May 1991, vol. 95(5), pp. 715–718.

Platelet Studies in the Pathogenesis of Thrombocytopenia in May-Hegglin Anomaly: E.R. Burns; Am. J. Pediatr. Hematol. Oncol., Winter 1991, vol. 13(4), pp. 431–436.

Birth Defects Encyclopedia: M.L. Buyse, ed.-in-chief; Blackwell Scientific Publications, 1990, p. 1052.

Dictionary of Medical Syndromes, 3rd ed.: S.I. Magalini, et al., eds.: J.B. Lippincott Company, 1990, p. 580.

Hematology, 4th ed.: W.J. Williams, et al., eds.; McGraw-Hill, 1990, p. 768.

# MULTIPLE MYELOMA

**Description** Multiple myeloma is a rare malignant neoplasm that develops in bone marrow and is characterized by neoplastic proliferation of plasma cells in the marrow of various bones, especially the skull, spine, rib cage, pelvis, and legs. Subdivisions of the disease are known as plasma cell leukemia, nonsecretory myeloma, osteosclerotic myeloma, smoldering myeloma, extramedullary plasmacytoma, and solitary plasmacytoma of bone (see under Related Disorders, below).

**Synonyms**

> Kahler Disease
>
> Myelomatosis
>
> Plasma Cell Myeloma

**Signs and Symptoms** The features most often seen in multiple myeloma are bone pain, anemia, and renal insufficiency. Body movements trigger pain in the bones of the chest or back, which may be followed by pallor, anemia, fatigue, weakness, complications in the kidneys, hepatosplenomegaly, compressed nerves in the spinal column, and greater susceptibility to bacterial infections (especially pneumonia). Results of blood studies show increased levels of suppressor T cells and decreased levels of helper T cells.

**Etiology** While the precise etiology of this cancer is not known, scientists have implicated a number of possible causes, including such environmental factors as exposure to asbestos, radiation, and toxic chemicals used in agriculture and industry, as well as viruses and a genetic disposition to the disease.

**Epidemiology** Twice as many men as women are affected by multiple myeloma, and symptoms usually occur between the ages of 40 and 70. This cancer makes up 1 percent of all cancers and fully 10 percent of all malignant blood disorders.

**Related Disorders** See *Amyloidosis; Waldenström Macroglobulinemia.*

A group of disorders known as **heavy chain diseases** are related to multiple myeloma in that they are characterized by an excessive number of plasma cells or lymphocytes that look like plasma cells, in the lymph nodes and bone marrow. These proliferative disorders are of 3 types: **alpha, gamma,** and **mu heavy chain diseases.** In the alpha form, patients have progressive weight loss, malabsorption of nutrients, steatorrhea, and diarrhea. In the gamma form, patients have anemia, amino acid deficiencies, hepatosplenomegaly, and lymphadenoma. In the mu form, patients have chronic lymphocytic leukemia or lymph gland neoplasms and gammaglobulinemia.

In addition, a number of disorders are secondary to multiple myeloma and considered subdivisions of the disease. However, they do not have to be present for differential diagnosis of multiple myeloma.

The 1st is **plasma cell leukemia,** which is marked by plasma cell hyperplasia in the blood. Thirty percent of these patients have documented multiple myeloma, although initially patients present with signs of leukemia.

The 2nd is **nonsecretory myeloma,** in which multiple myeloma patients fail to produce M protein in their blood or urine.

The 3rd is **osteosclerotic myeloma,** which is a chronic inflammatory disease marked by very low numbers of plasma cells (5 percent or less of normal), osteosclerotic lesions, and sometimes lytic lesions. It causes motor deficiencies, poor motor nerve conduction, high levels of protein in spinal fluid, clubbing of the fingers, fluid retention, hepatosplenomegaly, and skin discoloration.

The 4th is **smoldering myeloma,** in which atypical plasma cells are present in bone marrow in unusually high numbers but without signs of disease. However, protein is present in the urine of many patients.

The 5th is **extramedullary plasmacytoma,** which is marked by the presence of plasma cell neoplasms in places other than bone marrow, most notably in the upper respiratory tract but also in almost every other organ of the body.

Finally, the 6th and last is **solitary plasmacytoma of bone,** which is marked by the presence of only one bone lesion and no evidence of multiple myeloma in the marrow.

**Treatment—Standard** Analgesic drugs and chemotherapy are usually given to relieve pain. Interferon is sometimes administered along with chemotherapy. Fluid administration may be necessary if the kidneys are affected. Radiation therapy may be given to shrink any bone masses that develop. Allogeneic bone marrow transplantation should be considered in patients under the age of 55.

**Treatment—Investigational** Plasmapheresis has been used experimentally and has potential benefit; however, more research is needed. Sandoglobulin is also under investigation as a treatment to reduce infections, but its safety and efficacy have not yet been determined. The Food and Drug Administration is studying the orphan product malphalan (alkeran for injection) as a treatment for patients who cannot take oral medication. Burroughs Wellcome is the sponsor.

Please contact the agencies listed under Resources, below, for the most current information. Addresses and telephone numbers of these agencies, as well as of individual experts and research centers, may be found in the Master Resources List.

### Resources

**For more information on multiple myeloma:** National Organization for Rare Disorders (NORD); American Cancer Society; American Kidney Fund; NIH/National Cancer Institute Physician Data Query Phoneline; National Kidney Foundation.

### References

Internal Medicine, 3rd ed.: J.H. Stein, ed.-in-chief; Little, Brown and Company, 1990, pp. 1146–1149.

Effects of Plasmapheresis on the Plasma Concentration of Proteins Used to Monitor the Disease Process in Multiple Myeloma: A. Wahlin, et al.; Acta Med. Scand., 1988, vol. 223(3), pp. 263–267.

Interferon in the Treatment of Multiple Myeloma: M.R. Cooper, et al.; Cancer, February 1987, vol. 59(3 suppl.), pp. 594–600.

The Use of Interferon in the Treatment of Multiple Myeloma: J.J. Costanzi, et al.; Semin. Oncol., June 1987, vol. 14(2 suppl. 2), pp. 24–28.

# MYCOSIS FUNGOIDES

**Description** Mycosis fungoides is a chronic lymphocyte disorder that arises in the skin and is characterized by progressive infiltration by malignant lymph cells. In the late stages, the patient may have lymph-node infiltrations and ulcerated tumors that resemble mushrooms. In addition to skin, the malignant cells may infiltrate other parts of the body, such as the brain, spleen, liver, and gastrointestinal tract. One type of this disorder is called Vidal-Brocq mycosis fungoides.

### Synonyms

Granuloma Fungoides

**Signs and Symptoms Stage I:** The first signs of mycosis fungoides usually resemble eczema or other skin disorders, such as psoriasis and lichen planus, and are marked by pruritus and pain in the dermal area affected. The patient has scattered erythematous patches on the skin of the trunk and extremities. The patient may also suffer from insomnia.

**Stage II:** Lymphoid cells infiltrate the skin, and bluish-red elevated plaques develop that are initially tiny but eventually grow larger and run together to look like exfoliative dermatitis. At this stage, lipomelanotic reticulosis may develop in the lymph nodes, and lymphadenitis can occur.

**Stage III:** Lobulated tumors develop that resemble mushrooms. They are bluish or red-brown ulcerated lesions measuring 1 to 15 cm in diameter. The dermis may thicken, and atypical lymphoid cells may infiltrate the upper dermis in bands and the clear spaces of the lower dermis, causing necrosis.

**Stage IV:** The final stage is marked by generalized spread of diseased lymphocytes throughout the body, accompanied by anemia, weight loss, fever, gastrointestinal tract involvement with or without intestinal ulceration, and hepatosplenomegaly. Cardiac muscle may also be involved, and dysphagia and coughing may occur. When the brain is affected, the patient may lose clear vision and experience eye pain.

**Etiology** While the precise etiology of this disorder is unknown, researchers believe that the cause is probably a lymphoma arising in the skin or reticulum.

**Epidemiology** Mycosis fungoides generally occurs in patients over 40 years, and twice as often in men as in women.

**Related Disorders** See *Leprosy; Lymphocytic Infiltrate of Jessner.*

**Chronic lymphocytic leukemia** is a related disorder characterized by an abnormal buildup of lymph cells that infiltrate bone marrow and cause deficiencies in blood cell development.

In **Sézary syndrome (Sézary reticulosis syndrome; Sézary erythroderma),** reticular cells infiltrate the skin, causing patches to fall off in scales. Patients have intense pruritus, hair loss, hyperkeratosis, and swelling.

**Treatment—Standard** The standard treatments for mycosis fungoides are electron beam radiation and local administration of the drugs psoralen and mechlorethamine, followed by exposure to long-wavelength ultraviolet light or sunlight.

**Treatment—Investigational** Clinical trials of intramuscular injections of high-dose recombinant leukocyte α-interferon for advanced stages of the disease are under way with positive initial results. Lowering the dosage can reduce side effects, but more research into safety and effectiveness is needed.

While cyclosporine has potential benefit in the treatment of mycosis fungoides and a number of other dermatologic disorders, its side effects can be life-threatening and its use must be limited. It remains an experimental drug for even the most extreme cases, and its long-term effects are not known.

The orphan drug methotrexate USP (Whitby Research) with laurocapram has received approval for testing in the treatment of mycosis fungoides.

Please contact the agencies listed under Resources, below, for the most current information. Addresses and telephone numbers of these agencies, as well as of individual experts and research centers, may be found in the Master Resources List.

**Resources**

**For more information on mycosis fungoides:** National Organization for Rare Disorders (NORD); American Cancer Society; Skin Cancer Foundation; NIH/National Cancer Institute Physician Data Query Phoneline.

**References**

Combined Total Body Electron Beam Irradiation and Chemotherapy for Mycosis Fungoides: I.M. Braverman, et al.; J. Am. Acad. Dermatol., January 1987, vol. 16(1 pt. 1), pp. 45–60.

Alpha-Interferon Treatment of Cutaneous T-Cell Lymphoma and Chronic Lymphocytic Leukemia: K.A. Foon, et al.; Semin. Oncol., December 1986, vol. 13(4 suppl. 5), pp. 35–39.

Cutaneous Malignancies and Metastatic Squamous Cell Carcinoma Following Topical Therapies for Mycosis Fungoides: E.A. Abel, et al.; J. Am. Acad. Dermatol., June 1986, vol. 14(6), pp. 1029–1038.

# Myelofibrosis-Osteosclerosis (MOS)

**Description** MOS is a bone marrow condition characterized by proliferation of fibrous tissue to repair or replace damaged bone marrow, and by generalized anemia and splenomegaly.

**Synonyms**

Agnogenic Myeloid Metaplasia

Myelofibrosis

Myelofibrosis and Myeloid Metaplasia

Osteosclerosis

**Signs and Symptoms** About 30 percent of patients are asymptomatic. The rest experience the signs and symptoms of anemia, such as pallor, weakness, fatigue, dizziness, and headache. Splenomegaly occurs in almost all patients, and hepatomegaly in about 50 percent. Other features include drowsiness, irritability, sweating, gastrointestinal complaints, jaundice, weight loss, and amenorrhea. The patient usually suffers bouts of severe pain in the abdomen, bones, and joints.

**Etiology** MOS is thought to be a connective tissue reaction to several different types of injury that destroy bone marrow tissue. One cause of MOS is metastasis to bone marrow of primary tumors in the breast, prostate, kidney, lung, or adrenal or thyroid glands. A rare cause of MOS in children is osteopetrosis. Tuberculosis and exposure to such toxic substances as benzene, fluoride, or phosphorus are often associated with secondary MOS.

**Epidemiology** MOS occurs in both sexes, usually during midlife, and rarely in children. The disorder is seen in about 2:100,000 persons, slightly more often in whites.

**Treatment—Standard** If the cause of MOS is known, therapy involves treating the underlying cause. If the cause is not known, therapy involves treating the symptoms. If anemia produces cardiovascular symptoms, blood transfusions are effective. Moderate success has been achieved in treating primary MOS with androgens or corticosteroids or both to increase erythrocyte production and decrease their destruction. Allogeneic bone marrow transplantation is indicated in children with severe osteopetrosis.

**Treatment—Investigational** Please contact the agencies listed under Resources, below, for the most current information. Addresses and telephone numbers of these agencies, as well as of individual experts and research centers, may be found in the Master Resources List.

**Resources**

**For more information on myelofibrosis-osteosclerosis:** National Organization for Rare Disorders (NORD); American Cancer Society; NIH/National Cancer Institute Physician Data Query Phoneline; NIH/National Heart, Lung and Blood Institute.

**References**

Internal Medicine, 3rd ed.: J.H. Stein, ed.-in-chief; Little, Brown and Company, 1990, pp. 1126–1128.

# Nevoid Basal Cell Carcinoma Syndrome

**Description** Nevoid basal cell carcinoma syndrome is a malignant neoplastic disease marked by lesions in the epidermis or mucous membranes of the patient's mouth, as well as bony formations and multiple cysts on the head and face. The syndrome may also involve the nervous and vascular systems and connective tissue. The epidermal lesions do not usually have external causes and are limited in size but unlimited in number.

**Synonyms**

Basal Cell Nevus Syndrome
Gorlin-Goltz Syndrome
Herzberg-Wiskemann Phakomatosis
Nevus, Epitheliomatosis Multiplex with Jaw Cysts

**Signs and Symptoms** Multiple lesions appear on the patient's face, neck, chest, and back; they increase in number with age. Onset usually occurs after puberty. Multiple cysts can cause mandibular swelling and frontal bossing. Other manifestations include mental retardation, cataracts, coloboma of the choroid and optic nerve, vertebral defects, scoliosis, bifid ribs, calcification of the falx cerebri, and late eruption of teeth in children.

**Etiology** While the precise cause of nevoid basal cell carcinoma is not known, it is believed that patients may have a genetic predisposition to the disease, which is inherited as an autosomal dominant trait.

**Epidemiology** Equal numbers of males and females are affected by this disorder.

**Related Disorders** See *Malignant Melanoma.*

**Squamous cell carcinoma** is a common epithelial neoplasm that often occurs in sun-exposed skin. The carcinoma may also develop in mucous membranes and elsewhere on the body. Cutaneous squamous cell carcinoma is a red, scaly, sharply outlined keratosis that may develop on normal tissue or on precancerous leukoplakia. There may be satellite nodules. The tumor can reach to the lower reticular dermis. The most common cause of cutaneous squamous cell carcinoma is exposure to the sun. The cancer may also arise on the site of preexisting lesions such as a scar from a burn or from trauma, or a lesion of systemic lupus erythematosus.

**Basal cell carcinoma** is a common skin cancer characterized by hard and shiny nodules, hardened scarlike patches that hemorrhage, or ulcerated and encrusted lesions.

**Treatment—Standard** The lesions are usually removed surgically, although their numbers and locations make this difficult. If the lesions cannot be completely removed by surgery, chemotherapy is also given. Many patients benefit from the chemotherapeutic drug etretinate, which has been shown to destroy the lesions and prevent the formation of new tumors. Patients and their families should receive genetic counseling. Other treatments depend on symptoms.

**Treatment—Investigational** Oral isotretinoin is under investigation as a treatment for this disease, but more research is needed to determine its long-term safety and efficacy.

Please contact the agencies listed under Resources, below, for the most current information. Addresses and telephone numbers of these agencies, as well as of individual experts and research centers, may be found in the Master Resources List.

**Resources**

**For more information on nevoid basal cell carcinoma:** National Organization for Rare Disorders (NORD); Skin Cancer Foundation; American Cancer Society; NIH/National Cancer Institute Physician Data Query Phoneline.

**References**

Mendelian Inheritance in Man, 9th ed.: V.A. McKusick; The Johns Hopkins University Press, 1990, pp. 120–122.

Etretinate Treatment of the Nevoid Basal Cell Carcinoma Syndrome: Therapeutic and Chemopreventive Effect: E. Hodak, Int. J. Dermatol., November 1987, vol. 26(9), pp. 606–609.

Long-Term Retinoid Therapy Is Needed for Maintenance of Cancer Chemopreventative Effect: G.L. Peck; Dermatologica, 1987, vol. 175(suppl. 1), pp. 138–144.

Aromatic Retinoid in the Chemoprevention of the Progression of Nevoid Basal-Cell Carcinoma Syndrome: M. Cristofolini; J. Dermatol. Surg. Oncol., October 1984, vol. 10(10), pp. 778–781.

# NEZELOF SYNDROME

**Description** Nezelof syndrome is an immune deficiency disorder that impairs cellular immunity against infections, especially opportunistic infections. The syndrome also includes some abnormalities in humoral immunity. In a subgroup of about 12 patients, immune deficiency appears to be due to a lack of purine nucleoside phosphorylase **(PNP).**

**Synonyms**

Cellular Immunodeficiency with Abnormal Immunoglobulin Synthesis

**Signs and Symptoms** Patients suffer frequent and severe infections from birth, including oral candidiasis, diarrhea, skin infections, septicemia, urinary tract infections, measles, pulmonary infections, and vaccinia. *Pneumocystis carinii* pneumonia and chronic diarrhea are characteristic of the syndrome. Cytomegalovirus, rubeola, *Pseudomonas,* and mycobacterial infections may also occur. The patient's growth is retarded and general wasting is evident.

Impairment of cellular immunity results in delayed cutaneous anergy, an inability to reject foreign tissue grafts, potentially fatal reactions to vaccination, and a high incidence of malignant tumors. Patients are susceptible to graft-versus-host disease, which causes fever, skin reactions, hepatitis, and gastrointestinal disturbances, such as diarrhea, vomiting, intestinal obstruction, and malabsorption. Patients with PNP deficiency show progressive neurologic deterioration characterized by spastic paralysis of all limbs, autoimmune hemolytic anemia, and thrombocytopenic purpura.

Low T-cell counts and lymphopenia are common laboratory findings in Nezelof syndrome patients. Leukocytes may show a reduced number of neutrophils and high concentrations of eosinophils. Lymph glands shrink in size. The patient's thymus gland is small and histologically abnormal. All classes of antibodies are present, often in normal concentrations, and the patient sometimes has a selective IgA deficiency and substantial elevations of IgE and/or IgD antibodies. Patients with PNP deficiency have very low uric acid levels in the blood and urine.

**Etiology** While the means of transmission and pathophysiology are not clear, Nezelof syndrome is thought to be hereditary, either through an autosomal or a sex-linked gene. The gene that causes PNP deficiency is on the long arm of chromosome 14. A dysfunction of the thymus gland is suspected in most cases. In patients with PNP deficiency, researchers think that the PNP substrate accumulates because of enzyme deficiency and is then preferentially taken up by T lymphocytes. High concentrations of the substrate molecule inhibit DNA synthesis and impair cell function.

**Epidemiology** This extremely rare syndrome affects both males and females.

**Related Disorders** See *Acquired Immune Deficiency Syndrome; Severe Combined Immunodeficiency; DiGeorge Syndrome; Wiskott-Aldrich Syndrome; Ataxia Telangiectasia.*

**Treatment—Standard** Each infection must be treated vigorously according to symptoms, with antifungal, antibiotic, and supportive measures. In several cases, bone marrow transplants taken from immunologically compatible siblings have been successful in treating the disease.

*Pneumocystis carinii* pneumonia is particularly resistant to treatment. Trimethoprim-sulfamethoxazole and the orphan drug pentamidine isethionate are usually used. Idoxuridine, floxuridine, or cytarabine are preferred in the treatment of cytomegalovirus and generalized herpes simplex infections. Amphotericin B therapy has been successful in treating severe infections from *Candida* and related fungi.

For patients with PNP deficiency, researchers have tried to replace the missing enzyme or at least dilute the excess purine bases by giving blood transfusions, but with little success. Also unsuccessful has been deoxycytidine therapy. Patients have to be protected from exposure to infectious agents, including live viral vaccines. They should not be given corticosteroids or immunosuppressant drugs, nor should they undergo splenectomy. If blood transfusions become necessary, the blood must be irradiated to avoid graft-versus-host disease. The prognosis for survival beyond childhood is poor unless matched sibling bone marrow transplants are successful.

**Treatment—Investigational** Please contact the agencies listed under Resources, below, for the most current information. Addresses and telephone numbers of these agencies, as well as of individual experts and research centers, may be found in the Master Resources List.

**Resources**

**For more information on Nezelof syndrome:** National Organization for Rare Disorders (NORD); NIH/National Institute of Allergy and Infectious Diseases; Immune Deficiency Foundation; NIH/National Cancer Institute Physician Data Query Phoneline; American Cancer Society.

**For genetic information and genetic counseling referrals:** March of Dimes Birth Defects Foundation; Alliance of Genetic Support Groups.

**References**

Cecil Textbook of Medicine, 19th ed.: J.B. Wyngaarden, et al., eds.; W.B. Saunders Company, 1992, p. 1450.

Mendelian Inheritance in Man, 10th ed.: V.A. McKusick; The Johns Hopkins University Press, 1992, pp. 1477–1478.

Nelson Textbook of Pediatrics, 14th ed.: R.E. Behrman, ed.-in-chief; W.B. Saunders Company, 1992, p. 554.

Pruine Nucleoside Phosphorylase Deficiency: M.L. Markert; Immunodefic. Rev., 1991, vol. 3(1), pp. 45–81.

Birth Defects Encyclopedia: M.L. Buyse, ed.-in-chief; Blackwell Scientific Publications, 1990, pp. 956–957.

Dictionary of Medical Syndromes, 3rd ed.: S.I. Magalini, et al., eds.: J.B. Lippincott Company, 1990, p. 633.

Immunodeficiency: R.H. Buckley; J. Allergy Clin. Immunol., December 1983, vol. 72(6), pp. 627–641.

Metabolic Defects in Immunodeficiency Diseases: R.D. Webster; Clin. Exp. Immunol., July 1982, vol. 49(1), pp. 1–10.

Combined Immunodeficiency and Thymic Abnormalities: R.D. Webster; J. Clin. Pathol., 1979, vol. 13(suppl.), pp. 10–14.

# PAGET DISEASE OF THE BREAST

**Description** Paget disease of the breast is a rare type of breast cancer characterized by eczema of the nipple and areola. When it spreads to the epidermis of the genitals and rectum, it is called extramammary Paget disease. Paget disease of the breast, not to be confused with Paget disease of the bones, often signals the existence of other internal cancers.

**Synonyms**

>Nipple Cancer
>Adenocarcinoma of the Nipple
>Paget Disease of the Nipple
>Mammary or Extramammary Paget Disease
>Extramammary Paget Disease

**Signs and Symptoms** Paget disease of the breast is characterized by scaling, oozing, and sharply defined inflamed patches on the nipple and areola. This disorder occurs in both men and women. Nearly always associated with adenocarcinoma of the breast, it is called extramammary Paget disease if it spreads to the genitals and rectum where it causes itchy, patchy, crusty areas with well-defined borders. In women, the lower abdominal wall, naval area, vagina, and rectum may be affected. In men, the rectum, prostate, urethra and other parts of the genitourinary tract may be involved. If detected early and if only the nipple is involved, the cure rate for Paget disease of the breast is very high. However, when extramammary tissue is involved, the prognosis is less.

**Etiology** The exact cause of Paget disease of the breast and extramammary Paget disease is not known. Since the disorder arises from epidermotropic cancer cells in the parenchyma of the breast, some scientists believe that this type of cancer may be an early warning sign of more common breast cancers or other internal forms of cancer.

**Epidemiology** Paget disease of the breast affects both males and females, but the ratio is much higher in women than in men, and onset is usually after the age of 50.

**Related Disorders** See ***Bowen Disease; Malignant Melanoma; Mycosis Fungoides.***

**Treatment—Standard** Treatment depends on identifying the type of Paget disease; antikeratin antibody staining may prove helpful. If nipple disease is present but the lymph nodes are unaffected, excision of the affected area is usually indicated. Radiation or chemotherapy with or without surgery may also be necessary. If the lymph nodes are involved, a simple or radical mastectomy and radiation are indicated. If Paget disease of the breast accompanies an underlying cancer of the breast, then the underlying cancer is treated first and the Paget treatment is determined by the type of breast cancer found. When the patient has extramammary Paget disease, the treatment is determined by the organs affected.

A mammogram may not indicate the presence of a malignancy because often no mass is formed in the breast. In this situation, a nipple wedge biopsy may show Paget disease of the nipple as well as intraductal carcinoma of the breast.

Other treatment is symptomatic and supportive.

**Therapies–Investigational** Please contact the agencies listed under Resources, below, for the most current information. Addresses and telephone numbers of these agencies, as well as of individual experts and research centers, may be found in the Master Resources List.

**Resources**

**For more information on Paget disease of the breast:** National Organization for Rare Disorders (NORD); Skin Cancer Foundation; American Cancer Society; NIH/National Cancer Institute Physician Data Query Phoneline.

**References**

The Histogenesis of Mammary and Extramammary Paget's Disease: R.R. Jones, et al.; Histopathology, April 1989, vol. 14(4), pp. 409–416.

Mammography in the Symptomatic Woman: S. Edeiken; Cancer, April 1989, vol. 63(7), pp. 1412–1414.

Radiotherapy for Paget's Disease of the Nipple: A Conservative Alternative: A.D. Stockdale, et al.; Lancet, September 16, 1989, vol. 2(8664), pp. 664–666.

Paget's Disease of the Breast: J.A. Sanchez, et al.; Am. Fam. Physician, August 1987, vol. 36(2), pp. 145–147.

# PHEOCHROMOCYTOMA

**Description** Pheochromocytoma is a rare neoplastic disorder marked by usually benign chromaffinoma derived from tumors in the adrenal medullary tissue and characterized by hypertension that does not respond to usual treatment.

**Synonyms**

>Adrenal Tumor
>Chromaffin Cell Tumor

**Signs and Symptoms** The patient's hypertension may be associated with heart palpitations, angina, rapid breathing, profuse sweating, headache, pallor, cold and clammy skin, nausea, stomach pain, vomiting, constipation, tingling sensations, and visual disturbances.

Diagnosis is by urine testing, magnetic resonance imaging, and lack of response to hypertension medication.

**Etiology** Pheochromocytoma results from tumors growing in adrenal glands and possibly along certain nerve pathways as well. In some cases, it has been shown to appear without an apparent cause, while in other cases it has been linked to an autosomal dominant gene whose penetrance is incomplete.

**Epidemiology** Symptoms usually appear before the patient reaches age 50, but pheochromocytoma can strike at any age. Equal numbers of women and men are affected.

**Related Disorders** See *Neurofibromatosis; von Hippel–Lindau Disease.*

**Sipple syndrome** is a related disorder marked by adrenal tumors associated with other endocrine gland tumors.

**Treatment—Standard** The standard treatment is removal of the neoplasm by surgery. Other treatments depend on symptoms. When pheochromocytoma is shown to occur in families, genetic counseling is recommended.

**Treatment—Investigational** Please contact the agencies listed under Resources, below, for the most current information. Addresses and telephone numbers of these agencies, as well as of individual experts and research centers, may be found in the Master Resources List.

**Resources**

**For more information on pheochromocytoma:** National Organization for Rare Disorders (NORD); American Cancer Society; NIH/National Cancer Institute Physician Data Query Phoneline.

**For genetic information and genetic counseling referrals:** March of Dimes Birth Defects Foundation; Alliance of Genetic Support Groups.

**References**

Localization of Ectopic Pheochromocytomas by Magnetic Resonance Imaging: J.E. Schmedt, et al.; Am. J. Med., October 1987, vol. 83(4), pp. 770–772.

Clinically Unsuspected Pheochromocytomas: Experience at Henry Ford Hospital and a Review of the Literature: N.K. Krane; Arch. Intern. Med., January 1986, vol. 146(1), pp. 54–57.

Diagnosis and Management of Pheochromocytoma: G.W. Gifford, et al.; Cardiology, 1985, vol. 72(suppl. 1), pp. 126–130.

# POLYCYTHEMIA VERA

**Description** A chronic proliferative disorder involving bone marrow, polycythemia vera is characterized by an increase in the number of erythrocytes and a rise in the concentration of hemoglobin in the blood.

**Synonyms**

Erythremia

**Signs and Symptoms** Patients experience fatigue, malaise, difficulty in concentrating, headache, drowsiness, dizziness, and forgetfulness. Pruritis occurs in about 50 percent of cases, especially after a hot bath. The patient's skin is sometimes erythematous, or it may be normal in color and have only dusky redness in the mucous membranes. Retinal veins may be dark red, full, and tortuous, and the spleen is generally palpable. Osteonecrosis may occur. Some patients are symptomless.

**Etiology** The cause is unknown.

**Related Disorders** Leukemia is a related disorder.

**Treatment—Standard** Phlebotomy is the most common treatment. Three to 6 phlebotomies are usually required to return the number of erythrocytes in the blood to normal by reducing the hematocrit level to less than 50 percent. However, repeated phlebotomy usually causes iron-deficiency anemia, and the treatment is not as effective in patients with high iron absorption rates or greatly elevated platelet counts. It is not convenient in patients with poor veins. If the patient is elderly and has advanced arteriosclerosis or a heart condition, less blood should be removed with each phlebotomy.

The patient should not be given supplemental iron when phlebotomy is the only therapy because the iron tends to accelerate hemoglobin production. Neither should the patient eat foods rich in iron, such as clams, oysters, liver, and legumes.

Almost all patients treated by phlebotomy followed by radiophosphorus ($32_p$) therapy experience clinical and hematologic remission that usually lasts 18 months but can vary from 6 months to several years. Most patients so treated usually have no immediate side effects, but approximately 10 percent of patients treated with $32_p$ develop acute leukemia that usually occurs after more than 10 years of treatment. Chemotherapy for polycythemia vera increases the risk of acute leukemia.

Patients suffer hyperuricemia that requires treatment with allopurinol. Acute gouty arthritis can develop; it should be treated with colchicine or nonsteroidal anti-inflammatory drugs. Although corticosteroids can produce rapid and complete remission in some patients, they are generally used only when other drugs are not effective.

**Treatment—Investigational** The Food and Drug Administration has approved the experimental use of the orphan drug anagrelide (Roberts Pharmaceutical Corporation) for treatment of polycythemia vera.

Please contact the agencies listed under Resources, below, for the most current information. Addresses and telephone numbers of these agencies, as well as of individual experts and research centers, may be found in the Master Resources List.

**Resources**

**For more information on polycythemia vera:** National Organization for Rare Disorders (NORD); Myelo-proliferative Disease Research Center; NIH/National Heart, Lung and Blood Institute.

**References**

A New Treatment for Polycythemia Vera: Recombinant Interferon Alpha: R.T. Silver; Blood, August 1990, vol. 76(4), pp. 664–665.

Cecil Textbook of Medicine, 18th ed.: J.B. Wyngaarden and L.H. Smith, Jr., eds.; W.B. Saunders Company, 1988, pp. 973, 980–984.

# PSEUDOMYXOMA PERITONEI

**Description** Pseudomyxoma peritonei is a slow-growing malignancy that originates from appendiceal, intestinal, or ovarian neoplasm and settles in the peritoneal cavity.

**Synonyms**

> Malignant Appendiceal Tumor
> Malignant Large Cystadenocarcinoma
> Malignant Large Peritoneal Carcinomatosis

**Signs and Symptoms** Onset is usually marked by pain in the lower abdomen that suggests appendicitis. Upon examination the abdomen is found to be swollen but not painful to the touch. Surgery to remove the appendix reveals ascites and mucinous tumors, often in great numbers. However, the small bowel is usually spared, allowing for removal of much of the tumorous growth. Serious consequences of the disorder may be loss of intestinal function and intestinal obstruction.

**Etiology** Pseudomyxoma peritonei is generally thought to develop slowly from the spread of appendiceal, large bowel, or ovarian cancer to the abdominal area. The mucinous tumor fills the abdomen with an "omental cake," resulting in a condition known as "jelly belly."

**Epidemiology** Because it usually develops from an ovarian tumor, pseudomyxoma peritonei affects women more often than men, at a 4:1 ratio. The mean age is 57. Approximately 450 cases have been reported.

**Related Disorders** See *Carcinoid Syndrome.*

**Adenocarcinoma of the appendix** is the most common form of appendiceal malignancy and is often difficult to distinguish from noncancerous mucoceles. Both disorders cause appendicitis.

**Treatment—Standard** Presurgical CT and ultrasound scans can often show if mucinous cells have produced large amounts of mucus in the abdominal cavity. Surgery along with intraperitoneal chemotherapy (mitomycin-C and 5-fluorouracil) can often increase life expectancy if the cancer has not spread from another location.

**Treatment—Investigational** For more information on surgical and medicinal ways of treating pseudomyxoma peritonei, contact Dr. Paul H. Sugarbaker at The Cancer Institute, Washington, D.C.

Please contact the agencies listed under Resources, below, for the most current information. Addresses and telephone numbers of these agencies, as well as of individual experts and research centers, may be found in the Master Resources List.

**Resources**

**For more information on pseudomyxoma peritonei:** National Organization for Rare Disorders (NORD); American Cancer Society; NIH/National Cancer Institute Physician Data Query Phoneline.

**References**

Cancer of the Appendix and Pseudomyxoma, *in* Current Therapy in Colon and Rectal Surgery: P.H. Sugarbaker; B.C. Decker, 1990.

Pseudomyxoma Peritonei Presenting As a Scrotal Mass: W.C. Baker, et al.; J. Urol., April 1988, vol. 139(4), pp. 821–822.

A 25-Year Review of Adenocarcinoma of the Appendix: A Frequently Perforating Carcinoma: M.A. Cerame; Dis. Colon Rectum, February 1988, vol. 31(2), pp. 145–150.

Malignant Pseudomyxoma Peritonei of Colonic Origin: Natural History and Presentation of a Curative Approach to Treatment: P.H. Sugarbaker, et al.; Dis. Colon Rectum, October 1987, vol. 30(10), pp. 772–779.

# PURE RED CELL APLASIA

**Description** A rare blood disorder that affects only erythrocytes, pure red cell aplasia is marked by a sudden decline in the number of red blood cells produced by the bone marrow.

**Signs and Symptoms** Pallor, weakness, and lethargy are seen, with the course determined by the degree of aplasia. Patients have a deficient number of erythroblasts despite elevated levels of erythropoietin.

**Etiology** Believed to be an autoimmune disorder, pure red cell aplasia is one of a group of syndromes related to bone marrow failure. The possible causes of this disorder are viral infection, a neoplasm in the thymus gland, or certain drugs, such as the sulfonylureas, anesthetic halothane, gold used in the treatment of arthritis, and antiepileptic drugs (e.g., phenobarbital, phenytoin, and penicillin).

**Epidemiology** This rare disorder affects equal numbers of adult males and females.

**Related Disorders** See *Anemia, Aplastic.*

**Treatment—Standard** When drugs are the cause of pure red cell aplasia and those drugs are discontinued, the disorder usually goes into remission.

The anti-inflammatory drugs prednisone and antithymocyte globulin are used to treat patients under 30, while older patients are treated with cytotoxic immunosuppressants (e.g., azathioprine, cyclophosphamide, and 6-mercaptopurine). Antihuman thymocyte gammaglobulin is used for patients resistant to conventional immunosuppressive agents. All patients may require blood transfusions periodically until the drugs take effect. If the drugs lead to remission, they are discontinued.

Surgical removal of the thymus gland often results in remission.

**Treatment—Investigational** Please contact the agencies listed under Resources, below, for the most current information. Addresses and telephone numbers of these agencies, as well as of individual experts and research centers, may be found in the Master Resources List.

**Resources**

**For more information on pure red cell aplasia:** National Organization for Rare Disorders (NORD); NIH/National Heart, Lung and Blood Institute; Aplastic Anemia Foundation of America.

**References**

New Therapies for Aplastic Anemia: S.B. Krantz; Amer. J. Med. Sciences, 1986, vol. 291, pp. 371–379.

Pure Red Cell Aplasia Characterized by Erythropoietic Maturation Arrest: Response to Anti-Thymocyte Globulin: A.D. Jacobs, et al.; Amer. J. Med., March 1985, vol. 78(3), pp. 515–517.

Diphenylhydantoin-Induced Pure Red Cell Aplasia: E.N. Dessypris, et al.; Blood, 1985, vol. 65, pp. 789–794.

# PURPURA, IDIOPATHIC THROMBOCYTOPENIC (ITP)

**Description** ITP is a platelet disorder characterized by abnormal hemorrhaging into the skin and mucous membranes without an apparent cause or underlying disease. Anemia may result.

**Synonyms**

> Purpura Hemorrhagica
> Werlhof Disease

**Signs and Symptoms** The signs of hemorrhaging from the mucous membranes are epistaxis and gastrointestinal, genitourinary, and vaginal bleeding. Hemarthrosis and bleeding into the central nervous system are less common features. Anemia produces weakness, fatigue, or signs of congestive heart failure. Fever and splenomegaly may also occur.

**Etiology** Although the cause of ITP is not known, symptoms are sometimes preceded by an acute viral infection. There is evidence to support an immunologic basis for the disorder, since antiplatelet antibodies have been identified in most patients. Bone marrow samples show the presence of a large number of inactive or nonproductive megakaryocytes.

**Epidemiology** ITP affects children and young adults most frequently and occurs in females more often than males. Pregnant women who have systemic lupus erythematosus are particularly vulnerable to ITP.

**Related Disorders Allergic purpura** is acute or chronic vasculitis that involves the skin, joints, and gastrointestinal and renal systems.

**Treatment—Standard** Corticosteroids (hydrocortisone or prednisone) are effective in about 15 percent of ITP patients. About one-half of those who do not respond to steroid therapy or who have recurrence when steroids are discontinued respond well to splenectomy. Immunosuppressive drugs, such as cyclophosphamide and azathioprine, have been effective in some patients who did not respond to steroids or splenectomy. The antineoplastic drug vincristine has sometimes been therapeutic.

While platelet concentrates can be transfused to control hemorrhaging until more specific therapy has time to be effective, the short survival time of platelets limits the usefulness of this treatment. Patients also risk an immune reaction to repeated platelet transfusions.

The Food and Drug Administration has approved the use of intravenous immunoglobulin for short periods in patients (especially children) who have an acute form of ITP. Chronic ITP may require frequent use of intravenous immunoglobulin.

**Treatment—Investigational** The orphan products presently under investigation as treatment for ITP include the following: the drug defibrotide, which is available from Crinos International in Italy on an experimental basis; and the product Rho(d) immune globulin (human) (trade name Winrho SD), which is manufactured by RH Pharmaceuticals, Canada.

Children with ITP have shown good response when treated with anti-D immune globulin, which is less expensive and has fewer side effects than other products. More research is needed to determine its safety and efficacy.

Please contact the agencies listed under Resources, below, for the most current information. Addresses and telephone numbers of these agencies, as well as of individual experts and research centers, may be found in the Master Resources List.

### Resources
**For more information on idiopathic thrombocytopenic purpura:** National Organization for Rare Disorders (NORD); NIH/National Heart, Blood and Lung Institute.

### References
Combination Chemotherapy in Refractory Immune Thrombocytopenic Purpura: M. Figueroa, et al; N. Engl. J. Med., April 1993, vol. 328(17), pp. 1226–1229.

Cecil Textbook of Medicine, 18th ed.: J.B. Wyngaarden and L.H. Smith, Jr., eds.; W.B. Saunders Company, 1988, pp. 1050–1051.

# PURPURA, SCHOENLEIN-HENOCH

**Description** Schoenlein-Henoch purpura is a capillary disorder characterized by purpural skin lesions and internal hemorrhaging. The disorder can also affect the joints, gastrointestinal tract, kidneys, and, rarely, the central nervous system.

If the skin and joints are affected, but not the gastrointestinal tract, the disorder is termed **Schoenlein purpura.** If the patient has skin purpura and acute abdominal problems without joint disease, the disorder is termed **Henoch purpura.**

### Synonyms
Allergic Purpura
Anaphylactoid Purpura
Hemorrhagic Capillary Toxicosis
Henoch-Schoenlein Purpura
Nonthrombocytopenic Idiopathic Purpura
Peliosis Rheumatica
Rheumatic Purpura

**Signs and Symptoms** Initially, the patient's skin reddens, swells, and develops hives, which are associated with capillary inflammation or hemorrhaging beneath the skin that produces a reddish-brown or reddish-purple appearance. In most patients, hives appear on the buttocks and lower extremities first and may then spread or worsen.

Patients may also experience fever and a general feeling of discomfort or weakness. Acute local pain can result if blood and plasma accumulate in the joints or abdomen. Gastrointestinal hemorrhaging may cause iron-deficiency anemia and other gastrointestinal disturbances, such as vomiting or blood in the stool.

Approximately 10 percent of patients have kidney inflammation or lesions that can appear at any time and signify a more severe form of the disorder. When the central nervous system is affected, the patient may suffer headaches, perceptual changes, and seizures.

**Etiology** Although the cause is not known, it is suggested that the disorder may be an extreme allergic reaction to certain foods, such as chocolate, milk, eggs, or beans; various drugs; or insect bites. Upper respiratory tract infection or rubella sometimes precedes the disease, but a causal link to viral infections has not been proved.

**Epidemiology** Schoenlein-Henoch purpura can occur at any age, but it most commonly occurs in childhood. Males are apparently affected slightly more often than females; one study showed a 35:25 male-to-female ratio.

**Related Disorders Common purpura** is the most prevalent type of purpura, occurring most often in women over age 50. Where there has been no injury, purpural lesions occur more often than subcutaneous bleeding. However, following surgery or even minor injury, blood vessel fragility results in excessive bleeding. The bleeding may be reduced by short-term corticosteroid therapy and, in postmenopausal women, estrogen.

**Scurvy,** a type of purpura, results from a deficiency of vitamin C in the diet. Patients suffer weakness, anemia, spongy gums, and a tendency to subcutaneous and mucous membrane hemorrhaging.

**Gardener-Diamond syndrome,** sometimes called painful bruising syndrome, is also a type of purpura that chiefly occurs in young women. An autoimmune association has been suggested.

**Treatment—Standard** If the cause of the disorder is found to be an allergic reaction, the patient should avoid the precipitant. Other therapy depends on symptoms. Mild childhood cases tend to improve spontaneously with age. Some studies indicate that early steroid treatment may reduce risk of renal damage. Hemodialysis has been found to benefit some patients with renal failure. In most patients, the disease has a limited course and the prognosis is good.

**Treatment—Investigational** Adults with severe cases of this disorder have been experimentally treated with combination therapy of anticoagulants (heparin and acenocoumarol), corticosteroids, and immunosuppressants.

Cyclophosphamide has been successfully used alone in a few patients. Plasmapheresis has been tried, but more research is needed.

Intravenous immunoglobulin (IVGG) has been used to treat children with severe abdominal pain associated with this disorder. Other studies are under way to determine if such therapy with or without azathioprine is effective for severe IgA nephropathy. In patients who received heparin intravenously for 3 days, renal involvement was significantly reduced compared to the control group. Further research is needed for all 3 treatments to determine their safety and efficacy.

Please contact the agencies listed under Resources, below, for the most current information. Addresses and telephone numbers of these agencies, as well as of individual experts and research centers, may be found in the Master Resources List.

### Resources

**For more information on Schoenlein-Henoch purpura:** National Organization for Rare Disorders (NORD); National Kidney Foundation; American Kidney Fund; NIH/National Institute of Allergy and Infectious Diseases; NIH/National Heart, Lung and Blood Institute.

### References

Henoch-Schonlein Purpura: I.S. Szer; Curr. Opin. Rheumatol., January 1994, vol. 6(1), pp. 25–31.

Henoch-Schonlein Purpura: Four Cases and a Review: A.L. Causey, et al.; J. Emerg. Med., May–June 1994, vol. 12(3), pp. 331–341.

High-Dose Immunoglobulin Therapy for Severe IgA Nephropathy and Henoch-Schonlein Purpura: G. Rostoker, et al.; Ann. Intern. Med., March 1994, vol. 120(6), pp. 476–484.

Henoch-Schonlein Purpura: K.M. Tapson; Am. Fam. Physician, February 15, 1993, vol. 47(3), pp. 633–638.

Intravenous Immunoglobulin in Henoch-Schonlein Purpura: F.J. Heldrich, et al.; Md. Med. J., June 1993, vol. 42(6), pp. 577–579.

Cecil Textbook of Medicine, 19th ed.: J.B. Wyngaarden, et al., eds.; W.B. Saunders Company, 1992, pp. 556, 1538.

Classification of Purpura: B.A. Michel; Curr. Opin. Rheumatol, February 1992, vol. 4(1), pp. 3–8.

Crescentic Glomerulonephritis in Children: H.M. Jardim, et al.; Pediatr. Nephrol., May 1992, vol. 6(3), pp. 231–235.

Effectiveness of Early Prednisone Treatment in Preventing the Development of Nephropathy in Anaphylactoid Purpura: F. Mollica, et al.; Eur. J. Pediatr., February 1992, vol. 151(2), pp. 140–144.

Nelson Textbook of Pediatrics, 14th ed.: R.E. Behrman, ed.-in-chief; W.B. Saunders Company, 1992, p. 627–628.

Textbook of Dermatology, 5th ed.: R.H. Champion, et al., eds.: Blackwell Scientific Publications, 1992, pp. 1918–1920.

Harrison's Principles of Internal Medicine, 12th ed.: J.D. Wilson, et al., eds.; McGraw-Hill, 1991, p. 334–336.

Dictionary of Medical Syndromes, 3rd ed.: S.I. Magalini, et al., eds.: J.B. Lippincott Company, 1990, p. 795.

Hematology, 4th ed.: W.J. Williams, et al., eds.; McGraw-Hill, 1990, pp. 1443–1448.

Clinical Aspects of the Nephropathy in Schoenlein-Henoch Syndrome: E. Verrina, et al.; Pediatr. Med. Chir., May–June 1986, vol. 8(3), pp. 317–320.

Neurological Manifestations of Schoenlein-Henoch Purpura: Report of Three Cases and Review of the Literature: A.L. Belman, et al.; Pediatrics, April 1985, vol. 75(4), pp. 687–692.

Schoenlein-Henoch Syndrome in Adults: D.A. Roth, et al.; Q. J. Med., May 1985, vol. 55(217), pp. 145–152.

# PURPURA, THROMBOTIC THROMBOCYTOPENIC (TTP)

**Description** TTP is a rare blood disease characterized by an abnormally small number of platelets in the blood, abnormal destruction of erythrocytes, kidney dysfunction, nervous system disturbances, fever, and the presence of purpura in the skin and mucous membranes.

### Synonyms

Moschowitz Disease

**Signs and Symptoms** Onset is often sudden, severe, and persistent. Normal blood flow may be blocked by platelets clotting the blood vessels of many of the patient's organs. Headaches, arthralgias, slight or partial paresis, changes in the patient's mental condition, seizures, and coma may also occur, as well as proteinuria, hematuria, and fever. Hemorrhaging in mucous membranes and skin causes purpura. Pallor, fatigue, weakness, nausea, vomiting, and abdominal pain are further signs and symptoms. Increased levels of creatinine are found in the blood of 50 percent of these patients.

Ten percent of patients suffer acute kidney failure. Urine flow decreases to a very low level, followed by shortness of breath, swelling of feet, fever, and headache. High blood pressure, heart and lung congestion, and brain metabolism alterations result from retention of salt and water in the blood. Irregular heartbeat can result from hyperkalemia.

Retinal abnormalities sometimes occur in women patients who take oral contraceptives, but clarity of vision is generally not affected. Female TTP patients may also have severe complications while they are pregnant.

**Etiology** While the precise cause is not known, studies have implicated some kind of autoimmune reaction or infectious agent. It has also been shown that the disease may be inherited in some cases, with TTP occurring in members of the same family many years apart. Other studies have shown a hormonal influence on the disease and that oral contraceptives and the menstrual cycle (**cyclic TTP**) may affect relapses. **AIDS** (acquired immunodeficiency syndrome), **ARC** (the AIDS-related complex), and **HIV** infection (human immunodeficiency virus) have also been shown to be causative factors.

**Epidemiology** TTP affects 1:1,00,000 persons every year, two-thirds of them women who are mostly between the ages of 20 and 50. Individuals with HIV infection are more often affected. Pregnant women and persons with collagen-vascular diseases may occasionally develop TTP.

**Related Disorders** See *Hemolytic-Uremic Syndrome; Purpura, Idiopathic Thrombocytopenic; Purpura, Schoenlein-Henoch; Thrombocytopenia, Essential.*

The combination of TTP and hemolytic-uremic syndrome has been called **thrombotic microangiopathy** or **TTP-HUS complex.** Some researchers suggest that the 2 are really variations of the same disease.

**Treatment—Standard** Immediate diagnosis and treatment are important to the outcome. Prednisone is used as an anti-inflammatory and immunosuppressant. Treatment also includes plasmapheresis or infusions of fresh-frozen plasma.

Patients and families genetically affected by this disorder should receive genetic counseling. Other treatments depend on symptoms.

**Treatment—Investigational** Whole-blood exchange and splenectomy are being investigated as therapies. The immuno-suppressive drug vincristine has been used for patients who do not respond to other therapy, as have the vasodilator dipyridamole and aspirin. Antiplatelet drugs have shown some promise, but their safety and efficacy are not yet known. An Italian pharmaceutical company has developed the orphan drug defibrotide for experimental use. For information, contact Crinos International, Via Belvedere 1, 22079 Villa Guardia, Como, Italy.

Please contact the agencies listed under Resources, below, for the most current information. Addresses and telephone numbers of these agencies, as well as of individual experts and research centers, may be found in the Master Resources List.

**Resources**

**For more information on thrombotic thrombocytopenic purpura:** National Organization for Rare Disorders (NORD); NIH/National Heart, Lung and Blood Institute.

**For genetic information and genetic counseling referrals:** March of Dimes Birth Defects Foundation; Alliance of Genetic Support Groups.

**References**

Internal Medicine, 3rd ed.: J.H. Stein, ed.-in-chief; Little, Brown and Company, 1990, pp. 1046–1047, 897.

Thrombotic Thrombocytopenic Purpura: A Review: S.J. Sierakow and E.J. Kucharz; Cor. Vasa., 1988, vol. 30(1), pp. 60–72.

Thrombotic Thrombocytopenic Purpura in Patients with the Acquired Immunodeficiency Syndrome (AIDS)-Related Complex: A Report of Two Cases: J.M. Nair, et al.; Ann. Intern. Med., August 1, 1988, vol. 109(3), pp. 209–212.

# SHWACHMAN SYNDROME

**Description** Shwachman syndrome is a digestive and respiratory disorder characterized by insufficient digestive enzymes and abnormally low leukocyte counts. Onset is usually in infancy or early childhood. Because the infant does not digest nutrients properly, short stature, other problems with bone growth, and chronic diarrhea may result. The patient usually suffers persistent respiratory and skin infections as well.

**Synonyms**

Burke Syndrome

Metaphyseal Dysostosis (Type B IV)

Neutropenia-Pancreatic Insufficiency

Shwachman-Diamond Syndrome

**Signs and Symptoms** The initial symptom of this syndrome is usually diarrhea. Affected infants frequently have respiratory and skin infections and tend to bleed easily. Some infants may fail to thrive or suffer anemia because of insufficient absorption of nutrients. One-third of patients are short of stature. Bone deformities that can impair walking occur in some.

**Etiology** While the exact cause of the spectrum of this disease is not known, studies have shown that the digestive and respiratory effects are due to insufficient amounts of digestive enzymes and leukocytes.

**Epidemiology** The syndrome begins to manifest itself in infancy or early childhood. Males and females appear to be equally affected.

**Related Disorders** See *Agranulocytosis, Acquired.*

The respiratory and digestive symptoms of Shwachman syndrome may mimic those of cystic fibrosis.

**Treatment—Standard** Antibiotics are used to treat infections; pancreatic enzymes are administered to correct enzyme deficiencies; and the patient is fed a diet high in protein, calories, and vitamins. Other therapy depends on symptoms.

**Treatment—Investigational** Severe, chronic neutropenia responds to treatment with granulocyte-colony stimulating factor.

A drug (LF1695) that restores the immune system in children with Hodgkin disease, Shwachman syndrome, and Chagas disease is being developed by the French manufacturer Fournier.

The DNA of families affected by Shwachman syndrome is being analyzed by researchers at the Hospital for Sick Children, Toronto, in order to identify the gene responsible.

Please contact the agencies listed under Resources, below, for the most current information. Addresses and telephone numbers of these agencies, as well as of individual experts and research centers, may be found in the Master Resources List.

### Resources

**For more information on Shwachman syndrome:** National Organization for Rare Disorders (NORD); NIH/National Diabetes, Digestive and Kidney Diseases Information Clearinghouse; Shwachman Syndrome Support; Cystic Fibrosis Foundation; American Lung Association.

### References

Pancreatic Lipomatosis in the Shwachman-Diamond Syndrome: Identification by Sonography and CT-Scan: E. Robberecht, et al.; Pediatr. Radiol., 1985, vol. 15(5), pp. 348–349.

Chronic Diarrhea and Neutropenia Not Associated with Pancreatic Insufficiency: A Non-Shwachman-Diamond Entity: L.R. Marino, et al.; J. Pediatr. Gastroenterol. Nutr., 1983, vol. 2(3), pp. 559–562.

Cystic Fibrosis "Factor(s)": Present Also in Sera of Shwachman's Pancreatic Insufficiency: G. Banchini, et al.; Pediatr. Res., July 1981, vol. 15(7), pp. 1073–1075.

# THALASSEMIA MAJOR

**Description** Characterized by a marked increase in F hemoglobin and decreased synthesis of the β-polypeptide chains in the hemoglobin molecule, thalassemia major is the most severe form of chronic familial hemolytic anemias found originally in persons living in the Mediterranean basin. Patients also have a decreased number of erythrocytes.

### Synonyms

> Cooley Anemia
> Erythroblastotic Anemia of Childhood
> Hemolytic Anemia
> Hereditary Leptocytosis
> Mediterranean Anemia
> Target Cell Anemia
> Thalassemia
> β-Thalassemia Major

**Signs and Symptoms** Symptoms, which occur insidiously and generally in infancy or early childhood, include generalized weakness, malaise, dyspepsia, and palpitations. Patients may be jaundiced and suffer from leg ulcers, hepatomegaly, splenomegaly, cholelithiasis, and an enlarged abdomen. Hyperactive bone marrow growth may result in thickened cranial bones and prominent cheek bones. Osteoporosis may occur in the long bones, and pathologic fractures are common. Patients may be underdeveloped and short in stature for their age. Iron deposits in the cardiac muscle can cause cardiac dysfunction and eventual cardiac failure. Patients may show mental deterioration. Intercurrent infections may cause additional complications.

**Etiology** Thalassemia major is a congenital disorder inherited as an autosomal recessive trait. Homozygotic individuals are more severely afflicted than heterozygotic ones. The disorder is more prevalent among those families who intermarry and in those whose parents both have genes for thalassemia minor.

**Epidemiology** Thalassemia major most commonly occurs in individuals of Mediterranean ancestry, especially Italians and Greeks, and in an area that extends from northern Africa and southern Europe to Thailand, including Iran, Iraq, Indonesia, and southern China.

**Treatment—Standard** Patients are treated for severe anemia; chronic blood transfusions are necessary to maintain the hemoglobin above 10 gm percent and to allow for normal growth. Splenectomy may help patients with splenomegaly by reducing the number of blood transfusions required. To avoid iron overload, children should be given daily administration of deferoxamine.

**Treatment—Investigational** Several iron chelating compounds are being clinically investigated for thalassemia major therapy. Bone marrow transplantation is also under investigation.

Several drugs are being developed to treat thalassemia major. Vertex Pharmaceuticals is investigating the orphan products arginine butyrate, isobutyramide, VX-105 and oral VX-366. The latter 2 seem to reactivate the gene that controls production of hemoglobin F. Researchers at Johns Hopkins Hospital, Children's Medical and Surgical Center, are studying the effect on sickling diseases of the orphan drug sodium phenylbutyrate.

Please contact the agencies listed under Resources, below, for the most current information. Addresses and telephone numbers of these agencies, as well as of individual experts and research centers, may be found in the Master Resources List.

## Resources

**For more information on thalassemia major:** National Organization for Rare Disorders (NORD); AHEPA Cooley's Anemia Foundation; Cooley's Anemia Foundation; NIH/National Heart, Lung and Blood Institute.

**For genetic information and genetic counseling referrals:** March of Dimes Birth Defects Foundation; Alliance of Genetic Support Groups.

## References

Mendelian Inheritance in Man, 11th ed.: V.A. McKusick; The Johns Hopkins University Press, 1994, p. 1069.

Cecil Textbook of Medicine, 19th ed.: J.B. Wyngaarden, et al., eds.; W.B. Saunders Company, 1992, pp. 883–884.

Beta-Thalassemia Major and Sickle Cell Disease: R.B. Butler; NAACOGS Clin. Issu. Perinat. Women's Health Nurs., 1991, vol. 2(3), pp. 349–356.

Management of Thalassemia Major (Cooley's Anemia): S. Piomelli; Hematol. Oncol. Clin. North Am., June 1991, vol. 5(3), pp. 557–569.

Birth Defects Encyclopedia: M.L. Buyse, ed.-in-chief; Blackwell Scientific Publications, 1990, pp. 1658–1661.

Hematology, 4th ed.: W.J. Williams, et al., eds.; McGraw-Hill, 1990, pp. 510–534.

# THALASSEMIA MINOR

**Description** A relatively mild form of anemia that is both congenital and familial, thalassemia minor is the heterozygous state of a thalassemia gene.

## Synonyms

Hereditary Leptocytosis

Heterozygous β-Thalassemia

Thalassemia

β-Thalassemia Minor

**Signs and Symptoms** Persistent fatigue may be the only sign of this disorder. However, if anemia becomes severe, the patient may have slight splenomegaly and pallor and occasionally complain of pain in the left upper quadrant of the abdomen. The life span of patients is normal. The disease may be exacerbated when the patient is under stress, suffers infections or malnutrition, or is pregnant.

**Etiology** Thalassemia minor is inherited as an autosomal recessive trait.

**Epidemiology** The disorder most commonly occurs in persons of Mediterranean or southern Chinese descent. The occurrence rate in some Italian populations is as high as 20 percent.

**Related Disorders** See *Thalessemia Major.*

**Treatment—Standard** Treatment is generally not necessary. Iron therapy is ineffective and might be detrimental; prolonged administration of parenteral iron could result in excess iron storage. Pregnant women might require blood transfusions during pregnancy to maintain hemoglobin levels.

**Treatment—Investigational** Saul Brusilow, M.D., at Johns Hopkins Hospital, is studying the orphan drug sodium phenylbutyrate for the treatment of thalassemia minor and other blood disorders.

Please contact the agencies listed under Resources, below, for the most current information. Addresses and telephone numbers of these agencies, as well as of individual experts and research centers, may be found in the Master Resources List.

## Resources

**For more information on thalassemia minor:** National Organization for Rare Disorders (NORD); Sickle Cell Disease Association of America, Cooley's Anemia Foundation; NIH/National Heart, Lung and Blood Institute.

**For genetic information and genetic counseling referrals:** March of Dimes Birth Defects Foundation; Alliance of Genetic Support Groups.

## References

Mendelian Inheritance in Man, 11th ed.: V.A. McKusick; The Johns Hopkins University Press, 1994, p. 496.

Cecil Textbook of Medicine, 19th ed.: J.B. Wyngaarden, et al., eds.; W.B. Saunders Company, 1992, p. 883.

Nelson Textbook of Pediatrics, 14th ed.: R.E. Behrman, ed.-in-chief; W.B. Saunders Company, 1992, pp. 1515–1516.

Birth Defects Encyclopedia: M.L. Buyse, ed.-in-chief; Blackwell Scientific Publications, 1990, pp. 1659–1661.

Hematology, 4th ed.: W.J. Williams, et al., eds.; McGraw-Hill, 1990, pp. 492–493, 511.

# THROMBASTHENIA

**Description** Thrombasthenia is an inherited coagulation disorder that causes hemorrhage due to abnormal functioning of platelets. A variety of genetic abnormalities may cause the disease. The condition is not progressive and seems to improve with age. However, if prolonged hemorrhaging is not treated successfully, the patient's life may be endangered.

**Synonyms**

> Diacyclothrombopathia
> Glanzmann Disease
> Glanzmann-Naegeli Syndrome

**Signs and Symptoms** Beginning at birth or shortly thereafter, thrombasthenia patients tend to bleed easily and profusely, particularly after injury and during surgery, and are susceptible to developing bruises and large purplish spots on the skin that are caused by subcutaneous bleeding. They may also suffer nosebleeds, unusually heavy menstrual flow, and irregular uterine bleeding with varying degrees of severity. Laboratory results show that platelets are abnormal in appearance, deficient of certain proteins (GPIIa/GPIIIb), fail to aggregate normally, and evidence unusual retraction of clots.

**Etiology** Thrombasthenia is a congenital disorder transmitted either through autosomal dominant or recessive genes. The gene responsible for the disorder, glycoprotein IIB (IIb/IIIa complex), is located on the long arm of chromosome 17 (17q21.32). Researchers have found 4 different genetic abnormalities that they associate with thrombasthenia.

**Epidemiology** Males and females are affected in equal numbers. The disorder occurs more frequently among children of consanguineous parents.

**Related Disorders** Related disorders of abnormal platelet function are Bernard-Soulier syndrome, May-Hegglin anomaly, Chédiak-Higashi syndrome, the gray platelet syndrome, and various defects related to collagen-induced platelet aggregation. See **Bernard-Soulier Syndrome; May-Hegglin Anomaly; Chédiak-Higashi Syndrome.**

Platelet disorders have also been linked with such congenital conditions as Wiskott-Aldrich syndrome, Down syndrome, thrombocytopenia with absent radius syndrome, and von Willebrand disease.

**Treatment—Standard** When hemorrhaging is severe, the standard therapy is transfusion of platelets from a normal donor.

**Treatment—Investigational** Please contact the agencies listed under Resources, below, for the most current information. Addresses and telephone numbers of these agencies, as well as of individual experts and research centers, may be found in the Master Resources List.

**Resources**

**For more information on thrombasthenia:** National Organization for Rare Disorders (NORD); NIH/National Heart, Lung and Blood Institute.

**For genetic information and genetic counseling referrals:** March of Dimes Birth Defects Foundation; Alliance of Genetic Support Groups.

**References**

Mendelian Inheritance in Man, 11th ed.: V.A. McKusick; The Johns Hopkins University Press, 1994, pp. 1072, 1722–1723.

Platelet-Derived Microparticle Formation Involves Glycoprotein IIb-IIIa: Inhibition by RGDS and Glanzmann's Thrombasthenia Defect: C.H. Gemmel, et al.; J. Biol. Chem., July 1993, vol. 268(20), pp. 14586–14589.

Cecil Textbook of Medicine, 19th ed.: J.B. Wyngaarden, et al., eds.; W.B. Saunders Company, 1992, pp. 1056–1057.

Delivery of Infants with Glanzmann Thrombasthenia and Subsequent Blood Transfusions Requirements: A Follow-up of 39 Patients: A.S. Awidi; Am. J. Hematol., May 1992, vol. 40(1), pp. 1–4.

Diagnosis of Glanzmann's Thrombasthenia and Carrier Detection Using Monoclonal Antibodies to Platelet Glycoprotein IIb and IIIb in Immunoglotting: P. Perutelli, et al.; Haemostasis, 1992, vol. 22(6), pp. 330–333.

Nelson Textbook of Pediatrics, 14th ed.: R.E. Behrman, ed.-in-chief; W.B. Saunders Company, 1992, p. 1281.

Studies of the Platelet Fibronogen Receptor in Glanzmann Patients and Uremic Patients: T.L. Lingahl, et al.; Thromb. Res., August 1992, vol. 67(4), pp. 457–466.

A Deletion in the Gene for Glycoprotein IIb Associated with Glanzmann Thrombasthenia: C.D. Burk, et al.; J. Clin. Invest., January 1991, vol. 87(1), pp. 270–276.

Hemostasis in Glanzmann's Thrombasthenia (GT): GT Platelets Interfere with the Aggregation of Normal Platelets: L.K. Jennings, et al.; Am. J. Pediatr. Hematol. Oncol., Spring 1991, vol. 13(1), pp. 84–90.

Birth Defects Encyclopedia: M.L. Buyse, ed.-in-chief; Blackwell Scientific Publications, 1990, pp. 1664–1665.

Dictionary of Medical Syndromes, 3rd ed.: S.I. Magalini, et al., eds.; J.B. Lippincott Company, 1990, pp. 350–351.

Hematology, 4th ed.: W.J. Williams, et al., eds.; McGraw-Hill, 1990, pp. 1409–1410.

# THROMBOCYTHEMIA, ESSENTIAL

**Description** Essential thrombocythemia is a rare blood platelet disorder characterized by abnormally increased circulating platelets and associated thrombosis, hemorrhaging, and splenomegaly.

**Synonyms**

>Essential Hemorrhagic Thrombocythemia
>Essential Thrombocytosis
>Idiopathic Thrombocythemia
>Primary Thrombocythemia

**Signs and Symptoms** Bleeding occurs in two-thirds of patients as a result of abnormal platelet function. These patients may experience epistaxis, easy bruising, or bleeding in the gastrointestinal tract. Thrombosis may produce peripheral vascular ischemia such as pulmonary emboli and deep vein thrombosis as well as digital ischemia, or central nervous system ischemia that includes transient ischemic attacks **(TIAs),** headache, and dizziness. Splenomegaly is present in about one-half of patients.

**Etiology** While the precise cause of this disorder is not known, some patients have been shown to have inherited it as an autosomal dominant genetic trait.

**Epidemiology** Men and women are affected in equal numbers, usually in their 50s or 60s, although symptoms can occur at any age.

**Related Disorders** See *Thrombocytopenia, Essential.*

**Treatment—Standard** Hydroxyurea is the treatment of choice, since other effective agents (e.g., radioactive phosphorus) have been associated with risk of neoplasms.

Other therapy depends on symptoms. In cases of genetic transmission, patients and their families should receive genetic counseling.

**Treatment—Investigational** The orphan drug anagrelide (Roberts Pharmaceutical Corporation) is being tested for treatment of essential thrombocythemia.

Plateletpheresis is also being used experimentally to treat this disorder, but its safety and effectiveness over the long term have not yet been determined.

Please contact the agencies listed under Resources, below, for the most current information. Addresses and telephone numbers of these agencies, as well as of individual experts and research centers, may be found in the Master Resources List.

**Resources**

**For more information on essential thrombocythemia:** National Organization for Rare Disorders (NORD); Myeloproliferative Disease Research Center; NIH/National Heart, Lung and Blood Institute.

**For genetic information and genetic counseling referrals:** March of Dimes Birth Defects Foundation; Alliance of Genetic Support Groups.

**References**

Mendelian Inheritance in Man, 9th ed.: V.A. McKusick; The Johns Hopkins University Press, 1990, pp. 910–911.

Internal Medicine, 3rd ed.: J.H. Stein, ed.-in-chief; Little, Brown and Company, 1990, p. 1128.

Clinical Presentation and Natural History of Patients with Essential Thrombocythemia and the Philadelphia Chromosome: D.B. Stoll, et al.; Am. J. Hematol., February 1988, vol. 27(2), pp. 77–83.

Essential Thrombocythemias: Clinical Evolutionary and Biological Data: S. Bellucci, et al.; Cancer, December 1986, vol. 58(11), pp. 2440–2447.

Essential Thrombocythemia and Leukemic Transformation: S. M. Sedlacek, et al.; Medicine (Baltimore), November 1986, vol. 65(6), pp. 353–364.

# THROMBOCYTOPENIA, ESSENTIAL

**Description** Essential thrombocytopenia is a rare blood platelet disorder characterized by an abnormally small number of circulating platelets (less than 150 x 109 per liter) that survive for a shorter than normal time (10 days). Excessive hemorrhaging in the mucous membranes or skin, especially at the time of menstruation, also is characteristic.

**Signs and Symptoms** Excessive hemorrhaging is the chief symptom, especially purpura under the skin, in the eyes, and in the mucous membranes of the mouth, and, in extreme cases, hemorrhaging in the skull. Patients bruise easily and have sudden nosebleeds. Tiny petechiae form in mild cases around the ankles and feet but become more widespread and enlarged in more severe cases. Uncontrolled hemorrhaging causes anemia, fatigue, weakness, and symptoms of congestive heart failure. However, the massive extravasation that happens in hemophilia does not occur in thrombocytopenia.

**Etiology** The major causes of thrombocytopenia are decreased platelet production, increased platelet destruction, and platelet sequestration by the spleen.

Platelet production can be impaired as a result of vitamin B12 or folate deficiency, generalized disease in the bone marrow, viral infections, a toxic reaction or hypersensitivity to drugs, systemic infections, malignant disease, or aplastic anemia.

Increased platelet destruction can be immune-mediated; can be induced by drugs such as hydrocortisone, aspirin, thiazide diuretics, quinine, cyclophosphamide, prednisone, azathioprine, tricyclic antidepressants, indomethacin, phenylbutazone, antihistamines, vincristine, or phenothiazines; or there may be alloantibody or autoantibody precipitants. Nonimmune-related platelet destruction may result from disorders such as thrombotic thrombocytopenic purpura or disseminated intravascular coagulation, or be related to extracorporeal circulation or prosthetic intravascular devices.

Sequestration of platelets by the spleen causes thrombocytopenia and results in splenomegaly.

**Epidemiology** Both males and females are equally affected by this disorder.

**Related Disorders** See *Chédiak-Higashi Syndrome; Anemia, Fanconi; Hemophilia; May-Hegglin Anomaly; von Willebrand Disease; Thrombocytopenia–Absent Radius Syndrome.*

**Kasabach-Merritt syndrome** is characterized by hemorrhages in the eyes and skin, hemangiomas, and some cutaneous features of thrombocytopenic purpura.

**Treatment—Standard** Transfusions of normal platelets are given to control hemorrhage, and intravenous injections of immune globulin are given to stimulate platelet production. In rare instances, splenectomy is performed. When the underlying cause of thrombocytopenia is another disease, platelet production improves with successful treatment of that disease. Patients should avoid drugs that inhibit platelet function, such as anti-inflammatory agents and certain salicylates.

**Treatment—Investigational** Plasmapheresis has been used experimentally for extreme cases, but its safety and efficacy are still being investigated. The orphan drug anagrelide (Roberts Pharmaceutical Corporation) is also being tried experimentally to treat essential thrombocytopenia. Low-dose radiation of the spleen has resulted in short-term improvement in the platelet count among some patients, but more research is necessary. WinRho SD, a new anti-Rh immune globulin, is being developed by Univax Biologics to reduce platelet counts.

Please contact the agencies listed under Resources, below, for the most current information. Addresses and telephone numbers of these agencies, as well as of individual experts and research centers, may be found in the Master Resources List.

### Resources

**For more information on essential thrombocytopenia:** National Organization for Rare Disorders (NORD); NIH/National Heart, Lung and Blood Institute.

**For more information on thrombocytopenia–absent radius syndrome only, not other forms of thrombocytopenia:** Thrombocytopenia–Absent Radius Syndrome Association.

**For genetic information and genetic counseling referrals:** March of Dimes Birth Defects Foundation; Alliance of Genetic Support Groups.

### References

Internal Medicine, 3rd ed.: J.H. Stein, ed.-in-chief; Little, Brown and Company, 1990, pp. 1044–1048.

Splenectomy for Thrombocytopenia Due to Secondary Hypersplenism: W.W. Coon; Arch. Surg., March 1988, vol. 148(3), pp. 369–371.

Successful Conservative Management of Thrombocytopenia in Adult Hemophiliacs: J.C. Goldsmith, et al.; Transfusion, January–February 1988, vol. 28(1), pp. 68–69.

Successful Intravenous Immune Globulin Therapy for Human Immunodeficiency Virus-Associated Thrombocytopenia: A.N Pollak, et al.; Arch. Intern. Med., March 1988, vol. 148(3), pp. 695–697.

# TONGUE CARCINOMA

**Description** Tongue carcinoma is a malignant oral neoplasm characterized by an ulcerating squamous cell tumor. It is usually located on the side of the tongue and can metastasize to the same side of the neck.

### Synonyms

Cancer of the Tongue

**Signs and Symptoms** The lesion bleeds easily, fails to heal, and may become painful. The pain may eventually spread throughout the side of the face. Movement of the patient's tongue may become restricted. About one-half of patients experience ipsilateral lymph-node enlargement if the tumor metastasizes to the neck.

**Etiology** Increased risk for tongue carcinoma is associated with excessive alcohol consumption, excessive use of tobacco, syphilis, herpes simplex virus, and human papillomavirus. Leukoplakia and erythroplasia are precancerous lesions that may progress to carcinoma.

**Epidemiology** Tongue carcinoma is rare. Males are affected more often than females, although the number of females affected has risen in recent years. Age at onset is generally between 40 and 60, and the incidence tends to increase with age.

**Related Disorders Carcinoma of the floor of the mouth,** another rare malignant neoplasm, is characterized by a hard tumor often felt with the tip of the patient's tongue. Symptoms include increased salivation, ear pain, difficulty in speaking, and, ultimately, bleeding. Lymph nodes in the neck are frequently affected. Poor oral hygiene and tobacco use are suspected causes.

**Carcinoma of the cheek (mouth or buccal mucosa)** is a malignant neoplasm marked by a buccal lesion, trismus, pain, mucosal bleeding, and difficulty in chewing. The neoplasm can metastasize to lymph glands beneath the jaw.

**Treatment—Standard** Treatment may be by surgical excision of the lingual muscle and cervical lymph nodes, possibly combined with pre- or postoperative radiation therapy. Interstitial irradiation and chemotherapy may also be beneficial. Twenty-eight percent of patients survive 5 years. Early diagnosis and treatment are keys to survival, particularly if the patient is under 20 years of age.

**Treatment—Investigational** Please contact the agencies listed under Resources, below, for the most current information. Addresses and telephone numbers of these agencies, as well as of individual experts and research centers, may be found in the Master Resources List.

**Resources**

**For more information on tongue carcinoma:** National Organization for Rare Disorders (NORD); American Cancer Society; NIH/National Cancer Institute Physician Data Query Phoneline.

**References**

Harrison's Principles of Internal Medicine, 12th ed.: J.D. Wilson, et al., eds.; McGraw-Hill, 1991, pp. 245–248.

Surgical Treatment of Early-Stage Carcinoma of the Oral Tongue: Would Wound Adjuvant Treatment Be Beneficial?: Head Neck Surg., July–August 1986, vol. 8(6), pp. 401–408.

What You Need to Know About Cancer of the Mouth: U.S. Department of Health and Human Services, Public Health Service, National Institutes of Health, National Cancer Institute; March 1985.

Changing Trends in the Management of Squamous Carcinoma of the Tongue: C.D. Callery, et al.; Am. J. Surg., October 1984, vol. 148(4), pp. 449–454.

# VON WILLEBRAND DISEASE

**Description** An inherited coagulation disease that usually arises in infancy or early childhood, von Willebrand disease is characterized by prolonged bleeding and abnormally slow blood-clotting time due to a deficiency of factor VIII and von Willebrand factor protein combined with a morphologic defect of platelets.

**Synonyms**

>Angiohemophilia
>Constitutional Thrombopathy
>Minot–von Willebrand Disease
>Pseudohemophilia
>Vascular Hemophilia
>Willebrand-Juergens Disease

**Signs and Symptoms** Prolonged bleeding usually occurs in the nose or gastrointestinal tract. Patients bruise easily and bleed excessively after injury, menstruation, childbirth, surgery, and some dental procedures. Hemarthrosis also occurs, but rarely.

**Etiology** Inheritance is both autosomal dominant and recessive; an X-linked form has also been reported. Abnormal coagulation and excessive bleeding result from deficiency in the production of factor VIII and von Willebrand factor plus a platelet abnormality. A similar disorder, acquired in adulthood, results from overproduction of von Willebrand factor antibodies. Associated disorders include certain renal diseases, congenital cardiac disease that involves a defective heart valve, and one type of leukemia.

**Epidemiology** Onset is usually in infancy or early childhood, although some nonhereditary forms can be acquired in adulthood. The disease tends to affect more females than males.

**Related Disorders** See *Hemophilia.*

**Treatment—Standard** Intravenous injections of frozen or stored plasma or whole blood are administered to increase the levels of factor VIII and von Willebrand factor in the patient's blood to aid coagulation. Transfusions of blood or plasma before childbirth or surgery or after an accident or unexplained bleeding are given to reduce the risk of hemorrhage. Patients with mild cases have been given daily doses of the synthetic blood agent desmopressin acetate (**DDAVP**) before surgery to shorten clotting time by stimulating the release of factor VIII molecules from cells that line the blood vessels. Injectable DDAVP, which is an antidiuretic peptide, is available from

Rorer Pharmaceutical Corp., Fort Washington, Pennsylvania. DDAVP nasal spray has been approved by the Food and Drug Administration for treatment of mild to moderate (type I) von Willebrand disease.

Cryoprecipitates may be given to control excess bleeding in some cases, but careful monitoring of dosage is required. For severe cases, cryoprecipitates are the most effective means of replacing factor VIII. Aminocaproic acid can also be given to reduce bleeding.

Patients are advised to wear a medical identification bracelet that includes information about the medications used to treat the disease. Patients should also avoid drugs that prolong bleeding, aspirin, and any activities that are likely to result in injury. Most patients can lead a normal life if they receive proper treatment and take the necessary precautions. Generally, the bleeding tendencies will decrease with age. Patients and their families should receive genetic counseling.

**Treatment—Investigational** The use of coagglutinin is being studied by Marjorie Read, Ph.D., at the University of North Carolina in Chapel Hill, under a grant from the Food and Drug Administration. The Food and Drug Administration has approved the orphan drug antihemophilic factor (human) (Humate P) for testing; it is manufactured by Behringwerke Aktiengesellschaft, Collegeville, Pennsylvania. In addition, Novo-Nordisk A/S, Copenhagen, is testing the orphan drug NovoSeven (factor VIIa) (recombinant DNA origin) for patients without antibodies against factor VIII/IX.

Please contact the agencies listed under Resources, below, for the most current information. Addresses and telephone numbers of these agencies, as well as of individual experts and research centers, may be found in the Master Resources List.

**Resources**

**For more information on von Willebrand disease:** National Organization for Rare Disorders (NORD); NIH/National Heart, Lung and Blood Institute.

**Although von Willebrand disease is not a form of hemophilia, national health agencies providing information, referrals, and support groups for von Willebrand disease are organizations that are primarily concerned with hemophilia:** National Hemophilia Foundation; Canadian Hemophilia Society; World Federation of Hemophilia; Haemophilia Society.

**For genetic information and genetic counseling referrals:** March of Dimes Birth Defects Foundation; Alliance of Genetic Support Groups.

**References**

Nasal Spray Desmopressin (DDAVP) for Mild Hemophilia A and von Willebrand Disease: E.H. Rose, et al.; Ann. Intern. Med., April 1991, vol. 114, pp. 563–568.

Mendelian Inheritance in Man, 9th ed.: V.A. McKusick; The Johns Hopkins University Press, 1990, pp. 972–976, 1530–1531, 1732.

A Human Myeloma-Produced Monoclonal Protein Directed Against the Active Subpopulation of von Willebrand Factor: E.G. Bovill, et al.; Am. J. Clin. Pathol., January 1986, vol. 85(1), pp. 115–123.

Von Willebrand Syndrome: I. Scharrer; Behring Inst. Mitt., February 1986, vol. 79, pp. 12–23.

Von Willebrand's Disease and Pregnancy: Management During Delivery and Outcome of Offspring: J.R. Chédiak, et al.; Am. J. Obstet. Gynecol., September 1986, vol. 155(3), pp. 618–624.

# WEGENER GRANULOMATOSIS

**Description** Wegener granulomatosis is a multisystem disease characterized primarily by necrotizing vasculitis of the lung and upper respiratory tract, and by glomerulonephritis. There is a range of symptom severity. The disease can affect one or more systems.

**Synonyms**

> Lethal Midline Granuloma
> Necrotizing Respiratory Granulomatosis
> Pathergic Granulomatosis

**Signs and Symptoms** Upper respiratory tract involvement is usually the initial presentation, with sinusitis and bloody, purulent discharge that do not respond to antibiotics. Other early symptoms and signs include fever, malaise, and weight loss. Nasal mucosal ulceration may be present, with septal deterioration that results in saddle-nose deformity.

The eyes may be involved, with findings that include conjunctivitis, episcleritis, optic neuritis, ciliary vessel vasculitis, and occlusion of the retinal artery. Aseptic meningitis and cranial nerve lesions have been reported. Cardiac involvement includes pericarditis and myocardial infarctions due to coronary arteritis. Skin lesions occur in a variety of forms that include papules, a purpuric rash, and ulcers. Arthralgias occur in about one-half of cases. Pulmonary cavitations are seen on x-ray.

Renal disease, present in 85 percent of patients, is the gravest development. Hematuria, proteinuria, and red cell casts may be seen initially, but without treatment the initial mild glomerulonephritis progresses to rapid renal failure.

Some patients with the limited form of the disorder have only nasal and pulmonary lesions, with little or no systemic involvement.

**Etiology** The cause has not been determined. Delayed hypersensitivity and immune complex mediation seem to be associated. No viral, bacterial, or other causative agent has been identified.

**Epidemiology** Wegener granulomatosis can occur at any age. Males are affected twice as often as females.

**Related Disorders** These include glomerulonephritis, the other vasculitides, Goodpasture syndrome, and some granulomatous diseases.

**Treatment—Standard** Early diagnosis and treatment are important because of the possible rapid progression to renal failure. Cyclophosphamide is the drug of choice, but azathioprine and chlorambucil are useful also. Today, 90 percent of those treated with cyclophosphamide and prednisone experience complete remission.

Duration of therapy depends on the patient's response. Leukocytes are monitored closely, and therapeutic dosages are reduced gradually to prevent leukopenia. When the patient has been free of symptoms for 1 year, attempts should be made to discontinue therapy. When medications are being reduced or discontinued, careful monitoring for relapse of the kidney disease should be conducted. Complete long-term remissions are often achieved with drug therapy, even in cases of advanced disease. Kidney transplantation has been successful in cases with kidney failure.

For nonrenal symptoms, corticosteroids can be used intermittently in conjunction with cytotoxic drugs. Pulmonary symptoms may improve or worsen spontaneously.

**Treatment—Investigational** The National Institute of Allergy and Infectious Diseases is studying treatment for Wegener granulomatosis. NIH will pay for treatment and travel for patients who are at least 14 years old and who have recently developed symptoms. For more information, contact Gary S. Hoffman, M.D., or Randi Y. Levitt, M.D., at NIH/National Institute of Allergy and Infectious Diseases.

Please contact the agencies listed under Resources, below, for the most current information. Addresses and telephone numbers of these agencies, as well as of individual experts and research centers, may be found in the Master Resources List.

**Resources**

**For more information on Wegener granulomatosis:** National Organization for Rare Disorders (NORD); Wegener's Granulomatosis Support Group; NIH/National Heart, Lung and Blood Institute; National Kidney Foundation; American Lung Association.

**References**

Harrison's Principles of Internal Medicine, 12th ed.: J.D. Wilson, et al., eds.; McGraw-Hill, 1991, pp. 1460–1461.

# WILMS TUMOR

**Description** Wilms tumor, the most common malignant renal neoplasm in children, is characterized by abdominal pain and swelling. Current therapy results in a long-term survival rate of close to 80 percent of patients, depending on the child's general health and his or her age at the time of detection.

**Synonyms**

> Embryoma of Kidney
> Embryonal Adenomyosarcoma of Kidney
> Embryonal Carcinosarcoma of Kidney
> Embryonal Mixed Tumor of Kidney
> Nephroblastoma

**Signs and Symptoms** Initially, patients are usually asymptomatic, but in later stages of the disease, pallor, appetite loss, weight loss, low-grade fever, lethargy, hematuria, and abdominal swelling occur, along with pain that may be sudden or sharp, or intermittent and slight. The child may also have developmental anomalies, including hemihypertrophy (in approximately 3 percent of patients), genitourinary defects (in about 5 percent), and aniridia (in about 10 percent).

**Etiology** While the cause of Wilms tumor is unknown, evidence suggests that both hereditary and nonhereditary forms exist. It is believed that the hereditary type affects both kidneys or several areas of one kidney, with onset at an early age due to a genetic abnormality that results in a fetal kidney defect. Studies suggest a link between the growth of Wilms tumor and a deleted section of chromosome 11 (p13); the location of the gene that controls this growth is still being sought.

**Epidemiology** Wilms tumor comprises 6 to 8 percent of all malignant neoplasms in children; it strikes about 1:10,000 children in the United States. The disease affects equal numbers of boys and girls, who are mainly under age 7 and most frequently between ages 1 and 4.

**Treatment—Standard** Surgery (including nephrectomy) combined with radiation therapy and chemotherapy has proved to be successful in treating most patients. The antineoplastic drugs vincristine and actinomycin D are used to reduce the tumors. Two-year survival without recurrence of disease is considered a cure; 70 to 80 percent of treated patients survive for 2 years or more. The outlook is less promising, however, for a small number of children who have aggressive or widespread forms of the disease, but intensive therapy can lead to long-term survival.

**Treatment—Investigational** The National Cancer Institute has funded The National Wilms Tumor Study in a group of hospitals and clinics nationwide. Findings of this study are the basis for treatment standards for this disease. Present research is investigating ways to improve care for patients with metastatic disease or who are at high risk because they have certain cell types.

Please contact the agencies listed under Resources, below, for the most current information. Addresses and telephone numbers of these agencies, as well as of individual experts and research centers, may be found in the Master Resources List.

### Resources

**For more information on Wilms tumor:** National Organization for Rare Disorders (NORD); National Kidney Foundation; American Cancer Society; NIH/National Cancer Institute Physician Data Query Phoneline.

**For genetic information and genetic counseling referrals:** March of Dimes Birth Defects Foundation; Alliance of Genetic Support Groups.

### References

Drug Evaluations Subscription, vol. 3: Division of Drugs and Toxicology; Amer. Med. Assoc., 1994, p. ONC-1:27.

Adult Kidney Cancer and Wilms' Tumor. Research Report: U.S. Department of Health and Human Services, Public Health Service, National Cancer Institute, National Institutes of Health.

# X-LINKED LYMPHOPROLIFERATIVE (XLP) SYNDROME

**Description** A rare genetic disease, XLP syndrome is a life-threatening condition of the immune system in males that exposes them to death from mononucleosis caused by Epstein-Barr virus.

### Synonyms

Duncan Disease

Epstein-Barr Infection, Familial Fatal

Immunodeficiency 5

**Signs and Symptoms** Patients are usually asymptomatic until they are infected with the Epstein-Barr virus. Symptoms include fever, pharyngitis, lymphadenopathy, and hepatosplenomegaly. The mononucleosis can be life-threatening, and the patients are vulnerable to other potentially fatal disorders, such as hypogammaglobulinemia and lymphoma. Death can result in 60 to 75 percent of XLP patients after they contract one of these diseases.

**Etiology** A rare inherited recessive defect on the X chromosome is believed to be the cause; however, scientists have not yet found the precise location of the defect. Only males who carry the defect and are infected by Epstein-Barr virus are affected.

**Related Disorders** See *Agammaglobulinemias, Primary.*

**Infectious mononucleosis** is caused by the Epstein-Barr virus. It is characterized by extreme fatigue, fever, swollen lymph glands, and an unusual proliferation of leukocytes in the blood. Tests are sometimes necessary to distinguish these leukocytes from certain leukemia cells. Mild forms are difficult to diagnose. Patients usually recover after 6 to 8 weeks or longer without treatment.

**Malignant lymphoma** is a malignant neoplasm that arises from the normal sites containing lymphoreticular cells, such as the spleen and lymph nodes. The disease may infiltrate the blood and mimic leukemia or it can be found in virtually any part of the body. The different varieties of lymphoma are distinguished by their nodular pattern, degrees of differentiation, and cell type.

**Treatment—Standard** Treatment depends on symptoms. Gammaglobulin is given to boost the patient's immune system when hypogammaglobulinemia occurs. Patients and their families should receive genetic counseling.

**Treatment—Investigational** Interferon-γ is under investigation as a treatment, but further study is necessary. DNA probes are being used to try to determine the location of the defective gene.

Please contact the agencies listed under Resources, below, for the most current information. Addresses and telephone numbers of these agencies, as well as of individual experts and research centers, may be found in the Master Resources List.

### Resources

**For more information on X-linked lymphoproliferative syndrome:** National Organization for Rare Disorders (NORD); NIH/National Institute of Allergy and Infectious Diseases.

**For information on participation in genetic studies:** James Skare, M.D., Boston University School of Medicine, Center for Human Genetics, Boston, Massachusetts.

**For genetic information and genetic counseling referrals:** March of Dimes Birth Defects Foundation; Alliance of Genetic Support Groups.

## References

Mendelian Inheritance in Man, 9th ed.: V.A. McKusick; The Johns Hopkins University Press, 1990, pp. 1654–1655.

Interferon-Gamma in a Family with X-Linked Lymphoproliferative Syndrome with Acute Epstein-Barr Virus Infection: M. Okano, et al.; J. Clin. Immunol., January 1989, vol. 9(1), pp. 48–54.

Markers Mapped for Life-Threatening Disorder: J. Skare, Research Resources Reporter, National Institutes of Health, June 1989, vol. XIII(6), pp. 6–7.

X-Linked Lymphoproliferative Disease: A Karyotype Analysis: A. Harris, et al.; Cytogenet. Cell Genet., 1988, vol. 47(1–2), pp. 92–94.

Epstein-Barr Virus Infections in Males with the X-Linked Lymphoproliferative Syndrome: H. Grierson, et al.; Ann. Intern. Med., April 1987, vol. 106(4), pp. 538–545.

Malignant Lymphoma in the X-Linked Lymphoproliferative Syndrome: D.S. Harrington, et al.; Cancer, April 15, 1987, vol. 59(8), pp. 1419–1429.

# 6 | IMMUNOLOGIC DISORDERS AND INFECTIOUS DISEASES
### By Robert Fekety, M.D.

The approach to the diagnosis of rare infectious and immunologic diseases is no different from that of other diseases. Taking a complete history from the patient and doing a thorough physical examination will usually point to the salient features of the illness. The differential diagnosis can then be built around those features. Attention to the family and social history may provide additional important clues. Where has the patient traveled? What pets, wild animals, birds, chemicals, or toxic substances has the patient encountered? What "recreational" or prescribed drugs has the patient used? What is the sexual history, and what specific kinds of sexual behavior have been practiced? Parenthetically, the importance of an expert, detailed, and above all sensitive and nonjudgmental sexual history cannot be overemphasized, not only for the elicitation of specific information, but also because it provides an opportunity to demonstrate your empathy, sensitivity, and trustworthiness to the patient. For example, patients should not be asked whether they are gay or homosexual, but instead whether they have sexual relations with members of the same or the opposite sex, or both.

The travel history may suggest infectious diseases indigenous and unique to certain countries, and may also indicate whether the patient traveled to the areas of risk in those countries. Going into the bush poses a very different risk to the traveler than does staying in cities with modern conveniences. A good, up-to-date textbook of tropical and geographic medicine, or an up-to-date book on rare diseases (such as this one!), is useful for browsing through once a few likely diseases have come to mind. What other diseases are listed under differential diagnosis for those diseases that are being considered? Do they occur in the countries visited by the patient, and are they a high risk only to persons engaged in certain activities? Did the patient engage in those activities? What other diseases are known to occur in that area? Are there variants of that disease that resemble the patient's illness? Above all, remember that if the disease is common in the foreign country the patient visited, even if rare in the country where *you* are, it should be considered a common disease for that patient.

Armed with the clues generated by the workup outlined above, one can peruse the standard texts for more information on the most likely conditions. The clinician can then begin to order pertinent, simple, and readily available laboratory tests and radiologic studies, or even begin empiric therapy for those conditions that are most likely and for which treatment is likely to be beneficial and safe, depending on the patient's condition.

Fortunately, a few rare diseases, such as meningococcemia, are well known to lay persons as well as to physicians. They are often lethal if untreated and are usually readily treated if the diagnosis is entertained early enough. They must be high on the differential diagnosis list for every patient with an acute illness characterized by fever and a petechial or purpuric rash.

Other "rare" diseases are the "new" diseases, discovered or detected by advances in laboratory methodology, often by the astute application of new serologic, cultural, or molecular methods. They are exemplified by *Helicobacter pylori* (originally named *Campylobacter pyloridis*), an organism that has been observed microscopically on the gastric mucosa of humans for decades, but never grown from it, by pathologists who had accepted the dogma that these organisms were dead, having been killed by the acid contents of the stomach, even though the organisms appeared to be morphologically intact. In 1982, with the use of appropriate media and other conditions (a microaerophilic atmosphere and prolonged incubation), *Helicobacter pylori* was isolated for the first time by Barry Marshall, a gastroenterologist in training; Robin Warren, a pathologist; and their microbiologist colleagues, Helen Royce and Frank Kosaris, from a gastric biopsy specimen taken from a patient with gastritis.[1,2] Remarkably, it has subsequently been shown that these organisms are the most common cause not only of gastritis, but also of peptic ulcers, and that they also appear to cause many gastric carcinomas and certain lymphomas of the gastric mucosa that are cured after the institution of antimicrobial therapy appropriate for eradication of *H. pylori!* Consequently, a disease that was formerly considered not only very rare but frankly nonexistent, namely, duodenal ulcers caused specifically by bacterial infection, was found to be extremely common, despite initial ridicule and skepticism as to the validity, relevance, and importance of the scientific evidence! Incidentally, it is entirely possible that this organism would not have been discovered had it not been for the advances in antimicrobial therapy that made it possible to prevent stomach contaminants from overgrowing the culture media and obscuring the presence of *H. pylori.*

Another important advance leading to the discovery of new and rare diseases was the development of the polymerase chain reaction (**PCR**), which made it possible to demonstrate, using enormously sophisticated techniques and reasoning, that *Bartonella henselae*, an organism closely related to *Rochalimeae quintana*, the cause of trench fever in Word War I, is the cause not only of bacillary angiomatosis and peliosis hepatis in patients with acquired immune deficiency syndrome (**AIDS**), but also of cat-scratch disease in healthy children and young adults.

Recently, using PCR to characterize the DNA of the organism, it was found that Whipple disease, a rare disease long suspected of being caused by a bacillary agent, is caused by a newly discovered organism that has been given the name *Tropherema whipplei*, even though it has not yet actually been cultivated! This is undoubtedly a portent of things to come.

A special plea should be made at this point for obtaining a "curbside consult" from clinical microbiology or clinical immunology laboratory personnel when laboratory tests are being ordered to help in making the diagnosis of a rare or unusual infectious disease. The first reason for this is that these persons can often suggest an additional diagnosis or two for further consideration. The second and more important reason is that if these personnel know what diseases are being considered, they can help you to obtain laboratory studies in the most appropriate way, by incubating cultures in appropriate media and atmospheric conditions, for an appropriate time, and at the proper temperature. With a mixed culture or with one contaminated by virtue of being obtained from a normally unsterile body site, the organism is less likely to be overlooked if it is suspected beforehand.

Laboratory personnel may also be able to recommend the best serologic test to use in diagnosing the disease in question. Laboratory tests to diagnose rare or newly discovered infectious diseases are often available only by special request to a reference laboratory, and clinical microbiology laboratory personnel frequently are more knowledgeable about specific ways to obtain the best tests than are clinicians.

In many cases, it may be necessary to obtain one or more biopsy specimens to confirm diagnosis. The surgical pathologist should be given all the pertinent information so that he or she can become a close collaborator in the elucidation of the problem.

Patients with eosinophilia often have immunologic or parasitic diseases. Proper ways to obtain and transport stool specimens are critical in making many of these diagnoses. The Parasitology Branch of the United States Public Health Service's Centers for Disease Control in Atlanta, Georgia, can provide a battery of special serologic tests designed to aid in the diagnosis of diseases causing eosinophilia. Their help may be invaluable. Of course, it goes without saying that an infectious diseases consultant may provide invaluable help in the diagnosis and management of these patients.

The first reason for enlisting the informed aid of these clinical support scientists mentioned above is that they can often suggest an additional diagnosis or two. Another more important reason is that if they know what diseases are being considered, they will be more able to help you obtain laboratory studies in the most appropriate way by incubating cultures in appropriate media for an appropriate time and at proper temperature and atmospheric conditions. And they also will get more fun and pleasure out of doing their jobs, because they will realize how interesting their work really is and also how much they have helped a sick person who was a diagnostic problem.

Empiric therapy is usually a poor way to reach a diagnosis of a rare disease. Even if the patient responds, it may be because he or she has a different disease than the one you suspected, but one that can be treated in the same way. Furthermore, coincidental improvement after therapy is begun is surprisingly common. As an example, one of my patients with fever of unknown origin was treated empirically with antituberculous therapy for suspected retroperitoneal tuberculosis (which was not an unreasonable thing to do at that point), and responded dramatically to it. Later it was found out that he had Hodgkin disease, and studies for tuberculosis during life and later at postmortem examination remained negative for *M. tuberculosis*. "Gut reactions" and "shotgun therapy" are discouraged.

It has been said, "You don't have to be smart to be a good doctor." If you are not brilliant, and even if you are, what you should do with a problem patient is apply to the diagnostic problem the simple system for working up a patient that is taught in every medical school. That is what is outlined above. If you use it, "The System" will make the diagnosis for you, often by isolation of an unsuspected rare and unusual organism in a culture of blood or other normally sterile body specimen, or sometimes by a surprising biopsy or serologic test result. Everyone will then think you are brilliant, but you will *know* you are just a good doctor, which is a pretty good thing to be! Try it.

### References

1. Unidentified Curved Bacilli on Gastric Epithelium in Active Chronic Gastritis: J.R. Warren and B. Marshall; Lancet, vol. 1, 1983, pp. 1273–1275.
2. History of the Discovery of *C. pylori:* B. Marshall; *in Campylobacter pylori* in Gastritis and Peptic Ulcer Disease: M.J. Blaser, ed.; Igaku Shoin, 1989, pp. 7–23.

# IMMUNOLOGIC DISORDERS AND INFECTIOUS DISEASES

*Listings in This Section*

# ACANTHOCHEILONEMIASIS

**Description** Acanthocheilonemiasis is a mild parasitic infection caused by the tissue nematode *Acanthocheilonema perstans.* It is found most commonly in Africa.

**Synonyms**
> Dipetalonemiasis

**Signs and Symptoms** Infection with *A. perstans* is usually asymptomatic. Symptoms appear to be more frequent in visitors to endemic regions rather than in native populations. One common presentation in a tourist on return from an endemic region is asymptomatic eosinophilia.

When symptoms occur, they may include pruritis, abdominal pain, chest pain, myalgias, and subcutaneous swellings. Physical examination may reveal hepatosplenomegaly, and eosinophilia is the rule. The adult worm lodges in the subserous tissues of the abdomen and thorax, where local inflammatory and immune reactions give rise to pleuritis, pericarditis, and the symptoms described above.

Microfilariae of *A. perstans* can be isolated from the blood. The usual means of diagnosis is examination of a thick blood smear for these organisms.

**Etiology** The causative organism is a filarial worm, *Acanthocheilonema perstans,* also referred to as *Dipetalonema perstans.* It is transmitted by a small black midge, *A. cailicoides.*

**Epidemiology** *A. perstans* is common in central Africa and in some areas of South America. Males and females are affected equally.

**Related Disorders** See *Filariasis.*

**Treatment—Standard** Diethylcarbamazine is the treatment of choice. Surgical removal of large adult worms is occasionally necessary. Mild cases do not require treatment.

**Treatment—Investigational** Please contact the agencies listed under Resources, below, for the most current information. Addresses and telephone numbers of these agencies, as well as of individual experts and research centers, may be found in the Master Resources List.

**Resources**

**For more information on acanthocheilonemiasis:** National Organization for Rare Disorders (NORD); NIH/National Institute of Allergy and Infectious Diseases; Centers for Disease Control.

**References**

Experimental Chemotherapy of Filariasis: Comparative Evaluation of the Efficacy of Filaricidal Compounds in Mastomys Coucha Infected with *Litomosoides carinii, Acanthocheilonema viteae, Burgua Malayi* and *B. Pahangi:* H. Zahner; Acta Trop., January 1993, vol. 52(4), pp. 221–266.

Cecil Textbook of Medicine, 19th ed.: J.B. Wyngaarden, et al., eds.; W.B. Saunders Company, 1992, pp. 2017–2018.

Intensity and Efficiency of Transmission and the Development of Microfilaraemia and Disease: Their Relationship on Lymphatic Filariasis: B.A. Southgate; J. Trop. Med. Hyg., February 1992, vol. 95(1), pp. 1–12.

Hematology, 4th ed.: W.J. Williams, et al., eds.; McGraw-Hill, 1990, p. 1706.

# ACQUIRED IMMUNE DEFICIENCY SYNDROME (AIDS)

**Description** AIDS is an immunosuppressive disorder caused by infection with the human immunodeficiency virus **(HIV).** The immune deficiency results from viral infection and destruction of specific T cells. HIV infection is characterized initially by a long asymptomatic period. This may be followed by the development of generalized lymphadenopathy. Eventually most patients experience a syndrome of constitutional symptoms (fatigue, weight loss, rashes), which has been referred to as the AIDS-related complex or **ARC.** The end-stage of HIV infection is marked by progressive depression of T-cell immunity; opportunistic infections, particularly *Pneumocystis carinii* pneumonia; neoplasms; and a wide variety of neurologic abnormalities, most notably the AIDS dementia complex, which appears to be a direct result of HIV nervous system infection.

**Signs and Symptoms** HIV infection is usually acquired years before signs of immunodeficiency appear. There are usually no symptoms at the time the infection is acquired, but in some patients an acute mononucleosis-like illness can be clearly identified a few weeks after exposure.

Most infected individuals experience a long asymptomatic period of variable length. At 10 years from exposure, 50 percent of patients have developed some type of symptoms, although only one-third manifest the full-blown immunosuppressive syndrome. Some develop persistent generalized lymphadenopathy without evidence of superinfection. Later, a constitutional syndrome of wasting, fatigue, fever, oral thrush, and rashes develops which is considered by some investigators to represent a manifestation of full-blown AIDS, and by others to be an AIDS-related complex (ARC).

The best-known stage of HIV infection is characterized by superinfection with opportunistic organisms. However, patients with HIV infection appear to be unusually susceptible to certain infections before they reach this stage, most notably candida and tuberculosis.

Thrombocytopenia is common, and infection may initially be manifested by symptoms of idiopathic thrombocytopenic purpura.

The final stages of HIV infection are marked by superinfection, malignant neoplasms, and neurologic disease. Superinfection, the hallmark of the disease, results from progressive destruction of the T4 helper cell population. Most commonly, the infected individual succumbs to one or more opportunistic infections, particularly *Pneumocystis carinii*. These infections are frequently difficult to treat and impossible to eradicate, and consequently recurrences are the rule. They may be due to viral, bacterial, fungal, or protozoan agents:

**Viral:** cytomegalovirus **(CMV);** herpes simplex virus, types I and II; Epstein-Barr virus; varicella zoster; papovavirus.

**Bacterial:** *Mycobacterium tuberculosis; Mycobacterium avium-intracellulare; Legionella pneumophila; Klebsiella pneumoniae; Salmonella* species.

**Fungal:** *Candida albicans; Cryptococcus neoformans; Aspergillus* species; *Histoplasma capsulatum.*

**Protozoan:** *Pneumocystis carinii; Toxoplasma gondii; Entamoeba histolytica; Giardia lamblia; Cryptosporidium; Isospora belli.*

Many infections due to the agents listed above present differently in patients with HIV infection than in immunocompetent individuals.

The most common opportunistic infection in patients with AIDS is an interstitial pneumonia caused by *Pneumocystis carinii*. The symptoms, fever and dyspnea, usually develop gradually over several weeks. Also very common is CMV infection, especially CMV retinitis and enteritis. Tuberculosis, particularly with extrapulmonary manifestations, is common in AIDS. Often the tubercle bacilli are resistant to standard therapeutic agents. Common central nervous system infections include cryptococcal meningitis, and toxoplasmosis, which usually presents as a mass lesion with focal signs or seizures.

Malignant neoplasms are also characteristic of AIDS. Kaposi sarcoma is especially common in homosexual males with AIDS, occurring in as many as 37 percent of these patients. It is much less frequent in heterosexuals because it is transmitted best during anal intercourse. It is also seen in homosexual males lacking HIV infection. In this type of cancer, the skin, and often the viscera, develop small purple plaques and nodules representing vascular tumors. Patients who have only Kaposi sarcoma have a somewhat better prognosis than those with other opportunistic infections, apparently because their immune systems have retained slightly better function up to that point. Other cancers associated with AIDS include certain malignant lymphomas and primary B-cell lymphoma of the brain.

There are a variety of neurologic manifestations of AIDS that may become apparent before the immunodeficiency is recognized. The most devastating neurologic complication is HIV encephalopathy, or AIDS-related dementia complex. Recent research suggests that as many as 60 percent of AIDS patients develop dementia that cannot be attributed to superinfection. Ataxia, spastic paraplegia, and peripheral neuropathies have also been recognized as neurologic complications of AIDS.

Peripheral neuropathy may affect 10 percent or more of patients with AIDS, but the clinical and pathologic features are not completely characterized. The spectrum of symptom complexes includes sensory and motor neuropathies and multiple mononeuropathy.

Developmental abnormalities in children with AIDS, characterized by loss of cognitive ability and progressive long-tract signs, are now encountered with increasing frequency. An AIDS-associated dysmorphic syndrome in children, the result of intrauterine infection, has also been described (see ***Acquired Immunodeficiency Dysmorphic Syndrome).***

**Etiology** AIDS is caused by a human T-cell lymphotrophic virus (originally called HTLV-III) known as **HIV** (human immunodeficiency virus). It is a retrovirus. There are now known to be 2 human immunodeficiency viruses, HIV-1 and HIV-2. HIV-1 causes the vast majority of AIDS cases worldwide. HIV-2 occurs primarily in West Africa and may be less virulent than HIV-1.

**Epidemiology** Several populations are at risk for HIV infection, the 2 major ones being homosexuals and intravenous drug abusers. Other groups at risk include recipients of blood transfusion and blood products (including hemophiliacs), although the risk of new infection should be dramatically reduced since the advent of blood screening. Finally, sexual partners and children of individuals in high-risk groups are also at risk for acquiring HIV infection.

There are 3 major routes of transmission: sexual contact, blood-borne transmission, and perinatal transmission. Worldwide, sexual contact is the most common mode of transmission; in the United States, this accounts for the spread of disease among homosexuals. In central Africa, sexual transmission occurs primarily in heterosexuals.

The next most common means of spread worldwide is the blood-borne route, which includes transfusions of blood and blood products, needlestick and other occupational accidents among health care workers, and intravenous drug abuse that involves sharing contaminated needles. The high incidence of the disease among hemophiliacs is due to their need for factor VIII concentrate, which is derived from pooled plasma. Blood screening for HIV antibody, which began in 1985, has drastically reduced the risk of acquiring AIDS through transfusions and blood products.

HIV-infected mothers may transmit the virus in utero and perinatally, through breast milk and possibly delivery. The majority of pediatric AIDS cases result from perinatal transmission, the mothers being either intravenous drug abusers or sexual partners of drug abusers. The risk of a child's acquiring infection by this route is estimated to be about 30 to 40 percent. By 1990, approximately 2,000 cases of AIDS had been reported in children under the age of 13 in the United States.

In young children, the incubation period of HIV infection is much shorter than in adults. Most develop symptoms within 2 years.

About 55 percent of the homosexual population in certain communities have been found to have antibodies to HIV, suggesting that, although exposure to it has been widespread, some other cofactors may be necessary for HIV infection to develop. Coinfection with other microbial agents has been postulated as a cofactor.

Kaposi sarcoma, immunologic evidence of exposure or infection with HIV, and AIDS-like syndromes are exceptionally common among both sexes in central Africa, where the disease is thought to have originated. Here the major route of transmission is sexual contact between heterosexuals.

In the United States, transmission through heterosexual intercourse is thought to account for about 5 percent of all cases. Intravenous drug addicts and their sexual partners are the primary sources of AIDS infection among heterosexuals. Four out of 5 cases reported among this group are women. The proportion attributed to heterosexual contact in Africa is much higher than that in the United States. Three percent of cases seem to be idiopathic, but there are questions as to accurate admission by these patients of past drug use and/or sexual practices. Transmission of AIDS by a Florida dentist seems to have been caused by insufficient sterilization of instruments, but this was an extraordinarily rare way for the virus to be spread.

Data from blood donors screened from April through December 1985 in New York City revealed that 0.08 percent had antibodies to the AIDS virus. Further investigation revealed 90 percent of those with the virus belonged to one of the high-risk groups mentioned above. In only 11 cases could the source of infection not be identified.

In tests of military applicants in New York City from October 1985 through July 1986, 1.06 percent of men and 0.83 percent of women had evidence of AIDS infection. Most of these infections could be traced to homosexual contact or drug use, and the proportion attributed to heterosexual relations was "minor." Heterosexual transmission has been steadily increasing in frequency in the United States.

The exact risk of virus transmission between males and females during intercourse is unclear. Two studies on risks of unprotected intercourse with a virus carrier have described a higher rate of transmission (50 to 80 percent over months to years) than was previously thought possible for ordinary vaginal intercourse. In addition, one of these studies describes 2 cases of transmission from an infected male despite the use of condoms. This may be attributed to oral sex with semen discharge. It is clear that the risk of heterosexual transmission from a man to a woman is much greater than from a woman to a man.

Some studies find inconsistent rates of transmission through intercourse, depending on how the first partner became infected. One study found that drug abusers were much more effective transmitters than persons infected through contaminated blood products. In addition, rates of infection may vary among individuals or in the same person over time.

Available evidence indicates that the likelihood of viral transmission in a single heterosexual encounter is less than 1 percent. The virus probably spreads more easily in anal intercourse, which more often involves tearing of tissue, with resultant entry of the virus into the bloodstream. Promiscuity also increases risk.

Recent evidence suggests the AIDS virus can survive in insect hosts such as mosquitoes and other blood-sucking insects. However, there is no evidence that these insects can propagate the virus and transfer it to humans. To date, no case of AIDS has been linked to an insect bite in the United States.

There is currently a worldwide epidemic of AIDS and HIV infection. Areas with a high incidence include North America, central Africa, western Europe, and South America, particularly Brazil. Although there is a high incidence in Haiti, Haitians in the United States are not a high-risk group.

In the United States, over 1 million persons are thought to be infected, with the major cities having the highest reporting rates. Given this prevalence rate, AIDS can no longer be regarded as a disease restricted to certain populations.

**Diagnosis** The diagnosis of HIV infection usually begins with the screening test, the enzyme-linked immunosorbent assay **(ELISA),** for antibody to HIV. Because this test has a fairly high rate of false-positive results, any positive test should be repeated and confirmed by the Western blot test for specific viral antibodies.

These tests will miss those cases of HIV infection where antibody is absent or undetectable, which may be the case in the first few months of infection. Rare cases have been reported in which antibody took years to develop in infected individuals. Detection of these cases requires a test for the virus itself; such tests are currently under investigation.

The diagnosis of AIDS, rather than HIV infection, is made on the basis of documented HIV infection and the presence of one of the clinical syndromes discussed above, opportunistic infection, neoplasm, and neurologic disease being the major categories.

**Treatment—Standard** The treatment of choice for AIDS is the orphan drug zidovudine (**ZDV**), brand name Retrovir (formerly known as azidothymidine or **AZT**). It is currently used for patients, symptomatic or not, with CD4+ lymphocytes at levels of less than 500 cells per microliter. The drug appears to slow the progression of AIDS (and in some cases allows the immune system to rebuild itself) by inhibiting production of an essential enzyme necessary for the AIDS virus to replicate. In 1990, AZT was approved by the Food and Drug Administration for treatment of pediatric AIDS patients as young as 6 months old. The drug was approved in 1987 for patients 13 years of age and older. Treatment of infected pregnant women with ZDV can prevent infection of the fetus in utero.

A variety of nucleoside analogues have been under investigation for the treatment of HIV infection, including dideoxyinosine (**ddI**), dideoxycytydine (**ddC**), and others. Initial reports indicate that while ddC may reduce viral antigen levels, AZT remains the only drug that improves long-term survival. It has been reported that ddI can cause pancreatitis in about 10 percent of patients with AIDS, and that it is fatal in about 10 percent of cases. Therefore, patients taking ddI should avoid alcoholic beverages and seek medical help immediately if they have abdominal pain, nausea, or vomiting.

Treatment of the HIV infection with suramin, interleukin-2 to promote T lymphocyte growth, and various types of interferon (an antiviral protein), have not been effective, nor has treatment with acyclovir, vidarabine, various other drugs, white cell transfusions, thymic factors, and thymus and bone marrow transplants.

Many of the infections associated with AIDS respond to antibiotics, antifungals, etc., although recurrences are very common. Nystatin, clotrimazole, and ketoconazole are used to control episodes of esophageal and oral candidiasis. Severe candidiasis, as well as the other major fungal infection of AIDS, cryptococcal meningitis, will respond to amphotericin B or fluconazole. 5-Fluorocytosine may be used in combination with amphotericin in cryptococcal disease. Herpes simplex has responded to a course of treatment with acyclovir. Toxoplasmosis may be controlled with sulfadiazine and pyrimethamine, although these drugs have side effects that can limit their usefulness. Cryptosporidiosis may be treated symptomatically with tincture of opium, diphenoxylate, or cholestyramine. Spiramycin, an antibiotic used in Canada and Europe but not yet approved in the United States, may diminish diarrhea associated with cryptosporidiosis. (See Orphan and Experimental Drugs, below, for further mention of spiramycin.) A combination of quinine and clindamycin has also been reported to be effective.

*Pneumocystis carinii* pneumonia is more difficult to treat. At present, trimethoprim-sulfamethoxazole, pentamidine, atovaquone, and clindomycin plus primaquine are known to be effective. Intravenous pentamidine has been associated with serious side effects, including hypoglycemia, hyperglycemia, hypocalcemia, hypotension, and renal and hepatic dysfunction. These functions must be monitored very closely in any patient on pentamidine. Currently, aerosolized pentamidine is recommended for prophylaxis against *P. carinii* infection. Patients with very low CD4+ counts (under 200 cells per microliter), as well as patients who have had one episode of *P. carinii* pneumonia, are recommended to receive aerosolized pentamidine on a monthly basis. Pentamidine is commercially available in the United States from Lyphomed, in inhalant (NebuPent) and injectable (Pentam 300) forms. (See under Treatment—Investigational, below, for information on other studies of pentamidine.) The drug atovaquone (Mepron) may be a useful alternative for treatment of pneumocystis pneumonia because it appears to have fewer side effects than trimethoprim and sulphamethoxazole (Septra, Bactrim).

Effective treatment has recently been found for *Mycobacterium avium-intracellulare* (clarithromycin, rifabutin), CMV, and Epstein-Barr virus. The drug ganciclovir (dihydroxypropoxymethyl guanine—**DHPG**) is effective against CMV retinitis in AIDS patients. The patient's eyesight often can be protected by this treatment, which is, however, complicated by toxic reactions, usually hematologic.

Kaposi sarcoma sometimes responds to chemotherapy. Drugs have included vinblastine, etoposide, doxorubicin, bleomycin, and combinations of these. α-Interferon in high doses is moderately effective in treating Kaposi sarcoma. Also reportedly effective in this cancer is vincristine, which has antitumor activity without causing further immunosuppression due to bone marrow suppression. Radiation therapy may also be used to palliate the lesions of Kaposi sarcoma. Generally, however, treatment is not recommended for Kaposi sarcoma unless the lesions are cosmetically unacceptable to the patient or are producing significant symptoms.

Prevention is the key to slowing the AIDS epidemic. Among the precautions against HIV transmission recommended by the Public Health Service are the following:

1) The use of condoms during sexual contact. 2) Sexual contact with persons known or suspected to be HIV carriers should be avoided. Multiple sex partners increase the probability of acquiring infection. 3) No members of high-risk groups should donate blood or blood products. 4) Blood transfusions should only be performed when absolutely necessary. 5) Screening procedures for plasma or blood likely to transmit AIDS have been developed,

and safer blood products are available for hemophilia patients. 6) Health care personnel, laboratory workers, and others in frequent contact with AIDS patients should take great care with needles and similar sharp objects, and with blood-soiled materials.

**Treatment—Investigational** (See above under Treatment—Standard for a comparison of some investigational therapies with AZT.)

Tests to identify individuals infected with HIV before they develop AIDS have shown an increase in virus-infected white blood cells in the year before AIDS symptoms become apparent. Present methods to detect these cells (peripheral blood mononuclear cells or monocytes) are time-consuming and expensive, and simpler tests are currently under development. Treatment of asymptomatic infection, when identified early enough, may be more effective than treating the disease after symptoms appear, but this is controversial.

The Food and Drug Administration gave a 1987 orphan drug research grant to John E. Conte, Jr., M.D., for studies on pentamidine pharmacokinetics related to AIDS patients on hemodialysis. Another grant was given for studies on the drug diethyldithiocarbamate for treatment of AIDS to Evan M. Hersh, M.D., of the University of Arizona.

Various vaccines are currently under investigation for the prevention of HIV infection.

**Orphan and experimental drugs (see also the Orphan Drug Directory elsewhere in the Guide):** Patients and doctors wishing to apply for admission into clinical trials of any AIDS drug should call the Food and Drug Administration at 1-800-TRIALS-A (see under Resources, below, for further information on this service).

Clinical trials are being conducted on the following orphan drugs for treatment of AIDS: diethyldithiocarbamate (Imuthiol), by Merieux Institute; and 2'3'-dideoxycytidine, by the National Cancer Institute.

Experimental orphan drugs for the treatment of AIDS include HPA-23, and others. For additional information about HPA-23, contact Rhone-Poulenc Pharmaceuticals. (See below for a further listing of experimental drugs and their indications and manufacturers.)

Two orphan drugs are undergoing clinical trials for treatment of AIDS-related Kaposi sarcoma: interferon alfa-nf (Wellferon), Burroughs Wellcome Company; and interferon alfa-2b (Intron A), Schering Corporation. Other drugs being investigated for treating Kaposi sarcoma include lymphoblastoid interferon and piritrexim isethionate, Burroughs Wellcome Company; doxorubicin, National Institute of Allergy and Infectious Diseases; tumor necrosis factor, Genentech; and menogaril, National Cancer Institute.

Reports that cyclosporine might be an effective treatment for AIDS were released prematurely from researchers in France in 1985. This drug is commonly used for immunosuppression in patients who have received a transplanted organ. The French reports were issued after the drug had been used for only 6 days on a very limited number of patients, all of whom died after transient initial improvement.

More than 80 ongoing human studies have been approved by the Food and Drug Administration to test potential drug treatments for opportunistic infections and cancers often found in AIDS patients, based on investigational new drug **(IND)** applications. They are listed below by what they are designed to treat, their names, and the manufacturers, respectively.

### Anti-infective agents

#### For *Pneumocystis carinii* pneumonia:
aerosol pentamidine, Fisons Corporation and the National Institute of Allergy and Infectious Diseases; dapsone, Jacobus Pharmaceutical Co.; diethyldithiocarbamate (Imuthiol), Merieux Institute; eflornithine (DMFO), Merrell Dow Pharmaceuticals; pentamidine isethionate, Rhone Poulenc Pharmaceuticals; piritrexim, Burroughs Wellcome Company; trimetrexate, Warner-Lambert Company and the National Institute of Allergy and Infectious Diseases;

#### For CMV retinitis:
foscarnet sodium IV (Foscavir), Astra Pharmaceutical Products and the National Institute of Allergy and Infectious Diseases;

#### For *Mycobacterium avium-intracellulare:*
ansamycin, also called rifabutin (no brand name as yet established), in combination with other drugs, Adria Laboratories; clofazimine (Lamprene-Geigy Pharmaceuticals), San Francisco General Hospital;

#### For cryptosporidiosis:
spiramycin, Rhone-Poulenc Pharmaceuticals;

#### For opportunistic infections:
immune globulin IG-IV, Sandoz Pharmaceuticals Corporation; Alpha Therapeutic Corporation; and Miles. Also involved are the National Institutes of Health and the National Institute of Child Health and Human Development.

## Experimental antineoplastic agents
### For primary lymphoma:
M-BACOD (**m**ethotrexate; **b**leomycin; **A**driamycin [doxorubicin]; **c**yclophosphamide; **O**ncovin [vincristine]; **d**examethasone), National Institute of Allergy and Infectious Diseases (NIAID).
## Other experimental agents
### For oral candidiasis prevention:
nystatin, E.R. Squibb and Sons;
### For AIDS-related diarrhea:
octreotide acetate (Sandostatin), Sandoz Pharmaceuticals Corporation;
### For cryptosporidial diarrhea:
diclazuril, Janssen Pharmaceutica;
### For toxoplasmic encephalitis:
clindamycin, Mark Jacobson, M.D., San Francisco, CA;
### For toxoplasmosis prevention:
pyrimethamine (Daraprim), Burroughs Wellcome Company;
### For histoplasmosis:
itraconazole (Sporanox), Janssen Pharmaceutica.

Please contact the agencies listed under Resources, below, for the most current information. Addresses and telephone numbers of these agencies, as well as of individual experts and research centers, may be found in the Master Resources List.

### Resources

**For more information on acquired immune deficiency syndrome:** National Organization for Rare Disorders (NORD); American Foundation for AIDS Research; National Gay Task Force (NGTF—provides a handbook listing support groups, fund-raising organizations, etc.); National Gay Task Force Crisis Line; National Hemophilia Foundation; NIH/National Institute of Allergy and Infectious Diseases; Centers for Disease Control; National Sexually Transmitted Diseases Hotline; AIDS Information Clearinghouse; NIH/National Cancer Institute Physician Data Query Phoneline; AIDSLINE—National Library of Medicine.

Information on privately funded clinical trials of drugs and biologics used to treat AIDS and AIDS-related illnesses is now available through a toll-free telephone service **(1-800-TRIALS-A).** This service is staffed by specially trained information specialists, including some who speak Spanish. Service for the hearing-impaired is also available, at **(800) 243-7012.** Callers can find out where studies are located and the eligibility criteria for participants, the name of the product being studied and the purpose of the study, and a contact person and phone number for the company sponsoring the clinical trials. All inquiries are kept confidential. Information from the phone service is also accessible through AIDSLINE, the National Library of Medicine's online computer database, available from MEDLARS management section.

### References

DDI and DDC Show Similar Benefits in Advanced Disease: New Options for People Who Cannot Take or Who No Longer Benefit from AZT: National Institute of Allergy and Infectious Diseases; January 22, 1993.

HIV Infection and AIDS: Are You at Risk?: Department of Health and Human Services, Centers for Disease Control; February 1993, D539.

Cecil Textbook of Medicine, 19th ed.: J.B. Wyngaarden, et al., eds.; W.B. Saunders Company, 1992, pp. 1908–1970.

FDA Talk Paper: Food and Drug Administration, U.S. Department of Health and Human Services; October 5, 1992, T92–45.

FDA Talk Paper: Food and Drug Administration, U.S. Department of Health and Human Services; December 23, 1992, T92–71.

HHS News: U.S. Department of Health and Human Services, December 23, 1992, P92–41.

Nelson Textbook of Pediatrics, 14th ed.: R.E. Behrman, ed.-in-chief; W.B. Saunders Company, 1992, pp. 496, 676.

Recommendations for Prophylaxis Against Pneumocystis carinii Pneumonia for Adults and Adolescents Infected with Human Immunodeficiency Virus: Centers for Disease Control Morbidity and Mortality Weekly Report; April 10, 1992, vol. 41(RR–4).

Update: Early Use of AZT Reduces Risk of Death: National Institute of Allergy and Infectious Diseases; April 15, 1992.

Voluntary HIV Counseling and Testing: Facts, Issues, and Answers: Department of Health and Human Services, Centers for Disease Control; September 1991, D545.

AZT Therapy for Early HIV Infection: National Institute of Allergy and Infectious Diseases; J. Clin. Courier, April 1990, vol. 8(5).

Clinical Dermatology, 2nd ed.; T.P. Habif, ed.; C.V. Mosby Company, 1990, pp. 256–266.

Hematology, 4th ed.: W.J. Williams, et al., eds.; McGraw-Hill, 1990, pp. 973–993.

Principles of Neurology, 4th ed.; R.D. Adams and M.Victor, eds.; McGraw-Hill, 1989, pp. 611–614.

Pulmonary Diseases and Disorders, 2nd ed.: A.P. Fishman, ed.; McGraw-Hill, 1988, pp. 1687–1692.

Justification of Appropriation Estimates for Committee on Appropriations: Public Health Service Supplementary Budget Data (Moyer Material) A Through L: Fiscal Year 1986, vol. VII. This publication contains information on all AIDS research being funded by NIH.

Treatment of Kaposi's Sarcoma and Thrombocytopenia with Vincristine in Patients with the Acquired Immunodeficiency Syndrome: D.M. Mintzer, et al.; Ann. Intern. Med., February 1985, vol. 102(2), pp. 200–202.

The Acquired Immune Deficiency Syndrome: A.J. Pinching; Clin. Exp. Immunol., April 1984, vol. 56(1), pp. 1–13.

Acquired Immunodeficiency Syndrome: A.M. Macher; Am. Fam. Phys., December 1984, vol. 30(6), pp. 131–144.

Treatment of Intestinal Cryptosporidiosis with Spiramycin: D. Portnoy, et al.; Ann. Intern. Med., August 1984, vol. 101(2), pp. 202–204.

Acquired Immune Deficiency Syndrome: An Update and Interpretation: C.B. Daul, et al.; Ann. Allergy, September 1983, vol. 51(3), pp. 351–361.

Acquired Immunodeficiency Syndrome: Epidemiologic, Clinical, Immunologic, and Therapeutic Considerations: A.S. Fauci, et al.; Ann. Intern. Med., January 1983, vol. 100(1), pp. 92–106.

National Institutes of Health Conference. Acquired Immunodeficiency Syndrome: Epidemiologic, Clinical, Immunologic, and Therapeutic Considerations: A.S. Fauci, et al.; Ann. Intern. Med., January 1983, vol. 100(1), pp. 92–106.

Reports on AIDS have been published in the Morbidity and Mortality Weekly Report from June 1981 through the present by the Centers for Disease Control.

# ACQUIRED IMMUNODEFICIENCY DYSMORPHIC SYNDROME

**Description** AIDS dysmorphic syndrome is a constellation of craniofacial anomalies accompanied by developmental delay. The syndrome has been reported in some infants with intrauterine human immunodeficiency virus (**HIV**) infection. HIV is thought to be transmitted transplacentally by an infected woman who may or may not have symptoms of AIDS. Children with AIDS dysmorphic syndrome are infected with HIV and hence are prone to develop all the other manifestations of AIDS.

**Synonyms**

> AIDS Dysmorphic Syndrome
> Dysmorphic Acquired Immune Deficiency Syndrome
> Embryopathy

**Signs and Symptoms** Signs of AIDS dysmorphic syndrome become apparent before 1 year of age. It is characterized by growth failure, microcephaly, and dysmorphic craniofacial features, including wide-set eyes, prominent boxlike forehead, flat nasal bridge, mild upward or downward slant of the eyes, long eyelid fissures, a blue tinge to the whites of the eyes, a shortened nose, a triangular groove in the upper lip, and patulous lips. These features vary in severity and may not be noticeable until the child is a few months old.

The degree of physical and mental developmental delay in affected children varies.

The typical infections of pediatric AIDS usually develop later in infancy. Affected infants are highly susceptible to infections such as *Pneumocystis carinii* pneumonia, meningitis, urinary infections, or soft tissue infections.

**Etiology** The syndrome is thought to be caused by intrauterine transmission of the HIV virus from an AIDS-infected mother.

**Epidemiology** Dysmorphic AIDS usually becomes apparent among affected children between 3 weeks and 23 months of age. The disorder affects males and females in equal numbers.

**Treatment—Standard** Fetal HIV infection can be diagnosed prenatally by testing for the presence of the HIV virus in the fetus after the 14th week of pregnancy. Blood from the umbilical cord may also be tested for the virus. After birth, HIV antibody is present, but it is likely to have been passively transferred from the mother.

In children with dysmorphic AIDS, treatment with intravenous immunoglobulin (**IG-IV**) helps restore the immune system, thus decreasing the chance of infections. Treatment with zidovudine (formerly known as AZT) may help prevent developmental delay. The long-term outcome of these treatments is unknown at this time.

**Treatment—Investigational** Please contact the agencies listed under Resources, below, for the most current information. Addresses and telephone numbers of these agencies, as well as of individual experts and research centers, may be found in the Master Resources List.

**Resources**

**For more information on acquired immunodeficiency dysmorphic syndrome:** National Organization for Rare Disorders (NORD); American Foundation for AIDS Research; Computerized AIDS Information Network; NIH/National Institute of Allergy and Infectious Diseases; Centers for Disease Control.

**References**

AIDS in Children: B.J. Proujan; Research Resources Reporter, January 1988, vol. 12(1), pp. 1–5.

Fetal AIDS Syndrome Score: R.W. Marion, et al.; Am. J. Dis. Child., 1987, vol. 141, pp. 429–431.

Human T-Cell Lymphotropic Virus Type III (HTLV-III) Embryopathy: R.W. Marion, et al.; Am. J. Dis. Child., July 1986, vol. 140(7), pp. 638–640.

Intravenous Gamma-Globulin in Infant Acquired Immunodeficiency Syndrome: T.A. Calvelli, et al.; Pediatr. Infect. Dis., 1986, vol. 5, pp. S207–S210.

Pediatric AIDS: A. Rubinstein; Curr. Probl. Pediatr., 1986, vol. 16, pp. 364–409.

# ANAPHYLAXIS

**Description** Anaphylaxis is a type I IgE-mediated hypersensitivity reaction. It is an immediate systemic response triggered by IgE-antigen interaction, and mediated by mast cells, basophils, and their products. Major symptoms may include pruritis, urticaria, flushing, angioedema, vomiting, diarrhea, dyspnea, and shock.

**Synonyms**

>Anaphylactic Reaction
>Anaphylactic Shock
>Generalized Anaphylaxis

**Signs and Symptoms** Anaphylaxis is mediated by prostaglandins and histamine, substances that can evoke angioedema, urticaria, bronchiolar constriction, laryngeal edema, and vascular collapse. The respiratory symptoms may include wheezing, chest tightness, stridor, and dyspnea. Urticarial eruptions may be local or generalized, and are very pruritic. Angioedema represents edema and reaction at deeper layers of the skin, and includes the subcutaneous tissue. It is generally not pruritic but may be accompanied by a burning sensation.

Anaphylactic reactions occur within seconds or minutes and can be rapidly fatal. When death occurs, it may be due to upper airway obstruction, or shock, or both.

The diagnosis is made on the basis of the history and clinical appearance of the patient.

**Etiology** Anaphylaxis is a hypersensitivity reaction to an antigen. The most common triggers include penicillin, insect venom, pollen extracts, fish, shellfish, and nuts. Various other foods, drugs, radiographic dyes, food additives (particularly sulfites), and chemicals are known to cause anaphylactic reactions in hypersensitive individuals.

**Epidemiology** The sexes and all age groups are affected equally. There are approximately 50 to 100 deaths from anaphylaxis caused by insect stings each year in the United States.

**Related Disorders** Other hypersensitivity reactions that are IgE-mediated include atopy and urticaria. Repeated contact with a particular antigen may result in more serious reactions at a later time. See *Arachnoiditis.*

**Atopic dermatitis,** a common, chronic form of eczematous dermatitis, is usually seen in persons with a history of allergy. This disorder is characterized by itching with cutaneous erythema, and crusted, scaling, and oozing lesions. Lichenification is often present. The irritants that trigger atopic dermatitis are many and include harsh soaps, detergents, medications, extremes of heat and cold, wool and silk clothing, and emotional stress. Distribution of skin lesions to the flexor surfaces of the arms and legs, neck, and face is common.

**Contact dermatitis** is an inflammatory reaction in the skin in response to irritants and allergens. It may be acute or chronic and is marked by inflamed skin and, possibly, blisters at the site of contact with an offending agent. If acute, the area may be edematous, crusty, scaly, and exudative. The patient complains of burning pain and, as a rule, pruritus. Irritating the site by scratching or rubbing may cause lichenification.

**Treatment—Standard** The major drug used in the treatment of anaphylaxis is epinephrine. It should be given as early as possible and may be required in repeated doses. Bronchospasm may benefit from aminophylline in addition to epinephrine, and supplemental oxygen will be required in most cases where there is respiratory compromise. Diphenhydramine may be used to treat urticarial and angioedematous reactions. Desensitization may reduce hypersensitivity to some substances.

**Treatment—Investigational** Please contact the agencies listed under Resources, below, for the most current information. Addresses and telephone numbers of these agencies, as well as of individual experts and research centers, may be found in the Master Resources List.

**Resources**

**For more information on anaphylaxis:** National Organization for Rare Disorders (NORD); NIH/National Institute of Allergy and Infectious Diseases; Asthma and Allergy Foundation of America.

**References**

Anaphylaxis: An Allergic Reaction That Can Kill: M. Segal; FDA Consumer, May 1989, pp. 21–23.

Anaphylactic Shock: Guidelines for Immediate Diagnosis and Treatment: A.J. Costa; Postgrad. Med., March 1988, vol. 83(4), pp. 368–369, 372–373.

Fatal Food-Induced Anaphylaxis: J.W. Yunginger, et al.; JAMA, September 9, 1988, vol. 260(10), pp. 1450–1452.

Internal Medicine, 2nd ed.: J.H. Stein, ed.-in-chief; Little, Brown and Company, 1987, pp. 1249–1250.

# ANTIPHOSPHOLIPID SYNDROME

**Description** Antiphospholipid syndrome is an autoimmune disorder characterized by recurring thromboses before age 45. It may also be associated with repeated spontaneous abortions in young women.

**Synonyms**

Antiphospholipid Antibody Syndrome

**Signs and Symptoms** The clots characteristic of antiphospholipid syndrome appear in veins and arteries usually before age 45 and often cause strokes or transient ischemic attacks as well as repeated spontaneous abortions. Coagulation and abnormal bleeding may occur in many organs or parts of the body, especially the arms, legs, and gastrointestinal tract. Other symptoms include myocardial infarction as a result of inflammation and thickening of the heart valves. In individuals who have had coronary artery bypass surgery, thromboses may block the new bypass grafts. Clots infrequently cause cardiomyopathy.

If the neurologic system is involved, symptoms may include migraine headaches, chorea, and encephalopathy.

Skin disorders include livedo reticularis, livedoid vasculitis, necrotic gangrene, and, rarely, Degos disease.

Infrequently, antiphospholipid syndrome may cause ophthalmic problems such as blood clots within the eye, hemorrhages, and retinopathy.

**Etiology** Antiphospholipid syndrome is an autoimmune disorder affecting blood coagulation. It is found in association with other disorders or may be present by itself. Rarely, multiple cases have been reported in one family.

**Epidemiology** Antiphospholipid syndrome affects males and females equally. Some teenage cases have been reported, but most cases begin before the age of 45, with all age groups and ethnic backgrounds represented.

**Related Disorders** See *Polyarteritis Nodosa; Arteritis, Takayasu; Arteritis, Giant Cell; Lupus Erythematosus, Systemic; Thrombocytopenia, Essential.*

**Therapies Standard** The diagnosis of antiphospholipid syndrome is usually confirmed by laboratory tests that detect antiphospholipid and/or anticardiolipin antibodies. Other tests may include ELISA, Ouchterlony, inhibition experiments, and Western blot tests. Frequently a false positive reading for syphilis is reported in individuals with antiphospholipid syndrome.

Heart damage associated with antiphospholipid syndrome may be evaluated by magnetic resonating imaging and echocardiogram. A CT scan of the brain frequently shows areas of damage due to inadequate blood supply.

Steroid drugs (e.g., prednisone) constitute the usual treatment for antiphospholipid syndrome. Aspirin, heparin, or coumadin may be given to prevent coagulation.

When antiphospholipid syndrome affects the eyes, skin, and other organs, treatment is symptomatic and supportive. People who have suffered a stroke may require physical therapy.

**Treatment—Investigational** Immunosuppressive drugs are under investigation as a treatment for antiphospholipid syndrome. More study is needed to determine their long-term safety and effectiveness.

Plasmapheresis may be of benefit in some cases of antiphospholipid syndrome. More research is needed, however, before it can be recommended in all but the most severe cases.

Please contact the agencies listed under Resources, below, for the most current information. Addresses and telephone numbers of these agencies, as well as of individual experts and research centers, may be found in the Master Resources List.

**Resources**

**For more information on antiphospholipid syndrome:** National Organization for Rare Disorders (NORD); American Autoimmune Related Disease Association; Lupus Foundation of America; NIH/National Heart, Lung and Blood Institute Information Center.

**References**

Antiphospholipid Syndrome: R.A. Asherson, et al.; J. Invest. Dermatol., January 1993, vol. 100(1), pp. 21S–27S.

The Antiphospholipid Syndrome: Ten Years On: G.R.V. Hughes; Lancet, August 1993; vol. 342(8867), pp. 341–344.

A Comparison of Cardiac Valvular Involvement in the Primary Antiphospholipid Syndrome Versus Anticardiolipin-Negative Systemic Lupus Erythematosus: C.B. Gleason, et al.; Am. Heart J., April 1993, vol. 1256(4), pp. 1123–1129.

Different Manifestations of the Antiphospholipid Antibody Syndrome in a Family with Systemic Lupus Erythematosus: K.P. May, et al.; Arthritis Rheum., April 1993, vol. 36(4), pp. 528–533.

Neurobehavioral Presentations of the Antiphospholipid Antibody Syndrome: D.G. Gorman, et al.; J. Neuropsychiatry Clin. Neurosci., Winter 1993, vol. 5(1), pp. 37–42.

Antiphospholipid Antibodies and Arterial Thrombosis: Case Reports and a Review of the Literature: G.S. McGee, et al.; Arch. Surg., March 1992, vol. 127(3), pp. 342–346.

Antiphospholipid Antibody Syndrome: L.R. Sammaritano, et al.; Clin. Lab. Med., March 1992, vol. 12(1), pp. 41–59.

Primary Antiphospholipid Syndrome with Multiorgan Arterial and Venous Thromboses: R.E. Perez, et al.; J. Rheumatol., August 1992, vol. 19(8), pp. 1289–1292.

Repeated Fetal Losses Associated with Antiphospholipid Antibodies: A Collaborative Randomized Trial Comparing Prednisone with Low-Dose Heparin Treatment: F.S. Cowchock, et al.; Am. J. Obstet. Gynecol., May 1992, vol. 166(5), pp. 1318–1323.

Vascular Disease in the Antiphospholipid Syndrome: A Comparison with the Patient Population with Atherosclerosis: C.K. Shortell, et al.; J. Vasc. Surg., January 1992, vol. 15(1), pp. 158–165.

Cutaneous Histopathologic Findings in Antiphospholipid Syndrome: Correlation with Disease, Including Human Immunodeficiency Virus Disease: K.J. Smith, et al.; Arch. Dermatol., September 1990, vol. 126 (9), pp. 1176–1183.

# APECED SYNDROME

**Description** APECED ([**A**]utoimmune [**P**]oly[**E**]ndocrinopathy, [**C**]andidiasis, [**E**]ctodermal [**D**]ysplasia) syndrome is a genetic immunosuppressive disorder characterized by a combination of at least 2 of the following: hypoparathyroidism, adrenocortical failure, and candidiasis. Three types of polyglandular autoimmune syndrome (**PGA**) have been recognized: PGA I, characterized by the presence of 2 or 3 endocrine diseases and candidiasis; PGA II, in which autoimmune thyroid disease and Addison disease and/or insulin-dependent diabetes are present without candidiasis or hypoparathyroidism; and PGA III, in which thyroid disease and another autoimmune disease are present, but Addison disease is not.

**Synonyms**
> Autoimmune Polyendocrinopathy–Candidiasis–Ectodermal Dystrophy
> Polyglandular Autoimmune Syndrome, Type I

**Signs and Symptoms** In childhood, candidiasis of either the mouth or nails is an early sign of APECED syndrome. Hypoparathyroidism is often diagnosed before adrenal insufficiency. Malabsorption of nutrients results in diarrhea. Anemia, autoimmune thyroid disease, and loss or delay of sexual development may also occur. Enamel dystrophy, alopecia, vitiligo, and keratopathy are common. Patients may develop liver disease or insulin-dependent diabetes.

**Etiology** APECED syndrome is inherited as an autosomal recessive trait.

**Epidemiology** APECED syndrome affects males and females equally. Childhood onset is most common, but the disease can develop as late as the 5th decade. The majority of those affected are of Finnish descent.

**Related Disorders** See *Addison Disease*.

**Hypoparathyroidism** causes insufficient amounts of calcium and phosphate in the blood. It is characterized by weakness, muscle cramps, and abnormal sensations, such as tingling, burning, and numbness of the hands. Excessive nervousness, loss of memory, headaches, and uncontrollable cramping muscle movements of the hands and feet may also occur.

**Candidiasis** is usually a benign yeast infection of the mouth, intestinal tract, skin, nails, and genitalia. It is caused by *Candida albicans*. In those with weakened immune systems, it can spread throughout the body.

The **ectodermal dysplasias** are hereditary and nonprogressive. They affect the skin and other organs that develop from the ectodermal germ layer during gestation. Respiratory infection is a common serious complication that develops because those affected tend to exhibit a weakened immune system and impaired respiratory mucous glands.

**Treatment—Standard** Treatment of APECED syndrome is directed toward the specific diseases apparent in each patient.

Addison disease is treated with hydrocortisone and fluorocortisone to replace the missing cortisol and aldosterone.

Hypoparathyroidism is treated with calcium, ergocalciferol, or dihydrotachysterol (forms of vitamin D).

In chronic mucocutaneous candidiasis, amphotericin B, nystatin, clotrimaxole, miconazole, or 5-fluorocytosine is used.

There is no known cure for ectodermal dysplasia. Treatment is directed at symptoms. Over-the-counter creams may relieve skin discomfort. Dentures, hearing aids, etc., may be required. Heat and strenuous exercise are to be avoided due to impairment of sweat glands. Surgery is usually indicated for cleft lip, cleft palate, syndactyly, and other limb deformations. Other treatment is symptomatic and supportive.

Genetic counseling is important for APECED patients and their relatives, especially if the patient is of Finnish descent.

**Treatment—Investigational** Please contact the agencies listed under Resources, below, for the most current information. Addresses and telephone numbers of these agencies, as well as of individual experts and research centers, may be found in the Master Resources List.

**Resources**

**For more information on APECED syndrome:** National Organization for Rare Disorders (NORD); National Foundation for Ectodermal Dysplasias; National Adrenal Disease Foundation; NIH/National Digestive Diseases Information Clearinghouse.

**For genetic information and genetic counseling referrals:** March of Dimes Birth Defects Foundation; Alliance of Genetic Support Groups.

### References

Clinical Variation of Autoimmune Polyendocrinopathy–Candidiasis–Ectodermal Dystrophy (APECED): P. Ahonen, et al.; N. Engl. J. Med., June 1990, vol. 322(26), pp. 1829–1836.

Mendelian Inheritance in Man, 8th ed.: V.A. McKusick; The Johns Hopkins University Press, 1986, pp. 1263–1264.

Autoimmune Polyendocrinopathy–Candidosis–Ectodermal Dystrophy (APECED): Autosomal Recessive Inheritance: P. Ahone; Clin. Genet., June 1985, vol. 27(6), pp. 535–542.

# ASPERGILLOSIS

**Description** Aspergillosis is an infection with a species of the fungus *Aspergillus,* the most common pathogen being *A. fumigatus.* Infections may be focal or systemic and most commonly occur in the lung; the brain and sinuses are also common sites. There are several distinct types of *Aspergillus* infection that occur in different circumstances; these are allergic bronchopulmonary aspergillosis, aspergilloma, and invasive aspergillosis. Immunosuppressed patients, particularly acute leukemics, are prone to fulminant invasive forms of aspergillosis. Other types of aspergillus infection include endocarditis, skin ulcers, and bone involvement.

**Signs and Symptoms Allergic bronchopulmonary aspergillosis (ABPA)** is one of the syndromes associated with pulmonary infiltrates and eosinophilia (**PIE** syndrome). It occurs in patients with asthma and is characterized by infiltrates on chest x-ray, eosinophilia, elevated serum IgE, and serum precipitins to *A. fumigatus.* This form of aspergillosis is not invasive but may lead to central bronchiectasis. Patients complain of worsening asthma, cough, and expectorating mucous plugs.

Pulmonary mycetoma, also known as **aspergilloma** or "fungus ball," is a form of noninvasive aspergillosis that often occurs as a result of fungal colonization of a pulmonary cavity. This may complicate tuberculosis, sarcoidosis, histoplasmosis, and many chronic pulmonary diseases. The patient's symptoms are usually referrable to the underlying lung disease rather than to the fungus, but complications can occur. These include hemoptysis, bronchopleural fistula, and bacterial superinfection. Fungus balls are usually diagnosed on chest x-ray.

**Invasive aspergillosis** commonly originates in the lung or the sinuses and tends to occur in immunosuppressed patients, particularly those with severe neutropenia. *Aspergillus* pneumonia is a rapidly progressive infection with fever, pulmonary symptoms, and rapidly enlarging infiltrates on chest x-ray. Hematogenous spread throughout the body is common, and the patient usually succumbs. A fulminant, invasive sinusitis can also occur in immunosuppressed patients, particularly acute leukemics.

The diagnosis of invasive aspergillosis is rarely made on blood culture. Since *Aspergillus* is ubiquitous, positive sputum and nasal cultures may represent contamination, colonization, or invasion; the interpretation rests on the clinical appearance of the patient.

*Aspergillus* is also a cause of infective endocarditis, and Madura foot.

**Etiology** There are several pathogenic species of *Aspergillus,* the most frequent being *A. fumigatus,* followed by *A. flavus,* and others. *Aspergillus* infection or colonization is acquired by inhalation. The spores of this fungus are ubiquitous and may be found in decaying vegetable matter, grains, grass, leaves, soil, wet paint, air conditioning systems, and construction and fireproofing materials, and on refrigerator walls. Nosocomial infections may be associated with potted plants in the patient's room, and hospital construction.

**Epidemiology** Aspergillosis affects males and females in equal numbers. It is seen more often in those people who have chronic respiratory problems or whose immune system has been weakened.

**Related Disorders** Related diseases include other fungal infections of the lung, including histoplasmosis, cryptococcosis, blastomycosis, and coccidioidomycosis. *Aspergillus* infections of the sinus and nasal cavity may resemble rhinocerebral mucormycosis.

ABPA is one of the PIE syndromes; the others are eosinophilic pneumonia, ***Churg-Strauss Syndrome,*** Loeffler disease, and the hypereosinophilic syndrome. ABPA may be distinguished by its association with asthma, elevated serum IgE, and serum precipitins and skin reactions to *A. Fumigatus.* ABPA may precede the development of bronchiectasis.

**Treatment—Standard** The treatment of ABPA is with systemic steroids. Amphotericin B or itraconazole (by mouth) are used for invasive disease. Surgery is often indicated in cases of aspergillus endocarditis, as well as invasive disease of the sinuses and brain. Aspergillomas do not ordinarily require treatment, except if life-threatening hemoptysis complicates the picture. Surgical excision is the treatment of choice in these cases.

**Treatment—Investigational** Studies are currently being conducted on the effectiveness of the therapeutic agents itraconazole, imidazole, ketoconazole, and fluconazole in aspergillosis.

Paul Greenberger, M.D., at Northwestern University, is conducting clinical trials to study antibodies in aspergillosis.

Please contact the agencies listed under Resources, below, for the most current information. Addresses and telephone numbers of these agencies, as well as of individual experts and research centers, may be found in the Master Resources List.

### Resources

**For more information on aspergillosis:** National Organization for Rare Disorders (NORD); NIH/National Institute of Allergy and Infectious Diseases; Centers for Disease Control.

### References

Aspergillosis: S. Levitz; Infect. Dis. Clin. North Am., March 1989, vol. 3(1), pp. 1–18.

Allergic Bronchopulmonary Aspergillosis: P. Bock; Am. Fam. Phys., January 1988, vol. 37(1), pp. 177–182.

Cecil Textbook of Medicine, 18th ed.: J.B. Wyngaarden and L.H. Smith, Jr., eds.; W.B. Saunders Company, 1988, p. 1850.

Aspergilloma in Sarcoid and Tuberculosis: J. Tomlinson, et al.; September 1987, vol. 92(3), pp. 505–508.

Internal Medicine, 2nd ed.: J.H. Stein, ed.-in-chief; Little, Brown and Company, 1987, p. 1765.

Invasive Aspergillosis in Children: E. Golladay, et al.; J. Pediatr. Surg., June 1987, vol. 22(6), pp. 504–505.

Rapid Diagnosis of Candidiasis and Aspergillosis: J. Bennett; Rev. Infect. Dis., March–April 1987, vol. 9(2), pp. 398–402.

Pulmonary Diseases and Disorders, vol. 2, 2nd ed.: A.P. Fishman, ed.-in-chief; McGraw-Hill, 1980, p. 1639.

# BABESIOSIS

**Description** Babesiosis is primarily a disease of animals that is caused by protozoan organisms of the genus *Babesia*. The disease is similar to malaria in its pathophysiology and symptoms. Those who have had a splenectomy or who have an impaired immune system develop fulminant, frequently fatal infection.

**Signs and Symptoms** Most human *Babesia* infections are probably asymptomatic. Patients who experience symptoms tend to be younger than 12 or older than 50, asplenic, or immunodeficient.

Babesiosis has a 1- to 3-week incubation period, after which patients complain of fever, malaise, fatigue, and myalgias. Nausea, vomiting, and abdominal pain are also common. Laboratory examination reveals evidence of hemolytic anemia; thrombocytopenia and leukopenia may also be seen. In severe cases jaundice and renal failure may occur. In very rare cases babesiosis may be responsible for adult respiratory distress syndrome (**ARDS**).

The diagnosis of babesiosis is made by examination of thick and thin blood smears for parasitic forms inside the erythrocytes. The diagnosis may also be serologically confirmed by indirect immunofluorescent antibody testing.

**Etiology** *Babesia* are protozoa. There are many species, but only 3 are pathogenic in man: *B. microti, B. bovis,* and *B. divergens*. Of these, the first is the major cause of babesiosis in the United States, whereas the other 2 have been found in European infection. *Babesia* are erythrocytic parasites, like the *Plasmodium* species that causes malaria. Both have a reproductive cycle inside the red blood cell, with cell rupture and subsequent hemolysis. Unlike most species of *Plasmodium, Babesia* do not rupture in a synchronous fashion, and so periodic paroxysms do not occur.

**Epidemiology** Babesiosis is transmitted by the *Ixodes dammini* tick, which also transmits Lyme disease. In the United States, most cases are confined to the Northeastern coast. The disease has been reported in a small number of recipients of blood transfusions. The disease is rare; only about 200 cases were reported in the United States in the 1980s.

**Related Disorders** Babesiosis is closely related to malaria, although the 2 are easily distinguished by the geographic history of the patient. Symptoms of Lyme disease and toxoplasmosis often mimic those of babesiosis.

**Treatment—Standard** Most cases of babesiosis will resolve spontaneously. Severe disease is treated with a regimen of clindamycin and quinine. These 2 drugs alone or in combination with others are required to treat patients with impaired immune systems.

**Treatment—Investigational** Please contact the agencies listed under Resources, below, for the most current information. Addresses and telephone numbers of these agencies, as well as of individual experts and research centers, may be found in the Master Resources List.

### Resources

**For more information on babesiosis:** National Organization for Rare Disorders (NORD); NIH/National Institute of Allergy and Infectious Diseases; Centers for Disease Control; World Health Organization.

### References

Babesiosis: An Underdiagnosed Disease of Children: P.J. Krause, et al.; Pediatrics, June 1992, vol. 89(Pt. 1), pp. 1045–1048.

Cecil Textbook of Medicine, 19th ed.: J.B. Wyngaarden, et al., eds.; W.B. Saunders Company, 1992, pp. 871–1997.

Human Babesiosis In New York State: An Epidemiological Description of 136 Cases: S.C. Meldrum; Clin. Infect. Dis., December 1992, vol. 15(6), pp. 1019–1023.

Babesiosis: Diagnostic Pitfalls: J.M. Carr, et al.; Am. J. Clin. Pathol., June 1991, vol. 95(6), pp. 774–777.

Tick-Borne Diseases: L. Doan-Wiggins; Emerg. Med. Clin. North Am., May 1991, vol. 9(2), pp. 303–325.

Transfusion-Transmitted Babesiosis: A Case Report from a New Endemic Area: E.D. Mintz; Transfusion, May 1991, vol. 31(4), pp. 365–368.

Transmission of Parasitic and Bacterial Infections Through Blood Transfusions Within the U.S.: I.A. Shulman; Crit. Rev. Clin. Lab. Sci., 1991, vol. 28(5–6), pp. 447–459.

Babesia: J.A. Gelfand; in Principles and Practice of Infectious Diseases: G.L. Mandell, et al., eds.; Churchill Livingstone, 1990, pp. 2119–2121.

Hematology, 4th ed.: W.J. Williams, et al., eds.; McGraw-Hill, 1990, pp. 22, 664, 813, 898, 1705.

Self-Limited Babesiosis in a Splenectomized Child: H.O. Mathewson, et al.; Pediatr. Infect. Dis. J., March–April 1990, vol. 3(2), pp. 66–67.

Pulmonary Diseases and Disorders, 2nd ed.; A.P. Fishman, ed.; McGraw-Hill, 1988, pp. 2204, 2206.

Report of the Committee on Infectious Diseases, 21st ed.: G. Peter, et al., eds.; American Academy of Pediatrics, 1988, p. 131.

Tick Exposure and Related Infections: R. Jacobs; Pediatr. Infect. Dis. J., September 1988, vol. 7(8), pp. 342–346.

# BALANTIDIASIS

**Description** Balantidiasis is an intestinal infection with *Balantidium coli*, a ciliated protozoan parasite that frequently infects pigs. On the rare occasions it is transmitted to man, it may produce a disease that resembles amebic dysentery.

**Synonyms**

> Balantidial Dysentery
> Ciliary Dysentery

**Signs and Symptoms** *B. coli* infection may be asymptomatic or mild, or the patient may be acutely ill with fever, nausea, vomiting, abdominal pain, and bloody diarrhea. The symptoms are caused by mucosal invasion of the intestinal wall, creating ulcers. In fulminating infections, perforation through the ulcer occurs, resulting in peritonitis.

In dysentery, the trophozoite form of the organism is usually recoverable from the stool. Another diagnostic method involves scraping the ulcer base and examining the scrapings for trophozoites.

**Etiology** Balantidiasis is caused by the ciliated protozoan parasite *B. coli*.

**Epidemiology** This disease occurs in tropical regions such as Brazil, New Guinea, and southern Iran. It is primarily a disease of people in close contact with pigs. Transmission is fecal-oral, through direct contact with pig feces, or indirectly from contaminated drinking water.

**Related Disorders** Balantidiasis must be distinguished from amebic dysentery, *Shigella* dysentery, and ulcerative colitis. Symptoms are also similar to the following:

**Crohn disease** is an inflammatory disorder of the intestine. Symptoms include nausea, vomiting, fever, night sweats, loss of appetite, malaise, abdominal pain, diarrhea, and rectal bleeding.

**Chronic erosive gastritis** is an inflammatory disorder characterized by a burning or heavy feeling in the stomach, mild nausea, vomiting, loss of appetite, and malaise. Gastric bleeding occurs in severe cases and can result in anemia.

**Treatment—Standard** The treatment of choice is tetracycline. Alternatives include iodoquinol or metronidazole. Prevention is accomplished by good hygiene.

**Treatment—Investigational** Please contact the agencies listed under Resources, below, for the most current information. Addresses and telephone numbers of these agencies, as well as of individual experts and research centers, may be found in the Master Resources List.

**Resources**

**For more information on balantidiasis:** National Organization for Rare Disorders (NORD); NIH/National Institute of Allergy and Infectious Diseases; Centers for Disease Control; World Health Organization.

**References**

Cecil Textbook of Medicine, 19th ed.: J.B. Wyngaarden, et al., eds.; W.B. Saunders Company, 1992, p. 1996.

Human Balantidiasis: A Case Report: A.R. Currie; S. Afr. J. Surg., March 1990, vol. 28(1), pp. 23–25.

Gastrointestinal Disease, 4th ed.; M.H. Sleisenger, et al.; W.B. Saunders Company, 1989, pp. 1171–1172.

Invasive Balantidiasis Presented As Chronic Colitis and Lung Involvement: S.D. Lucas; Dig. Dis. Sci., October 1989, vol. 34(10), pp. 1621–1623.

# BARTONELLOSIS

**Description** Bartonellosis is a disease caused by *Bartonella bacilliformis* and transmitted by sandflies. It is characterized by fever, hemolytic anemia, and a chronic skin rash. It is now recognized that an organism called *Bartonella henselae* can produce cat-scratch disease (see **Cat-Scratch Disease**).

**Synonyms**

> Carrion Disease

Oroya Fever

Verruga Peruana

**Signs and Symptoms** There are 2 phases of *B. bacilliformis* infection. In the first, called Oroya fever, there is fever, anemia, headache, and severe bone and joint pain. Physical examination reveals hepatosplenomegaly and generalized lymphadenopathy. The anemia is hemolytic and results from parasitization of erythrocytes by the bacteria, with subsequent rupture. Neurologic involvement may also occur, with meningoencephalitis. The mortality of untreated disease is high and often due to superinfection with *Salmonella* and other microorganisms.

The 2nd phase of infection, referred to as verruga peruana, usually but not necessarily follows the Oroya fever phase. It is characterized by fever, pains, and an eruption on the skin. The rash consists of multiple small nodular lesions, usually on the face and extremities. Lesions may also appear in the gastrointestinal and genitourinary tracts, where they occasionally make their presence known by bleeding.

The diagnosis of bartonellosis during the first phase is made on microscopic examination of a peripheral blood smear; the bacteria may be seen inside the red blood cells. During the 2nd phase of illness, organisms may be seen on a smear of material from a skin lesion.

**Etiology** The cause of bartonellosis is the gram-negative bacterium, *Bartonella bacilliformis.* This organism parasitizes erythrocytes, cells of the reticuloendothelial system, and the endothelial cells of blood vessels. Invasion of the skin and subcutaneous tissues characterizes the verruga peruana phase.

**Epidemiology** The geography of bartonellosis is limited by the range of its mosquito vector, which lives at certain altitudes in the Andes. The populations of Peru, Ecuador, Colombia, Chile, and Guatemala may be affected, particularly in the spring.

**Related Disorders** Symptoms of malaria and toxoplasmosis can be similar to those of bartonellosis. See also ***Cat-Scratch Disease.***

**Treatment—Standard** The treatment of choice is chloramphenicol. Preventive measures include the use of mosquito netting, adequate clothing, and insect repellents.

**Treatment—Investigational** Please contact the agencies listed under Resources, below, for the most current information. Addresses and telephone numbers of these agencies, as well as of individual experts and research centers, may be found in the Master Resources List.

**Resources**

**For more information on bartonellosis:** National Organization for Rare Disorders (NORD); NIH/National Institute of Allergy and Infectious Diseases; Centers for Disease Control.

**References**

Cecil Textbook of Medicine, 19th ed.: J.B. Wyngaarden, et al., eds.; W.B. Saunders Company, 1992, pp. 1729, 1732.

Dendrocytes in Verruga Peruana and Bacillary Angiomatosis: J. Arrese Estrada, et al.; Dermatology, 1992, vol. 184(1), pp. 22–25.

Bartonellosis: An Immunodepressive Disease and the Life of Daniel Alcides Carrion: U. Garcia, et al.; Am. J. Clin. Pathol., April 1991, vol. 95(4:1), pp. S58–66.

An Epidemic of Oroya Fever in the Peruvian Andes: G.C. Gray, et al.; Am. J. Trop. Med. Hyg., March 1990, vol. 42(3), pp. 215–221.

Hematology, 4th ed.: W.J. Williams, et al., eds.; McGraw-Hill, 1990, pp. 1705–1706.

Manson's Tropical Diseases, 19th ed.: P.E.C. Manson-Bahr and D.R. Bell; Ballière Tindall, 1987, pp. 246–251.

# BEJEL

**Description** Bejel is a treponemal disease that is very similar to syphilis but is not transmitted sexually. Also referred to as **endemic syphilis,** bejel is a disease of stages, the late stage being the most clinically significant. The disease consists of skin and bone lesions.

**Synonyms**

Dichuchwa

Endemic Syphilis

Frenga

Njovera

Nonvenereal Syphilis

Siti

Treponematosis, Bejel Type

**Signs and Symptoms** The primary lesion is an ulcer on a mucous membrane, frequently inside the mouth. It usually occurs in childhood and is rarely noticed. Secondary disease involves adenopathy, ulcers, and a rash, generally on the trunk, arms, and legs. Lesions may also be concentrated in the axilla, groin, and rectum. The late lesion is the gumma, which appears in the skin and bones. The diagnosis is based on the geographic history of the patient, with darkfield examination of material from the lesions, or serology (Venereal Disease Research Laboratory [**VDRL**] test; the fluorescent treponemal antibody-absorption [**FTA-ABS**] test).

**Etiology** Bejel is caused by a spirochete, *Treponema pallidum II*. It is morphologically indistinguishable from the agent that causes syphilis.

**Epidemiology** Males and females are affected in equal numbers. Transmission is by direct, nonsexual contact, or indirectly, through shared eating utensils. It is rare in the United States, but occurs in the Middle East; Africa; parts of Europe, particularly Yugoslavia; Southeast Asia; and Australia.

**Related Disorders** Bejel is a treponematosis, and as such is related to syphilis, pinta, and yaws. These organisms are morphologically similar, but their epidemiologies and clinical characteristics differ.

**Treatment—Standard** Bejel is treated with benzathine penicillin G. Doxycycline or tetracycline are alternatives for patients allergic to penicillin.

**Treatment—Investigational** Please contact the agencies listed under Resources, below, for the most current information. Addresses and telephone numbers of these agencies, as well as of individual experts and research centers, may be found in the Master Resources List.

**Resources**

For more information on bejel: National Organization for Rare Disorders (NORD); NIH/National Institute of Allergy and Infectious Diseases; Centers for Disease Control; World Health Organization.

**References**

Cecil Textbook of Medicine, 19th ed.; J.B. Wyngaarden, et al., eds.; W.B. Saunders Company, 1992, p. 1770–1771.

Epidemiology of Endemic Non-Venereal Treponematoses: S. Talhari; Bull. Mem. Acad. R. Med. Belg., 1992, vol. 147(3–5), pp. 149–161.

Nelson Textbook of Pediatrics, 14th ed.: R.E. Behrman, ed.-in-chief; W.B. Saunders Company, 1992, p. 781.

Late Endemic Syphilis: Case Report of Bejel with Gummatous Laryngitis: J.L. Pace; Genitourin. Med., June 1988, vol. 64(3), pp. 202–204.

# BLASTOMYCOSIS

**Description** Blastomycosis is a systemic fungal infection caused by *Blastomyces dermatitidis*. The lungs, skin, bones, and genitourinary tract are most frequently involved.

**Synonyms**

Gilchrist Disease

North American Blastomycosis

**Signs and Symptoms** The initial infection is pulmonary. Fever, chills, headaches, chest pain, weight loss, night sweats, myalgia, articular pain, cough, and dyspnea may occur; alternatively, the acute pulmonary infection may be asymptomatic. The chronic phase of blastomycosis may involve the lung, skin, bones, joints, genitourinary tract, or central nervous system.

Involvement of the skin is most common; papulopustular and verrucous lesions are common. The color may be violaceous, and microabscesses may form around the periphery of the lesion. Subcutaneous nodules may appear, usually accompanied by active pulmonary disease.

Chronic pulmonary disease usually takes the form of chronic pneumonia. Consolidation or cavitation may be evident on chest x-ray.

Bone lesions commonly involve the long bones, ribs, and vertebrae, the most frequent lesion being a painless lytic lesion that may present with an overlying abscess or sinus.

Genitourinary tract involvement is common in men; prostate and epididymal disease is seen in up to one-third of cases.

Involvement of the central nervous system, liver, spleen, gastrointestinal tract, thyroid, adrenals, and other organs has been reported.

The diagnosis of blastomycosis is initially made by direct microscopic examination of infected material (pus, sputum, urine, or biopsy material). Preparation with potassium hydroxide usually renders the yeast cells easily visible. Culture will confirm the diagnosis. Skin testing and serologic tests are not helpful.

**Etiology** Blastomycosis is caused by the dimorphic fungus *Blastomyces dermatitidis*. It grows in the yeast form at body temperature, and the mycelial form at room temperature.

**Epidemiology** Blastomycosis affects males and females in equal numbers and is endemic in the south central and southeastern United States. It is also found around the perimeter of the Great Lakes, and along the St. Lawrence River in Canada. Elsewhere, blastomycosis has been reported in Mexico, South and Central America, Africa, and India.

The natural habitat of this fungus is unclear but may be in the soil. Farmers, construction workers, and others who work with soil appear to be at increased risk.

**Related Disorders** Pulmonary blastomycosis may be mistaken for malignancy, and bronchoscopy may be required to confirm the diagnosis. Cutaneous blastomycosis may also resemble malignancy.

**Treatment—Standard** Oral itraconazole is now the treatment of choice for all but severe cases of blastomycosis.

Fluconazole and ketoconazole also appear to be effective for treatment of mild or moderate cases. When the central nervous system is involved, amphotericin B is required.

**Treatment—Investigational** Please contact the agencies listed under Resources, below, for the most current information. Addresses and telephone numbers of these agencies, as well as of individual experts and research centers, may be found in the Master Resources List.

**Resources**

**For more information on blastomycosis:** National Organization for Rare Disorders (NORD); Centers for Disease Control; NIH/National Institute of Allergy and Infectious Diseases; World Health Organization.

**References**

Current Therapy of Major Fungal Diseases of the Lung: P. Johnson, et al.; Infect. Dis. Clin. North Am., September 1994, vol. 5(3), pp. 635–645.

Blastomycosis in Immunocompromised Patients: P.G. Pappas, et al.; Medicine, September 1993, vol. 72(5), pp. 311–325.

A Clinician's View of Blastomycosis: R.W. Bradsher; Curr. Trop. Med. Mycol., 1993, vol. 5, pp. 181–200.

Blastomycosis: R.W. Bradsher; Clin. Infect. Dis., March 1992, vol. 14(suppl. 1), pp. 282–290.

Blastomycosis in Patients with the Acquired Immunodeficiency Syndrome: P.G. Pappas, et al.; Ann. Intern. Med., May 1992, vol. 116(10), pp. 847–853.

Case Report: Treatment of Blastomycosis with Fluconazole: G.J. Pearson, et al.; Am. J. Med. Sci., May 1992, vol. 393(5), pp. 313–315.

Cecil Textbook of Medicine, 19th ed.: J.B. Wyngaarden, et al., eds.; W.B. Saunders Company, 1992, pp. 1892–1893.

Cutaneous Blastomycosis: M.G. Mercurio, et al.; Cutis, December 1992, vol. 50(6), pp. 422–424.

Infectious Diseases: S.L. Gorbach, ed.; W.B. Saunders Company, 1992, pp. 499, 1928–1930.

Itraconazole Therapy for Blastomycosis and Histoplasmosis: Niaid Mycoses Study Group: W.E. Dismukes, et al.; Am. J. Med., November 1992, vol. 93(5), pp. 487–497.

Nelson Textbook of Pediatrics, 14th ed.: R.E. Behrman, ed.-in-chief; W.B. Saunders Company, 1992, pp. 866–867.

Tropical Mycoses: M.A. Bayles; Chemotherapy, 1992, vol. 38(suppl. 1), pp. 27–34.

Harrison's Principles of Internal Medicine, 12th ed.: J.D. Wilson, et al., eds.: McGraw-Hill, 1991, pp. 744–745.

Hyperendemic Urban Blastomycosis: A.C. Manetti; Am. J. Public Health, May 1991, vol. 81(5), pp. 633–636.

North American Blastomycosis: J. Weingardt, et al.; Am. Fam. Physician, April 1991, vol. 43(4), pp. 1245–1248.

Systemic Fungal Infections: An Overview: G. Medoff, et al.; Hosp. Pract., February 1991, vol. 26(2), pp. 41–52.

Blastomyces Dermatitidis: S.W. Chapman; in Principles and Practice of Infectious Diseases: G.L. Mandell, et al., eds.; Churchill Livingstone, 1990, pp. 1999–2007.

Pulmonary Diseases and Disorders, 2nd ed.: A.P. Fishman, ed.; McGraw-Hill, 1988, pp. 315–316.

# BOTULISM

**Description** Botulism is a paralytic syndrome caused by an enterotoxin elaborated by *Clostridium botulinum.* There are 3 different forms: food-borne, in which food containing the toxin is ingested; wound botulism, where the wound becomes contaminated with *C. botulinum,* which then produces the toxin; and infant botulism, in which food contaminated with the bacteria is ingested, and the toxin is elaborated after ingestion. The toxin produces symptoms by blocking transmission at the neuromuscular junction.

**Signs and Symptoms** In **food-borne botulism,** the most common form, food containing preformed toxin is ingested. Symptoms start approximately 12 to 36 hours later, although the incubation period varies from 4 hours to 8 days. The initial manifestations are nonspecific, including weakness, headache, and dizziness. There may be gastrointestinal symptoms such as nausea, vomiting, diarrhea, and abdominal pain.

When neurotransmission in the autonomic system is blocked, extreme dryness of the mouth and pharynx occurs. The same pathophysiologic process may give rise to urinary retention, ileus, and constipation.

The neurologic manifestations of botulism may accompany the anticholinergic symptoms, or may be delayed as long as 3 days. When neurologic symptoms begin, they do so in a descending fashion, starting with the cranial nerves. Patients may experience blurred vision and photophobia, then dysarthria and dysphagia, followed by variable degrees of muscle weakness, descending down the body. When death occurs, it is usually a result of respiratory muscle paralysis.

Physical examination usually reveals a fully conscious patient. Fever is generally absent. Postural hypotension is a relatively frequent finding. The pupils are dilated and fixed, and a variety of cranial nerve abnormalities may be present. The pharynx may be so erythematous and dry that bacterial pharyngitis is suspected. Neurologic examination reveals muscle weakness with variable deep tendon reflexes and normal sensation.

Recovery is generally slow, and some symptoms, such as constipation, dry mouth, and intermittent diplopia have been known to persist for months.

The diagnosis of botulism is made on the clinical features described above, although a characteristic electromyographic picture supports the diagnosis. Diagnosis may be confirmed by demonstrating the toxin in the blood, stool, or gastric contents.

**Wound botulism** generally appears 4 to 14 days after the injury. It is characterized by the same neurologic symptoms as food-borne botulism; however, gastrointestinal symptoms are absent, and wound infection may be associated with fever.

**Infant botulism** is seen most often between the ages of 2 and 3 months. Constipation occurs initially in approximately two-thirds of cases. This may be followed by varying degrees of neuromuscular paralysis—the so-called floppy infant syndrome. The diagnosis is made by demonstrating the organism in the stool.

Milk is not usually the source of infant botulism. Cases have been related to the ingestion of honey, vacuum cleaner dust, and soil.

**Etiology** Botulism is the result of ingestion and absorption of toxin produced by the anaerobic bacillus *Clostridium botulinum*. The toxin blocks neurotransmission at the neuromuscular junction by inhibiting the release of the neurotransmitter acetylcholine.

There are 8 distinct types of the toxin, but human poisoning is usually caused by only 3: types A, B, and E. Wound and infant botulism tend to be associated only with types A and B.

*Clostridium botulinum* spores are highly resistant to heat and may survive for several hours at 100° C (212° F), but not at 120° C (248° F). On the other hand, the toxins are readily destroyed by heat; cooking at 80° C (176° F) for 30 minutes protects against botulism.

**Epidemiology** Home-canned food is the most common source of botulism; however, commercially prepared foods have been implicated in about 10 percent of cases. A wide variety of foods may cause botulism, including vegetables, fish, fruits, beef, milk products, pork, and poultry.

The different types of toxins have different geographic distributions. Type A is the most common in the United States, and is the most frequent type west of the Mississippi River. Type B is more frequent in the eastern states, and type E is more prevalent in Alaska and the Great Lakes region. Worldwide, type E is frequent in northern latitudes and Japan.

**Treatment—Standard** Botulism requires careful attention to respiratory status. Monitoring, with frequent determinations of vital capacity, is recommended, and early institution of mechanical ventilation may be lifesaving.

A trivalent antitoxin (A, B, E) is available through the Centers for Disease Control. Antitoxin is also available for outbreaks due to types C, D, and F. Treatment should be initiated as soon as possible; it may still be beneficial even weeks after toxin ingestion. However, the risks of treatment must be weighed against potential benefits. The antitoxins are made from horse serum and may cause serious allergic reactions. Patients should be tested for hypersensitivity and desensitized if necessary prior to administration of the antitoxin.

The antitoxin does not reverse preexisting neurologic impairment although it may slow or halt further progression of disease.

Guanidine has been advocated by some in the treatment of botulism; it is thought to enhance release of acetylcholine at the synapse. However, results have been inconsistent, and the effectiveness of the drug remains unproved.

**Treatment—Investigational** Stephen S. Amon, M.D., of the California Department of Health Services, Berkeley, is conducting clinical trials of human botulism globulin (**BIG**).

Please contact the agencies listed under Resources, below, for the most current information. Addresses and telephone numbers of these agencies, as well as of individual experts and research centers, may be found in the Master Resources List.

**Resources**

**For more information on botulism:** National Organization for Rare Disorders (NORD); NIH/National Institute of Allergy and Infectious Diseases; Centers for Disease Control; Food and Drug Administration.

**References**

Clostridium Botulinum (Botulism): W. Schaffner; *in* Principles and Practice of Infectious Diseases: G.L. Mandell, et al., eds.; Churchill Livingstone, 1990, pp. 1847–1849.

Cecil Textbook of Medicine, 18th ed.: J.B. Wyngaarden and L.H. Smith, Jr., eds.; W.B. Saunders Company, 1988, pp. 1633–1634, 1663, 1666.

# BRUCELLOSIS

**Description** Brucellosis is an infection of livestock that may be transmitted to humans. It is caused by different species of the genus *Brucella*. It is worldwide in its distribution. Initial infection may result in an acute flulike illness or may evolve insidiously over months. Untreated cases may take months to resolve, and some cases become chronic.

**Synonyms**

Bang Disease

Cyprus Fever

Febris Melitensis
Febris Sudoralis
Febris Undulans
Fievre Caprine
Gibraltar Fever
Goat Fever
Maltese Fever
Mediterranean Fever
Melitensis Septicemia
Melitococcosis
Neapolitan Fever
Rock Fever
Undulant Fever

**Signs and Symptoms** Brucellosis has a very wide range of manifestations. Asymptomatic infection occurs, particularly in children. Acute brucellosis is a flulike illness without localizing symptoms. Typically there is gradual onset of fever, weakness, headache, myalgias, night sweats, and fatigue. Examination generally reveals few abnormalities; occasionally there may be lymphadenopathy, splenomegaly, or hepatomegaly. In untreated cases, the symptoms may persist intermittently for several weeks. Occasionally, chronic disease develops, with repeated waves of fever (the so-called undulant fever) recurring for more than a year.

Localized forms of brucellosis may occur anywhere in the body. The most frequent focal infections are osteomyelitis (usually of the lumbar vertebrae), splenic abscess, orchitis, endocarditis, and lung infection. Renal and ophthalmic abnormalities, in addition to neuritis, may also be present.

Endocarditis is an uncommon complication but is the most frequent cause of death. A wide variety of central nervous system complications may also occur.

Laboratory tests are not distinctive and generally do not help to distinguish brucellosis from other conditions with similar symptoms.

The diagnosis of brucellosis is occasionally made by isolating the organism from the blood, bone marrow, or other sites (lymph nodes, spleen, liver). However, *Brucella* is hazardous to culture in the laboratory, and only certain laboratories will undertake the task. Most infections are confirmed serologically using agglutination tests. A fourfold rise in antibody titer of specimens drawn a few weeks apart is diagnostic of acute infection. The presence of IgG antibodies against *Brucella* may be used to indicate ongoing infection, since with effective treatment they should disappear.

**Etiology** *Brucella* are small gram-negative coccobacilli. There are several species, but human brucellosis is caused by only 4 of these: *B. abortus* (carried by cattle), *B. suis* (carried by hogs), *B. melitensis* (transmitted by sheep and goats), and *B. canis,* carried by dogs. Of these, *B. melitensis* is the most frequent pathogen and causes the most severe disease.

**Epidemiology** Domestic livestock are the major source of human infection. As an infection of livestock, brucellosis occurs worldwide. There are 2 major routes of transmission. Direct contact with infected secretions may transmit the disease, as may occur with veterinarians, abattoir employees, meat packers, and farmers. More commonly, infection occurs by ingestion of unpasteurized milk or milk products.

Brucellosis is rare in the United States, since pasteurization of milk is routine and cattle are vaccinated against the disease. It is much more common in Russia, Africa, South America, and the Middle East. Less than 200 cases are reported annually in the United States, most cases being either imported from endemic regions or related to consumption of unpasteurized goat's milk or cheese.

**Related Disorders** Symptoms for toxoplasmosis may mimic those of brucellosis.

See *Cat-Scratch Disease; Psittacosis; Q Fever.*

**Treatment—Standard** The treatment of choice for brucellosis is a combination of doxycycline and rifampin. Trimethoprim/sulfamethoxazole is an adequate alternative, but it is not as effective. The combination of tetracycline and streptomycin is not longer considered the treatment of choice. In serious infections, such as meningitis or endocarditis, rifampin may be added to the regimen. Endocarditis generally warrants valve replacement in addition to antibiotic therapy.

Relapse of brucellosis is experienced in less than 10 percent of patients after antibiotic therapy. For toxemia, steroids may be administered; for severe spinal pain, codeine may be required.

Human infection can be prevented by a variety of measures. A vaccine is available for cattle, sheep, and goats. Workers handling meat or milk products that are likely to be infected should use protective clothing and gloves. Finally, pasteurization kills the bacteria.

**Treatment—Investigational** Please contact the agencies listed under Resources, below, for the most current information. Addresses and telephone numbers of these agencies, as well as of individual experts and research centers, may be found in the Master Resources List.

## Resources

**For more information on brucellosis:** National Organization for Rare Disorders (NORD); Centers for Disease Control; Food and Drug Administration; World Health Organization.

## References

Southwestern Internal Medicine Conference: Brucellosis: Don't Let It Get Your Goat!: J.D. Radolf; Am. J. Med. Sci., January 1994, vol. 307(1), pp. 64–75.

Brucellar Sacroilitis: Findings in 63 Episodes and Current Relevance: J. Ariza, et al.; Clin. Infect. Dis., June 1993, vol. 16(6), pp. 761–765.

Current Aspects of Brucellosis: F. Janbon; Rev. Med. Interne, May 1993, vol. 14(5), pp. 307–312.

Open, Randomized Therapeutic Trial of Six Antimicrobial Regimens in the Treatment of Human Brucellosis: J.M. Montejo, et al.; Clin. Infect. Dis., May 1993, vol. 16(5), pp. 671–676.

Treatment of Childhood Brucellosis: Result of a Prospective Trial on 113 Children: N.A. Khuri-Bulos, et al.; Pediatr. Infect. Dis. J., May 1993, vol. 12(5), pp. 377–381.

Cecil Textbook of Medicine, 19th ed.: J.B. Wyngaarden, et al., eds.; W.B. Saunders Company, 1992, pp. 1727–1729.

Infectious Diseases: S.L. Gorbach, ed.; W.B. Saunders Company, 1992, pp. 1513–1521.

Nelson Textbook of Pediatrics, 14th ed.: R.E. Behrman, ed.-in-chief; W.B. Saunders Company, 1992, pp. 741–742.

Harrison's Principles of Internal Medicine, 12th ed.: J.D. Wilson, et al., eds.: McGraw-Hill, 1991, pp. 625–626.

Brucella Species: A.J. Mikolich; *in* Principles and Practice of Infectious Diseases: G.L. Mandell, et al., eds.; Churchill Livingstone, 1990, pp. 1735–1742.

# CAT-SCRATCH DISEASE

**Description** Cat-scratch disease is a self-limiting infectious disease characterized by regional lymphadenitis. In most cases a scratch, bite, or lick of a cat is the source of the infection.

**Synonyms**

Cat-Scratch Adenitis
Cat-Scratch Fever
Debre Syndrome
Foshay-Mollaret Cat-Scratch Fever
Lymphadenitis, Regional Nonbacterial
Lymphoreticulosis, Benign Inoculation
Petzetakis Syndrome

**Signs and Symptoms** The major symptoms of cat-scratch disease may not appear for several days or weeks after exposure. A macule may appear at the infection site, and a papule may appear 3 to 5 days after exposure. The papule is painless, does not itch, may fill with fluid, then crust over and heal with a scar similar to those of chickenpox. The papule persists for 1 to 3 weeks, but may go unnoticed or be attributed to an injury.

A primary symptom of cat-scratch disease is regional lymphadenopathy near the bite or scratch, usually about 2 weeks after initial exposure. Lymphanginitis does not typically occur. Suppuration may develop in the involved lymph nodes, which then become very tender; the skin surface appears red and feels hot to the touch.

Loss of appetite, fatigue, low-grade fever, and/or malaise are common. In some cases, chills, backache, abdominal pain, encephalitis, and convulsions have been reported.

If the site of infection is on the eyelid, cat-scratch-oculoglandular syndrome (Parinaud syndrome) may develop, which includes preauricular lymphadenopathy, palpebral conjunctivitis, and/or fever.

A more severe systemic form of cat-scratch disease has been reported. Major symptoms include prolonged fever, arthralgia, rash, weight loss, and/or splenomegaly.

In some rare cases, symptoms include swelling of the parotid gland, osteolytic lesions, neuroretinitis, hepatitis or splenitis, and/or abscesses of the spleen. In very rare cases, cat-scratch disease has been associated with atypical pneumonia, encephalitis, erythema nodosum, and/or thrombocytopenia purpura.

**Etiology** Cat-scratch disease is thought to be caused by the bacterium *Bartonella henselae* (formerly *Rochalimaea henselae*). The great majority of cases are the result of a lick, scratch, or bite from a cat or kitten. A deep puncture wound, such as from a thorn or splinter, may also introduce infection. Bites from dogs and monkeys have been reported to cause the disease. Fleas and mites have been implicated in the transmission of cat-scratch disease. Animals that are carrying the disease are not ill and exhibit no symptoms, even though the organism may be in their blood. Not every person exposed to the carrier animal will develop cat-scratch disease, and in most cases the symptoms are transient and mild.

**Epidemiology** Cat-scratch disease affects more males than females. Approximately 80 percent of cases occur in people under 20 years of age, and about 95 percent have a history of a scratch from a cat or exposure to cats. In the United States, an estimated 22,000 cases are diagnosed every year, with significant rises in September and February.

**Related Disorders** Symptoms of the following disorders can be similar to those of cat-scratch disease. Comparisons may be useful for a differential diagnosis.

**Adenitis** (bacterial, fungal, pyogenic, and tuberculous) is an inflammatory disease characterized by lymphadenopathy. Differential diagnosis may be accomplished through skin testing and/or microscopic examination of the involved lymph nodes.

**Atypical mycobacterial infections** are caused by nontuberculous mycobacteria but can be very difficult to distinguish from tuberculosis. When lymphadenopathy is caused by nontuberculous mycobacteria, biopsy may be necessary for diagnosis.

**Lymphogranuloma venereum** is a sexually transmitted infection characterized by a primary skin lesion at the site of infection. The papule may heal spontaneously or go unnoticed. Acute pain and uni- or bilateral lymphadenopathy ensue. The site of the first infection or lesion determines the region affected.

**Sarcoidosis** is a rare multisystem disorder characterized by tubercles of granulomatous tissue. Symptoms, which may be absent, slight, or severe, depend on the severity of the disease, how much of the body is affected, and the site of involvement. Peripheral lymphadenopathy is common. Both enlarged and normal-sized lymph nodes may contain the characteristic sarcoid tubercles.

**Tularemia**, an infectious disease primarily of rodents but also of humans, is transmitted by the bites of deer flies, fleas, and ticks, and/or as a result of handling contaminated animals or their products, inhaling the responsible microorganism, or ingesting contaminated food or water. Ulceroglandular tularemia begins as a painful papule that fills with pus and may rupture to form a shallow ulcer. Mild, generalized pain and lymphadenopathy, splenomegaly, hepatomegaly, and/or pneumonia are associated disorders.

See also *Brucellosis.*

In addition to atypical pneumonia and encephalitis, the following disorders may be associated with cat-scratch disease as secondary characteristics. They are not necessary for a differential diagnosis.

**Erythema nodosum** is an inflammatory reaction to infection characterized by multiple tender nodules or bumps on the shins. Young women are affected most often. Symptoms of acute erythema nodosum include fever, malaise, and arthralgia.

**Thrombocytopenia purpura** is a disorder in which the blood platelet count is decreased. It may be either primary or secondary to another disorder. Symptoms may include petechiae and a tendency to bruise easily.

**Treatment—Standard** The diagnosis of cat-scratch disease is dependent on a history of contact with animals (usually a cat), a positive serum antibody test, a positive skin test for cat-scratch disease, examination of fluid extracted from an involved lymph node, and/or characteristic changes in the involved lymph nodes.

Cat-scratch disease may subside without any treatment within 4 to 8 weeks. Therapy is symptomatic and supportive. The prognosis is very good, with no long-term health effects. When secondary disorders (e.g., encephalitis) develop, they are usually resolved when the lymphadenopathy and associated symptoms are resolved.

The effectiveness of antimicrobial therapy has not been established in the treatment of cat-scratch disease. Some reports, however, show that erythromycin or drugs such as ciprofloxacin, gentamicin, and/or a combination of trimethoprim and sulfamethoxazole may be useful in the treatment of systemic symptoms secondary to cat-scratch disease. Antibiotic therapy may speed the resolution of the primary symptoms.

If the lymph node suppurates and becomes large and/or painful, aspiration is preferrable to making an incision. Usually one aspiration is sufficient to relieve discomfort.

**Treatment—Investigational** A new test to detect antibodies to *Bartonella henselae* in serum is available from the Centers for Disease Control. A high level of these antibodies in the blood is indicative of the disease. New techniques to culture and grow this bacteria are also being investigated.

Please contact the agencies listed under Resources, below, for the most current information. Addresses and telephone numbers of these agencies, as well as of individual experts and research centers, may be found in the Master Resources List.

**Resources**

**For more information on cat-scratch disease:** National Organization for Rare Disorders (NORD); Centers for Disease Control; NIH/National Institute of Allergy and Infectious Diseases.

**References**

Cat-Scratch Disease in Connecticut: K.M. Zangwill, et al.; N. Engl. J. Med., July 1993, vol. 329(1), pp. 8–13.

Antimicrobial Therapy for Parinaud's Oculoglandular Syndrome: M. Jackson, et al.; Pediatr. Infect. Dis. J. [CD ROM], February 1992, vol. 2(2), p. 402.

Nelson Textbook of Pediatrics, 14th ed.: R.E. Behrman, ed.-in-chief; W.B. Saunders Company, 1992, pp. 863–864.

Diseases of the Nose, Throat, Ear, Head and Neck, 14th ed.: J.J. Ballenger; Lea and Febiger, 1991, p. 302.

Ophthalmology: Principles and Concepts, 7th ed.: F.W. Newell; Mosby Year Book, 1991, p. 230.

Successful Treatment of Cat-Scratch Disease with Ciproflaxin: H.P. Holley, Jr.; JAMA, March 1991, vol. 265(12), pp. 1563–1565.

Clinical Dermatology, 2nd ed.: T.P. Habif, ed.; C.V. Mosby Company, 1990, p. 396.

Dictionary of Medical Syndromes, 3rd ed.: S.I. Magalini, et al., eds.: J.B. Lippincott Company, 1990, pp. 670, 684–685.

Antibiotic Therapy for Cat-Scratch Disease?: C.W. Bogue, et al.; JAMA, August 1989, vol. 262(6), pp. 813–816.

Cat-Scratch Adenitis: C.M. Ginsberg; Pediatr. Infect. Dis. J. [CD ROM], September–October 1984, vol. 3(5), p. 209.

# CHAGAS DISEASE

**Description** Chagas disease is a systemic parasitic infection caused by *Trypanosoma cruzi* and transmitted by the bite of an insect or by blood transfusion. Acute infection is usually contracted in childhood and is a mild illness. However, this is generally followed by chronic, low-grade parasitemia, and in 10 to 30 percent of patients, chronic Chagas disease develops. The heart and gastrointestinal systems are most frequently involved; heart failure, megaesophagus, and megacolon are the most common features of end-stage disease.

**Synonyms**

American Trypansomiasis

Brazilian Trypansomiasis

**Signs and Symptoms** Acute Chagas disease initially becomes manifest with a local reaction at the inoculation site, referred to as a chagoma. Occasionally the parasite enters through the conjunctiva of the eye, which produces a periorbital swelling referred to as Romana's sign. This is followed by fever, malaise, and facial and leg edema. Physical examination may reveal generalized lymphadenopathy and hepatosplenomegaly. Severe cases may be complicated by meningoencephalitis or myocarditis, either of which may be fatal, but in the vast majority of cases symptoms resolve spontaneously without treatment.

*T. cruzi* infection then enters an indeterminate, or asymptomatic, phase. During this phase, parasitemia persists and the organisms may be transmitted by blood transfusion.

Many years after initial infection, the symptoms of chronic Chagas disease develop, which may be worse in patients with compromised immune systems. The heart is the organ most commonly involved; it becomes dilated as a result of atrophy of the myocardial cells and diffuse fibrosis. The symptoms are those of a dilated cardiomyopathy: arrhythmia; thromboembolism; congestive heart failure; edema of the face, arms, and legs; syncope; bradycardia; and dyspnea.

Esophageal involvement, or megaesophagus, presents with dysphagia, chest pain, regurgitation, and aspiration. Megacolon generally produces constipation and abdominal pain and may be complicated by obstruction or volvulus.

In the acute stage, Chagas disease is diagnosed by microscopic examination of fresh anticoagulated blood, or thick and thin blood smears. Chronic infection may be confirmed serologically by either enzyme-linked immunosorbent assay **(ELISA),** or complement fixation tests.

**Etiology** Chagas disease is caused by the protozoan *Trypanosoma cruzi*.

**Epidemiology** *T. cruzi* is transmitted in nature by reduviid bugs. The bug bites the host; then its feces, which contain the trypanosomes, contaminate the bite wound. Reduviid bugs tend to live in thatched and mud houses in rural areas of Latin America. The acute disease is mostly seen in children living in such environments, but the organism is also transmitted by blood transfusion, and this is its major route of spread in urban areas.

*T. cruzi* infection is very common in Central and South America; it has been estimated that 24 million people are parasitemic in these regions. Infection does not occur in the United States through reduviid bug transmission, but transfusion-associated cases have been reported. With increasing numbers of immigrants from endemic areas, transfusion-associated Chagas disease may become a more significant problem in the United States.

**Related Disorders** There are 2 species of trypanosomes that are pathogenic in man. *T. brucei* causes African trypanosomiasis. There are several subspecies, each of which causes different disease syndromes in different regions of Africa. The best known is African sleeping sickness, which is transmitted by the tsetse fly.

**Treatment—Standard** Acute Chagas disease may be treated with nifurtimox (a derivative of nitrofurazone) or with benzimidazole, which reduces the morbidity and mortality of the acute illness. In most cases, however, the parasite survives and chronic parasitemia ensues. There are no satisfactory antimicrobial drugs for the treatment of the indeterminate and chronic stages of Chagas disease.

Amiodarone helps control arrhythmias, and anticoagulation therapy may be of benefit in preventing thromboemboli.

Chagas disease can be prevented by eliminating the insect that transmits the disease. Various insecticides can be used to spray houses. Improvements in housing are also helpful in preventing transmission.

**Treatment—Investigational** Allopurinol riboside is currently undergoing clinical trials. For more information, physicians can contact Burroughs Wellcome Company.

A French pharmaceutical manufacturer, Fournier Labs, is developing the drug LF1695, for the treatment of Chagas and other diseases.

Please contact the agencies listed under Resources, below, for the most current information. Addresses and telephone numbers of these agencies, as well as of individual experts and research centers, may be found in the Master Resources List.

## Resources

**For more information on Chagas disease:** National Organization for Rare Disorders (NORD); Centers for Disease Control; NIH/National Institute of Allergy and Infectious Diseases; World Health Organization.

### References

Cardiac Arrhythmias in Chagas Heart Disease: M.V. Elizari, et al.; J. Cardiovasc. Electrophysiol., October 1993, vol. 4(5), pp. 596–608.

Chagas Disease: American Trypanosomiasis: L.V. Kirchhoff; Infect. Dis. Clin. North Am., September 1993, vol. 7(3), pp. 487–502.

Chagas Disease and Blood Transfusion: A New World Problem?: S. Wendel, et al.; Vox Sang., 1993, vol. 64(1), pp. 1–12.

Chagas Disease Diagnosis: Evaluation of Several Tests in Blood Bank Screening: M.R. Carvalho, et al.; Transfusion, October 1993, vol. 33(10), pp. 830–834.

The Challenge of Chagas Disease Chemotherapy: An Update of Drugs Assayed Against Trypanosoma Cruzi: S.K. de Castro; Acta Trop., April 1993, vol. 53(2), pp. 83–98.

Trypanosoma Cruzi: Mechanisms for Entry into Host Cells: B.F. Hall; Semin. Cell Biol., October 1993, vol. 4(5), pp. 323–333.

Autonomic Neuropathy and Immunological Abnormalities in Chagas Disease: A. Fernandaz, et al.; Clin. Auton. Res., December 1992, vol. 2(6), pp. 409–412.

Cecil Textbook of Medicine, 19th ed.: J.B. Wyngaarden, et al., eds.; W.B. Saunders Company, 1992, pp. 1978–1982.

Chagas Disease: H.B. Tanowitz, et al.; Clin. Microbiol. Rev., October 1992, vol. 5(4), pp. 400–419.

Infectious Diseases: S.L. Gorbach, ed.; W.B. Saunders Company, 1992, pp. 1987–1991.

Nelson Textbook of Pediatrics, 14th ed.: R.E. Behrman, ed.-in-chief; W.B. Saunders Company, 1992, pp. 879–883.

Use of Recombinant Antigens for the Accurate Immunodiagnosis of Chagas Disease: M.A. Krieger, et al.; Am. J. Trop. Med. Hyg., April 1992, vol. 46(4), pp. 427–434.

Harrison's Principles of Internal Medicine, 12th ed.: J.D. Wilson, et al., eds.: McGraw-Hill, 1991, pp. 791–793.

Laboratory Diagnosis of Trypanosomiasis: P. Cattand, et al.; Clin. Lab. Med., December 1991, vol. 11(4), pp. 899–908.

Mimicry in Trypanosoma Cruzi: Fantasy and Reality: H. Eisen, et al.; Curr. Opin. Immunol., August 1991, vol. 3(4), pp. 507–510.

Purine Analogs As Chemotherapeutic Agents in Leishmaniasis and American Trypanosomiasis: J.J. Marr; J. Lab. Clin. Med., August 1991, vol. 118(2), pp. 111–119.

Gastrointestinal Disease, 4th ed.; M.H. Sleisenger, et al.; W.B. Saunders Company, 1989, pp. 1187–1188.

Is *Trypanosoma cruzi* a New Threat to Our Blood Supply? L.V. Kirschoff; Ann. Int. Med., November 1989, vol. 110(10), pp. 773–774.

The Heart, 3rd ed.; E. Braunwald; W.B. Saunders Company 1988, pp. 1445–1448.

# CHIKUNGUNYA

**Description** Chikungunya is one of several arthropod-borne viral diseases characterized by a rash, fever, and severe arthralgias. (Others include o'nyong-nyong fever, Ross River virus, and Mayaro virus disease.)

**Signs and Symptoms** Clinical disease begins with fever, headache, and arthralgias that may be so severe as to immobilize the patient. The joints involved include the knees, elbows, wrists, ankles, and fingers. Photophobia, sore throat, anorexia, vomiting, backache, and a rash are also common. Occasionally conjunctivitis and lymphadenopathy are present. The fever usually abates before the 10th day, but the joint symptoms may take several weeks to resolve. Permanent joint damage does not occur.

**Etiology** Chikungunya is caused by a virus belonging to the group A arboviruses.

**Epidemiology** Chikungunya affects mostly children and young adults in Africa, Southeast Asia, and India. It is transmitted by various species of mosquitoes. Monkeys may also be infected.

**Treatment—Standard** Diagnosis is confirmed by an ELISA test. Chikungunya resolves spontaneously. There is no specific treatment, but bed rest and anti-inflammatory agents may be useful.

**Treatment—Investigational** Please contact the agencies listed under Resources, below, for the most current information. Addresses and telephone numbers of these agencies, as well as of individual experts and research centers, may be found in the Master Resources List.

## Resources

**For more information on chikungunya:** National Organization for Rare Disorders (NORD); Centers for Disease Control; NIH/National Institute of Allergy and Infectious Diseases.

### References

Cecil Textbook of Medicine, 19th ed.: J.B. Wyngaarden, et al., eds.; W.B. Saunders Company, 1992, pp. 1870–1871.

Development of a Simple Indirect Enzyme-Linked Immunosorbent Assay for the Detection of Immunoglobulin M Antibody in Serum from Patients Following an Outbreak of Chicungunya Virus Infection in Yangon, Myanmar: S. Thein, et al.; Trans. R. Soc. Trop. Med. Hyg., July–August 1992, vol. 86(4), pp. 438–443.

Nelson Textbook of Pediatrics, 14th ed.: R.E. Behrman, ed.-in-chief; W.B. Saunders Company, 1992, 850–851.

# CHOLERA

**Description** Cholera is an acute illness caused by *Vibrio cholerae,* which colonizes but does not invade the small intestine. The major symptom, massive watery diarrhea, results from a bacterial enterotoxin that stimulates the intestinal cells to secrete fluid. There are several strains of *V. cholerae,* which differ somewhat in their virulence.

Cholera is not difficult to treat; most patients recover well with appropriate oral hydration alone. Without treatment, it can be a rapidly fatal disease.

**Synonyms**

>Asiatic Cholera
>Epidemic Cholera

**Signs and Symptoms** The symptoms of cholera vary in severity. Infection may be symptomatic, or the patient may only experience a few days of mild diarrhea. Alternatively, the initial fluid loss may be so great that the patient develops shock and dies within hours of onset.

The initial symptoms consist of a sudden painless diarrhea associated with vomiting. The diarrhea becomes progressively watery, and large volumes of fluid, sodium, chloride, potassium, and bicarbonate are lost. Subsequent symptoms are all a result of dehydration and electrolyte imbalance. Intense thirst, decreased urine output, muscle cramps, and weakness can develop. Hypotension and hypokalemia are common; acidosis and shock may intervene if treatment is not provided. Renal failure may develop, but this generally responds to fluid replacement.

**Etiology** Cholera is caused by *Vibrio cholerae,* a gram-negative rod with several variably virulent biotypes. The symptoms represent the effects of a bacterial toxin.

**Epidemiology** Cholera is endemic in India and parts of the Middle East, Asia, and Africa. In these areas children, especially those under the age of 5, are affected most often, with outbreaks occurring during the warmest part of the year. In addition, it occasionally spreads to Europe, Japan, Australia, and South America, where epidemics can occur at any time of the year and affect persons of all ages equally.

Cholera is primarily a waterborne disease. During epidemics, spread may be particularly rapid as increasing numbers of individuals excrete large volumes of infected stool. If sanitation standards are less than optimal, drinking, washing, and cooking water becomes rapidly contaminated.

**Related Disorders** Cholera is one of several enterotoxigenic diarrheal diseases. *Escherichia coli* and some salmonella and shigella infections also produce similar clinical features. Other bacteria of the *Vibrio* genus that cause gastroenteritis include *V. parahaemolyticus.*

**Pancreatic cholera** is not a bacterial disease but a result of pancreatic dysfunction leading to severe diarrhea.

**Treatment—Standard** In mild cases, cholera resolves spontaneously within 3 to 6 days of onset, and the bacteria disappear within 2 weeks. Most cases will require fluid replacement, and if started early, the majority of patients can do this orally. Intravenous fluids are necessary in very severe cases (when stool output exceeds 7 liters a day), for patients in shock, and in cases where vomiting prohibits oral intake. Various solutions containing salts, bicarbonate, and glucose are available in packet form and can be administered easily without medical personnel.

Antibiotics will shorten the course of the disease. Tetracycline is the drug of choice, and ampicillin is an acceptable substitute for pregnant women and children. Furazolidone is effective against resistant strains.

The most important methods of prevention and control are a clean water supply and adequate sewage disposal. Boiling all water and food prior to consumption is also effective but is expensive and impractical in many areas of the world where the disease is endemic.

Vaccines are available but are not 100 percent effective and require booster injections every 6 months. Tetracycline may be used prophylactically to protect against cholera if a patient is exposed to contaminated food or water.

Persons living in endemic areas usually develop immunity. Travelers to endemic regions should be vaccinated against this disorder.

**Treatment—Investigational** Please contact the agencies listed under Resources, below, for the most current information. Addresses and telephone numbers of these agencies, as well as of individual experts and research centers, may be found in the Master Resources List.

**Resources**

**For more information on cholera:** National Organization for Rare Disorders (NORD); Centers for Disease Control; NIH/National Institute of Allergy and Infectious Diseases.

**References**

Cholera: Developments in Prevention and Cure: F.P. van Loon; Trop. Geogr. Med., 1993, vol. 45(6), pp. 293–315.

Epidemiology of Cholera in the Americas: P.A. Blake; Gastroenterol. Clin. North Am., September 1993, vol. 22(3), pp. 639–660.

Bacterial Enteric Infections and Vaccine Development: J. Holmgren, et al.; Gastroenterol. Clin. North Am., June 1992, vol. 21(2), pp. 283–302.

Cecil Textbook of Medicine, 19th ed.: J.B. Wyngaarden, et al., eds.; W.B. Saunders Company, 1992, pp. 1699–1702.

Cholera As a Model for Research on Mucosal Immunity and Development of Oral Vaccines: J. Holmgren, et al.; Curr. Opin. Immunol., August 1992, vol. 4(4), pp. 387–391.

Cholera Vaccines: C.O. Tacket, et al.; Biotechnology, 1992, vol. 20, pp. 53–68.

The Diagnosis and Treatment of Cholera: M.F. Keen, et al.; Nurse Pract., December 1992, vol. 17(12), pp. 53–56.

Immunizations for Foreign Travel: D.R. Hill; Yale J. Biol. Med., July–August 1992, vol. 65(4), pp. 293–315.

Infectious Diseases: S.L. Gorbach, ed.; W.B. Saunders Company, 1992, pp. 605–611.

Nelson Textbook of Pediatrics, 14th ed.: R.E. Behrman, ed.-in-chief; W.B. Saunders Company, 1992, pp. 736–738.

Pathogenesis and Ecology: The Case of Cholera: B.S. Drasar; J. Trop. Med. Hyg., December 1992, vol. 95(6), pp. 365–372.

Recent Progress in Cholera Vaccination: P.G. Pierre, et al.; Acta Gastroenterol., September–December 1992, vol. 55(5–6), pp. 430–436.

The Treatment of Cholera: Clinical Science at the Bedside: C.C. Carpenter; J. Infect. Dis., July 1992, vol. 166(1), pp. 2–14.

Cholera and Cholera-like Diarrhoeal Diseases: Why the Difference in Severity?: S.A. Abdulkadir; Med. Hypotheses, March 1991, vol. 35(3), pp. 278–281.

Harrison's Principles of Internal Medicine, 12th ed.: J.D. Wilson, et al., eds.: McGraw-Hill, 1991, pp. 632–633.

Gastrointestinal Disease, 4th ed.; M.H. Sleisenger, et al.; W.B. Saunders Company 1989, pp. 1192–1194.

# COWPOX

**Description** Cowpox, a viral disease normally affecting the udders and teats of cows, is occasionally transmitted to man, in whom it produces a characteristic rash and enlarged lymph nodes. Cowpox also produces an immunity to smallpox, a fact that was massively exploited in the 19th century through widespread use of the virus, or virus-infected material, in vaccination programs. As a result, smallpox has been eradicated. The cause of cowpox, now called vaccinia virus, has been noted to produce systemic reactions in certain individuals following vaccination. This is referred to as generalized vaccinia.

**Synonyms**

Bovine Smallpox

Vaccinia

**Signs and Symptoms** The rash characteristic of human cowpox infection consists of numerous vesicles that may become inflamed or may bleed or ulcerate. The rash occurs on exposed skin (i.e., the face and extremities), and may be accompanied by lymphadenopathy.

When an immunosuppressed individual (particularly with agammaglobulinemia or chronic lymphocytic leukemia) is inadvertently vaccinated, a more severe form of infection may occur. Called vaccinia necrosum, vaccinia gangrenosum, or progressive vaccinia, this syndrome is characterized by progressive necrosis of the vaccination site, and a generalized eruption of metastatic lesions. It can be fatal.

Patients with severe eczema may also experience a generalized vaccinia eruption on vaccination or on contact with someone recently vaccinated.

A mild form of generalized vaccinia occurs in normal individuals following vaccination. Typically, a vesicular rash develops 7 to 12 days after vaccination; there are no other symptoms, and the rash resolves spontaneously.

Other complications of smallpox vaccination include bacterial superinfection of vesicular lesions, postinfectious encephalitis, myocarditis, pericarditis, and arthritis.

**Etiology** Cowpox is caused by vaccinia virus.

**Epidemiology** Cowpox can be transmitted to humans directly by handling the udders of infected cows. It can also result from vaccination against smallpox, or, in some cases, from contact with a person with a vaccination lesion.

Currently, disease resulting from vaccination has become rare because the eradication of smallpox has rendered vaccination unnecessary, and it is no longer routine. However, vaccinia is being considered as a vector for immunization against other types of infectious agents; more widespread use of this virus will increase the prevalence of its adverse reactions.

**Related Disorders Smallpox,** caused by the variola virus, is a far more severe and disfiguring disease. Smallpox no longer occurs, although the virus is still retained in a few laboratories.

**Treatment—Standard** As in the case of most viral infections, there is no specific treatment for most cases. Vaccinia hyperimmune globulin is used to treat some complications of vaccinia. Other complications are treated symptomatically.

**Treatment—Investigational** Please contact the agencies listed under Resources, below, for the most current information. Addresses and telephone numbers of these agencies, as well as of individual experts and research centers, may be found in the Master Resources List.

**Resources**

**For more information on vaccinia:** National Organization for Rare Disorders (NORD); Centers for Disease Control; NIH/National Institute of Allergy and Infectious Diseases.

**References**

Cowpox Infection Causing a Generalized Eruption in a Patient with Atopic Dermatitis: S. Blackford, et al.; Br. J. Dermatol., November 1993, vol. 129(5), pp. 628–629.

Cecil Textbook of Medicine, 19th ed.: J.B. Wyngaarden, et al., eds.; W.B. Saunders Company, 1992, p. 1844.

# CRYOGLOBULINEMIA, ESSENTIAL MIXED

**Description** Essential mixed cryoglobulinemia is an autoimmune disorder that affects the blood and various other body systems. Major symptoms include unusual response to cold, skin abnormalities, weakness, and blood problems. There may also be renal, joint, and vascular problems.

**Signs and Symptoms** Essential mixed cryoglobulinemia is characterized by numbness in the hands or feet when exposed to the cold, purpura, inflamed kidneys, proteinuria, and hematuria. Joint pain, myalgia, and problems with the central nervous system are common. Liver and spleen may be affected. Gastrointestinal symptoms usually occur, and chronic diarrhea may be a sign of colon involvement.

**Etiology** Essential mixed cryoglobulinemia is idiopathic, but an autoimmune disorder is suspected.

**Epidemiology** Essential mixed cryoglobulinemia is usually not apparent until middle age, and it affects females more often than males.

**Related Disorders** See *Raynaud Disease and Phenomenon; Wegener Granulomatosis.*

**Treatment—Standard** Protection from cold temperatures is requisite for patients with essential mixed cryoglobulinemia. A combination of drugs, including steroids and cyclophosphamide, is effective in altering the immune system and alleviating symptoms. Other therapies include plasmapheresis and cryofiltration.

**Treatment—Investigational** Please contact the agencies listed under Resources, below, for the most current information. Addresses and telephone numbers of these agencies, as well as of individual experts and research centers, may be found in the Master Resources List.

**Resources**

   **For more information on essential mixed cryoglobulinemia:** National Organization for Rare Disorders (NORD); NIH/National Heart, Lung and Blood Institute Information Center.

**References**

Cecil Textbook of Medicine, 19th ed.: J.B. Wyngaarden, et al., eds.; W.B. Saunders Company, 1992, p. 601.

Chronic Diarrhea in Essential Mixed Cryoglobulinemia: A Manifestation of Visceral Vasculitis?: M.P. Jones, et al.; Am. J. Gastroenterol., April 1991, vol. 86(4), pp. 522–524.

The Kidney, 4th ed.; B.M. Brenner and F.C. Rector, Jr., eds.; W.B. Saunders Company, 1991, pp. 1311–1312.

Rapid Improvement in a Patient with Leukocytoclastic Vasculitis with Secondary Mixed Cryoglobulinemia Treated with Cryofiltration: K. Sawada, et al.; J. Rheumatol., January 1991, vol. 18(1), pp. 91–94.

Hematology, 4th ed.: W.J. Williams, et al., eds.; McGraw-Hill, 1990, p. 1437.

# CRYPTOCOCCOSIS

**Description** Cryptococcosis is a systemic fungal infection caused by *Cryptococcus neoformans.* It is a common infection in patients with AIDS, and occasionally occurs in immunocompetent individuals. The most frequent systems involved are the central nervous system and the lungs.

**Synonyms**

   Busse-Buschke Disease

   European Blastomycosis

   Torulosis

**Signs and Symptoms** The most common presentation is meningoencephalitis. The onset is usually gradual, and symptoms often are mild. The usual complaints include headache, confusion, nausea, dizziness, irritability, gait abnormalities, and behavioral changes.

   There may be few specific findings on physical examination. Fever is frequently absent, as is meningismus. Papilledema is present in about one-third of cases, and even fewer patients have cranial nerve deficits. Other neurologic findings are rare.

   The diagnosis is made on lumbar puncture. The cerebrospinal fluid usually shows elevated protein levels, low glucose levels, and a leukocytosis. An india ink stain of the fluid will reveal the organism in about 50 percent of cases. However, approximately 90 percent of samples will contain the cryptococcal capsular antigen.

Pulmonary infection is frequently inapparent. Chest pain and cough occur occasionally. The chest x-ray picture frequently resembles a malignancy. Diagnosis of pulmonary cryptococcosis often requires a biopsy, since sputum cultures are frequently negative and are difficult to interpret when positive (many patients with other types of lung disease may be colonized).

*C. neoformans* may also cause skin lesions and osteolytic bone lesions. Cryptococcal pyelonephritis, chorioretinitis, endocarditis, adrenalitis, and hepatitis have also been reported, but these are rare.

**Etiology** Cryptococcosis is caused by the fungus *Cryptococcus neoformans.*

**Epidemiology** Cryptococcosis occurs worldwide. It is found in the soil and in pigeon feces, although patients generally have no history of exposure to pigeons. Transmission is thought to be by inhalation. Most patients with cryptococcosis have an underlying immunodeficiency, such as AIDS or lymphoma. The disease tends to occur more often in males than females.

**Treatment—Standard** The antibiotic regimen used to treat cryptococcal meningoencephalitis includes amphotericin B, either alone or in combination with flucytosine. Fluconazole is a useful alternative to amphotericin B and may be substituted for it after the patient has responded well to amphotericin B.. Hematologic side effects and rashes are very common in AIDS patients on flucytosine, unless the dose and serum levels are monitored. The time course of therapy is determined by repeated lumbar puncture and cultures. Patients with AIDS are notoriously difficult to cure and may require some form of suppressive treatment for life, such as weekly intravenous injections of amphotericin B, or regular doses of fluconazole or flucytosine orally.

Other forms of cryptococcal disease are also treated with amphotericin B, with or without flucytosine or fluconazole. Some forms in immunocompetemt individuals may not require treatment, or may respond to surgical excision alone.

**Treatment—Investigational** Please contact the agencies listed under Resources, below, for the most current information. Addresses and telephone numbers of these agencies, as well as of individual experts and research centers, may be found in the Master Resources List.

**Resources**

**For more information on cryptococcosis:** National Organization for Rare Disorders (NORD); NIH/National Institute of Allergy and Infectious Diseases; Centers for Disease Control; NIH/National Institute of Neurological Disorders and Stroke.

**References**

Cryptococcal Meningitis: R. Biniek, et al.; Nervenarzt, 1986, vol. 57(1), pp. 47–55.

Cryptococcal Meningitis: T.L. Tjia, et al.; J. Neurol. Neurosurg. Psychiatry, 1985, vol. 48(9), pp. 853–858.

Clinical Spectrum of Infections in Patients with HTLV-III–Associated Diseases: J.W. Gold; Cancer Res., 1985, vol. 45(9 suppl.), pp. 4652s–4654s.

# CYSTICERCOSIS

**Description** Cysticercosis is one type of infection with the pork tapeworm, *Taenia solium.* Humans may be infected with 2 different stages of *T. solium,* and each produces a different syndrome.

In the life cycle of this parasite, pork containing encysted *T. solium* larvae are ingested by humans, and the larvae develop into mature worms in the intestinal tract. This results in a tapeworm infection, which is usually mild or asymptomatic. The adult passes eggs in the stool, and these are ingested by the pig, develop into larvae, and the cycle continues. If humans ingest the eggs (not the larvae), these will penetrate into the bloodstream and disseminate throughout various tissues of the body, where they encyst, resulting in cysticercosis.

Once in the tissues, they develop into cysticerci, which evoke a granulomatous reaction until they start to die. Dying cysts stimulate an acute inflammatory response that can produce tissue damage. While the cysticerci may appear anywhere in the body, preferred sites are the skeletal muscles, the eye, and brain. Other less common sites include the liver, heart, and lungs. Eventually, larvae will calcify.

**Signs and Symptoms** Cysts outside the brain and eye are generally asymptomatic. Cerebral cysticercosis causes seizures, which may be focal or generalized. Less common manifestations include headache, transient neurologic deficits, and psychosis. Ocular symptoms include visual disturbances, uveitis, and retinitis. Rarely, muscular infection may produce the symptoms of a myopathy.

Once the larvae calcify, they may be easily seen on skull x-rays, as well as CT scan. The radiologic appearance is diagnostic in some cases, and in others the disease may be confirmed serologically, although a large number of patients have false negative tests. Surgery is often necessary to provide a definitive diagnosis.

**Etiology** Cysticercosis develops when the eggs of the pork tapeworm *T. solium* are ingested. Egg ingestion occurs through consumption of food or water contaminated with human feces, and may occur by autoingestion. This results when the patient harbors the adult worm in the intestine; the eggs are passed in the feces, and through poor hygiene are transferred to the mouth of the same individual.

**Epidemiology** Cysticercosis is common in Mexico, Africa, and South America.

**Related Disorders** Tapeworms can be acquired from various uncooked meats, including beef *(Taenia saginata)* and fish *(Diphyllobothrium latum)*, but *T. solium* appears to be the only tapeworm that produces larvae capable of invading human muscle and forming cysts. The roundworm *Trichinella spiralis* also has a larval stage that invades the tissues and encysts; the resulting disease, trichinosis, is predominantly characterized by a diffuse myositis.

**Treatment—Standard** Praziquantel is the treatment of choice for both adult and larval stages of *T. solium*. Niclosamide may be used as an alternative. Steroids may be necessary to control edema surrounding cerebral lesions. Surgery may be required in some cases.

**Treatment—Investigational** Please contact the agencies listed under Resources, below, for the most current information. Addresses and telephone numbers of these agencies, as well as of individual experts and research centers, may be found in the Master Resources List.

**Resources**

For more information on cysticercosis: National Organization for Rare Disorders (NORD); Centers for Disease Control; NIH/National Institute of Allergy and Infectious Diseases.

**References**

Cecil Textbook of Medicine, 18th ed.: J.B. Wyngaarden and L.H. Smith, Jr., eds.; W.B. Saunders Company, 1988, p. 1892.

Manson's Tropical Diseases, 19th ed.: P.E.C. Manson-Bahr and D.R. Bell; Ballière Tindall, 1987, pp. 536–540.

# DENGUE FEVER

**Description** Dengue fever is an acute viral illness primarily consisting of fever, severe myalgias, and a rash. It is caused by a flavivirus and transmitted by mosquitoes. A severe form of dengue fever, known as dengue hemorrhagic fever, is characterized by thrombocytopenia, bleeding, and shock.

**Synonyms**

Breakbone Fever
Dandy Fever
Duengero
Seven-Day Fever

**Signs and Symptoms** Dengue fever begins abruptly after an incubation period of 5 to 8 days. Symptoms include fever, weakness, prostration, severe headache, retro-orbital pain, and severe myalgias. The temperature rises rapidly, sometimes to as high as 40° C (104° F), and may be accompanied by a relative bradycardia. There may be lymphadenopathy and a maculopapular rash on physical examination. The rash typically begins on the trunk and spreads peripherally. The symptoms usually persist for 7 days.

**Dengue hemorrhagic fever** appears to occur in individuals already immunized against one dengue virus serotype, who are infected with another. It usually begins with fever, nausea, vomiting, and abdominal pain. Then thrombocytopenia develops, accompanied by petechiae, purpura, epistaxis, gastrointestinal hemorrhage, and, in severe cases, shock **(dengue shock syndrome)**. Fibrinogen and clotting factors V, VII, IX, and X are also reduced.

The diagnosis of dengue fever may be confirmed by virus isolation from the blood, or by serologic testing.

**Etiology** The dengue fever virus is a flavivirus. There are several distinct serotypes.

**Epidemiology** Dengue fever occurs mainly in the subtropical or tropical regions of southern Asia, South America (particularly Brazil), and the Caribbean, including Puerto Rico and the U.S. Virgin Islands. Dengue fever virus has also been imported into the United States by tourists from endemic areas.

Severe forms of dengue fever, including dengue hemorrhagic fever and dengue shock syndrome, usually occur in young children who have previously been infected with a different serotype. Infants may also develop the severe forms; they acquire immunity to one serotype passively either transplacentally or through breast milk. Infection with a new serotype produces the severe disease. Massive outbreaks have occurred when a new serotype is introduced to a susceptible population.

Dengue is transmitted by the *Aedes aegypti* mosquito.

**Related Disorders** There are a number of viral hemorrhagic fevers. The best known is yellow fever. Others include Lassa fever, Machupo fever (Bolivian hemorrhagic fever), Junin fever (Argentinian hemorrhagic fever), lymphocytic choriomeningitis, Marburg virus (hemorrhagic fever), and Ebola virus (hemorrhagic fever). Most of these can be distinguished on epidemiologic grounds.

**Treatment—Standard** There is no specific treatment for dengue fever, or dengue hemorrhagic fever. Supportive care, particularly intravenous fluid administration, may be lifesaving in severe cases. Transfusions of packed red blood cells or platelets may control bleeding.

**Treatment—Investigational** Interferon has been under investigation for the treatment of dengue hemorrhagic fever. In addition, there have been attempts to develop a vaccine.

Please contact the agencies listed under Resources, below, for the most current information. Addresses and telephone numbers of these agencies, as well as of individual experts and research centers, may be found in the Master Resources List.

**Resources**

**For more information on dengue fever:** National Organization for Rare Disorders (NORD); Centers for Disease Control; NIH/National Institute of Allergy and Infectious Diseases.

**References**

Dengue and Hepatic Failure: M.E. Alvarez, et al.; Amer. J. Med., 1985, vol. 79(5), pp. 670–674.

Dengue Virus Type 2 Vaccine: Reactogenicity and Immunogenicity in Soldiers: W.H. Bancroft, et al.; J. Infect. Dis., 1984, vol. 149(6), pp. 1005–1010.

Effect of Interferons on Dengue Virus Multiplication in Cultured Monocytes/Macrophages: H. Hotta, et al.; Biken Journal, 1984, vol. 27(4), pp. 189–193.

Dengue Fever in the United States: A Report of a Cluster of Imported Cases and Review of the Clinical, Epidemiologic, and Public Health Aspects of the Disease: M.D. Malison, et al.; JAMA, 1983, vol. 249(4), pp. 496–500.

# Dracunculiasis

**Description** Dracunculiasis is an infection caused by the tissue nematode *Dracunculus medinensis,* the guinea worm. Infection begins by drinking water containing infected crustaceans. Once in the stomach, the larvae are released and pass into the intestine. From there they migrate into the retroperitoneum where they mature. The adult females migrate out into the subcutaneous tissues and produce ulcers in the overlying skin. On contact with water, larvae are discharged from the ulcer.

**Synonyms**

Dracontiasis

Dracunculosis

Fiery Serpent Infection

Guinea Worm Infection

**Signs and Symptoms** Dracunculiasis is characterized by chronic skin ulcers in which the worms may be visible. Skin involvement begins with a painful, stinging papule on the skin, usually on the legs. This may be accompanied by nausea, vomiting, and diarrhea. Later the papule ulcerates and the female worm discharges her larvae. Gradually the worm is extruded over several weeks and then the ulcers heal.

Diagnosis of dracunculiasis is made on finding the larvae during microscopic examination of ulcer fluid.

**Etiology** Dracunculiasis is caused by swallowing water containing small, barely visible water fleas that carry the larva of the parasitic guinea worm, *Dracunculus medinensis.*

**Epidemiology** Dracunculiasis affects people in regions of Africa, the Middle East, and India, where drinking water is contaminated with *D. medinensis.*

**Treatment—Standard** This disorder is treated with niridazole, or the antihelmintic drugs thiabendazole or metronidazole. Treatment with these drugs promptly relieves symptoms and reduces the inflammation, but does not affect the worms. However, once the inflammation has subsided, the worms can be easily removed.

Chlorination, boiling, and straining of contaminated drinking water in areas of the world with poor sanitation can prevent transmission of dracunculiasis.

**Treatment—Investigational** Please contact the agencies listed under Resources, below, for the most current information. Addresses and telephone numbers of these agencies, as well as of individual experts and research centers, may be found in the Master Resources List.

**Resources**

**For more information on dracunculiasis:** National Organization for Rare Disorders (NORD); NIH/National Institute of Allergy and Infectious Diseases; Centers for Disease Control.

**References**

Dracunculus Orchitis: A Case Report: A.K. Pendse, et al.; J. Trop. Med. Hyg., 1987, vol. 90(3), pp. 153–154.

The Comparative Study of Patterns of Guinea Worm Prevalence As a Guide to Control Strategies: S.J. Watts, et al.; Soc. Sci. Med., 1986, vol. 23(10), pp. 975–982.

Controlled Comparative Trial of Thiabendazole and Metronidazole in the Treatment of Dracontiasis: O.O. Kale, et al.; Ann. Trop. Med. Parasitol., 1983, vol. 77(2), pp. 151–157.

# ELEPHANTIASIS

**Description** Elephantiasis is characterized by massive hypertrophy of a limb. It is caused by lymphatic obstruction. In tropical regions, it is most commonly associated with filariasis (**elephantiasis filariensis**). In temperate regions, it has been reported rarely in individuals with recurrent streptococcal infections (**elephantiasis nostras**).

**Synonyms**

      Elephantiasis Nostras

**Signs and Symptoms** The patient provides a history of recurrent streptococcal lymphangitis and cellulitis. There may have been initially an episode of thrombophlebitis. With successive infections, the impairment to lymphatic drainage worsens, and the edema progresses. The skin and subcutaneous tissue become thickened and fibrotic. The skin becomes darkened, thickened, and firm, and ulcerations may develop. Ultimately, the skin becomes pebbly and verrucous in appearance. The reason for the skin's responding in this way to chronic lymphedema is unclear.

In filariasis the external genitalia may also be involved.

**Etiology Elephantiasis nostras** is the end result of a cycle of repeated streptococcal infections, each followed by progressive edema, occurring over many years. Impairment of lymphatic drainage is known to be a risk factor for streptococcal infection, and while the initial insult to the lymphatics may have been noninfectious, each bout of infection worsens the lymphatic obstruction, and therefore continues the cycle.

**Tinea pedis** has been associated with streptococcal infection of the leg. First reported in men following saphenous vein resection for coronary bypass surgery, the lesions of tinea pedis are thought to be the portal of entry for the streptococcus. The combination of superficial foot wound and lymphatic obstruction sets the stage for infection. However, in spite of the prevalence of minor degrees of lymphatic obstruction in the population, progression to elephantiasis nostras is very rare.

**Epidemiology** Elephantiasis is most common in Africa, where filariasis is the usual cause. Elephantiasis nostras occurs very rarely in temperate climates.

**Related Disorders**

**Hereditary lymphedema** is a genetic disorder of the lymphatic system in which the lymphatic channels are obstructed or underdeveloped.

**Filariasis** is the most common cause of elephantiasis worldwide.

**Treatment—Standard** The infections are treated with penicillin. Erythromycin is the major alternative in penicillin-allergic patients. Once elephantiasis develops, surgery may be necessary to remove excess tissue.

**Treatment—Investigational** Please contact the agencies listed under Resources, below, for the most current information. Addresses and telephone numbers of these agencies, as well as of individual experts and research centers, may be found in the Master Resources List.

**Resources**

**For more information on elephantiasis:** National Organization for Rare Disorders (NORD); NIH/National Institute of Allergy and Infectious Diseases; Centers for Disease Control.

**References**

Elephantiasis Nostras—A Case Report: S.A. Baughman et al.; Angiology, February 1988, vol. 39(2), pp. 164–168.

Elephantiasis Nostras: An Eight-Year Observation of Progressive Nonfilarial Elephantiasis of the Lower Extremity: L.J. Sanders, et al.; Cutis, November 1988, vol. 42(5), pp. 406–411.

# ENCEPHALITIS, HERPETIC

**Description** Herpetic encephalitis is caused by herpes simplex virus (**HSV**), and is the most common form of acute, sporadic encephalitis in the United States. It is characterized clinically by fever, headache, and focal neurologic symptoms, usually due to a focus of infection in the temporal lobe.

**Synonyms**

      Herpes Encephalitis

      Herpes Simplex Encephalitis

      Herpetic Meningoencephalitis

**Signs and Symptoms** The onset of herpetic encephalitis is usually abrupt, with fever, headache, behavioral disturbances, personality changes, and focal seizures. In some cases there is a prodrome of malaise, fever, anorexia, and other nonspecific symptoms. Focal neurologic deficits may occur, including hemiparesis, dysphasia, and cranial nerve deficits, and later in the course of illness stupor and coma may develop.

The cerebrospinal fluid characteristically shows elevated protein levels, lymphocytosis, and the presence of red blood cells. The most common electroencephalographic abnormality is a diffuse slowing over the involved temporal lobe. CT scanning may reveal swelling in the temporal lobe. None of these is diagnostic, and brain biopsy has been the method of choice for confirming the diagnosis of herpetic encephalitis. Assays for HSV antigens in the cerebrospinal fluid are under investigation, and should they become available, the diagnosis may require only a lumbar puncture.

**Etiology** The vast majority of cases of herpetic encephalitis are caused by HSV-1. Encephalitis may result from primary HSV infection, or more commonly there is evidence of past mucocutaneous infection.

**Epidemiology** Herpetic encephalitis usually occurs during childhood or early adulthood. There is no seasonal variation.

**Related Disorders** The differential diagnosis of herpetic encephalitis includes other viral encephalitides, meningitis, and focal intracerebral processes such as abscess, tumor, and vascular accidents.

**Treatment—Standard** The treatment of choice for herpetic encephalitis is intravenous acyclovir. This improves survival but does not always correct all neurologic deficits; significant residual neurologic impairment is common. Vidarabine (arabinosyl adenine, Ara-A) is also useful but is less effective than acyclovir.

**Treatment—Investigational** Several new antiviral agents are currently under investigation.

Please contact the agencies listed under Resources, below, for the most current information. Addresses and telephone numbers of these agencies, as well as of individual experts and research centers, may be found in the Master Resources List.

**Resources**

**For more information on herpetic encephalitis:** National Organization for Rare Disorders (NORD); NIH/National Institute of Allergy and Infectious Diseases; Centers for Disease Control; NIH/National Institute of Neurological Disorders and Stroke.

**References**

Herpetic Encephalitis: Prognostic Elements in Adults and Children (49 Cases): A. Foucher, et al.; Rev. Electroencephalogr. Neurophysiol. Clin., 1985, vol. 15(2), pp. 185–193.

Ocular Infection with Herpes Simplex Virus Type 1: Prevention of Acute Herpetic Encephalitis by Systemic Administration of Virus-Specific Antibody: W.B. Taylor, et al.; J. Infect. Dis., 1979, vol. 140(4), pp. 534–540.

# ENCEPHALITIS, JAPANESE

**Description** Japanese encephalitis is caused by a flavivirus, the Japanese B encephalitis virus (**JBEV**), and transmitted by mosquitoes in certain areas of the world, particularly Asia. This disorder most commonly affects children and tends to be more actively spread during the summer.

**Synonyms**

Japanese B Encephalitis

Russian Autumnal Encephalitis

Summer Encephalitis

**Signs and Symptoms** Most JBEV infections are mild or asymptomatic, but in a small percentage of cases, severe encephalitis occurs. After an incubation period of 4 to 14 days, the patient is suddenly stricken with fever, headache, nausea, vomiting, behavioral changes, and neurologic deficits. The patient may be stuporous or comatose by the 4th day. The mortality rate is high, particularly in the elderly, and residual neurologic deficits are common among those who survive.

The cerebrospinal fluid may be normal, or may show a pleocytosis and elevated protein. The diagnosis may be confirmed serologically, using complement fixation or hemagglutination inhibition tests.

**Etiology** Japanese encephalitis is caused by a flavivirus (group B arbovirus). Symptoms are due to viral invasion and destruction of neurons. Necrosis is most marked in the thalamus and substantia nigra.

**Epidemiology** Japanese encephalitis afflicts approximately 20,000 people annually. Epidemics occur during the summer months in India, Bangladesh, the eastern part of Russia, China, Korea, Nepal, Burma, Vietnam, and northern Thailand. In tropical areas of southeast Asia, southern India, southern Thailand, and Sri Lanka, the disease is present year-round. Sporadic outbreaks occur throughout the year until the tropical rainy season, when the illness can be transmitted in epidemic proportions.

The virus is transmitted by mosquitoes that breed in rice fields. Pigs and birds are the major reservoirs.

**Related Disorders** The symptoms of Japanese encephalitis are similar to those of other viral encephalitides. JBEV is antigenically related to the viruses of Murray Valley encephalitis and St. Louis encephalitis, and to West Nile virus.

**Murray Valley encephalitis,** also known as **Australian X disease,** is a severe encephalitis that is found in Australia and New Guinea. Like Japanese encephalitis, the Murray Valley type is also transmitted by mosquitoes. Cases among children tend to be most severe, and permanent brain damage may result.

**St. Louis encephalitis** is less severe. Caused by a group B arbovirus and transmitted by mosquitoes, this type of encephalitis occurs in sporadic outbreaks in urban areas of Missouri, Arizona, Colorado, Nevada, Texas, Indiana, Illinois, Kentucky, Florida, New Jersey, Pennsylvania, and the Ohio Valley. It tends to be more prevalent from midsummer to early fall. The symptoms are typical of encephalitis.

**West Nile encephalitis,** also known as **West Nile fever,** is characterized by severe headaches, high fever, enlargement of the lymph nodes, and meningismus. Symptoms of this disorder may last only a few weeks, but it may cause permanent neurologic damage.

**Treatment—Standard** In Asian nations, an effective vaccination is available for Japanese encephalitis. In the United States, the vaccination is available for travelers to areas at risk. For information on availability of vaccines against Japanese encephalitis, please contact the Division of Vector-Borne Viral Diseases, Department of Health and Human Services, Public Health Service, Centers for Disease Control. Short-term travelers to Asian urban centers are at low risk to contract this disorder. The mosquitoes that transmit the virus are most concentrated in rural areas where there is standing water. They feed at sunset. Precautions include adequate clothing, sleeping in screened quarters under mosquito netting, and the use of insect repellents on exposed skin. Repellents containing over 30 percent active ingredient N,N-diethyl-meta-toluamide (**DEET**) are recommended.

**Treatment—Investigational** The antiviral agent carboxymethylacridanone (**CMA**) is currently under investigation for the treatment of Japanese encephalitis. It has shown benefit in JBEV-infected laboratory animals. More research is needed before it can be recommended for use in humans.

Please contact the agencies listed under Resources, below, for the most current information. Addresses and telephone numbers of these agencies, as well as of individual experts and research centers, may be found in the Master Resources List.

**Resources**

**For more information on Japanese encephalitis:** National Organization for Rare Disorders (NORD); Centers for Disease Control; World Health Organization.

**References**

The Pathogenesis of Acute Viral Encephalitis and Postinfectious Encephalomyelitis: R.T. Johnson; J. Infect. Dis., 1987, vol. 155(3), pp. 359–364.

Clinical Aspects of Japanese B Encephalitis in North Vietnam: D.H. Le; Clin. Neurol. Neurosurg., 1986, vol. 88(3), pp. 189–192.

Trial of Inactivated Japanese Encephalitis Vaccine in Children with Underlying Diseases: A. Yamada, et al.; Vaccine, 1986, vol. 4(1), pp. 32–34.

# ENCEPHALITIS, RASMUSSEN

**Description** Rasmussen encephalitis is a rare central nervous system disorder characterized by seizures, progressive hemiparesis, and mental deterioration.

**Synonyms**

Chronic Encephalitis and Epilepsy
Chronic Localized Encephalitis
Epilepsy, Hemiplegia, and Mental Retardation

**Signs and Symptoms** Rasmussen encephalitis usually begins in childhood. Some cases are thought to follow viral infections such as influenza and measles. Typically, the child develops seizures that are usually focal but may become generalized. Hemiparesis and mental retardation generally have their onset early in childhood and progress slowly.

The diagnosis of encephalitis may not be made until surgery is performed or postmortem brain tissue is examined.

**Etiology** The etiology of Rasmussen encephalitis is unknown. It may be a postviral phenomenon or a slow viral infection.

**Epidemiology** Fewer than 30 cases of Rasmussen encephalitis have been described in the medical literature since this disorder was first identified in 1958. The number of unidentified cases may be much higher.

**Related Disorders** See *Subacute Sclerosing Panencephalitis;* its course and symptoms may be similar to those of Rasmussen encephalitis.

**Treatment—Standard** Treatment consists of anticonvulsants and other symptomatic measures.

**Treatment—Investigational** Surgery is currently under investigation for the treatment of Rasmussen encephalitis. The procedure involves resection of the areas of the brain affected by encephalitis, in an attempt to control the seizures and progressive neurologic degeneration. For more information, please contact Ben Carson, M.D., at Johns Hopkins Hospital.

Researchers at Duke University Medical School and the University of Utah are studying the behavior of antibodies on surface brain cells in patients with Rasmussen encephalitis in hopes of finding both a treatment and a blood test to screen children.

Please contact the agencies listed under Resources, below, for the most current information. Addresses and telephone numbers of these agencies, as well as of individual experts and research centers, may be found in the Master Resources List.

### Resources

**For more information on Rasmussen encephalitis:** National Organization for Rare Disorders (NORD); NIH/National Institute of Neurological Disorders and Stroke; Centers for Disease Control; The Arc (a national organization on mental retardation); Theodore Rasmussen, M.D., Montreal Neurological Hospital; Ben Carson, M.D., Johns Hopkins Hospital.

### References

Smoldering Encephalitis in Children: P.C. Gupta, et al.; Neuropediatrics, 1984, vol. 15(4), pp. 191–197.

Further Observations on the Syndrome of Chronic Encephalitis and Epilepsy: T. Rasmussen; Appl. Neurophysiol., 1978, vol. 41, pp. 1–12.

# ENCEPHALOMYELITIS, MYALGIC (ME)

**Description** ME is a disorder that affects the central, peripheral, and autonomic nervous systems and the muscles. It is thought to be infectious in nature, possibly viral, but the exact etiology is unknown. The major symptoms include fatigue, headache, myalgias, weakness, and emotional lability.

### Synonyms

Akureyri Disease
Benign Myalgic Encephalomyelitis
Epidemic Myalgic Encephalomyelitis
Epidemic Neuromyasthenia
Iceland Disease
Raphe Nucleus Encephalopathy
Royal Free Disease
Tapanui Flu

**Signs and Symptoms** There may be a prodromal phase consisting of one or more of the following symptoms: headache, fatigue, sore throat, coughing, diarrhea or vomiting, malaise, and depression. These symptoms may persist up to 3 weeks. Then myalgias and arthralgias may develop, with or without a low-grade fever. Mental symptoms such as emotional lability, memory loss, depression, and difficulty in concentrating may be present. Other symptoms may include visual disturbances and paresthesias, urinary retention, and respiratory symptoms. Symptoms may be aggravated by strenuous exercise or emotional stress.

The aches and pains may subside after several days but can persist intermittently for months or years.

Physical examination may reveal hepatomegaly, hyperactive tendon reflexes, muscle twitching, sensory loss, and cranial nerve paralysis. Certain laboratory abnormalities have been reported, such as an elevated lactic dehydrogenase (**LDH**), abnormal lymphocytes, and an elevated cerebrospinal fluid protein level.

**Etiology** The etiology of ME is unknown. It is thought to be a viral illness, possibly related to Epstein-Barr virus (**EBV**), although this relationship is unproved.

**Epidemiology** ME occurs most often in the summer. It affects young adults and is more common in females than in males. Epidemics have been reported worldwide, but sporadic cases are the rule.

**Related Disorders** Symptoms of the following disorders can be similar to ME. Comparisons may be useful for a differential diagnosis.

**Chronic EBV infection,** the protracted form of infectious mononucleosis that occurs in some patients, resembles ME in many respects.

See *Multiple Sclerosis,* which may manifest itself in a similar fashion to ME, with intermittent neurologic deficits. MS has a characteristic picture on nuclear magnetic resonance scanning that will easily distinguish it from ME.

See *Polymyalgia Rheumatica,* which is also characterized by muscle pain and may be accompanied by fever, fatigue, and depression. Polymyalgia rheumatic, however, usually occurs in older individuals.

**Treatment—Standard** The treatment of ME is supportive. Antidepressant drugs may be helpful. Drugs such as pizotifen and carbamazepine may alleviate headache and myalgias.

**Treatment—Investigational** Research is under way to determine if a coxsackie B virus and tryptophan deficiency may be etiologic factors in ME.

Please contact the agencies listed under Resources, below, for the most current information. Addresses and telephone numbers of these agencies, as well as of individual experts and research centers, may be found in the Master Resources List.

**Resources**

**For more information on myalgic encephalomyelitis:** National Organization for Rare Disorders (NORD); Myalgic Encephalomyelitis Association; NIH/National Institute of Allergy and Infectious Diseases; Centers for Disease Control; Chronic Fatigue Syndrome Society; National Chronic Fatigue Syndrome Association.

**References**

Raphe Nucleus Encephalopathy (Myalgic Encephalomyelitis, Epidemic Neuromyasthenia): C.P. Maurizi; Med. Hypotheses, 1985, vol. 16(4), pp. 351–354.

Epidemiological Approaches to 'Epidemic Neuromyasthenia': Syndromes of Unknown Etiology (Epidemic Myalgic Encephalopathies): M. Thomas; Postgrad. Med. J., 1978, vol. 54(637), pp. 768–770.

# ERYSIPELAS

**Description** Erysipelas is a streptococcal infection of the face, arms, or legs.

**Synonyms**

Saint Anthony Fire

Cellulitis

**Signs and Symptoms** Erysipelas first appears as a localized, tender red lesion with a raised, spreading, sharply demarcated border that rapidly becomes bright red, shiny, hot, and painful. The skin may resemble the peel of an orange (peau d'orange). High fever, chills, headache, nausea, and malaise are accompanying symptoms.

In both children and adults, the face, legs, and arms are common sites of infection. Infants may develop erysipelas of the umbilical cord stump. Infection can occur at sites of minor surgery or trauma, or be a complication of lymphatic obstruction or edema.

**Etiology** Erysipelas is caused by group A streptococcal bacteria.

**Epidemiology** Erysipelas affects males and females of all ages. It is most common in infants, young children, and the elderly.

**Related Disorders** See *Angioedema, Hereditary.*

**Orbital cellulitus** is a bacterial infection of the eye. Symptoms include pain in the eye socket, exophthalmos, chemosis, impaired motility of the eye, edema, lid swelling, and fever.

**Herpes zoster** is a viral infection of the peripheral nervous system. It is characterized by the eruption of vesicles, neuralgia, and severe itching.

**Contact dermatitis** is an inflammatory reaction in the skin in response to irritants and allergens. It may be acute or chronic and is marked by inflamed skin and, possibly, blisters at the site of contact with an offending agent. If acute, the area may be edematous, crusty, scaly, and exudative. The patient complains of burning pain and, as a rule, pruritus. Irritating the site by scratching or rubbing may cause lichenification.

**Treatment—Standard** Erysipelas is usually treated with oral antibiotics, such as penicillin or erythromycin. Cold packs, aspirin, and pain relievers may be prescribed to relieve local discomfort. Bacteremia and the sepsis syndrome may occur. Hospitalization may be required for intravenous administration of antibiotics if the infection is extensive or severe.

**Treatment—Investigational** Please contact the agencies listed under Resources, below, for the most current information. Addresses and telephone numbers of these agencies, as well as of individual experts and research centers, may be found in the Master Resources List.

**Resources**

**For more information on erysipelas:** National Organization for Rare Disorders (NORD); NIH/National Institute of Allergy and Infectious Disease.

**References**

Changes in the Pattern of Infection Caused by Streptococcus Pyogenes: E. Gaworzewska, et al.; Epidemiol. Infect., April 1988, vol. 100(2), pp. 257–269.

Cellulitis and Related Skin Infections: S.J. Suss, et al.; Am. Fam. Physician, September 1987, vol. 36(3), pp. 126–136.

Erysipelas and Group G Streptococci: M. Hugo-Persson, et al.; Infection, May–June 1987, vol. 15(3), pp. 184–187.

Internal Medicine, 2nd ed.: J.H. Stein, et al., eds.; Little, Brown and Company, 1987, p. 1508.

# FASCIOLIASIS

**Description** Fascioliasis is caused by the liver fluke, *Fasciola hepatica.* The clinical syndrome is caused by parasitization of the bile ducts. A subtype of fascioliasis **(Halzoun syndrome)** affects the pharynx.

**Signs and Symptoms** Initial symptoms may include fever, epigastric pain, arthralgias, diarrhea, pruritis, and jaundice. There may be hepatosplenomegaly and facial edema, and eosinophilia is evident on laboratory examination. In untreated cases, cirrhosis may occur, but only after very prolonged infection. Subclinical infections are probably common in some parts of the world.

The diagnosis rests on finding the parasite ova in the feces.

**Etiology** The cause of fascioliasis is infection with *F. hepatica.*

**Epidemiology** *F. hepatica* infection is a zoonosis; sheep are the usual host. Consequently, fascioliasis is most common in sheep-raising areas, particularly in South America, Australia, China, and Africa. Infection has been reported in the southern and western United States. The intermediate host is the snail, and encysted forms of the parasite may be found attached to aquatic plants. Humans usually acquire infection by ingestion of contaminated plants. Adequate cooking is generally sufficient to prevent infection.

**Related Disorders** Other liver flukes capable of producing infection in humans are *Clonorchis sinensis,* and the *Opisthorchis* species.

**Halzoun syndrome,** a variant of fascioliasis, affects the throat. It is caused by *F. hepatica, F. gigantica,* or other parasites known as linguatulid larvae.

**Treatment—Standard** Praziquantel, emetine, and choroquine have been used to treat fascioliasis, although recent studies show that bithionol (see Treatment—Investigational, below) may be more effective. Preventive measures include boiling vegetables and water purification.

**Treatment—Investigational** Studies of bithionol are being conducted by the Centers for Disease Control **(CDC).** Although this drug is available for experimental use through the CDC, its long-term effectiveness and toxicity have yet to be determined.

The drug Niclofolan, a biphenyl anthelmintic compound, is being investigated in Germany as a treatment for fascioliasis. Further testing is needed to determine effectiveness and possible side effects of this drug.

Please contact the agencies listed under Resources, below, for the most current information. Addresses and telephone numbers of these agencies, as well as of individual experts and research centers, may be found in the Master Resources List.

**Resources**

**For more information on fascioliasis:** National Organization for Rare Disorders (NORD); American Liver Foundation; United Liver Association; Children's Liver Foundation; NIH/National Institute of Allergy and Infectious Diseases; Centers for Disease Control.

**References**

Treatment of Human Fascioliasis with Niclofolan: T. Eckhardt, et al.; Gastroenterology, October 1981, vol. 81(4), pp. 795–798.

# FILARIASIS

**Description** The term *filariasis* usually refers to disease caused by either the *Wuchereria bancrofti* or *Brugia malayi* worms. It is characterized by lymphadenopathy and chronic lymphatic obstruction, which, over prolonged periods, may result in elephantiasis (see *Elephantiasis),* especially of the legs and genitalia.

The larval forms of the pathogen are inoculated by the mosquito. These make their way to the lymphatics, where they mature and reproduce microfilariae. Disease is primarily a response to adult worms, which elicit a granulomatous inflammatory reaction. The chronic inflammation progresses to fibrosis and obstruction of the lymph flow.

**Synonyms**

> Bancroftian Filariasis
> Filarial Elephantiasis
> Filariasis Malayi
> Malayi Tropical Eosinphilia
> Wuchereriasis

**Signs and Symptoms** Filariasis may be asymptomatic. Alternatively, there may be bouts of lymphangitis with fever, aches, and pain in the involved lymph nodes. Edema of the involved limb may occur, but it resolves after the attack. Acute funiculitis, epididymitis, and orchitis may accompany these attacks. Characteristically, eosinophilia may be found during acute episodes, but when the inflammation subsides, the eosinophil count returns to normal.

Another common presentation of filariasis is chronic lymphadenopathy without other findings.

Long-standing lymphatic obstruction has several consequences. These include hydrocele, chyluria (due to rupture of lymph into the urinary tract), lymph varices, and progressive edema of the scrotum, vulva, breast, or limbs, i.e., elephantiasis. Chronic edema is ultimately accompanied by a thickened, warty appearance of the skin.

The diagnosis of filariasis requires examination of a blood smear for microfilariae. Since parasitemia tends to occur at night, the specimen is best obtained at night. When parasitemia cannot be demonstrated, the adult worms may occasionally be found in a lymph node biopsy. In the late stages of disease, the diagnosis is often made by exclusion.

**Etiology** Filariasis is caused by the tissue nematodes *W. bancrofti* and *B. malayi*. Symptoms result primarily from inflammatory reactions to the adult worms, as described above. Hypersensitivity reactions to the microfilariae may also develop.

**Epidemiology** Filariasis is common in tropical regions of the world. *W. bancrofti* is widely distributed throughout Africa, Asia, China, and South America. *B. malayi* is found in southern and southeast Asia. The disease does not occur in North America, although cases are occasionally imported from tropical regions. The infection is transmitted by several tropical mosquito species that transfer the larval stage (microfilariae) from one host to another.

**Related Disorders** The term *filariasis* has been used here in its narrower sense. In its broad sense, filariasis refers to infections with various species of nematodes, whose adult forms have a hairlike appearance. In addition to the lymphatic filariasis described in this entry, there are subcutaneous types (onchocerciasis and loiasis) and those associated with serous cavity infection, chiefly acanthocheilonemiasis (see ***Acanthocheilonemiasis).*** Others include dirofilariasis. All of these, except dirofilariasis, are common tropical diseases.

**Treatment—Standard** Diethylcarbamazine is the most effective agent for filariasis. It removes microfilariae from the circulation and kills or impairs the reproductive capacity of the adult worms. The somewhat less effective drug levamisole and the drug ivermectin have also been investigated. The elimination of adult worms must be undertaken with care because the dead worms can provoke dangerous allergic reactions and abscesses. Antihistamines and corticosteroids are used to control such hypersensitivity reactions. Surgery may be used to treat hydrocele, or to remove the remains of adult worms and calcifications developing around them.

**Treatment—Investigational** Please contact the agencies listed under Resources, below, for the most current information. Addresses and telephone numbers of these agencies, as well as of individual experts and research centers, may be found in the Master Resources List.

**Resources**

**For more information on filariasis:** National Organization for Rare Disorders (NORD); Centers for Disease Control; NIH/National Institute of Allergy and Infectious Diseases; World Health Organization.

**References**

Filarial Infections: E.A. Ottesen; Infect. Dis. Clin. North Am., September 1993, vol. 7(3), pp. 619–633.

Cecil Textbook of Medicine, 19th ed.: J.B. Wyngaarden, et al., eds.; W.B. Saunders Company, 1992, pp. 2015–2020.

Intensity of Efficiency of Transmission and the Development of Microfilaraemia and Disease: Their Relationahip in Lymphatic Filariasis: B.A. Southgate; J. Trop. Med. Hyg., February 1992, vol. 95(1), pp. 1–12.

Nelson Textbook of Pediatrics, 14th ed.: R.E. Behrman, ed.-in-chief; W.B. Saunders Company, 1992, pp. 901–903.

Immune Responses to Filarial Parasites: R.M. Maizels, et al.; Immunol. Lett., October 1991, vol. 30(2), pp. 249–254.

Laboratory Analysis of Filariasis: M.L. Eberhard, et al.; Clin. Lab. Med., December 1991, vol. 11(4), pp. 977–1010.

The Vector Host Link in Filariasis: P. Wenk; Ann. Trop. Med. Parasitol., February 1991, vol. 85(1), pp. 139–147.

Recent Advances in Research on Filariasis: Chemotherapy: L.G. Goodwin; Trans. R. Soc. Trop. Med. Hyg., 1984, vol. 78(suppl.), pp. 1–8.

Tropical Diseases of Importance to the Traveler: K.R. Brown, S.M. Phillips; Adv. Intern. Med., 1984, vol. 29, pp. 59–84.

Efficacy of the Vermectins Against Filarial Parasites: A Short Review: W.C. Campbell; Vet. Res. Commun., May 1982, vol. 5(3), pp. 251–262.

Tropical Eosinophilia: C.J. Spry, V. Kumaraswami; Semin. Hematol., April 1982, vol. 19(2), pp. 107–115.

Use of Levamisole in Parasitic Infections: M.J. Miller; Drugs, August 1980, vol. 20(2), pp. 122–130.

Diethylcarbamazine and New Compounds for the Treatment of Filariasis: F.Hawking; Adv. Pharmacol. Chemother., 1979, vol. 16, pp. 129–194.

# FITZ-HUGH-CURTIS SYNDROME

**Description** Fitz-Hugh-Curtis syndrome is a complication of pelvic inflammatory disease. The bacterium *Chlamydia trachomatis* can cause infection and ensuing adhesions between the liver and other sites in the peritoneum, but *Neisseria gonorrhoeae* is also a cause of the syndrome. Symptoms can mimic those of hepatitis. Severe pain in the upper quadrant is common.

**Synonyms**

Gonococcal Perihepatitis

Perihepatitis Syndrome

**Signs and Symptoms** Fitz-Hugh-Curtis syndrome is characterized by the sudden onset of severe pain in the upper right abdomen, which is often confused with the development of hepatitis. Scar tissue develops between the abdominal wall and the liver, which causes severe right-side pain. Other clinical findings include fever, liver tenderness and dysfunction, and blood irregularities.

**Etiology** Fitz-Hugh-Curtis syndrome is caused by infection with the bacteria *Chlamydia trachomatis* and is usually associated with pelvic inflammatory disease. Other causes for severe right-side pain, such as cholecystitis, pancreatitis, and hepatitis, must be ruled out in order to diagnose this disease.

**Epidemiology** Fitz-Hugh-Curtis syndrome can affect sexually active women of any age group or nationality who are infected with *Chlamydia trachomatis.*

**Related Disorders Primary sclerosing cholangitis** is a rare collagen disorder involving inflammation and blockage of the bile duct, liver ducts, and gallbladder. Episodes of pain and discomfort in the right upper quadrant may gradually become prolonged.

**Treatment—Standard** Confirmation of diagnosis of Fitz-Hugh-Curtis syndrome is made through the use of ultrasound or laparoscopy and a positive test for *Chlamydia trachomatis.* Tetracyclines, ofloxacin, and other antibiotics are the drugs of choice. Surgery to remove the stringlike scar tissue may be indicated.

**Treatment—Investigational** The drug azithromycin is under investigation for treating the infection associated with Fitz-Hugh-Curtis syndrome. This antibiotic is given in a single dose, however, its long-term safety and efficacy have yet to be proved.

Please contact the agencies listed under Resources, below, for the most current information. Addresses and telephone numbers of these agencies, as well as of individual experts and research centers, may be found in the Master Resources List.

**Resources**

**For more information on Fitz-Hugh-Curtis syndrome:** National Organization for Rare Disorders (NORD); NIH/National Institute of Allergy and Infectious Diseases; Centers for Disease Control; American Social Health Association; National Sexually Transmitted Diseases Hotline; Council on Sex Information and Education.

**References**

Cecil Textbook of Medicine, 19th ed.: James B. Wyngaarden, et al., eds.; W.B. Saunders Company, 1992, pp. 834, 1708.

Laparoscopic Treatment of Painful Perihepatic Adhesions in Fitz-Hugh-Curtis Syndrome: S. Owens, et al.; Obstet. Gynecol., September 1991, vol. 78(3 pt. 2), pp. 542–543.

An Atypical Presentation of the Fitz-Hugh-Curtis Syndrome: M. McCormick, et al.; J. Emerg. Med., January–February 1990, vol. 8(1), pp. 55–58.

# GIARDIASIS

**Description** Giardiasis is an infection of the duodenum and jejunum caused by the protozoan *Giardia lamblia.* The primary manifestation of symptomatic infection is malabsorption, but many infections are asymptomatic.

**Synonyms**

Beaver Fever

Lambliasis

**Signs and Symptoms** Within 3 weeks of exposure, crampy abdominal discomfort, watery diarrhea, flatulence, and foul-smelling stools may appear. Acute attacks usually last approximately 3 or 4 days, although symptoms may persist for several weeks.

In long-term infestation, patients may experience chronic diarrhea, malabsorption of nutrients, weight loss, epigastric cramping, anorexia, nausea, and vomiting. Children with chronic giardiasis may experience growth retardation.

The diagnosis of giardiasis is usually made by demonstrating the parasites in the stool. Occasionally a duodenal aspirate or jejunal biopsy is required.

**Etiology** Giardiasis is caused by the protozoan parasite known as *Giardia lamblia.* Humans are infected by the parasites in the cyst stage.

**Epidemiology** This disorder occurs worldwide. Epidemics in the United States have been linked to the excretion of cysts into public water reservoirs by infected beavers. Outbreaks have also occurred in daycare centers and custodial institutions, such as prisons and long-term care facilities, where transmission occurs directly from person to person.

Other populations at risk include homosexuals practicing anilingus, immunocompromised individuals, travelers from endemic areas, and campers who drink untreated water.

**Related Disorders** Related disorders include other parasitic infections of the intestine: amebiasis, hookworm infection, and strongyloidiasis. Disorders with similar symptoms include those that produce malabsorption.

**Amebiasis** is a disease of the intestinal tract caused by the protozoan parasite *Entamoeba histolytica*. It is transmitted from person to person and by food- and waterborne routes. The organism invades the colon and rectum, producing ulcers and inflammation. Symptoms begin gradually, with an increasing number of stools reaching as many as 15 per day. Stools may be semisolid to liquid and may be bloody. Abdominal pain is common, but fever is unusual. In the United States, amebiasis primarily affects visitors returning from countries with poor sanitation. Treatment with the drug metronidazole is often effective in eliminating the disorder.

**Hookworm** is a parasitic organism that penetrates the skin and migrates to the intestines, where it attaches and sucks blood. Abdominal pain may occur, but the most prominent symptoms are those related to chronic blood loss: iron deficiency anemia and hypoalbuminemia. Approximately 25 percent of the world population may be infected with hookworms. Infection is acquired by walking barefoot in soil contaminated with parasites that penetrate the skin.

**Strongyloidiasis** is a parasitic intestinal disorder that, when severe, produces epigastric pain and tenderness, vomiting, and diarrhea. The causative agent is the intestinal nematode *Strongyloides stercoralis*. This disorder is usually found in the tropics in areas of poor sanitation. It can exist in crowded, unsanitary institutions anywhere, persisting for decades and recrudescing in fulminant form should the host become immunocompromised. Treatment with thiabendazole is often effective for patients with strongyloidiasis.

**Treatment—Standard** The treatment of choice for giardiasis patients is quinacrine or metronidazole (the latter is not yet approved for giardiasis in the United States). Furazolidone is especially useful in the treatment of children. The most important factor for preventing this disorder is proper treatment of infected water. Chlorination may not kill cysts; sedimentation, flocculation, and filtration should also be performed. Water can be boiled for 1 minute or mixed with halazone or iodine to eliminate contamination. Travelers to areas with contaminated water should drink only boiled or treated water and should not consume uncooked fruit or vegetables.

**Treatment—Investigational** Treatment with tinidazole or ornidazole for giardiasis may be effective. However, these medications have not yet been approved for use in the United States for this condition.

Please contact the agencies listed under Resources, below, for the most current information. Addresses and telephone numbers of these agencies, as well as of individual experts and research centers, may be found in the Master Resources List.

**Resources**

**For more information on giardiasis:** National Organization for Rare Disorders (NORD); NIH/National Institute of Allergy and Infectious Diseases; Centers for Disease Control.

**References**

Internal Medicine, 2nd ed.: J.H. Stein, ed.-in-chief; Little, Brown and Company, 1987, pp. 1785–1786.

Treatment of Intestinal *E. histolytica* and *G. lamblia* with Metronidazole, Tinidazole and Ornidazole: A Comparative Study: S. Bassily, et al.; J. Trop. Med. Hyg., 1987, vol. 90(1), pp. 9–12.

Management of Giardiasis: E.D. Gorski; Am. Fam. Phys., 1985, vol. 32(5), pp. 157–164.

Selective Primary Health Care: Strategies for Control of Disease in the Developing World. XIX. Giardiasis: D.P. Stevens; Rev. Infect. Dis., 1985, vol. 7(4), pp. 530–535.

# GRAFT-VERSUS-HOST DISEASE (GVHD)

**Description** GVHD is caused by the response of donor cells against a host with an impaired immune system. It strikes those patients who have undergone a bone marrow transplant or other immunosuppressed individuals who have received blood transfusions. Onset can be acute or chronic. Symptoms include dermatitis, intestinal problems similar to colitis, and liver dysfunction.

**Signs and Symptoms** The most frequent signs of both acute and chromic GVHD occur after a blood transfusion or bone marrow transplant.

**Acute GVHD** usually occurs in the first 100 days after blood transfusion or bone marrow transplant. The first symptoms are usually mild dermatitis, liver dysfunction, and intestinal problems; alternatively, severe dermatitis, diarrhea, nausea, abdominal pain, and hepatopathy may be present.

**Chronic GVHD** usually persists long after a transfusion or bone marrow transplant. In addition to the symptoms for acute GVHD, chronic GVHD may involve the eyes, mouth, lungs, and musculoskeletal system.

**Etiology** GVHD is the result of an immunosuppressed recipient's inability to respond properly to the lymphoid cells in the donor's blood. Immunosuppression can occur as a result of certain drugs, radiation, or certain diseases.

**Epidemiology** GVHD affects about 60 percent of all bone marrow transplant and transfusion patients whose immune system was suppressed before treatment. Males and females of all ages are affected equally. In cases of bone marrow transplants, the recipient usually undergoes radiation to destroy their own diseased bone marrow, thereby weakening their immune system. Cancer patients undergoing chemotherapy are also at high risk of getting GVHD from blood transfusions. Cancer patients and organ transplant recipients often use drugs that suppress their immune systems.

**Related Disorders Lichen planus** is a recurrent, itchy, inflammatory eruption of the skin characterized by small separate, angular spots that may join together into rough scaly patches. It is often accompanied by oral lesions. The initial attack persists for weeks or months, and intermittent recurrences may be noted for years. Moderate to severe itching may be present and is often refractory.

**Ulcerative colitis** is an inflammatory disease of the bowel characterized by chronic ulcers in the colon. The chief characteristic of this disorder is bloody diarrhea. Colitis may involve only the left side of the colon or may eventually extend to involve the entire bowel. However, in some cases it may attack most of the large bowel simultaneously. The disease is usually chronic, with repeated periods of exacerbation and remission.

**Treatment—Standard** Treatment of GVHD usually consists of steroid therapy and a combination of cyclosporine and methotrexate. In some cases where GVHD is resistant to steroids, treatment with anti-interleukin-2 receptor monoclonal antibody has been used. To prevent GVHD from developing, the above methods may be employed prior to a blood transfusion or bone marrow transplant, or the blood may be treated before being given to the recipient.

**Treatment—Investigational** In patients unable to tolerate steroids or who have a poor response to them, the orphan drug thalidomide (Andrulis Research Corp.) is being tested. Because of thalidomide's severe side effects on a developing fetus, extreme care must be taken in choosing test subjects. Georgia B. Vogelsang, M.D., of Johns Hopkins University is studying the immunosuppressive properties of thalidomide as a first line therapy in patients with GVHD and other serious diseases. Further investigation is needed to determine the long-term safety and effectiveness of this treatment. Thalidomide is available in England under special license from Penn Pharmaceuticals of Tredegar, South Wales.

Interleukin-1 antagonist, human recombinant (Antril) is being sponsored by Synergen, Boulder, CO, as an investigational therapy for GVHD in transplant patients.

The orphan drug humanized antitac (Hoffmann–La Roche) is being tested as a treatment to prevent GVHD following bone marrow transplantation.

In a recent clinical trial, doctors found that when patients received the standard drugs cyclosporine and prednisone following bone marrow transplantation, 23 percent of them developed serious GVHD. But when the anticancer drug methotrexate was added, the rate dropped to 9 percent.

Please contact the agencies listed under Resources, below, for the most current information. Addresses and telephone numbers of these agencies, as well as of individual experts and research centers, may be found in the Master Resources List.

**Resources**

**For more information on graft-versus-host disease:** National Organization for Rare Disorders (NORD); Caitlin Raymond International Registry of Bone Marrow Donor Banks; NIH/National Heart, Lung and Blood Institute Information Center.

**References**

Cyclosporine, Methotrexate, and Prednisone Compared with Cyclosporine and Prednisone for Prophylaxis of Acute Graft-Versus-Host Disease: N.J. Chao, et al., N. Engl. J. Med., October 1993, vol. 329(17), pp. 1225–1230.

A Retrospective Analysis of Therapy for Acute Graft-vs-Host Disease: Initial Treatment: P.J. Martin, et al.; Blood, October 1990, vol. 76(8), pp. 1464–1472.

Transfusion-Associated Graft-vs-Host Disease in Patients with Malignancies: Report of Two Cases and Review of the Literature: S.D. Decoste, et al.; Arch. Dermatol., October 1990, vol. 126(10), pp. 1324–1329.

Cecil Textbook of Medicine, 18th ed.: J.B. Wyngaarden and L.H. Smith, Jr., eds.; W.B. Saunders Company, 1988, pp. 950, 1040.

Gastrointestinal Inflammation After Bone Marrow Transplantation: Graft-vs-Host Disease or Opportunistic Infection?: B. Jones, et al.; AJR Am. J. Roentgenol., February 1988, vol. 150(2), pp. 277–281.

# HAND-FOOT-MOUTH SYNDROME

**Description** Hand-foot-mouth syndrome is a relatively common mild viral disease that occurs in young children. It is characterized by a vesicular rash that appears on the hands and feet and in the mouth. It is usually caused by coxsackieviruses.

**Synonyms**

Vesicular Stomatitis with Exanthem

**Signs and Symptoms** The most prominent feature of the syndrome is a rash, which begins as a macular or papular eruption. The lesions become vesicular and ulcerate. The intraoral lesions are ulcerative and painful and occur on the tongue and buccal mucosa. The lesions on the hands and feet, usually vesicular, occur most often dorsally.

Occasionally lesions appear on the buttocks as well. The rash generally resolves in a week, but chronic and recurrent forms occur. The rash may be accompanied by fever, malaise, and headache. Hand-foot-mouth syndrome may be epidemic in certain geographic areas.

More severe forms of hand-foot-mouth syndrome have been associated with enterovirus 71; these may be complicated by central nervous system involvement (aseptic meningitis or encephalitis).

Hand-foot-mouth syndrome is generally diagnosed clinically, and usually can be distinguished from other exanthems by its distribution.

**Etiology** Hand-foot-mouth syndrome is caused by a virus, the coxsackievirus A16 or enterovirus 71.

**Epidemiology** The syndrome affects males and females in equal numbers and is common in young children.

**Related Disorders** The differential diagnosis of hand-foot-mouth syndrome includes chickenpox, herpangina, and exanthems caused by coxsackie- and echoviruses.

**Herpangina** is an acute viral infection that usually affects infants and young children. Fever is often the initial complaint. Sore throat, anorexia, and diffuse myalgias may occur, as well as vomiting and convulsions. In the first 24 hours, a small number (average, 5) of small lesions appear in the oropharangeal area. These lesions eventually become shallow ulcers and will heal within 5 days. In contrast to hand-foot-mouth syndrome, the extremities are generally not involved.

The skin lesions of **chickenpox** may resemble hand-foot-mouth syndrome, but the distributions are quite different. The rash of chickenpox is more extensive and more centrally located.

Echoviruses and coxsackieviruses are also associated with vesicular eruptions, although the distributions are more central.

**Encephalitis** may be associated with hand-foot-mouth syndrome. It can also be caused by viruses such as the St. Louis, western equine, California, mumps, ECHO, and several coxsackieviruses.

**Treatment—Standard** Treatment is supportive. Calamine lotion and acetaminophen (not aspirin in children) may be helpful.

**Treatment—Investigational** At the present time, a study is being conducted on the effectiveness of murine interferon as a treatment for coxsackievirus type A 16 **(CA 16)** or enterovirus type 71 **(EV 71).** More research must be conducted to determine long-term safety and effectiveness of this drug.

Please contact the agencies listed under Resources, below, for the most current information. Addresses and telephone numbers of these agencies, as well as of individual experts and research centers, may be found in the Master Resources List.

**Resources**

**For more information on hand-foot-mouth syndrome:** National Organization for Rare Disorders (NORD); Centers for Disease Control; NIH/National Institute of Allergy and Infectious Diseases.

**References**

Outbreak of Enterovirus 71 Infection in Victoria, Australia, with a High Incidence of Neurological Involvement: G. Gilbert, et al.; Pediatr. Infect. Dis. J., 1988, vol. 7(7), pp. 484–488.

Internal Medicine, 2nd ed.: J.H. Stein, ed.-in-chief; Little, Brown and Company, 1987, p. 1569.

Protective Effect of Interferon on Infections with Hand, Foot and Mouth Disease Virus in Newborn Mice: D. Sasaki, et al.; J. Infect. Dis., 1986, vol. 153(3), pp. 498–502.

# HANTAVIRUS PULMONARY SYNDROME

**Description** Hantavirus pulmonary syndrome is a lung infection with the Sin Nombre (Muerto Canyon) hantavirus, which is frequently found in the deer mouse *(Peromyscus maniculatus)*. Symptoms progress rapidly, and hypotension, shock, and respiratory failure may occur.

**Synonyms**

Four Corners Hantavirus **(FCV)**

Hantavirus-Associated Respiratory Distress Syndrome **(HARDS)**

**Signs and Symptoms** The initial symptoms most commonly associated with hantavirus pulmonary syndrome are fever, myalgias, headache, and cough. Chills, abdominal pain, diarrhea, and malaise may also be present. Other symptoms include shortness of breath, tachypnea, tachycardia, dizziness, arthralgia, sweating, and back and/or chest pain. These are followed by thrombocytopenia, hypoxemia, and pulmonary, interstitial, and bilateral alveolar edema. Accumulation of infiltrates may also occur. The disease progresses rapidly and may cause hypotension, shock, and/or respiratory distress. Patients infrequently report inflammation of the tympanic membrane, sinusitis, inflamed throat, conjunctivitis, and/or rhinorrhea.

**Etiology** Hantavirus pulmonary syndrome is caused by the Sin Nombre (Muerto Canyon) hantavirus. This newly identified virus within the *Bunyaviridae* family is carried by rodents, usually by the deer mouse *(Peromyscus man-*

*iculatus*), common to all parts of the United States except the Southeast. Not all deer mice are infected, and those that do carry the virus do not appear to be affected by any associated disease. Humans become infected on direct or indirect contact with waste products or saliva from an infected rodent. Inhaling dust or dried particles that carry saliva or waste products of an infected rodent is the most common mode of transmission.

**Epidemiology** Hantavirus pulmonary syndrome appears to affect males and females in equal numbers. Approximately half of reported cases are Native American, and most of the remainder are white. Geographic location and exposure to rodent droppings, rather than ethnic background, seem to play the determining role.

**Related Disorders** In general, the symptoms of severe, generalized pneumonia are similar to those of hantavirus pulmonary syndrome. Only diagnostic testing can determine which disease is affecting an individual.

**Interstitial pneumonia** involves an abnormal increase in the interstitial tissue and a decrease and induration of other lung tissue. Major symptoms include shortness of breath on exertion, cough, and loss of appetite. Symptoms vary from mild to severe. The patient is often afebrile, but occasionally the onset may be rapid, with fever present, suggesting an acute respiratory infection.

**Eosinophilic pneumonia** is characterized by an inflammation of the lungs and an abnormal increase in eosinophils in the lymph nodes, lungs, and blood. This disorder is usually associated with allergic conditions and various parasitic infections. Onset is sudden, and symptoms range from mild to severe and may be accompanied by weight loss and increased pulse rate. Low-grade fever, cough with the possibility of blood in the phlegm, wheezing, and labored breathing are common. There may also be chills, sweating, chest pain, and/or malaise.

**Treatment—Standard** Preventive measures include avoiding areas such as storage sheds, basements, and woodpiles where deer mice leave their droppings; and wearing a face mask that covers both nose and mouth, as well as rubber gloves, when exposure is unavoidable. The area should be sanitized with disinfectant. *People who exhibit flulike symptoms after exposure to mouse droppings require immediate medical attention, because of the aggressive nature of this disorder.* If the hantavirus pulmonary syndrome is strongly suspected, the patient should be hospitalized at once.

Diagnosis depends on symptoms, a history of contact with rodents (especially deer mice) or exposure to areas where rodents live, the lack of any alternative diagnosis, and/or laboratory tests, which may show atypical lymphocytes, thrombocytopenia, a higher than normal white blood cell count, and hypoxemia.

The diagnosis is confirmed upon laboratory results that reveal the presence and/or increased levels of Hantavirus IgM and/or a rising IgG titer. The polymerase chain reaction (**PCR**) may be used to implicate a hantavirus and identify which strain has caused the infection.

Treatment of hantavirus pulmonary syndrome involves intensive care, including the monitoring of respiratory status, fluid balances, electrolyte balances, and blood pressure. Hypoxemia may require the administration of oxygen. Shock and hypotension associated with hantavirus pulmonary syndrome may be treated with drugs (e.g., dopamine and norepinephrine) to increase blood flow and thus improve blood and oxygen delivery to organs.

**Treatment—Investigational** The antiviral drug ribavirin is being tested on hantavirus pulmonary syndrome, but its safety and efficacy are questionable. The development of a vaccine is also being investigated.

Please contact the agencies listed under Resources, below, for the most current information. Addresses and telephone numbers of these agencies, as well as of individual experts and research centers, may be found in the Master Resources List.

**Resources**

**For more information on hantavirus pulmonary syndrome:** National Organization for Rare Disorders (NORD); Centers for Disease Control; NIH/National Institute of Allergy and Infectious Diseases.

**References**

Hantavirus Pulmonary Syndrome—United States, 1993: MMWR Morb. Mortal. Wkly. Rep., January 28, 1994, vol. 43(3), pp. 45–48.

A Novel Hantavirus Associated with an Outbreak of Fatal Respiratory Disease in the Southwestern United States: Evolutionary Relationships to Known Hantaviruses: J. Virol., February 1994, vol. 68(2), pp. 592–596.

A New Hantavirus: A Videotape for Health Professionals: Centers for Disease Control and Prevention; December 1993, Videotape Graphics Booklet, pp. 1–26.

Update: Hantavirus Pulmonary Syndrome—United States, 1993: MMWR Morb. Mortal. Wkly. Rep., October 29, 1993, vol. 42(42), pp. 816–820.

# HEPATITIS, NEONATAL

**Description** Neonatal hepatitis is one of several cholestatic disorders that present in the first month of life. It is the most common cause of neonatal intrahepatic cholestasis. The histologic picture is characterized by diffuse hepatocellular disease with giant cell transformation of the hepatocytes.

**Synonyms**

> Congenital Liver Cirrhosis
> Giant Cell Cirrhosis of Newborn
> Giant Cell Disease
> Giant Cell Hepatitis
> Idiopathic Neonatal Hepatitis

**Signs and Symptoms** The symptoms of neonatal hepatitis usually become apparent 2 to 4 weeks after birth. The clinical picture is that of bile duct obstruction, with jaundice, pale stools, dark urine, and hepatomegaly. By the age of 2 to 3 months, slow growth, irritability from pruritus, and signs of portal hypertension may be present. These signs and symptoms do not differentiate neonatal hepatitis from other causes of neonatal cholestasis.

The first step in establishing a diagnosis depends on the finding of conjugated hyperbilirubinemia, indicating the presence of cholestasis. Following this, infectious causes of cholestasis (such as sepsis) should be ruled out, as well as specific inherited metabolic diseases ($\alpha$-1-antitrypsin deficiency, tyrosinemia, Gaucher disease, galactosemia, and others). Ultrasonography and hepatobiliary scintigraphy help to distinguish neonatal hepatitis from biliary atresia and other forms of extrahepatic biliary obstruction. Liver biopsy is frequently diagnostic. Occasionally laparotomy with intraoperative cholangiography is necessary.

**Etiology** The cause of neonatal hepatitis is unknown in the majority of cases.

**Epidemiology** Infants of both sexes may be affected by neonatal hepatitis.

**Related Disorders** The clinical syndrome of neonatal cholestasis may be produced by a wide variety of diseases including infections (most commonly sepsis or a viral infection such as cytomegalovirus [**CMV**]), and inherited metabolic disorders, but the most common cause is either biliary atresia or idiopathic neonatal hepatitis. Spur-cell anemia, characterized by spikelike cells filled with cholesterol and thereby unable to carry oxygen, occurs in infants with neonatal hepatitis.

Related disorders include intrahepatic bile duct hypoplasia or paucity, Alagille syndrome, and Zellweger syndrome. The latter 2 syndromes usually have associated congenital anomalies. See ***Alagille Syndrome; Zellweger Syndrome.***

**Treatment—Standard** Cholestyramine, which binds bile salts in the intestine, can be administered if pruritis is suspected. Malabsorption of long-chain triglycerides can be corrected by special formulas containing medium-chain triglycerides, and fat-soluble vitamins should be replaced.

With progression of disease, portal hypertension, ascites, and cirrhosis develop. Transplantation is the treatment of choice for signs of impending liver failure.

**Treatment—Investigational** Please contact the agencies listed under Resources, below, for the most current information. Addresses and telephone numbers of these agencies, as well as of individual experts and research centers, may be found in the Master Resources List.

**Resources**

**For more information on neonatal hepatitis:** National Organization for Rare Disorders (NORD); American Liver Foundation; NIH/National Digestive Diseases Information Clearinghouse; United Liver Association; Children's Liver Foundation.

**References**

Cecil Textbook of Medicine, 19th ed.: J.B. Wyngaarden, et al., eds.; W.B. Saunders Company, 1992, pp. 775–778.

Fate of Infants with Neonatal Hepatitis: Pediatric Surgeons' Dilemma: S. Suita, et al.; J. Pediatr. Surg., June 1992, vol. 27(6), pp. 696–699.

Mendelian Inheritance in Man, 10th ed.: V.A. McKusick; The Johns Hopkins University Press, 1992, p. 1440.

Nelson Textbook of Pediatrics, 14th ed.: R.E. Behrman, ed.-in-chief; W.B. Saunders Company, 1992, pp. 1010–1013.

Polymerase Chain Reaction to Detect Human Cytomegalovirus in Livers of Infants with Neonatal Hepatitis: M.H. Chang, et al.; Gastroenterology, September 1992, vol. 103(3), pp. 1022–1025.

Harrison's Principles of Internal Medicine, 12th ed.: J.D. Wilson, et al., eds.: McGraw-Hill, 1991, pp. 1537–1538.

Birth Defects Encyclopedia: M.L. Buyse, ed.-in-chief; Blackwell Scientific Publications, 1990, p. 91.

Gastrointestianl Disease, 4th ed.; M.H. Sleisenger, et al.; W.B. Saunders Company, 1989, pp. 1640–1641.

Diagnositic Utility of Hepatobiliary Scintigraphy with 99mTc-Disida in Neonatal Cholestasis: W. Spivak, et al.; J. Pediatr., June 1987, vol. 110(6), pp. 855–861.

Neonatal Hepatitis: A Follow-up Study: M.G. Chang, et al.; J. Pediatr. Gastroenterol. Nutr., March–April 1987, vol. 6(2), pp. 203–207.

Niemann-Pick Variant Lipidosis Presenting As "Neonatal Hepatitis.": L.A. Semeraro, et al.; J. Pediatr. Gastroenterol. Nutr., May–June 1986, vol. 5(3), pp. 492–500.

# HEPATITIS, NON-A, NON-B (HEPATITIS C)

**Description** Non-A, non-B hepatitis is currently thought to consist of 2 distinct viral illnesses that will hereafter be referred to as hepatitis C and hepatitis E. Hepatitis C is caused by the hepatitis C virus (**HCV**) and is a blood-borne infection. **HEV** is transmitted enterically like hepatitis A.

Hepatitis C resembles hepatitis B clinically, but the risk of progression to chronic hepatitis is much higher. As with HBV infection, a carrier state, chronic active hepatitis and cirrhosis may occur.

**Synonyms**

Hepatitis

Hepatitis C

**Signs and Symptoms** Symptoms of hepatitis C and B are indistinguishable, although hepatitis C tends to be less severe in the acute phase. Flulike symptoms (fever, aches, eye-ear-nose-throat involvement, weakness, nausea, vomiting, etc.) and jaundice usually occur. The incubation period of this form of hepatitis is usually from 4 to 25 weeks. A carrier form of HCV infection (asymptomatic) occurs more frequently than in HBV infection, and the rate of progression to chronic hepatitis is almost 50 percent.

A specific antibody test is available for diagnosis of hepatitis C. However, this test may not become positive until up to 3 months after infection. An alternative method, diagnosis by exclusion, can be used by testing for HBsAg, IgM antiHBc, and IgM antiHAV. If all of these are negative, then HCV infection is more likely.

**Etiology** Hepatitis C is caused by a DNA virus transmitted predominantly by blood transfusion, inoculation, medical procedures that involve penetration of the skin, and other percutaneous routes (intravenous drug abuse).

**Epidemiology** To date, there are approximately 170,000 cases of hepatitis C in the United States each year, according to the Centers for Disease Control. Approximately 6 to 10 percent of these cases are due to transfusions of infected blood. (In 1990, the Food and Drug Administration approved an antibody test for hepatitis C, which is now used to screen blood for transfusion.) The vast majority of persons are infected through other types of contact, including intravenous drug use or sexual contact. Hemodialysis patients are also at risk. Half of all cases of hepatitis C develop chronic liver inflammation, and 10 percent develop cirrhosis of the liver. This disease occurs worldwide and affects males and females of all age groups equally.

**Related Disorders** Many aspects of hepatitis A, D, and E; fulminant hepatitis; anicteric hepatitis; recrudescent hepatitis; cholestatic hepatitis; bridging necrosis; δ-hepatitis; chronic active hepatitis; hepatitis induced by long-term alcoholism; and toxic, drug, or chemically induced hepatitis are related to hepatitis C. See also ***Hepatitis, Neonatal.***

**Treatment—Standard** Treatment for acute hepatitis C is symptomatic and supportive. Personal hygiene should be carefully maintained, and blood precautions are appropriate. The Food and Drug Administration has approved interferon alfa-2b (Intron-A) for treatment of non-A, non-B (C) hepatitis and chronic hepatitis B. Liver function returns to near normal, but patients may relapse when therapy ceases.

**Treatment—Investigational** Effective immunization against hepatitis C does not exist at this time. Biogen is sponsoring the development of the orphan product β-interferon (recombinant human) for the treatment of non-A, non-B hepatitis.

Please contact the agencies listed under Resources, below, for the most current information. Addresses and telephone numbers of these agencies, as well as of individual experts and research centers, may be found in the Master Resources List.

**Resources**

**For more information on non-A, non-B hepatitis (hepatitis C):** National Organization for Rare Disorders (NORD); National Sexually Transmitted Diseases Hotline; Centers for Disease Control; American Liver Foundation; Children's Liver Foundation; United Liver Association; NIH/National Institute of Allergy and Infectious Diseases; American Social Health Association; Council for Sex Information and Education.

**References**

Recombinant Interferon Alfa Therapy for Chronic Hepatitis C: A Randomized, Double-Blind, Placebo Controlled Trial: Di Bisceglie, M. Adrian, et al.; N. Engl. J. Med., 1989, vol. 321(2), pp. 1406–1410.

Treatment of Chronic Hepatitis C with Recombinant Interferon Alfa: A Multicenter Randomized, Controlled Trial: G.L. Davis, et al.; N. Engl. J. Med., 1989, vol. 321(221), pp. 1501–1506.

Hepatitis in Clinical Practice: D.K. Sarver; Postgrad. Med., 1986, vol. 79(4), pp. 229–230.

Non-A, Non-B Hepatitis: An Update: J.A. Hellings; Vox Sang., 1986, vol. 51(suppl. 1), pp. 63–66.

Non-A, Non-B Hepatitis: Evolving Epidemiologic and Clinical Perspective: J.L. Dienstag, et al.; Semin. Liver Dis., 1986, vol. 6(1), pp. 67–81.

Weighing the Risks of the Raw Bar: C. Ballantine; FDA Consumer, 1986, vol. 90(1), pp. 150–157.

# JOB SYNDROME

**Description** Job syndrome is a congenital disorder of the immune system characterized by cold staphylococcal abscesses and granulocyte chemotactic defect.

**Synonyms**

HIE Syndrome

Hyper-IgE Syndrome
Hyperimmunoglobulin E–Recurrent Infection Syndrome
Hyperimmunoglobulin E Syndrome
Hyperimmunoglobulinemia E–Staphylococcal Abscess Syndrome
Job-Buckley Syndrome

**Signs and Symptoms** The primary symptoms of Job syndrome are cold staphylococcal abscesses of the skin and also of the mastoid, joints, gums, bronchi, and lung; granulocyte chemotactic defect; chronic eczema; hyperimmunoglobulinemia E; and mild eosinophilia. Secondary symptoms include mucocutaneous candidiasis; coarse facial features (broad nasal bridge, prominent nose, and irregularly proportioned cheeks and jaws); fair skin; and reddish hair.

**Etiology** Job syndrome is thought to be inherited as an autosomal recessive trait.

**Epidemiology** Job syndrome affects males and females in equal numbers. Symptoms of this disorder are present at birth or in early childhood.

**Related Disorders** See *Granulomatous Disease, Chronic; Wiskott-Aldrich Syndrome.*

**Treatment—Standard** The most effective treatment for Job syndrome is antibiotics. Trimethoprim/sulfamethoxazole is given continuously or intermittently, depending on the longevity of the infections. Patients often experience repeated infections.

For treatment of chronic mucocutaneous candidiasis, amphotericin B, nystatin, clotrimazole, miconizole, or 5-fluorocytosine are beneficial. Antifungal and immune system–stimulating substances, such as transfer factor, thymosin, thymus epithelial cell transplantation, and levamisole, are also useful.

Genetic counseling may be of benefit for patients and their families.

Other treatment is symptomatic and supportive.

**Treatment—Investigational** The effects of interferon gamma on excessive immunoglobulin E production in patients with Job syndrome (HIE-hyperimmunoglobulinemia E) are being studied. Long-term safety and effectiveness of this treatment is still under investigation.

Please contact the agencies listed under Resources, below, for the most current information. Addresses and telephone numbers of these agencies, as well as of individual experts and research centers, may be found in the Master Resources List.

**Resources**

**For more information on Job syndrome:** National Organization for Rare Disorders (NORD); Immune Deficiency Foundation; NIH/National Institute of Allergy and Infectious Diseases.

**For genetic information and genetic counseling referrals:** March of Dimes Birth Defects Foundation; Alliance of Genetic Support Groups.

**References**

Use of Recombinant Human Interferon Gamma to Enhance Neutrophil Chemotactic Responses in Job Syndrome of Hyperimmunoglobulinemia E and Recurrent Infections: J.D. Jeppson, et al.; J. Pediatr., March 1991, vol. 118(3), pp. 383–387.

Clinical Dermatology, 2nd ed.; T.P. Habif, ed.; C.V. Mosby Company, 1990, pp. 200–201.

Hematology, 4th ed.: W. J. Williams, et al., eds.; McGraw-Hill, 1990, pp. 823, 826.

The Hyperimmunoglobulinemia E and Recurrent Infections Syndrome in the Adult: J.P. L'Huillier, et al.; Thorax, September 1990, vol. 45(9), pp. 707–708.

Mendelian Inheritance in Man, 9th ed.: V.A. McKusik; The Johns Hopkins University Press, 1990, pp. 1281–1282.

Regulation of Immunoglobulin Production in Hyperimmunoglobulin E Recurrent Infection Syndrome by Interferon Gamma: C.L. King, et al.; Proc. Natl. Acad. Sci. USA, December 1989, vol. 86(24), pp. 10085–10089.

# LEPROSY

**Description** Leprosy is a progressive, chronic infection caused by *Mycobacterium leprae.* It affects the peripheral nerves, skin, mucous membranes, and eyes. In severe cases, sensory loss, disfigurement, and blindness may result. Leprosy occurs in several forms: tuberculoid (minor and major; benign Hansen disease); lepromatous (malignant Hansen disease); dimorphous (borderline leprosy); and indeterminate leprosy.

**Synonyms**

Elephantiasis Graecorum
Hansen Disease
Lepra

**Signs and Symptoms** Leprosy is a slowly progressive disease that involves the nerves and skin of the face, hands, lower legs, and feet. Symptoms of nerve involvement include paresthesias, anesthesia, weakness, paralysis, and muscular atrophy. Nerve lesions tend to occur in the skin and along the nerve trunks. Skin lesions include macules, plaques (which may be erythematous or hypopigmented), papules, and nodules.

Leprosy is classified into the subtypes **lepromatous** and **tuberculoid,** and **intermediate subtypes** between these two. The most limited subtype is the tuberculoid, which is manifested by large plaques that are anesthetic, dry, and hairless. The intermediate or borderline subtype is characterized by more numerous skin lesions but less sensory loss. Patients with intermediate or borderline disease tend to progress toward either the tuberculoid or the lepromatous form over time.

Lepromatous disease also has less severe sensory loss, but both skin and nerve involvement are more extensive and invasive. Nodular skin lesions are characteristic of this subtype. Complications, with eye involvement and deformities of the face, hands, and feet, may occur. Facial deformities are a direct result of mycobacterial destruction of the nasal septum, cartilage, and other facial tissues. In addition, the eyebrows and eyelashes are usually lost, and the earlobes enlarge. In the hands and feet, deformities result from repeated trauma sustained in the face of sensory loss.

Ocular complications include conjunctivitis, keratitis, and iridocyclitis that may lead to cataract formation. Corneal anesthesia, due to trigeminal nerve involvement, may lead to inadvertent corneal injury and blindness.

Another serious complication of lepromatous leprosy is erythema nodosum leprosum **(ENL).** This is a syndrome of high fever, necrosis of skin nodules, and a painful neuritis. This may be associated with polyarthralgias and glomerulonephritis.

Some patients with intermediate or tuberculoid leprosy experience a worsening of disease while on therapy (reversal reaction). Pathologically, this appears to be a local immune reaction. Clinically, the lesions become indurated and may ulcerate, and associated neurologic symptoms may deteriorate.

Amyloidosis is a complication of leprosy, although its prevalence varies from one geographic region to another.

The pathologic lesion of leprosy is the granuloma. These may be seen in the dermis, lymph nodes, liver, and spleen. The diagnosis is made on skin biopsy, and it is important to examine a fairly large specimen in order to be certain of the diagnosis. An excisional biopsy is preferred over a punch biopsy.

**Etiology** Leprosy is caused by the bacterium *Mycobacterium leprae.* This is an acid-fast bacillus that grows only in vivo.

**Epidemiology** The mode of transmission is not clear. Spread may be by direct skin contact, or by inhalation, but prolonged exposure is usually necessary. Breast feeding and vector transmission by insects have also been implicated.

Worldwide, 12 million to 15 million people are affected. Children are more susceptible. Leprosy is a major problem in tropical regions of Asia, Africa, and South America, and is also prevalent in some islands of the South Pacific. In the United States, native leprosy occurs in the south (i.e., around the Gulf of Mexico), but the majority of cases are imported. North American Indians appear to be immune.

The incidence of leprosy is currently rising in the United States, a result of large waves of immigrants from endemic regions, particularly Southeast Asia. The exact incidence is unknown, since many patients may not seek or have access to health care.

**Related Disorders** Symptoms of the following disorders can be similar to those of leprosy. Comparisons may be useful for a differential diagnosis.

**Lupus miliaris disseminatus faciei** is a chronic skin infection caused by *Mycobacterium tuberculosis.* It is characterized by soft, brownish-red papules that may appear singularly or in clusters. The face, neck, mouth, and nose may be involved. Healing is slow, and scarring is common.

**Lupus vulgaris,** another cutaneous form of tuberculosis, is a progressive infection that may cause scarring and deformities of the face. The lesions are small, soft, yellowish-brown tubercles and crusted ulcers. Lupus vulgaris is more common in children and young adults.

See also *Mycosis Fungoides; Lymphocytic Infiltrate of Jessner.*

**Treatment—Standard** The treatment of leprosy may include the use of dapsone, rifampin, ethionamide, and the orphan drug clofazimine (Lamprene). Combination therapy is currently recommended. A typical regimen would include dapsone, rifampin, and clofazimine. Therapy must be continued for 2 years in all cases, and longer in some. Reversal reactions and ENL are treated with steroids.

Corneal dryness is treated with eye drops and ophthalmic mucin substitutes. Ocular complications of ENL must be treated promptly to prevent permanent damage to the eyes. Local atropine and hydrocortisone may be used to keep the pupils dilated and reduce the inflammation until the reaction subsides. Supportive care is important. Anesthetic areas (eyes and limbs) must be protected from injury and infection.

**Treatment—Investigational** Solasulphone, acedapsone, and fluoroquinolones such as ofloxacin are currently under investigation. Vaccines are also being studied. Progress is hampered by the inability to culture the organism in vitro.

Thalidomide (Pediatric Pharmaceuticals) is being tested for use in treatment of leprosy except in women of childbearing age, because of the possibility of serious birth defects. Vaccines from armadillos and monkeys are also under investigation.

Please contact the agencies listed under Resources, below, for the most current information. Addresses and tele-

phone numbers of these agencies, as well as of individual experts and research centers, may be found in the Master Resources List.

**Resources**

**For more information on leprosy:** National Organization for Rare Disorders (NORD); National Hansen Disease Center; NIH/National Institute of Allergy and Infectious Diseases; Centers for Disease Control.

**References**

Cecil Textbook of Medicine, 19th ed.: J.B. Wyngaarden, et al., eds.; W.B. Saunders Company, 1992, pp. 1745–1751.

Leprosy: W.M. Meyers; Dermatol. Clin., January 1992, vol. 10(1), pp. 73–96.

Clofazimine: A Review of Its Use in Leprosy and Mycobacterium Avium Complex Infection: J.C. Garrelts; DICP, May 1991, vol. 25(5), p. 5.

Inside the Skin: The Local Immune and Inflammatory Milieu in Leprosy: D.M. Scollard; Am. J. Trop. Med. Hyg., April 1991, vol. 44(4.2), pp. 17–23.

Internal Medicine, 3rd ed.: J.H. Stein, ed.-in-chief; Little, Brown and Company, 1990, pp. 1552–1556.

Principles of Neurology, 4th ed.; R.D. Adams and M. Victor, eds.; McGraw-Hill, 1989, p. 1054.

# LEPTOSPIROSIS

**Description** Leptospirosis is an acute systemic disease of domestic and wild animals that is caused by spirochetes of the genus *Leptospira*. Human leptospirosis is rare. The disease usually occurs in 2 stages: the 1st, a leptospiremic phase with flulike symptoms; and the 2nd, a widespread vasculitis thought to be of immune etiology. The most severe form of leptospirosis is referred to as **Weil Syndrome.**

**Synonyms**

>Canefield Fever
>Canicola Fever
>Field Fever
>Mud Fever
>Seven-Day Fever
>Spirochetosis
>Swineherd Disease

**Signs and Symptoms** Leptospirosis is characteristically a biphasic illness. The first phase begins after an incubation period of 2 to 20 days, with fever, severe headache, myalgias, chills, coughing, chest pain, and gastrointestinal symptoms, including nausea, vomiting, and abdominal pain. The symptoms last a week or less and then abate. After an afebrile period of 1 to 2 days, the 2nd phase begins, with severe headache, myalgias, nausea, vomiting, and abdominal pain. In severe cases there is jaundice, hepatic and renal dysfunction, and vascular collapse; this is called Weil syndrome (see **Weil Syndrome).**

Physical examination frequently reveals signs of meningitis, hepatosplenomegaly, muscle tenderness, and conjunctival hemorrhage. Except in severe cases, fever is minimal. Rashes and uveitis may also be seen. The cerebrospinal fluid generally shows a pleocytosis, normal glucose, and elevated protein levels. The bacteria cannot be isolated from either blood or cerebrospinal fluid; at this stage, however, antibodies appear in the serum. The diagnosis of leptospirosis is usually made by serology. Agglutination tests, and an enzyme-linked immunosorbent assay **(ELISA)** are available for diagnosis. The spirochetes may be found in the blood and cerebrospinal fluid, but only in the early phase of illness. They may also be found in the urine for up to a month.

**Etiology** Leptospirosis is caused by spirochetes of the genus *Leptospira.* There is one species, *L. interrogans,* that has several serotypes.

**Epidemiology** Leptospirosis is distributed worldwide. It is primarily a disease of animals. In the United States, dogs, cats, livestock, and rodents are the usual sources of human infection. Infected animals may pass leptospira in the urine for many months, which can contaminate soil and water.

Approximately 75 percent of cases occur in young men and may be related to occupational or recreational transmission (e.g., swimming in contaminated water). At particular risk are farmers, veterinarians, and abattoir and sewer workers.

Leptospirosis may occur in people of all ages. Breaks in the skin and exposed mucous membranes (such as the conjunctiva, nose, or mouth) are the usual portals of entry.

**Related Disorders Aseptic meningitis** may be caused by a variety of viruses.

See **Weil Syndrome,** a severe icteric form of leptospirosis that appears to be due to extensive vasculitis.

**Treatment—Standard** The treatment of leptospirosis is doxycycline, intravenous penicillin, or ampicillin, but this must be started by the 4th day of illness if it is to have any effect. Mild cases may be treated with tetracycline, which has the added advantage of eradicating the bacteria in the urine, which the penicillins do not. Intensive supportive care, including ventilatory assistance, dialysis, and other measures may be required in severe cases.

A vaccine is available for domestic animals, but it is not very effective.

**Treatment—Investigational** Please contact the organizations listed under Resources, below, for the most current information. Addresses and telephone numbers of these agencies, as well as of individual experts and research centers, may be found in the Master Resources List.

**Resources**

**For more information on leptospirosis:** National Organization for Rare Disorders (NORD); Centers for Disease Control; NIH/National Institute of Allergy and Infectious Diseases.

**References**

Leptospiral Exposure in Detroit Rodent Control Workers: R.Y. Demers; Am. J. Pub. Health, 1985, vol. 75(9), pp. 1090–1091.

# LISTERIOSIS

**Description** Listeriosis is an infection caused by *Listeria monocytogenes.* This organism produces several different clinical syndromes, depending on various host factors. In pregnant women, and probably in other immunocompetent hosts, asymptomatic infection, or mild nonspecific illness occurs. Transplacental transmission is associated with a severe disseminated disease known as granulomatosis infantiseptica. Two additional *Listeria* syndromes, primary *Listeria* sepsis and meningoencephalitis, occur in immunosuppressed adults and in neonates. Focal infections with *L. monocytogenes* have also been reported, but these are very rare.

**Signs and Symptoms** The majority of listeria infections are mild. The major disease syndromes of listeriosis will be described individually here.

**Listeriosis of pregnancy** may be asymptomatic or may be marked only by a fever and back pain. It is most common in the last trimester, when it may be mistaken for pyelonephritis. The diagnosis can be confirmed by blood culture. If untreated, the fetus is at risk for developing granulomatous infantiseptica.

**Granulomatous infantiseptica** is a fetal listeria infection that results from transplacental transmission. This form of listeriosis is characterized by widespread abscesses and granulomas, usually involving the liver, spleen, kidneys, lungs, skin, eyes, and brain. Such infants should be extensively cultured, including lumbar puncture, and treated immediately, but even with treatment the prognosis is poor.

**Listeria sepsis** may occur in infants infected during vaginal delivery or postnatally, and in immunosuppressed adults. Such patients show all the signs of bacterial sepsis, and shock may intervene. There are no focal signs and few clues as to the exact nature of the illness. Blood cultures confirm the diagnosis.

**Listeria meningoencephalitis** can occur in immunosuppressed patients or newborns. Predisposing factors include cirrhosis, malignancy, and organ transplantation, and cases also occur in immunocompetent individuals. Unlike most cases of bacterial meningoencephalitis, listeria often presents in a subtle or subacute fashion, with anorexia, lethargy, behavioral changes, and/or low-grade fever. Focal neurologic signs, such as cranial nerve palsies, may be present, as well as other signs of meningitis and encephalitis. The cerebrospinal fluid shows variable abnormalities. The organism may not be seen on a Gram stain, which may be misleading, but cultures are diagnostic.

**Localized listeria infection** may follow direct contact with *L. monocytogenes* on the skin or conjunctiva. Other cases may result from the bacteremia. In these cases, arthritis, osteomyelitis, endocarditis, or peritonitis may occur.

**Etiology** Listeriosis is caused by *Listeria monocytogenes,* a gram-positive, aerobic bacillus.

**Epidemiology** *L. moncytogenes* appears to be ubiquitous. It is found worldwide in soil, water, and dust, and in the meat of many wild and domestic animals. It has also been isolated from the feces of normal humans, and it has been cultured from the vagina and the urethra.

Several epidemics have been traced to ingestion of contaminated food products, such as improperly pasteurized milk, cheese, unwashed vegetables, and raw meat. An epidemic in California in 1985 affected nearly 200 persons and was attributed to contaminated cheese manufactured in Mexico. Other cases have been transmitted through contact with other infected persons or animals, but most patients have no history of such contact.

Listeriosis occurs most often in the summer months. According to the Centers for Disease Control, approximately 1,850 cases are reported annually in the United States, of which 425 are fatal.

**Related Disorders** Listeria sepsis resembles gram-negative sepsis. Similarly, listeria meningoencephalitis is usually clinically indistinguishable from other types of meningitis or encephalitis. (See also Signs and Symptoms, above.)

**Treatment—Standard** The treatment of choice for listeriosis usually includes high-dose intravenous penicillin G, or ampicillin with or without an aminoglycoside. Alternative drugs include trimethoprim/sulfamethoxazole, tetracycline, erythromycin, or chloramphenicol. Supportive therapy is important in severe cases.

**Treatment—Investigational** DNA probes that can detect the presence of *L. monocytogenes* in food samples are currently under investigation. This technique is much faster than conventional culture techniques, and may be useful in controlling food-borne outbreaks of listeriosis. New pasteurization procedures to eliminate the presence of *L. monocytogenes* in milk and milk products are also under study.

Please contact the agencies listed under Resources, below, for the most current information. Addresses and telephone numbers of these agencies, as well as of individual experts and research centers, may be found in the Master Resources List.

**Resources**

**For more information on listeriosis:** National Organization for Rare Disorders (NORD); NIH/National Institute of Allergy and Infectious Diseases; Centers for Disease Control; Food and Drug Administration.

**References**

Listeria: Battling Back Against One 'Tough Bug': K.J. Skinner; FDA Consumer, July–August 1988, pp. 12–15.

Clinical Manifestations of Epidemic Neonatal Listeriosis: A.J. Teberg, et al.; Pediatr. Infect. Dis. J., September 1987, vol. 6(9), pp. 817–820.

Perinatal Listeriosis (Early-Onset): Correlation of Antenatal Manifestations and Neonatal Outcome: M. Boucher, et al.; Obstet. Gynecol., 1986, vol. 68(5), pp. 593–597.

# MENINGITIS, MENINGOCOCCAL

**Description** Meningococcal meningitis is caused by *Neisseria meningitidis*. It can be either acute or subacute and is characterized by inflammation of the meninges. Early signs are respiratory illness or a sore throat. Skin rash occurs in about half of all patients.

**Synonyms**

      Bacterial Meningococcal Meningitis

      Epidemic Cerebrospinal Meningitis

**Signs and Symptoms** In its acute form, meningococcal meningitis progresses more rapidly than any other bacterial meningitis. It is often preceded by a sore throat or a respiratory illness and is quickly followed or accompanied by fever, a stiff neck, headache, and vomiting. *Adults may become seriously ill within hours, and children, even sooner.*

A central nervous system disorder, meningococcal meningitis is 1 of the 3 most common types of bacterial meningitis. Symptoms among older children and adults may progress from irritability to confusion, drowsiness, and stupor, sometimes leading to coma. Skin rashes of a petechial or purpuric nature occur in about half of all patients. Cerebral edema, ventriculitis, or hydrocephalus may also occur. Other symptoms include chills, sweating, weakness, loss of appetite, myalgia of the lower back or legs, or photophobia. Dehydration often occurs, and vascular collapse may lead to shock (Waterhouse-Friderichsen syndrome) when the meningococcal infection becomes septicemic and the adrenal glands become hemorrhagic and necrotic. Later symptoms include hemiparesis, hearing loss, or other neurologic abnormalities.

The course of meningococcal meningitis is less predictable among infants between 3 months and 2 years of age. Fever, refusal to feed, vomiting, irritability, and convulsions usually occur. A high-pitched cry and a fontanel bulge may be present. Subdural effusions may occur after several days. A brain abscess or subdural pus accumulation may also occur. Hydrocephalus, deafness, and slowed mental and physical development are possible consequences of meningitis. Since the incidence of most types of meningitis is highest among this age group, any unexplained fever needs to be closely watched.

**Etiology** Meningococcal meningitis is caused by the bacteria *Neisseria meningitidis;* serogroups A, B, C, and Y are responsible for most meningococcal diseases.

**Epidemiology** Meningococcal meningitis primarily affects infants, children, and young adults. Males are affected slightly more than females. Between 1984 and 1986, 2,400 to 2,700 cases of meningococcal infection were reported annually in the United States, where most cases seem to occur in the winter or spring and involve infants and military recruits infected with serogroup B.

**Related Disorders** See *Rocky Mountain Spotted Fever.*

**Encephalitis** is an acute inflammatory disorder, usually of viral origin. Symptoms include headache, drowsiness, hyperactivity, and general malaise. Some symptoms mimic those of meningitis, such as a stiff neck, altered reflexes, confusion, speech disorders, convulsions, paralysis and coma.

**Treatment—Standard** Diagnosis is made by examination of the cerebrospinal fluid. Testing for meningococcal meningitis also includes CT scans or magnetic resonance imaging. Blood and/or skin cultures may be performed.

Penicillin G, ampicillin, or ceftriaxone are usually the drugs of choice. Alternative drugs include chloramphenicol, cefuroxime, cefotaxime, or ceftizoxime. Family members of those infected can be treated prophylactically with rifampin; however, for pregnant women, ceftriaxone is recommended.

Epidemics caused by serogroups A, C, Y, or W135 among military personnel and students in dormitories can be controlled with vaccines.

**Treatment—Investigational** Please contact the agencies listed under Resources, below, for the most current information. Addresses and telephone numbers of these agencies, as well as of individual experts and research centers, may be found in the Master Resources List.

**Resources**

**For more information on meningococcal meningitis**: National Organization for Rare Disorders (NORD); NIH/National Institute of Allergy and Infectious Diseases; Centers for Disease Control.

**References**

Bacterial Meningitis in Older Children: W.A. Bonadio, et al.; Am. J. Dis. Child, April 1990, vol. 144(4), pp. 463–465.

Gd-DTPA-Enhanced MR Imaging of the Brain in Patients with Meningitis: Comparison with CT: K.H. Chang, et al.; AJR Am. J. Roentgenol., April 1990, vol. 154(4), pp. 809–816.

Cecil Textbook of Medicine, 18th ed.: J.B. Wyngaarden and L.H. Smith, Jr., eds.; W.B. Saunders Company, 1988, pp. 65, 1604–1621.

Ceftriaxone Alone Compared to Ampicillin and Chloramphenicol in the Treatment of Bacterial Meningitis: N.I. Girgis; Chemotherapy, 1988, vol. 34(suppl. 1), pp. 16–20.

Control of an Outbreak of Group C Meningococcal Meningitis with a Polysaccharide Vaccine: R.G. Masterton, et al.; J. Infect., September 1988, vol. 17(2), pp. 177–182.

Internal Medicine, 2nd ed.: J.H. Stein, ed.-in-chief; Little, Brown and Company, 1987, pp. 1494–1502, 1666–1669.

# MENINGITIS, TUBERCULOUS

**Description** Tuberculous meningitis is a subacute disorder of the central nervous system caused by *Mycobacterium tuberculosis*.

**Signs and Symptoms** Headaches and behavioral changes often dominate the onset. Other clinical findings include fever, headache, a stiff neck, and vomiting. Symptoms among older children and adults progress from irritability to confusion, drowsiness, and stupor, and may lead to coma.

Diagnosis is confirmed upon examination of the cerebrospinal fluid. Testing for tuberculous meningitis also includes chest x-rays, CT scans, and magnetic resonance imaging. Untreated, this disorder can lead to seizures, communicating hydrocephalus, deafness, mental retardation, hemiparesis, other neurologic abnormalities, and death.

**Etiology** Tuberculous meningitis occurs as a result of exposure to *Mycobacterium tuberculosis*.

**Epidemiology** Tuberculous meningitis is a rare complication of tuberculosis, especially miliary tuberculosis. It also occurs in individuals who were infected with *Mycobacterium tuberculosis*. It is usually found in children aged 1 to 5, although it may occur at any age.

**Related Disorders** Meningitis in general is characterized by inflammation of the meninges and is a result of bacterial, viral, or fungal infection; malignant tumor; or reaction to certain spinal injections.

**Encephalitis** is an acute inflammatory disorder, usually of viral origin. Symptoms include headache, drowsiness, hyperactivity, and general malaise. Some symptoms mimic those of meningitis, such as stiff neck, altered reflexes, confusion, speech disorders, convulsions, paralysis, and coma.

**Treatment—Standard** Meningitis is usually treated with antibiotics such as isoniazid, rifampin, streptomycin, and ethambutol for at least 9 months to 1 year. Recently, some strains of the organism have been found to be resistant to 5 or more of the antimicrobials used in treatment. Corticosteroid drugs such as prednisone may be of benefit when the patient is receiving effective chemotherapy.

**Treatment—Investigational** Please contact the agencies listed under Resources, below, for the most current information. Addresses and telephone numbers of these agencies, as well as of individual experts and research centers, may be found in the Master Resources List.

**Resources**

**For more information on tuberculous meningitis**: National Organization for Rare Disorders (NORD); The Arc (a national organization on mental retardation); NIH/National Institute of Allergy and Infectious Diseases; Centers for Disease Control.

**References**

Gd-DTPA-Enhanced MR Imaging of the Brain in Patients with Meningitis: Comparison with CT: K.H. Chang, et al.; AJR Am. J. Roentgenol., April 1990, vol. 154(4), pp. 809–816.

Tuberculous Meningitis in Children: Treatment with Isoniazid and Rifampicin for Twelve Months: P. Visudhiphan, et al.; J. Pediatr., May 1989; vol. 114(5), pp. 875–879.

Cecil Textbook of Medicine, 18th ed.: J.B. Wyngaarden and L.H. Smith, Jr., eds.; W.B. Saunders Company, 1988, pp. 1497, 1502.

Internal Medicine, 2nd ed.: J.H. Stein, ed.-in-chief; Little, Brown and Company, 1987, pp. 1497, 1502.

# MENINGOCOCCEMIA

**Description** Meningococcemia is an acute infection caused by *Neisseria meningitidis*. Some patients experience a chronic or subacute illness that waxes and wanes. Although rare, epidemics of the disease have occurred. Major symptoms include upper respiratory tract infection, fever, skin rash and lesions, eye and ear problems, and possibly shock.

**Synonyms**

> Meningococcal Disease
>
> Meningococcemia Meningitis

**Signs and Symptoms** Meningococcemia is characterized by sudden, intense headache; nausea; fever; vomiting; skin rash; and, in cases associated with meningitis, stiff neck. Initial complaint of an upper respiratory infection is quickly followed by chills, a skin rash on the arms or legs and trunk, and possibly diarrhea. The rash may become widespread or develop into petechiae, ecchymoses, or purpura. There may be associated swelling, myalgia, skin deterioration, or gangrene in the arms and legs. In the immunosuppressed patient, pneumonia may also develop.

In cases where meningitis accompanies meningococcemia, the patient may manifest the above symptoms along with headache, confusion, stiff neck, and muscle pain from meningismus.

**Fulminant meningococcemia,** or **Waterhouse-Friderichsen syndrome,** is the most severe form of the disorder. Onset is sudden and the progression rapid. In less than a few hours, the patient has very high fever, chills, weakness, vomiting, and severe headache. A red rash appears on the arms and legs and quickly spreads over the entire body, including the eyes and nose. Both blood pressure and fever may drop dramatically. The patient may go into shock. *Without immediate medical treatment this disorder can be life-threatening.*

**Chronic meningococcemia** is a rarer form of the disease characterized by fever, muscle and joint pain with headache, as well as a skin rash, all of which occur intermittently over a period of weeks or months. Some patients experience splenomegaly.

**Etiology** Meningococcemia is caused by infection with the bacteria *Neisseria meningitidis,* which are gram-negative diplococci bacteria. The disease varies according to the strain responsible: A, B, C, D, X, Y, Z, 29E, or W135. The bacteria reside in either the nose or throat and are transmitted by inhalation or close contact. The carrier may spread the infection for weeks or months if not diagnosed and treated.

**Epidemiology** Meningococcemia affects males and females equally. Most cases develop in persons 20 years of age or younger, and half of these are in children under 5. In the United States, 1.2 cases per 100,000 occur annually. Winter and spring are the most common seasons during which cases are reported. Epidemics occur under crowded conditions and at 20- to 30-year intervals. In other parts of the world, epidemics are usually caused by the group A strain of the bacteria. During epidemics, rates of 5 to 24 cases per 100,000 persons have occurred. In Sao Paulo, Brazil, the epidemic rate in 1974 was 370 per 100,000 persons infected with meningococcemia. In the United States, the most prevalent group strains of the bacteria are B, C, Y, and W-135.

**Related Disorders** See *Rocky Mountain Spotted Fever; Purpura, Shoenlein-Henoch; Rheumatic Fever; Toxic Shock Syndrome.*

**Acute infective endocarditis** usually has a very sudden onset. Lower back pain, arthralgia, or myalgia are common in the early stages of the disease, and occasionally they are the only initial symptoms. Fever, night sweats, chills, headache, and loss of appetite may also occur. Hematuria, petechiae of the upper trunk, and pale, oval spots on the retina are common.

**Treatment—Standard** Penicillin, ampicillin, and ceftriaxone are the usual drugs of choice in treating meningococcemia. In adults penicillin G is administered intravenously. In children, however, other organisms must be ruled out before treatment is begun. For patients unable to take penicillin, antibiotics such as cefuroxime, cefotaxime, or ceftriaxone are indicated.

In patients who survive severe meningococcal septicemia, venous and arterial problems may be ongoing. Serious orthopedic problems may develop. If gangrene occurs, amputation may be required.

During epidemics, chemoprophylaxis in the form of rifampin, ciprofloxacin, or ceftriaxone has been shown to be effective in protecting exposed persons against meningococcemia.

**Treatment—Investigational** To prevent and treat purpura fulminans in meningococcemia, Immuno Clinical Research Corporation has developed a new orphan product called protein C concentrate (human) vapor heated, immuno.

Please contact the agencies listed under Resources, below, for the most current information. Addresses and telephone numbers of these agencies, as well as of individual experts and research centers, may be found in the Master Resources List.

**Resources**

**For more information on meningococcemia:** National Organization for Rare Disorders (NORD); NIH/National Institute of Allergy and Infectious Diseases; Centers for Disease Control.

**References**

Cecil Textbook of Medicine, 19th ed.: James B. Wyngaarden, et al., eds.; W.B. Saunders Company, 1992, pp. 1611–1617.

Clinical Dermatology, 2nd ed.; T.P. Habif, ed.: C.V. Mosby Company, 1990, pp. 210–211.

Chondro-Osseous Growth Abnormalities After Meningococcemia: A Clinical and Histopathological Study: D.P. Grogan, et al.; J. Bone Joint Surg. Am., July 1989, vol. 71(6), pp. 920–928.

# Mesenteritis, Retractile

**Description** Retractile mesenteritis (mesenteric panniculitis) is a poorly understood inflammatory disorder of the mesentery. It appears to begin with lipodystrophy in the mesenteric fat, and then progresses to inflammation and marked fibrosis. The major symptoms include abdominal pain, nausea, vomiting, and fever, and the major complication is intestinal obstruction.

**Synonyms**

> Mesenteric Panniculitis
> Nodular Mesenteritis
> Nonspecific Sclerosing Mesenteritis
> Sclerosing Panniculitis

**Signs and Symptoms** The onset of retractile mesenteritis is characterized by malaise, fever, vague abdominal pain, nausea, vomiting, and weight loss. As the inflammation progresses, the mesentery becomes thickened and may distort and retract the intestines, which eventually may lead to obstruction of the lymphatics, veins, or the intestines themselves. Ultimately, malabsorption, steatorrhea, ascites, and symptoms of partial or complete intestinal obstruction complicate the picture.

The diagnosis of retractile mesenteritis is usually made at laparotomy, and biopsy is confirmatory.

**Etiology** The exact cause of retractile mesenteritis is not known.

The mesentery initially develops lipodystrophy, then becomes infiltrated with inflammatory cells. Fibrosis, scarring, and calcifications follow. The initial insult may be infectious, vascular, or related to another underlying process.

**Epidemiology** Retractile mesenteritis is more common in the elderly, and in men.

**Related Disorders** See *Weber-Christian Disease,* which is characterized by fever and the development of subcutaneous nodules. The pathology of these nodules is similar to that found in the mesentery in retractile mesenteritis, and for this reason, retractile mesenteritis is also called mesenteric Weber-Christian disease. However, Weber-Christian disease has a different epidemiology; it usually affects young adult women.

**Treatment—Standard** The treatment of retractile mesenteritis most often consists of prednisone and immunosuppressants such as azathioprine. Surgery is usually necessary for complete intestinal obstruction. Other treatment is symptomatic and supportive.

**Treatment—Investigational** Please contact the agencies listed under Resources, below, for the most current information. Addresses and telephone numbers of these agencies, as well as of individual experts and research centers, may be found in the Master Resources List.

**Resources**

**For more information on retractile mesenteritis:** National Organization for Rare Disorders (NORD); NIH/National Digestive Diseases Information Clearinghouse.

**References**

Retractile Mesenteritis Involving the Colon: Barium Enema, Sonographic, and CT Findings: F.J. Perez-Fontan, et al.; AJR, 1986, vol. 147(5), pp. 937–940.

Sclerosing Mesenteritis: Response to Cyclophosphamide: R.W. Bush, et al.; Arch. Intern. Med., 1986, vol. 146(3), pp. 503–505.

Successful Treatment of a Patient with Retractile Mesenteritis with Prednisone and Azathioprine: G.N. Tytgat, et al.; Gastroenterology, 1980, vol. 79(2), pp. 352–356.

# Neutropenia, Chronic

**Description** Chronic neutropenia is a blood disorder in which bone marrow does not produce adequate numbers of granulocytic white blood cells (neutrophils), which causes susceptibility to fungal and bacterial infections. Chronic neutropenia can last for months or years. It affects both children and adults.

**Signs and Symptoms** Symptoms vary greatly depending on the level of neutrophils in the bone marrow. In general, the fewer the neutrophils, the more susceptible is the patient to infection. Common characteristics include normal or nearly normal counts of lymphocytes, erythrocytes, reticulocytes, and platelets. The levels of monocytes and immunoglobulin are elevated or normal. There is no apparent cause for the neutropenia. There may be an increase in the ratio of immature cells to mature cells, indicating an imbalance in cellular regeneration.

Fever, splenomegaly, and infection may be present. However, if diagnosed very early, patients may be treated before infections occur. Inflammation of the gums, pneumonia, and lung abscesses are characteristic of chronic neutropenia. In rare cases, chronic neutropenia may develop into aplastic anemia or leukemia.

Subtypes of chronic neutropenia include **familial neutropenia, chronic benign neutropenia,** and **familial benign neutropenia** in children. The adult form of this disorder is referred to as **chronic idiopathic neutropenia.**

**Etiology** Chronic neutropenia is the result of impaired production of blood cells in the bone marrow. The cause is often unknown, but some cases are due to drug therapy. Some drugs may cause chronic neutropenia as a side effect, while other drugs cause neutropenia in a way that is not related to the dosage or duration.

Familial neutropenia and familial benign neutropenia are both thought to be inherited as autosomal dominant traits.

Chronic benign neutropenia (in children) usually has no family history, so it does not appear to be genetic.

Chronic idiopathic neutropenia is usually found in adults, having lain dormant since childhood.

**Epidemiology** Chronic neutropenia affects males and females equally. Both children and adults are affected. The most severe cases tend to occur during adulthood.

**Related Disorders** See *Chronic Granulomatous Disease; Myelofibrosis-Osteosclerosis.*

**Vitamin B12 deficiency** causes changes in the blood and the central nervous system. Symptoms are delayed and include anemia, splenomegaly and hepatomegaly, anorexia, intermittent constipation and diarrhea, and abdominal pain. The first symptom is usually a burning sensation in the mouth.

**Treatment—Standard** The infections associated with chronic neutropenia are usually managed with antibiotics. Some patients may benefit from glucocorticoids. Intravenous immunoglobulin is usually prescribed to control this disorder. The orphan drug Neupogen (manufactured by Amgen) has been approved by the Food and Drug Administration for use in the treatment of chronic neutropenia.

Genetic counseling may be of benefit for patients and their families if they have the familial type of chronic neutropenia.

**Treatment—Investigational** Colony-stimulating factor is undergoing clinical trials. Granulocyte macrophage colony stimulating factor **(GM-CSF),** a protein derived from bacteria, yeast, and mammalian cells, is being developed by Schering Plough and Sandoz Pharmaceuticals under the brand name Leucomax. Plasmapheresis, whose long-term effectiveness is still under investigation, should be reserved for only the most severe cases of chronic neutropenia.

Please contact the agencies listed under Resources, below, for the most current information. Addresses and telephone numbers of these agencies, as well as of individual experts and research centers, may be found in the Master Resources List.

**Resources**

**For more information on chronic neutropenia:** National Organization for Rare Disorders (NORD); NIH/National Heart, Lung and Blood Institute Information Center.

**For genetic information and genetic counseling referrals:** March of Dimes Birth Defects Foundation; Alliance of Genetic Support Groups.

**References**

Hematology, 4th ed.: W.J. Williams, et al., eds.; McGraw-Hill, 1990, pp. 273, 803, 809–810.

Internal Medicine, 2nd ed.: J.H. Stein, ed.-in-chief; Little, Brown and Company, 1987, pp. 974–975.

Mendelian Inheritance in Man, 8th ed.: V.A. McKusick; The Johns Hopkins University Press, 1986, p. 660.

# NOCARDIOSIS

**Description** Nocardiosis is an infectious disease caused by *Nocardia asteroides,* now classified as a bacterium. This organism typically produces chronic, smoldering infections, most frequently in the lung, though the brain, soft tissues, and many other organs may be involved.

**Signs and Symptoms** Pulmonary infection is the most common form of nocardiosis. Pneumonia, cavitation, and abscess are common presentations. Frequent complications include empyema and extension into the chest wall. In most patients, infection is chronic and dominated by nonspecific symptoms: weight loss, anorexia, weakness, cough, chest pain, and, occasionally, hemoptysis. In the immunocompromised host, the course tends to be more acute.

Hematogenous spread is common, resulting in brain abscesses in about one-third of cases, or, less frequently, abscesses in the kidney, intestines, or other organs. Symptoms associated with brain abscesses may include severe headache and focal neurologic deficits.

Skin abscesses occur in approximately one-third of all cases of nocardiosis. Iliopsoas, ischiorectal, and perirectal abscesses are also relatively common forms of nocardial infection.

Nocardiosis may last from several months to years, but it is not difficult to diagnose. A Gram stain and modified acid-fast stains of pus or sputum are often diagnostic.

**Etiology** Nocardiosis is caused by *Nocardia asteroides*. While it is classified as a bacterium, it is able to grow in filaments like fungi.

**Epidemiology** Nocardiosis occurs worldwide. It is most common in the southern United States and in South America. It is more common in males than in females, and it is increasingly seen in patients with underlying diseases, such as malignancy, chronic obstructive pulmonary disease, cirrhosis, ulcerative colitis, and other chronic diseases. Transplant recipients and patients on steroids and other forms of immunosuppressive therapy are also at risk.

**Related Disorders** The clinical features of nocardiosis may resemble tuberculosis, actinomycosis, and malignancy. See *Tuberculosis.*

The hallmark of **actinomycosis** is the draining sinus. The organism produces small abscesses that spread without regard for anatomic boundaries. Pulmonary and abdominal disease may occur, and chronic smoldering infections are frequent.

**Treatment—Standard** Nocardia organisms are usually resistant to penicillin. Sulfonamides are the drugs of choice for nocardiosis; sulfisoxazole or trimethoprim-sulfamethoxazole are the most commonly used. Minocycline and cycloserine have also been used to treat this infection. Usually treatment must be continued for 6 to 12 months. In addition, surgery is often required to drain abscesses or empyema.

**Treatment—Investigational** Please contact the agencies listed under Resources, below, for the most current information. Addresses and telephone numbers of these agencies, as well as of individual experts and research centers, may be found in the Master Resources List.

**Resources**

**For more information on nocardiosis:** National Organization for Rare Disorders (NORD); American Lung Association; NIH/National Institute of Allergy and Infectious Diseases; Centers for Disease Control.

**References**

Nocardiosis: A Neglected Chronic Lung Disease in Africa: G.G. Baily, et al.; Thorax, 1988, vol. 43(11), pp. 905–910.

Pleuropulmonary Manifestations of Actinomycosis and Nocardiosis: J.E. Heffner; Semin. Respir. Infect., 1988, vol. 3(4), pp. 352–361.

Presumed Intraocular Nocardiosis in a Cardiac-Transplant Patient: N. Mamalis, et al.; Ann. Ophthalmol., 1988, vol. 20(7), pp. 271–273, 276.

# PARACOCCIDIOIDOMYCOSIS (PCM)

**Description** PCM is a chronic, systemic infection caused by the fungus *Paracoccidioides brasiliensis*. The initial infection is in the lungs, but dissemination to the skin, mucous membranes, and reticuloendothelial system is common.

**Synonyms**

> Lutz-Splendore-Almeida Disease
> Paracoccidioidal Granuloma
> South American Blastomycosis

**Signs and Symptoms** After a prolonged incubation period of at least 5 years, patients present with one or more types of disease. Mucocutaneous PCM involves the mouth and nose most frequently, with ulcerative granulomatous lesions.

In pulmonary PCM, the patient commonly notes cough, dyspnea, and chest pain. The chest x-ray may show areas of patchy infiltration. In older patients, fibrosis and emphysema are evident, with progression to cor pulmonale in some cases.

In the lymphatic form of PCM, there is generalized lymphadenopathy, most prominent in the neck. Suppuration may occur, with sinus tract formation.

Other visceral lesions may occur in the liver, spleen, intestines, and adrenals.

The diagnosis is made by examination of infected material. Sputum or pus may be examined with potassium hydroxide and found to reveal the fungus. Biopsy specimens may also be diagnostic. Cultures are confirmatory.

Serologic tests are useful but cannot distinguish between active and past infection. Skin tests are available but are unreliable. Chest x-rays may show infiltration.

**Etiology** The cause of PCM is the dimorphic fungus, *Paracoccidioides brasiliensis*.

**Epidemiology** This disease is largely limited to the state of Sao Paolo in Brazil. Sporadic cases have occurred in other regions of South and Central America. Men between the ages of 20 and 50 are affected about 10 times as frequently as women.

**Related Disorders** PCM may resemble and even coexist with *Tuberculosis.*

**Treatment—Standard** The most effective therapy for PCM is amphotericin B. Sulfonamides have also been used; these halt the progress of the disease but do not eliminate the fungus.

**Treatment—Investigational** Ketoconazole, fluconazole, and itraconazole are currently under investigation for the treatment of PCM and other systemic mycoses. They seem to be as effective as amphotericin B in most reported series.

Studies involving an antigen, Gp43, common to those infected with paracoccidioides brasiliensis are ongoing in an effort to improve diagnostic serologic tests.

Please contact the agencies listed under Resources, below, for the most current information. Addresses and telephone numbers of these agencies, as well as of individual experts and research centers, may be found in the Master Resources List.

**Resources**

**For more information on paracoccidioidomycosis:** National Organization for Rare Disorders (NORD); Centers for Disease Control; NIH/National Institute of Allergy and Infectious Diseases; World Health Organization.

**References**

Factors Associated with Paracoccidioides Brasiliensis Infection Among Permanent Residents of Three Endemic Areas in Colombia: D. Cadavid, et al.; Epidemiol. Infect., August 1993, vol. 111(1), pp. 121–133.

Paracoccidioidomycosis: An Update: E. Brummer, et al.; Clin. Microbiol. Rev., April 1993, vol. 6(2), pp. 89–117.

Recovery of Adrenal Function After Treatment of Paracoccidioidomycosis: A.C. DoValler, et al.; Am. J. Trop. Hyg., May 1993, vol. 48(5), pp. 626–629.

Cecil Textbook of Medicine, 19th ed.: J.B. Wyngaarden, et al., eds.; W.B. Saunders Company, 1992, pp. 1893–1894.

A Pan-American 5-Year Study of Fluconazole Therapy for Deep Mycoses in the Immunocompetent Host: Pan-American Study Group: M. Diaz, et al.; Clin. Infect. Dis., March 1992, vol. 14(suppl. 1), pp. S68–76.

Oral Manifestations of Paracoccidioidomycosis (South American Blastomycosis): O.P. de Almeida, et al.; Oral Surg. Oral Med. Oral Pathol., October 1991, vol. 72(4), pp. 430–435.

Manson's Tropical Diseases, 19th ed.: P.E.C. Manson-Bahr and D.R. Bell; Baillière Tindall, 1987, pp. 708–712.

# PERTUSSIS

**Description** Pertussis is an acute respiratory disease caused by *Bordetella pertussis*. The illness has 3 stages: catarrhal, paroxysmal, and convalescent. The paroxysmal phase is characterized by a cough with an inspiratory whoop, which gives the disease its common name, whooping cough. With widespread use of the DPT (Diphtheria, Pertussis, Tetanus) vaccine, the incidence of pertussis has diminished substantially.

**Synonyms**

Whooping Cough

**Signs and Symptoms** The incubation period is 7 to 10 days. Following this, the catarrhal stage begins with the nonspecific symptoms of the common cold: malaise, rhinorrhea, sneezing, and lacrimation. Low-grade fever may or may not be present. Toward the end of this phase, a cough appears, becoming increasingly persistent.

The paroxysmal stage is characterized by recurrent bouts of coughing. A paroxysm consists of a series of coughs in rapid succession, with inadequate attempts at inspiration between them. Typically, the patient expectorates copious amounts of thick mucus, which may induce vomiting. This phase is associated with very high white blood cell counts, predominantly lymphocytosis.

The convalescent stage of pertussis begins approximately 4 weeks after onset. By then paroxysms are less frequent and severe, but occasionally they will recur sporadically for months. Complications include epistaxis and scleral hemorrhage, due to sudden increases in venous pressure associated with a paroxysm. Other complications associated with paroxysms include seizures, atelectasis, bronchiectasis, subcutaneous emphysema, and inguinal hernia. Bacterial superinfection and, rarely, encephalitis may occur.

The diagnosis of pertussis is confirmed by isolating the organism from the sputum. Samples are best obtained using a swab placed through the nose into the posterior pharynx.

**Etiology** Pertussis is caused by the gram-negative coccobacillus, *Bordetella pertussis*.

**Epidemiology** Pertussis occurs most frequently in young children. In adolescents and adults, the symptoms are much less severe and the disease may not be recognized as pertussis. The disease has a worldwide distribution.

**Related Disorders** Bronchitis and influenza often resemble pertussis in the catarrhal stage.

**Treatment—Standard** Antibiotic therapy for pertussis rapidly clears the bacteria but does not change the symptoms. Erythromycin is the drug of choice and is routinely given because it halts transmission of the disease to others. Trimethoprim-sulfamethoxazole is an alternative. Exposed contacts are also given erythromycin if nasopharyngeal cultures grow the organism.

Human hyperimmune pertussis globulin is recommended by some, but its efficacy is the subject of controversy.

Intensive supportive care may be lifesaving in severe cases, particularly in infants. Meticulous pulmonary toilet and prompt ventilatory assistance are critical, as is adequate nutrition.

The pertussis vaccine has been in widespread use since the late 1940s. Since then, the incidence of pertussis has fallen from 250,000 to less than 3,000 cases annually. The vaccine is not 100 percent effective in preventing disease; in outbreaks, susceptibility to infection rises with time elapsed since immunization.

Adverse reactions have been associated with vaccination, and the risk rises with age. Vaccination is contraindicated over the age of 7 years in most circumstances. Adverse reactions may be local or systemic. Local reactions include pain, erythema, and swelling. Fever is a common systemic reaction. Rarely, fever over 40.5° C (104.9° F), seizures, encephalopathy, shock, and severe hypersensitivity reactions occur. The Centers for Disease Control estimate the risk of serious complications to be 1:100,000 to 1:300,000 for the vaccine, and 1:9,500 for the disease. Unfortunately, local outbreaks of pertussis have occurred because parents have refused vaccination.

**Treatment—Investigational** Acellular pertussis vaccines are currently under investigation in Sweden and Japan. Their success rates are not as high as was initially hoped.

Please contact the agencies listed under Resources, below, for the most current information. Addresses and telephone numbers of these agencies, as well as of individual experts and research centers, may be found in the Master Resources List.

**Resources**

**For more information on pertussis:** National Organization for Rare Disorders (NORD); NIH/National Institute of Allergy and Infectious Diseases; Centers for Disease Control; Dissatisfied Parents Together; World Health Organization.

**References**

The 1993 Epidemic of Pertussis in Cincinnati: Resurgence of Disease in a Highly Immunized Population of Children: C.D.C. Christie, et al.; N. Engl. J. Med., July 1994, vol. 331(1), pp. 16–21.

Answers to Questions About the Acellular Pertussis Vaccine: S.R. Kimmel, et al.; Am. Fam. Physician, June 1993, vol. 47(8), pp. 1825–1832.

Immunizations in Children: A. Nicoll, et al.; Curr. Opin. Pediatr., February 1993, vol. 5(1), pp. 60–67.

Cecil Textbook of Medicine, 19th ed.: J.B. Wyngaarden, et al., eds.: W.B. Saunders Company, 1992, pp. 1674–1676.

Control of Pertussis in the World: A. Galazka; World Health Stat. Q., 1992, vol. 45(2–3), pp. 238–247.

Epidemiological Features of Pertussis in the United States, 1980–1989: K.M. Farizo, et al.; Clin. Infect. Dis., March 1992, vol. 14(3), pp. 708–719.

Epidemiology of Pertussis and Reactions to Pertussis Vaccine: S.L. Hodder, et al.; Epidemiol. Rev., 1992, vol. 14, pp. 243–267.

Infectious Diseases: S.L. Gorbach, ed.; W.B. Saunders Company, 1992, pp. 1538–1543.

Nelson Textbook of Pediatrics, 14th ed.: R.E. Behrman, ed.-in-chief; W.B. Saunders Company, 1992, pp. 724–725.

Pertussis in Adults: T. Aoyama, et al.; Am. J. Dis. Child., February 1992, vol. 146(2), pp. 163–166.

Progress Towards the Development of New Vaccines Against Whooping Cough: R. Rappuoli, et al.; Vaccine, 1992, vol. 10(14), pp. 1027–1032.

Harrison's Principles of Internal Medicine, 12th ed.: J.D. Wilson, et al., eds.: McGraw-Hill, 1991, pp. 620–622.

Vaccine-Preventable Respiratory Infections in Childhood: K.K. Connelly, et al.; Semin. Respir. Infect., December 1991, vol. 6(4), pp. 204–216.

Pulmonary Diseases and Disorders, 2nd ed.; A.P. Fishman, ed.; McGraw-Hill, 1988, pp. 1497–1498.

# PINTA

**Description** Pinta, a skin disease caused by the spirochete *Treponema carateum*, is characterized by rashes and skin discoloration.

**Synonyms**

Azul

Carate

Empeines

Iota

Mal del Pinto

Tina

**Signs and Symptoms** The earliest lesions are small papules that occur at the site of inoculation. Within several months, secondary lesions appear; these are small, reddish or purplish, and psoriatic (pintids). They occur most often on the face, hands, and feet. Gradually the color of these lesions changes to slate blue. These colored patches eventually undergo depigmentation and become vitiligoid. The skin on the soles and palms may become somewhat thickened.

The lesions are susceptible to secondary infection by other organisms, but the skin is the only organ affected.

The diagnosis of pinta may be made on darkfield examination of fluid from the skin lesions, which usually reveals spirochetes. Serologic tests (VDRL; fluorescent treponemal antibody absorption—FTA-ABS) usually become positive after the secondary lesions appear.

**Etiology** Pinta is caused by the spirochete *Treponema carateum*.

**Epidemiology** Predominantly a disease of remote rural areas, pinta is common in the tropical lowlands of South and Central America, such as Mexico and Colombia. It is rare in the United States. Transmission is by direct, nonsexual contact with pinta lesions.

**Related Disorders** See *Yaws; Bejel.* The treponematoses—bejel (endemic syphilis), venereal syphilis, pinta, and yaws—are caused by identical-looking treponemes and are capable of producing chronic disease syndromes. However, their clinical and epidemiologic characteristics are quite distinct.

**Treatment—Standard** The lesions of pinta respond to antibiotics such as benzathine penicillin G, given in a single dose of 1.2 million units. Alternatives include tetracyclines and chloramphenicol.

**Treatment—Investigational** Please contact the agencies listed under Resources, below, for the most current information. Addresses and telephone numbers of these agencies, as well as of individual experts and research centers, may be found in the Master Resources List.

**Resources**

For more information on pinta: National Organization for Rare Disorders (NORD); Centers for Disease Control; NIH/National Institute of Allergy and Infectious Diseases; World Health Organization.

**References**

Nonvenereal Treponematoses: Yaws, Endemic Syphilis, and Pinta: A.B. Koff, et al.; J. Am. Acad. Dermatol., October 1993, vol. 29(4), pp. 519–535.

Cecil Textbook of Medicine, 19th ed.: J.B. Wyngaarden, et al., eds.; W.B. Saunders Company, 1992, p. 1770.

Nelson Textbook of Pediatrics: 14th ed.: R.E. Behrman, ed.-in-chief; W.B. Saunders Company, 1992, p. 781.

Endemic Treponematoses, Part II: Pinta and Endemic Syphilis: H.F. Engelkens, et al.; Int. J. Dermatol., April 1991, vol. 30(4), pp. 231–238.

Clinical Dermatology, 2nd ed.: T.P. Habif, ed.; C.V. Mosby Company 1990, p. 223.

Specificity of Antibodies from Patients with Pinta for Antigens of Treponema Pallidum: M.J. Fohn, et al.; J. Infect. Dis., January 1988, vol. 157(1), pp. 32–37.

# POEMS Syndrome

**Description** POEMS ([p]olyneuropathy, [o]rganomegaly, [e]ndocrinopathy, [M] protein, [s]kin changes) syndrome is a constellation of anomalies accompanied by hypothroidism.

**Synonyms**

> Crow-Fukase Syndrome
> PEP Syndrome
> Shimpo Syndrome
> Takatsuki Syndrome

**Signs and Symptoms** Polyneuropathy causes tingling, numbness, burning pain, deficiencies in perception, and vibratory sensations usually in the limbs. Organomegaly may cause splenomegaly or hepatosplenomegaly. Adenopathy may also occur. Hypothyroidism and hypoadrenocorticism are examples of the endocrinopathy. Sexual functioning may be affected. Serum levels of M protein or other abnormal proteins are usually elevated. Skin manifestations may include hyperpigmentation and thickened skin resembling scleroderma. Ascites, anasarca, and edema in other tissues may also occur. Most patients have signs and symptoms resembling those of multiple myeloma.

**Etiology** The exact cause of POEMS syndrome is not known. An autoimmune disorder has been suggested. Abnormal proteins from the myeloma-like tumor is another possible cause.

**Epidemiology** Males and females are affected in equal numbers.

**Related Disorders** See *Castleman Disease; Scleroderma.*

**Treatment—Standard** Melphalan and prednisone have proved effective in the treatment of POEMS syndrome.

**Treatment—Investigational** Plasmapheresis may be of benefit in some cases of POEMS syndrome. Its safety and effectiveness is still under investigation. More research is needed before plasmapheresis can be recommended for use in all but the most severe cases of POEMS syndrome.

Please contact the agencies listed under Resources, below, for the most current information. Addresses and telephone numbers of these agencies, as well as of individual experts and research centers, may be found in the Master Resources List.

**Resources**

For more information on POEMS syndrome: National Organization for Rare Disorders (NORD); NIH/National Arthritis, Musculoskeletal and Skin Diseases Information Clearinghouse.

**References**

POEMS Syndrome Presenting As Systemic Sclerosis: Clinical and Pathologic Study of a Case with Microangiopathic Glomerular Lesions: J.P. Viard, et al.; Am. J. Med., March 1988, vol. 84(3 pt. 1), pp. 524–528.

The Skin Changes in the Crow-Fukase (POEMS) Syndrome: A Case Report: W.B. and E.D. Shelley; Arch. Dermatol., January 1987, vol. 123(1), pp. 85–87.

# PSITTACOSIS

**Description** Psittacosis is a common infectious disorder found in birds, some poultry, and mammals. Among humans it can spread and become epidemic. The most prominent symptom is usually pneumonia. Other clinical findings include chills, fever, headache, nausea, vomiting, and muscle pain in the neck and back. Because these symptoms can mimic those of many other diseases, a high suspicion of the diagnosis is prerequisite to treatment.

**Synonyms**
> Ornithosis
> Parrot Fever

**Signs and Symptoms** Symptoms of psittacosis are usually those of pneumonia, including tachypnea, fatigue, and pain when breathing. However, the illness can mimic influenza or mononucleosis, or the symptoms may be more severe, suggesting a serious lung problem. The patient may cough and spit up bloody mucus, in addition to experiencing severe headache, vomiting, anorexia, severe muscle pain, chills, and fever. In serious cases, pericarditis and irregular or forceful heartbeat appear, along with splenomegaly or hepatomegaly. Diagnosis is confirmed by a rise in serum antibodies and by x-rays that show a ground-glass-like shadow, most often in the right inferior lobe of the lung.

**Etiology** Psittacosis is caused in humans by exposure to *Chlamydia psittaci,* which is transmitted from infected birds and poultry. Most instances of infection occur from handling infected birds themselves or by working in areas where birds are kept or butchered. Another source of infection is the dried feces and the dust from feathers and cages.

The birds themselves are often asymptomatic, spreading the disease for months before it becomes fatal. Not only pet birds but domestic fowls, feral birds, city pigeons, and sparrows are known carriers of psittacosis.

**Epidemiology** Psittacosis affects males and females in equal numbers. Poultry and pet store workers are at a very high risk, as are bird breeders and pigeon keepers. Poultry workers handling the viscera of butchered turkeys run a high risk of contracting the disease. However, pet birds can also carry the organism and infect their owners. Since the disease can become epidemic in animals as well as in humans, discovery of a single case of the disease should be reported to local public health authorities.

**Related Disorders** See *Q Fever; Brucellosis.*

**Legionnaire disease** causes a similar pneumonia, including a shaking chill, sharp pain in the involved side of the chest, cough with sputum or phlegm production, fever of up to 105° F, and, in some cases, rapid and painful respiration. Abdominal pain, diarrhea, and neurologic signs, such as headache, confusion, lethargy, or agitation, may also be present.

**Treatment—Standard** Treatment of psittacosis in humans usually consists of antibiotic drug therapy. Tetracycline or doxycycline are the drugs most commonly used, but minocycline, floxacin, and erythromycin have also proved beneficial.

Treatment of psittacosis in birds includes injecting oxytetracycline into the muscle, followed by injections just under the skin of the bird with the same drug every 2 to 3 days. Alternatively, daily feedings of food and water treated with antibiotics may cure the disease. Macaws and other large birds may be treated by adding chlortetracycline to their food. Protective gloves and masks can often prevent transmission of the disease to pet store workers.

**Treatment—Investigational** Please contact the agencies listed under Resources, below, for the most current information. Addresses and telephone numbers of these agencies, as well as of individual experts and research centers, may be found in the Master Resources List.

**Resources**

**For more information on psittacosis:** National Organization for Rare Disorders (NORD); NIH/National Institute of Allergy and Infectious Disease; Centers for Disease Control.

**References**

Potential Use of Long-Acting Injectable Oxytetracycline for Treatment of Chlamydiosis in Goffin's Cockatoos: K. Flammer et al.; Avian Dis., January–March 1990, vol. 34 (1), pp. 228–234.

Genetic, Immunologic, and Pathologic Characterization of Avian Chlamydial Strains: A.A. Anderson, et al.; J. Am. Vet. Med. Assoc., December 1989, vol. 195(11), pp. 1512–1516.

An Outbreak of Psittacosis in Minnesota Turkey Industry Workers: Implications for Modes of Transmission and Control: K. Hedberg, et al.; Am. J. Epidemiol., September 1989, vol. 130(30), pp. 569–577.

Psittacosis Pneumonia, R. Stubbs, et al.; J. Tenn. Med. Assoc. , April 1989, vol. 82(4), pp. 189–190.

Cecil Textbook of Medicine, 18th ed.: J.B. Wyngaarden and L.H. Smith, Jr., eds.; W.B. Saunders Company, 1988, pp. 1564, 1735–1737.

# Q FEVER

**Description** Q fever is a rickettsial disease that primarily occurs in animals and is caused by *Coxiella burnetti*. It is most commonly an acute febrile illness with headache, chills, and myalgias. Pneumonia, hepatitis, and endocarditis may also occur.

**Synonyms**

Q Fever Pneumonia

**Signs and Symptoms** Q fever usually begins with sudden severe headache and high fever. Chills and myalgias are also common. Occasionally, gastrointestinal symptoms are prominent, with nausea, vomiting, and diarrhea. Examination frequently shows hepatosplenomegaly.

Q fever has a wide variety of clinical manifestations. In addition to the above, patients may present with pneumonitis, hepatitis, or endocarditis. Q fever endocarditis is a chronic infection with symptoms characteristic of infective endocarditis: fatigue, fever, and cardiac murmurs, typically of the aortic valve.

The diagnosis of Q fever is based on the clinical picture and the history of possible exposure. Unlike other rickettsia, *C. burnetti* does not produce a positive Weil-Felix reaction. Diagnosis may be confirmed retrospectively by demonstrating a rise in antibody titer.

**Etiology** The cause of Q fever is the rickettsia *Coxiella burnetti.*

**Epidemiology** Q fever is primarily a disease of cattle, sheep, and goats, although infection has been reported in cats, rats, rabbits, and ticks. The organism is distributed worldwide, but human infection usually occurs only in those with occupational exposure to animals. Infection is usually transmitted by inhalation of aerosolized organisms from contaminated urine, feces, milk, or dust. These are most concentrated in the placenta and milk of an infected animal. Those at risk include veterinarians, abattoir workers, farmers, wool sorters, dairy workers, and researchers working in close proximity to the organism. Infection can also occur through a tick bite.

**Related Disorders** Related disorders include other rickettsioses and diseases with similar presentations. Mild forms of Q fever without significant focal symptoms (such as those of pneumonitis or hepatitis) resemble viral illness. Q fever pneumonia is an atypical pneumonia and must be distinguished from *Mycoplasma* pneumonia, legionellosis, **Psittacosis**, and viral pneumonias. Q fever endocarditis should be suspected in cases of culture-negative subacute endocarditis.

Other rickettsioses include **Rocky Mountain Spotted Fever;** endemic, epidemic, and scrub typhus; and rickettsialpox. These differ from Q fever in that they are associated with rashes, arthropod transmission, and a positive Weil-Felix reaction.

**Treatment—Standard** Q fever is treated with tetracyclines or chloramphenicol. Endocarditis may require treatment for years, as it is rarely cured without surgery. A vaccine is available for individuals with occupational risk of contracting Q fever.

**Treatment—Investigational** Please contact the agencies listed under Resources, below, for the most current information. Addresses and telephone numbers of these agencies, as well as of individual experts and research centers, may be found in the Master Resources List.

**Resources**

**For more information on Q fever:** National Organization for Rare Disorders (NORD); NIH/National Institute of Allergy and Infectious Diseases; Centers for Disease Control.

**References**

Poker Player's Pneumonia: An Urban Outbreak of Q Fever Following Exposure to a Parturient Cat: Joanne M. Langley, et al.; N. Engl. J. Med., August 1988, vol. 319(6), pp. 354–56.

Q Fever: Current Concepts: L.A. Sawyer, et al.; Rev. Infect. Dis., September–October 1987, vol. 9(5), pp. 935–946.

# RABIES

**Description** Rabies is an infectious disease that can affect all warm-blooded animals, including man. It is caused by the virus *Neurotropic lyssavirus,* which is found in the salivary glands and the central nervous system of infected animals. The symptoms may lead to serious complications if the virus is not treated immediately.

**Synonyms**

Hydrophobia

Lyssa

**Signs and Symptoms** The symptoms of rabies usually develop within 20 to 60 days after a bite or scratch from an animal infected with the rabies virus. The incubation period is usually shorter when the inoculation site is close to the brain. The initial symptoms include a general feeling of discomfort or uneasiness, nervousness, anxiety, insomnia, depression, loss of appetite, fever, chills, cough, sore throat, headache, nausea, vomiting, and pain at the site of exposure. Serious neurologic symptoms usually present themselves 2 to 10 days after the initial symptoms. Two types of syndromes may develop during this period: **furious** or **paralytic**.

The hyperactive, or furious, syndrome is usually characterized by thrashing, agitation, biting, spasms of the pharynx and larynx, choking, gagging, hydrophobia, hyperventilation, and cardiac arrhythmias. In about 20 percent of patients, a paralytic syndrome occurs, characterized by paralysis and its upward movement at the inoculation site, increased blood pressure, rapid heart rate, confusion, hallucinations, and disorientation. During this time the patient may have increased periods of hyperactivity, stiffness in the back of the neck, and an abnormal increase in the number of cells in the cerebrospinal fluid, ending with the onset of coma or respiratory failure.

**Etiology** Rabies is caused by a lyssovirus that affects the saliva and nervous system. In humans, a bite or scratch from an infected animal is the mode of transmission. In at least 2 known cases, rabies has been transmitted by breathing the air of caves of infected bats. Six recorded cases of rabies in humans were transmitted as a result of cornea transplants from donors who had undiagnosed rabies.

**Epidemiology** Rabies in humans has been almost completely eliminated in most developed countries. The vaccinations of domesticated animals and elimination of stray dogs has helped control this problem. In the 1980s, the Centers for Disease Control reported one case per year. In the United States, rabies is found primarily among wild animals, such as skunks, foxes, bats, and raccoons. There were 49 cases of human rabies reported in the United States between 1960 and 1986. Only 7 of the 49 cases were acquired by exposure to rabid domesticated animals. The remainder were the result of contact with wild animals.

**Related Disorders** See *Typhoid Fever; Encephalitis, Herpetic.*

**Cerebral malaria** is a serious complication of falciparum malaria in infants, pregnant women, and travelers not immune to indigenous parasites. It is caused by a communicable parasite and is spread through the bite of the anopheles mosquito. The symptoms may be fever of up to 104° F, severe headache, drowsiness, confusion, or delirium.

**Tetanus (lockjaw)** is a neurologic syndrome caused by the microorganism *Clostridium tetani,* which enters the body through wounds, injections, or skin ulcers. The incubation period is usually 7 to 21 days. Symptoms usually last for 3 to 4 weeks and include a tightly closed mouth (lockjaw), low-grade fever, fear, restlessness, difficulty swallowing, stiffness, heartbeat irregularities, muscle spasms, and convulsions. Although tetanus is a treatable disease, preventive vaccination is recommended during infancy and every few years thereafter.

**Treatment—Standard** The most effective treatment for rabies is immediate cleansing of the wound with soap and water followed by immunization with the rabies vaccine and hyperimmune globulin. If the wound has broken the skin, a tetanus shot should be given. If the patient has been bitten by a wild animal that has escaped, or a domestic animal that shows signs of rabies, a series of vaccinations to prevent rabies is prescribed before the onset of symptoms. Once the disease presents itself in the patient, there is no effective treatment to stop the progression.

**Treatment—Investigational** In 1988, a vaccine absorbed into an aluminum salt for both preexposure and postexposure to rabies was licensed in Michigan. This vaccine is produced and distributed by the Michigan Department of Public Health. Distribution in other states is under investigation.

Please contact the agencies listed under Resources, below, for the most current information. Addresses and telephone numbers of these agencies, as well as of individual experts and research centers, may be found in the Master Resources List.

**Resources**

**For more information on rabies:** National Organization for Rare Disorders (NORD); NIH/National Institute of Allergy and Infectious Diseases; Centers for Disease Control.

**References**

Controlling Rabies: Mad Dogs and Friendly Skunks: K. Flieger; FDA Consumer, June 1990, pp. 23–26.

Drug Evaluations Subscriptions, Vol. 3: Department of Drugs, Division of Drugs and Toxicology; American Medical Association, 1990, Immu. Ch. 4, pp. 27–30.

Principles of Neurology, 4th ed.: R.D. Adams and M. Victor, eds.: McGraw-Hill, 1989, pp. 605–606.

Cecil Textbook of Medicine, 18th ed.: J.B. Wyngaarden and L.H. Smith, Jr., eds.: W.B. Saunders Company, 1988, pp. 2200–2202.

Internal Medicine, 2nd ed.: J.H. Stein, ed.-in-chief; Little, Brown and Company, 1987, pp. 1587–1589.

# REYE SYNDROME

**Description** Reye syndrome is a childhood disease characterized by acute hepatic failure, encephalopathy, and hypoglycemia. It usually follows a viral infection, typically influenza or varicella, and is associated with the use of salicylates. In addition to these factors, deficiencies of urea cycle enzymes have been implicated as contributing factors in the development of Reye syndrome.

**Synonyms**

Fatty Liver with Encephalopathy

**Signs and Symptoms** Reye syndrome usually follows an upper respiratory tract infection and begins with vomiting. In very young children (under 2 years of age), diarrhea and/or hyperventilation may be the first signs of illness. The initial stage is rapidly followed by signs of central nervous system involvement: listlessness, somnolence, irritability, and other behavioral changes. The neurologic disturbance progresses quickly to involve seizures, stupor, and then coma, usually within 3 to 5 days of onset. These symptoms are due to cerebral edema, which is a prominent feature of the disease. Hepatomegaly is usually seen on physical examination, but jaundice is minimal.

Laboratory data usually reveal elevated serum aminotransferases, prolonged prothrombin time, hypoglycemia, hyperammonemia, and metabolic acidosis.

The mortality rate of Reye syndrome is very high, but complete recovery is possible. Residual brain damage may occur.

**Etiology** Reye syndrome may be caused by a mitochondrial insult, precipitated by certain toxins, specifically salicylates, in individuals with a deficiency of urea cycle enzymes. The use of aspirin is contraindicated in children with viral illnesses. The Food and Drug Administration has also warned that antiemetics such as the phenothiazines may increase the severity of Reye syndrome or mask its early symptoms.

Reye syndrome may occur in the absence of salicylate ingestion; however, one recent study indicated that 90 percent of affected children had taken salicylate-containing drugs during the preceding viral illness.

**Epidemiology** Reye syndrome occurs almost exclusively in children under the age of 16 years with a recent viral upper respiratory tract illness (most frequently, chickenpox or influenza). It has also been reported in newborns and the middle-aged. The incidence of Reye syndrome in teenagers has been rising in recent years, possibly because of self-medication with aspirin.

The incidence of Reye syndrome varies with the pattern of influenza virus activity from year to year, according to the National Reye Syndrome Surveillance System. However, in 1984, the incidence of influenza rose, while reported cases of Reye syndrome in children under 10 years of age decreased. There were decreases in both influenza- and varicella-associated cases.

**Related Disorders** See ***Medium-Chain Acyl-CoA Dehydrogenase Deficiency,*** a very rare metabolic disorder with clinical features similar to those of Reye syndrome. The enzyme medium-chain acyl-CoA dehydrogenase is important in triglyceride metabolism. Hypoglycemia and central nervous system involvement (lethargy and possibly coma) occur, associated with fatty changes in the liver. During hypoglycemic periods, tests usually show massive urinary levels of dicarboxylic acid.

**Treatment—Standard** There is no specific treatment for Reye syndrome; however, intensive supportive measures addressing both the hepatic failure and the cerebral edema have improved survival. Permanent neurologic sequelae, such as mental impairment, have been reported.

**Treatment—Investigational** Please contact the agencies listed under Resources, below, for the most current information. Addresses and telephone numbers of these agencies, as well as of individual experts and research centers, may be found in the Master Resources List.

**Resources**

**For more information on Reye syndrome:** National Organization for Rare Disorders (NORD); Reye Syndrome Society; NIH/National Institute of Neurological Disorders and Stroke; Centers for Disease Control; Food and Drug Administration.

**References**

Cecil Textbook of Medicine, 19th ed.: J.B. Wyngaarden, et al., eds.; W.B. Saunders Company, 1992, pp. 2194–2195.

Investigation of Metabolic Disorders Resembling Reye's Syndrome: A. Green; Arch. Dis. Child., October 1992, vol. 67(10), pp. 1313–1317.

Nelson Textbook of Pediatrics, 14th ed.: R.E. Behrman, ed.-in-chief; W.B. Saunders Company, 1992, pp. 1020–1021.

Fatty Acid Composition of Hepatic Triglycerides in Reye's Syndrome: Implications for Hepatic Desaturase Abnormalities: E.S. Kang; Clin. Chim. Acta, December 1991, vol. 31(204), pp. 167–177.

Interrelationships of Liver and Brain with Special Reference to Reye Syndrome: J.K. Brown; J. Inherit. Metab. Dis., 1991, vol. 14(4), pp. 438–458.

A Sibling-Controlled Study of Intelligence and Academic Performance Following Reye Syndrome: J. Duffy, et al.; Dev. Med. Child. Neurol., September 1991, vol. 33(9), pp. 811–815.

Dictionary of Medical Syndromes, 3rd ed.: S.I. Magalini, et al., eds.: J.B. Lippincott Company, 1990, pp. 760–761.

Principles of Neurology, 4th ed.; R.D. Adams and M. Victor, eds.; McGraw-Hill, 1989, pp. 855–856.

Reye Syndrome: D.C. DeVivio; Neurol. Clin., 1985, vol. 3, pp. 95–115.

# RHEUMATIC FEVER

**Description** Rheumatic fever is an inflammatory syndrome that appears to represent an inappropriate immune response to streptococcal infection. It is characterized by symptoms known as the Jones criteria; the major criteria include carditis, polyarthritis, chorea, a skin rash referred to as erythema marginatum, and subcutaneous nodules. Of these, the cardiac manifestations are ultimately the most serious, since damage inflicted on the cardiac valves during a bout of rheumatic fever continues chronically, long after the acute episode. Affected individuals are susceptible to recurrent attacks with each subsequent streptococcal infection; they are also at risk for infective endocarditis with any episode of bacteremia, such as might occur during a dental procedure. These patients require prophylactic antibiotics for recurrent streptococcal infections, as well as infective endocarditis.

**Synonyms**
> Acute Rheumatic Fever
> Inflammatory Rheumatism
> Rheumatic Arthritis

**Signs and Symptoms** Acute rheumatic fever **(ARF)** follows an episode of streptococcal pharyngitis, which is usually, but not always, symptomatic. (In as many as one-third of cases, the preceding streptococcal infection may be either asymptomatic or so mild that the patient does not seek medical attention.) Approximately 1 to 5 weeks later, the attack of ARF begins, usually with polyarthritis and fever. Arthralgias or arthritis may develop, classically with a migratory pattern.

Other common manifestations include carditis, which may only be evident by the appearance of a new murmur, or may be symptomatic. Endocarditis, myocarditis, or pericarditis may occur, alone or in combination. In severe cases, congestive heart failure may occur, which can be fatal.

Serious disease of the cardiac valves may evolve over the years following the acute episode. Inflammation of the valves, most frequently the mitral valve, is followed by scarring, turbulent flow, and further damage. The end result may not be evident for 20 or 30 years, when the patient presents with symptoms of progressive valvular dysfunction. Because the initial insult may have been silent, this end result may be the first sign of a problem.

Chorea is much less common. It consists of involuntary, abrupt, purposeless movements, and inappropriate crying or laughter. It typically persists for 2 to 4 months.

Rashes and subcutaneous nodules are also less common. The characteristic rash, erythema marginatum, occurs mainly on the trunk and may only last for hours. Subcutaneous nodules are small and painless. They appear on bony prominences.

The diagnosis of ARF is made on clinical grounds by a set of criteria. The Jones criteria include major and minor manifestations of ARF. The diagnosis is considered highly probable if the patient meets either 2 major, or 1 major and 2 minor, criteria, and has evidence of a recent streptococcal infection (positive throat culture; elevated titers of anti-streptococcal antibodies, such as antistreptolysin-O).

The major criteria are carditis, polyarthritis, chorea, erythema marginatum, and subcutaneous nodules. The minor criteria include fever, arthralgia, elevated C-reactive protein **(CRP)** or erythrocyte sedimentation rate **(ESR),** a prolonged PR interval on electrocardiogram, and a history of rheumatic fever in the past.

**Etiology** Although rheumatic fever is clearly linked to Group A streptococcal infections, the exact mechanism causing the disorder is not well understood. It is thought to be an autoimmune phenomenon, triggered by cross-reactivity between streptococcal antigens and host tissue, but this is not proved.

Certain strains of *Streptococcus pyogenes* are known to be more rheumatogenic than others and have been associated with outbreaks. However, only a small percentage of patients with pharyngitis will develop ARF. Why this occurs in some individuals and not in others remains a mystery.

Following a primary episode of ARF, recurrences develop with each subsequent streptococcal infection. These are progressively more severe and are preventable with antibiotic prophylaxis.

**Epidemiology** Rheumatic fever is epidemic in India, the Middle East, and regions of South America and Africa, where it accounts for a major percentage of heart disease. In the United States, the incidence of ARF has declined steadily in the 20th century, but outbreaks were reported in the mid-1980s, apparently related to a resurgence of the rheumatogenic serotypes of *S. pyogenes.*

Rheumatic fever usually affects children between 5 and 15 years of age, but may occur among young adults as well. In the United States the delayed sequelae of ARF generally do not appear before the 4th or 5th decade; in the developing world, where recurrences are common, these sequelae may become evident much earlier.

**Related Disorders** There are a number of diseases that may be manifested by fever and polyarthritis, and several may resemble ARF. Juvenile rheumatoid arthritis (Still disease), is associated with fever, arthritis, and skin rash, as may be rheumatoid arthritis and other autoimmune disorders. These may often be distinguished from ARF by the appearance of rheumatoid factor and antinuclear antigens, which do not occur in ARF, as well as by their symptom evolution.

**Treatment—Standard** There is no specific therapy for ARF. It can be prevented by timely treatment of streptococcal pharyngitis, although, as stated above, this will only prevent those cases that are preceded by a symptomatic pharyngitis.

When rheumatic fever first develops, a course of penicillin is recommended to ensure eradication of any remaining streptococci. Following this, patients require long-term antibiotic prophylaxis, such as a monthly injection of 1.2 million units of benzathine penicillin G. Exactly how long such a regimen should be continued is controversial; some argue that it should be lifelong. Antibiotic prophylaxis against infective endocarditis is also necessary for any instrumental procedure with a risk of bacteremia.

Arthritic symptoms may be treated with anti-inflammatory and analgesic drugs. When carditis is present, steroids may be prescribed, although their benefit has yet to be demonstrated by controlled clinical trials. Chorea does not respond to steroids or anti-inflammatory drugs. Sedatives may be useful.

**Treatment—Investigational** Researchers at Rockefeller University have identified 2 monoclonal antibodies that have the potential to be used as a screen to detect those at risk for rheumatic fever. It is hoped that when fully developed, this screen might be used to select candidates for immunization against streptococcal pharyngitis.

Please contact the agencies listed under Resources, below, for the most current information. Addresses and telephone numbers of these agencies, as well as of individual experts and research centers, may be found in the Master Resources List.

**Resources**

**For more information on rheumatic fever:** National Organization for Rare Disorders (NORD); NIH/National Institute of Allergy and Infectious Diseases; Centers for Disease Control.

**References**

Resurgence of Acute Rheumatic Fever in the Intermountain Area of the United States: L.G. Veasy, et al.; N. Engl. J. Med., 1987, vol. 316(8), pp. 421–427.

Rheumatic Fever: Down but Not Out: E. Zamula; FDA Consumer, July–August 1987, pp. 26–28.

Rheumatic Fever in the Eighties: M. Markowitz; Pediatr. Clin. North Am., 1986, vol. 33(5), pp. 1141–1150.

# ROCKY MOUNTAIN SPOTTED FEVER (RMSF)

**Description** RMSF is an acute disease caused by a rickettsia and transmitted by ticks. The illness is initially manifested by fever and rash, but progresses to multisystem involvement. Pathologically, it is a diffuse vasculitis. Early diagnosis and treatment are vital to avoid serious complications, but the disease lacks distinctive features in the early stages, frequently thwarting early diagnosis.

**Synonyms**

> Black Fever
> Black Measles
> Blue Disease
> Blue Fever
> Mexican Spotted Fever
> Sao Paulo Fever
> Tobia Fever

**Signs and Symptoms** The incubation period of RMSF is 2 to 12 days, with an average of 7 days. The usual clinical picture then begins suddenly, with fever, severe headache, and myalgias. Nausea, vomiting, and abdominal pain may accompany these early symptoms. On about the 4th day, a rash develops, classically beginning on the wrists and ankles and spreading centrally. The rash is the most helpful diagnostic sign, but it may not occur in as many as 10 percent of cases, and in fulminant cases, death may intervene before the rash develops. The lesions are macular at the outset, but the rash generally becomes petechial within a few days. As the disease progresses, the skin lesions may become purpuric, ulcerative, necrotic, and finally gangrenous in severe cases.

Extensive vasculitis may occur throughout the body, with subsequent capillary leak syndrome. As fluid leaks out into the tissue, edema becomes prominent in the face, hands, and feet. Pulmonary edema may also develop. Other manifestations seen in severe cases include myocarditis and renal and liver dysfunction. Capillary leakage also results in hypotension, which compounds the ischemic effect of vasculitis and may progress to shock.

The central nervous system manifestations of RMSF include delirium, agitation, and meningismus, which frequently leads to a diagnosis of meningitis. Seizures and coma can occur in severe cases.

Laboratory data usually reveal a normal white blood cell count and thrombocytopenia. Signs of disseminated intravascular coagulation (**DIC**) may be present.

**Etiology** The cause of RMSF is the rickettsial organism *Rickettsia rickettsii.* It is transmitted by ticks, specifically *Dermacentor variabilis* in the eastern United States, and *Dermacentor andersoni* in the west.

**Epidemiology** RMSF was initially reported in the Rocky Mountains, the region that gave rise to its name, but it has subsequently been reported in almost all 50 states. Currently, the areas of greatest prevalence are in the eastern states. RMSF is a disease that concentrates in certain specific localities, such as Cabarrus and Rowan counties in North Carolina, Cape Cod in Massachusetts, and Long Island, New York. While it is normally thought of as a rural disease, an epidemic was reported in New York City in 1988, related to tick infestation of a park in the Bronx.

The tick that transmits RMSF has a marked preference for crevices in the skin, such as the axilla and gluteal regions. It attaches, feeds for several hours, and only then does it release the rickettsia into the bite wound.

Approximately 1,000 cases are reported in the United States each year, with the greatest number occurring in the spring and summer. By law, all cases of RMSF must be reported to the Centers for Disease Control.

**Related Disorders** Related disorders include other rickettsial diseases and other infections that may resemble RMSF. The differential diagnosis commonly includes measles, meningococcemia, meningitis, Ehrlichiosis, typhoid fever, and other riskettsial diseases, particularly epidemic typhus. A wide variety of other illnesses may occasionally resemble RMSF: thrombotic thrombocytopenic purpura (**TTP**), septic shock, rubella, leptospirosis, and typhoid fever, to mention a few.

*Meningococcemia* may resemble RMSF, but the purpuric rash of this disease occurs very early in its course, whereas in RMSF the rash does not become petechial or purpuric until several days after onset of the illness.

Measles and epidemic typhus frequently are the most similar. In children, measles is a common misdiagnosis, which can be disastrous since no specific treatment is given for measles. The rash of measles characteristically starts on the neck and face, and there is also often a history of measles exposure; these features may distinguish it from RMSF.

Epidemic, or louse-borne typhus, caused by *Rickettsia prowazecki,* begins similarly to RMSF. A rash appears on the trunk on about the 5th day. Multisystem involvement occurs, as in RMSF, although it is usually not as severe.

Typhus and RMSF may be distinguished epidemiologically. Typhus is rare in the United States, and recent cases have been either recrudescent cases, initially acquired outside the United States, or in association with flying squirrels.

Typhus and RMSF may also be distinguished by the Weil-Felix reaction, a test for rickettsial antigens.

The diagnosis of RMSF is based on the clinical picture. The Weil-Felix reaction provides supportive evidence of RMSF, but the test is considered insufficiently sensitive to be confirmatory. A direct immunofluorescence test for skin biopsy specimens is available in some laboratories, and this may reveal rickettsia in the specimen by the 3rd or 4th day of illness.

The diagnosis of RMSF is generally confirmed by serologic testing, comparing acute and convalescent antibody titers. Obviously this is not useful in the acute illness.

**Treatment—Standard** Rocky Mountain spotted fever is treated with tetracycline, doxycycline, or chloramphenicol. Tetracyclines are preferred except in pregnant women and young children.

Preventive measures include the use of protective clothing, insect repellents, and regular hourly checks for ticks.

**Treatment—Investigational** A vaccine is currently under investigation.

Please contact the agencies listed under Resources, below, for the most current information. Addresses and telephone numbers of these agencies, as well as of individual experts and research centers, may be found in the Master Resources List.

**Resources**

**For more information on Rocky Mountain spotted fever:** National Organization for Rare Disorders (NORD); NIH/National Institute of Allergy and Infectious Diseases; Centers for Disease Control.

**References**

Rocky Mountain Spotted Fever: C.A. Kamper, et al.; Clin. Pharm., 1988, vol. 7(2), pp. 109–116.

Cloned Gene of Rickettsia Rickettsii Surface Antigen: Candidate Vaccine for Rocky Mountain Spotted Fever: G.A. McDonald, et al.; Science, 1987, vol. 235(4784), pp. 83–85.

*Staphylococcus aureus* Septicemia Mimicking Fulminant Rocky Mountain Spotted Fever: M.R. Milunski, et al.; Am. J. Med., 1987, vol. 83(4), pp. 801–803.

Rocky Mountain Spotted Fever Presenting As Thrombotic Thrombocytopenic Purpura: R.C. Turner, et al.; Am. J. Med., 1986, vol. 81(1), pp. 153–157.

The Sensitivity of Various Serologic Tests in the Diagnosis of Rocky Mountain Spotted Fever: J.E. Kaplan, et al.; Am. J. Trop. Med. Hyg., 1986, vol. 35(4), pp. 840–844.

# RUBELLA, CONGENITAL

**Description** When rubella is contracted during pregnancy, the virus may be transmitted transplacentally. Congenital rubella is associated with a wide variety of birth defects as well as fetal demise.

**Synonyms**

>   Congenital German Measles
>   Expanded Rubella Syndrome

**Signs and Symptoms** The symptoms of congenital rubella may be transient or permanent. Among the transient symptoms are low birth weight, thrombocytopenia, hepatosplenomegaly, and meningoencephalitis. The permanent symptoms include deafness, cataracts, microphthalmia, retinopathy, cardiac malformations, mental retardation, and microcephaly. Infants who appear to be asymptomatic at birth may manifest symptoms, such as hearing loss and psychomotor retardation, later in childhood.

The diagnosis of congenital rubella is confirmed by serologic testing. The presence of IgM antibody to rubella in the fetus indicates that transplacental infection occurred. Also, rising rubella titers in the infant suggest that active rubella infection, rather than passive antibody transfer, has occurred.

**Etiology** Congenital rubella results from the transplacental transmission of the rubella virus, an RNA virus of the *Togaviridae* family.

**Epidemiology** Not all maternal infections are transmitted transplacentally. The risk of fetal infection is highest early in pregnancy, as is the risk of severe manifestations. There is a 40 to 60 percent risk of infection with multiple sequelae in the first 8 weeks of gestation; however, by the 16th week the risk has declined to 10 percent. The risks of fetal defects with infection at 8, 12, 13 to 20, and over 20 weeks of gestation are 85, 50, 15, and 0 percent, respectively.

Widespread vaccination against rubella has dramatically reduced the incidence of the congenital disease. There have been no epidemics since vaccination has become routine.

**Treatment—Standard** There is no treatment for either maternal or congenital rubella. Vaccination is currently required at the age of 15 months. Because the vaccine is a live virus vaccine, there is a theoretical risk of developing congenital rubella following vaccination in pregnancy. Currently, vaccination is contraindicated during pregnancy, and conception should be avoided for at least 3 months following vaccination.

**Treatment—Investigational** Please contact the agencies listed under Resources, below, for the most current information. Addresses and telephone numbers of these agencies, as well as of individual experts and research centers, may be found in the Master Resources List.

**Resources**

**For more information on congenital rubella:** National Organization for Rare Disorders (NORD); NIH/National Institute of Child Health and Human Development.

**For genetic information and genetic counseling referrals:** March of Dimes Birth Defects Foundation; Alliance of Genetic Support Groups.

**References**

Rubella Virus: A.A. Gershon; *in* Principles and Practice of Infectious Diseases, 3rd ed.: G.L. Mandell, et al., eds.; Churchill Livingston, 1990, pp. 1242–1247.

Rubella; Public Health Education Information Sheet: March of Dimes Birth Defects Foundation, 1984.

# SEVERE COMBINED IMMUNODEFICIENCY (SCID)

**Description** SCID comprises a group of congenital syndromes in which there appears to be little or no specific cellular or humoral immune response. Thus, the patient is susceptible to recurrent infections with bacteria, viruses, fungi, and other infectious agents. Untreated, SCID results in frequent, severe infections, growth retardation, and a short life span. Several causes and types of SCID have been identified: autosomal recessive, X-linked recessive, adenosine deaminase deficiency (**ADA**), bare lymphocyte syndrome, SCID with leukopenia (reticular dysgenesis), and Swiss-type agammaglobulinemia.

**Signs and Symptoms** Maternal antibodies usually continue to protect young infants with SCID in the first few months of life. Afterwards, however, infections occur and recur frequently, e.g., pneumonia, sepsis, otitis media, diarrhea, and skin infections. Weight loss, weakness, and drastic growth retardation ensue. Opportunistic organisms that may cause fatal infections include *Candida albicans*, vaccinia, varicella, measles, cytomegalovirus, and the live bacteria in the **BCG** (bacille Calmette-Guérin) vaccine against tuberculosis. The pneumonia caused by *Pneumocystis carinii* is a common complication and is very difficult to treat.

The fact that SCID patients do not reject foreign tissue has several effects. Immunocompetent cells introduced into the patient's body (e.g., by a blood transfusion) may cause *Graft-versus-Host Disease,* reacting primarily against the recipient's skin, liver, gut, and bone marrow. However, since transplants are not rejected, bone marrow transplantation, one of the only effective treatments in this disorder, is facilitated. After immunization, antibodies are not formed; if immunization is with a live vaccine, fatal infections may result. Patients do not have cutaneous reactions to antigens and do not develop allergic reactions.

In SCID patients, T and B lymphocytes and serum immunoglobulins are usually severely reduced in number or are absent; even if present, function is severely impaired. The thymus is small and underdeveloped; lymph nodes are lacking in lymphocytes; and tonsils, adenoids, and other lymphoid organs are poorly developed or absent.

In SCID with leukopenia (reticular dysgenesis), granulocytes are also absent or greatly reduced in number. These patients also have virtually no means of removing invading organisms from the body.

**Etiology** Hereditary SCID occurs in autosomal recessive and X-linked recessive forms. Approximately 50 percent of autosomal recessive cases of SCID have adenosine deaminase (**ADA**) deficiency. This results in high levels of adenosine in the plasma. Lymphocytes trap unusually high levels of this adenosine. Intracellularly, adenosine and its metabolites interfere with a variety of cell functions.

In the bare lymphocyte syndrome, clinical SCID is associated with a lack of histocompatibility antigens and B2 microglobulin on the lymphocytes. In the absence of these proteins, T cells cannot be activated.

**Epidemiology** SCID is estimated to occur with a frequency of about 1:100,000 to 1:500,000 live births.

**Related Disorders** Various other forms of immunodeficiency exist. They include the acquired immune deficiency syndrome, isolated defects of T-cell function, and various antibody disorders. (See *Acquired Immune Deficiency Syndrome [AIDS]*).

**Treatment—Standard** Bone marrow transplantation, which can cure this disorder if an identical donor match can be found, has been facilitated greatly by the use of haplo-identical bone marrow cells, treated to remove those cells likely to cause graft-versus-host disease but to leave stem cells intact.

Fetal liver grafts, which contain lymphoid and white blood stem cells, have sometimes been effective in restoring T-cell function, but not antibody production. Fetal thymus grafts have usually been unsuccessful.

In isolated cases, agents such as transfer factor, thymosin, and levamisole may augment existing cellular immunity.

In 1990 the Food and Drug Administration approved PEG-ADA, an orphan drug that replaces the ADA enzyme deficiency in SCID. Children taking PEG-ADA through a weekly injection have had a normal immune system restored, and they are recovering from infections that might previously have been deadly. For more information on PEG-ADA, please contact Enzon.

Infections in persons with SCID must be treated vigorously with antifungal, antibiotic, and supportive measures. *P. carinii* pneumonia can be particularly difficult to treat; the 2 drugs used are usually trimethoprim-sulfamethoxazole and the orphan drug pentamidine idethionate. (For further information on treatment of *P. carinii* pneumonia, see *Acquired Immune Deficiency Syndrome [AIDS]).* Cytomegalovirus and generalized herpes simplex infections are preferentially treated with gancyclovir, acyclovir, idoxuridine, or floxuridine. Severe candidiasis and other fungal infections usually respond to amphotericin B or fluconazole therapy.

Genetic counseling may be of benefit for patients with SCID and their families. Other treatment is symptomatic and supportive.

**Treatment—Investigational** Scientists at Johns Hopkins University are studying the use of thalidomide as a treatment for graft-versus-host disease. Preliminary studies indicate it may have beneficial side effects on skin and hair symptoms. The major side effects of thalidomide are sedation and teratogenesis. More research is necessary to determine long-term safety and effectiveness of this treatment for graft-versus-host disease.

Scientists at the National Institutes of Health are using an experimental gene therapy procedure in combination with the orphan drug PEG-ADA to enhance the immune system of children with ADA-deficient SCID. The procedure involves implanting the ADA gene into an activated virus. When the virus merges into the patient's cells, it manufactures the human enzyme. The corrected cells will be infused into the patient every few months. Patients interested in participating in this experimental protocol should ask their physicians to contact Dr. Nelson Wivel, Office of Recombinant DNA Activities, National Institutes of Health, Building 31, Room 4B11, Bethesda, MD 20892.

Researchers at the National Institutes of Health, National Heart, Lung and Blood Institute are studying a defect in the interleukin-2 receptor gene as a possible cause for X-linked SCID, in which this receptor may not be constructed properly.

The Food and Drug Administration Orphan Products Division awarded a grant in 1988 to Carol Michele Paradise, M.D., of Cetus Corporation, Emeryville, CA, for her treatment of SCID with interleukin-2.

Rebecca H. Buckley, M.D., and Michael Hershfield, M.D., at Duke University Medical Center, are conducting clinical trials to study genetically determined immunodeficiency diseases.

Please contact the agencies listed under Resources, below, for the most current information. Addresses and tele-

phone numbers of these agencies, as well as of individual experts and research centers, may be found in the Master Resources List.

## Resources

**For more information on severe combined immunodeficiency:** National Organization for Rare Disorders (NORD); Immune Deficiency Foundation; Rebecca H. Buckley, M.D., and Michael Hershfield, M.D., Duke University Medical Center; NIH/National Institute of Allergy and Infectious Diseases.

**For genetic information and genetic counseling referrals:** March of Dimes Birth Defects Foundation; Alliance of Genetic Support Groups.

## References

InterLeukin-2 Receptor Gamma Chain Mutation Results in X-Linked Severe Combined Immunodeficiency in Humans: M. Noguchi; Cell, April 1993, vol. 73(1), pp. 147–157.

Antibody Responses to Bacteriophage Phi X174 in Patients with Adenosine Deaminase Deficiency: H.D. Ochs; Blood, September 1992, vol. 80(5), pp. 1163–1171.

Cecil Textbook of Medicine, 19th ed.: J.B. Wyngaarden, et al., eds.; W.B. Saunders Company, 1992, pp. 1450–1451.

Mendelian Inheritance in Man, 10th ed.: V.A. McKusick; The Johns Hopkins University Press, 1992, pp. 1960.

Nelson Textbook of Pediatrics, 14th ed.: R.E. Behrman, ed.-in-chief; W.B. Saunders Company, 1992, pp. 554–555.

Severe Combined Immunodeficiencies: A. Fisher; Immunodefic. Rev., 1992, vol. 3(2), pp. 83–100.

Birth Defects Encyclopedia: M.L. Buyse, ed.-in-chief; Blackwell Scientific Publications, 1990, p. 949–951, 959–961.

Hematology, 4th ed.: W.J. Williams, et al., eds.; McGraw-Hill, 1990, pp. 967–969.

The Metabolic Basis of Inherited Disease, 6th ed.: C.R. Scriver, et al., eds.; McGraw-Hill, 1989, pp. 1045–1047.

Immunodeficiency: Buckley, R.H.; J. Allergy Clin. Immunol., 1983, vol. 72(6), pp. 627–641.

Metabolic Defects in Immunodeficiency Diseases: A.D.B. Webster; Clin. Exp. Immunol., 1982, vol. 49(1), pp. 1–10.

Combined Immunodeficiency and Thymic Abnormalities; A.D.B. Webster; J. Clin. Pathol., 1979, vol. 13(suppl.), pp. 10–14.

# SIMIAN B VIRUS INFECTION

**Description** Simian B virus is a type of herpesvirus that causes infection in monkeys. Human infections have occurred through monkey bites and laboratory accidents. In humans, the virus produces a severe encephalitis.

## Synonyms

Herpesvirus Simiae, B Virus
Herpesvirus Simiae Encephalomyelitis
Monkey B Virus

**Signs and Symptoms** Infection with simian B virus produces the clinical picture of severe encephalitis, with fever, headache, malaise, vomiting, and meningismus. Associated neurologic abnormalities may include neuromuscular dysfunction, visual disturbances, cranial nerve dysfunction, psychiatric symptoms, seizures, paralysis, and coma. Respiratory function may be affected.

Encephalomyelitis and meningitis may occur. The mortality rate is high.

**Etiology** This disease is caused by the simian B virus, a herpesvirus.

**Epidemiology** Simian B virus infection occurs in laboratory workers who are bitten or scratched by infected monkeys, or accidentally exposed to virus-infected simian tissue cultures. It is rare; it has been estimated that 24 cases of the disorder occurred in the United States between 1932 and 1972.

**Related Disorders** The symptoms of simian B virus infection are common to the viral encephalitides. The epidemiologic setting of simian B virus infection is the major diagnostic clue to the nature of the disease. The syndrome of acute disseminated encephalomyelitis may also be caused by viruses other than simian B virus.

**Treatment—Standard** Protective clothing is recommended for those working with infected monkeys or tissues. Once a laboratory worker is bitten or scratched, there is some evidence that transmission may be prevented by intravenous acyclovir. Intravenous acyclovir may also be helpful once the disease has developed. Otherwise, treatment is supportive.

**Treatment—Investigational** A vaccine is under investigation, but it is not yet available for general use.

Please contact the agencies listed under Resources, below, for the most current information. Addresses and telephone numbers of these agencies, as well as of individual experts and research centers, may be found in the Master Resources List.

## Resources

**For more information on simian B virus infection:** National Organization for Rare Disorders (NORD); NIH/National Institute of Allergy and Infectious Diseases; Centers for Disease Control.

## References

B Virus, Herpesvirus Simiae: Historical Perspective: A.E. Palmer; J. Med. Primatol., 1987, vol. 16(2), pp. 99–130.

The Spectrum of Antiviral Activities of Acyclovir in Vitro and in Vivo: P. Collins; J. Antimicrob. Chemother., September 1983, vol. 12(suppl. B), pp. 19–27.

Successful Treatment of Experimental B Virus (Herpesvirus Simiae) Infection with Acyclovir: E.A. Boulter, et al.; Br. Med. J., March 8, 1980, vol. 280(6215), pp. 681–683.

# STEVENS-JOHNSON SYNDROME

**Description** Stevens-Johnson syndrome is the most severe form of erythema multiforme and is characterized by bullous lesions on the skin and mucous membranes.

**Synonyms**

> Dermatostomatitis
> Ectodermosis Erosiva Pluriorificialis
> Erythema Multiforme Major
> Febrile Mucocutaneous Syndrome
> Herpes Iris

**Signs and Symptoms** Typical Stevens-Johnson syndrome affects the mucous membranes of the oral cavity, pharynx, nares, eyes, and anogenital region. It may or may not be associated with erythema multiforme elsewhere on the body. The bullous lesions are generally painful; oropharyngeal lesions may be so intolerable as to prevent eating. A painful conjunctivitis occurs, frequently with a purulent discharge, and can lead to corneal scarring and loss of vision. In addition to the mucous membrane lesions, fever and prostration are usual.

Approximately one-third of patients have pulmonary involvement, with cough and patchy infiltrates on chest x-ray. In fatal cases, renal failure and pneumonia may occur.

The diagnosis of Stevens-Johnson syndrome is usually based on the clinical appearance and distribution of the lesions.

**Etiology** Stevens-Johnson syndrome has been associated with a variety of infectious and pharmacologic agents. Coxsackie-, echo-, and, most commonly, herpes simplex viruses, as well as mycoplasma, have precipitated the syndrome. Vaccines, such as those for tuberculosis, smallpox, and polio have also been implicated. Penicillin, sulfonamides, anticonvulsants, and barbiturates are the most frequently associated drugs. In approximately 50 percent of cases, no cause can be identified.

**Epidemiology** Stevens-Johnson syndrome is more frequent in children and young adults but occurs in patients of all ages. Males are affected more frequently than females.

**Related Disorders** See *Behçet Syndrome.* Other diseases that may resemble Stevens-Johnson syndrome include the following.

**Allergic stomatitis** is characterized by an intense, painful erythema that may be related to food or cosmetic hypersensitivity. **Herpetic stomatitis** is characterized by pruritis followed by the appearance of small, tense blisters on a red base. **Mikulicz syndrome (aphthous stomatitis)** is also limited to the oral cavity; it consists of recurrent ulcerative lesions. The 3 diseases mentioned above tend not to have systemic manifestations.

**Treatment—Standard** Every attempt should be made to identify a precipitating agent and to remove it if possible. Antibiotics are appropriate if superinfection is suspected, or if bacterial disease, such as mycoplasma, is suspected to be the cause. Intensive supportive care is important in severe cases. Fluid replacement is often required, and meticulous oral hygiene is necessary to prevent superinfection. Examination by an ophthalmologist is recommended for patients with eye lesions so that precautions can be taken to avoid permanent eye damage.

**Treatment—Investigational** Please contact the agencies listed under Resources, below, for the most current information. Addresses and telephone numbers of these agencies, as well as of individual experts and research centers, may be found in the Master Resources List.

**Resources**

**For more information on Stevens-Johnson syndrome:** National Organization for Rare Disorders (NORD); NIH/National Institute of Allergy and Infectious Diseases; NIH/National Arthritis and Musculoskeletal and Skin Diseases Information Clearinghouse; NIH/National Eye Institute.

**References**

> Erythema Multiforme: W. Stewart, et al., eds.; *in* Dermatology, Diagnosis and Treatment of Cutaneous Disorders, 3rd ed.: C.V. Mosby Company, 1984.

# SUBACUTE SCLEROSING PANENCEPHALITIS (SSPE)

**Description** SSPE is a progressive neurologic disorder caused by an inappropriate immune response to the measles virus. Onset of SSPE often occurs 2 to 10 years after the original attack.

**Synonyms**

> Decerebrate Dementia

**Signs and Symptoms** SSPE is a disease of childhood or young adulthood. The first signs are behavioral changes: failing schoolwork, memory loss, and irritability. Myoclonic jerks, involuntary movements, and generalized seizures follow. The course is one of progressive dementia and neurologic deterioration. Spasticity, cortical blindness, and optic atrophy may occur. In advanced cases, signs of hypothalamic involvement are present, with hyperthermia and other disturbances of homeostasis.

The disease is usually fatal within 1 to 3 years, the terminal event often being pneumonia. Sometimes prolonged remissions occur.

Laboratory abnormalities include a characteristic EEG picture and high serum levels of measles antibody. The cerebrospinal fluid shows elevated levels of gammaglobulin and measles antibody. The diagnosis of SSPE is based on these abnormalities.

**Etiology** SSPE is thought to be a form of measles encephalitis, associated with an inappropriate immune response to rubeola (measles virus). Usually there is a history of measles 2 to 10 years prior to the onset. There have been cases in which patients have had contact with pets, such as monkeys, dogs, or kittens, that later died from the illness.

**Epidemiology** SSPE occurs in children and adolescents; almost all cases appear before the age of 20 years. Males are affected more often than females.

**Related Disorders Progressive multifocal leukoencephalopathy** is a polyoma virus infection of the brain seen in immunosuppressed patients. Symptoms include ataxia, paralysis, blindness, and, ultimately, coma.

**Inclusion-body encephalitis** is an infection with gradual onset, mostly in children under 12 years of age. Symptoms include behavioral changes, myoclonus of the trunk and extremities, and aphasia.

**Progressive rubella panencephalitis** is a rare, slowly progressive neurologic disorder caused by the rubella virus. It is the result of congenital rubella syndrome or childhood rubella infection (German measles). Behavioral changes, loss of previously acquired intellectual skills, ataxia, spasticity, and seizures are common.

**Treatment—Standard** There is no specific treatment for SSPE as yet. A number of antiviral agents have been investigated with little success. Isolated reports about the effectiveness of isoprinosine have not been confirmed by controlled clinical trials. Supportive measures and anticonvulsants are useful.

**Treatment—Investigational** Intrathecal α-interferon (**IFN**) delivered with and without the addition of oral inosiplex is under investigation. Approximately half of those treated have experienced an improvement in symptoms. However, the drug's safety and efficacy have yet to be proved.

Please contact the agencies listed under Resources, below, for the most current information. Addresses and telephone numbers of these agencies, as well as of individual experts and research centers, may be found in the Master Resources List.

### Resources

**For more information on subacute sclerosing panencephalitis:** National Organization for Rare Disorders (NORD); National Subacute Sclerosing Panencephalitis Registry; NIH/National Institute of Allergy and Infectious Diseases.

### References

The Effect of Inosiplex in Subacute Sclerosing Panencephalitis: A Clinical and Laboratory Study: B. Anlar, et al.; Eur. Neurol., 1994, vol. 34(1), pp. 44–47.

Combined Oral Isoprinosine-Intraventricular Alpha-Interferon Therapy for Subacute Sclerosing Panencephalitis: G. Gascon, et al.; Brain Dev., September–October 1993, vol. 15(5), pp. 346–355.

Principles of Neurology, 5th ed.; R.D. Adams and M. Victor, eds.; McGraw-Hill, 1993, pp. 656–657.

Cecil Textbook of Medicine, 19th ed.: J.B. Wyngaarden, et al., eds.; W.B. Saunders Company, 1992, pp. 2190–2191.

Infectious Diseases: S.L. Gorbach, ed.; W.B. Saunders Company, 1992, pp. 1754–1758.

Intraventricular Interferon and Oral Inosiplex in the Treatment of Subacute Sclerosing Panencephalitis: K. Yalaz, et al.; Neurology, March 1992, vol. 42(3 pt. 1), pp. 488–491.

Nelson Textbook of Pediatrics, 14th ed.: R.E. Behrman, ed.-in-chief; W.B. Saunders Company, 1992, pp. 843–845.

Progressive Rubella Panencephalitis: Follow-up EEG Study of a Case: A. Guizzaro, et al.; Acta Neurol., August–December 1992, vol. 14(4–6), pp. 485–492.

Virus-Induced Demyelination in Man: Models for Multiple Sclerosis: G.P. Rice; Curr. Opin. Neurol., Neurosurg., April 1992, vol. 5(2), pp. 188–194.

Apparent Response of Subacute Sclerosing Panencephalitis to Intrathecal Interferon Alpha: M. Miyazaki, et al.; Ann. Neurol., January 1991, vol. 29(1), pp. 97–99.

Harrison's Principles of Internal Medicine, 12th ed.: J.D. Wilson, et al., eds.: McGraw-Hill, 1991, pp. 191–192, 675, 706, 2035, 2064.

SSPE: But We Thought Measles Was Gone!: J. Frank, et al.; J. Pediatr. Nurs., April 1991, vol. 6(2), pp. 87–92.

Subacute Sclerosing Panencephalitis Presenting As Simple Partial Seizures: A.J. Kornberg, et al.; J. Child. Neurol., April 1991, vol. 6(2), pp. 146–149.

Dictionary of Medical Syndromes, 3rd ed.: S.I. Magalini, et al., eds.: J.B. Lippincott Company, 1990, pp. 229–230.

Fields Virology, 2nd ed.; B.N. Fields, ed.-in-chief; Raven Press, 1990, pp. 1015, 1032–1033.

# SUTTON DISEASE II

**Description** Sutton disease II, also known as recurrent aphthous stomatitis, is a disease of uncertain etiology characterized by recurrent painful episodes of aphthous stomatitis.

**Synonyms**

> Aphthous Ulcer
> Periadenitis Mucosa Necrotica
> Recurrent Aphthous Stomatitis
> Ulcerative Stomatitis
> von Mikulicz Aphthae
> von Zahorsky Disease

**Signs and Symptoms** This disease is marked by oral ulcers of varying size, often 7 to 15 mm. They may be numerous; as many as 15 may be present at any one time. At the start, they are shallow erosions covered with inflammatory exudate. As healing progresses, scarring may occur. Lesions heal in 1 to 2 weeks, but recurrence is the rule.

The diagnosis is based on the clinical appearance of the ulcers, as well as on the history of recurrence.

**Etiology** The precise etiology of Sutton disease II is unknown, but local disturbances in immunity may contribute. Iron, vitamin B12, and folic acid deficiencies increase susceptibility to the disease. Attacks are usually triggered by stress.

**Epidemiology** Before puberty, males and females are equally affected; after puberty, women are more often affected. The disease occurs most frequently in malnourished children and debilitated adults.

**Related Disorders** *Pemphigus* may resemble Sutton disease II. Herpetic oral ulcers are similar, but they occur mainly on the hard palate and immovable mucosa, while the aphthae of Sutton disease II rarely appear in these locations. Recurrent mouth ulcers also occur in the cyclic neutropenia syndrome and in B12, folate, and iron deficiency syndromes.

**Treatment—Standard** An anesthetic oral rinse and topical steroids give symptomatic relief, and a tetracycline oral suspension may reduce the lesions. However, use of antibiotics and steroids may promote the development of oral candidiasis. When therapy is begun promptly, relief is rapid. Subsequent attacks require renewed efforts at treatment.

**Treatment—Investigational** Zinc sulfate supplementation and the drug azathioprine are undergoing clinical trials in refractory cases of Sutton disease II. The safety and efficacy of these medications have yet to be proved, however.

Please contact the agencies listed under Resources, below, for the most current information. Addresses and telephone numbers of these agencies, as well as of individual experts and research centers, may be found in the Master Resources List.

**Resources**

**For more information on Sutton disease II:** National Organization for Rare Disorders (NORD); NIH/National Institute of Dental Research.

**References**

The Association of Menstrual Cycle, Pregnancy, and Menopause with Recurrent Oral Aphthous Stomatitis: A Review and Critique: B.E. McCartan, et al.; Obstet. Gynecol., September 1992, vol. 80(3 pt. 1), pp. 455–458.

Cecil Textbook of Medicine, 19th ed.: J.B. Wyngaarden, et al., eds.; W.B. Saunders Company, 1992, pp. 1863, 2325.

Nelson Textbook of Pediatrics, 14th ed.: R.E. Behrman, ed.-in-chief; W.B. Saunders Company, 1992, pp. 798–799, 1669.

Recurrent Aphthous Ulcers in Association with HIV Infection: L.A. MacPhail, et al.; Oral Surg. Oral Med. Oral Pathol., March 1992, vol. 73(3), pp. 283–288.

Effect of an Antimicrobial Mouthrinse on Recurrent Aphthous Ulcerations: T.F. Miller, et al.; Oral Surg. Oral Med. Oral Pathol., October 1991, vol. 72(4), pp. 425–429.

Harrison's Principles of Internal Medicine, 12th ed.: J.D. Wilson, et al., eds.: McGraw-Hill, 1991, p. 246.

Recurrent Aphthous Ulceration with Zinc Deficiency and Cellular Immune Deficiency: L. Endre; Oral Surg. Oral Med. Oral Pathol., November 1991, vol. 72(5), pp. 559–561.

Dictionary of Medical Syndromes, 3rd ed.: S.I. Magalini, et al., eds.: J.B. Lippincott Company, 1990, p. 852.

Gastrointestinal Disease, 4th ed.; M.H. Sleisenger, et al.; W.B. Saunders Company, 1989, p. 533.

# SYPHILIS, ACQUIRED

**Description** Syphilis is a chronic, infectious, sexually transmitted disease caused by *Treponema pallidum*. Congenital syphilis is acquired by the fetus in utero. When untreated, syphilis progresses through primary, secondary, and latent stages. Symptoms can remain dormant for years. Eventually any tissue or vascular organ in the body may be affected. With appropriate treatment, syphilis is curable.

**Synonyms**

Lues

Venereal Disease

**Signs and Symptoms** Untreated syphilis progresses through primary and secondary stages (which are infectious), and may end without further symptoms or continue to progress into a latent stage that may last for years.

**Primary syphilis** is characterized by chancres at the inoculation site, usually the skin, anus, vagina, or mouth, which present themselves from 10 to 90 days after the patient has been exposed to the organism. The lesions are usually painless and start as small, solid papules that gradually develop into raised, firm ulcers with a slight yellow discharge. When untreated, these lesions heal within 4 to 6 weeks and may leave scarring.

**Secondary syphilis** usually presents itself within 2 weeks to 6 months after the appearance of the primary lesions. This stage is characterized by infectious lesions of the skin and mucous membranes. These lesions may be pink or coppery in color, widespread, and symmetrical, and follow the lines of skin cleavage. Sites include the genitalia, palms, and soles of the feet. Symptoms, such as loss of appetite, sore throat, headache, low-grade fever, muscle aches, nasal discharge, and swollen lymph nodes, may occur. In 25 percent of untreated cases, a relapse occurs, most often in the first year. Secondary syphilis usually lasts 2 to 6 weeks, and some of the lesions may leave scarring.

**Latent syphilis** occurs when primary and secondary syphilis have gone untreated. The patient is asymptomatic, and the diagnosis can be made only through laboratory tests. Patients may relapse during the first 2 to 4 years of infection, and infectious secondary syphilis lesions may reappear. In about one-third of cases, the disease spontaneously cures itself. Another third will remain infected but show no signs of the disease. The final third will eventually develop late syphilis.

**Late syphilis** is not contagious and usually progresses slowly. Benign tumors of the skin and bones may develop on any part of the body. Cardiovascular problems, seizures, personality changes, impotence, bladder dysfunction, and eye problems, such as optic atrophy and Argyll Robertson pupils, may also be present with late syphilis. Dementia and blindness may result.

**Etiology** Syphilis is caused by the microorganism *Treponema pallidum* and acquired through sexual contact with an infected person. Occasionally health workers have become infected while examining patients with infectious lesions. It may also be acquired by kissing someone with oral infectious lesions. An infected mother can transmit syphilis to her fetus.

**Epidemiology** There are about 80,000 cases of syphilis reported each year in the United States. The highest rate is among 20- to 24-year-old men and women who have sexual contact with numerous partners. Males are currently affected 3 times more often than females. The recent dramatic increase in congenital syphilis is due to the use of "crack" cocaine and the increase in prostitution to support drug abuse.

**Related Disorders** See *Behçet Syndrome; Bejel; Syphilis, Congenital; Pinta; Yaws.*

**Candidiasis** *(Candida albicans)* is normally a harmless yeast infection found in the mouth, intestinal tract, and vagina. But in immunosuppressed patients, it spreads to other parts of the body. In severe cases it may affect the blood, the pericardium, or the meninges.

**Chancroid** is a sexually transmitted infection caused by the bacillus *Haemophilus ducreyi*. The incubation period is 2 to 14 days. Chancroid starts as an inflamed patch of skin that eventually becomes a painful ulcer. Lesions are usually single but may be multiple. In males they are usually found on the penis or around the anus. The lesions on females are normally found on the vagina, cervix, vulva, or around the anus. This infection is rare in the United States but common in Africa and Southeast Asia. Chancroid is usually treated with the antibiotic erythromycin.

**Herpes progenitalis** is a sexually transmitted infection of the genital skin caused by the herpes simplex virus. Lesions appear within 4 to 7 days after contact. These lesions start out as blisters and may have a watery discharge. Both men and women may experience headaches, muscle aches, and tender, swollen lymph nodes in the groin. The blisters crust over and heal without treatment. Symptoms may last about 3 weeks. The disorder is contagious for up to 2 weeks after the lesions appear. The virus may remain latent and then recur at any time. There is no cure for this infection, but lotions may relieve pain, and the drug acyclovir may prevent recurrent attacks.

**Therapies–Standard** Antibiotics, and penicillin especially, are used to treat acquired syphilis. Tetracycline or erythromycin may also be used. Preventive treatment should be given to anyone who has been in sexual contact with an infected person within 90 days. The patient's history (especially sexual) and a battery of tests are essential in determining the stage of syphilis.

**Treatment—Investigational** Please contact the agencies listed under Resources, below, for the most current information. Addresses and telephone numbers of these agencies, as well as of individual experts and research centers, may be found in the Master Resources List.

**Resources**

**For more information on acquired syphilis:** National Organization for Rare Disorders (NORD); Centers for Disease Control; American Social Health Association; National Sexually Transmitted Diseases Hotline; Council for Sex Information and Education; NIH/National Institute of Allergy and Infectious Diseases.

**For local testing and treatment facilities for venereal diseases:** Contact any state or local health department listed in your area phone directory.

### References

Clinical Dermatology, 2nd ed.: T.P. Habif, ed.; C.V. Mosby Company, 1990, pp. 222–228.

Congenital Syphilis Presenting in Infants After the Newborn Period: D.H. Dorfman, et al.; N. Engl. J. Med., November 1990, vol. 323(19), pp. 1299–1302.

Cecil Textbook of Medicine, 18th ed.: J.B. Wyngaarden and L.H. Smith, Jr., eds.; W.B. Saunders Company, 1988, pp. 1713–1722.

Internal Medicine, 2nd ed.: J.H. Stein, ed.-in-chief; Little, Brown and Company, 1987, pp. 1719–1724.

# SYPHILIS, CONGENITAL

**Description** Congenital syphilis is a chronic infectious disease caused by *Treponema pallidum* acquired by the fetus in utero. Symptoms may not appear until weeks, months, or even years after birth. Symptoms of early congenital syphilis include fever, skin disorders, and low birth weight. In late congenital syphilis, symptoms do not usually become apparent until 2 to 5 years of age. In rare cases the disease remains latent until adulthood.

**Synonyms**

Lues, Congenital

**Signs and Symptoms** Pregnant women with syphilis show a reduction in estrogen, while serum progesterone levels may increase. Serologic tests may be seronegative during pregnancy. Symptoms may then show up when the infant is 3 to 14 weeks of age. In these cases the mother probably acquired the infection during the later part of her pregnancy.

Symptoms of **early congenital syphilis** usually appear at 3 to 14 weeks of age but may not appear until 5 years of age. Symptoms include inflammation and hardening of the umbilical cord, rash, fever, low birth weight, high levels of cholesterol at birth, aseptic meningitis, anemia, monocytosis, hepatomegaly, splenomegaly, jaundice, shedding of skin at the palms and soles, convulsions, mental retardation, periostitis, rhinitis with an infectious nasal discharge, hair loss, inflammation of the iris, and pneumonia.

Symptoms of **late congenital syphilis** usually present themselves after age 5 but may remain undiagnosed until well into adulthood. They include bone pain, retinitis pigmentosa, Hutchinson triad (interstitial keratitis, Hutchinson incisors, and labyrinthine disease), saddle nose, bony prominence of the forehead, high-arched palate, short upper jawbone, nerve deafness, and fissuring around the mouth and anus.

**Etiology** Congenital syphilis is a chronic infectious disease caused by the spirochete *Treponema pallidum* and transmitted through the umbilical cord from an infected mother to the fetus. The infant is more likely to contract congenital syphilis if the mother becomes infected during pregnancy, although it is possible for an infant to acquire the disease from a mother who was infected prior to becoming pregnant. Adults transmit syphilis through sexual contact.

**Epidemiology** The incidence of congenital syphilis in newborns under 1 year of age rose in the United States from 180 cases in 1957 to 422 in 1972. More recently there has been a dramatic increase, especially in urban areas, which has been attributed to the use of "crack" cocaine and the increase in prostitution to support drug abuse. In New York City alone, the number of cases rose from 57 in 1986 to 1,000 in 1989.

**Related Disorders** See *Bejel; Epidermolysis Bullosa; Pinta; Yaws.*

**Ectodermal dysplasias** are a group of hereditary, nonprogressive skin diseases. The skin, its derivatives, and some other organs are involved. A predisposition to respiratory infections, due to a somewhat depressed immune system and to defective mucous glands in the respiratory tract, is the most life-threatening characteristic. Symptoms include eczema, poorly functioning sweat glands, sparse or absent hair follicles, abnormal hair, disfigured nails, and difficulties with the nasal passages and ear canals. Skin is satiny smooth, prone to rashes, and slow to heal. Commonly, the teeth fail to develop properly. Other complications may include hearing deficit, loss of sight, mental retardation, limb abnormalities, cleft palate and lip, and urinary tract abnormalities. Allergies are common, as are bronchitis and pneumonia.

**Treatment—Standard** Congenital syphilis is preventable. It occurs in infants whose mothers have not been treated for the disease prior to or during pregnancy. If the infection is very recent, the disease may not be apparent in the neonate. Therefore, it is important to have the infant tested again later if the mother has been diagnosed with syphilis.

Penicillin is the drug of choice for treating syphilis in both mother and infant. Other antibiotics may also be used. Interstitial keratitis may be treated with corticosteroid drugs and atropine drops. An ophthalmologist should be consulted. If nerve deafness is present, a combination of penicillin and corticosteroids may be prescribed.

**Treatment—Investigational** Please contact the agencies listed under Resources, below, for the most current information. Addresses and telephone numbers of these agencies, as well as of individual experts and research centers, may be found in the Master Resources List.

**Resources**

**For more information on congenital syphilis:** National Organization for Rare Disorders (NORD); Centers for Disease Control; The Arc (a national organization on mental retardation); NIH/National Institute of Allergy and Infectious Diseases.

**For local testing and treatment facilities for venereal diseases:** Contact any state or local health department listed in your area phone directory.

**References**

Clinical Dermatology, 2nd ed.: T.P. Habif, ed.; C.V. Mosby Company, 1990, pp. 228–229.

Congenital Syphilis Presenting in Infants After the Newborn Period: D.H. Dorfman, et al.; N. Engl. J. Med., November 1990, vol. 323(19), pp. 1299–1302.

Umbilical Chord Schlerosi As an Indicator of Congenital Syphilis: S. Knowles, et al.; J. Clin. Pathol., November 1989, vol. 42(11), pp. 1157–1159.

Cecil Textbook of Medicine, 18th ed.: J.B. Wyngaarden and L.H. Smith, Jr., eds.; W.B. Saunders Company, 1988, pp. 1718–1719.

Congenital Syphilis in the Newborn: V. Chawla, et al.; Arch. Dis. Child, November 1988, vol. 63(11), pp. 1393–1394.

The Effects of Syphilis on Endocrine Function of the Fetoplacental Unit: C.R. Parker, Jr., et al.; Am. J. Obstet. Gynecol., December 1988, vol. 159(6), pp. 1327–1331.

Internal Medicine, 2nd ed.: J.H. Stein, ed.-in-chief; Little, Brown and Company, 1987, p. 1719.

Medical Aspects of Developmental Disabilities in Children Birth to Three: J.A. Blackman, ed.; University of Iowa, 1983, p. 72.

# TORCH SYNDROME

**Description** The term TORCH is a mnemonic referring to 4 infectious agents that are capable of causing serious intrauterine infection, leading to both disease and/or malformations. The agents are: (**TO**)*xoplasma gondii,* (**R**)ubella virus, (**C**)ytomegalovirus, and (**H**)erpes virus. The mnemonic is useful in the diagnostic workup of any neonate with hepatosplenomegaly, chorioretinitis, or fetal malformations; these 4 agents will rank high on the list of diagnostic possibilities.

**Synonyms**

Toxoplasmosis-Rubella-Cytomegalovirus-Herpes Syndrome

**Signs and Symptoms** Congenital toxoplasmosis may be asymptomatic or may be present at birth with a wide variety of symptoms, such as hepatosplenomegaly, chorioretinitis, jaundice, thrombocytopenia, and numerous central nervous system abnormalities. Those cases that are asymptomatic at birth may manifest evidence of infection at a later date.

The symptoms of congenital rubella are hepatosplenomegaly, thrombocytopenia, meningoencephalitis, microcephaly, cardiac malformations, cataracts, hearing loss, and mental retardation, to mention a few. (See **Rubella, Congenital.**)

Cytomegalovirus infection (**CMV**) is associated with hepatosplenomegaly, jaundice, petechiae, chorioretinitis, and a variety of central nervous system abnormalities. The clinical syndrome ranges in severity from asymptomatic to fulminant and fatal.

Neonatal herpes can be characterized by hepatosplenomegaly, jaundice, a bleeding diathesis, and central nervous system abnormalities. There is considerable variation in the severity of symptoms. Unlike the above disorders, herpes appears to be transmitted during delivery, by passage through an infected genital tract.

**Etiology** The etiologic agents are *Toxoplasma gondii,* rubella virus, cytomegalovirus, and herpes virus, usually herpes simplex virus, type II.

**Epidemiology** These infections occur worldwide. Transmission to the fetus is transplacental in rubella, toxoplasmosis, and cytomegalovirus, and appears to be at the time of delivery in the case of herpes.

**Treatment—Standard** Congenital toxoplasmosis may be treated with pyrimethamine and sulfadiazine, or spiramycin. There is some evidence that treatment reduces the chance of developing further symptoms during postnatal life.

There is no effective treatment for congenital rubella or congenital CMV, but ganciclovir may be of some benefit in the latter.

The first step in the approach to neonatal herpes is prevention; if the mother develops symptoms of herpes infection, or vaginal or cervical cultures done late in pregnancy show herpes virus, the fetus is best delivered by cesarean section. When this is not possible and infection results, acyclovir has been used with success in neonatal herpes.

**Treatment—Investigational** Please contact the agencies listed under Resources, below, for the most current information. Addresses and telephone numbers of these agencies, as well as of individual experts and research centers, may be found in the Master Resources List.

**Resources**
   **For more information on the TORCH diseases:** National Organization for Rare Disorders (NORD); NIH/National Institute of Allergy and Infectious Diseases; NIH/National Institute of Neurological Disorders and Stroke; Centers for Disease Control.
   **For genetic information and genetic counseling referrals:** March of Dimes Birth Defects Foundation; Alliance of Genetic Support Groups.

**References**
   TORCH: A Literature Review and Implications for Practice: L. Haggerty; J. Obstet. Gynecol. Nurs., 1985, vol. 14(2), pp. 124–129.
   The TORCH Syndrome: A Clinical Review: J.D. Fine and K.A. Arndt; J. Amer. Acad. Dermatol., 1985, vol. 12(4), pp. 2477–2478.

# TOXIC SHOCK SYNDROME (TSS)

**Description** TSS, produced by toxins elaborated by *Staphylococcus aureus*, is a multisystem disease with widespread manifestations. Characteristic features include high fever, vomiting, diarrhea, hypotension, and a skin rash that typically resembles a sunburn and desquamates during convalescence. Most, but not all, cases occur in menstruating females in association with the use of tampons. TSS also may develop as a consequence of relatively minor postoperative wound infections, sometimes in association with nasal packing.

**Signs and Symptoms** Onset of TSS is usually sudden. Initially, there is a high fever, accompanied by headache, sore throat, and conjunctivitis. The classic "sunburn" rash appears early and desquamates on the palms and soles over several days. Gastrointestinal involvement, with vomiting and diarrhea, is common. Central nervous system dysfunction may be noted, with disorientation. Hypotension is common, and frank shock occurs in severe cases. There may be acute renal failure, hepatic insufficiency, myositis, and disseminated intravascular coagulation, as well as development of adult respiratory distress syndrome.

   Diagnosis of toxic shock syndrome is based on clinical criteria that include fever, rash with desquamation, hypotension, and involvement of at least 3 organ systems (typically gastrointestinal, hepatic, renal, hematologic, muscular, or central nervous system). *S. aureus* may be isolated from the vagina or from focal lesions, but blood cultures are usually negative.

   The mortality rate is approximately 3 percent, though this figure may be excessive, reflecting heavy reporting of severe cases. Recurrences have occurred, chiefly during subsequent menses of women using tampons.

**Etiology** Toxic shock syndrome is caused by one or more toxins (**TSST-1**) elaborated by certain strains of *S. aureus*. Approximately 70 to 75 percent of cases are associated with vaginal infections of *S. aureus* and the use of hyperabsorbent tampons. Recent studies suggest that the tampons' polyester fibers absorb magnesium normally present in the vagina tissue and fluid, triggering the production of TSST-1. Other associated types of staphylococcal infection include postoperative and postpartum wound infections, abscesses, pneumonia, osteomyelitis, and skin infections.

**Epidemiology** The major risk group for toxic shock syndrome is menstruating women. The combination of vaginal *S. aureus* infection and continuous tampon use sets the stage for TSS. However, TSS has been reported in association with a wide variety of other infections occurring in nonmenstruating women, children, and men. The incidence is estimated to be 3 cases per 100,000 menstruating women. Cases have been reported from all 50 states and have declined since the mid-1980s.

   TSS has also been reported in association with the use of the vaginal contraceptive sponge. According to Food and Drug Administration reports, 12 cases have been confirmed out of an estimated 600,000 regular users, although none were fatal. To minimize the risk, it is recommended that the sponge not be worn for more than 30 hours continuously, and that it not be used during menstruation or during the first 3 months postpartum.

**Treatment—Standard** Aggressive fluid and electrolyte replacement is essential. In severe cases, intensive supportive care will be necessary to address pulmonary and renal insufficiency, hypotension, and other complications. In nonmenstrual TSS the wound, abscess, or other focus needs to be treated appropriately. The drug of choice is a β-lactamase–resistant antistaphylococcal penicillin.

   Prevention involves judicious use of tampons; intermittent use and avoidance of highly absorbent brands is advised.

**Treatment—Investigational** The role of antibiotics as a prophylaxis for recurring TSS is under investigation. More research is necessary to determine the safety and efficacy of such drugs.

   Please contact the agencies listed under Resources, below, for the most current information. Addresses and telephone numbers of these agencies, as well as of individual experts and research centers, may be found in the Master Resources List.

## Resources

**For more information on toxic shock syndrome:** National Organization for Rare Disorders (NORD); NIH/National Institute of Allergy and Infectious Diseases; Centers for Disease Control.

### References

Clinical Spectrum of Nonmenstrual Toxic Shock Syndrome (TSS): Comparison with Menstrual TSS by Multivariate Discriminant Analyses: K.C. Kain, et al.; Clin. Infect. Dis., January 1993, vol. 16(1), pp. 100–106.

Ehrlichiosis Presenting As a Life-Threatening Illness with Features of the Toxic Shock Syndrome: C.J. Fichtenbaum, et al.; Am. J. Med., October 1993, vol. 95(4), pp. 351–357.

Toxic Shock Syndrome: Are You Recognizing Its Changing Presentations?: L.J. Strausbaugh; Postgrad. Med., November 1993, vol. 94(6), pp. 107–108, 111–113, 117–118.

Cecil Textbook of Medicine, 19th ed.: J.B. Wyngaarden, et al., eds.: W.B. Saunders Company, 1992, pp. 780, 1629, 1650, 2301–2302.

Identification of HLA-DR Alpha Chain Residues Critical for Binding of the Toxic Shock Syndrome Toxin Superantigen: P. Panina-Bordignon, et al.; J. Exp. Med., December 1992, vol. 176(6), pp. 1779–1784.

Nelson Textbook of Pediatrics, 14th ed.: R.E. Behrman, ed.-in-chief; W.B. Saunders Company, 1992, pp. 708–709.

Toxic Shock Syndrome: A Complication of Continent Urinary Diversion: P.D. McCahill, et al.; J. Urol., March 1992, vol. 147(3), pp. 681–682.

Apparent Increase in the Incidence of Invasive Group A Beta-Hemolytic Streptococcal Disease in Children: L.B. Givner; J. Pediatr., March 1991, vol. 18, pp. 341–346.

Toxic Shock Syndrome and Tampons: A. Schuchat, et al.; Epidemiol. Rev., 1991, vol. 13, pp. 99–112.

Therapy of Toxic Shock Syndrome: J.K. Todd; Drugs, June 1990, vol. 39(6), pp. 856–861.

Toxic Shock Syndrome Associated with Use of Latex Nasal Packing: S.T. Allen, et al.; Arch. Intern. Med., December 1990, vol. 150(12), pp. 2587–2588.

Postinfluenza Toxic Shock Syndrome: G.C. Prechter, et al.; Chest, May 1989, vol. 95(5), pp. 1153–1154.

Recurrent Toxic Shock Syndrome: C.L. Bryner, et al.; Am. Fam. Physician, March 1989, vol. 39(3), pp. 157–164.

Toxic Shock Syndrome Caused by a Strain of *Staphylococcus aureus* That Produces Enterotoxin C But Not Toxic Shock Syndrome Toxin-1: M.F. Rizkallah, et al.; Am. J. Dis. Child., July 1989, vol. 143(7), pp. 848–849.

# TOXOCARIASIS

**Description** Toxocariasis is a systemic helminthic infection caused by the dog ascarid *Toxocara canis*.

**Synonyms**

Visceral Larva Migrans

**Signs and Symptoms** The majority of infections are probably asymptomatic, but severe and even fatal infection is possible. When symptoms occur, they vary with the migratory patterns of the parasite. Common complaints include fever, cough, wheezing, and abdominal pain. Involvement of the central nervous system, particularly the eye, occurs. Hepatomegaly is common, and lung examination frequently reveals rales and wheezes. The chest x-ray may be abnormal. Marked eosinophilia is the rule.

The diagnosis of toxocariasis is usually made on the clinical picture. An enzyme-linked immunosorbent assay **(ELISA)** may be used to confirm the diagnosis.

**Etiology** Toxocariasis is caused by the helminth *Toxocara canis*. Infection is acquired by eating the eggs of the organism. The larvae invade the tissues of the body where they elicit granuloma formation.

**Epidemiology** The adult worms inhabit the intestines of dogs, and the eggs are passed in the stool. Young children are at risk, particularly in areas where geophagia is common. Toxocariasis has been reported mostly in the United States (south central and southeastern regions) and in Europe.

**Related Disorders** Disorders that can produce symptoms similar to those of eosinophilia include other nematode infections, such as *Ascaris lumbricoides* and *Strongyloides stercoralis*, as well as schistosomes and hookworm. Ocular infection is unique to toxocariasis, but may require differentiation from other diseases of the eye, such as malignancy.

**Treatment—Standard** Toxocariasis may be treated with diethylcarbamazine or thiabendazole, but neither of these is uniformly effective. Most cases are self-limited and do not warrant specific therapy. Preventive measures consist of deworming dogs, preventing geophagia, and good hygiene. Retinal infection may be treated with laser photocoagulation.

**Treatment—Investigational** Please contact the agencies listed under Resources, below, for the most current information. Addresses and telephone numbers of these agencies, as well as of individual experts and research centers, may be found in the Master Resources List.

## Resources

**For more information on toxocariasis:** National Organization for Rare Disorders (NORD); NIH/National Institute of Allergy and Infectious Diseases; Centers for Disease Control.

### References

Human Toxocariasis. Review with Report of a Probable Case: P.D. Morris, et al.; Postgrad. Med., January 1987, vol. 81(1), pp. 263–267.

Internal Medicine, 2nd ed.: J.H. Stein, ed.-in-chief; Little, Brown and Company, 1987, pp. 1801–1802.

Serologic and Intradermal Test for Parasitic Infections: D.A. Bruckner; Pediatr. Clin. North Am., August 1985, vol. 32(4), pp. 1063–1075.

# TOXOPLASMOSIS

**Description** Toxoplasmosis is an infectious disease caused by the protozoan parasite, *Toxoplasma gondii*. The infection produces several different syndromes depending on host factors, and whether it occurs pre- or postnatally. Congenital toxoplasmosis produces a range of fetal abnormalities, including spontaneous abortion, central nervous system damage, hepatitis, and chorioretinitis. In immunocompetent adults, toxoplasmosis is usually a benign mononucleosis-like illness. Immunocompromised patients are more likely to develop a severe, disseminated form of infection that may be fatal.

**Synonyms**
>    Disseminated Toxoplasmosis
>    Lymphadenopathic Toxoplasmosis

**Signs and Symptoms** The 3 different syndromes of toxoplasmosis will be described separately.

The majority of **toxoplasma infections in immunocompetent individuals** are asymptomatic. In symptomatic cases the most frequent abnormality is lymphadenopathy, usually cervical; however, regional adenopathy in other locations, and generalized adenopathy, occur. Fever, malaise, hepatosplenomegaly, and laboratory features of a mononucleosis-like syndrome may also be present. The course is generally benign but may be protracted. Since toxoplasmosis often cannot be distinguished clinically from infectious mononucleosis, lymphoma, and other diseases, diagnosis should be confirmed by serologic testing.

**Toxoplasmosis in the immunosuppressed patient:** Patients with AIDS, hematologic malignancies, and organ transplants are at risk for a disseminated, more serious form of toxoplasmosis. Involvement of the central nervous system is the most common manifestation; mass lesions, encephalitis, and meningoencephalitis may occur. A common presentation is a generalized seizure, produced by a ring-enhancing lesion seen on CT scan. Brain biopsy may be necessary to distinguish cerebral toxoplasmosis from other lesions in the immunosuppressed host (lymphoma, tuberculoma, and others). Myocarditis and pneumonitis may also develop.

**Congenital toxoplasmosis** results from maternal infection, which is usually asymptomatic. When infection is acquired early in pregnancy, the risk of transmission to the fetus is lower, but the chance of severe fetal disease resulting from infection is higher. The manifestations of fetal toxoplasmosis may be evident before birth, with spontaneous abortion; may be evident at birth, in which case the disease is usually severe; or may be mild and not become evident until some time after birth. The clinical picture may include any of the following: microcephaly, hydrocephalus, chorioretinitis, blindness, mental retardation, seizures, anemia, jaundice, and a rash.

In cases where fetal infection is mild or asymptomatic at birth, early treatment can markedly reduce the risk of developing symptoms at a later date.

**Etiology** Toxoplasmosis is caused by an intracellular protozoan parasite, *T. gondii*. This organism is ubiquitous in nature. Its life cycle involves a sexual stage that occurs in cats. Humans become infected by cysts—either oocysts, which are excreted in cat feces, or tissue cysts, which are present in a variety of foodstuffs.

Infection may be asymptomatic but may persist in a latent form, only to be reactivated in the event of immunosuppression.

**Epidemiology** Toxoplasmosis affects men and women in equal numbers worldwide. The incidence varies widely from country to country, and within different regions of the United States. The incidence of congenital infection is 0.25:100,000 to 5.0:100,000 live births.

Toxoplasmosis is acquired transplacentally or by oral ingestion. Cysts may be present in lamb, pork, and eggs, and probably contaminate vegetables and other food products. As was mentioned above, cysts are also present in cat feces and may be transmitted during routine care of cat litter. Pregnant women are advised to avoid cat litter in order to minimize the risk of transmission.

**Related Disorders** The **mononucleosis** syndrome is most frequently caused by Epstein-Barr virus, or occasionally cytomegalovirus. Hepatitis B may produce a similar clinical picture (see ***Hepatitis B.***)

**Chorioretinitis** may also be caused by cytomegalovirus. Related congenital infections include those of the TORCH complex: toxoplasmosis-rubella-cytomegalovirus-herpes (see ***TORCH Syndrome.***)

**Treatment—Standard** Specific treatment of toxoplasmosis in immunocompetent individuals is rarely necessary. In pregnancy, spiramycin is the preferred drug, since pyrimethamine may be teratogenic. Immunocompromised patients are generally treated with pyrimethamine and sulfadiazine (clindamycin may be substituted for sulfadiazine); infected neonates may be treated with these or spiramycin. Since these drugs are associated with significant hematologic toxicity, periodic monitoring is recommended.

**Treatment—Investigational** The Food and Drug Administration has awarded a research grant to Rima McLeod, M.D., Michael Reese Hospital and Medical Center, Chicago, Illinois, for comparison studies on treatments for congenital toxoplasmosis. Included in the studies are pyrimethamine and sulfadiazine, spiramycin, and pyrimethamine and sulfadoxine.

Please contact the agencies listed under Resources, below, for the most current information. Addresses and telephone numbers of these agencies, as well as of individual experts and research centers, may be found in the Master Resources List.

### Resources

**For more information on toxoplasmosis:** National Organization for Rare Disorders (NORD); Centers for Disease Control; NIH/National Institute of Allergy and Infectious Diseases.

### References

Toxoplasma Gondii: R.E. McCabe and J.S. Remington; *in* Principles and Practice of Infectious Diseases: G.L. Mandell, et al., eds.; Churchill Livingstone, 1990, pp. 2090–2102.

# TUBERCULOSIS (TB)

**Description** TB is a bacterial disease caused by *Mycobacterium tuberculosis* or *Mycobacterium bovis*. Pathologically, the hallmark of TB is the granuloma. Clinically, typical TB is characterized by an initial asymptomatic infection followed by a latent period of years, with the possibility of reactivation in later adulthood.

TB is usually a chronic infection with protean manifestations. The lungs are most often affected, where the most common manifestation is cavitary pneumonia. The tubercle bacillus is remarkably adept at setting up infection in virtually any organ of the body.

**Signs and Symptoms** The signs and symptoms of TB depend on the site of infection. Tuberculosis is usually thought of as a disease that occurs in stages. The initial, or primary, infection is in the lungs. It frequently occurs in childhood and is most often asymptomatic. When symptomatic, the syndrome is one of lower lobe pneumonia. However, if primary infection does not occur until adulthood, the disease may progress so quickly that the clinical syndrome is indistinguishable from reactivation disease. In patients with AIDS, primary infections commonly progress relentlessly and spread to other parts of the body.

Reactivated or secondary TB is most commonly a chronic, slowly progressive disease that begins insidiously with nonspecific constitutional symptoms. Weight loss, night sweats, fever, and fatigue are prominent. In the lungs, a cavity usually develops, which may be seen on chest x-ray. The major symptom at this stage is coughing, and the secretions are infectious. Hemoptysis may also occur late in the disease.

Extrapulmonary TB is increasingly common because of a resurgence of tuberculosis in patients with AIDS. The organs most commonly affected are the pleura, genitourinary tract, kidney, meninges, bones, and pericardium. The symptoms vary with the organ involved.

Miliary TB may be a fulminant disease with severe lung disease and pleural, peritoneal, and meningeal involvement.

The diagnosis of TB requires demonstrating the organism in tissues or body fluids. The presence of a cavity on chest x-ray, with the appropriate clinical picture, points strongly to the diagnosis, and sputum smears for acid-fast bacilli are confirmatory. In the past, gastric aspirates have been used to obtain smears for microbiological staining, but these are regarded as unreliable.

Asymptomatic infection is diagnosed using the Mantoux, or tuberculin, test. This involves an intradermal injection of purified protein derivative (**PPD**) and observing for a reaction 48 to 72 hours later. A positive test is considered to be 10 mm or more induration (not erythema).

The diagnosis of extrapulmonary TB may require acid-fast staining of the cerebrospinal fluid and pleural, peritoneal, or bone marrow biopsy, depending on the site of suspected disease. Often cultures are necessary, particularly for determining antibiotic resistances. These are time-consuming, as growth of the organism in vitro requires 4 to 6 weeks.

**Etiology** In the United States today, *M. tuberculosis* is the most common cause of tuberculosis. This organism may also be referred to as the tubercle bacillus, or as acid-fast bacilli (**AFB**). In the past, the disease was often caused by *M. bovis,* which is transmitted through dairy products; in countries where milk pasteurization is not routine, *M. bovis* is still a principal source of infection.

**Epidemiology** TB is spread by droplets in the secretions from individuals with active cavitary disease. Patients with TB but without pulmonary cavities are generally regarded as noninfectious. TB is generally not highly contagious, and prolonged periods of close contact are usually required for spread of the disease.

TB is associated with advanced age, poverty, alcoholism, and AIDS. In the United States, it remains a serious health problem, particularly in urban areas with high concentrations of AIDS patients and immigrants from the third world. Recently, the southeast area of the United States and states bordering Mexico reported the highest number of TB cases. In addition, recent immigrants from Southeast Asia now constitute 3 to 5 percent of new cases.

Since 1984 the incidence of TB in the United States has been rising. In 1991, over 25,000 cases were reported, with approximately 2,000 deaths.

Worldwide, TB is a major health problem, with as many as 4 million new cases and 3 million deaths each year. The Centers for Disease Control currently estimate that 10 million people are infected worldwide, and while they are not all symptomatic, for each there is a lifelong risk of developing active TB.

**Related Disorders** See also *Nocardiosis* and *Paracoccidioidomycosis,* which may resemble TB.

Following is a list of the various subtypes of tuberculosis:

**Childhood tuberculosis (primary TB)** is the initial infection, and typically produces a lower lobe pneumonia in symptomatic cases.

**Disseminated hematogenous TB (miliary TB)** is a more fulminant form of TB occurring mostly during early childhood. Multisystem involvement is the rule.

**Tuberculous lymphadenitis** is only rarely associated with significant symptoms. Most patients have no sign of TB elsewhere in the body, and most have involvement of a single node. Lymph node biopsy is required for diagnosis.

**Cutaneous TB.** There are a variety of different skin lesions associated with tuberculous infection. Skin infection occurs through direct inoculation from an exogenous source, or through hematogenous or local spread from elsewhere in the body. Tuberculous warts and chancres are associated with inoculation; gummas, scrofuloderma, and many other lesions may result from endogenous infection.

**Bone involvement** is most frequent in the spine (Pott disease, tuberculous spondylitis). It produces a characteristic deformity (gibbus). If it spreads to the surrounding area, it may impinge on the spinal cord and cause paralysis. Other forms of bony involvement include osteomyelitis and arthritis, usually monoarticular.

**Central nervous system TB** may be manifested by meningitis, or by a tuberculoma in the brain, which behaves as a space-occupying lesion. Tuberculous meningitis is generally a problem of young children aged 1 to 5 years, although it may occur at any age. Approximately 25 percent of children will develop sequelae, including convulsive disorders, communicating hydrocephalus, mental retardation, and other neurologic abnormalities.

**Pleural TB** can occur in at least 2 forms, one in conjunction with active pulmonary TB, and the other shortly after primary infection. Stains of pleural fluid for AFB are not useful, although the yield on culture is higher. The diagnostic procedure of choice is a pleural biopsy. Surgical drainage may be required in addition to antituberculous drugs.

**Genitourinary TB** may involve the kidneys, bladder, seminal vesicles, prostate, fallopian tubes, or ovaries. In renal tuberculosis urinary symptoms usually, but not invariably, occur. The urinary sediment is abnormal in 90 percent of cases.

**Tuberculous peritonitis** may spread from the lymph nodes, gastrointestinal tract, or uterine tube and ovary to surrounding areas. Local tenderness, fever, and weight loss are symptomatic of this type of TB. In most cases the onset is insidious, but a more fulminant course resembling typical bacterial peritonitis may also occur. A peritoneal biopsy may be required for diagnosis.

**Tuberculous pericarditis** is usually due to spread from infected mediastinal nodes. Pericardiectomy is necessary in cases where the pericarditis becomes constrictive, or if the effusion threatens to progress to tamponade.

**Silicotuberculosis** is the result of TB infection in a patient with silicosis. Patients with silicosis run a much higher risk of contracting tuberculosis than the general population.

**Chronic hematogenous TB** is a blood-borne reactivated infection, usually spread from an extrapulmonary source. It occurs years after primary infection and tends to be superimposed on other chronic illness. The symptoms are vague and the diagnosis very difficult.

**Treatment—Standard** The tubercle bacillus is remarkably hardy and is capable of long periods of metabolic inactivity. Successful eradication requires multiple drugs administered over many months. Fortunately, infectivity is dramatically reduced after 10 to 14 days of effective therapy; and significant symptomatic improvement occurs in the first 2 to 3 weeks. Unfortunately, lengthy treatment regimens depend heavily on patient compliance for their success, and relapses are a problem in incompletely treated cases.

There are several currently recommended regimens. The precise regimen used initially depends on the likelihood of drug resistance, the likelihood of compliance, and other patient factors such as the presence of renal insufficiency or pregnancy.

The most effective regimen is isoniazid and rifampin for 9 months. Ethambutol is frequently added initially until the drug sensitivities of the organism are known. Less toxic, and recommended for pregnant women, is a regimen of isoniazid and ethambutol for 12 to 18 months.

In cases where the patient can be closely monitored and compliance is likely to be high, a short-course regimen may be suitable. There are several regimens, all starting with 2 months of isoniazid, rifampin, pyrazinamide, and a 4th drug (either streptomycin or ethambutol), followed by 4 to 6 months of double or triple drug therapy.

In all these regimens the drugs must be taken daily. When daily therapy over a long period is not a reasonable option, there is an effective regimen of twice weekly therapy, which may begin after the first month: isoniazid, at triple the usual dosage, and rifampin twice weekly for 8 months. Intermittent therapy of this type is best administered in a directly observed fashion, especially when noncompliance is a factor.

Patients with concurrent HIV infection are treated with the same regimens as other individuals, but because of their underlying immunodeficiency, the potential for relapse is probably lifelong in spite of therapy. In some large cities, patients with HIV are being infected with strains that are multidrug-resistant and unresponsive to intensive therapy. Patients with renal failure require significant dose reductions and close monitoring for toxicity.

Drug toxicity is an important factor in the choice and modification of treatment regimens. Hepatotoxicity is common to isoniazid, rifampin, and pyrazinamide, and when symptomatic hepatitis develops, the offending drugs should be discontinued. Monitoring liver enzymes has been recommended in the past but is no longer thought to be necessary.

**Prophylaxis:** Tuberculin-positive patients without evidence of active disease are recommended to take isoniazid daily for 1 year. Since the risk of hepatotoxicity rises with age, this recommendation is frequently limited to patients under the age of 35 years. Household contacts, particularly children, should be treated for 3 months. After 3 months, if their skin test is positive, treatment should continue for a full 12 months.

Surgery may be indicated for some skin manifestations of TB. Corticosteroid therapy in conjunction with antibiotics may be advantageous in refractory cases or in cases that concur with other diseases.

The vaccine for tuberculosis, the bacille Calmette-Guérin (**BCG**), has been widely used in some countries, but its efficacy is the subject of controversy. It is not currently recommended in the United States since not only is its protective value in doubt, but it interferes with the interpretation of the tuberculin skin test, the major test for detection of asymptomatic infections.

**Treatment—Investigational** The orphan drug Rifater (rifampin, isoniazid, pyrazinamide) is undergoing tests for short-course treatment of TB. Two orphan products, para-aminosalicylic acid and gabbromicina, are being developed for the treatment of TB. Thalidomide is undergoing tests in the treatment of clinical manifestations of mycobacterial infection caused by mycobacterial TB and non-TB mycobacteria.

Please contact the agencies listed under Resources, below, for the most current information. Addresses and telephone numbers of these agencies, as well as of individual experts and research centers, may be found in the Master Resources List.

### Resources

**For more information on tuberculosis:** National Organization for Rare Disorders (NORD); American Lung Association; NIH/National Institute of Allergy and Infectious Diseases; Centers for Disease Control.

### References

Mycobacterium Tuberculosis: R.M. Des Prez and C.R. Heim; *in* Principles and Practice of Infectious Diseases: G.L. Mandell, et al., eds.; Churchill Livingstone, 1990, pp. 1877–1905.

Curable, Preventable, but Still a Killer: Tuberculosis: Annabel Hecht; FDA Consumer, December 1986–January 1987, pp. 7–10.

# TYPHOID FEVER

**Description** Typhoid fever is an acute systemic infection caused by *Salmonella typhi.* Major symptoms reflect involvement of the gastrointestinal, hematologic, neurologic, and respiratory systems. Complications are common and may be life-threatening.

### Synonyms

Enteric Fever

**Signs and Symptoms** The symptoms of typhoid fever begin after an incubation period of 1 to 3 weeks. Onset is usually insidious, and the initial symptoms are characteristically vague, with fever, headache, myalgias, and malaise. Respiratory symptoms are common at this stage. By the end of the first week of illness, the fever is high and may be associated with a relative bradycardia. Diarrhea is common, but constipation may also occur. Neurologic symptoms may be present, such as seizures, psychosis, or delirium, the symptom for which the disease was originally named (*typhos,* Greek for cloud, referring to a clouded consciousness).

Physical examination may reveal a rash classically associated with typhoid fever: rose spots. These are erythematous lesions, usually 2 to 4 mm in size, that appear transiently on the upper abdomen. There may be rales on chest examination. The abdomen is tender and may be distended, and hepatosplenomegaly is common.

There are a number of laboratory abnormalities in typhoid fever. Anemia is common, as is neutropenia. There may be evidence of subclinical disseminated intravascular coagulation (**DIC**), and elevated hepatic enzymes.

Complications of typhoid fever include gastrointestinal hemorrhage and perforation, myocarditis, transient bone marrow suppression, and, rarely, hepatic failure. Relapses may occur in untreated cases.

*S. typhi* infection can persist in a chronic carrier state. In these cases there is asymptomatic shedding of bacteria in the stool or urine.

The diagnosis of typhoid fever is made by isolation of the bacteria from blood cultures. The majority of patients will have detectable bacteremia in the 1st week of illness, but the rate of blood culture positivity falls to 20 to 30 percent of untreated patients by the 3rd week. Stool cultures may be diagnostic in regions where the prevalence of asymptomatic carriers is extremely low. Bone marrow cultures may also be used to diagnose typhoid fever. Serologic tests, such as the Widal test for agglutinins against typhoid O antigen, are not sufficiently reliable for diagnosis.

**Etiology** Typhoid fever is caused by the gram-negative rod, *Salmonella typhi.*

**Epidemiology** Humans are the only reservoir for *S. typhi;* therefore infection is usually spread by contact with symptomatic individuals (carriers) or with food contaminated by a chronic carrier, or by sewage contamination of the water supply.

There are approximately 500 cases reported annually in the United States; the majority of these are imported from elsewhere, particularly Mexico and India. Outbreaks have occurred in the United States, and these are usually traced to a carrier involved in food preparation. Typhoid fever remains a serious health problem, with a mortality rate of 10 percent per year in many parts of the world (Central and South America, Asia, Africa, and the Middle East).

**Related Disorders** The differential diagnosis of typhoid fever varies with the stage and presenting symptoms of the illness. Depending on which symptoms are prominent, typhoid fever can resemble a respiratory illness, such as influenza or pneumonia; a neurologic infection, such as meningitis; an acute abdomen, such as appendicitis or intestinal infarction; or dysentery and other forms of infectious diarrhea. In long-standing untreated cases, the differential diagnosis may include brucellosis, bacterial endocarditis, inflammatory bowel disease, and malaria.

Related diseases include those caused by other species of *Salmonella,* including paratyphoid fever, which resembles typhoid fever but is usually milder, and acute enterocolitis. *Salmonella* species may also produce a primary bacteremia; patients with sickle cell anemia, hemolytic diseases, and AIDS are susceptible to this type of infection.

**Treatment—Standard** The treatment of typhoid fever involves administration of chloramphenicol, ampicillin, ceftriaxone, pefloxacin, or co-trimoxazole (trimethoprim-sulfamethoxazole). Vaccines are available but of debatable efficacy; and precautions regarding food and water are necessary when traveling in developing countries where typhoid fever is prevalent.

**Treatment—Investigational** Please contact the agencies listed under Resources, below, for the most current information. Addresses and telephone numbers of these agencies, as well as of individual experts and research centers, may be found in the Master Resources List.

**Resources**

**For more information on typhoid fever:** National Organization for Rare Disorders (NORD); Centers for Disease Control; NIH/National Institute of Allergy and Infectious Diseases.

**References**

Clinical Experience with Pefloxacin in the Therapy of Typhoid Fever: P. Christiano, et al.; Infection, March–April 1989, vol. 17(2), pp. 86–67.

Mary Mallon's Trail of Typhoid: C. Cary; FDA Consumer, April 1989, pp. 18–21.

Salmonella Typhi Infections in the United States, 1975–1984: Increasing Role of Foreign Travel: C.A. Ryan, et al.; Rev. Infect. Dis., January–February 1989, vol. 11(1), pp. 1–8.

Assessment on Antimicrobial Treatment of Acute Typhoid and Paratyphoid Fevers in Britain and the Netherlands 1971–1980: R.J. Fallon, et al.; J. Infect., March 1988, vol. 16(2), pp. 129–134.

Cefoperazone Compared with Chloramphenicol in the Treatment of Typhoid Fever: F. Paradisi; Chemotherapy, 1988, vol. 34(1), pp. 71–76.

Internal Medicine, 2nd ed.: J.H. Stein, ed.-in-chief; Little, Brown and Company, 1987, pp. 1664–1691, 1696.

# URTICARIA, CHOLINERGIC

**Description** Cholinergic urticaria is an immediate-type hypersensitivity disorder induced by heat, emotional stress, or exercise in susceptible individuals. It is characterized by the wheal-and-flare reaction and pruritus, and may be associated with systemic symptoms.

**Synonyms**

Physical Urticaria

**Signs and Symptoms** The disorder is characterized by pruritic, erythematous macules and hives (the wheal-and-flare reaction) that are usually 2 to 5 cm in diameter. These lesions may coalesce. The eyelids, lips, hands, and feet may become swollen, and this may be accompanied by abdominal cramps, diarrhea, faintness, weakness, and sweating.

The diagnosis may be established by provocative testing, such as an intradermal injection of methacholine. Heat, as in immersing an arm in warm water, or exercise may also be used provocatively to diagnose cholinergic urticaria.

**Etiology** Cholinergic urticaria is an IgE-mediated hypersensitivity reaction that may be produced by anything that raises the skin temperature, such as hot baths, warm rooms, physical exercise, and exposure to the sun. Irritants in products such as cosmetics or drugs may contribute to the reaction. Eating hot foods, excitement, sweating, and possibly hypersensitivity to acetylcholine, may also induce an urticarial reaction in this syndrome.

**Related Disorders** See *Dermatitis, Contact.*

**Treatment—Standard** Hydroxyzine is the drug of choice for cholinergic urticaria. Antihistamines may ameliorate the pruritis. Protective clothing, sunscreens, and avoiding direct sunlight may be helpful.

**Treatment—Investigational** Please contact the agencies listed under Resources, below, for the most current information. Addresses and telephone numbers of these agencies, as well as of individual experts and research centers, may be found in the Master Resources List.

**Resources**

    **For more information on cholinergic urticaria:** National Organization for Rare Disorders (NORD); Asthma and Allergy Foundation of America; NIH/National Institute of Allergy and Infectious Diseases.

**Reference**

    Cecil Textbook of Medicine, 18th ed.: J.B. Wyngaarden and L.H. Smith, Jr., eds.; W.B. Saunders Company, 1988, pp. 1948–1951, 2334–2335.

# URTICARIA, COLD

**Description** Cold urticaria is a chronic disorder in which exposure to cold precipitates urticaria and, in some cases, angioedema. It is a type of physical urticaria.

**Signs and Symptoms** In cold urticaria the skin develops pruritis, hives, and, in some cases, angioedema, when exposed to cold. Systemic manifestations, including fever, headache, anxiety, fatigue, and, sometimes, syncope, may occur. Palpitations and wheezing are other occasional complaints.

Familial cold urticaria is usually precipitated by generalized cold, rather than a local stimulus. It usually develops about 30 minutes after exposure, and may persist for up to 48 hours. It may be accompanied by systemic symptoms, including fever, headache, fatigue, and arthralgias, and leukocytosis may be evident on laboratory testing.

Acquired cold urticaria is classified into primary, secondary, delayed, localized, and reflex types.

**Primary acquired cold urticaria** occurs within minutes of exposure to cold. The reaction often develops during rewarming rather than during the cold phase itself. Usually the initial symptoms are pruritis and erythema, followed by a burning sensation and urticaria, which lasts 30 minutes. The systemic symptoms mentioned above may also occur.

In **delayed cold urticaria,** the reaction may be delayed for several hours after exposure.

**Localized cold urticaria** is similar to the primary type described above, except the reaction is limited to previous sites of immunologic challenge, such as ragweed injection sites or insect bites.

In **reflex cold urticaria,** generalized urticaria occurs when a local cold stimulus is applied (such as an ice pack). The local stimulus precipitates a fall in body temperature, which prompts the generalized response.

Secondary cold urticaria can occur in the presence of cryoglobulins and other cryoproteins, which may appear in association with lymphoproliferative disorders.

**Etiology** Cold urticaria can be idiopathic or it may rarely be transmitted as an autosomal dominant trait. It may also be associated with autoimmune disorders. Exposure to cold weather or water triggers mast cell degranulation in the dermis and subcutaneous tissue.

**Epidemiology** Cold urticaria affects males and females in equal numbers. The familial autosomal dominant form is rare.

**Related Disorders** See *Raynaud Disease and Phenomenon.* The symptoms of Raynaud disease, like those of cold urticaria, are precipitated by exposure to cold. However, the pathophysiology and symptoms themselves are different. Raynaud disease is a vasospastic disorder characterized by pain and pallor; urticaria is not a feature.

Other diseases in which symptoms are precipitated by cold include **cold agglutinin disease,** which may be associated with infectious mononucleosis, mycoplasma pneumonia, or lymphoproliferative disorders. The cold agglutinins are usually hemolytic; rarely they produce red cell agglutination with local cyanosis. They are not associated with urticaria. **Paroxysmal cold hemoglobinuria** is a rare disorder that can be associated with infectious diseases (syphilis, measles); it is a hemolytic disorder precipitated by exposure to cold. Urticaria may occur.

Urticaria should be distinguished from other skin lesions, such as contact dermatitis. The diagnosis is generally confirmed by attempting to elicit the symptoms with cold exposure (e.g., immersing the arm in cold water).

**Treatment—Standard** The treatment of cold urticaria includes the use of antihistamines and sympathomimetics: diphenhydramine, cyproheptadine, cetirizine, and epinephrine. Prevention involves the use of warm clothing during cold weather and avoiding cold environments, particularly swimming in cold water, since syncope, followed by drowning, may occur.

**Treatment—Investigational** Please contact the agencies listed under Resources, below, for the most current information. Addresses and telephone numbers of these agencies, as well as of individual experts and research centers, may be found in the Master Resources List.

**Resources**

**For more information on cold urticaria:** National Organization for Rare Disorders (NORD); NIH/National Institute of Allergy and Infectious Diseases; Asthma and Allergy Foundation of America.

**For information about Raynaud disease and phenomenon:** Raynaud's Association Trust.

**For genetic information and genetic counseling referrals:** March of Dimes Birth Defects Foundation; Alliance of Genetic Support Groups.

**References**

Inhibiting Effect of Cetirizine on Histamine-Induced and 48/80-Induced Wheals and Flares, Experimental Dermographism, and Cold-Induced Urticaria: L. Juhlin, et al.; J. Allergy Clin. Immunol., October 1987, vol. 80(4), pp. 599–602.

Internal Medicine, 2nd ed.: J.H. Stein, ed.-in-chief; Little, Brown and Company, 1987, pp. 945, 1058.

Clinical Characteristics of Cold-Induced Systemic Reactions in This Complication and a Proposal for a Diagnostic Classification of Cold Urticaria: A.A. Wanderer, et al.; J. Allergy Clin. Immunol., September 1986, vol. 78(3 pt. 1), pp. 417–423.

# VOGT-KOYANAGI-HARADA SYNDROME

**Description** Vogt-Koyanagi-Harada syndrome is a multisystem disease of unknown origin that affects the eyes, ears, skin, and meninges. The most noticeable symptom is a rapid loss of vision.

**Synonyms**

Alopecia-Poliosis-Uveitis-Vitiligo-Deafness-Cutaneous-Uveo-Oto Syndrome

Harada Syndrome

Uveomeningitis Syndrome

**Signs and Symptoms** Initial onset of Vogt-Koyanagi-Harada syndrome is characterized by severe headache, deep pain in the eye, vertigo, and nausea, followed in a few weeks by uveitis and vision loss. The other eye may become affected about 2 weeks later. The retina may detach, and hearing loss may become apparent. Facial nerve palsies and rigidity as well as gait disturbance can occur.

After treatment, sight and hearing usually return. However, there may be some permanent hair loss with associated depigmentation of the hair, eyelashes, and skin. Lasting visual effects include the development of secondary glaucoma and cataracts.

**Etiology** The exact cause of Vogt-Koyanagi-Harada syndrome is not known, but an immune response to a human leukocyte antigen **(HLA)** is suspected. Some researchers have found a genetic predisposition for the disease, since it has occurred in a brother and sister and in a set of twins.

**Epidemiology** Vogt-Koyanagi-Harada syndrome affects males and females equally. The disorder is more prevalent among Orientals and Native Americans than whites.

**Related Disorders** See *Alopecia Areata; Vitiligo.*

**Treatment—Standard** Confirmation of diagnosis is made by an ophthalmologist or neurologist using spinal tap, angiography, and ultrasound. High-dose systemic steroid drug therapy is the treatment of choice. Other treatment is symptomatic and supportive.

**Treatment—Investigational** Please contact the agencies listed under Resources, below, for the most current information. Addresses and telephone numbers of these agencies, as well as of individual experts and research centers, may be found in the Master Resources List.

**Resources**

**For more information on Vogt-Koyanagi-Harada syndrome:** National Organization for Rare Disorders (NORD); NIH/National Eye Institute.

**References**

A Case of Vogt-Koyanagi-Harada Syndrome: D.L. Hettler, et al.; J. Am. Optom. Assoc., February 1992, vol. 63(2), pp. 90–94.

Ophthalmology Principles and Concepts, 7th ed.; F.W. Newell; C.V. Mosby Company, 1992, p. 335.

Vogt-Koyanagi-Harada Syndrome in Patients with Cherokee Indian Ancestry: J.A. Martinez, et al.; Am. J. Ophthalmol., November 1992, vol. 114(5), pp. 615–620.

Variations in Clinical Features of the Vogt-Koyanagi-Harada Syndrome: J. Beniz, et al.; Retina, 1991, vol. 11(3), pp. 275–280.

Vogt-Koyanagi-Harada Syndrome: Clinical Course, Therapy, and Long-Term Visual Outcome: P.E. Rubsamen, et al.; Arch. Ophthalmol., May 1991, vol. 109(5), pp. 682–687.

Clinical Ophthalmology, 2nd ed.; J.J. Kanski, ed.; Butterworth-Heinemann, 1990, p. 150.

HLA Associations and Ancestry in Vogt-Koyanagi-Harada Disease and Sympathetic Ophthalmia: J.L. Davis, et al.; Ophthalmology, September 1990, vol. 97(9), pp. 1137–1142.

Principles of Neurology, 4th ed.; R.D. Adams and M. Victor, eds.; McGraw-Hill, 1989, pp. 560–561, 601.

# WALDENSTRÖM MACROGLOBULINEMIA

**Description** Waldenström macroglobulinemia is a malignant lymphocytic disorder in which the malignant lymphocytes secrete IgM. The major clinical manifestations are those of the hyperviscosity syndrome that results from macroglobulinemia.

**Synonyms**

> Hyperglobulinemic Purpura
> Macroglobulinemia
> Waldenström Purpura
> Waldenström Syndrome

**Signs and Symptoms** The clinical manifestations of Waldenström macroglobulinemia are weakness, fatigue, epistaxis, and a variety of neurologic symptoms, including visual disturbances, peripheral neuropathy, dizziness, and headache. Bleeding occurs because the high level of IgM interferes with platelet function. On examination there is usually hepatosplenomegaly and lymphadenopathy, and retinal examination may reveal segmentation of the veins due to hyperviscosity of the blood.

The initial complaint may be related to a peripheral neuropathy. Other neurologic manifestations include hearing loss, muscular atrophy, and leukoencephalopathy.

Anemia is common, and there is significant paraproteinemia (the serum M component). Cryoglobulins are often present, and these may be associated with Raynaud phenomenon.

The diagnosis of Waldenström macroglobulinemia is based on 2 findings: an elevated monoclonal IgM level (over 3 gm/dl), and histologic examination of the bone marrow aspirate.

**Etiology** Waldenström macroglobulinemia is a malignancy of plasma cells that produce IgM. The precise etiology is unknown.

**Epidemiology** The disorder is slightly more common in males than in females. Its frequency is highest in the 7th decade.

**Related Disorders** Waldenström macroglobulinemia is very similar to chronic lymphocytic leukemia, lymphocytic lymphoma, and multiple myeloma. The disease IgM myeloma differs only in that lytic bone lesions appear in myeloma.

Other entities associated with hypergammaglobulinemia include benign monoclonal gammopathy, and chronic cold agglutinin disease. It may not be possible to distinguish these from asymptomatic Waldenström macroglobulinemia; the diagnosis in this case can only be clarified later when symptoms appear.

**Treatment—Standard** This disease is commonly diagnosed while the patient is asymptomatic. These cases do not require treatment until symptoms appear. When symptomatic, patients are treated by plasmapheresis alone for those symptoms related directly to elevated IgM levels.

The standard chemotherapy of Waldenström macroglobulinemia consists of repeated courses of an alkylating agent, such as cyclophosphamide or chlorambucil, and prednisone. Treatment is administered every 4 to 6 weeks for 1 to 2 years, and doses are titrated against bone marrow toxicity.

**Treatment—Investigational** Please contact the agencies listed under Resources, below, for the most current information. Addresses and telephone numbers of these agencies, as well as of individual experts and research centers, may be found in the Master Resources List.

**Resources**

**For more information on Waldenström macroglobulinemia:** National Organization for Rare Disorders (NORD); American Cancer Society; NIH/National Cancer Institute Physician Data Query Phoneline; NIH/National Heart, Lung and Blood Institute.

**References**

Alleviation of Ocular Complications of the Hyperviscosity Syndrome in Waldenström Macroglobulinemia Using Plasma Exchange: F. Malecaze, et al.; J. Fr. Ophtalmol., 1986, vol. 9(5), pp. 367–371.

Polyneuropathy in Waldenström Macroglobulinemia: Reduction of Endoneural IgM Deposits After Treatment with Chlorambucil and Plasmapheresis: C. Meier, et al.; Acta Neuropathol. (Berl.), 1984, vol. 64(4), pp. 297–307.

Plasma Exchange and Moderate Dose of Cytostatics in Advanced Macro(cryo)-globulinemia: P. Pihlstedt; Acta Med. Scand., 1982, vol. 212(3), pp. 187–190.

# WEIL SYNDROME

**Description** Weil syndrome, the severe icteric form of leptospirosis, is characterized by hepatic and renal dysfunction, with alterations in consciousness, hemorrhage, and shock. Leptospirosis, a systemic spirochetal infection of animals occasionally transmitted to humans, is discussed in a separate chapter.

**Synonyms**

>   Fiedler Disease
>   Icterohemorrhagic Leptospirosis
>   Lancereaux-Mathieu-Weil Spirochetosis
>   Leptospiral Jaundice
>   Spirochetal Jaundice
>   Weil Disease

**Signs and Symptoms** Leptospirosis is typically a disease with 2 phases. The first phase consists of fever, headache, severe myalgias, nausea, vomiting, and abdominal pain. During this phase of the illness, spirochetes may be isolated from the blood.

The 2nd phase of leptospirosis, known as the immune phase, follows the 1st phase after an asymptomatic period of 1 to 3 days. Weil syndrome is a severe form of the 2nd phase; patients with this syndrome experience the 1st phase routinely. Weil syndrome is characterized by fever, jaundice, tender hepatomegaly, renal insufficiency with proteinuria and hematuria, thrombocytopenia, hemorrhage, and alterations of consciousness. Hepatic enzymes are moderately elevated, but the creatine phosphokinase is markedly elevated, which is characteristic of and of diagnostic importance. Cardiac involvement may occur with hemorrhagic myocarditis. Shock and adult respiratory distress syndrome may also occur. Hepatic and renal functions eventually return to normal if the patient survives.

The definitive diagnosis of leptospirosis requires isolation of the organism or a rise in antibody titer. Since isolation demands special techniques and media not found in many laboratories, specimens must be sent to the appropriate authorities.

The diagnosis of Weil syndrome is based on the clinical features described above, in the setting of leptospirosis.

**Etiology** Leptospirosis is caused by spirochetes of the genus *Leptospira*. Until recently there were thought to be several species of *Leptospira*, but these variants are currently considered to be serotypes of a single species, *L. interrogans*. Weil syndrome can be seen with any of the *Leptospira* serotypes.

Leptospirosis is a biphasic illness, as described above, in which the 1st phase is the septic phase, namely a direct result of bacterial action, and the 2nd phase is thought to be an immune reaction. Weil syndrome is a severe form of the 2nd phase and is probably due to diffuse vasculitis.

**Epidemiology** Leptospirosis is primarily a disease of animals. In the United States, human infection is usually contracted from livestock, dogs, rodents, and cats. Those at increased risk are veterinarians, abattoir workers, and farmers. Swimming in infected water has also been known to cause this infection.

**Related Disorders** Rickettsial diseases such as typhus, and viral diseases such as the hemorrhagic fever with renal syndrome (**HFRS**), as well as a host of bacterial diseases, particularly those progressing to septic shock, may resemble Weil syndrome.

**Treatment—Standard** The treatment of Weil syndrome itself is largely supportive. Dialysis, exchange transfusion, and other intensive measures may be appropriate.

Early treatment of leptospirosis may prevent its progression to Weil syndrome. The treatment of choice is doxycycline, intravenous penicillin, or ampicillin. Streptomycin, tetracyclines, chloramphenicol, and erythromycin have also been used effectively. A vaccine is available for animal use, but it is not 100 percent effective.

**Treatment—Investigational** Please contact the agencies listed under Resources, below, for the most current information. Addresses and telephone numbers of these agencies, as well as of individual experts and research centers, may be found in the Master Resources List.

**Resources**

**For more information on Weil syndrome:** National Organization for Rare Disorders (NORD); Centers for Disease Control; NIH/National Institute of Allergy and Infectious Diseases.

**References**

Leptospira Species (Leptospirosis): W.E. Farrar; *in* Principles and Practice of Infectious Diseases: G.L. Mandell, et al., eds.; Churchill Livingstone, 1990, pp. 1813–1815.

Adult Respiratory Distress Syndrome in Leptospira Icterohaemorrhagiae Infection: H.D. Chee, et al.; Intensive Care Med., 1985, vol. 11(5), pp. 254–256.

# WHIPPLE DISEASE

**Description** Whipple disease is a rare multisystem infectious disease that causes an abnormality in the metabolism and/or usage of fats (lipodystrophy) in the small intestine. The disorder is characterized by malabsorption, anemia, and joint pain. Whipple disease may also affect other organs of the body, including the heart, lungs, brain, and eyes.

**Synonyms**
> Intestinal Lipodystrophy
> Intestinal Lipophagic Granulomatosis
> Secondary Nontropical Sprue

**Signs and Symptoms** The major symptoms of Whipple disease include abdominal pain after eating, joint pain, bouts of diarrhea, cough, chest pain, general weakness, and night sweats. Typically, there is fat present in the stool (steatorrhea). Weight loss may occur because of a profound lack of appetite. Anemia may result due to insufficient levels of iron.

Other symptoms of Whipple disease include abnormally enlarged lymph nodes that are firm but usually not tender, splenomegaly, increased pigmentation of the skin, hypotension, and abnormally high fevers that come and go. Some people with this disorder may experience decreased intellectual abilities and impaired memory, judgment, and/or abstract thought. Occasionally, the loss of intellectual skills progresses to dementia. Eye movements may be impaired, and myoclonus may occur when Whipple disease has affected the brain or central nervous system.

The central nervous system is affected in the later stages of untreated Whipple disease. Symptoms of neurologic involvement include hearing loss, tinnitus, and impairment of vision and ocular movements. In rare cases, the heart may be affected, resulting in congestive heart failure and/or pericarditis or valvulitis.

If Whipple disease remains untreated and malabsorption from the small intestine is not reversed, hypokalemia and hypomagnesemia may occur, resulting in muscle cramps, convulsions, and tetany. Damage to the nerves, especially to those of the arms and legs (peripheral neuropathy), may also occur.

Whipple disease may be diagnosed by ultrasound tests and CT scan, which may reveal lymphadenopathy and/or a thickening of the lining of the small intestine. Biopsy samples of the small intestine reveal the presence of the PAS-positive bacteria that causes this disorder. Without proper antibiotic treatment, Whipple disease may result in life-threatening complications.

**Etiology** Whipple disease is caused by the intracellular rod-shaped gram-positive bacterium *Tropherema whipplei*. This bacterium cannot yet be cultured.

**Epidemiology** Whipple disease is a rare disorder that affects more males than females, at a ratio of 8:1. The symptoms typically begin between the ages of 30 and 60. Most cases have been diagnosed in Americans of European descent, although cases have been reported among American Indians and African-Americans. It has a tendency to occur in farmers.

**Related Disorders** See *Glucose-Galactose Malabsorption; Intestinal Pseudo-obstruction; Acquired Immune Deficiency Syndrome (AIDS); Gastritis, Chronic Hypertrophic.*

**Treatment—Standard** Treatment of Whipple disease includes the use of antibiotics. Many different types have been helpful (e.g., tetracycline, chlortetracycline, sulfasalizine, ampicillin, trimethoprim/sulfamethoxazole, penicillin, and ceftriaxone). Other patients may be treated with a combination of antibiotics, including tetracycline, streptomycin, and penicillin. Antibiotic therapy may be necessary for a few months to several years. In severe cases, corticosteroid drugs (e.g., prednisone) may be added to the antibiotic regimen.

Some patients with severe intestinal malabsorption may require the intravenous administration of fluids and electrolytes. Other patients may require iron, folate supplements, vitamin D, and calcium. Since most patients with this disorder suffer from malnutrition, the recommended diet is usually high in calories and protein. The diet should be monitored regularly by a physician.

While the symptoms of Whipple disease may improve rapidly with long-term antibiotic therapy, biopsy may reveal bacteria in the small intestine for up to 2 years. Whipple disease has been completely reversed by antibiotic therapy. The absence of bacilliform organisms in a biopsy sample of the small bowel typically suggests remission and possible cure.

**Treatment—Investigational** Please contact the agencies listed under Resources, below, for the most current information. Addresses and telephone numbers of these agencies, as well as of individual experts and research centers, may be found in the Master Resources List.

**Resources**

**For more information on Whipple disease:** National Organization for Rare Disorders (NORD); NIH/National Digestive Diseases Information Clearinghouse; Centers for Disease Control.

### References
Cecil Textbook of Medicine, 19th ed.: J.B. Wyngaarden, et al., eds.; W.B. Saunders Company, 1992, pp. 698, 1560.

Identification of the Uncultured Bacillus of Whipple's Disease: D.A. Relman; N. Engl. J. Med., July 30, 1992, vol. 327(5), pp. 293–301.

Short-Term Antibiotic Treatment in Whipple's Disease: J.C. Bai; J. Clin. Gastroenterol., June 1991, vol. 13(3), pp. 303–307.

Whipple's Disease, Familial Mediterranean Fever, and Adult-Onset Still's Disease: A. McMenemy; Curr. Opin. Rheumatol., August 1991, vol. 3(4), pp. 597–600.

Gastrointestinal Disease, 4th ed.: M.H. Sleisenger, et al.; W.B. Saunders Company, 1989, pp. 1302–1306.

# WISKOTT-ALDRICH SYNDROME

**Description** Wiskott-Aldrich syndrome is an X-linked hereditary disorder characterized by immune deficiency primarily affecting B cells, eczema, and thrombocytopenia. The course is variable, but those affected usually succumb to the complications of thrombocytopenia and immunodeficiency before adulthood.

**Synonyms**

Aldrich Syndrome

Immunodeficiency with Thrombocytopenia and Eczema

**Signs and Symptoms** Wiskott-Aldrich syndrome generally presents in infancy. Hemorrhage from circumcision or minor trauma is a common form of presentation. Gastrointestinal bleeding, which may be severe, also begins in infancy. Thrombocytopenic purpura and petechiae may be evident on examination. In addition, the skin shows a chronic eczematous eruption.

Affected boys have defects in both cell-mediated and humoral immunity, although the T-cell abnormalities are thought to be secondary. The most prominent defect is in the synthesis of antibody to polysaccharide antigens. Patients are highly susceptible to infections with encapsulated organisms, such as the pneumococcus and *Hemophilus influenzae*. Otitis media, pneumonia, meningitis, and sepsis are common problems.

Cell-mediated immunity becomes progressively dysfunctional with age; fungal and viral infections become significant later in the course of the disorder. *Pneumocystis carinii* and herpes virus infections are also common.

Additional features of the Wiskott-Aldrich syndrome include splenomegaly and anemia. There is a 10 percent incidence of malignancy, predominantly leukemia and lymphoma.

Serum antibody concentrations are normal, although the proportions between the different antibody classes are not, and, as was mentioned above, antibody function is distinctly abnormal. Platelet precursors appear normal, but circulating platelets have both structural and functional abnormalities.

**Etiology** Wiskott-Aldrich syndrome is hereditary. It is transmitted by an X-linked recessive mechanism. The defective gene is on the short arm of the X chromosome (p11.4–p11.21).

**Epidemiology** More males than females are affected, although females can be carriers.

**Related Disorders** Similar immune deficiency syndromes include ataxia telangiectasia, immunodeficiency with short-limbed short stature, and immunodeficiency with thymoma. See *Ataxia Telangiectasia.*

**Treatment—Standard** A lymphocyte-derived transfer factor has been used to restore hematologic and immunologic function. This factor, which also improves the eczema, is effective only in about 50 percent of cases. Bone marrow transplantation from a histocompatible sibling has also been used with some success.

Alternative forms of therapy for the platelet disorder include splenectomy and platelet transfusions. While effective in reducing the risk of bleeding, splenectomy further increases the risk of serious infection with encapsulated organisms, and most of such patients will require prophylactic antibiotics. Platelet transfusions are not without problems, since repeated transfusions are likely to stimulate the formation of platelet antibodies. Corticosteroids and immunosuppressant drugs have no role in the therapy of thrombocytopenia in Wiskott-Aldrich syndrome.

Intravenous gammaglobulin and antibiotics may be useful in preventing and combating infection.

Vincristine may be a useful drug in the treatment of malignancy in this disorder because it tends to improve platelet function and is not an immunosuppressant.

Infections require vigorous therapy with antifungal, antibiotic, and supportive measures. As in the case of AIDS, *P. carinii* pneumonia can be particularly difficult to treat; the 2 drugs usually used are trimethoprim-sulfamethoxazole and pentamidine isethionate. (For more information on treatment of *P. carinii* pneumonia, see *Acquired Immune Deficiency Syndrome [AIDS].)* Cytomegalovirus and generalized herpes simplex infections may be treated with acyclovir, ganciclovir **(DHPG),** idoxuridine, or floxuridine. Amphotericin B therapy remains the treatment of choice for severe fungal infections.

Prevention is important, and every attempt should be made to protect affected patients from infection. Immunization with live virus vaccines should probably be avoided.

Genetic counseling may be of benefit for patients and their families. Other treatment is symptomatic and supportive.

**Treatment—Investigational** Please contact the agencies listed under Resources, below, for the most current information. Addresses and telephone numbers of these agencies, as well as of individual experts and research centers, may be found in the Master Resources List.

**Resources**

**For more information on Wiskott-Aldrich syndrome:** National Organization for Rare Disorders (NORD); NIH/National Institute of Allergy and Infectious Diseases; Immune Deficiency Foundation; American Cancer Society; NIH/National Cancer Institute Physician Data Query Phoneline.

**For genetic information and genetic counseling referrals:** March of Dimes Birth Defects Foundation; Alliance of Genetic Support Groups.

**References**

Bone Marrow Transplantation for Genetic Disorders: J.A. Brochstein; Oncology, March 1992, vol. 6(3), pp. 51–58, 63–66.

Cecil Textbook of Medicine, 19th ed.: J.B. Wyngaarden, et al., eds.; W.B. Saunders Company, 1992, pp. 1451–1452, 1578.

Early Bone Marrow Transplantation in an Infant with Wiskott-Aldrich Syndrome: L.J. Beard; Am. J. Pediatr. Hematol. Oncol., Fall 1992, vol. 13(3), pp. 310–314.

Evidence for Defective Transmembrane Signaling in B Cells from Patients with Wiskott-Aldrich Syndrome: H.U. Simon; J. Clin. Invest., October 1992, vol. 90(4), pp. 1396–1405.

Mendelian Inheritance in Man, 10th ed.: V.A. McKusick; The Johns Hopkins University Press, 1992, pp. 1781–1783.

Nelson Textbook of Pediatrics, 14th ed.: R.E. Behrman, ed.-in-chief; W.B. Saunders Company, 1992, pp. 555, 1280.

Wiskott-Aldrich Syndrome: New Molecular and Biochemical Insights: M. Peacocke; J. Am. Acad. Dermatol., October 1992, vol. 27(4), pp. 507–519.

Birth Defects Encyclopedia: M.L. Buyse, ed.-in-chief; Blackwell Scientific Publications, 1990, p. 963–964.

Hematology, 4th ed.: W.J. Williams, et al., eds.; McGraw-Hill, 1990, p. 964–969.

Immunodeficiency: R.H. Buckley; J. Allergy Clin. Immunol., December 1983, vol. 72(6), pp. 627–641.

# YAWS

**Description** Yaws is an infectious disease caused by the spirochete *Treponema pertenue*. It is characterized by 3 stages of symptoms. The first stage consists of skin lesions; the later 2 stages, of bone, joint, and skin involvement. The late forms of the disease are known as gangosa (also referred to as ogo, or rhinopharyngitis mutilans) and goundou (henpue; henpuye; gundo; anakhre).

**Synonyms**

Bouba

Breda Disease

Charlouis Disease

Frambesia

Parangi

Pian

*(Note: Pian differs from pian bois [also called forest yaws, a form of leishmaniasis] and hemorrhagic pian [verruga peruana, one of the manifestations of bartonellosis].)*

**Signs and Symptoms** The first stage of yaws occurs in early childhood. A papillomatous lesion appears at the site of inoculation, usually on the leg or foot. The lesion grows, becomes crusted, and then heals slowly over several months, leaving a scar.

Stage 2 follows several weeks or months after the first. Similar skin lesions appear on the face, legs, and arms, and around the anus and genitals. Healing is slow, and relapses occur. On the soles of the feet, the lesions may become keratotic with painful cracks and ulcerations, resulting in a crablike gait called crab yaws.

The tertiary stage of yaws does not always occur. Several years after the initial stages, destructive lesions of the skin and bone may develop. Cutaneous plaques, nodules, and ulcers occur and can cause facial disfigurement. Painful, gummatous lesions of the bones develop, especially of the tibia. Painful and destructive nodules may appear around the joints.

Tertiary yaws may produce 2 distinct syndromes. **Goundou** is a painless but marked symmetrical paranasal swelling due to hypertrophic osteitis. It is accompanied by headache and nasal discharge. **Gangosa, or rhinopharyngitis mutilans,** consists of destruction of the nose, the pharynx, and the hard palate.

The diagnosis of stage 1 and 2 yaws is made by darkfield examination of material from the skin lesions. Tertiary yaws may be diagnosed by serologic tests (VDRL, treponemal antibodies), in the presence of the appropriate clinical picture.

**Etiology** Yaws is caused by the spirochete *Treponema pertenue*.

**Epidemiology** Yaws is common among children in tropical Africa, South and Central America, the West Indies, and the Far East, but is rare in the United States. It is usually transmitted by direct contact with infected skin lesions, but insect transmission occurs in some regions, and sexual transmission has been reported.

**Related Disorders** See *Bejel; Pinta.* The treponematoses—yaws, bejel (endemic syphilis), pinta, and venereal syphilis—are all caused by identical-looking spirochetes. While the organisms are related, the diseases they produce differ in distribution, mode of transmission, and clinical characteristics. The treponematoses do have 2 things in common: protracted chronic phases of illness, and response to penicillin.

**Treatment—Standard** Antimicrobial drugs such as benzathine penicillin G, given as a single dose of 1.2 million units, are very effective. Such drugs can also be used preventively for close contacts of affected individuals. There is no treatment for the destructive bony lesions, or for scars.

**Treatment—Investigational** Please contact the agencies listed under Resources, below, for the most current information. Addresses and telephone numbers of these agencies, as well as of individual experts and research centers, may be found in the Master Resources List.

**Resources**

For more information on yaws: National Organization for Rare Disorders (NORD); Centers for Disease Control; NIH/National Institute of Allergy and Infectious Diseases; World Health Organization.

**References**

The Localization of Treponemas and Characterization of the Inflammatory Infiltrates in Skin Biopsies from Patients with Primary or Secondary Syphilis, or Early Infectious Yaws: H.J. Engelkens, et al.; Genitourin. Med., April 1993, vol. 69(2), pp. 102–107.

Nonvenereal Treponematoses: Yaws, Endemic Syphilis, and Pinta: A.B. Koff, et al.; Am. J. Acad. Dermatol., October 1993, vol. 29(4), pp. 519–535.

Cecil Textbook of Medicine, 19th ed.: J.B. Wyngaarden, et al., eds.; W.B. Saunders Company, 1992, p. 1770.

Nelson Textbook of Pediatrics, 14th ed.: R.E. Behrman, ed.-in-chief; W.B. Saunders Company, 1992, p. 781.

# 7 | DERMATOLOGIC DISORDERS
### By Nancy Burton Esterly, M.D.

This section has been prepared to assist the physician in arriving at an accurate diagnosis of the rare dermatologic disorders. Based upon the presumptive diagnosis, the practitioner will be making selections of which descriptive passages to read, making decisions concerning referral to other physicians, and subjecting patients to diagnostic and therapeutic procedures.

The history may be particularly informative for rare disorders in this field. When was the dermatosis first observed? Was it present at birth? Was it first noticed in the neonatal period? At puberty? Are other family members similarly affected? Does the eruption persist, or is it only present periodically? Is it associated with exposure to environmental agents? Do physical elements such as sunlight, heat, or cold cause the eruption to worsen or remit? Is it associated with the ingestion of drugs or foods? Does the patient have any other significant medical illnesses or complaints?

The entire skin, including the epidermal appendages, should next be inspected. In a thorough examination, it is necessary to assess the scalp, nails, hair, mucous membranes, and body folds. It is not sufficient to look only at those portions of the uncovered skin that can be revealed by partially removing a skirt, blouse, or trousers. The patient must be completely undressed in order to determine the extent of the eruption and to assess the character of the individual lesions. What is the color and texture of the skin in general? Is jaundice, pallor, or cyanosis evident? Is the skin warm, moist, or cold to the touch?

Distribution of the lesions is important. Is the eruption bilateral and symmetrical? Does it localize to exposed or unexposed skin? Does it involve body folds? Intertriginous areas? Hairy skin? Mucous membranes? Do lesions occur in groups or clusters? In lines? In sites of previous trauma? In a dermatome? The following glossary of terms should be used to describe the pattern of lesions:

**distribution**—Where are the lesions located?

**arrangement**—Are the lesions grouped, single, linear, or follicular, or are they associated with body folds or a vascular or nerve distribution?

**size**—What are the dimensions of the lesions?

**margins**—Are the margins sharp or indistinct, and do they correspond to exposure to some environmental agent?

**shape**—Are the lesions round, gyrate, targetoid, polygonal, or polycyclic?

Careful assessment of a primary lesion is needed. There may be few such primary lesions, and therefore a complete examination may again be required. In addition, one must characterize secondary lesions that may have developed with the passage of time and represent a change from the primary lesion. Have lesions formed crusts, ulcers, or plaques? Do they coalesce? Do they hyper- or hypo-pigment or develop scars? It is appropriate to use precise adjectives, so that an accurate word picture of the skin eruption is presented.

The following glossary of terms should be used to describe individual lesions.

**atrophy**—Loss of cutaneous elements producing flaccid or sclerotic scars.

**bulla**—A large vesicle, tense or flaccid.

**crust**—Dried secretions on the surface of a lesion.

**erosion**—Loss of epidermal cells from the surface of the skin.

**excoriation**—Loss of skin secondary to scratching.

**fissure**—Linear separation or split in the skin.

**keratosis**—Firmly adherent, horny growth.

**macule**—A flat lesion with a different color from surrounding skin; may be brown, black, red, white; may have sharply defined or indistinct margins.

**nodule**—Large papule; a circumscribed lesion that represents a collection of inflammatory or neoplastic cells in the dermis.

**papule**—Elevated lesion caused by cellular proliferation or infiltration; 0.1 to 1.0 cm in diameter.

**pustule**—A vesicle containing purulent fluid.

**scale**—Desquamated epidermal cells.

**scar**—Permanent fibrous lesion of the skin secondary to resolution of a previous skin lesion.

**tumor**—A particularly large nodule that may be benign or malignant.

**ulcer**—Larger, deeper lesion than an erosion, caused by loss of epidermal and dermal skin cells.

**vesicle**—A small fluid-filled blister.

**wheal**—Transient raised lesion (these are also called hives), which represents extravasation of fluid from vessels into the perivascular skin; may be pink, red, or white.

The accuracy of dermatologic diagnosis is greatly enhanced by obtaining a specimen of skin from an appropriate lesion and subjecting the biopsy specimen to histopathologic examination. Other laboratory tests commonly used in dermatologic diagnosis include examination by Wood's light to enhance the evaluation of pigmentation, potassium hydroxide **(KOH)** preparations of scale to identify yeast and fungal elements, darkfield microscopy to identify spirochetal organisms, Gram stain to identify bacteria, and Giemsa stain to identify epidermal cells infected with virus (e.g., the herpes virus) or cells that have become separated from their neighbors because of the disease process (e.g., pemphigus).

Dermatophathology is a highly developed field, and diagnosis may require the use of one or more of several specialized techniques. Some of these diagnostic studies are performed routinely, but others are available only in certain laboratories or on an investigative basis. Electron microscopy has been invaluable in defining structural defects in certain skin disorders (e.g., epidermolysis bullosa), identifying specific cell types in infiltrative diseases (e.g., Langerhans cell histiocytosis), and documenting malfunctioning cellular components (e.g., albinism). Scanning electron microscopy is particularly useful for delineating hair shaft defects in a fashion that cannot be done in routine tissue sections or with transmission electron microscopy. Immunofluorescence microscopy studies are now considered standard care for all of the autoimmune diseases. Antibodies often can be detected both in skin (direct immunofluorescence) and in blood (indirect immunofluorescence); these antibody titers assist in establishing a diagnosis and provide a useful tool for monitoring the activity of the disease process. When needed, more precise localization of autoantibodies is possible by immunoelectron microscopy. Immunohistochemical stains are yet another way of distinguishing specific cell types and antigens and antibodies in tissue sections.

Finally, the application of modern techniques of molecular biology has produced an explosion of information in dermatology. The polymerase chain reaction (**PCR**) allows us to amplify small amounts of specific DNA, facilitating more accurate diagnosis of infectious diseases and genetic disorders and prenatal diagnosis of certain heritable conditions. Localization of particular genes and identification of specific mutations have helped us to understand the role of abnormal gene products in the pathogenesis of many skin disorders. Techniques for analyzing clonal proliferation of T and B lymphocytes and gene rearrangements in malignant cells can be used for detection of cutaneous tumors. These and other techniques will permit a greater understanding of rare diseases and improve our ability to treat, or even to prevent, many rare and devastating skin disorders.

# DERMATOLOGIC DISORDERS
*Listings in This Section*

# ACANTHOSIS NIGRICANS

**Description** Acanthosis nigricans is a disorder in which the skin in sites of predilection becomes hyperkeratotic and thickened with brown-gray pigmentation. Several forms are recognized, including a benign, inherited form; a benign form associated with many syndromes, including endocrine disorders with insulin resistance; a benign form associated with obesity (**pseudoacanthosis nigricans**); an adult form associated with an internal carcinoma (**malignant acanthosis**); and a drug-induced form.

**Synonyms**

Keratosis Nigricans

**Signs and Symptoms** The eruption is bilateral and symmetrical. Characteristic lesions are hyperpigmented, velvety, papillomatous, warty plaques with indistinct margins. Lesions appear in the skin of the face, neck, axillae, backs of hands, forearms, the area between the breasts, the inner thighs, and the groin. Other susceptible sites are the genitals, buttocks, and the perianal area. The oral and anal mucous membranes and other mucous membranes may be involved. In the inherited form, an increase in the number of lesions during adolescence is followed by regression after puberty. Regression is characteristic except in the adult types, in which the lesions tend to increase and the skin may become hairless and the fingernails may be affected. In the adult form related to malignancy, progression correlates with that of the neoplasm.

**Histology:** The epidermis is thickened and papillomatous, and may resemble that of a seborrheic keratosis.

**Etiology** The cause is unknown but may be related to increased response to trophic growth factors in connection with associated disorders. The inherited form is thought to be autosomal dominant. Pseudoacanthosis nigricans is associated with obesity. Another form is associated with genetic disorders and endocrinopathies, including pituitary adenoma, Addison disease, hypothyroidism, diabetes mellitus, and ovarian disorders such as Stein-Leventhal syndrome. The disorder may also be induced by certain drugs, including nicotinic acid, diethylstilbestrol, oral contraceptives, and glucocorticoids.

**Epidemiology** The inherited form may be present at birth. Pseudoacanthosis nigricans affects obese individuals. The malignant form is most common in patients with adenocarcinoma of the gastrointestinal tract, but it may occur with breast or lung cancers, as well.

**Related Disorders** See *Mycosis Fungoides; Epidermolysis Bullosa.*

**Treatment—Standard** Acanthosis nigricans responds to treatment of the underlying problem. Lesions usually regress as an obese patient loses weight, or a thyroid dysfunction or other endocrine disorder is brought under control. The adult form related to malignancy regresses upon remission or cure of the neoplastic disease.

A cream containing 12 percent lactic acid may be applied as needed to help soften lesions. Retinoic acid applied daily to affected areas may be helpful in reducing skin irritation. Oral isotretinoin may be useful in resolving skin lesions, which typically recur when the drug is discontinued.

**Treatment—Investigational** Please contact the agencies listed under Resources, below, for the most current information. Addresses and telephone numbers of these agencies, as well as of individual experts and research centers, may be found in the Master Resources List.

**Resources**

**For more information on acanthosis nigricans:** National Organization for Rare Disorders (NORD); NIH/National Arthritis and Musculoskeletal and Skin Diseases Information Clearinghouse.

**For genetic information and genetic counseling referrals:** March of Dimes Birth Defects Foundation; Alliance of Genetic Support Groups.

**References**

Acanthosis Nigricans—Decreased Extracellular Matrix Viscosity: Cancer, Obesity, Diabetes, Corticosteroids, Somatotrophin: O.J. Stone; Med. Hypotheses, March 1993, vol. 40, pp. 154–157.

Acanthosis Nigricans: D.L. Rogers; Semin. Dermatol., September 1992, vol. 10(3), pp. 160–163.

Cecil Textbook of Medicine, 19th ed.: J.B. Wyngaarden, et al., eds.; W.B. Saunders Company, 1992, p. 1048.

Lipoatrophic Diabetes: T. Sasaki, et al.; J. Dermatol., April 1992, vol. 19(4), pp. 246–249.

Mendelian Inheritance in Man, 10th ed.: V.A. McKusick; The Johns Hopkins University Press, 1992, p. 5.

Nelson Textbook of Pediatrics, 14th ed.: R.E. Behrman, ed.-in-chief; W.B. Saunders Company, 1992, pp. 1658–1659.

Prevalence and Significance of Acanthosis Nigricans in an Adult Obese Population: J.A.Hud, Jr., et al.; Arch. Dermatol., July 1992, vol. 128(7), pp. 941–944.

Textbook of Endocrinology, 8th ed.: J.D. Wilson and D.W. Foster, eds.; W.B. Saunders Company, 1992, p. 1562.

Birth Defects Encyclopedia: M.L. Buyse, ed.-in-chief; Blackwell Scientific Publications, 1990, pp. 1554–1555.

Clinical Dermatology, 2nd ed.: T.P. Habif, ed.: C.V. Mosby Company, 1990, p. 647.

Dictionary of Medical Syndromes, 3rd ed.: S.I. Magalini, et al., eds.; J.B. Lippincott Company, 1990, pp. 5–6, 593–594.

Acanthosis Nigricans: A Cutaneous Marker of Tissue Resistance to Insulin: M.J. Rendon, et al.; J. Am. Acad. Dermatol., 1989, vol. 21, p. 461.

# ACNE ROSACEA

**Description** Acne rosacea is a skin disorder in which flushing, acneiform pustules, erythema, and telangiectasia are seen on the central face.

**Synonyms**

Acne Erythematosa
Hypertrophic Rosacea
Rhinophyma
Rosacea

**Signs and Symptoms** In acne rosacea, the primary lesion is erythema distributed diffusely on the face. At the onset there is periodic flushing; but with time the skin of the forehead, nose, and cheeks becomes oily and progressively erythematous, and telangiectasia develops. Small papules and perifollicular pustules develop in the affected areas. In very severe cases, rhinophyma, conjunctivitis, and keratitis may be found.

**Etiology** The cause is not known, although a genetic predisposition is believed to exist. Vasodilatory symptoms can be intensified by hot liquids, spicy foods, vitamin deficiencies, alcohol consumption, heat and vigorous exercise, certain endocrine disturbances, and emotional stress. Reactions to the follicular mite, *Demodex folliculorum,* have been implicated.

**Epidemiology** Onset usually is between 30 and 50 years of age. Females are affected more often than males, but males may be more severely affected.

**Related Disorders Acne vulgaris** is primarily a disease of the follicular structure and is not related. In the common form of adolescent acne, the skin eruptions primarily appear on the face, upper back, and chest.

**Acne conglobata** is a severe chronic variant of acne vulgaris in which many skin eruptions become abscessed and cysts form, often containing purulent liquid. Scarring is common. The eruptions occur most often on the neck and upper trunk; they also occur on the upper arms, lower back, buttocks, and thighs. Acne conglobata is seen most often in males, with onset usually at puberty but continuing in later years. This form of acne resists treatment with systemic antibiotics. In some cases symptoms may be controlled by the use of isotretinoin.

**Acne fulminans** is a rare variant of acne seen mostly in adolescent males. The skin lesions initially are similar to mild acne vulgaris but progress to severely inflamed and painful ulcerations on the upper trunk and occasionally the face. Systemic symptoms and signs may be associated, e.g., fever, weight loss, polyarthritis, leukocytosis, anemia, and elevated erythrocyte sedimentation rate. Treatment usually involves isotretinoin, with or without systemic corticosteroid drugs and antibiotics.

**Excoriated acne** results from excessive manipulation of acne lesions, with resulting increased scarring. Although it is often found among young women, it can be seen in any age group and both sexes.

**Chloracne** is a skin eruption that resembles acne and may occur as a result of exposure to chlorinated hydrocarbons. Treatment must include removal of the irritating substance from the environment.

**Atypical acneiform eruptions** may result from certain drugs (corticosteroids, androgens, progesterone, diphenylhydantoin, and lithium), ingestion of iodine or bromine salts, or skin contact with certain machine oils. These eruptions can occur in any age group and are not always limited to sebaceous glands.

**Treatment—Standard** There is no cure for acne rosacea. Topical and systemic antibiotics can reduce microbial flora. Mild topical steroids can reduce inflammation. The orphan drug metronidazole (Metrogel—Curatek Pharmaceuticals of Elk Village, Illinois) was approved in 1988 by the Food and Drug Administration for treatment of acne rosacea.

In rhinophyma, carbon dioxide laser and conventional surgery are used to remove excess skin growth. Argon lasers have been effective in reducing erythema in the nose area in mild cases that have not progressed to rhinophyma. Other treatment is symptomatic and supportive.

**Treatment—Investigational** Please contact the agencies listed under Resources, below, for the most current information. Addresses and telephone numbers of these agencies, as well as of individual experts and research centers, may be found in the Master Resources List.

**Resources**

**For more information on acne rosacea:** National Organization for Rare Disorders (NORD); NIH/National Arthritis and Musculoskeletal and Skin Diseases Information Clearinghouse.

**References**

Dermatology, 3rd ed.: S.L. Moschella and H.J. Hurley, eds.; W.B. Saunders Company, 1992.
Textbook of Dermatology, 5th ed.: R.H. Champion, et al., eds.; Blackwell Scientific Publications, 1992.
Dermatology, 3rd ed.: O. Braun-Falco, et al.; Springer-Verlag, 1991.
Internal Medicine, 3rd ed.: J.H. Stein, ed.-in-chief; Little, Brown and Company, 1990, p. 1840.
Combined Carbon Dioxide Laser Excision and Vaporization in the Treatment of Rhinophyma: R.G. Wheeland, et al.; J. Dermatol. Surg. Oncol., February 1987, vol. 13(2), pp. 172–177.

Dermatology in General Medicine: Textbook and Atlas, 3rd ed.: T.B. Fitzpatrick, et al., eds.; McGraw-Hill, 1987.
Topical Metronidazole Therapy for Rosacea: P.A. Bleicher, et al.; Arch. Dermatol., May 1987, vol. 123(5), pp. 609–614.
Surgical Treatment of Rhinophyma with the Shaw Scalpel: R.F. Eisen, et al.; Arch. Dermatol., March 1986, vol. 122(3), pp. 307–309.
Treatment of Rosacea with Isotretinoin: E. Hoting, et al.; Int. J. Dermatol., December 1986, vol. 25(10), pp. 660–663.
Treatment of the Red Nose with the Argon Laser: C.H. Dicken; Mayo Clin. Proc., November 1986, vol. 61(11), pp. 893–895.

# ACRODERMATITIS ENTEROPATHICA (AE)

**Description** AE is characterized by dermatitis, diarrhea, and alopecia. The disorder may be either inherited or acquired.

**Synonyms**
> Brandt Syndrome
> Danbolt-Closs Syndrome
> Zinc Deficiency, Congenital

**Signs and Symptoms** Minor or significant chronic diarrhea and steatorrhea in infancy are hallmarks of inherited AE. Onset is gradual, usually occurring during weaning. A vesicobullous dermatitis appears around the mouth, genitalia, anus, eyes, and nails; also affected is the skin on the elbows, knees, hands, and feet. Initially the skin is blistered, but eventually drying produces lesions resembling those of psoriasis. Inflammatory lesions around the nail may result in chronic paronychia and nail dystrophy. Alopecia involving the scalp, eyelids, and eyebrows may occur. Conjunctivitis is usually present.

When the disorder is acute, atrophy of the cerebral cortex may lead to irritability and mental disturbances.

Long remissions of congenital AE are common, usually beginning at puberty. Rarely, the disorder may recur during pregnancy. With treatment, patients may enjoy a normal life.

**Etiology** Inherited AE is an autosomal recessive disorder in which the serum alkaline phosphatase is deficient and the serum zinc is also low because of faulty absorption of zinc. This is presumed to be due to lack of a carrier protein (ligand).

Acquired AE is the result of a nutritional lack of zinc.

**Epidemiology** The congenital form is rare. Males and females are affected in equal numbers. Women with inherited AE who breast-feed their infants have milk that is deficient in this factor. Consequently, healthy infants may become zinc-deficient and symptomatic.

Acquired AE occurs in an endemic form in individuals of all ages on total parenteral nutrition, in premature infants, and in patients with diseases of the liver and pancreas.

**Related Disorders** See *Celiac Sprue.*

**Treatment—Standard** Zinc sulfate supplements are indicated upon diagnosis of inherited AE and must be continued throughout life. Iodoquinol obtains a response within a week but is no longer commonly used. Genetic counseling is suggested.

For acquired AE, the addition of zinc supplements to the nutritional regimen is both prophylactic and therapeutic.

**Treatment—Investigational** Please contact the agencies listed in Resources, below, for the most current information. Addresses and telephone numbers of these agencies, as well as of individual experts and research centers, may be found in the Master Resources List.

**Resources**

**For more information on acrodermatitis enteropathica:** National Organization for Rare Disorders (NORD); NIH/National Digestive Diseases Information Clearinghouse; Research Trust for Metabolic Diseases in Children.

**For genetic information and genetic counseling referrals:** March of Dimes Birth Defects Foundation; Alliance of Genetic Support Groups.

**References**
Dermatology, 3rd ed.: S.L. Moschella and H.J. Hurley, eds.; W.B. Saunders Company, 1992.
Textbook of Dermatology, 5th ed.: R.H. Champion, et al., eds.; Blackwell Scientific Publications, 1992.
Dermatology, 3rd ed.: O. Braun-Falco, et al.; Springer-Verlag, 1991.
Mendelian Inheritance in Man, 9th ed.: V.A. McKusick; The Johns Hopkins University Press, 1990, pp. 999–1000.
Dermatology in General Medicine: Textbook and Atlas, 3rd ed.: T.B. Fitzpatrick, et al., eds.; McGraw-Hill, 1987.
Abnormal Immune Responses During Hypozincaemia in Acrodermatitis Enteropathica: P.H. Anttila, et al., Acta Paediatr. Scand., November 1986, vol. 75(6), pp. 988–992.
Ocular Histopathology of Acrodermatitis Enteropathica: J.D. Cameron, et al.; Br. J. Ophthalmol., September 1986, vol. 70(9), pp. 662–667.

# ALBINISM

**Description** Albinism comprises a cluster of syndromes with the common denominator of the congenital absence of pigmentation in the skin, hair, and eyes. Associated with the disorders are several ocular defects. The syndromes are primarily categorized as **oculocutaneous albinism** (of which there are several types), **albinoidism,** and **ocular albinism.**

**Synonyms**
>Albinismus
>Congenital Achromia
>Hypomelanosis
>Hypopigmentation

**Signs and Symptoms** In **oculocutaneous albinism,** the integument and the eyes are affected. The tyrosinase-negative and -positive forms are similar at birth, with pinkish-white skin, white hair, and pink, light gray, blue, or hazel eyes. However, those children who are tyrosinase-positive will develop some pigmentation in the skin, hair, and eyes as they grow. Children with both forms of oculocutaneous albinism (tyrosinase-positive and tyrosinase-negative) may have nystagmus, astigmatism, strabismus, and myopia; photophobia will be a problem. Squamous cell carcinomas may develop in these patients.

**Albinoidism** is characterized by hypomelanism of the skin and hair and certain pigmentation abnormalities of the eyes, but without other visual defects such as nystagmus.

In **ocular albinism,** the skin and hair are relatively normal but are fair. Photophobia and the ocular abnormalities of oculocutaneous albinism are present, and there may be retinal mosaicism.

The various forms of oculocutaneous albinism have distinctive characteristics. In Hermansky-Pudlak syndrome, for example, lipid- and platelet-storage abnormalities are associated with pulmonary fibrosis, granulomatous colitis, and recurrent infections. Chédiak-Higashi syndrome is marked by leukocytic disease, proneness to infections, and a high rate of lymphoreticular malignancies.

Types of ocular albinism include Nettleship-Falls syndrome (X-linked), and Forsius-Eriksson syndrome (X-linked).

**Etiology** A lack of tyrosinase, which catalyzes the incorporation of tyrosine to melanin, explains the pigmentary aspect of albinism. There is even distribution of the melanocytes per se, but the melanosomes, which normally become filled with melanin prior to transfer to keratinocytes, are empty. Most of the oculocutaneous forms are autosomal recessive; an autosomal dominant form has been described. Ocular types may be autosomal dominant, recessive, or X-linked. The defective gene thought to cause Forsius-Eriksson syndrome has been located on the short arm of the X chromosome (position 21). The defective gene that is responsible for tyrosinase-positive oculocutaneous albinism has been located on the long arm of chromosome 15 (15q11–q13). The defective gene responsible for ocular albinism has been mapped to chromosome 15 (15q11.2–q12).

**Epidemiology** The incidence of all forms of albinism is approximately 1:10,000. The disorder is more common in some isolated communities, such as the Amish or Mennonite groups in the United States.

**Related Disorders** See *Hermansky-Pudlak Syndrome; Chédiak-Higashi Syndrome.*

See also *Vitiligo* for discussion of an unrelated depigmenting disorder.

**Treatment—Standard** The basic metabolic abnormality in albinism is incurable. Protection from sunlight, especially for those patients with oculocutaneous syndromes, is essential. Sunglasses, protective clothing, and sun-protective lotions are beneficial. Visual aids may be helpful. Surgery for strabismus provides cosmetic improvement but none in vision; the optic decussation is abnormal. Treatment of other disorders of the syndromes is symptomatic. In Chédiak-Higashi syndrome, it is reported that high doses of ascorbic acid may lessen some of the consequences of the lipid storage abnormalities.

**Treatment—Investigational** Please contact the agencies listed under Resources, below, for the most current information. Addresses and telephone numbers of these agencies, as well as of individual experts and research centers, may be found in the Master Resources List.

**Resources**

**For more information on albinism:** National Organization for Rare Disorders (NORD); National Organization for Albinism and Hypopigmentation; NIH/National Institute of Child Health and Human Development.

**For genetic information and genetic counseling referrals:** March of Dimes Birth Defects Foundation; Alliance of Genetic Support Groups.

**References**

Mutations of the P Gene in Oculocutaneous Albinism, Ocular Albinism, and Prader-Willi Syndrome Plus Albinism: S.T. Lee, et al.; N. Engl. J. Med., February 1994, vol. 8(330), pp. 529–534.

Cecil Textbook of Medicine, 19th ed.: J.B. Wyngaarden, et al., eds.; W.B. Saunders Company, 1992, pp. 2322–2323.

Dermatology, 3rd ed.: S.L. Moschella and H.J. Hurley, eds.; W.B. Saunders Company, 1992.

Mendelian Inheritance in Man, 10th ed.: V.A. McKusick; The Johns Hopkins University Press, 1992, pp. 1202–1207.

Textbook of Dermatology, 5th ed.: R.H. Champion, et al., eds.; Blackwell Scientific Publications, 1992.

Albinism: J.W. Harfemeyer; J. Ophthalmic Nurs. Technol., March–April 1991, vol. 10(2), pp. 55–62.

Dermatology, 3rd ed.: O. Braun-Falco, et al.; Springer-Verlag, 1991.

Birth Defects Encyclopedia: M.L. Buyse, ed.-in-chief; Blackwell Scientific Publications, 1990, pp. 69–81.

A Frequent Tyrosinase Gene Mutation in Classic, Tyrosinase-Negative (Type IA) Oculocutaneous Albinism: L.B. Giebel, et al.; Proc. Natl. Acad. Sci. USA, May 1990, vol. 87(9), pp. 3255–3258.

Genetic Mapping of X-Linked Albinism-Deafness Syndrome (ADFN) to Xq26.3–q27: I.Y. Shiloh, et al.; Am. J. Hum. Genet., July 1990, vol. 47(1), pp. 20–27.

The Metabolic Basis of Inherited Disease, 6th ed.: C.R. Scriver, et al., eds.; McGraw-Hill, 1989, pp. 2915–2922.

Thioredoxin Reductase Activity in Hermansky-Pudlak Syndrome: A Method for Identification of Putative Heterozygotes: K.U. Schallreuter and C.J. Witkop; J. Invest. Dermatol., March 1988, vol. 90(3), pp. 372–377.

Dermatology in General Medicine: Textbook and Atlas, 3rd ed.: T.B. Fitzpatrick, et al., eds.; McGraw-Hill, 1987.

# ALOPECIA AREATA

**Description** Alopecia areata is marked by the development of nontender patches of hair loss. As a rule, the bald patches are limited to the scalp and facial hair, but they may involve the entire scalp (**alopecia totalis**) or be generalized (**alopecia universalis**).

**Synonyms**
>Alopecia Celsi
>Alopecia Circumscripta
>Cazenave Vitiligo
>Celsus Vitiligo
>Jonston Alopecia
>Porrigo Decalvans
>Vitiligo Capitis

**Signs and Symptoms** Onset is frequently sudden; oval or round hairless areas develop, usually on the head. These are painless, are not inflamed, and do not itch. The bald spots appear pale and smooth and slowly enlarge. New patches may abut existing bald spots, and this joining of the bald spots may occur during regrowth in established bald spots. Loss of hair may be permanent in patients, however. While hair follicles enter a resting phase, the sebaceous glands usually remain stable. This condition is nonscarring. A few patients may become totally bald. When alopecia areata develops in children, it is likely to be more severe and more refractory to treatment than that which starts in adulthood.

**Etiology** Alopecia areata is idiopathic, but there are microscopic signs of inflammation. An autoimmune disorder is suggested. In addition, some cases are associated with an endocrine disorder.

**Epidemiology** Males and females are affected in equal numbers in either childhood or adulthood. A 1983 study at the Mayo Clinic in Rochester, Minnesota, estimated there were 2 million cases in the United States at that time.

**Related Disorders** The following conditions may be confused with alopecia areata but are not related:

In **congenital alopecia (congenital baldness),** the newborn is hairless. Congenital alopecia is hereditary and either dominant or recessive. Frequently, there are other ectodermal abnormalities.

**Alopecia medicamentosa,** characterized by significant hair loss (usually of the scalp), occurs in individuals who are hypersensitive or allergic to a drug. Chemotherapy is another cause.

**Alopecia mucinosa (follicular mucinosis)** appears in children and young adults as roseate, discrete plaques under the bald spots. Histologically, there are deposits of mucinous material in the hair follicles. Small scales may form on the face, scalp, trunk, arms, or legs. Plaque growth may be accompanied by numbness in the area. The disorder is idiopathic; it may be due to a cutaneous inflammation. Prognosis is guarded. Resolution is frequently spontaneous within a few months. In some patients, however, this is an early sign of a lymphoma.

**Scarring alopecias:** In contrast to alopecia areata, the bald skin is scarred or atrophic. Scarring alopecias develop after many types of inflammatory conditions of the scalp, including infections from bacteria or fungi. Among the noninfectious causes of scarring alopecias are lichen planopilaris (related to lichen planus); systemic lupus erythematosus; pseudopelade (of Brocq); and sarcoidosis.

**Androgenetic alopecia:** Both males and females, with age, develop gradual hair loss, the extent of which is genetically determined. Because it sometimes starts at a young age, it may be confused with some of the pathologic conditions mentioned in this list. In males, the pattern is usually patchy, involving the temporal, frontal, or occipital scalp. In females, the pattern of alopecia is usually diffuse. Treatment with topical minoxidil may be useful.

In **trichotillomania,** patches of hair loss caused by hair pulling are a manifestation of psychological disturbance. Prognosis is good in young children and in older children for whom counseling is sought.

**Telogen effluvium:** Temporary hair loss, often very extensive, is associated with an acute febrile illness, surgery, administration of certain medicines, severe psychological stress, and the postpartum period.

**Treatment—Standard** Many cases of alopecia areata are self-limited. The goal of treatment is regrowth of hair. Systemic corticosteroids may achieve this, but a long-term course may have unacceptable side effects. Triamcinolone acetonide suspension administered sublesionally is usually effective for discrete patches. Application of potent topical steroids is sometimes useful. Wigs and hairpieces may be indicated.

**Treatment—Investigational** A combination of 8-methoxypsoralen ointment and ultraviolet light exposure has been tried; it may not be effective in every patient. Some investigators consider that ultraviolet light may produce immunomodulation, which might control hair loss.

Synthetic immunomodulator drugs such as isoprinosine and diphencyprone are also being studied. Minoxidil was ineffective in a trial with patients with alopecia areata. Other tests compared dinitrochlorobenzene ointment with squaric acid dibutylester, but the former is not recommended because some study participants developed undesirable side effects.

Cyclosporine may have potential in treating alopecia areata, but the possibly dangerous side effects must be considered. Relapse may occur upon stopping the drug.

Please contact the agencies listed under Resources, below, for the most current information. Addresses and telephone numbers of these agencies, as well as of individual experts and research centers, may be found in the Master Resources List.

**Resources**

**For more information on alopecia areata:** The National Organization for Rare Disorders (NORD); National Alopecia Areata Foundation; Alopecia Areata International Research; NIH/National Arthritis and Musculoskeletal and Skin Diseases Information Clearinghouse.

**References**
Dermatology, 3rd ed.: S.L. Moschella and H.J. Hurley, eds.; W.B. Saunders Company, 1992.

Textbook of Dermatology, 5th ed.: R.H. Champion, et al., eds.; Blackwell Scientific Publications, 1992.

Dermatology, 3rd ed.: O. Braun-Falco, et al.; Springer-Verlag, 1991.

Dermatology in General Medicine: Textbook and Atlas, 3rd ed.: T.B. Fitzpatrick, et al., eds.; McGraw-Hill, 1987.

Low-Dose Spironolactone in the Treatment of Female Hirsutism: Int. J. Fertil., January–February 1987, vol. 32(1), pp. 41–45.

Clinical and Immunologic Response to Isoprinosine in Alopecia Areata and Alopecia Universalis: Association with Autoantibodies: M. Lowy, et al.; J. Am. Acad. Dermatol., January 1985, vol. 12(1 pt. 1), pp. 78–84.

Topical Photochemotherapy for Alopecia Areata: A.J. Mitchell, et al.; J. Am. Acad. Dermatol., April 1985, vol. 12(4), pp. 644–649.

# APLASIA CUTIS CONGENITA

**Description** Aplasia cutis congenita is characterized by a congenital absence of skin on the scalp, trunk, and/or extremities. The affected area may be ulcerated, healed as a scar, or covered with a thin, transparent membrane. The skull and underlying areas may be visible. This disorder may be found alone or as a feature of several other disorders.

**Synonyms**
>Congenital Absence of Skin
>Congenital Defect of the Skull and Scalp
>Scalp Defect, Congenital

**Signs and Symptoms** Individuals with aplasia cutis congenita are born with an absence of one or several small to large areas of skin. Some patients may just have skin involvement, while others may also have abnormal development of the underlying structures. This disorder is found most often on the scalp but can also be found on the trunk and/or extremities. Numerous defects, but particularly limb anomalies, have been found in some patients with this disorder.

Aplasia cutis congenita may also occur as one of the findings in the following disorders: Adams-Oliver syndrome, epidermolysis bullosa, and Johanson-Blizzard syndrome. It may also occur with placental infarcts or death of a twin fetus.

**Etiology** Aplasia cutis congenita is an uncommon disorder that can be inherited as an autosomal dominant or autosomal recessive trait.

**Epidemiology** Males and females are affected in equal numbers.

**Related Disorders** See *Adams-Oliver Syndrome.*

**Johanson-Blizzard syndrome** is a form of ectodermal dysplasia that is characterized by nose, scalp, and hair defects, as well as by hypodontia, deafness, short stature, lack of motor development, and malabsorption problems. The most striking feature of this syndrome is the beaklike appearance of the nose. Three-fourths of patients have a protrusion over the posterior fontanelle of the skull at birth, which gets thick and hard as the child grows. Patients have peg-shaped teeth and thin hair, which sweeps up from the forehead. There is marked hearing loss from birth, as well as motor and mental retardation. Bone growth is delayed, and there may be associated intestinal, absorption, and genital defects.

**Treatment—Standard** Treatment of aplasia cutis congenita may consist of surgery when the affected areas do not heal spontaneously. Other treatment is symptomatic and supportive. Genetic counseling may be of benefit for patients and their families.

**Treatment—Investigational** Please contact the agencies listed under Resources, below, for the most current information. Addresses and telephone numbers of these agencies, as well as of individual experts and research centers, may be found in the Master Resources List.

**Resources**

**For more information on aplasia cutis congenita:** National Organization for Rare Disorders (NORD); NIH/National Arthritis and Musculoskeletal and Skin Diseases Information Clearinghouse.

**For genetic information and genetic counseling referrals:** March of Dimes Birth Defects Foundation; Alliance of Genetic Support Groups.

**References**

Birth Defects Encyclopedia: M.L. Buyse, ed.-in-chief; Blackwell Scientific Publications, 1990, p. 171.

Clinical Dermatology, 2nd ed.: T.P. Habif, ed.: C.V. Mosby Company, 1990, p. 614.

Mendelian Inheritance in Man, 9th ed.: V.A. McKusick; The Johns Hopkins University Press, 1990, pp. 88, 1037.

Aplasia Cutis: A Clinical Review and Proposal for Classification: I.S. Frieden; J. Am. Acad. Dermatol., 1986, vol. 14, p. 646.

# BOWEN DISEASE

**Description** Bowen disease, often referred to as squamous cell carcinoma in situ, is a psoriasiform squamous cell carcinoma of the skin with the potential for invasion. Its advance is slow, and it may appear anywhere on the skin or in the mucous membranes.

**Synonyms**

Intraepidermal Squamous Cell Carcinoma

**Signs and Symptoms** The initial sign of Bowen disease is an irregular, sharply demarcated scaly patch. Irregularly formed pink or brown crusty papules develop. An exudative red surface lies under the crust. Misdiagnosis of the disorder as psoriasis, actinic keratosis, or other dermatitis is possible.

**Etiology** Bowen disease is idiopathic. Frequent exposure to the sun may be a contributing factor. Arsenic exposure has also been implicated, especially when the lesion occurs in body areas protected from light or in the mucous membranes. Human papillomavirus 16 DNA has been isolated from the lesions and may be significant in etiology.

**Epidemiology** Bowen disease affects both males and females at any age, but it is very seldom seen in children. In women, the incidence of the disorder in the genital area is 3 times that of men.

**Related Disorders** See *Malignant Melanoma; Paget Disease of the Breast.*

**Squamous cell carcinoma** is a common epithelial neoplasm that often occurs in sun-exposed skin. The carcinoma may also develop in mucous membranes and elsewhere on the body. Squamous cell carcinoma is a red, scaly, sharply outlined nodule that may develop in normal tissue or in precancerous leukoplakia. There may be satellite nodules. The tumor can reach to the lower reticular dermis.

**Treatment—Standard** Treatment commonly requires surgical removal of the cutaneous carcinoma. Carbon dioxide lasers are being utilized as are other destructive modes of treatment for skin lesions. For other types of tumors, various surgical procedures are indicated. Otherwise, therapy is symptomatic and supportive.

**Treatment—Investigational** Please contact the agencies listed under Resources, below, for the most current information. Addresses and telephone numbers of these agencies, as well as of individual experts and research centers, may be found in the Master Resources List.

**Resources**

**For more information on Bowen disease:** National Organization for Rare Disorders (NORD); The Skin Cancer Foundation; American Cancer Society; NIH/National Cancer Institute Physician Data Query Phoneline; NIH/National Institute of Arthritis and Musculoskeletal and Skin Diseases Information Clearinghouse.

**References**

Dermatology, 3rd ed.: S.L. Moschella and H.J. Hurley, eds.; W.B. Saunders Company, 1992.

Textbook of Dermatology, 5th ed.: R.H. Champion, et al., eds.; Blackwell Scientific Publications, 1992.

Dermatology, 3rd ed.: O. Braun-Falco, et al.; Springer-Verlag, 1991.

Bowen's Disease and Internal Malignant Diseases: A Study of 581 Patients: F. Reymann, et al.; Arch. Dermatol., May 1988, vol. 124(5), pp. 677–679.

Bowen's Disease of the Feet: Presence of Human Papillomavirus 16 DNA in Tumor Tissue: M.S. Stone, et al.; Arch. Dermatol., November 1987, vol. 123(11), pp. 1517–1520.

Dermatology in General Medicine: Textbook and Atlas, 3rd ed.: T.B. Fitzpatrick, et al., eds.; McGraw-Hill, 1987.
Bowenoid Papulosis in a Three-Year-Old Girl: C. Halsz, et al.; J. Am. Acad. Dermatol., February 1986, vol. 14(2 pt. 2), pp. 326–330.

# BOWENOID PAPULOSIS

**Description** Bowenoid papulosis is a rare sexually transmitted disorder characterized by lesions on the genitals of males and females.

**Signs and Symptoms** The genital lesions are small, solid, raised, reddish brown or violet in color (darker in females), and sometimes velvety. They may last from 2 weeks to several years. In females, the vagina, clitoris, groin folds, labia majora, labia minora, and/or anus may be affected. Males may be affected on the glans, shaft, and/or foreskin of the penis, as well as the anus.

Many patients with bowenoid papulosis often have other types of viral infections that precede this condition. Herpes simplex, human papillomavirus, viral warts, and HIV infection have been found in some patients with this disorder. When viewed under a microscope, the bowenoid papulosis tissue looks like preinvasive squamous cell carcinoma. In some cases, bowenoid papulosis has become malignant.

**Etiology** Bowenoid papulosis is a sexually transmitted disorder thought to be caused by human papilloma virus **(HPV)** type 16. Other viruses as well as a suppressed immune system may also play a role in patients who contract bowenoid papulosis.

**Epidemiology** Bowenoid papulosis affects males and females in equal numbers. This disorder is seen in sexually active adults, with the average ages being 30 for males and 32 for females. However, bowenoid papulosis has been found in patients ranging from ages 3 to 80. Worldwide, the incidence is increasing.

**Related Disorders** See *Bowen Disease*

**Condyloma** is a common infectious venereal disease that is caused by the human papilloma virus and is usually transmitted by direct sexual contact. The lesions found in this disorder are small, soft, moist, pink or red elevations (warts) on the skin or mucous membranes of the genitals, mouth, anus, or rectum. Typically, the lesions form in clusters.

**Lichen planus** is a recurrent, pruritic, inflammatory eruption of the skin that is characterized by small, separate, angular spots that may grow together, forming rough scaly patches. It is often accompanied by oral lesions. Women are most commonly affected by this disorder. The lesions are most commonly found on the joint surfaces of the wrists and on the legs, trunk, glans penis, and mucous membrane of the mouth and vagina. It is not sexually transmitted.

**Treatment—Standard** In some cases bowenoid papulosis may heal spontaneously. Sexual activity should be limited to avoid infecting other people during the contagious stages of this disorder. Electrosurgery, cryosurgery, and/or laser surgery may be used to remove the lesions. In milder cases, the use of 5-Fluorouracil has been successful.

**Treatment—Investigational** Please contact the agencies listed under Resources, below, for the most current information. Addresses and telephone numbers of these agencies, as well as of individual experts and research centers, may be found in the Master Resources List.

**Resources**

**For more information on bowenoid papulosis:** National Organization for Rare Disorders (NORD); American Social Health Association (ASHA/HRC); Council for Sex Information and Education; National Sexually Transmitted Diseases Hotline; NIH/National Institute of Allergy and Infectious Diseases; Centers for Disease Control.

**References**

Clinical Dermatology, 2nd ed.: T.P. Habif, ed.: C.V. Mosby Company, 1990, p. 246.
Bowenoid Papulosis: T.T. Rogozinski, et al.; Am. Fam. Physician, July 1988, vol. 38(1), pp. 161–164.
Bowenoid Papulosis: J.W. LaVoo; Dis. Colon Rectum, January 1987, vol. 30(1), pp. 62–64.
Bowenoid Papulosis of the Male and Female Genetalia: S. Obalek, et al.; J. Am. Acad. Dermatol., March 1986, vol. 14(3), pp. 433–444.
Bowenoid Papulosis: Presence of Human Papillomavirus (HPV) Structural Antigens and of HPV 16-Related DNA Sequences: G. Gross, et al.; Arch. Dermatol., July 1985, vol. 121(7), pp. 858–863.
Bowenoid Papulosis: Demonstration of Human Papillomavirus (HPV) with Anti-HPV Immune Serum: G.Y. Guillet, et al.; Arch. Dermatol., April 1984, vol. 120(4), pp. 514–516.

# CAVERNOUS HEMANGIOMA

**Description** Cavernous hemangioma, a vascular tumor composed of large blood-filled spaces, can occur at any site in the body and is present at birth or shortly thereafter. It grows rapidly and, after several years, spontaneously regresses or disappears.

**Synonyms**

> Cavernomas
> Cavernous Angioma
> Congenital Vascular Cavernous Malformations
> Hemangioma, Familial
> Nevus Cavernosus
> Vascular Erectile Tumor

**Signs and Symptoms** In the skin, lesions vary in size from 1 to 50 cm or more. They are red, purple-red, or gray, depending upon their depth and state of regression. The most common extracutaneous site for cavernous hemangioma is the liver, but these lesions have been found in the rectum, kidney, eyes, nerves, spinal cord, and brain as well.

**Etiology** Most cases are spontaneous and nonheritable and arise for unknown reasons. Growth factors may be responsible for the proliferation of vascular tissue.

**Epidemiology** Males and females of all ages are affected equally.

**Related Disorders Arteriovenous malformations of the brain** may cause headaches, seizures, strokes, or bleeding into the brain. They may affect arteries, veins, and midsized blood vessels.

See *Moyamoya Disease; Blue Rubber Bleb Nevus; von Hippel-Lindau Disease.*

**Treatment—Standard** Because these lesions usually disappear spontaneously, treatment is often not necessary. If, however, they impinge upon body orifices or cause bleeding, treatment may be required.

Various imaging diagnostic methods such as magnetic resonance imaging, computed tomography scans, and x-rays are useful in determining the extent of the lesions. There is some question as to the effectiveness of surgical treatment of hemangioma. Cryotherapy, systemic corticosteroids, and radiotherapy have their places in treatment of hemangiomas. Lasers are often useful for small superficial lesions.

**Treatment—Investigational** Please contact the agencies listed under Resources, below, for the most current information. Addresses and telephone numbers of these agencies, as well as of individual experts and research centers, may be found in the Master Resources List.

**Resources**

For more information on cavernous hemangioma: National Organization for Rare Disorders (NORD); NIH/National Heart, Lung and Blood Institute Information Center.

For genetic information and genetic counseling referrals: March of Dimes Birth Defects Foundation; Alliance of Genetic Support Groups.

**References**

Dermatology, 3rd ed.: S.L. Moschella and H.J. Hurley, eds.; W.B. Saunders Company, 1992.

Textbook of Dermatology, 5th ed.: R.H. Champion, et al., eds.; Blackwell Scientific Publications, 1992.

Dermatology, 3rd ed.: O. Braun-Falco, et al.; Springer-Verlag, 1991.

Mendelian Inheritance in Man, 9th ed.: V.A. McKusick; The Johns Hopkins University Press, 1990, p. 391.

Cavernous Angiomas of the Spinal Cord: G.R. Cosgrove, et al.; J. Neurosurg., January 1988, vol. 68(1), pp. 31–36.

Cavernous Hemangioma of the Liver: Role of Percutaneous Biopsy: J.J. Cronan, et al.; Radiology, January 1988, vol. 166(1 pt. 1), pp. 135–138.

Cavernous Hemangioma of the Optic Nerve: N. Maruoka, et al.; J. Neurosurg., August 1988, vol. 69(2), pp. 292–294.

Colorectal Hemangioma: Radiologic Findings: A.H. Dachman, et al.; Radiology, April 1988, vol. 167(1), pp. 31–34.

Dermatology in General Medicine: Textbook and Atlas, 3rd ed.: T.B. Fitzpatrick, et al., eds.; McGraw-Hill, 1987.

# CUTIS LAXA

**Description** Cutis laxa is a congenital or acquired connective tissue disorder marked by limp or slack skin. The affected areas of skin may be thickened and dark.

**Synonyms**

> Chalasodermia
> Dermatochalasia
> Dermatolysis
> Dermatomegaly
> Elastorrhexis

**Signs and Symptoms Congenital cutis laxa** is diagnosed at birth or during an infant's early months. Transient edema is often an initial sign. The skin is inelastic, and folds appear in the areas of loose skin. These are most apparent on the face, giving the infant a sad expression. When cutis laxa affects the tissue around the eyes, symptoms may include burning, itching, redness, photosensitivity, and loss of the eyebrows and eyelashes. The disease advances during infancy and is less noticeable in postpuberty. The voice may deepen because of vocal cord laxity.

As a rule, patients develop normally, but in some males the genitalia may remain immature into adulthood and the patient may be impotent. Cardiorespiratory complications (e.g., cor pulmonale, emphysema) can be severe. Other complications include inguinal hernia, and diverticula of the gastrointestinal tract and the urinary bladder.

The onset of **acquired cutis laxa** is slow. It may not manifest until puberty or later. Transient angioedema and inflammation are frequent precursors. Skin changes emerge slowly and may be generalized or localized to the face, body, or neck. Blood vessels are subject to rupture, and purpura results. Potential dangers are aortic rupture, pulmonary complications, respiratory insufficiency due to emphysema, or gastroenteric problems.

**Etiology** The autosomal recessive form of cutis laxa is the most common, but autosomal dominant and X-linked forms exist. Congenital cutis laxa is usually more severe when it is inherited as an autosomal recessive trait. When cutis laxa is inherited as an autosomal dominant trait, the skin problems may be minimal. The X-linked form of cutis laxa has also been classified as Ehlers-Danlos syndrome type IX. Acquired cutis laxa may develop following a severe illness involving fever, polyserositis, and erythema multiforme. The patient is frequently a child or an adolescent. Acquired cutis laxa also may have an autoimmune association.

**Epidemiology** Males and females are affected in equal numbers.

**Related Disorders** See *Ehlers-Danlos Syndromes; De Barsy Syndrome.*

**Treatment—Standard** No specific treatment exists. Plastic surgery may be indicated as a cosmetic measure in patients with the congenital form. The surgery may be less effective in patients with the acquired form. Otherwise, treatment is confined to that for any cardiorespiratory or other complications that may develop.

**Treatment—Investigational** Please contact the agencies listed under Resources, below, for the most current information. Addresses and telephone numbers of these agencies, as well as of individual experts and research centers, may be found in the Master Resources List.

**Resources**

**For more information on cutis laxa:** National Organization for Rare Disorders (NORD); NIH/National Arthritis and Musculoskeletal and Skin Diseases Information Clearinghouse.

**For genetic information and genetic counseling referrals:** March of Dimes Birth Defects Foundation; Alliance of Genetic Support Groups.

**References**

Acquired Cutis Laxa with Dermatitis Herpetoformis and Sarcoidosis: F.M. Lewis; J. Am. Acad. Dermatol., November 1993, vol. 29(5 pt. 2), pp. 846–848.

Congenital Cutis Laxa: A Case Report and Review of Loose Skin Syndromes: W.O. Thomas, et al.; Ann. Plast. Surg., March 1993, vol. 30(3), pp. 252–256.

Dermatochalasis and Dry Eye: S.D. Vold, et al.; Am. J. Ophthalmol., February 1993, vol. 115(2), pp. 216–220.

Cecil Textbook of Medicine, 19th ed.: J.B. Wyngaarden, et al., eds.; W.B. Saunders Company, 1992, pp. 1122–1124.

Dermatology, 3rd ed.: S.L. Moschella and H.J. Hurley, eds.; W.B. Saunders Company, 1992.

Mendelian Inheritance in Man, 10th ed.: V.A. McKusick; The Johns Hopkins University Press, 1992, pp. 286–287, 1307–1308, 1810.

Nelson Textbook of Pediatrics, 14th ed.: R.E. Behrman, ed.-in-chief; W.B. Saunders Company, 1992, pp. 1660–1661.

Textbook of Dermatology, 5th ed.: R.H. Champion, et al., eds.; Blackwell Scientific Publications, 1992, pp. 1769–1771.

Cutis Laxa: Autosomal Dominant Inheritance in Five Generations: A. Damkier, et al.; Clin. Genet., May 1991, vol. 39(5), pp. 321–329.

Dermatology, 3rd ed.: O. Braun-Falco, et al.; Springer-Verlag, 1991.

Harrison's Principles of Internal Medicine, 12th ed.: J.D. Wilson, et al., eds.; McGraw-Hill, 1991, p. 924.

Birth Defects Encyclopedia: M.L. Buyse, ed.-in-chief; Blackwell Scientific Publications, 1990, pp. 473–474.

Dictionary of Medical Syndromes, 3rd ed.: S.I. Magalini, et al., eds.; J.B. Lippincott Company, 1990, pp. 218–219.

Syndromes of the Head and Neck, 3rd ed.: R.J. Gorlin, et al; Oxford University Press, 1990, pp. 422–425.

Dermatology in General Medicine: Textbook and Atlas, 3rd ed.: T.B. Fitzpatrick, et al., eds.; McGraw-Hill, 1987.

# Cutis Marmorata Telangiectatica Congenita

**Description** Cutis marmorata telangiectatica congenita is a rare disorder characterized by unusual discolored patches of skin (livedo reticularis) caused by dilated surface blood vessels (telangiectases). This condition gives the skin a reddish-blue marbling or fishnet appearance.

**Signs and Symptoms** In addition to the mottling of the skin, large, craterlike skin ulcers are also apparent in a few individuals. The skin abnormalities may improve with age.

Over 50 percent of patients have other associated abnormalities, including a red or reddish-purple benign vascular malformation (nevus flammeus or port-wine stain); atrophy of one side of the body; glaucoma; complete or partial absence of a limb, bone, or bones (transverse limb defects); unbalanced body development; hypertrophy of one leg; or a larger than normal brain.

A few individuals may have other abnormalities, such as a detached retina, syndactyly, and/or growth retardation.

**Etiology** The cause of cutis marmorata telangiectatica congenita is unknown and usually is idiopathic. In a few affected families, the disorder may be inherited as an autosomal dominant genetic trait. However, within affected families, defects may vary.

**Epidemiology** Cutis marmorata telangiectatica congenita affects males and females in equal numbers. There have been fewer than 70 cases of this disorder reported in the medical literature.

**Related Disorders Cutis marmorata** is a transient skin disorder in which the skin has a bluish-red marbling pattern when exposed to cold temperatures. This condition is found most often in infants but may also affect adults. When the skin is warmed, the condition disappears. Cutis marmorata is very common in premature infants and usually disappears completely in infancy.

**Rothmund-Thomson syndrome** is a rare disorder inherited as an autosomal recessive genetic trait. The most common symptoms of this disorder are an abnormal redness of the skin caused by congested capillaries, small stature, and tissue wasting.

**Treatment—Standard** Treatment of cutis marmorata telangiectatica congenita is symptomatic and supportive. The associated skin abnormalities disappear in approximately 50 percent of affected individuals. When port-wine stains are present, treatment with the flash pump dye laser is often effective. Because it is relatively painless and eliminates any lasting effects on the skin, the flash pump dye laser can be used on children as young as 1 month of age. Individuals with transverse limb defects may benefit from surgery and/or a prosthesis. When other family members are affected, genetic counseling may be of benefit.

**Treatment—Investigational** Please contact the agencies listed under Resources, below, for the most current information. Addresses and telephone numbers of these agencies, as well as of individual experts and research centers, may be found in the Master Resources List.

**Resources**

**For more information on cutis marmorata telangiectatica congenita:** National Organization for Rare Disorders (NORD); Sturge-Weber Foundation; Nevus Network; NIH/National Arthritis and Musculoskeletal and Skin Diseases Information Clearinghouse; The Arc (a national organization on mental retardation).

**For genetic information and genetic counseling referrals:** March of Dimes Birth Defects Foundation; Alliance of Genetic Support Groups.

**References**

Localized Cutis Marmorata Telangiectatica Congenita: S.M. Suarez, et al.; Pediatr. Dermatol., December 1991, vol. 8(4), pp. 329–331.

Birth Defects Encyclopedia: M.L. Buyse, ed.-in-chief; Blackwell Scientific Publications, 1990, pp. 476–477.

Mendelian Inheritance in Man, 9th ed.: V.A. McKusick, The Johns Hopkins University Press, 1990, pp. 1308–1309.

Cutis Marmorata Telangiectatica Congenita: Report of 22 Cases: D.D. Picascia, et al.; J. Am. Acad. Dermatol., June 1989, vol. 20(6), pp. 1098–1104.

Scalp and Limb Defects with Cutis Marmorata Telangiectatica Congenita: Adams-Oliver Syndrome?: H.V. Toriello, et al.; Am. J. Med. Genet., February 1988, vol. 29(2), pp. 269–276.

Cutis Marmorata Telangiectatica Congenita with Multiple Congenital Anomalies: S.M. Deln Giudice, et al.; Arch. Dermatol., September 1986, vol. 122(9), pp. 1060–1061.

Cutis Marmorata Telangiectatica Congenita: A Case Report: A.R. Altman, et al.; Pediatr. Dermatol., January 1984, vol. 1(3), pp. 223–225.

Cutis Marmorata Telangiectatica Congenita: M. Rogers, et al.; Arch. Dermatol., November 1982, vol. 118(11), pp. 895–899.

# DARIER DISEASE

**Description** Darier disease is a gradually progressive, hereditary skin disorder characterized by widespread keratotic papules on the skin and mucous membranes, and by nail dystrophy.

**Synonyms**

Dyskeratosis Follicularis

White-Darier Disease

**Signs and Symptoms** The onset of Darier disease is gradual, beginning with burning and itching of the skin in the seborrheic areas, and extending elsewhere. Papules appear, becoming larger and darker and covered with gray-brown scales or crusts. The enlarging papules eventually coalesce to form larger patches. Sites of predilection include the scalp, forehead, trunk, and extremities. The hyperkeratotic plaques are often foul-smelling as a result of bacterial colonization. Nails show longitudinal ridging, splits, and subungual keratoses. Hyperkeratotic white plaques in the oral cavity are characteristic. Patients complain of severe pruritus. Symptoms tend to be more severe during periods of emotional stress and with exposure to sunlight, and may decrease during the winter. Some but not all patients are mentally retarded.

**Etiology** Darier disease is inherited as a dominant trait. The cause is unknown. Histologically there is suprabasal acantholysis with evidence of premature cornification of individual keratinocytes.

**Epidemiology** Onset usually is during childhood, but the disease may appear as late as the 7th decade of life. Males are more commonly affected. In Denmark the incidence has been estimated at 1:10,000 persons.

**Related Disorders Acrokeratosis verruciformis of Hopf** is a dominant, hereditary skin disorder typified by flat or convex, smooth, firm papules distributed symmetrically on the backs of the hands, feet, wrists, and ankles. The number, size, and coloration of the papules vary. Other symptoms include hyperkeratosis of the palms and soles, and nail abnormalities such as opacity and brittleness.

**Hyperkeratosis follicularis in cutem penetrans (Kyrle disease)** is a rare dermatologic disorder occurring mostly in female adults. It is characterized by painful, scattered eruptions with hornlike, cone-shaped plugs on the extremities, buttocks, and cheeks.

**Keratosis pilaris (follicular ichthyosis)** is a common skin disorder of adolescence that is characterized by mild erythema and the development of irregularly distributed keratotic papules. The thighs and arms also may have the appearance of gooseflesh.

**Treatment—Standard** The cutaneous manifestations of Darier disease sometimes respond to etretinate. *(This drug should not be taken by pregnant women.)* Surgical debridement may be helpful in certain cases. Keratolytics and antibiotics are useful.

**Treatment—Investigational** Please contact the agencies listed under Resources, below, for the most current information. Addresses and telephone numbers of these agencies, as well as of individual experts and research centers, may be found in the Master Resources List.

**Resources**

**For more information on Darier disease:** National Organization for Rare Disorders (NORD); Foundation for Ichthyosis and Related Skin Types; NIH/National Arthritis and Musculoskeletal and Skin Diseases Information Clearinghouse.

**For genetic information and genetic counseling referrals:** March of Dimes Birth Defects Foundation; Alliance of Genetic Support Groups.

**References**

Dermatology, 3rd ed.: S.L. Moschella and H.J. Hurley, eds.; W.B. Saunders Company, 1992.

Textbook of Dermatology, 5th ed.: R.H. Champion, et al., eds.; Blackwell Scientific Publications, 1992.

Dermatology, 3rd ed.: O. Braun-Falco, et al.; Springer-Verlag, 1991.

Dermatology in General Medicine: Textbook and Atlas, 3rd ed.: T.B. Fitzpatrick, et al., eds.; McGraw-Hill, 1987.

Genetically Transmitted, Generalized Disorders of Cornification: The Ichthyoses: M.L. Williams, et al.; *in* Dermatologic Clinics, January 1987, vol. 5(1), pp. 173–175.

The Surgical Treatment of Hypertrophic Darier's Disease: R.G. Wheeland, et al.; J. Dermatol. Surg. Oncol., April 1985, vol. 11(4), pp. 420–423.

Etretinate: Effect of Milk Intake on Absorption: J.J. DiGiovanna, et al.; J. Invest. Dermatol., June 1984, vol. 82(6), pp. 636–640.

# DERMATITIS HERPETIFORMIS (DH)

**Description** A chronic disorder, DH is marked by groups of severely itching blisters and papules and is often associated with gluten-sensitive enteropathy.

**Synonyms**

> Brocq-Duhring Disease
> Dermatitis Multiformis
> Duhring Disease
> Gluten-Sensitive Enteropathy

**Signs and Symptoms** A slow onset is typical in adult life, but children can be affected also. Small blisters, discrete papules, and itchy, smooth lesions resembling hives appear symmetrically on the head, elbows, knees, lower back, and buttocks. Quite often blisters and papules occur on the face and neck. Itching and burning may be almost intolerable, and the need to scratch irresistible. Over three-quarters of patients have a gluten-sensitive, gastrointestinal atrophy similar to that in celiac disease. Malabsorption generally does not occur.

The direct immunofluorescence test for IgA in normal skin is positive.

**Etiology** Dermatitis herpetiformis is idiopathic, but several immunologic abnormalities have been detected. The presence in lesions of IgA and complement components supports an immunoregulatory disturbance. Iodide and other halides can cause a flare. Approximately 90 percent of patients test positive for HLA B8-DR3, suggesting a genetic predisposition to the disease.

**Epidemiology** Onset may be at any age, but it usually occurs in middle adult life; it is rare in the pediatric group. Males are affected more often than females (3:2).

**Related Disorders** See *Pemphigoid, Bullous; Pemphigus; Erythema Multiforme; Epidermolytic Hyperkeratosis; Epidermolysis Bullosa.*

**Linear IgA disease (linear IgA dermatosis)** is a rare chronic skin disease characterized by the development of groups of pruritic blisters and papules. It is not associated with gluten-sensitive enteropathy. Blisters and hives develop on the skin, especially on the arms, legs, lower back, and/or buttocks. The skin may become very red and extremely itchy.

**Treatment—Standard** Dapsone frequently treats the rash successfully and brings symptomatic relief within 1 or 2 days. The urgent need to scratch usually abates in 1 to 3 days. Dapsone can be associated with severe hematologic disturbances and must be closely monitored. Sulfapyridine may be used as an alternative to dapsone, especially in patients who also have coronary disease. Topical corticosteroids may help to relieve pruritus. However, the administration of oral nonsteroidal anti-inflammatory drugs usually aggravates symptoms. Some patients who also have gluten-sensitive enteropathy may be able to discontinue drug therapy if they follow a strict gluten-free diet for at least 6 to 12 months.

**Treatment—Investigational** Russell P. Hall, III, M.D., of Duke University, is exploring the relationship between the skin and the function of the digestive system in people with dermatitis herpetiformis and other similar dermatologic disorders.

Please contact the agencies listed under Resources, below, for the most current information. Addresses and telephone numbers of these agencies, as well as of individual experts and research centers, may be found in the Master Resources List.

**Resources**

**For more information on dermatitis herpetiformis:** National Organization for Rare Disorders (NORD); Gluten Intolerance Group of North America; NIH/National Arthritis and Musculoskeletal and Skin Diseases Information Clearinghouse.

**References**

Dermatitis Herpetiformis and Established Coeliac Disease: D.J. Gawkrodger, et al.; Br. J. Dermatol., December 1993, vol. 129(6), pp. 694–695.

Diet and Dermatology: The Role of Dietary Manipulation in the Prevention and Treatment of Cutaneous Disorders: S.C. Rackett, et al.; J. Am. Acad. Dermatol., September 1993, vol. 29(3), pp. 447–461.

Cecil Textbook of Medicine, 19th ed.: J.B. Wyngaarden, et al., eds.; W.B. Saunders Company, 1992, pp. 1478, 2308.

Dermatology, 3rd ed.: S.L. Moschella and H.J. Hurley, eds.; W.B. Saunders Company, 1992.

The Incidence and Prevalence of Dermatitis Herpetiformis in Utah: J.B. Smith, et al.; Arch. Dermatol., December 1992, vol. 128(12), pp. 1608–1610.

Serologic Markers of Gluten-Sensitive Enteropathy in Bullous Diseases: V. Kumar, et al.; Arch. Dermatol., November 1992, vol. 128(11), pp. 1474–1478.

Textbook of Dermatology, 5th ed.: R.H. Champion, et al., eds.; Blackwell Scientific Publications, 1992, pp. 1658–1659.

Vesiculobullous Diseases with Prominent Immunologic Features: E.E. Boh, et al.; JAMA, November 25, 1992, vol. 268(20), pp. 2893–2898.

Dermatology, 3rd ed.: O. Braun-Falco, et al.; Springer-Verlag, 1991.

The Effect of an Elemental Diet with and Without Gluten on Disease Activity in Dermatitis Herpetiformis: D.P. Kadunce, et al.; J. Invest. Dermatol., August 1991, vol. 97(2), pp. 175–182.

Harrison's Principles of Internal Medicine, 12th ed.: J.D. Wilson, et al., eds.; McGraw-Hill, 1991, pp. 318–320.

Small Intestinal Function and Dietary Status in Dermatitis Herpetiformis: D.J. Gawrodger, et al.; Gut, April 1991, vol. 32(4), pp. 377–382.

Clinical Dermatology, 2nd ed.: T.P. Habif, ed.; C.V. Mosby Company, 1990, pp. 406–411.

Dictionary of Medical Syndromes, 3rd ed.: S.I. Magalini, et al., eds.; J.B. Lippincott Company, 1990, pp. 266–267.

Internal Medicine, 3rd ed.: J.H. Stein, ed.-in-chief; Little, Brown and Company, 1990, p. 1831.

Dermatology in General Medicine: Textbook and Atlas, 3rd ed.: T.B. Fitzpatrick, et al., eds.; McGraw-Hill, 1987.

# DYSKERATOSIS CONGENITA

**Description** Dyskeratosis congenita is a rare disorder in which 3 groups of symptoms occur: hyper- and/or hypopigmentation; progressive nail dystrophy; and leukoplakia in the anus, urethra, lips, mouth, and/or eye. Other symptoms found in some patients with this syndrome may be pancytopenia, overgrowth of skin on the palms of the hands and soles of the feet, excessive sweating of the palms and soles, sparse or absent hair, fragile bones, underdeveloped testes, and dental abnormalities.

**Synonyms**

Dyschromatosis Universalis Hereditaria

Zinsser-Cole-Engman Syndrome

**Signs and Symptoms** The main symptoms of dyskeratosis congenita are:

1. **Hyper- and hypopigmentation:** Hyperpigmentation in dyskeratosis congenita has a netlike pattern of distribution that is brownish gray in color. Hypopigmentation is a lack of skin color that is intermixed. These skin discolorations may be present at birth but usually are progressive and appear later.

2. **Progressive nail dystrophy** may lead to loss of nails on the fingers or toes. This condition is not apparent at birth.

3. **Mucosal leukoplakia:** a slowly developing change in normal mucous membrane tissue. This condition may be found in the mucous membranes of the anus, urethra, lips, mouth, and/or eyes. This condition should be monitored closely and the leukoplakic lesions removed before they can become malignant.

The following conditions are often, but not always, present in patients with dyskeratosis congenita:

4. **Pancytopenia:** a reduction in the normal number of red and white blood cells and platelets caused by bone marrow failure.

5. **Hyperkeratosis:** the overgrowth of skin on the palms of the hands and the soles of the feet. This condition often causes a lack of finger- and footprints.

6. **Hyperhidrosis:** excessive sweating of the palms of the hands and the soles of the feet.

7. **Atresia of the lacrimal puncta:** absence of the tiny opening in the edge of each eyelid that drains the tears. This condition causes chronic tearing.

The following conditions are sometimes associated with dyskeratosis congenita and have been found in some patients with this disorder:

8. **Alopecia:** absence of hair from skin areas where it is normally present. The hair is often fine and sparse, and there may be premature graying.

9. **Dental abnormalities:** displacement of teeth from a normal position in the dental arch. Teeth may also be lost at an early age.

10. **Osteoporosis:** Patients with dyskeratosis congenita may also have a fragile build and a slow growth pattern.

11. **Testicular atrophy.** The penis may also be underdeveloped.

12. **Thrombocytopenia.**

13. **Microcephaly.**

14. **Mental retardation or reduced intelligence.**

15. **Cirrhosis of the liver.**

16. **Dysphagia**.

17. **Acrocyanosis:** hands and/or feet that are blue, cold, and sweaty. This is caused by spasms of the blood vessels and usually occurs when the patient is cold or under stress.

18. **Cataracts.**

**Etiology** Most cases of dyskeratosis congenita have an X-linked recessive inheritance, although cases have been reported of autosomal recessive and autosomal dominant inheritance. A significant number of cases have also occurred sporadically. Dyskeratosis congenita has been mapped to the Xq27–q28 gene.

**Epidemiology** Dyskeratosis congenita affects males most often, with the ratio of affected males to females 10:1. This disorder is usually detected between the ages of 5 and 15, although mucous membrane (mouth) and nail abnormalities may be present earlier. There have been only 120 cases of dyskeratosis congenita reported. The disease has occurred in all races.

**Related Disorders** See *Anemia, Fanconi.*

**Treatment—Standard** Treatment of dyskeratosis congenita is symptomatic and supportive. Leukoplakic lesions should be surgically removed to prevent malignancy. Dental abnormalities require dental intervention. Genetic counseling may be of benefit for patients and their families.

**Treatment—Investigational** Please contact the agencies listed under Resources, below, for the most current information. Addresses and telephone numbers of these agencies, as well as of individual experts and research centers, may be found in the Master Resources List.

**Resources**

**For more information on dyskeratosis congenita:** National Organization for Rare Disorders (NORD); National Foundation for Ectodermal Dysplasias; The Arc (a national organization on mental retardation); NIH/National Institute of Child Health and Human Development; NIH/National Heart, Lung and Blood Institute Information Center.

**For genetic information and genetic counseling referrals:** March of Dimes Birth Defects Foundation; Alliance of Genetic Support Groups.

**References**

Birth Defects Encyclopedia: M.L. Buyse, ed.-in-chief; Blackwell Scientific Publications, 1990, pp. 567–568.

Enhanced G2 Chromatid Radiosensitivity to Dyskeratosis Congenita Fibroblasts: D.M. DeBauche, et al.; Am. J. Hum. Genet., February 1990, vol. 46(2), pp. 350–357.

Mendelian Inheritance in Man, 9th ed.: V.A. McKusick; The Johns Hopkins University Press, 1990, pp. 275, 1154, 1586.

Etiologic Heterogeneity in Dyskeratosis Congenita: G.S. Pai, et al.; Am. J. Med. Genet., January 1989, vol. 32(1), pp. 63–66.

Dyskeratosis Congenita: Report of a Case and Review of the Literature: G.R. Ogden, et al.; Oral Surg. Oral Med. Oral Pathol., May 1988, vol. 65(5), pp. 586–591.

Smith's Recognizable Patterns of Human Malformation, 4th ed.: K.L. Jones, ed.; W.B. Saunders Company, 1988, p. 474.

Diagnostic Recognition of Genetic Diseases: W. Nyhan and N.O. Sakati, eds.; Lea and Febiger, 1987, pp. 600, 672.

# DYSPLASTIC NEVUS SYNDROME

**Description** Dysplastic nevus syndrome is characterized by the appearance in adolescence or young adulthood of typical nevi or moles having variation in size, shape, and color. They are considered by many people to be precursors of melanoma. Sporadic, multiple heritable, and multiple nonheritable forms exist.

**Synonyms**
> B-K Mole Syndrome
> Familial Atypical Mole–Malignant Melanoma Syndrome

**Signs and Symptoms** Dysplastic nevi have irregular edges and are pink to reddish brown in color. They appear in variable numbers, especially on the trunk. Histologically, these nevi have marked atypical melanocytic hyperplasia. When frankly malignant histologic features are present, dysplastic nevi are then said to be melanomas.

**Etiology** The cause is unknown. Heritable forms are transmitted as autosomal dominant genes.

**Epidemiology** Symptoms usually first appear in young adulthood. Males and females are affected in equal numbers.

**Treatment—Standard** Periodic examination of lesions for change suggesting malignancy is indicated. Questionable lesions should be excised. Patients should use sunscreen and avoid sunburn.

**Treatment—Investigational** Please contact the agencies listed under Resources, below, for the most current information. Addresses and telephone numbers of these agencies, as well as of individual experts and research centers, may be found in the Master Resources List.

**Resources**

   **For more information on dysplastic nevus syndrome:** National Organization for Rare Disorders (NORD); Skin Cancer Foundation; American Cancer Society; NIH/National Cancer Institute Physician Data Query Phoneline; Nevus Network; Giant Congenital Pigmented Nevus Support Group; Nevus Support Group; American Cancer Society.

   **For genetic information and genetic counseling referrals:** March of Dimes Birth Defects Foundation; Alliance of Genetic Support Groups.

**References**
Dermatology, 3rd ed.: S.L. Moschella and H.J. Hurley, eds.; W.B. Saunders Company, 1992.

Textbook of Dermatology, 5th ed.: R.H. Champion, et al., eds.; Blackwell Scientific Publications, 1992.

Dermatology, 3rd ed.: O. Braun-Falco, et al.; Springer-Verlag, 1991.

The Efficacy of Histopathological Criteria Required for Diagnosing Dysplastic Naevi: P.M. Steijlen, et al.; Histopathology, March 1988, vol. 12(3), pp. 289–300.

Mendelian Inheritance in Man, 8th ed.: V.A. McKusick; The Johns Hopkins University Press, 1988, pp. 485–486.

Dermatology in General Medicine: Textbook and Atlas, 3rd ed.: T.B. Fitzpatrick, et al., eds.; McGraw-Hill, 1987.

Dysplastic Nevus Syndrome: Ultraviolet Hypermutability Confirmed in Vitro by Elevated Sister Chromatid Exchanges: E.G. Jung, et al.; Dermatologica, 1986, vol. 173(6), pp. 297–300.

Role of Topical Tretinoin in Melanoma and Dysplastic Nevi: F.L. Meyskens Jr., et al.; J. Am. Acad. Dermatol., October 1986, vol. 15(4 pt. 2), pp. 822–825.

# EPIDERMAL NEVUS SYNDROME

**Description** Epidermal nevus syndrome is a rare disorder characterized by distinctive nevi on the skin, often on the face. Neurologic and skeletal abnormalities may also occur. This disorder is often associated with seizures, mental deficiency, eye problems, bone malformations, and atrophy of the brain.

**Synonyms**
> Linear Sebaceous Nevus Syndrome
> Linear Sebaceous Nevus Sequence
> Nevus Sebaceus of Jadassohn
> Ichthyosis Hystrix Gravior
> Inflammatory Linear Nevus Sebaceus Syndrome
> Lambert Type Ichthyosis
> Linear Nevus Sebaceus Syndrome
> Porcupine Man
> Sebaceous Nevus Syndrome

**Signs and Symptoms** The most visible sign of epidermal nevus syndrome is the skin lesions, which may be apparent at birth. These lesions tend to form in a line and have excessive pigmentation. Singular or multiple forms of the 5 major types of epidermal nevi may emerge: raised wartlike streaks; polyplike masses forming in lines; dark, velvety spots; scaly streaks; and an orange, hairless, velvety patch covering part of the face, nose, eyelids, and scalp.

The sebaceous glands tend to overgrow, causing the abnormal changes in the outer layer of skin. These discolored lesions are usually found in the middle of the face, extending from the forehead down the nose and onto the scalp. Less commonly, the lesions may be found on the trunk and limbs.

When the patient reaches puberty, the lesions start to resemble wartlike elevations, and there is an increase in the cell growth of the sebaceous glands, sometimes causing the growth of tumors. The growth and severity of these lesions usually become stable by the end of puberty.

Other symptoms associated with epidermal nevus syndrome may be skeletal abnormalities, such as excessive development of bones, backward or lateral curvature of the spine, and deformities of the foot and ankle. Mental retardation, cysts, seizures, and abnormalities of the eyes may also occur.

**Etiology** The exact cause of epidermal nevus syndrome is not known. Approximately two-thirds of cases appear to be inherited as an autosomal dominant trait.

**Epidemiology** Epidermal nevus syndrome is a very rare disorder affecting males and females in equal numbers. There have been approximately 450 cases of epidermal nevus syndrome reported.

**Related Disorders** See *Sturge-Weber Syndrome; Tuberous Sclerosis.*

**Treatment—Standard** Treatment is symptomatic and supportive. Small nevi may be removed surgically, but removal of larger lesions often does not improve the appearance.

Topical application of a dilute solution of propylene glycol combined with lactic acid may result in slight improvement of appearance. Retinoic acid solution applied topically may also be used, but this treatment also results only in slight improvement.

Abnormalities of the eyes, bones, and other organs may require medical attention. Genetic counseling may be of benefit for patients and their families.

**Treatment—Investigational** Monolaurin (glylorin) is being tested for the treatment of epidermal nevus syndrome. The product is manufactured by Cellegy Pharmaceuticals.

Please contact the agencies listed under Resources, below, for the most current information. Addresses and telephone numbers of these agencies, as well as of individual experts and research centers, may be found in the Master Resources List.

**Resources**

**For more information on epidermal nevus syndrome:** National Organization for Rare Disorders (NORD); Nevus Network; Giant Congenital Pigmented Nevus Support Group; Nevus Support Group; Foundation for Ichthyosis and Related Skin Types; The Arc (a national organization on mental retardation); NIH/National Arthritis and Musculoskeletal and Skin Diseases Information Clearinghouse.

**For genetic information and genetic counseling referrals:** March of Dimes Birth Defects Foundation; Alliance of Genetic Support Groups.

**References**

Birth Defects Encyclopedia: M.L. Buyse, ed.-in-chief; Blackwell Scientific Publications, 1990, pp. 1251–1252.
Mendelian Inheritance in Man, 9th ed.: V.A. McKusick; The Johns Hopkins University Press, 1990, p. 662.
Smith's Recognizable Patterns of Human Malformation, 4th ed.: K.L. Jones, ed.; W.B. Saunders Company, 1988, p. 446.
Epidermal Nevus Syndrome: A.S. Paller; Neuro. Clin., August 1987, vol. 5(3), pp. 451–457.
The Epidermal Nevus Syndrome: Case Report and Review: L.H. Goldberg, et al.; Pediatr. Dermatol., May 1987, vol. 4(1), pp. 27–33.

# EPIDERMOLYSIS BULLOSA (EB)

**Description** EB refers to a group of more than 20 rare hereditary skin diseases characterized by fragile skin in which bullae and vesicles develop following minor trauma. In some forms of EB the mucous membranes are involved. Healing is impaired in some forms, causing chronic exudative plaques, mutilating scars, or contractures.

**Synonyms**

> Dowling-Meara Syndrome
> Hallopeau-Siemens Disease
> Herlitz Syndrome
> Koebner Disease
> Localized Epidermolysis
> Weber-Cockayne Disease

**Signs and Symptoms** Classification of the major types of EB depends upon the depth of the blisters.

In **EB simplex (nonscarring),** the blisters occur within the epidermis. The **Weber-Cockayne form** of EB simplex is characterized by the development of blisters following minor trauma to the hands and feet and other friction points. It is autosomal dominant. In **EB herpetiformis (Dowling-Meara),** which is another form of EB simplex, there is extensive blistering and much of the body may be affected. It is also autosomal dominant. The mucous membranes are seldom involved. Blisters usually heal without scars; secondary infection is the primary complication. Warm weather may aggravate the condition. Patients with the simplex form usually have normal mental and physical development.

In **junctional EB,** the blisters occur within the lamina lucida of the basement membrane zone. The **Herlitz type (EB lethalis)** has extensive blisters of skin and mucous membranes and is usually fatal in infancy. In other junctional forms of EB, such as the generalized junctional form, there may be extensive facial erosions and loss of nails. All junctional forms are probably autosomal recessive diseases.

**EB dystrophic (scarring)** is characterized by blisters that develop beneath the basement membrane zone of the skin. All forms cause scarring. There are both autosomal dominant and recessive types. The **recessive dystrophic form (Hallopeau-Siemens)** is the most severe. Blisters appear on extremities and are widespread, affecting mucous membranes and skin. Blisters leave scars and miliary cysts after healing. The tongue, eyes, and esophagus are often affected; teeth may be malformed. Nails may be lost. Scars leave mitten deformities of the digits. In some cases, hair follicles may be destroyed and alopecia develops. Malnutrition, anemia, and growth retardation can result from chronic blood loss and poor food intake.

**Etiology** Various forms of epidermolysis bullosa are inherited as either autosomal dominant or recessive traits (see Signs and Symptoms, above). The mechanism involved may be related to structural abnormalities of keratin and collagen and/or to defects with the reparative dermal enzyme, collagenase. In EB simplex, genes on chromosomes 12 and 17 have been found to be involved in causing the disorder. The gene associated with the Weber-Cockayne form of EB simplex has been mapped to chromosome 17 (17q12–q21). The gene associated with the Herlitz type has been mapped to chromosome 1 (1q25–q31). The gene for EB dystrophic has been located on chromosome 3.

**Epidemiology** About 25,000 to 50,000 persons in the United States are thought to be affected by all forms of epidermolysis bullosa.

**Related Disorders** See *Syphilis, Congenital; Ichthyosis.*

**Treatment—Standard** Therapy is symptomatic and supportive. Antibiotics are useful, and a high-protein diet is helpful in cases where malnutrition develops. A cool environment is usually more comfortable for patients suffering from this disease.

**Treatment—Investigational** Research is ongoing in the areas of orphan drugs, wound-healing antibiotics, and the inhibition of blister formation. Phenytoin blocks collagenase in vitro, but has not proved to be clinically useful in reducing blistering.

Sucralfate suspension (Naska Pharmacal Company) is being tested as a treatment of oral ulcerations and dysphagia in EB patients. Studies are also under way to explore the effectiveness of cyclosporine, as well as cyclosporine in conjunction with prednisone.

Epidermal cells cultured to form sheets of skin have been successfully transplanted onto the damaged skin of patients with epidermolysis bullosa. Approximately 50 percent of the grafted tissue attached successfully, with no sign of infection, rejection, or recurrent blistering during a 4-year follow-up period.

Please contact the agencies listed under Resources, below, for the most current information. Addresses and telephone numbers of these agencies, as well as of individual experts and research centers, may be found in the Master Resources List.

**Resources**

**For more information on epidermolysis bullosa:** National Organization for Rare Disorders (NORD); Dystrophic Epidermolysis Bullosa Research Association; Eugene Bauer, M.D., Stanford University School of Medicine, Department of Dermatology; NIH/National Arthritis and Musculoskeletal and Skin Diseases Information Clearinghouse.

**For genetic information and genetic counseling referrals:** March of Dimes Birth Defects Foundation; Alliance of Genetic Support Groups.

**References**

Human Genetics Disorders: The Journal of NIH Research, August 1994, vol. 6(8), pp. 115–134.

Dermatology, 3rd ed.: S.L. Moschella and H.J. Hurley, eds.; W.B. Saunders Company, 1992.

Inherited and Acquired Blistering Diseases: S.I. Katz; N. Engl. J. Med., July 16, 1992, vol. 327(3), pp. 196–197.

Nelson Textbook of Pediatrics, 14th ed.: R.E. Behrman, ed.-in-chief; W.B. Saunders Company, 1992, pp. 1642–1643.

Textbook of Dermatology, 5th ed.: R.H. Champion, et al., eds.; Blackwell Scientific Publications, 1992.

Dermatology, 3rd ed.: O. Braun-Falco, et al.; Springer-Verlag, 1991.

Clinical Dermatology, 2nd ed.: T.P. Habif, ed.; C.V. Mosby Company, 1990, pp. 419–421.

Mendelian Inheritance in Man, 9th ed.: V.A. McKusick; The Johns Hopkins University Press, 1990, pp. 303–305.

Dermatologic Clinics: The Genodermatoses: J. Alper, ed.; W.B. Saunders Company, 1987, vol. 5(1), pp. 27–30.

Dermatology in General Medicine: Textbook and Atlas, 3rd ed.: T.B. Fitzpatrick, et al., eds.; McGraw-Hill, 1987.

# EPIDERMOLYTIC HYPERKERATOSIS

**Description** Epidermolytic hyperkeratosis is a hereditary skin disorder characterized by hyperkeratosis and erythroderma.

**Synonyms**

Bullous Congenital Ichthyosiform Erythroderma

**Signs and Symptoms** Symptoms are present at birth and may range from mild to severe. The skin appears warty, blistery, and thickened over most of the body surface, and particularly in the skin creases over joints. There is degeneration of the granular layer, increased epidermal proliferation and reduced epidermal transit time. The disorder can be detected by amniocentesis.

**Etiology** Epidermolytic hyperkeratosis is transmitted by an autosomal dominant gene (the keratin K1 gene) thought to be located on chromosome 12.

**Epidemiology** Males and females are affected in equal numbers.

**Related Disorders** See *Ichthyosis Congenita; Ichthyosis Hystrix, Curth-Macklin Type; Darier Disease; Sjögren-Larsson Syndrome; Netherton Syndrome.*

**Treatment—Standard** Symptoms can be alleviated by the application of keratolytics and emollients, including plain petroleum jelly. This can be especially effective after bathing while the skin is still moist. Salicylic acid gel, applied under occlusion, is useful in some instances for removal of scales. Lactate lotion also can be an effective keratolytic. Topical and systemic retinoids can be beneficial in some cases but must be used with caution because of adverse side effects including those to fetal development in pregnant women. Long-term antibiotic treatment (e.g., benzathine penicillin or oral erythromycin) may be required to prevent formation of pustules from secondary bacterial infection.

**Treatment—Investigational** Please contact the agencies listed under Resources, below, for the most current information. Addresses and telephone numbers of these agencies, as well as of individual experts and research centers, may be found in the Master Resources List.

**Resources**

**For more information on epidermolytic hyperkeratosis:** National Organization for Rare Disorders (NORD); Foundation for Ichthyosis and Related Skin Types; NIH/National Arthritis and Musculoskeletal and Skin Diseases Information Clearinghouse; Ervin H. Epstein, Jr., M.D., University of California, San Francisco; Robert D. Goldman, M.D., Northwestern University Medical School; Leonard Milstone, M.D., Yale University Medical School.

**For genetic information and genetic counseling referrals:** March of Dimes Birth Defects Foundation; Alliance of Genetic Support Groups.

**References**

Dermatology, 3rd ed.: S.L. Moschella and H.J. Hurley, eds.; W.B. Saunders Company, 1992.

Textbook of Dermatology, 5th ed.: R.H. Champion, et al., eds.; Blackwell Scientific Publications, 1992.

Dermatology, 3rd ed.: O. Braun-Falco, et al.; Springer-Verlag, 1991.

Dermatology in General Medicine: Textbook and Atlas, 3rd ed.: T.B. Fitzpatrick, et al., eds.; McGraw-Hill, 1987.

Genetically Transmitted, Generalized Disorders of Cornification: The Ichthyoses: M.L. Williams, et al.; Dermatol. Clin., January 1987, vol. 5(1), pp. 155–178.

Therapeutic Activity of Lactate 12% Lotion in the Treatment of Ichthyosis: Active Versus Vehicle and Active Versus a Petroleum Cream: M. Buxman, et al.; J. Am. Acad. Dermatol., December 1986, vol. 15(6), pp. 1253–1258.

# ERYTHEMA MULTIFORME

**Description** Erythema multiforme is a hypersensitivity inflammatory skin disorder, caused by various agents, producing characteristic lesions that develop on the skin and mucous membranes.

**Synonyms**

Erythema Multiforme Major

Erythema Multiforme Minor

Stevens-Johnson Syndrome

**Signs and Symptoms** Usually the initial lesions are erythematous macules or papules, possibly with vesicular centers and progressing to bullae. Target or iris lesions are characteristic. Mild pruritus may be present. Distribution of the lesions is usually on the hands, forearms, and feet, and the mucous membranes of the mouth, nose, and genitals. The skin lesions are bilateral and symmetrical and tend to resolve in 2 to 6 weeks, but may recur.

Systemic symptoms include fever, arthralgia, malaise, cough, and sore throat.

See *Stevens-Johnson Syndrome,* which is a severe, bullous form of erythema multiforme.

**Etiology** Several infectious agents have been identified as the cause of erythema multiforme. These include viruses (e.g., herpes simplex, coxsackie, and echo) and other agents (e.g., *Mycoplasma pneumoniae, Histoplasma capsulatum,* and *Coccidioides immitis).*

The disorder can also be induced by drugs (e.g., sulfonamides, penicillins, phenytoin, and barbiturates), by occult malignancies, and by radiation therapy in persons being treated for malignancies.

**Epidemiology** Individuals of both sexes and any ages can be affected.

**Related Disorders** There are many disorders producing blisters that are to be distinguished from erythema multiforme. See ***Pemphigoid, Bullous; Dermatitis Herpetiformis; Pemphigus.***

**Treatment—Standard** The underlying cause should be identified and treated. Other therapy for mild erythema multiforme is symptomatic. Systemic corticosteroids may be required for severe cases, although care should be used if there is a danger of respiratory infections. Systemic antibiotics may be needed in some cases.

**Treatment—Investigational** Thalidomide is being tested as a treatment for erythema multiforme. *This drug should not be taken by pregnant women because it can cause severe birth defects.* For more information, contact Pediatric Pharmaceutical.

Please contact the agencies listed under Resources, below, for the most current information. Addresses and telephone numbers of these agencies, as well as of individual experts and research centers, may be found in the Master Resources List.

**Resources**

**For more information on erythema multiforme:** National Organization for Rare Disorders (NORD); NIH/National Arthritis and Musculoskeletal and Skin Diseases Information Clearinghouse.

**References**

Dermatology, 3rd ed.: S.L. Moschella and H.J. Hurley, eds.; W.B. Saunders Company, 1992.

Textbook of Dermatology, 5th ed.: R.H. Champion, et al., eds.; Blackwell Scientific Publications, 1992.

Dermatology, 3rd ed.: O. Braun-Falco, et al., eds.; Springer-Verlag, 1991.

Harrison's Principles of Internal Medicine, 12th ed.: J.D. Wilson, et al., eds.; McGraw-Hill, 1991, p. 331.

Dermatology in General Medicine: Textbook and Atlas, 3rd ed.: T.B. Fitzpatrick, et al., eds.; McGraw-Hill, 1987.

# ERYTHROKERATODERMIA SYMMETRICA PROGRESSIVA

**Description** Erythrokeratodermia symmetrica progressiva is a rare hereditary skin disorder characterized by sharply marginated, red, hyperkeratotic plaques with hyperpigmented margins.

**Signs and Symptoms** The hyperkeratotic plaques are distributed symmetrically and may appear on the head, arms, legs, and buttocks. The lesions may be pruritic. Usually, this disorder stabilizes after 1 to 2 years, and partially regresses during puberty. Palms and soles are spared.

**Etiology** This disorder is probably transmitted through an autosomal dominant gene.

**Epidemiology** Males and females are affected in equal numbers.

**Related Disorders** See ***Ichthyosis; Ichthyosis Congenita; Ichthyosis Hystrix, Curth-Macklin Type; Ichthyosis, Lamellar Recessive; Ichthyosis, X-Linked; Darier Disease; Epidermolytic Hyperkeratosis; Netherton Syndrome; Sjögren-Larsson Syndrome.***

**Treatment—Standard** Symptoms can be alleviated by the application of keratolytic and emollient ointments, including plain petroleum jelly. These can be especially effective after bathing while the skin is still moist. Salicylic acid gel applied under occlusive dressings is useful in some instances for removal of scales. Lactate lotion can also be an effective keratolytic agent. Topical and systemic retinoids can be beneficial in some cases but must be used with caution because of adverse side effects including those to fetal development in pregnant women.

**Treatment—Investigational** Monolaurin (glylorin) is being tested for treatment of erythrokeratodermia symmetrica progressiva. The product is manufactured by Cellegy Pharmaceuticals.

The National Institute of Arthritis and Musculoskeletal and Skin Diseases is seeking ichthyosis patients to participate in a study aimed at mapping the genes responsible for the various forms of the disease. For more information, contact Sherri Bale, M.D.

Please contact the agencies listed under Resources, below, for the most current information. Addresses and telephone numbers of these agencies, as well as of individual experts and research centers, may be found in the Master Resources List.

**Resources**

**For more information on erythrokeratodermia symmetrica progressiva:** National Organization for Rare Disorders (NORD); Foundation for Ichthyosis and Related Skin Types; NIH/National Arthritis and Musculoskeletal and Skin Diseases Information Clearinghouse.

**For genetic information and genetic counseling referrals:** March of Dimes Birth Defects Foundation; Alliance of Genetic Support Groups.

### References

Dermatology, 3rd ed.: S.L. Moschella and H.J. Hurley, eds.; W.B. Saunders Company, 1992.

Textbook of Dermatology, 5th ed.: R.H. Champion, et al., eds.; Blackwell Scientific Publications, 1992.

Dermatology, 3rd ed.: O. Braun-Falco, et al.; Springer-Verlag, 1991.

Dermatology in General Medicine: Textbook and Atlas, 3rd ed.: T.B. Fitzpatrick, et al., eds.; McGraw-Hill, 1987.

Genetically Transmitted, Generalized Disorders of Cornification: The Ichthyoses: M.L. Williams, et al.; Dermatol. Clin., January 1987, vol. 5(1), pp. 155–178.

Progressive Symmetric Erythrokeratodermia: Histological and Ultrastructural Study of Patient Before and After Treatment with Etretinate: V. Nazzaro, et al.; Arch. Dermatol., April 1986, vol. 122(4), pp. 434–440.

Therapeutic Activity of Lactate 12% Lotion in the Treatment of Ichthyosis: Active Versus Vehicle and Active Versus a Petroleum Cream: M. Buxman, et al.; J. Am. Acad. Dermatol., December 1986, vol. 15(6), pp. 1253–1258.

# ERYTHROKERATODERMIA VARIABILIS

**Description** Erythrokeratodermia variabilis is a rare form of ichthyosis characterized by sharply marginated erythematous scaling plaques with a shifting configuration, and by fixed hyperkeratotic plaques.

**Synonyms**

    Keratosis Rubra Figurata

    Mendes Da Costa Syndrome

**Signs and Symptoms** The eruption begins early in childhood and persists throughout life. The erythematous areas may develop after exposure to heat, cold, or wind, or as a result of emotional upset, and they may rapidly change shape or position. The keratotic plaques usually are limited to small areas but in some cases appear over the entire body surface, including the palms and soles. The disorder may improve in the summer.

**Etiology** The disorder appears to be transmitted by an autosomal dominant gene.

**Epidemiology** Erythrokeratodermia variabilis affects males and females in equal numbers.

**Related Disorders** See *Ichthyosis; Ichthyosis Congenita; Ichthyosis, Harlequin Type; Ichthyosis Hystrix, Curth-Macklin Type; Ichthyosis, Lamellar Recessive; Ichthyosis Vulgaris; Darier Disease; Epidermolytic Hyperkeratosis; Erythrokeratodermia Symmetrica Progressiva; Erythrokeratolysis Hiemalis; Multiple Sulfatase Deficiency; Netherton Syndrome; Refsum Syndrome; Sjögren-Larsson Syndrome.*

**Treatment—Standard** Symptoms can be alleviated by the application of emollient and keratolytic ointments, including plain petroleum jelly. This can be especially effective after bathing while the skin is still moist. Salicylic acid gel and lactate lotions are useful in some instances for removal of scales, especially when used under occlusion. The retinoids, topically or systemically, and topical steroids may be indicated but must be used with caution to avoid side effects.

**Treatment—Investigational** Monolaurin (glylorin) is being tested for treatment of erythrokeratodermia variabilis. The product is manufactured by Cellegy Pharmaceuticals.

The National Institute of Arthritis and Musculoskeletal and Skin Diseases is seeking ichthyosis patients to participate in a study aimed at mapping the genes responsible for the various forms of the disease. For more information, contact Sherri Bale, M.D.

Please contact the agencies listed under Resources, below, for the most current information. Addresses and telephone numbers of these agencies, as well as of individual experts and research centers, may be found in the Master Resources List.

**Resources**

    **For more information on erythrokeratodermia variabilis:** National Organization for Rare Disorders (NORD); Foundation for Ichthyosis and Related Skin Types; NIH/National Arthritis and Musculoskeletal and Skin Diseases Information Clearinghouse.

    **For genetic information and genetic counseling referrals:** March of Dimes Birth Defects Foundation; Alliance of Genetic Support Groups.

**References**

Dermatology, 3rd ed.: S.L. Moschella and H.J. Hurley, eds.; W.B. Saunders Company, 1992.

Textbook of Dermatology, 5th ed.: R.H. Champion, et al., eds.; Blackwell Scientific Publications, 1992.

Dermatology, 3rd ed.: O. Braun-Falco, et al.; Springer-Verlag, 1991.

Mendelian Inheritance in Man, 9th ed.: V.A. McKusick; The Johns Hopkins University Press, 1990, pp. 311–312.

Dermatology in General Medicine: Textbook and Atlas, 3rd ed.: T.B. Fitzpatrick, et al., eds.; McGraw-Hill, 1987.

Erythrokeratodermia Variabilis: Immunohistochemical and Ultrastructural Studies of the Epidermis: N. McFadden, et al.; Acta Derm. Venereol. (Stockh.), 1987, vol. 67(4), pp. 284–288.

Genetically Transmitted, Generalized Disorders of Cornification: The Ichthyoses: M.L. Williams, et al.; Dermatol. Clin., January 1987, vol. 5(1), pp. 155–178.

Erythrokeratodermia Variabilis Treated with Isotretinoin: A Clinical, Histologic, and Ultrastructural Study: I.P. Rappaport, et al.; Arch. Dermatol., April 1986, vol. 122(4), pp. 441–445.

Progressive Symmetric Erythrokeratodermia: Histological and Ultrastructural Study of Patient Before and After Treatment with Etretinate: V. Nazzaro, et al.; Arch. Dermatol., April 1986, vol. 122(4), pp. 434–440.

# ERYTHROKERATOLYSIS HIEMALIS

**Description** Erythrokeratolysis hiemalis is a heritable eruption of the palms and soles with recurrent episodes in cold weather of scaling erythematous plaques that peel from the center outwards.

**Synonyms**

Keratolytic Winter Erythema

Oudtshoorn Skin

**Signs and Symptoms** Lesions are symmetrical red scaling, peeling plaques. In most cases only the palms and soles are affected, but in severe cases the plaques may involve the skin of the back or elsewhere. Appearance of new plaques may be precipitated by fever or surgery. Onset of symptoms ranges from infancy to adolescence.

**Etiology** The disorder is inherited as an autosomal dominant trait.

**Epidemiology** The syndrome primarily affects descendants of farmers from the Oudtshoorn district in South Africa. Males and females are affected in equal numbers. The ratio of affected individuals is 1:100,000.

**Related Disorders** See *Ichthyosis; Ichthyosis Congenita; Ichthyosis, X-Linked; Ichthyosis Hystrix, Curth-Macklin Type; Epidermolytic Hyperkeratosis; Darier Disease; Netherton Syndrome; Sjögren-Larsson Syndrome.*

**Treatment—Standard** None is curative. Symptoms can be alleviated by the application of keratolytic and emollient ointments, including plain petroleum jelly. This can be especially effective after bathing while the skin is still moist. Salicylic acid gel and lactate lotion, applied under occlusion, are useful in some instances for removal of scales. Topical and systemic retinoids can be beneficial in some cases but must be used with caution because of adverse side effects including those to fetal development in pregnant women.

**Treatment—Investigational** Monolaurin (glylorin) is being tested for treatment of erythrokeratolysis hiemalis. The product is manufactured by Cellegy Pharmaceuticals.

The National Institute of Arthritis and Musculoskeletal and Skin Diseases is seeking ichthyosis patients to participate in a study aimed at mapping the genes responsible for the various forms of the disease. For more information, contact Sherri Bale, M.D.

Please contact the agencies listed under Resources, below, for the most current information. Addresses and telephone numbers of these agencies, as well as of individual experts and research centers, may be found in the Master Resources List.

**Resources**

**For more information on erythrokeratolysis hiemalis:** National Organization for Rare Disorders (NORD); Foundation for Ichthyosis and Related Skin Types; NIH/National Arthritis and Musculoskeletal and Skin Diseases Information Clearinghouse.

**For genetic information and genetic counseling referrals:** March of Dimes Birth Defects Foundation; Alliance of Genetic Support Groups.

**References**

Dermatology, 3rd ed.: S.L. Moschella and H.J. Hurley, eds.; W.B. Saunders Company, 1992.

Textbook of Dermatology, 5th ed.: R.H. Champion, et al., eds.; Blackwell Scientific Publications, 1992.

Dermatology, 3rd ed.: O. Braun-Falco, et al.; Springer-Verlag, 1991.

Dermatology in General Medicine: Textbook and Atlas, 3rd ed.: T.B. Fitzpatrick, et al., eds.; McGraw-Hill, 1987.

Genetically Transmitted, Generalized Disorders of Cornification: The Ichthyoses: M.L. Williams, et al.; Dermatol. Clin., January 1987, vol. 5(1), pp. 155–178.

Therapeutic Activity of Lactate 12% Lotion in the Treatment of Ichthyosis: Active Versus Vehicle and Active Versus a Petroleum Cream: M. Buxman, et al.; J. Am. Acad. Dermatol., December 1986, vol. 15(6), pp. 1253–1258.

# ERYTHROMELALGIA

**Description** Erythromelalgia is characterized by episodes of severe burning pain and increased temperature in the extremities. It occurs both as a primary disorder and secondarily to organic disease.

**Synonyms**

Gerhardt Disease

Mitchell Disease

Weir-Mitchell Disease

**Signs and Symptoms** The patient complains of burning pain and redness of the feet, which worsen during hot weather; less frequently, the hands may be involved. Severity of symptoms may increase over the years, with eventual disability for the patient.

**Etiology** Primary erythromelalgia may be inherited as an autosomal dominant trait.

The underlying disorder in secondary erythromelalgia may be proliferative bone marrow disease, polycythemia vera, diabetes mellitus, venous insufficiency, or hypertension. The condition has been attributed to intravascular platelet aggregation and to disturbances in prostaglandin metabolism, but the cause is unknown.

**Epidemiology** Males are affected more often than females.

**Related Disorders Causalgia syndrome (traumatic erythromelalgia)** is associated with persistent diffuse burning pain, particularly in the palms and the soles. Friction, heat, and other minor stimuli intensify the discomfort.

**Treatment—Standard** Cold packs or immersion in ice water, rest, and elevation of the extremity can relieve symptoms. In primary erythromelalgia, aspirin may be beneficial, as may ephedrine, propranolol, or methysergide. In the secondary form, the primary disorder is treated.

**Treatment—Investigational** IV sodium nitroprusside (sodium nitroferricyanide) has been used, but its potential side effects are severe.

Please contact the agencies listed under Resources, below, for the most current information. Addresses and telephone numbers of these agencies, as well as of individual experts and research centers, may be found in the Master Resources List.

**Resources**

**For more information on erythromelalgia:** National Organization for Rare Disorders (NORD); Erythromelalgia and Related Disorders Association of America.

**For genetic information and genetic counseling referrals:** March of Dimes Birth Defects Foundation; Alliance of Genetic Support Groups.

**References**

Dermatology, 3rd ed.: S.L. Moschella and H.J. Hurley, eds.; W.B. Saunders Company, 1992.

Textbook of Dermatology, 5th ed.: R.H. Champion, et al., eds.; Blackwell Scientific Publications, 1992.

Dermatology, 3rd ed.: O. Braun-Falco, et al.; Springer-Verlag, 1991.

Mendelian Inheritance in Man, 9th ed.: V.A. McKusick; The Johns Hopkins University Press, 1990, p. 309.

Dermatology in General Medicine: Textbook and Atlas, 3rd ed.: T.B. Fitzpatrick, et al., eds.; McGraw-Hill, 1987.

Sodium Nitroprusside Treatment in Erythromelalgia: S. Ozsoylu, et al.; Euro. J. Pediatr., 1984, vol. 141, pp. 185–187.

# FOCAL DERMAL HYPOPLASIA

**Description** Focal dermal hypoplasia is a rare form of ectodermal dysplasia found primarily in females. This disorder is characterized by skin abnormalities in which there are underdeveloped areas of skin that form streaks or lines and tumorlike herniations of fat in the skin. Skeletal, facial, dental, ocular, and soft tissue defects are also present.

**Synonyms**

> Combined Mesoectodermal Dysplasia
> Ectodermal and Mesodermal Dysplasia, Congenital
> Ectodermal and Mesodermal Dysplasia with Osseous Involvement
> Focal Dermato-Phalangeal Dysplasia
> Goltz-Gorlin Syndrome
> Goltz Syndrome

**Signs and Symptoms** Focal dermal hypoplasia is characterized by skin lesions that look streaked, underdeveloped, or "punched-out." Papillomas are typically found on the gums, tongue, lips, vulva, and anus. There may be inflammation, pruritus, reddening, blistering, and crusting of the skin. Skin may be absent, discolored, or lack pigmentation in some areas. Overgrowth of tissue may be found on the palms of the hands and soles of the feet. Hyper- or hypohydrosis is often present on the palms of the hands and soles of the feet. The hair may be sparse, brittle, or missing.

Eye abnormalities include ptosis, corneal clouding, a cleft along the edge of the eyeball (colobomas), nystagmus, absence of an eye (anophthalmia), wide spacing between the eyes, more than one color within the iris (heterochromia), dislocation of the lens, strabismus, and/or exposure of the lining of the eyelid (ectropion).

Patients with focal dermal hypoplasia may also have a variety of skeletal abnormalities. Curvature of the spine, fused vertebrae, ectrodactyly, polydactyly, syndactyly, clinodactyly, camptodactyly, and/or fusion of the bones of the fingers and toes may be present. Other skeletal malformations may include a small skull, an underdeveloped jaw, a forward projection of the jaw, and/or uneven development of the face, limbs, or trunk.

Failure of the teeth to develop properly often occurs in patients with focal dermal hypoplasia. The teeth may be missing, underdeveloped, unusually small, or improperly spaced. Missing enamel may result in the development of cavities.

Abnormalities of the gums, tongue, lips, ears, heart, and kidneys may also be present. Mental retardation is found in some patients with focal dermal hypoplasia.

**Etiology** Focal dermal hypoplasia is thought to be inherited as an X-linked dominant genetic trait.

**Epidemiology** Focal dermal hypoplasia is found primarily in females. It is thought that when expressed fully, it is lethal in males. Affected males frequently die before birth. As a result, the reported ratio of affected females to males is 150:11. In those males who survive, the condition is always more severe than in females. Focal dermal hypoplasia occurs in many areas of the world.

**Related Disorders** See *Oculocerebrocutaneous Syndrome.*

**Ectrodactyly–ectodermal dysplasia–clefting syndrome,** a form of ectodermal dysplasia, is a genetic disorder characterized by an absence of fingers and/or toes; an absence of tear ducts; cleft lip and/or palate; and sparse scalp hair, lashes, and eyebrows. This disorder may be inherited as an autosomal dominant genetic trait.

**Treatment—Standard** Treatment for patients with focal dermal hypoplasia is symptomatic. Dermatologic creams may relieve skin discomfort. Dentures and hearing aids may be required. Heat and overexercise should be avoided. Limb deformities may be treated with surgery. Genetic counseling may be of benefit for patients and their families.

**Treatment—Investigational** The National Institute of Dental Research in Bethesda, MD, is conducting a research project to evaluate dental treatment of individuals who have ectodermal dysplasias. Treatment will consist of either conventional removable dentures or fixed dentures supported by dental implants. The project is designed to evaluate the effect of dental implants on such things as satisfaction with treatment, the ability to chew foods, and maintenance of the bone that supports the dentures. To be eligible to participate in this study, individuals must have one of the ectodermal dysplasias, be missing several teeth, and be between the ages of 12 and 70 years. A complete oral and dental examination will be provided to determine if an individual qualifies for the 5-year study. Financial aid is expected to be available to help defray travel and lodging expenses for trips to Bethesda, Maryland. For additional information, contact Albert D. Guckes, M.D.

Please contact the agencies listed under Resources, below, for the most current information. Addresses and telephone numbers of these agencies, as well as of individual experts and research centers, may be found in the Master Resources List.

**Resources**

**For more information on focal dermal hypoplasia:** National Organization for Rare Disorders (NORD); National Foundation for Ectodermal Dysplasias; NIH/National Institute of Dental Research; The Arc (a national organization on mental retardation); NIH/National Arthritis and Musculoskeletal and Skin Diseases Information Clearinghouse.

**For genetic information and genetic counseling referrals:** March of Dimes Birth Defects Foundation; Alliance of Genetic Support Groups.

**References**

Birth Defects Encyclopedia: M.L. Buyse, ed.-in-chief; Blackwell Scientific Publications, 1990, pp. 516–517.

Mendelian Inheritance in Man, 9th ed.: V.A. McKusick, The Johns Hopkins University Press, 1990, pp. 1592–1593.

Cutaneous Defects of Focal Dermal Hypoplasia: An Ectomesodermal Dysplasia Syndrome: J.B. Howell, et al.; J. Cutan. Pathol., October 1989, vol. 16(5), pp. 237–258.

Smith's Recognizable Patterns of Human Malformation, 4th ed.: K.L. Jones; W.B. Saunders Company, 1988, p. 472.

Variable Expression in Focal Dermal Hypoplasia: An Example of Different X-Chromosome Inactivation: M.A. Wechsler, et al.; Am. J. Dis. Child., March 1988, vol. 142(3), pp. 297–300.

Focal Dermal Hypoplasia Syndrome: Case Report and Literature Review: E.H. Hall, et al.; J. Am. Acad. Dermatol., September 1983, vol. 9(3), pp. 443–451.

# FOX-FORDYCE DISEASE

**Description** Fox-Fordyce disease is a rare disorder that occurs most often in women. It is characterized by the development of intense pruritus, usually in the axillae, in the pubes, and around the nipple of the breast. It results from obstruction and rupture of the ducts of the apocrine sweat gland and is a form of sweat retention. Skin in the area may become darkened and dry; raised papules develop. Hair is often sparse in affected areas.

**Synonyms**

    Apocrine Duct Occlusion

    Sweat Retention Disease

**Signs and Symptoms** Fox-Fordyce disease is characterized by plaques of dry papules in the axillary, pubic, and nipple area of the body. Perspiration that is trapped in the apocrine gland or in the surrounding skin produces intense pruritus, inflammation, and swelling of the gland. There is also obstruction of the gland duct. The disease can cause loss or breakage of hair follicles in these areas. The disorder usually affects women after puberty and around the time of menstruation.

**Etiology** The abnormal functioning of the apocrine sweat glands characteristic of Fox-Fordyce disease may have a hormonal cause.

**Epidemiology** Fox-Fordyce disease is a rare disorder that affects females on a 10:1 ratio. It usually begins after puberty. In women, the disorder may be more severe at the time of menstruation and tends to disappear during pregnancy.

**Related Disorders** See *Hidradenitis Suppurativa.*

**Miliaria,** commonly called heat rash, occurs when the sweat gland is blocked and fluid is trapped in the surrounding area. Miliaria does not involve the hair follicle and does not result in hair loss and inflammatory conditions. Cooling the affected areas with water or compresses usually results in the disappearance of the rash.

**Treatment—Standard** Treatments have included contraceptive pills, estrogen, and intralesional corticosteroid. Other treatments may involve topical application of a form of vitamin A and clindamycin in an alcohol propylene glycol solution.

**Treatment—Investigational** The antiandrogen cyproterone acetate with or without estrogen therapy is being tested as a treatment for Fox-Fordyce disease.

Please contact the agencies listed under Resources, below, for the most current information. Addresses and telephone numbers of these agencies, as well as of individual experts and research centers, may be found in the Master Resources List.

**Resources**

**For more information on Fox-Fordyce disease:** National Organization for Rare Disorders (NORD); NIH/National Arthritis and Musculoskeletal and Skin Diseases Information Clearinghouse.

**References**

Fox-Fordyce Disease: Successful Treatment with Topical Clindamycin in Alcoholic Propylene Glycol Solution: R. Feldmann, et al.; Dermatology, 1992, vol. 184(4), pp. 310–313.

Clinical Dermatology, 2nd ed.: T.P. Habif, ed.: C.V. Mosby Company, 1990, pp. 139–140.

The Therapeutic Uses of Topical Vitamin A Acid: J.R. Thomas, et al.; J. Am. Acad. Dermatol., May 1981, vol. 4(5), pp. 505–513.

# GIANOTTI-CROSTI SYNDROME

**Description** Gianotti-Crosti syndrome is an inflammatory condition affecting children in which there are a lichenoid papular skin eruption, enlarged lymph nodes, and an intercurrent viral infection, sometimes with hepatitis B.

**Synonyms**

> Acrodermatitis, Infantile Lichenoid
> Acrodermatitis, Papular Infantile
> Crosti-Gianotti Syndrome

**Signs and Symptoms** Onset of Gianotti-Crosti syndrome, often preceded by a viral infection, is usually between ages 9 months and 9 years. Infections with Epstein-Barr and hepatitis B viruses and coxsackie- and cytomegalovirus, and vaccination with a live virus, may be precursors. Large flat papules appear, most commonly on the face, buttocks, arms, and legs. The papules may not be pruritic, and their usual duration is 20 to 25 days; recurrence is uncommon. Upon palpation, enlarged lymph nodes are often found in the truncal area. Patients may have a slight fever.

**Etiology** The cause is unknown. The trigger is considered to be a reaction to a prior viral infection, but the mechanism is not known. In many countries the precursor is most frequently infection with the hepatitis B virus. In North America other viruses are more commonly involved.

**Epidemiology** Boys and girls are affected in equal numbers.

**Related Disorders Coxsackievirus infections** are summer-associated illnesses. Young children, especially boys, are most prone to the disease. Characteristic are fever, sore throat, vomiting, headache, respiratory signs and symptoms, diarrhea, abdominal pain, rash, and earache.

**Infectious mononucleosis,** caused by the Epstein-Barr virus, has an incubation period of 30 to 50 days in young adults, and a briefer one in children. Symptoms include flulike malaise for a few days, headache, fever, and sore throat, with marked fatigue. Signs include generalized lymphadenopathy, eyelid and orbital edema, and perhaps rash. Tonsillitis, anorexia, photosensitivity, and hepato- and splenomegaly may be present. Other organs in the body may become involved.

**Treatment—Standard** Spontaneous resolution, usually within 20 to 25 days, is the rule. Meanwhile, treatment is symptomatic and supportive.

**Treatment—Investigational** Please contact the agencies listed under Resources, below, for the most current information. Addresses and telephone numbers of these agencies, as well as of individual experts and research centers, may be found in the Master Resources List.

**Resources**

**For more information on Gianotti-Crosti syndrome:** National Organization for Rare Disorders (NORD); NIH/National Arthritis and Musculoskeletal and Skin Diseases Information Clearinghouse; NIH/National Institute of Allergy and Infectious Disease; Centers for Disease Control.

**References**

Dermatology, 3rd ed.: S.L. Moschella and H.J. Hurley, eds.; W.B. Saunders Company, 1992.

Textbook of Dermatology, 5th ed.: R.H. Champion, et al., eds.; Blackwell Scientific Publications, 1992.

Dermatology, 3rd ed.: O. Braun-Falco, et al.; Springer-Verlag, 1991.

Dermatology in General Medicine: Textbook and Atlas, 3rd ed.: T.B. Fitzpatrick, et al., eds.; McGraw-Hill, 1987.

Gianotti-Crosti Syndrome: A Study of 26 Cases: A. Taieb, et al.; Br. J. Dermatol., July 1986, vol. 115(1), pp. 49–59.

Gianotti-Crosti Syndrome: A Review of Ten Cases Not Associated with Hepatitis-B: K.L. Spear, et al.; Arch. Dermatol., July 1984, vol. 120(7), pp. 891–896.

# GRANULOMA ANNULARE

**Description** Granuloma annulare is a benign dermatologic disease characterized by ringlike papules or nodules that may be confined to certain areas or disseminated over a large part of the body. It may be self-limited or chronic and recurrent.

**Synonyms**

Pseudorheumatoid Nodules

**Signs and Symptoms** The circular lesions are indurated and reddish brown, yellow, or flesh-colored, with centers of normal or slightly depressed skin. Usually the lesions appear on the dorsa of the hands and feet, and on the ankles, knees, or elbows. The disorder's chronicity may have a pattern of remissions and recurrence.

The diagnosis is established histopathologically where there are granulomas with necrobiotic destruction of collagen resembling rheumatoid nodules. A disseminated form may be associated with sun exposure.

**Etiology** Granuloma annulare is idiopathic, and the cause is unknown. The disseminated form may occur in diabetes mellitus.

**Epidemiology** Both children and adults may develop the disorder. Females are affected more often than males.

**Related Disorders** The condition must be distinguished from sarcoidosis and syphilis. Also to be differentiated is **eruptive xanthoma,** marked by groups of tiny yellow or yellow-brown elevated spots, perhaps ringed in red, in generalized distribution.

**Treatment—Standard** Spontaneous remission is common. PUVA, isotretinoin, and dapsone have been used in the chronic, generalized form of the disorder. *(Care should be taken in prescribing these drugs for pregnant and nursing women.)*

**Treatment—Investigational** Please contact the agencies listed under Resources, below, for the most current information. Addresses and telephone numbers of these agencies, as well as of individual experts and research centers, may be found in the Master Resources List.

**Resources**

**For more information on granuloma annulare:** National Organization for Rare Disorders (NORD); NIH/National Arthritis and Musculoskeletal and Skin Diseases Information Clearinghouse.

**References**

Dermatology, 3rd ed.: S.L. Moschella and H.J. Hurley, eds.; W.B. Saunders Company, 1992.

Textbook of Dermatology, 5th ed.: R.H. Champion, et al., eds.; Blackwell Scientific Publications, 1992.

Dermatology, 3rd ed.: O. Braun-Falco, et al.; Springer-Verlag, 1991.

Dermatology in General Medicine: Textbook and Atlas, 3rd ed.: T.B. Fitzpatrick, et al., eds.; McGraw-Hill, 1987.

Resolution of Disseminated Granuloma Annulare Following Isotretinoin Therapy: S.M. Schleicher, et al.; Cutis, August 1985, vol. 36(2), pp. 147–148.

Sulfone Treatment of Granuloma Annulare: A. Steiner, et al.; J. Am. Acad. Dermatol., December 1985, vol. 13(6), pp. 1004–1008.

Localized Granuloma Annulare Associated with Insulin-Dependent Diabetes Mellitus: M.F. Muhlemann, et al., Brit. J. Dermatol., September 1984, vol. 111(3), pp. 325–329.

# GROVER DISEASE

**Description** Grover disease is a rare, temporary skin disorder that consists of small, firm, raised red lesions on the skin. Microscopic examination reveals the presence of acantholysis. Small blisters containing a watery liquid are also present.

**Synonyms**

Transient Acantholytic Dermatosis

**Signs and Symptoms** Signs of Grover disease are small, solid, raised bumps on the skin; acantholysis; and pruritus. Patients with this disorder often have, within the affected area, blisters containing a thin, watery liquid with a central hair follicle. The skin eruptions are found in groups and have a swollen red border around them. Hyperkeratosis occurs above the blisters. The eruptions in Grover disease are usually found on the back, chest, and sometimes on the sides of the extremities and can last from a few weeks to many months.

**Etiology** The exact cause of Grover disease is not known. It may be related to the fragility of aged, sun-damaged skin. It may also be related to heat and sweating. There have been multiple cases of this disorder associated with hot tubs, hot-water bottles, electric blankets, steam baths, and prolonged confinement to a bed. At least one case of this disorder has been associated with follicle mites.

**Epidemiology** Grover disease is a rare skin disorder seen mainly in males over the age of 40, although it has also been found in females.

**Related Disorders** See *Darier Disease; Dermatitis Herpetiformis; Pemphigus.*

**Treatment—Standard** Decreased bathing and topical lubrication is usually beneficial. Topical steroids and antihistamines may provide temporary relief of itching. Antibiotics are often helpful. Topical treatment with selenium sulfide has been effective in clearing up the lesions on some patients. Isotretinoin has also been effective in the treatment of lesions in some patients with Grover disease. In some cases, prolonged therapy may be necessary to treat multiple recurrences.

**Treatment—Investigational** Please contact the agencies listed under Resources, below, for the most current information. Addresses and telephone numbers of these agencies, as well as of individual experts and research centers, may be found in the Master Resources List.

**Resources**

**For more information on Grover disease:** National Organization for Rare Disorders (NORD); NIH/National Arthritis and Musculoskeletal and Skin Diseases Information Clearinghouse.

**References**

Myelodysplastic Syndrome and Transient Acantholytic Dermatosis: P.F. Rockley, et al.; Cleve. Clin. J. Med., September 1990, vol. 57(6), pp. 575–577.

Demodicidosis Mimicking Granulomatous Rosacea and Transient Acantholytic Dermatosis (Grover's Disease): A. Lindmaier, et al.; Dermatologica, 1987, vol. 175(4), pp. 200–204.

Rapid Response of Transient Acantholytic Dermatosis to Selenium Sulfide Treatment for Pityriasis Versicolor: R. Segal, et al.; Dermatologica, 1987, vol. 175(4), pp. 205–207.

Erythematous Plaque Variant of Transient Acantholytic Dermatosis: Y. Horiuchi, et al.; Cutis, July 1986, vol. 38(1), pp. 48–49.

Grover's Disease Treated with Isotretinoin: Report of Four Cases: R.J. Helfman; J. Am. Acad. Dermatol., June 1985, vol. 12(6), pp. 981–984.

Transient Acantholytic Dermatosis (Grover's Disease): A Skin Disorder Related to Heat and Sweating: E.M. Farber, et al.; Arch. Dermatol., November 1985, vol. 121(11), pp. 1439–1441.

# HAIRY TONGUE

**Description** Hairy tongue is a disorder characterized by discoloration of the tongue and excessive growth of the filiform papillae.

**Synonyms**

Black Hairy Tongue

Lingua Nigra

**Signs and Symptoms** The tongue appears yellow, brown, black, or blue, and the papillae form a V shape at its rear. These signs may disappear spontaneously and, in some cases, recur. There is often a bad taste in the mouth.

**Etiology** The disorder may result from changes in the oral flora caused by antibiotics or be due to poor hygiene, with resultant elongation of the filiform papillae. Some cases seem to be the result of reduced saliva or of fever. Tobacco can stain the papillae.

**Epidemiology** Onset and duration of hairy tongue are variable. The disorder can affect both males and females, and is seen in children and adults.

**Related Disorders** Differential diagnosis includes the following disorders.

**Glossitis (inflammation of the tongue)** may occur in association with candidiasis, anemia, diabetes mellitus, latent nutritional deficiencies, and malignancies.

**Geographic tongue** is characterized by migratory lesions of smooth, sore, and sometimes itchy patches on the tongue. Episodes typically may remit and then recur. The cause is unknown; the disorder may be familial.

In **Moeller glossitis** the tongue is slick, glossy, or glazed. The lesions are often a concomitant sign of pernicious anemia. They can cause great discomfort and are persistent.

**Severe acute glossitis** can occasionally be the result of local infection, burns, or injury to the tongue, with ensuing pain and tenderness, and swelling that in severe cases blocks air passages.

In **burning tongue (burning mouth) syndrome** patients experience a burning sensation. There is no obvious clinical evidence of inflammation. The disorder may be one of the first signs of vitamin B12 deficiency. A *Candida albicans* infection or denture irritation may also be responsible. Other suggested etiologies include allergic reactions to pollen, cereals, and metals, and materials used in the manufacture of dentures. The disorder may be a hysterical symptom and an early sign of depression in middle-aged or older women.

**Treatment—Standard** Treatment includes avoidance of irritants and substances that can sensitize the tongue, and encouraging desquamation by brushing with a soft-bristled brush. Discontinuation of antibiotics or mouthwashes usually results in disappearance of symptoms as normal oral flora regenerate. In some cases the symptoms disappear spontaneously.

**Treatment—Investigational** Please contact the organizations listed under Resources, below, for the most current information. Addresses and telephone numbers of these agencies, as well as of individual experts and research centers, may be found in the Master Resources List.

**Resources**

**For more information on hairy tongue:** National Organization for Rare Disorders (NORD); NIH/National Institute of Dental Research; Smell and Taste Research Center, University of Pennsylvania Hospital; Chemosensory Clinical Research Center of Connecticut, University of Connecticut Health Center.

**References**

Dermatology, 3rd ed.: S.L. Moschella and H.J. Hurley, eds.; W.B. Saunders Company, 1992.

Textbook of Dermatology, 5th ed.: R.H. Champion, et al., eds.; Blackwell Scientific Publications, 1992.

Dermatology, 3rd ed.: O. Braun-Falco, et al.; Springer-Verlag, 1991.

Dermatology in General Medicine: Textbook and Atlas, 3rd ed.: T.B. Fitzpatrick, et al., eds.; McGraw-Hill, 1987.

# HAY-WELLS SYNDROME

**Description** Hay-Wells syndrome is one of a group of rare genetic skin disorders known as the ectodermal dysplasias. Major characteristics of this disorder include cleft lip and/or palate; fusion of one or both eyelids; absent or defective nails; coarse, sparse, or wiry hair; diminished ability to sweat; and missing, widely spaced, or cone-shaped teeth.

**Synonyms**

AEC Syndrome

Ankyloblepharon–Ectodermal Defects–Cleft Lip/Palate

**Signs and Symptoms** The main features of Hay-Wells syndrome are:

1. **Congenital ectodermal dysplasia:** a skin condition in which the patient is born with abnormal growth or development of the skin, its derivatives, and some organs. The affected tissue derives primarily from the ectodermal germ layer. Hair and teeth are also abnormal.

2. **Cleft lip and/or palate.**

3. **Ankyloblepharon filiforme adnatum:** bands of tissue causing the eyelids to adhere or fuse together. This may occur in one or both eyes.

4. **Mild hypohidrosis:** a condition in which the patient has a diminished capacity to sweat due to abnormal or partial sweat glands.

5. **Dystrophic nails:** a condition in which the nails of the fingers and toes do not develop normally.

6. **Abnormal hair:** patients with Hay-Wells syndrome have coarse, sparse, wiry hair and may experience partial or total alopecia.

7. **Hypodontia:** a condition in which the patient is born with less than the normal number of teeth. Patients with Hay-Wells syndrome may also have widely spaced, cone-shaped teeth with insufficient enamel.

8. **Velopharyngeal incompetence:** a birth defect in the opening structure of the throat. The part of the mouth under the nasal passages is not completely closed. This condition may cause food to spit up through the nose and a speech impairment. In some cases, velopharyngeal incompetence may occur instead of cleft lip and/or palate.

Some, but not all, of the following additional symptoms may be present in patients with Hay-Wells syndrome:

9. **Maxillary hypoplasia:** a condition in which the upper jaw is smaller than normal.
10. **Infections or erosions of the scalp.**
11. **Oval-shaped face and broad nasal bridge.**
12. **Palmoplantar keratoderma:** a horny skin condition appearing on the palms of the hands and soles of the feet. This condition often occurs during adulthood.
13. **Hyperpigmentation.**
14. **Dry skin.**
15. **Photophobia.**
16. **Blepharitis.**
17. **Lacrimal puncta:** one or more of the upper or lower duct openings of the eye are absent or under-developed.
18. **Cupped Ears.**
19. **Stenosis of the ear canal.**
20. **Hearing loss**

**Etiology** Hay-Wells syndrome may be inherited as an autosomal dominant trait.

**Epidemiology** Hay-Wells syndrome is a very rare disorder that affects males and females in equal numbers. Of the 12 reported cases of this syndrome, all were from the United States, Canada, and Great Britain.

**Related Disorders** See *Hallerman-Streiff Syndrome.*

**Christ-Siemens-Touraine syndrome** is a form of ectodermal dysplasia that is characterized by hypodontia; reduced ability to sweat, resulting in heat intolerance; and alopecia. The face may have a bulging forehead and chin; sunken cheeks; broad, flat nose; thick lips; and fine, wrinkled skin around the eyes.

**Johanson-Blizzard syndrome** is a form of ectodermal dysplasia that is characterized by nose, scalp, and hair defects, as well as hypodontia, deafness, short stature, lack of motor development, and malabsorption problems. The most striking feature of this syndrome is the beaklike appearance of the nose. Three-fourths of patients have a protrusion over the posterior fontanelle of the skull at birth, which gets thick and hard as the child grows. Patients have peg-shaped teeth and thin hair, which sweeps up from the forehead. There is marked hearing loss from birth, as well as motor and mental retardation. Bone growth is delayed, and there may be associated intestinal, absorption, and genital defects.

**Jorgenson syndrome** is another form of ectodermal dysplasia characterized by the inability to sweat properly, a lack of hair and tooth growth, and unusual skin problems. These patients do sweat, but the amount is very slight. There is a lack of growth of eyebrows and eyelashes, and the patient is usually bald by the teen years. The skin is dry with fine fingerprints (dermal ridges) on the hands and feet. There are abnormal amounts of cavities in the baby teeth, and a lack of development of some of the permanent teeth. The patient usually has a long, thin nose; a thin upper lip; and a long space between the nose and mouth.

**Rapp-Hodgkins syndrome** is another form of ectodermal dysplasia. The main characteristics of this disorder are absence of the ability to sweat in combination with cleft lip and palate, dental abnormalities, and alopecia. Corneal opacities and other eye defects, with a tendency to develop eye infections, are often present. The ears may be large, malformed, and prone to infections. Hearing and speech problems may also be associated with this disorder.

**Zanier-Roubicek syndrome** is a form of ectodermal dysplasia that is often associated with severe overheating due to the inability to sweat. There is usually normal sweating, however, on the palms of the hands and soles of the feet. The patient usually shows a lack of hair on the head but normal eyebrows and eyelashes. Patients have hypodontia, with yellow discoloration of the teeth. The nails are brittle. Lacrimation may be lacking, and there may be underdevelopment of the breasts. This syndrome is transmitted as an autosomal recessive trait.

**Treatment—Standard** There is no known cure for any of the ectodermal dysplasias. Treatment is directed at the symptoms. Certain skin creams may relieve skin discomfort. Dentures and hearing aids may be required. Heat and overexertion are avoided. Vaccines and anti-infectious agents are used to reduce infections of the skin and respiratory tract. Treatment of a person with cleft lip and/or palate requires the coordination efforts of a team of specialists. Pediatricians, dental specialists, surgeons, speech pathologists, and psychologists must work together in planning the child's treatment and rehabilitation. Genetic counseling may be of benefit for patients and their families. Other treatment is symptomatic and supportive.

**Treatment—Investigational** The palate of cleft palate patients is closed during early childhood, but difficulties may persist if the palate is excessively short in relation to the pharynx. Researchers are studying a Teflon-glycerine paste that is applied to the rear of the pharynx in a minor surgical procedure. A rounder bump or ledge is formed, bringing the pharynx and palate into the proper relationship with each other. The hardened paste remains in place indefinitely; no side effects have been observed. Children as young as 8 years old have been treated with this procedure. For further information on this procedure, contact William N. Williams, D.D.S., of the University of Florida College of Dentistry.

The National Institute of Dental Research in Bethesda, MD, is conducting a research project to evaluate dental treatment of individuals who have ectodermal dysplasias. Treatment will consist of either conventional removable dentures or fixed dentures supported by dental implants. The project is designed to evaluate the effect of dental implants on such things as satisfaction with treatment, the ability to chew foods, and maintenance of the bone that supports the dentures. To be eligible to participate in this study, individuals must have one of the ectodermal dysplasias, be missing several teeth, and be between the ages of 12 and 70 years. A complete oral and dental examination will be provided to determine if an individual qualifies for the 5-year study. Financial aid is expected to be available to help defray travel and lodging expenses for trips to Bethesda, MD. For additional information, contact Albert D. Guckes, M.D.

Please contact the agencies listed under Resources, below, for the most current information. Addresses and telephone numbers of these agencies, as well as of individual experts and research centers, may be found in the Master Resources List.

## Resources

**For more information on Hay-Wells syndrome:** National Organization for Rare Disorders (NORD); National Foundation for Ectodermal Dysplasias; NIH/National Arthritis and Musculoskeletal and Skin Diseases Information Clearinghouse; American Cleft Palate Cranial Facial Association.

**For genetic information and genetic counseling referrals:** March of Dimes Birth Defects Foundation; Alliance of Genetic Support Groups.

## References

Birth Defects Encyclopedia: M.L. Buyse, ed.-in-chief; Blackwell Scientific Publications, 1990, pp. 599–600.

Mendelian Inheritance in Man, 9th ed.: V.A. McKusick; The Johns Hopkins University Press, 1990, p. 71.

Smith's Recognizable Patterns of Human Malformation, 4th ed.: K.L. Jones, ed.; W.B. Saunders Company, 1988, p. 254.

Variable Expression in Ankyloblepharon-Ectodermal Defects: Cleft Lip and Palate Syndrome: S.L. Green, et al.; Am. J. Med., May 1987, vol. 27(1), pp. 207–212.

AEC Syndrome: Ankyloblepharon, Ectodermal Defects, and Cleft Lip and Palate: Report of Two Cases: J. Spiegel, et al.; J. Am. Acad. Dermatol., May 1985, vol. 12(5 pt. 1), pp. 810–815.

Ectodermal Dysplasias: A Clinical and Genetic Study: N. Freire-Maia, et al.; Alan R. Liss, 1984, p. 47.

# HIDRADENITIS SUPPURATIVA

**Description** Hidradenitis suppurativa is a chronic inflammatory process with scarring associated with bacterial infection of the apocrine gland follicles. Subcutaneous nodules in the involved area are similar to furuncles.

## Synonyms

Apocrinitis

Hidrosadenitis Axillaris

**Signs and Symptoms** Patients commonly complain of pain in the involved sites, which are usually axillary or inguinal but are sometimes anogenital. Examination shows subcutaneous inflamed nodules that resemble boils. Tenderness and a purulent exudate are present. Patients may be febrile and lose weight. Eventually, scarring of tissue in inflamed sites may produce a tender, bound-down mass. The lesions may recur.

**Etiology** Hidradenitis is idiopathic, and the cause for destruction of the apocrine glands is unknown. Hidradenitis suppurativa has been associated with endocrine disorders and the use of depilatories or deodorants.

**Epidemiology** Onset is commonly during puberty. Men and women are affected in equal numbers. Familial cases have been described.

**Related Disorders** Differential diagnosis includes the following disorders.

**Furunculosis,** the common boil, usually stems from a staphylococcal infection of hair follicles or the sebaceous glands. The erythematous, painful nodules may burst and emit pus, and they may recur. Among the settings in which they occur are inadequate hygiene, obesity, diabetes mellitus, blood disorders, poor health, and malnutrition.

**Aural furunculosis** can develop from a scratch in the ear or discharge of pus from the middle ear. Frequently the patient has boils elsewhere, has diabetes mellitus, or is in poor health. Symptoms include mild hearing impairment, a feeling of pressure on the ear from a swollen mass, and fever. The mass eventually ruptures and drains. When treated, lasting injury to the ear is unlikely.

**American cutaneous leishmaniasis** is due to the bite of a sandfly (*Phlebotomus*), which is indigenous to Central and South America. The lesions itch intensely, and are accompanied by joint pain, weight loss, and poor health.

**Pyoderma gangrenosum, cutaneous inflammatory bowel disease (Crohn disease),** and **actinomycosis** may also resemble hidradenitis suppurativa.

**Treatment—Standard** The patient should avoid antiperspirants or other skin irritants such as depilatories. Rest and local moist heat are helpful. Oral antibiotic therapy is required. Excision and/or plastic surgery may be necessary in the most persistent cases.

Recurrence at the same location after surgical removal is likely. Recurrences are fewer when excision is followed by split skin grafting or local skin flap cover.

**Treatment—Investigational** An antiandrogen (cyproterone acetate) in combination with estrogen therapy is being tried in women with long-standing severe cases of hidradenitis suppurativa. At times, cyproterone acetate alone has achieved control.

Please contact the agencies listed under Resources, below, for the most current information. Addresses and telephone numbers of these agencies, as well as of individual experts and research centers, may be found in the Master Resources List.

**Resources**

**For more information on hidradenitis suppurativa:** National Organization for Rare Disorders (NORD); NIH/National Institute of Allergy and Infectious Diseases; NIH/National Arthritis and Musculoskeletal and Skin Diseases Information Clearinghouse.

**References**

Dermatology, 3rd ed.: S.L. Moschella and H.J. Hurley, eds.; W.B. Saunders Company, 1992.

Textbook of Dermatology, 5th ed.: R.H. Champion, et al., eds.; Blackwell Scientific Publications, 1992.

Dermatology, 3rd ed.: O. Braun-Falco, et al.; Springer-Verlag, 1991.

Dermatology in General Medicine: Textbook and Atlas, 3rd ed.: T.B. Fitzpatrick, et al., eds.; McGraw-Hill, 1987.

Control of Hidradenitis Suppurativa in Women Using Combined Antiandrogen (Cyproterone Acetate) and Oestrogen Therapy: R.S. Sawers, et al.: Br. J. Dermatol., September 1986, vol. 115(3), pp. 269–274.

Hidradenitis Suppurativa: A Clinical Review: J.D. Watson; Br. J. Plast. Surg., October 1985, vol. 38(4), pp. 567–569.

# HYPERHIDROSIS

**Description** This condition is characterized by constitutional hyperactivity of the eccrine sweat glands. The disorder may be generalized and consist of excessive body sweating, or localized, with sweating confined to the palms, soles, armpits, groin, and under the breasts.

**Synonyms**

      Excessive Perspiration

      Excessive Sweating

      Genuine Hyperhidrosis

**Signs and Symptoms** As a rule, onset is in childhood or during puberty. Patients experience a heightened reaction to sweating stimuli such as anxiety, pain, exercise, tension, caffeine, and nicotine. The sweat-prone areas may be localized or generalized. When the palms and soles are involved, the skin may appear pink or blue-white, and may even macerate, crack, or scale, particularly on the feet. Patients often experience spontaneous relief in adult life.

**Etiology** The cause is unknown. In very rare cases, hyperhidrosis of the palms and soles is thought to be inherited as an autosomal dominant genetic trait. One must distinguish idiopathic hyperhidrosis from excess sweating due to malfunction of the thyroid or pituitary gland, infection, diabetes mellitus, tumors, gout, and menopause.

**Epidemiology** The disorder affects males and females in equal numbers.

**Related Disorders** See *Frey Syndrome.*

**Greither disease** is a rare inherited skin disorder characterized by keratosis of the skin on the palms and soles. The major symptom of this disorder is excessive sweating of the palms and soles. Areas of keratosis may extend to the top of the feet and hands.

**Treatment—Standard** Before treating generalized hyperhidrosis, a primary disorder must be ruled out.

For patients with palmar-plantar-type hyperhidrosis, cotton socks and shoes that promote the circulation of air prevent overheating of the feet. Alternating footwear is helpful. Applications of medicated powder formulated to hamper bacterial growth and absorb moisture may be beneficial.

For refractory cases, topical agents, such as aluminum chloride in ethyl alcohol, may be indicated. Short-term courses of anticholinergic drugs are also useful in severely afflicted patients, but the side effects of dry mouth, drowsiness, and constipation frequently occur.

Sympathectomy will not completely overcome the excessive sweating, and recurrence is not unlikely. Furthermore, the sequela may be Horner syndrome, in which nerve paralysis results in ptosis. Endoscopic sympathectomy seems to eliminate the risk of Horner syndrome.

Biofeedback has met with varying degrees of success.

**Treatment—Investigational** Iontophoresis, in which ions are electrically driven into the skin, is being used to treat the condition.

Please contact the agencies listed under Resources, below, for the most current information. Addresses and telephone numbers of these agencies, as well as of individual experts and research centers, may be found in the Master Resources List.

## Resources

**For more information on hyperhidrosis:** National Organization for Rare Disorders (NORD); NIH/National Institute of Diabetes, Digestive and Kidney Diseases.

## References

Hyperhidrosis: A Case History: J.A. Rosenblum, et al.; Angiology, January 1994, vol. 45(1), pp. 61–64.

Transthoracic Endoscopic Sympathectomy in the Treatment of Palmar Hyperhidrosis: H.J. Chen, et al.; Arch. Surg., June 1994, vol. 129(6), pp. 630–633.

Keratosis Extremitatum (Greither's Disease): Clinical Features, Histology, Ultrastructure: R. Fluckiger, et al.; Dermatology, 1993, vol. 187(4), pp. 309–311.

Principles of Neurology, 5th ed.: R.D. Adams and M. Victor, eds.; McGraw-Hill, 1993, p. 472.

Thoracoscopy for Autonomic Disorders: G. Claes, et al.; Ann. Thorac. Surg., September 1993, vol. 56(3), pp. 715–716.

Cecil Textbook of Medicine, 19th ed.: J.B. Wyngaarden, et al.., eds.; W.B. Saunders Company, 1992, p. 2094.

Dermatology, 3rd ed.: S.L. Moschella and H.J. Hurley, eds.; W.B. Saunders Company, 1992.

Endoscopic Transthoracic Sympathectomy in the Treatment of Hyperhidrosis: R.A. Edmondson, et al.; Ann. Surg., March 1992, vol. 215(3), pp. 289–293.

Mendelian Inheritance in Man, 10th ed.: V.A. McKusick; The Johns Hopkins University Press, 1992, p. 568.

Telford's Operation for Primary Palmar Hyperhidrosis: D. Gyftokostas, et al.; Angiology, April 1992, vol. 43(4), pp. 336–341.

Textbook of Dermatology, 5th ed.: R.H. Champion, et al., eds.; Blackwell Scientific Publications, 1992, pp. 1752–1755.

Dermatology, 3rd ed.: O. Braun-Falco, et al.; Springer-Verlag, 1991.

Surgical Management of Primary Hyperhidrosis: K.T. Moran, et al.; Br. J. Surg., March 1991, vol. 78(3), pp. 279–283.

Clinical Dermatology, 2nd ed.: T.P. Habif, ed.; C.V. Mosby Company, 1990, p. 704.

Dictionary of Medical Syndromes, 3rd ed.: S.I. Magalini, et al., eds.; J.B. Lippincott Company, 1990, pp. 435–436.

Dermatology in General Medicine: Textbook and Atlas, 3rd ed.: T.B. Fitzpatrick, et al., eds.; McGraw-Hill, 1987.

Sweating It Out: The Problem of Profuse Perspiration: D. Farley, FDA Consumer, December 1985–January 1986, pp. 21–25.

# HYPOMELANOSIS OF ITO

**Description** Hypomelanosis of Ito is characterized by hypopigmentation of many areas of the body.

**Synonyms**

Incontinenti Pigmenti Achromians

**Signs and Symptoms** The most distinctive characteristic of hypomelanosis of Ito is the patterned hypopigmentation that may appear on any area of the body except the palms, soles, and scalp. The patterning of the eruption gives it a marbled appearance. Initially, during childhood, the hypopigmentation may progress. These areas may darken in color later in life. A decreased amount of melanin causes the discoloration.

Over half of those affected by hypomelanosis of Ito have abnormalities in addition to hypopigmentation. Seizures and mental retardation are found most frequently. Dental abnormalities, strabismus, myopia, a cleft along the edge of the eyeball (coloboma), megalocephaly, microcephaly, and/or an inability to sweat in the areas of hypopigmentation have also been found in some affected individuals.

**Etiology** Hypomelanosis of Ito may be idiopathic or rarely may be inherited as an autosomal dominant genetic trait. It is thought that the sporadic cases of this disorder may be the result of chromosomal mosaicism.

**Epidemiology** There have been approximately 100 cases of hypomelanosis of Ito reported in the medical literature. This disorder affects females more often than males. Most cases of hypomelanosis are detected during childhood.

**Related Disorders** See *Albinism; Vitiligo.*

**Treatment—Standard** The areas of hypopigmentation tend to darken with time without treatment. Anticonvulsant agents such as phenytoin, valproic acid, phenobarbital, clonazepam, ethusuximide, primidone, corticotropin, and corticosteroid drugs help to prevent and control seizures when present. When strabismus is present, surgery, corrective lenses, or the orphan drug oculinum may be beneficial. Genetic counseling may be of benefit for patients and their families. Other treatment is symptomatic and supportive.

**Treatment—Investigational** Experimental anticonvulsant agents such as nimodipine, praziquantel, clomiphene, and lorazepam are being investigated.

Please contact the agencies listed under Resources, below, for the most current information. Addresses and telephone numbers of these agencies, as well as of individual experts and research centers, may be found in the Master Resources List.

## Resources

**For more information on hypomelanosis of Ito:** National Organization for Rare Disorders (NORD); The Arc (a national organization on mental retardation); Epilepsy Foundation of America; NIH/National Arthritis and Musculoskeletal and Skin Diseases Information Clearinghouse.

**For genetic information and genetic counseling referrals:** March of Dimes Birth Defects Foundation; NIH/National Institute of Child Health and Human Development.

## References

Hypomelanosis of Ito Associated with Chromosomal Translocation Involving Xp11: M.S. Lungarotti, et al.; Am. J. Med. Genet., September 15, 1991, vol. 40(4), pp. 447–448.

Birth Defects Encyclopedia: M.L. Buyse, ed.-in-chief; Blackwell Scientific Publications, 1990, pp. 925–926.

Chromosome Mosaicism in Hypomelanosis of Ito: C.L. Ritter, et al.; Am. J. Med. Genet., January 1990, vol. 35(1), pp. 14–17.

Hypomelanosis of Ito: A Nonspecific Marker of Somatic Mosaicism: D. Chitayat, et al.; Am. J. Med. Genet., March 1990, vol. 35(3), pp. 422–424.

Mendelian Inheritance in Man, 9th ed.: V.A. McKusick, The Johns Hopkins University Press, 1990, p. 503.

Hypomelanosis of Ito: Spectrum of the Disease: M.T. Glover, et al.; J. Pediatr., July 1989, vol. 115(1), pp. 75–80.

# ICHTHYOSIS

**Description** The ichthyoses are a group of cutaneous disorders of keratinization.

**Signs and Symptoms** Ichthyosis is characterized by dry, scaly, itchy, erythematous skin, often over large areas of the body. Symptoms range from mild to severe, and remissions can occur.

**Etiology** Most known forms of ichthyosis are inherited, some as dominant traits, some as recessive.

**Epidemiology** Most ichthyoses are present at birth and affect males and females in equal numbers. X-linked ichthyosis affects only males.

**Related Disorders** See *Ichthyosis Congenita; Ichthyosis, Harlequin Type; Ichthyosis Hystrix, Curth-Macklin Type; Ichthyosis, Lamellar Recessive; Ichthyosis Vulgaris; Ichthyosis, X-Linked.*

See also *Conradi-Hünermann Syndrome; Darier Disease; Epidermolytic Hyperkeratosis; Erythrokeratodermia Symmetrica Progressiva; Erythrokeratodermia Variabilis; Erythrokeratolysis Hiemalis; Keratosis Follicularis Spinulosa Decalvans; Sjögren-Larsson Syndrome; Tay Syndrome; Netherton Syndrome.*

**Treatment—Standard** Symptoms can be alleviated by application of keratolytics and emollients, including plain petroleum jelly. This can be especially effective after bathing while the skin is still moist. Salicylic acid gel, applied under occlusion, is useful in some instances for removal of scales. Lactate lotion can also be an effective keratolytic. Topical and systemic retinoids can be beneficial in some cases but must be used with caution because of adverse side effects, including those to fetal development in pregnant women.

**Treatment—Investigational** Monolaurin (glylorin) is being tested for treatment of ichthyosis. The product is manufactured by Cellegy Pharmaceuticals.

The National Institute of Arthritis and Musculoskeletal and Skin Diseases is seeking ichthyosis patients to participate in a study aimed at mapping the genes responsible for the various forms of the disease. For more information, contact Sherri Bale, M.D.

Please contact the agencies listed under Resources, below, for the most current information. Addresses and telephone numbers of these agencies, as well as of individual experts and research centers, may be found in the Master Resources List.

**Resources**

**For more information on ichthyosis:** National Organization for Rare Disorders (NORD); Foundation for Ichthyosis and Related Skin Types; NIH/National Arthritis and Musculoskeletal and Skin Diseases Information Clearinghouse.

**For genetic information and genetic counseling referrals:** March of Dimes Birth Defects Foundation; Alliance of Genetic Support Groups.

## References

Dermatology, 3rd ed.: S.L. Moschella and H.J. Hurley, eds.; W.B. Saunders Company, 1992.

Textbook of Dermatology, 5th ed.: R.H. Champion, et al., eds.; Blackwell Scientific Publications, 1992.

Dermatology, 3rd ed.: O. Braun-Falco, et al.; Springer-Verlag, 1991.

Dermatology in General Medicine: Textbook and Atlas, 3rd ed.: T.B. Fitzpatrick, et al., eds.; McGraw-Hill, 1987.

Genetically Transmitted, Generalized Disorders of Cornification: The Ichthyoses: M.L. Williams, et al., Dermatol. Clin., January 1987, vol. 5(1), pp. 155–178.

Therapeutic Activity of Lactate 12% Lotion in the Treatment of Ichthyosis: Active Versus Vehicle and Active Versus a Petroleum Cream: M. Buxman, et al., J. Am. Acad. Dermatol., December 1986, vol. 15(6), pp. 1253–1258.

# ICHTHYOSIS CONGENITA

**Description** Ichthyosis congenita comprises a group of inherited skin disorders characterized by dry, rough, and erythematous skin of various degrees of severity.

**Synonyms**

Collodion Baby

Congenital Ichthyosiform Erythroderma
Desquamation of Newborn

**Signs and Symptoms** The skin over most of the body typically is red, dry, and rough, and also may be scaly and itchy. The skin on the palms of the hands and soles of the feet may be abnormally thick.

**Etiology** The ichthyosis congenita syndromes are all probably transmitted as autosomal recessive inherited disorders, with some forms being sex-linked.

**Epidemiology** The ichthyosis congenita syndromes are rare. Symptoms onset is pre- or postnatal.

**Related Disorders** See *Ichthyosis Vulgaris; Ichthyosis, X-Linked; Epidermolytic Hyperkeratosis.*

**Treatment—Standard** The symptoms may be alleviated by application of keratolytics and emollients, including plain petroleum jelly. This can be especially effective after bathing while the skin is still moist. Because the skin barrier is defective, topical agents must be chosen with care. Lactate lotion can be an effective keratolytic. Topical and systemic retinoids can be beneficial in some cases but must be used with caution because of potentially adverse side effects.

**Treatment—Investigational** Investigational approaches include the local application of cholesterol and of therapeutic agents that can hydrolyze the cholesterol sulfate bond.

Monolaurin (glylorin) is being tested for treatment of ichthyosis congenita. The product is manufactured by Cellegy Pharmaceuticals.

The National Institute of Arthritis and Musculoskeletal and Skin Diseases is seeking ichthyosis patients to participate in a study aimed at mapping the genes responsible for the various forms of the disease. For more information, contact Sherri Bale, M.D.

Please contact the agencies listed under Resources, below, for the most current information. Addresses and telephone numbers of these agencies, as well as of individual experts and research centers, may be found in the Master Resources List.

**Resources**

**For more information on ichthyosis congenita:** National Organization for Rare Disorders (NORD); Foundation for Ichthyosis and Related Skin Types; NIH/National Arthritis and Musculoskeletal and Skin Diseases Information Clearinghouse; The Eczema Association for Science and Education.

**For genetic information and genetic counseling referrals:** March of Dimes Birth Defects Foundation; Alliance of Genetic Support Groups.

**References**

Dermatology, 3rd ed.: S.L. Moschella and H.J. Hurley, eds.; W.B. Saunders Company, 1992.
Textbook of Dermatology, 5th ed.: R.H. Champion, et al., eds.; Blackwell Scientific Publications, 1992.
Dermatology, 3rd ed.: O. Braun-Falco, et al.; Springer-Verlag, 1991.
Mendelian Inheritance in Man, 9th ed.: V.A. McKusick; The Johns Hopkins University Press, 1990, p. 1272.
Cecil Textbook of Medicine, 18th ed.: J.B. Wyngaarden and L.H. Smith, Jr., eds.; W.B. Saunders Company, 1988, pp. 2326–2329.
Dermatology in General Medicine: Textbook and Atlas, 3rd ed.: T.B. Fitzpatrick, et al., eds.; McGraw-Hill, 1987.

# ICHTHYOSIS, HARLEQUIN TYPE

**Description** This rare, autosomal recessive skin disorder is characterized by the appearance at birth of very large, thick skin plates causing facial distortion and various other constricting deformities.

**Synonyms**

Harlequin Fetus
Ichthyosis Congenita, Harlequin Fetus Type

**Signs and Symptoms** Newborns with the disease have massive, thick scales on the skin. The top layer of skin reveals an abnormally large number of squames, thought to be caused by a defect in the metabolism of the corneocytes. There is marked ectropion of the eyelids and lips and flexion deformities at the joints. Constriction of the chest and abdomen causes respiration and feeding difficulties. Until recently, the disorder was considered lethal.

Harlequin-type ichthyosis can be detected by fetoscopy.

**Etiology** The disorder is transmitted through autosomal recessive genes that cause formation of abnormal keratins.

**Epidemiology** The disorder is evident in utero. Males and females are affected in equal numbers. The ratio of affected individuals is 1:500,000.

**Related Disorders** See *Ichthyosis; Ichthyosis Congenita; Ichthyosis Hystrix, Curth-Macklin Type; Ichthyosis, Lamellar Recessive.*

See also *Epidermolytic Hyperkeratosis; Netherton Syndrome; Sjögren-Larsson Syndrome.*

**Treatment—Standard** Treatment is only palliative. Symptoms can be alleviated by application of keratolytics and emollients, including plain petroleum jelly. This can be especially effective after bathing while the skin is still moist.

Despite the thick scales, the skin barrier is defective; topical agents must be chosen with care. Lactate lotion also can be an effective keratolytic. Systemic retinoids (etretinate) have been lifesaving in several cases.

**Treatment—Investigational** Monolaurin (glylorin) is being tested for treatment of harlequin type ichthyosis. The product is manufactured by Cellegy Pharmaceuticals.

The National Institute of Arthritis and Musculoskeletal and Skin Diseases is seeking ichthyosis patients to participate in a study aimed at mapping the genes responsible for the various forms of the disease. For more information, contact Sherri Bale, M.D.

Please contact the agencies listed under Resources, below, for the most current information. Addresses and telephone numbers of these agencies, as well as of individual experts and research centers, may be found in the Master Resources List.

### Resources

**For more information on harlequin type ichthyosis:** National Organization for Rare Disorders (NORD); Foundation for Ichthyosis and Related Skin Types; NIH/National Arthritis and Musculoskeletal and Skin Diseases Information Clearinghouse.

**For genetic information and genetic counseling referrals:** March of Dimes Birth Defects Foundation; Alliance of Genetic Support Groups.

### References

Dermatology, 3rd ed.: S.L. Moschella and H.J. Hurley, eds.; W.B. Saunders Company, 1992.

Textbook of Dermatology, 5th ed.: R.H. Champion, et al., eds.; Blackwell Scientific Publications, 1992.

Dermatology, 3rd ed.: O. Braun-Falco, et al.; Springer-Verlag, 1991.

Harlequin Baby Treated with Etretinate: M. Rogers, et al.; Pediatr. Dermatol., 1989, vol. 6, p. 216.

Dermatology in General Medicine: Textbook and Atlas, 3rd ed.: T.B. Fitzpatrick, et al., eds.; McGraw-Hill, 1987.

Genetically Transmitted, Generalized Disorders of Cornification: The Ichthyoses: M.L. Williams, et al.; Dermatol. Clin., January 1987, vol. 5(1), pp. 155–178.

Therapeutic Activity of Lactate 12% Lotion in the Treatment of Ichthyosis: Active Versus Vehicle and Active Versus a Petroleum Cream: M. Buxman, et al.; J. Am. Acad. Dermatol., December 1986, vol. 15(6), pp. 1253–1258.

# ICHTHYOSIS HYSTRIX, CURTH-MACKLIN TYPE

**Description** Ichthyosis hystrix, Curth-Macklin type, is a rare inherited skin disorder characterized by ichthyosis that can range from mild to severe. Keratoderma may be limited to the palms and soles or may extend to other parts of the body surface.

**Signs and Symptoms** In ichthyosis hystrix, Curth-Macklin type, the skin on the soles of the feet and the palms of the hands is abnormally thick and hard. In some cases, widespread hyperkeratosis is also seen. Microscopic examination reveals many corneocytes with 2 nuclei and prominent nuclear shells.

**Etiology** The disorder is transmitted by autosomal dominant genes.

**Epidemiology** Onset is at birth. Males and females are affected in equal numbers.

**Related Disorders** See *Ichthyosis Congenita; Ichthyosis Vulgaris; Epidermolytic Hyperkeratosis.*

**Treatment—Standard** The cutaneous symptoms of ichthyosis hystrix, Curth-Macklin type, can be alleviated by the application of keratolytics and emollient ointments, including plain petroleum jelly. This can be especially effective after bathing while the skin is still moist. Salicylic acid gel and lactate lotion can be useful. Topical and systemic retinoids are beneficial in some cases but must be used with caution because of potentially adverse side effects.

**Treatment—Investigational** Monolaurin (glylorin) is being tested for treatment of ichthyosis hystrix, Curth-Macklin type. The product is manufactured by Cellegy Pharmaceuticals.

The National Institute of Arthritis and Musculoskeletal and Skin Diseases is seeking ichthyosis patients to participate in a study aimed at mapping the genes responsible for the various forms of the disease. For more information, contact Sherri Bale, M.D.

Please contact the agencies listed under Resources, below, for the most current information. Addresses and telephone numbers of these agencies, as well as of individual experts and research centers, may be found in the Master Resources List.

### Resources

**For more information on ichthyosis hystrix, Curth-Macklin type:** National Organization for Rare Disorders (NORD); Foundation for Ichthyosis and Related Skin Types; NIH/National Arthritis and Musculoskeletal and Skin Diseases Information Clearinghouse.

**For genetic information and genetic counseling referrals:** March of Dimes Birth Defects Foundation; Alliance of Genetic Support Groups.

### References

Dermatology, 3rd ed.: S.L. Moschella and H.J. Hurley, eds.; W.B. Saunders Company, 1992.

Textbook of Dermatology, 5th ed.: R.H. Champion, et al., eds.; Blackwell Scientific Publications, 1992.

Dermatology, 3rd ed.: O. Braun-Falco, et al.; Springer-Verlag, 1991.

Mendelian Inheritance in Man, 9th ed.: V.A. McKusick; The Johns Hopkins University Press, 1990, p. 507.

Dermatology in General Medicine: Textbook and Atlas, 3rd ed.: T.B. Fitzpatrick, et al., eds.; McGraw-Hill, 1987.

Genetically Transmitted, Generalized Disorders of Cornification: The Ichthyoses: M.L. Williams, et al.; Dermatol. Clin., January 1987, vol. 5(1), pp. 155–178.

Therapeutic Activity of Lactate 12% Lotion in the Treatment of Ichthyosis: Active Versus Vehicle and Active Versus a Petroleum Cream: Buxman, et al.; J. Am. Acad. Dermatol., December 1986, vol. 15(6), pp. 1253–1258.

Ichthyosis Hystrix (Curth-Macklin): Light and Electron Microscopic Studies Performed Before and After Etretinate Treatment: L. Kanerva, et al.; Arch. Dermatol., September 1984, vol. 120(9), pp. 1218–1223.

# ICHTHYOSIS, LAMELLAR RECESSIVE

**Description** Lamellar recessive ichthyosis is characterized by extreme hyperkeratosis over the entire body surface.

**Synonyms**

Congenital Ichthyosiform Erythroderma, Nonbullous Type

**Signs and Symptoms** Large, dark, platelike scales appear over the entire body surface. Ectropion of the eyelids and lips may be present. Erythroderma may underlie the scales, and keratoderma may occur on the palms of the hands and soles of the feet. Lamellar recessive ichthyosis in a newborn may be manifest by the collodion baby type of ichthyosis congenita. Sweating is impaired, and patients may develop secondary bacterial infections in their skin. Lipid analysis of the stratum corneum shows increased free sterols and ceramides but normal hydrocarbon content.

**Etiology** The disorder is transmitted through autosomal recessive genes. There is also an autosomal dominant type of lamellar ichthyosis. The recessive type is due to mutations on the transglutaminase 1 gene (chromosome 14).

**Epidemiology** Lamellar recessive ichthyosis is very rare, affecting fewer than 1:200,000 births. Males and females are affected in equal numbers.

**Related Disorders** See *Ichthyosis Congenita; Ichthyosis Hystrix; Epidermolytic Hyperkeratosis; Sjögren-Larsson Syndrome.*

**Treatment—Standard** The discomfort of the dry, scaly skin can be alleviated by application of keratolytics and emollients, including plain petroleum jelly. This can be especially effective after bathing while the skin is still moist. Salicylic acid gel is useful in older patients for removal of scales. Lactate lotion also can be an effective keratolytic. Topical and systemic retinoids can be beneficial in some cases but must be used with caution because of potentially adverse side effects. Surgical correction of the ectropion is of some benefit in severe cases. Topical and systemic antibiotics may be useful.

**Treatment—Investigational** Monolaurin (glylorin) is being tested for treatment of lamellar recessive ichthyosis. The product is manufactured by Cellegy Pharmaceuticals.

The National Institute of Arthritis and Musculoskeletal and Skin Diseases is seeking ichthyosis patients to participate in a study aimed at mapping the genes responsible for the various forms of the disease. For more information, contact Sherri Bale, M.D.

Please contact the agencies listed under Resources, below, for the most current information. Addresses and telephone numbers of these agencies, as well as of individual experts and research centers, may be found in the Master Resources List.

**Resources**

**For more information on lamellar recessive ichthyosis:** National Organization for Rare Disorders (NORD); Foundation for Ichthyosis and Related Skin Types; NIH/National Arthritis and Musculoskeletal and Skin Diseases Information Clearinghouse.

**For genetic information and genetic counseling referrals:** March of Dimes Birth Defects Foundation; Alliance of Genetic Support Groups.

**References**

Linkage of Autosomal Recessive Lamellar Ichthyosis to Chromosome 14q: L.J. Russell, et al.; Am. J. Hum. Genet., 1994, vol. 55, p. 1146.

Dermatology, 3rd ed.: S.L. Moschella and H.J. Hurley, eds.; W.B. Saunders Company, 1992.

Textbook of Dermatology, 5th ed.: R.H. Champion, et al., eds.; Blackwell Scientific Publications, 1992.

Dermatology, 3rd ed.: O. Braun-Falco, et al.; Springer-Verlag, 1991.

Mendelian Inheritance in Man, 9th ed.: V.A. McKusick; The Johns Hopkins University Press, 1990, p. 507.

Dermatology in General Medicine: Textbook and Atlas, 3rd ed.: T.B. Fitzpatrick, et al., eds.; McGraw-Hill, 1987.

Genetically Transmitted, Generalized Disorders of Cornification: The Ichthyoses: M.L. Williams, et al.; Dermatol. Clin., January 1987, vol. 5(1), pp. 155–178.

Therapeutic Activity of Lactate 12% Lotion in the Treatment of Ichthyosis: Active Versus Vehicle and Active Versus a Petroleum Cream: Buxman, et al.; J. Am. Acad. Dermatol., December 1986, vol. 15(6), pp. 1253–1258.

Autosomal Dominant Lamellar Ichthyosis: A New Skin Disorder: H. Traupe, et al.; Clin. Genet., 1984, vol. 26, p. 457.

Ichthyosis Hystrix (Curth-Macklin): Light and Electron Microscopic Studies Performed Before and After Etretinate Treatment: L. Kanerva, et al.; Arch. Dermatol., September 1984, vol. 120(9), pp. 1218–1223.

# ICHTHYOSIS VULGARIS

**Description** Ichthyosis vulgaris is an inherited disorder characterized by firmly adherent scales on the skin.

**Synonyms**
Ichthyosis Simplex

**Signs and Symptoms** Symptoms usually begin during the first year of life, and may vary from mild to severe. Features of this disorder include hyperkeratosis and the development of fish-scale-like skin on the back and over extensor surfaces. Pronounced palm and sole markings are commonly seen. In approximately 50 percent of patients, atopic dermatitis also is observed. Hay fever, asthma, or eczema may be present. Symptoms tend to improve with age and change of season, and in moist, warm climates.

**Etiology** The disorder is transmitted through autosomal dominant inheritance. The cause is unknown, but epidermal proliferation rate and transit time are normal. Thus, the symptoms are thought to be due to abnormal retention and decreased shedding of scales.

**Epidemiology** Ichthyosis affects approximately 1:250 persons in the United States. The disorder occurs in males and females in equal numbers.

**Related Disorders** See *Ichthyosis Congenita; Ichthyosis Hystrix, Curth-Macklin Type; Epidermolytic Hyperkeratosis; Netherton Syndrome; Sjögren-Larsson Syndrome.*

**Treatment—Standard** Cutaneous symptoms can be alleviated by application of keratolytics and emollient ointments, including plain petroleum jelly. This can be especially effective after bathing while the skin is still moist. Salicylic acid gel and lactate lotion are also effective. Topical and systemic retinoids can be beneficial in some cases but must be used with caution because of potentially adverse side effects.

**Treatment—Investigational** Monolaurin (glylorin) is being tested for treatment of ichthyosis vulgaris. The product is manufactured by Cellegy Pharmaceuticals.

The National Institute of Arthritis and Musculoskeletal and Skin Diseases is seeking ichthyosis patients to participate in a study aimed at mapping the genes responsible for the various forms of the disease. For more information, contact Sherri Bale, M.D.

Please contact the agencies listed under Resources, below, for the most current information. Addresses and telephone numbers of these agencies, as well as of individual experts and research centers, may be found in the Master Resources List.

**Resources**
**For more information on ichthyosis vulgaris:** National Organization for Rare Disorders (NORD); Foundation for Ichthyosis and Related Skin Types; NIH/National Arthritis and Musculoskeletal and Skin Diseases Information Clearinghouse.

**For genetic information and genetic counseling referrals:** March of Dimes Birth Defects Foundation; Alliance of Genetic Support Groups.

**References**
Dermatology, 3rd ed.: S.L. Moschella and H.J. Hurley, eds.; W.B. Saunders Company, 1992.

Textbook of Dermatology, 5th ed.: R.H. Champion, et al., eds.; Blackwell Scientific Publications, 1992.

Dermatology, 3rd ed.: O. Braun-Falco, et al.; Springer-Verlag, 1991.

Dermatology in General Medicine: Textbook and Atlas, 3rd ed.: T.B. Fitzpatrick, et al., eds.; McGraw-Hill, 1987.

Genetically Transmitted, Generalized Disorders of Cornification: The Ichthyoses: M.L. Williams, et al.; Dermatol. Clin., January 1987, vol. 5(1), pp. 155–178.

Therapeutic Activity of Lactate 12% Lotion in the Treatment of Ichthyosis: Active Versus Vehicle and Active Versus a Petroleum Cream: M. Buxman, et al.; J. Am. Acad. Dermatol., December 1986, vol. 15(6), pp. 1253–1258.

# ICHTHYOSIS, X-LINKED

**Description** X-linked ichthyosis is a genetic skin disorder of males linked to an inborn error of metabolism. This is a retention hyperkeratosis with normal epidermal proliferation rate and transit times. The condition is associated with a deficiency of steroid sulfatase, resulting in several biochemical alterations in keratocyte biology and in steroid sex hormone metabolism. Maternal estrogen production is diminished in late pregnancy in carrier females. Cholesterol sulfate may accumulate in the blood and skin.

**Synonyms**

Steroid Sulfatase Deficiency

**Signs and Symptoms** Symptoms usually begin between 1 and 3 weeks of age with development of large, tightly adherent brownish scales. These are most prominent on the skin covering extensor surfaces, but the flexor surfaces may also be involved. The back of the neck is almost always scaly, and the skin in the hollows of the elbows and knees is less commonly affected. The trunk may be involved, but the face, scalp, palms, and soles are usually spared.

Symptoms often greatly improve in the summer.

Clouding of the cornea occurs in approximately 50 percent of adult men with X-linked ichthyosis. Affected males have cryptorchidism in about 12 to 25 percent of cases, and may also be at increased risk of testicular malignancies. Normal functioning of sex hormones does not appear to be affected.

Diminished estrogen production may occur if a female carrier is pregnant with an affected male, and there may be a delay in labor and difficulties with cervical dilation. The disorder can be detected by amniocentesis.

**Etiology** X-linked genes transmit the disorder.

**Epidemiology** X-linked ichthyosis is rare, affecting slightly more than 1:6,000 males. Female carriers are usually asymptomatic but may have mild scaling and clouding of corneas.

**Related Disorders** See *Ichthyosis Congenita; Ichthyosis Hystrix, Curth-Macklin Type; Ichthyosis, Lamellar Recessive; Darier Disease; Epidermolytic Hyperkeratosis; Netherton Syndrome; Sjögren-Larsson Syndrome.*

**Treatment—Standard** Cutaneous manifestations of X-linked ichthyosis can be alleviated by the application of keratolytics and emollients, including plain petroleum jelly. This can be especially effective after bathing while the skin is still moist. Salicylic acid gel, lactate lotion, and propylene glycol products are also effective. Topical and systemic retinoids can be beneficial in some cases but must be used with caution because of potentially adverse side effects.

**Treatment—Investigational** Monolaurin (glylorin) is being tested for treatment of recessive X-linked ichthyosis. The product is manufactured by Cellegy Pharmaceuticals.

The National Institute of Arthritis and Musculoskeletal and Skin Diseases is seeking ichthyosis patients to participate in a study aimed at mapping the genes responsible for the various forms of the disease. For more information, contact Sherri Bale, M.D.

Please contact the agencies listed under Resources, below, for the most current information. Addresses and telephone numbers of these agencies, as well as of individual experts and research centers, may be found in the Master Resources List.

**Resources**

**For more information on X-linked ichthyosis:** National Organization for Rare Disorders (NORD); Foundation for Ichthyosis and Related Skin Types; NIH/National Arthritis and Musculoskeletal and Skin Diseases Information Clearinghouse.

**For genetic information and genetic counseling referrals:** March of Dimes Birth Defects Foundation; Alliance of Genetic Support Groups.

**References**

Dermatology, 3rd ed.: S.L. Moschella and H.J. Hurley, eds.; W.B. Saunders Company, 1992.

Textbook of Dermatology, 5th ed.: R.H. Champion, et al., eds.; Blackwell Scientific Publications, 1992.

Dermatology, 3rd ed.: O. Braun-Falco, et al.; Springer-Verlag, 1991.

Dermatology in General Medicine: Textbook and Atlas, 3rd ed.: T.B. Fitzpatrick, et al., eds.; McGraw-Hill, 1987.

Genetically Transmitted, Generalized Disorders of Cornification: The Ichthyoses: M.L. Williams, et al.; Dermatol. Clin., January 1987, vol. 5(1), pp. 155–178.

Therapeutic Activity of Lactate 12% Lotion in the Treatment of Ichthyosis: Active Versus Vehicle and Active Versus a Petroleum Cream: M. Buxman, et al.; J. Am. Acad. Dermatol., December 1986, vol. 15(6), pp. 1253–1258.

Topical Cholesterol Treatment of Recessive X-Linked Ichthyosis: G. Lykkesfeldt, et al.; Lancet, December 1983, vol. 2(8363), pp. 1337–1338.

# INCONTINENTIA PIGMENTI

**Description** The disorder is characterized by unusual patterns of discolored, hyperpigmented skin caused by excessive deposits of melanin. Developmental abnormalities are sometimes seen; oral, visual, and neurologic symptoms may occur.

**Synonyms**

Bloch-Siemens-Sulzberger Syndrome
Bloch-Sulzberger Syndrome

**Signs and Symptoms** There are 4 stages of progression in incontinentia pigmenti. Onset of **stage 1** is typically between birth and 6 months. The skin is inflamed and red, with spiral or linear patterns of small fluid-filled blisters. The white cell count, especially eosinophils, is usually elevated.

The skin in **stage 2** is characterized by rough, warty growths, sometimes including pustules, following the same patterns as the blisters in the first stage. The lesions more commonly are found on the arms and legs, less often on the head or trunk. These lesions generally may persist for 6 to 12 months. Some babies are born with stage 2 skin changes, suggesting that stage 1 occurs before birth.

**Stage 3** generally begins between 3 and 6 months, often as the lesions of the first 2 stages are resolving. Abnormal deposits of melanin cause spots of discoloration that may be brown or gray. These spots appear in linear or whorl patterns in areas previously affected. This stage generally begins to fade by adolescence, although the condition persists into adulthood in occasional cases.

**Stage 4** sometimes occurs, consisting of loss of pigmentation and atrophy in areas of discoloration. Hair loss and scarring are seen rarely.

Approximately 50 percent of affected persons also have nondermatologic symptoms and signs. These include dental abnormalities such as absence or malformation of teeth, delayed tooth eruption, a fibrovascular proliferation in the infant retina resembling retinopathy of prematurity, and neurologic findings such as abnormal migration of gray matter of the brain, seizures, or developmental delay.

Developmental abnormalities may accompany incontinentia pigmenti but are not typical: short stature, clubfoot, spina bifida, skull and ear deformities, cleft lip or palate, hemiatrophy, chondrodystrophy, syndactyly, and congenital dislocation of the hip.

**Etiology** The specific cause is unknown. In familial cases, the disorder is inherited as an X-linked dominant trait that is lethal in males. At least one-third of cases are isolated and appear to represent new mutations on X.

**Epidemiology** Approximately 600 cases have been reported in this century. The condition affects females almost exclusively.

**Related Disorders** See *Hypomelanosis of Ito.*

**Naegeli-Franceschetti-Jadassohn syndrome,** inherited as an autosomal dominant trait, is characterized by reticulated skin pigmentation in childhood that resembles incontinentia pigmenti. However, there are no inflammatory skin changes. Skin may thicken on the hands and feet, the ability to sweat may become impaired, and yellow mottling of the teeth may occur.

**Treatment—Standard** The cutaneous abnormalities generally resolve without treatment by adolescence or adulthood. The other aspects of the condition can usually be treated effectively by the appropriate specialist (ophthalmologist, neurologist, geneticist). Treatment is otherwise symptomatic and supportive, and genetic counseling may be of benefit.

**Treatment—Investigational** Families with this disorder having living affected individuals should contact Richard A. Lewis, M.D., of Baylor College of Medicine, who is conducting genetic research on incontinentia pigmenti.

Please contact the agencies listed under Resources, below, for the most current information. Addresses and telephone numbers of these agencies, as well as of individual experts and research centers, may be found in the Master Resources List.

**Resources**

**For more information on incontinentia pigmenti:** National Organization for Rare Disorders (NORD); Incontinentia Pigmenti Network; NIH/National Arthritis and Musculoskeletal and Skin Diseases Information Clearinghouse.

**For genetic information and genetic counseling referrals:** March of Dimes Birth Defects Foundation; Alliance of Genetic Support Groups.

**References**
De Novo Mutation in Three Families with Multigenerational Incontinentia Pigmenti: A. Scheuerle, et al.; Am. J. Hum. Genet., 1994, vol. 55, pp. 1279–1281.

The Gene for the Familial Form of Incontinentia Pigmenti (IP2) Maps to the Distal Part of Xq28: A. Smahi, et al.; Hum. Mol. Genet., 1994, vol. 3, pp. 273–278.

Retinal and Other Manifestations of Incontinentia Pigmenti (Bloch-Sulzberger Syndrome): M.F. Goldberg, et al.; Ophthalmology, 1993, vol. 100, pp. 1645–1654.

Dermatology, 3rd ed.: S.L. Moschella and H.J. Hurley, eds.; W.B. Saunders Company, 1992.

Textbook of Dermatology, 5th ed.: R.H. Champion, et al., eds.; Blackwell Scientific Publications, 1992.

Dermatology, 3rd ed.: O. Braun-Falco, et al.; Springer-Verlag, 1991.

Dermatology in General Medicine: Textbook and Atlas, 3rd ed.: T.B. Fitzpatrick, et al., eds.; McGraw-Hill, 1987.

Dominant Disorders with Multiple Organ Involvement: M.F. Kegel; in Dermatologic Clinics, January 1987, vol. 5(1), pp. 210–214.

Ocular Findings in Incontinentia Pigmenti: S.I. Rosenfield, et al.; Ophthalmology, 1985, vol. 92, pp. 543–546.

# KERATITIS-ICHTHYOSIS-DEAFNESS (KID) SYNDROME

**Description** KID syndrome is a very rare disorder that is characterized by inflammation of the cornea; plaques on the extremities and face; thick, hardened skin on the palms and the soles; and deafness.

**Synonyms**

> Disorder of Cornification 15, Keratitis Deafness Type
> Ichthyosiform Erythroderma–Corneal Involvement–Deafness

**Signs and Symptoms** KID syndrome is present at birth. The cornea is usually inflamed. A red, diffusely thickened skin rash is usually shed during the first week of life. Fixed, hardened skin plaques, often with a red base, usually occur on the extremities and face, producing an aged or lionlike appearance. Some patients have hyperkeratosis and prominent hair follicles over much of the body surface. In others, the involvement may be limited to the face and extremities. Hyperkeratosis around the hair follicles on the scalp may result in significant baldness. The nails may be abnormal or underdeveloped, and teeth may be small and susceptible to decay. Hardening and thickening of the outer skin layer of the palms and the soles (keratoderma palmoplantare) makes them appear pebbly. Some patients develop recurrent skin infections, including candidiasis, multiple abscesses, and uncommon granulomatous fungus infections. Squamous cell skin cancers may occur in some cases.

Nerve deafness, which may be severe in some cases, usually occurs. Eye involvement includes inflammation of the cornea and the conjunctiva, which may progress to abnormal formation of tiny vessels in the cornea.

Growth may be impaired in patients with this syndrome.

**Etiology** KID syndrome occurs for no apparent reason in the majority of cases. Several cases of this disorder have been linked to an autosomal recessive trait.

**Epidemiology** KID syndrome appears to affect females slightly more often then males. This syndrome usually starts during infancy. However, symptoms may begin as late as the 2nd decade of life.

**Related Disorders** See *Darier Disease; Ichthyosis; Ichthyosis Congenita; Ichthyosis, X-Linked; Sjögren-Larsson Syndrome; Netherton Syndrome; Ichthyosis Hystrix, Curth-Macklin Type; Ichthyosis, Lamellar Recessive; Refsum Syndrome; Conradi-Hünermann Syndrome; Epidermolytic Hyperkeratosis.*

**Treatment—Standard** Symptoms can be alleviated by application of keratolytics and emollients, including plain petroleum jelly. This can be especially effective after bathing while the skin is still moist. Salicylic acid gel, applied under occlusion to limited areas, is useful in some instances for removal of scales. Lactate lotion can also be an effective keratolytic. Topical and systemic retinoids can be beneficial in some cases but must be used with caution because of adverse side effects, including those to fetal development in pregnant women.

Genetic counseling may be of benefit for patients and their families. Other treatment is symptomatic and supportive.

**Treatment—Investigational** Monolaurin (glylorin) is being tested for treatment of ichthyosis. The product is manufactured by Cellegy Pharmaceuticals.

The National Institute of Arthritis and Musculoskeletal and Skin Diseases is seeking ichthyosis patients to participate in a study aimed at mapping the genes responsible for the various forms of the disease. For more information, contact Sherri Bale, M.D.

Please contact the agencies listed under Resources, below, for the most current information. Addresses and telephone numbers of these agencies, as well as of individual experts and research centers, may be found in the Master Resources List.

**Resources**

For more information on keratitis-ichthyosis-deafness syndrome: National Organization for Rare Disorders (NORD); Foundation for Ichthyosis and Related Skin Types; NIH/National Arthritis and Musculoskeletal and Skin Diseases Information Clearinghouse; National Eye Institute; Schepens Eye Research Institute.

For genetic information and genetic counseling referrals: March of Dimes Birth Defects Foundation; Alliance of Genetic Support Groups.

**References**

Birth Defects Encyclopedia: M.L. Buyse, ed.-in-chief; Blackwell Scientific Publications, 1990, pp. 935–936.

Mendelian Inheritance in Man, 9th ed.: V.A. McKusick; The Johns Hopkins University Press, 1990, p. 1272.

Genetically Transmitted, Generalization Disorders of Cornification: The Ichthyoses: M.L. Williams, et al.; Dermatol. Clin., January 1987, vol. 5(1), pp. 155–178.

Therapeutic Activity of Lactate 12% Lotion in the Treatment of Ichthyosis: Active Versus Vehicle and Active Versus a Petroleum Cream: M. Buxman, et al.; J. Am. Acad. Dermatol., December 1986, vol. 15(6). pp. 1253–1258.

KID Syndrome (Keratitis, Ichthyosis, And Deafness) and Chronic Mucocutaneous Candidiasis: Case Report and Review of the Literature: M. Harms, et al,; Pediatr. Dermatol., July 1984, vol. 2(1), pp. 1–7.

# KERATOSIS FOLLICULARIS SPINULOSA DECALVANS

**Description** The disorder is characterized by keratosis of the hair follicles, which leads to progressive scarring and alopecia.

**Synonyms**

Siemens Syndrome

**Signs and Symptoms** Keratosis around the hair follicles results in scarring and baldness. Atopy, photophobia, and keratitis may occur.

**Etiology** The disorder is inherited as an X-linked trait.

**Epidemiology** Female carriers usually have a milder form of the disease than affected males.

**Related Disorders** See *Ichthyosis Congenita; Ichthyosis, X-Linked.*

**Treatment—Standard** Symptoms can be alleviated by applications of keratolytics and emollients, including plain petroleum jelly. This can be especially effective after bathing while the skin is still moist. Salicylic acid gel is useful in some instances for removal of scales. Lactate lotion can also be an effective keratolytic. Topical and systemic retinoids may be beneficial in some cases but must be used with caution because of potentially adverse side effects.

**Treatment—Investigational** Monolaurin (glylorin) is being tested for treatment of keratosis follicularis spinulosa decalvans. The product is manufactured by Cellegy Pharmaceuticals.

The National Institute of Arthritis and Musculoskeletal and Skin Diseases is seeking ichthyosis patients to participate in a study aimed at mapping the genes responsible for the various forms of the disease. For more information, contact Sherri Bale, M.D.

Please contact the agencies listed under Resources, below, for the most current information. Addresses and telephone numbers of these agencies, as well as of individual experts and research centers, may be found in the Master Resources List.

**Resources**

**For more information on keratosis follicularis spinulosa decalvans:** National Organization for Rare Disorders (NORD); Foundation for Ichthyosis and Related Skin Types; NIH/National Arthritis and Musculoskeletal and Skin Diseases Information Clearinghouse.

**For genetic information and genetic counseling referrals:** March of Dimes Birth Defects Foundation; Alliance of Genetic Support Groups.

**References**

Dermatology, 3rd ed.: S.L. Moschella and H.J. Hurley, eds.; W.B. Saunders Company, 1992.

Textbook of Dermatology, 5th ed.: R.H. Champion, et al., eds.; Blackwell Scientific Publications, 1992.

Dermatology, 3rd ed.: O. Braun-Falco, et al.; Springer-Verlag, 1991.

Dermatology in General Medicine: Textbook and Atlas, 3rd ed.: T.B. Fitzpatrick, et al., eds.; McGraw-Hill, 1987.

Genetically Transmitted, Generalized Disorders of Cornification: The Ichthyoses: M.L. Williams, et al.; Dermatol. Clin., January 1987, vol. 5(1), pp. 155–178.

Therapeutic Activity of Lactate 12% Lotion in the Treatment of Ichthyosis: Active Versus Vehicle and Active Versus a Petroleum Cream: M. Buxman, et al.; J. Am. Acad. Dermatol., December 1986, vol. 15(6), pp. 1253–1258.

Trichostasis Spinulosa: M.C. Young, et al.; Int. J. Dermatol., November 1985, vol. 24(9), pp. 575–580.

Keratosis Spinulosa Decalvans: Report of Two Cases and Literature Review: Arch. Dermatol., January 1983, vol. 119(1), pp. 22–26.

# LEINER DISEASE

**Description** Leiner disease is a skin disorder that typically appears during early infancy as seborrheic dermatitis and extends to erythroderma. A reddish patch of thickened skin appears on the buttocks, then spreads and is accompanied by scaling, peeling, and itching. Symptoms usually decrease after a few weeks with treatment. Leiner disease probably represents several different entities.

**Synonyms**

Erythrodermia Desquamativa Leiner

Leiner-Moussous Desquamative Erythroderma

Severe Infantile Dermatitis

**Signs and Symptoms** The initial manifestation is the appearance of thick reddish skin on the buttocks. The erythema soon involves the entire body, and after a few days may be followed by the appearance of crusty, dry, moist, or greasy scaling on the scalp. Scaling may also appear behind the ears, on the nose or eyebrows, or around the mouth. In some cases, thin sheets of skin may peel from these areas. Loss of protein or electrolytes can result if skin infections are left untreated.

**Etiology** The etiology is unknown. Some infants have severe seborrheic dermatitis; others may have an immunodeficiency state. Netherton syndrome also presents in this way. A deficiency in C5 inhibitor has been suggested as another causative factor.

**Epidemiology** The disorder usually begins during the first 2 months of life. Breast-fed infants have a higher incidence. Males and females are affected in equal numbers.

**Related Disorders Staphylococcal scaled skin syndrome (Ritter disease; dermatitis exfoliativa neonatorum)** is a skin disorder of infants caused by a bacterial infection and characterized by erythematous skin that may peel, leaving raw areas that heal in dry, crusty yellow patches. This disorder may follow upper respiratory tract infections, impetigo, or other improperly treated staphylococcal infections.

**Treatment—Standard** Treatment may involve hospitalization to provide a controlled environment and to prevent nutritional deficiencies and skin infections. After a few weeks of careful treatment, redness and scaliness decrease and do not usually recur. However, 10 percent of cases may be fatal as a result of uncontrolled infection or severe electrolyte loss.

**Treatment—Investigational** Please contact the agencies listed under Resources, below, for the most current information. Addresses and telephone numbers of these agencies, as well as of individual experts and research centers, may be found in the Master Resources List.

**Resources**

   **For more information on Leiner disease:** National Organization for Rare Disorders (NORD); NIH/National Arthritis and Musculoskeletal and Skin Diseases Information Clearinghouse.

   **For genetic information and genetic counseling referrals:** March of Dimes Birth Defects Foundation; Alliance of Genetic Support Groups.

**References**

Dermatology, 3rd ed.: S.L. Moschella and H.J. Hurley, eds.; W.B. Saunders Company, 1992.

Textbook of Dermatology, 5th ed.: R.H. Champion, et al., eds.; Blackwell Scientific Publications, 1992.

Dermatology, 3rd ed.: O. Braun-Falco, et al.; Springer-Verlag, 1991.

Dermatology in General Medicine: Textbook and Atlas, 3rd ed.: T.B. Fitzpatrick, et al., eds.; McGraw-Hill, 1987.

Inherited Disorders of Complement: L. Guenther; J. Am. Acad. Dermatol., December 1983, vol. 9(6), pp. 815–839.

# LEOPARD SYNDROME

**Description** LEOPARD syndrome is a rare heritable disorder caused by an autosomal gene of variable expressivity whose characteristics include the presence of (**L**)entigenes, (**E**)lectrocardiogram abnormalities, (**O**)cular hypertelorism, (**P**)ulmonary stenosis, (**A**)nomalies of the genital organs, (**R**)etarded growth, and (**D**)eafness.

**Synonyms**

   Cardiomyopathic Lentiginosis

   Multiple Lentigines Syndrome

**Signs and Symptoms** LEOPARD syndrome is most visibly characterized by small, dark cutaneous spots (lentigines) that resemble freckles but are unrelated to exposure to the sun. The lentigines range between 1 and 5 mm in size; they are usually spread across the neck and torso but can occur anywhere on the skin. They tend to increase with age.

   Other abnormalities associated with LEOPARD syndrome include other cardiac defects, cardiomyopathy, prominent ears, winged scapulae, cryptorchidism, and late onset of adolescence. An impaired sense of smell, deafness, and ovarian and renal hypoplasia or agenesis are among other characteristics that may also be present.

**Etiology** The syndrome is inherited as an autosomal dominant trait.

**Epidemiology** Males and females are affected in equal numbers.

**Treatment—Standard** No specific therapy is available. Undescended testes may require surgery. Cardiac abnormalities must be monitored and treated as required. Other treatment is symptomatic and supportive. Genetic counseling may be beneficial.

**Treatment—Investigational** Please contact the agencies listed under Resources, below, for the most current information. Addresses and telephone numbers of these agencies, as well as of individual experts and research centers, may be found in the Master Resources List.

**Resources**

   **For more information on LEOPARD syndrome:** National Organization for Rare Disorders (NORD); NIH/National Institute of Child Health and Human Development.

   **For genetic information and genetic counseling referrals:** March of Dimes Birth Defects Foundation; Alliance of Genetic Support Groups.

**References**

Dermatology, 3rd ed.: S.L. Moschella and H.J. Hurley, eds.; W.B. Saunders Company, 1992.
Textbook of Dermatology, 5th ed.: R.H. Champion, et al., eds.; Blackwell Scientific Publications, 1992.
Dermatology, 3rd ed.: O. Braun-Falco, et al.; Springer-Verlag, 1991.
Mendelian Inheritance in Man, 9th ed.: V.A. McKusick, The Johns Hopkins University Press, 1990, pp. 565–566.
Smith's Recognizable Patterns of Human Malformation, 4th ed.: K.L. Jones; W.B. Saunders Company, 1988, pp. 470–471.
Dermatology in General Medicine: Textbook and Atlas, 3rd ed.: T.B. Fitzpatrick, et al., eds.; McGraw-Hill, 1987.

# Lichen Sclerosus et Atrophicus (LSA)

**Description** LSA is a chronic dermatologic disease characterized by the progressive development of white, atrophic skin lesions of the neck, arms, trunk, vulva, and other areas. LSA is not a premalignant disease.

**Synonyms**

Lichen Sclerosus

White Spot Disease

**Signs and Symptoms** LSA is characterized by the appearance in the skin of pale patches that become thin, shiny, and parchmentlike. On close inspection, the patches contain clusters of minute white lesions that coalesce. There may be a violaceous color to the borders. Fissures, cracks, and ecchymoses may appear. Distribution is on the neck, under the breast, in body folds, and in the perianal and vulvar areas. Patients may complain of pruritus. Atrophy and shrinkage of the skin of the vagina and vulva may cause painful sexual intercourse.

Females are affected most often. In cases of LSA in males, it is generally the foreskin that is affected, making retraction of the foreskin impossible. The condition is progressive and the atrophy does not regress. If leukoplakia is present, then squamous cell carcinoma must be suspected also. Some cases are associated with diabetes mellitus.

**Etiology** The cause is not known. LSA may be due to an autoimmune process or an injury. A genetic predisposition may exist.

**Epidemiology** The disorder most often affects females between the ages of 40 and 60, although cases involving younger females and males, including children, have been reported.

**Related Disorders** See *Scleroderma.*

Symptoms of **lichen planus** may be similar to those of LSA.

**Treatment—Standard** Treatment consists of topical applications of antipruritics, corticosteroids, and testosterone to the affected areas. Surgical removal of affected skin layers may be of benefit in severe cases.

**Treatment—Investigational** Etretinate is being evaluated as a treatment; the drug must not be used by pregnant women.

Please contact the agencies listed under Resources, below, for the most current information. Addresses and telephone numbers of these agencies, as well as of individual experts and research centers, may be found in the Master Resources List.

**Resources**

**For more information on lichen sclerosus et atrophicus:** National Organization for Rare Disorders (NORD); NIH/National Arthritis and Musculoskeletal and Skin Diseases Information Clearinghouse.

**References**

Dermatology, 3rd ed.: S.L. Moschella and H.J. Hurley, eds.; W.B. Saunders Company, 1992.
Textbook of Dermatology, 5th ed.: R.H. Champion, et al., eds.; Blackwell Scientific Publications, 1992.
Dermatology, 3rd ed.: O. Braun-Falco, et al.; Springer-Verlag, 1991.
Cecil Textbook of Medicine, 18th ed.: J.B. Wyngaarden and L.H. Smith, Jr., eds.; W.B. Saunders Company, 1988, pp. 1419, 2341.
Dermatology in General Medicine: Textbook and Atlas, 3rd ed.: T.B. Fitzpatrick, et al., eds.; McGraw-Hill, 1987.

# Mucha-Habermann Disease

**Description** Mucha-Habermann disease is an uncommon skin disorder characterized by a recurrent red rash. It occurs most often in young adults and children.

**Synonyms**

Pityriasis Lichenoides et Varioliformis Acuta

PLEVA

**Signs and Symptoms** The characteristic recurrent red rash is itchy and burning, with papules, pustules, and vesicles, some of which become hemorrhagic. These lesions usually become scaly and crusted and can ulcerate, leaving scars. Other symptoms associated with this disease may be headache, chills, malaise, and, rarely, arthralgia.

**Etiology** The exact cause is not known. There is some suggestion that it may be an autoimmune disorder or that it may be due to an infectious agent.

**Epidemiology** Mucha-Habermann disease affects males and females in equal numbers. It usually occurs in young adults, but it can affect children as well.

**Related Disorders** See *Gianotti-Crosti Syndrome; Erythema Multiforme.*

**Pityriasis rosea** is a self-limited, mild, inflammatory skin eruption characterized by scaly lesions found most commonly on the trunk. The disorder is possibly due to an unidentified infectious agent. It may occur at any age but is seen most frequently in young adults. In temperate climates, incidence is highest during the spring and autumn.

**Treatment—Standard** Tetracycline, erythromycin, corticosteroids, and cytotoxic drugs have provided relief to some people with this disease. Some patients respond to treatments with ultraviolet light. Other treatment is symptomatic and supportive.

**Treatment—Investigational** Please contact the agencies listed under Resources, below, for the most current information. Addresses and telephone numbers of these agencies, as well as of individual experts and research centers, may be found in the Master Resources List.

**Resources**

**For more information on Mucha-Habermann disease:** National Organization for Rare Disorders (NORD); NIH/National Arthritis and Musculoskeletal and Skin Diseases Information Clearinghouse.

**References**

Cecil Textbook of Medicine, 18th ed.: J.B. Wyngaarden and L.H. Smith, Jr., eds.; W.B. Saunders Company, 1988, p. 2328.

Clinical and Histologic Features in Pityriasis Lichenoides et Varioliformis Acuta in Children: J. Longley, et al.; Arch. Dermatol., October 1987, vol. 123(10), pp. 1335–1339.

Ultraviolet Light Treatment of a Patient with Pityriasis Lichenoides et Varioliformis Acuta (Mucha Haberman Disease): J. Mackinnon; Phys. Ther., October 1986, vol. 66(10), pp. 1542–1543.

Mucha-Habermann Disease in Children: The Association with Rheumatic Diseases: J. Ellsworth, et al.; J. Rheumatol., March–April 1982, vol. 9(2), pp. 319–324.

# NETHERTON SYNDROME

**Description** Netherton syndrome is a rare skin condition in which cornification leads to the distinctive circular scaling pattern of ichthyosis linearis circumflexa or less commonly to nonbullous congenital ichthyosiform erythroderma. Atopy and abnormalities of the hair are also associated with the syndrome.

**Synonyms**

Ichthyosis Linearis Circumflexa

Netherton Disease

**Signs and Symptoms** At birth, characteristic findings include generalized redness and the presence of a parchmentlike membrane that can be peeled off. Later, hyperkeratosis and shedding may lead to ichthyosis linearis circumflexa, or, in some cases, a rash similar to lamellar ichthyosis. Itching may be mild to severe.

Various allergic disorders often accompany the cutaneous findings, and lichenification on the arms and legs may be an allergic reaction.

Abnormalities of the hair that are characteristic of Netherton syndrome include trichorrhexis invaginata ("bamboo" hair), pili torti (twisted hair), and trichorrhexis nodosa.

**Etiology** The syndrome is transmitted through autosomal recessive genes.

**Epidemiology** Males and females are affected equally.

**Related Disorders** See *Ichthyosis Congenita; Ichthyosis, Lamellar Recessive; Tay Syndrome.*

**Treatment—Standard** Cutaneous symptoms can be alleviated by application of keratolytics and emollients, including plain petroleum jelly. This can be especially effective after bathing while the skin is still moist. Salicylic acid gel and lactate lotion are useful in some instances for removal of scales. Topical and systemic retinoids are beneficial in some cases but must be used with caution because of potentially adverse side effects.

Foods that are known to cause an allergic skin reaction should be avoided.

**Treatment—Investigational** Monolaurin (glylorin) is being tested for treatment of Netherton syndrome. The product is manufactured by Cellegy Pharmaceuticals.

The National Institute of Arthritis and Musculoskeletal and Skin Diseases is seeking ichthyosis patients to participate in a study aimed at mapping the genes responsible for the various forms of the disease. For more information, contact Sherri Bale, M.D.

Please contact the agencies listed under Resources, below, for the most current information. Addresses and tele-

phone numbers of these agencies, as well as of individual experts and research centers, may be found in the Master Resources List.

**Resources**

**For more information on Netherton syndrome:** National Organization for Rare Disorders (NORD); Foundation for Ichthyosis and Related Skin Types; NIH/National Arthritis and Musculoskeletal and Skin Diseases Information Clearinghouse.

**For genetic information and genetic counseling referrals:** March of Dimes Birth Defects Foundation; Alliance of Genetic Support Groups.

**References**

Dermatology, 3rd ed.: S.L. Moschella and H.J. Hurley, eds.; W.B. Saunders Company, 1992.

Textbook of Dermatology, 5th ed.: R.H. Champion, et al., eds.; Blackwell Scientific Publications, 1992.

Dermatology, 3rd ed.: O. Braun-Falco, et al.; Springer-Verlag, 1991.

Dermatology in General Medicine: Textbook and Atlas, 3rd ed.: T.B. Fitzpatrick, et al., eds.; McGraw-Hill, 1987.

Genetically Transmitted, Generalized Disorders of Cornification: The Ichthyoses: M.L. Williams, et al.; Dermatol. Clin., January 1987, vol. 5(1), pp. 155–178.

Therapeutic Activity of Lactate 12% Lotion in the Treatment of Ichthyosis: Active Versus Vehicle and Active Versus a Petroleum Cream: M. Buxman, et al.; J. Am. Acad. Dermatol., December 1986, vol. 15(6), pp. 1253–1258.

Netherton Syndrome: Report of a Case and Review of the Literature: S.L. Greene, et al.; J. Am. Acad. Dermatol., August 1985, vol. 13(2 pt. 2), pp. 329–337.

# PACHYDERMOPERIOSTOSIS

**Description** Pachydermoperiostosis is characterized by clubbing of the fingers and toes; periostosis; coarse facial features; thickening of the skin on the scalp and face, forming folds, depressions, or furrows (cutis verticis gyrata); and/or hyperhidrosis of the hands and feet.

**Synonyms**

Hypertrophic Osteoarthropathy

Touraine-Salente-Golé Syndrome

**Signs and Symptoms** This disorder typically appears during childhood or adolescence and progresses slowly for about 10 years. Patients with pachydermoperiostosis typically have coarse facial features with oily, thick, grooved skin on the face. In adolescence, the skin of the scalp and face thickens, resulting in depressions or grooves (cutis verticis gyrata). Joint pain, clubbing of the fingers and toes, and hyperhidrosis of the hands and feet may also be present. Periostosis, especially of the ends of the long bones, is present in patients with pachydermoperiostosis.

Other symptoms found in some patients with pachydermoperiostosis may include ptosis, seborrheic dermatitis, ulcers, and/or swelling of hair follicles related to large, open pores of the skin.

The symptoms in patients with pachydermoperiostosis vary in severity, with males typically having a more severe form of the disorder.

A variant of pachydermoperiostosis, **Rosenfeld-Kloepfer syndrome,** is characterized by enlarged bones of the jaw, and very large hands, feet, nose, lips, and tongue. Other features of this form of the disorder are a prominent upper forehead, cutis verticis gyrata, and corneal leukoma.

**Etiology** Pachydermoperiostosis is thought to be inherited as an autosomal dominant trait, with varying severity.

**Epidemiology** Pachydermoperiostosis is a rare disorder that affects males more often than females; the ratio of affected males to females is 7:1. However, this ratio may not be accurate, since the disease in females is often mild and may remain undetected until x-rays reveal the characteristic periostosis.

**Related Disorders** See *Acromegaly.*

**Hypertrophic pulmonary osteoarthropathy (Marie-Bamberger disease)** is a rare disorder in which there is expansion of the ends or the entire shaft of the long bones and often clubbing of the fingers and toes. This disorder occurs in chronic pulmonary disease, heart disease, and occasionally other acute and chronic disorders.

**Treatment—Standard** Vagotomy may alleviate joint pain and swelling. Gastric surgery may also be performed to reduce the release of gastric acid and the chance of developing a gastric ulcer. Plastic surgery may be performed to improve facial appearance. Other treatment is symptomatic and supportive. Genetic counseling may be of benefit for patients and their families.

**Treatment—Investigational** Please contact the agencies listed under Resources, below, for the most current information. Addresses and telephone numbers of these agencies, as well as of individual experts and research centers, may be found in the Master Resources List.

**Resources**

**For more information on pachydermoperiostosis:** National Organization for Rare Disorders (NORD); NIH/National Arthritis and Musculoskeletal and Skin Diseases Information Clearinghouse.

**For genetic information and genetic counseling referrals:** March of Dimes Birth Defects Foundation; Alliance of Genetic Support Groups.

### References

Birth Defects Encyclopedia: M.L. Buyse, ed.-in-chief; Blackwell Scientific Publications, 1990, pp. 1349–1350.

Mendelian Inheritance in Man, 9th ed.: V.A. McKusick, The Johns Hopkins University Press, 1990, p. 702.

Smith's Recognizable Patterns of Human Malformation, 4th ed.: K.L. Jones; W.B. Saunders Company, 1988, p. 488.

# PEMPHIGOID, BENIGN MUCOSAL

**Description** Benign mucosal pemphigoid is a rare chronic disease characterized by blisters and scarring of the mucous membranes. The oral cavity and the conjunctiva are the most commonly affected areas.

**Synonyms**

> Cicatricial Pemphigoid
>
> Mucous Membrane Pemphigoid

**Signs and Symptoms** Presenting symptoms may include erythema and blistering of the oral mucosa, or redness and inflammation of the eyes and conjunctiva. Conjunctival scarring may occur, with formation of scar tissue between the eyelid and eyeball. Blisters also may develop in the mucous membranes of the pharynx and esophagus, nose, urethra, and vulva, but are uncommon on the external skin.

Subepidermal blisters are seen histologically with deposits of immunoglobulins IgG and IgA and of C3 in the cutaneous basement membrane zone. The pattern resembles that of bullous pemphigoid.

Benign mucosal pemphigoid is a persistent condition that remits and recurs.

**Etiology** The cause is not known.

**Epidemiology** Middle-aged and elderly persons, males and females equally, are most often affected. However, cases involving children and adolescents have been reported.

**Related Disorders** See *Pemphigoid, Bullous; Pemphigus.*

**Localized cicatricial pemphigoid (Brunsting-Perry syndrome)** is a chronic scarring disease characterized by blisters on the head and neck that are caused by trauma or other factors.

**Vegetating mucous membrane pemphigoid** combines features of benign mucosal pemphigoid and **pemphigus vegetans** (a variation of **pemphigus vulgaris**). Blisters that are large and fast-growing are usually seen in the axillary and inguinal areas.

**Intermittent mucosal pemphigoid** is characterized by oral blisters that are sparse, occur only intermittently, and heal without forming scars.

**Epidermolysis bullosa acquisita** is an acquired autoimmune skin disorder in which blisters that leave scars occur on the skin of extensor areas, and sometimes the scalp. Eyes may also be affected. There usually is IgG activity around the blisters. Middle-aged and elderly persons are most often affected.

**Treatment—Standard** Treatment is not satisfactory. Topical corticosteroids such as fluocinonide can relieve inflammation and itching, and systemic corticosteroids such as prednisone relieve inflammation and can suppress the immune system. Immunosuppressive drugs such as cyclophosphamide or azathioprine may also be used. Dapsone may be given to relieve inflammation. *All of these drugs require careful monitoring.* Other treatment is symptomatic and supportive.

**Treatment—Investigational** Aldesulfonsodium is being investigated to treat childhood benign mucosal pemphigoid.

Please contact the agencies listed under Resources, below, for the most current information. Addresses and telephone numbers of these agencies, as well as of individual experts and research centers, may be found in the Master Resources List.

### Resources

**For more information on benign mucosal pemphigoid:** National Organization for Rare Disorders (NORD); NIH/National Institute of Arthritis and Musculoskeletal and Skin Diseases Information Clearinghouse.

### References

Dermatology, 3rd ed.: S.L. Moschella and H.J. Hurley, eds.; W.B. Saunders Company, 1992.

Textbook of Dermatology, 5th ed.: R.H. Champion, et al., eds.; Blackwell Scientific Publications, 1992.

Dermatology, 3rd ed.: O. Braun-Falco, et al.; Springer-Verlag, 1991.

Mucosal Involvement in Bullous and Cicatricial Pemphigoid: A Clinical and Immunopathological Study: V.A. Venning, et al.; Br. J. Dermatol., January 1988, vol. 118(1), pp. 7–15.

Dermatology in General Medicine: Textbook and Atlas, 3rd ed.: T.B. Fitzpatrick, et al., eds.; McGraw-Hill, 1987.

Ocular Cicatricial Pemphigoid with Granular IgG and Complement Deposition: A.D. Proia, et al.; Arch. Ophthalmol., November 1985, vol. 103(11), pp. 1669–1672.

Immunosuppressive Therapy in Ocular Cicatricial Pemphigoid: B.J. Mondino, et al.; Am. J. Opthalmol., October 1983, vol. 96(4), pp. 453–459.

# PEMPHIGOID, BULLOUS

**Description** A chronic, cutaneous, relatively benign blistering disease more common in elderly persons, bullous pemphigoid is marked by generalized subepidermal blisters. It usually subsides spontaneously in several months or years, but it may recur. Infrequently, potentially fatal complications such as pneumonia develop.

**Synonyms**

> Benign Pemphigus
> Old-Age Pemphigus
> Parapemphigus
> Pemphigoid
> Senile Dermatitis Herpetiformis

**Signs and Symptoms** The initial finding is erythema surrounding a lesion, scar, or the umbilicus. Within weeks bullae appear on the flexor surfaces, axillae, abdomen, and groin. The disorder usually spares mucous areas, such as the mouth; when these are affected, healing is rapid. The bullae are sizable and rigid, contain clear or blood-tinged fluid, and do not rupture easily. If rupture occurs, pain may result, but healing is rapid.

The white cell count rises, but the patient is not likely to have fever. Immunofluorescent microscopic examination of the skin reveals subepidermal blisters and binding of IgG to the basement membrane zone. The serum will reveal antibodies directed against the basement membrane in approximately 70 percent of patients. The significance of the antibody titer in relation to the degree of the symptoms is unknown, because titers do not correlate well with disease activity.

**Etiology** The disease is idiopathic; an autoimmune association has been suggested. Certain drug reactions can produce the picture of bullous pemphigoid.

**Epidemiology** Males and females are affected in equal numbers. The disease primarily affects the elderly.

**Related Disorders** See *Pemphigus; Erythema Multiforme; Pemphigoid, Benign Mucosal; Dermatitis Herpetiformis; Epidermolysis Bullosa; Epidermolytic Hyperkeratosis.*

**Treatment—Standard** Corticosteroids reduce the number of lesions, and doses required are lower than those needed in pemphigus. The drug (usually prednisone) can be discontinued in approximately 50 percent of cases because the patients go into remission. The balance of the patients need maintenance therapy. Some patients have a self-limited course and, because many are elderly, decisions about whether to treat with systemic steroids must be individualized.

**Treatment—Investigational** Immunosuppressive agents, e.g., azathioprine and methotrexate, have been used as adjuncts to corticosteroids. Cyclosporine may be useful in bullous pemphigoid.

W.R. Gammon, M.D., of the University of North Carolina, is conducting clinical trials to study possible new therapies for bullous pemphigoid.

Please contact the agencies listed under Resources, below, for the most current information. Addresses and telephone numbers of these agencies, as well as of individual experts and research centers, may be found in the Master Resources List.

**Resources**

**For more information on bullous pemphigoid:** National Organization for Rare Disorders (NORD); NIH/National Arthritis and Musculoskeletal and Skin Diseases Information Clearinghouse.

**References**

Cecil Textbook of Medicine, 19th ed.: J.B. Wyngaarden, et al., eds.; W.B. Saunders Company, 1992, pp. 2282, 2309.

Dermatology, 3rd ed.: S.L. Moschella and H.J. Hurley, eds.; W.B. Saunders Company, 1992.

Mendelian Inheritance in Man, 10th ed.: V.A. McKusick; The Johns Hopkins University Press, 1992, p. 171.

Textbook of Dermatology, 5th ed.: R.H. Champion, et al., eds.; Blackwell Scientific Publications, 1992.

Azathioprine in Dermatology: I.R. Younger, J. Am. Acad. Dermatol., August 1991, vol. 25(2 pt. 1), pp. 281–286.

Bullous Pemphigoid and Cicatricial Pemphigoid: G.J. Anhalt; J. Autoimmun., February 1991, vol. 4(1), pp. 17–35.

Dermatology, 3rd ed.: O. Braun-Falco, et al.; Springer-Verlag, 1991.

Clinical Dermatology, 2nd ed.: T.P. Habif, ed.: C.V. Mosby Company, 1990, pp. 415–416.

Bullous Pemphigoid: N. Korman; J. Am. Acad. Dermatol., May 1987, vol. 16(5 pt. 1), pp. 907–924.

Dermatology in General Medicine: Textbook and Atlas, 3rd ed.: T.B. Fitzpatrick, et al., eds.; McGraw-Hill, 1987.

Mechanism of Lesion Production in Pemphigus and Pemphigoid: W.M. Sams, Jr.; J. Am. Acad. Dermatol., April 1982, vol. 6(4 pt. 1), pp. 431–452.

Internal Disorders Associated with Bullous Disease of the Skin: A Critical Review: J.P. Callen; J. Am. Acad. Dermatol., August 1980, vol. 3(2), pp. 107–119.

# PEMPHIGUS

**Description** Pemphigus encompasses a group of autoimmune skin disorders characterized by the development of blisters in the epidermis and mucous membranes. The location and type of blisters vary according to the type of pemphigus. Untreated, pemphigus is often fatal.

**Signs and Symptoms** Blisters resulting from acantholysis (separation of epidermal cells from one another) are common to all types of pemphigus, explaining the development of intraepidermal blisters. The blisters generally occur on the neck, scalp, mucous membranes, and inguinal and axillary areas, and are usually flaccid. Most patients have deposits of IgG around keratinocytes in skin in the areas of the blisters. Antiepidermal antibodies are present in the serum. Diagnosis requires histologic identification of acantholytic blisters as well as detection of the IgG antibodies.

**Pemphigus vulgaris** may begin with isolated blisters on the scalp, and then in the mouth. These may persist for several months and then be followed by blistering of the skin, esophagus, nose, conjunctiva, and rectum. The blisters are soft, break easily, and heal poorly. Pressure on their borders causes them to spread. Pressure on normal-looking skin causes it to separate (**Nikolsky sign**). **Pemphigus vegetans** is a variation of pemphigus vulgaris. The blisters are large and fast-growing and have hypertrophic lesions that are usually located in the axillary and inguinal areas.

**Pemphigus foliaceus** is less severe and less common. Soft blisters occur closer to the surface of the skin, and when they break they ooze and become crusty, scaly, and susceptible to infection. They may occur on the scalp, face, upper chest, and back, but the mucous membranes are usually spared. Small, horny plugs attached to the undersurface of the affected skin also may be seen. Another type of pemphigus foliaceus occurs in South America, particularly Brazil and Colombia, and is called **fogo selvagem.**

When patients have features of both pemphigus foliaceus and systemic lupus erythematosus, they are said to have **pemphigus erythematosus.** Pemphigus may occur as an adverse reaction to drugs such as D-penicillamine and rifampin, with symptoms resembling those of pemphigus foliaceus rather than pemphigus vulgaris. Some research indicates that **pemphigus herpetiformis** is a discrete form of pemphigus with its own characteristic blisters, but blisters that form during a relapse may resemble those of pemphigus foliaceus.

In **benign familial pemphigus (Hailey-Hailey disease),** recurrent blisters are seen primarily on the neck, groin, and axillae. Precipitating factors include heat, sweating, skin infection, and ultraviolet radiation.

**Etiology** Most forms of pemphigus are generally considered to be autoimmune-related. Benign familial pemphigus (Hailey-Hailey disease) is inherited as an autosomal dominant trait.

Fogo selvagem (Brazilian pemphigus foliaceus) is an autoimmune disorder with blistering that is thought to be triggered by a substance transmitted by the bite of blackflies.

Pemphigus may also occur following x-ray exposure or as an adverse reaction to drugs such as D-penicillamine or rifampin.

**Epidemiology** Pemphigus is most common in the middle-aged and elderly, but cases involving children have been observed. It has been found in all ethnic groups and races, but is more common in persons of Jewish or Mediterranean origin. Pemphigus occurs once in every 100,000 live births, with males and females being affected equally.

Fogo selvagem occurs in Brazil in the central rural areas heavily infested with a species of blackfly.

**Related Disorders** See *Bullous Pemphigoid; Darier Disease; Epidermolysis Bullosa; Epidermolytic Hyperkeratosis; Erythema Multiforme; Dermatitis Herpetiformis.*

**Epidermolysis bullosa acquisita** is an autoimmune disorder affecting the middle-aged and elderly. Injuries may cause blisters on the skin of extensor areas such as hands, elbows, knees, pelvis, and buttocks, and on the scalp. Increased levels of IgG are usually found around the blisters, and scars remain after healing. Circulating antibasement membrane zone antibodies are commonly found.

**Treatment—Standard** Corticosteroids are widely used for treating pemphigus. Topical corticosteroids can relieve inflammation and itching, and systemic corticosteroids such as prednisone relieve inflammation and suppress the immune system.

Immunosuppressive drugs such as cyclosporine, cyclophosphamide, azathioprine, or methotrexate may be prescribed. Cytotoxic drugs are used to suppress the immune system. Gold compounds such as auranofin may be given to relieve inflammation and, possibly, to suppress the immune system. Dapsone is also given. *These drugs should be used with extreme caution.* To reduce immediate or long-term side effects, drug therapy may have to be stopped temporarily or changed.

Antibiotic drugs or creams may be given to manage infection and relieve inflammation. Silver sulfadiazine cream also may be used. Dusting the patient and the bedsheets with talcum powder may relieve the discomfort of raw skin. Other treatment is symptomatic and supportive. Genetic counseling may be beneficial for patients with hereditary pemphigus, and their families.

**Treatment—Investigational** Two methods of plasmapheresis are under investigation, as is the use of extracorporeal photopheresis.

Please contact the agencies listed under Resources, below, for the most current information. Addresses and telephone numbers of these agencies, as well as of individual experts and research centers, may be found in the Master Resources List.

**Resources**

**For more information on pemphigus:** National Organization for Rare Disorders (NORD); NIH/National Arthritis and Musculoskeletal and Skin Diseases Information Clearinghouse.

**For genetic information and genetic counseling referrals:** March of Dimes Birth Defects Foundation; Alliance of Genetic Support Groups.

**References**

Cecil Textbook of Medicine, 19th ed.: J.B. Wyngaarden, et al.; W.B. Saunders Company, 1992, p. 2309.

Dermatology, 3rd ed.: S.L. Moschella and H.J. Hurley, eds.; W.B. Saunders Company, 1992.

Mendelian Inheritance in Man, 10th ed.: V.A. McKusick; The Johns Hopkins University Press, 1992, pp. 835–836.

Textbook of Dermatology, 5th ed.: R.H. Champion, et al., eds.; Blackwell Scientific Publications, 1992.

Dermatology, 3rd ed.: O. Braun-Falco, et al.; Springer-Verlag, 1991.

Birth Defects Encyclopedia: M.L. Buyse, ed.-in-chief; Blackwell Scientific Publications, 1990, pp. 1373–1374.

Clinical Dermatology, 2nd ed.: T.P. Habif, ed.: C.V. Mosby Company, 1990, pp. 415–415.

The Pathogenic Effect of IgG 4 Autoantibodies in Endemic Pemphigus Foliaceus (Fogo Selvagem): J. Terblanche, et al.; N. Engl. J. Med., June 1989, vol. 320(22), pp. 1463–1469.

Pemphigus: N. Korman; J. Am. Acad. Dermatol., June 1988, vol. 18(6), pp. 1219–1238.

Dermatology in General Medicine: Textbook and Atlas, 3rd ed.: T.B. Fitzpatrick, et al., eds.; McGraw-Hill, 1987.

Dermatologic Clinics: The Genodermatoses: J.C. Alper, ed.; W.B. Saunders Company, 1987, vol. 5(1), pp. 160–161, 171–173.

Internal Medicine, 2nd ed.: J.H. Stein, ed.-in-chief; Little, Brown and Company, 1987, pp. 1368–1372.

# PITYRIASIS RUBRA PILARIS (PRP)

**Description** PRP is a chronic skin disorder characterized by pruritus and numerous coalescent, perifollicular papules that increase in size and eventually connect, producing large red scaling plaques.

**Signs and Symptoms** The follicular papules are itchy, sharply pointed, hornlike, and brownish red to rosy yellow or salmon in color. They usually occur on the scalp, axillae, forearms, elbows, wrists, hands, fingers, and knees. Over time the papules increase in size and connect, resulting in large dry, scaly, rough red plaques. Islands of normal skin may be present in so-called "skip" areas. Palms and soles may be severely affected with scaling. The nails may be gray and brittle and the scalp seborrheic. Ectropion of the eyelids may be present. The course can be limited to a few weeks or months or prolonged for many years. PRP can usually be distinguished from psoriasis.

**Etiology** The cause is unknown. An autosomal dominant inheritance is suspected in some families. An acquired form of the disease may be associated with a deficiency of vitamin A. Some cases are exacerbated by exposure to light.

**Epidemiology** Males and females of all ages are affected equally.

**Related Disorders** Symptoms of lichen planus, psoriasis, and pityriasis rosea may be similar to those of PRP.

**Treatment—Standard** Some cases resolve with only topical lubricants and topical corticosteroids. Patients with PRP may respond to treatment with oral vitamin A. Phototherapy must be considered cautiously because light exacerbates some cases.

**Treatment—Investigational** The disease has been treated successfully with retinoid drugs such as isotretinoin, and the antineoplastic drug methotrexate, but these agents must be used cautiously because of their toxic side effects.

Research on PRP is being conducted at New York University Medical Center. For information please contact Irwin M. Freedberg, M.D.

Please contact the agencies listed under Resources, below, for the most current information. Addresses and telephone numbers of these agencies, as well as of individual experts and research centers, may be found in the Master Resources List.

**Resources**

**For more information on pityriasis rubra pilaris:** National Organization for Rare Disorders (NORD); Foundation for Ichthyosis and Related Skin Types; NIH/National Institute of Arthritis and Musculoskeletal and Skin Diseases Information Clearinghouse.

**For genetic information and genetic counseling referrals:** March of Dimes Birth Defects Foundation; Alliance of Genetic Support Groups.

**References**

Dermatology, 3rd ed.: S.L. Moschella and H.J. Hurley, eds.; W.B. Saunders Company, 1992.

Textbook of Dermatology, 5th ed.: R.H. Champion, et al., eds.; Blackwell Scientific Publications, 1992.

Dermatology, 3rd ed.: O. Braun-Falco, et al.; Springer-Verlag, 1991.

Childhood-Onset Pityriasis Rubra Pilaris with Immunologic Abnormalities: D. Shvili, et al.; Pediatr. Dermatol., May 1987, vol. 4(1), pp. 21–23.

Dermatology in General Medicine: Textbook and Atlas, 3rd ed.: T.B. Fitzpatrick, et al., eds.; McGraw-Hill, 1987.

Isotretinoin Treatment of Pityriasis Rubra Pilaris: C.H. Dicken; J. Am. Acad. Dermatol., February 1987, vol. 16(2 pt. 1), pp. 297–301.

Pityriasis Rubra Pilaris, Vitamin A and Retinol-Binding Protein: A Case Study: P.C. van Voorst Vader, et al.; Acta Derm. Venereol. (Stockh.), 1984, vol. 64(5), pp. 430–432.

# PSEUDOXANTHOMA ELASTICUM (PXE)

**Description** Pseudoxanthoma elasticum describes a group of inherited connective tissue disorders involving the skin, eyes, and cardiovascular system.

**Synonyms**
> Elastosis Dystrophica Syndrome
> Groenblad-Strandberg Syndrome
> Systemic Elastorrhexis of Touraine

**Signs and Symptoms** Plaques and papules appear most often on the face and neck and in the axillary, antecubital, and inguinal areas. These areas are yellow or white in color. They thicken and become inelastic because of the connective tissue abnormalities. Skin folds may droop, and the surface resembles the plucked skin of a chicken. Retinal angioid streaks may be evident, and retinal hemorrhage and vision loss may develop. Vascular changes include peripheral, coronary, and cerebral arterial calcification and occlusion, which may be apparent on x-rays early in the course, even though other symptoms may appear years later. The condition is progressive, but in many cases progression is slow.

**Etiology** The cause is unknown. There is a generalized abnormality in elastic tissue with fragmentation in skin, eye, and vessels. Autosomal recessive inheritance is the most common pattern observed, although a dominant pattern has also been described.

**Epidemiology** The disease affects approximately 1:100,000 persons worldwide. It is estimated that there are 2,500 cases in the United States.

**Treatment—Standard** Only symptomatic treatment is available.

General therapeutic strategies include regular exercise, weight control, and avoidance of smoking, aspirin, and excessive calcium. Activities likely to cause head trauma (e.g., rough sports) should be avoided because of the danger of retinal bleeding.

Cosmetic surgery may be useful for improving the appearance of the skin. Laser coagulation may be required for retinal hemorrhage. Genetic counseling is recommended for patients and families.

**Treatment—Investigational** Please contact the agencies listed under Resources, below, for the most current information. Addresses and telephone numbers of these agencies, as well as of individual experts and research centers, may be found in the Master Resources List.

**Resources**

**For more information on pseudoxanthoma elasticum:** National Organization for Rare Disorders (NORD); National Association of Pseudoxanthoma Elasticum; NIH/National Arthritis and Musculoskeletal and Skin Diseases Information Clearinghouse; NIH/National Eye Institute.

**For information on clinical facilities:** Mark Lebwohl, M.D., Mount Sinai School of Medicine; Kenneth H. Nelder, M.D., Texas Tech University Health Sciences Center.

**For genetic information and genetic counseling referrals:** March of Dimes Birth Defects Foundation; Alliance of Genetic Support Groups.

**References**

Dermatology, 3rd ed.: S.L. Moschella and H.J. Hurley, eds.; W.B. Saunders Company, 1992.

Textbook of Dermatology, 5th ed.: R.H. Champion, et al., eds.; Blackwell Scientific Publications, 1992.

Dermatology, 3rd ed.: O. Braun-Falco, et al.; Springer-Verlag, 1991.

Cecil Textbook of Medicine, 18th ed.: J.B. Wyngaarden and L.H. Smith, Jr., eds.; W.B. Saunders Company, 1988, pp. 1181–1182.

Dermatology in General Medicine: Textbook and Atlas, 3rd ed.: T.B. Fitzpatrick, et al., eds.; McGraw-Hill, 1987.

# PYODERMA GANGRENOSUM

**Description** Pyoderma gangrenosum is an ulcerative skin disease of unknown etiology. It is not caused by cutaneous bacterial or other infection. It may occur sporadically alone or as a severe complication of one of a variety of underlying diseases.

**Signs and Symptoms** Pyoderma gangrenosum is characterized by an extremely painful, ulcerative, purplish skin lesion that may rapidly expand to 20 cm in size. The ulcers most frequently develop on the legs but may appear anywhere on the body. They can appear at sites of trauma (pathergy). Biopsy of these lesions reveals nonspecific inflammation; therefore the diagnosis of pyoderma gangrenosum is largely one of exclusion.

**Etiology** The cause is not known; an autoimmune etiology is suspected. Approximately 50 percent of all cases are idiopathic. The remainder are associated with an underlying disease; ulcerative colitis and Crohn disease are the most common. In these cases, the course of the skin lesion usually parallels the course of the bowel disease, but appearance during remission does occur. Other disorders associated with pyoderma gangrenosum include rheumatoid arthritis, chronic active hepatitis, and various hematologic malignancies such as acute and chronic myelogenous leukemia, polycythemia vera, and myeloma.

**Epidemiology** Males and females are affected equally. The disease is least common in children and most common in middle-aged women.

**Related Disorders** The ulcers of pyoderma gangrenosum may resemble those seen in necrotizing vasculitis, spider bites (such as those of the brown recluse spider), and certain deep fungal diseases.

**Treatment—Standard** Treatment is not satisfactory. Debridement, wet dressings, and topical application of disodium cromoglycate or zinc sulfate may be helpful. The skin must be protected from trauma, which could result in development of other ulcers. In severe cases, systemic steroids, antibiotics, and antimetabolites may be indicated.

**Treatment—Investigational** Thalidomide and clofazamine are being tested for treatment of pyoderma gangrenosum. Thalidomide, especially, is contraindicated in pregnancy because it causes severe birth defects. For information on the use of thalidomide, contact Pediatric Pharmaceutical.

Please contact the agencies listed under Resources, below, for the most current information. Addresses and telephone numbers of these agencies, as well as of individual experts and research centers, may be found in the Master Resources List.

**Resources**

**For more information on pyoderma gangrenosum:** National Organization for Rare Disorders (NORD); NIH/National Arthritis and Musculoskeletal and Skin Diseases Information Clearinghouse.

**For information about colitis or Crohn disease:** Crohn and Colitis Foundation of America.

**References**

Dermatology, 3rd ed.: S.L. Moschella and H.J. Hurley, eds.; W.B. Saunders Company, 1992.
Textbook of Dermatology, 5th ed.: R.H. Champion, et al., eds.; Blackwell Scientific Publications, 1992.
Dermatology, 3rd ed.: O. Braun-Falco, et al.; Springer-Verlag, 1991.
Dermatology in General Medicine: Textbook and Atlas, 3rd ed.: T.B. Fitzpatrick, et al., eds.; McGraw-Hill, 1987.
Internal Medicine, 2nd ed.: J.H. Stein, ed.-in-chief; Little, Brown and Company, 1987, pp. 1390–1392.
Pyoderma Gangrenosum Associated with Ulcerative Colitis: Treatment with Disodium Cromoglycate: D.R. Cave, et al.; Am. J. Gastroenterol., August 1987, vol. 82(8), pp. 802–804.
Pustular Pyoderma Gangrenosum Associated with Ulcerative Colitis in Childhood: Report of Two Cases and Review of the Literature: L. Barnes, et al.; J. Am. Acad. Dermatol., October 1986, vol. 15(4 pt. 1), pp. 608–614.
Pyoderma Gangrenosum Complicating Ulcerative Colitis: Successful Treatment with Methylprednisolone Pulse Therapy and Dapsone: E. Galun, et al.; Am. J. Gastroenterol., October 1986, vol. 81(10), pp. 988–989.

# SJÖGREN-LARSSON SYNDROME

**Description** Sjögren-Larsson syndrome is a rare autosomal recessive inherited disorder characterized by ichthyosis, ocular and speech abnormalities, seizures, spastic diplegia, and mental retardation.

**Signs and Symptoms** Onset of symptoms usually is in infancy. There is variably severe erythroderma accompanied by fine scales on the neck and lower abdomen; larger, thicker, platelike scales may appear later in infancy, developing into dark, nonerythematous lesions, especially in the flexures of the arms and legs. Speech abnormalities, mental retardation, and seizures usually begin in the first 2 or 3 years of life. Glistening spots in the fundus may be an early sign of the disorder. About half of patients have retinal pigmentary degeneration. Patients may be short in stature.

The syndrome can be detected in utero.

**Etiology** Sjögren-Larsson syndrome is transmitted through autosomal recessive genes. It is due to a deficiency of the enzyme fatty alcohol NAD oxidoreductase.

**Epidemiology** The syndrome occurs in approximately 8.3:100,000 persons in northern Sweden. It is less prevalent in the United States. Males and females are affected in equal numbers, and all races are affected.

**Related Disorders** See *Ichthyosis Congenita; Ichthyosis Hystrix, Curth-Macklin Type; Ichthyosis, Lamellar Recessive; Ichthyosis, X-Linked; Darier Disease; Epidermolytic Hyperkeratosis.*

**Treatment—Standard** Cutaneous symptoms can be alleviated by application of keratolytics and emollients, including plain petroleum jelly. This can be especially effective after bathing while the skin is still moist. Salicylic acid gel is useful in some instances for removal of scales. Lactate lotion can also be an effective keratolytic. Topical and systemic retinoids can be beneficial in some cases but must be used with caution because of adverse side effects.

Anticonvulsant medications may be needed to control seizures. Speech therapy and special education services may be helpful. Other treatment is symptomatic and supportive.

**Treatment—Investigational** Clinical improvement has been reported following limitation of dietary fat to medium-chain triglycerides.

Monolaurin (glylorin) is being tested for treatment of Sjögren-Larsson syndrome. The product is manufactured by Cellegy Pharmaceuticals.

The National Institute of Arthritis and Musculoskeletal and Skin Diseases is seeking ichthyosis patients to participate in a study aimed at mapping the genes responsible for the various forms of the disease. For more information, contact Sherri Bale, M.D.

Please contact the agencies listed under Resources, below, for the most current information. Addresses and telephone numbers of these agencies, as well as of individual experts and research centers, may be found in the Master Resources List.

**Resources**

**For more information on Sjögren-Larsson syndrome:** National Organization for Rare Disorders (NORD); Foundation for Ichthyosis and Related Skin Types; The Arc (a national organization on mental retardation); NIH/National Arthritis and Musculoskeletal and Skin Diseases Information Clearinghouse.

**For genetic information and genetic counseling referrals:** March of Dimes Birth Defects Foundation; Alliance of Genetic Support Groups.

**References**

Dermatology, 3rd ed.: S.L. Moschella and H.J. Hurley, eds.; W.B. Saunders Company, 1992.

Textbook of Dermatology, 5th ed.: R.H. Champion, et al., eds.; Blackwell Scientific Publications, 1992.

Dermatology, 3rd ed.: O. Braun-Falco, et al.; Springer-Verlag, 1991.

Mendelian Inheritance in Man, 9th ed.: V.A. McKusick; The Johns Hopkins University Press, 1990, p. 1478.

Sjögren-Larsson Syndrome: W.B. Rizzo, et al.; J. Clin. Invest., 1988, vol. 81, p. 738.

Dermatology in General Medicine: Textbook and Atlas, 3rd ed.: T.B. Fitzpatrick, et al., eds.; McGraw-Hill, 1987.

Genetically Transmitted, Generalized Disorders of Cornification: The Ichthyoses: M.L. Williams, et al.; Dermatol. Clin., January 1987, vol. 5(1), pp. 155–178.

Therapeutic Activity of Lactate 12% Lotion in the Treatment of Ichthyosis: Active Versus Vehicle and Active Versus a Petroleum Cream: M. Buxman, et al.; J. Am. Acad. Dermatol., December 1986, vol. 15(6), pp. 1253–1258.

Treatment of the Ichthyosis of the Sjögren-Larsson Syndrome with Etretinate (Tigason): S. Jagell, et al.; Acta Derm. Venereol. (Stockh.), 1983, vol. 63(1), pp. 89–91.

# SWEET SYNDROME

**Description** Sweet syndrome is a rare skin disorder characterized by the explosive appearance of multiform, painful erythematous lesions on the skin of the arms, face, neck, and legs, accompanied by fever and malaise.

**Synonyms**

Febrile Neutrophilic Dermatosis, Acute

**Signs and Symptoms** Malaise and other constitutional complaints including high fever accompany the widespread painful skin lesions. These may be up to 1 inch in diameter and are usually bluish red, sharply demarcated, indurated, and circular, and may be flat or raised. Tiny blisters or bacteria-free pustules may cover the plaques. Central clearing associated with a trailing collarette of scale is sometimes noted. Scarring may appear, especially in infants.

Sweet syndrome is usually preceded by a systemic febrile, infectious, or other inflammatory illness. Histologically, there is a massive neutrophilic infiltration in the dermis. A high ESR and leukocytosis with a predominance of neutrophils are present. Remission may occur after a few weeks, but recurrences are possible.

**Etiology** The cause is not known; an allergic reaction to an unknown infectious agent is often suspected. Leukemia may be associated, as may a skin injury such as vaccination or a scrape. An upper respiratory or skin infection may precede by 1 to 3 weeks the precipitation of the syndrome.

**Epidemiology** Sweet syndrome is seen most often in middle-aged females, but men, children, and infants have been affected in rare cases.

**Related Disorders** See *Erythema Multiforme; Leiner Disease.*

**Erythema elevatum diutinum** (possibly a variant of erythema multiforme) is a rare, chronic skin disorder usually seen in adults between ages 30 and 60. It may be associated with recurrent polyarthritis and is characterized by symmetrical nodules and plaques near the joints and on the backs of the hands and feet. The size of the lesions may vary over the course of a day.

**Treatment—Standard** Systemic corticosteroid drugs may produce dramatic improvement, but the syndrome may go into spontaneous remission after a few weeks without treatment.

**Treatment—Investigational** Dapsone has been used experimentally to treat the syndrome, but more research is needed to determine safety and effectiveness.

Please contact the agencies listed under Resources, below, for the most current information. Addresses and telephone numbers of these agencies, as well as of individual experts and research centers, may be found in the Master Resources List.

**Resources**

**For more information on Sweet syndrome:** National Organization for Rare Disorders (NORD); NIH/National Arthritis and Musculoskeletal and Skin Diseases Information Clearinghouse.

**References**

Dermatology, 3rd ed.: S.L. Moschella and H.J. Hurley, eds.; W.B. Saunders Company, 1992.

Textbook of Dermatology, 5th ed.: R.H. Champion, et al., eds.; Blackwell Scientific Publications, 1992.

Dermatology, 3rd ed.: O. Braun-Falco, et al.; Springer-Verlag, 1991.

Dermatology in General Medicine: Textbook and Atlas, 3rd ed.: T.B. Fitzpatrick, et al., eds.; McGraw-Hill, 1987.

Sweet's Syndrome: Histological and Immunohistochemical Study of 15 Cases: J.J. Going, et al.; J. Clin. Pathol., February 1987, vol. 40(2), pp. 175–179.

Acute Febrile Neutrophilic Dermatosis: Sweet's Syndrome: M.A. Bechtel, et al.; Arch. Dermatol., October 1981, vol. 117(10), pp. 664–666.

Skin Signs of Systemic Disease: I.M. Braverman; W.B. Saunders Company, 1981.

Acute Febrile Neutrophilic Dermatosis: Sweet's Syndrome: H. Chmel, et al.; South. Med. J., November 1978, vol. 71(11), pp. 1350–1352.

# TAY SYNDROME

**Description** Tay syndrome is a hereditary disorder characterized by erythroderma and ichthyosis, sparse and brittle hair, delayed physical development, mental retardation, and the look of progeria.

**Synonyms**

Congenital Ichthyosis with Trichothiodystrophy

Ichthyosiform Erythroderma with Hair Abnormality and Growth and Mental Retardation

Trichothiodystrophy with Congenital Ichthyosis

**Signs and Symptoms** Erythroderma may be present at birth.

Ichthyosis, characterized by fine, dark scales, covers most of the body. The hair (**trichothiodystrophy**) and nails are sulfur-deficient; the hair is sparse and brittle and the finger- and toenails dysplastic. Facial features include a beaked nose, receding chin, and protruding ears. Loss of subcutaneous fat results in a prematurely aged-looking face.

Low birth weight, short stature, and mental retardation are typical, and there may be an increased susceptibility to infection. Central nervous system abnormalities include neurosensory deafness, seizures, tremors, and ataxia. Cryptorchidism may be seen in males, and female genitalia may be underdeveloped. In women, normal nipple development may occur with absence of other breast tissue. Small cataracts and bone and teeth abnormalities may be found.

**Etiology** The syndrome is transmitted through autosomal recessive genes.

**Epidemiology** Abnormalities are usually present at birth. Males and females are affected in equal numbers.

**Related Disorders** See *Ichthyosis Congenita; Ichthyosis, Lamellar Recessive; Netherton Syndrome.*

**Amish brittle hair syndrome (hair-brain syndrome)** usually is found in persons of Amish descent. It is characterized by brittle hair, intellectual impairment, decreased fertility, and short stature. The condition lacks the skin and facial abnormalities of Tay syndrome.

**Pollitt syndrome (trichorrhexis nodosa syndrome)** is characterized by microcephaly, mental and physical retardation, and fragile hair (trichorrhexis nodosa). The skin is usually scaly and the nails are underdeveloped and spoon-shaped.

**Treatment—Standard** The discomfort of the dry, scaly skin can be alleviated by application of keratolytics and emollients, including plain petroleum jelly. This can be especially effective after bathing while the skin is still moist.

Salicylic acid gel is useful in some instances for removal of scales. Lactate lotion can also be an effective keratolytic. Topical and systemic retinoids can be beneficial in some cases, but must be used with caution.

Other treatment is symptomatic and supportive. Genetic counseling may be beneficial.

**Treatment—Investigational** Monolaurin (glylorin) is being tested for treatment of Tay syndrome. The product is manufactured by Cellegy Pharmaceuticals.

The National Institute of Arthritis and Musculoskeletal and Skin Diseases is seeking ichthyosis patients to participate in a study aimed at mapping the genes responsible for the various forms of the disease. For more information, contact Sherri Bale, M.D.

Please contact the agencies listed under Resources, below, for the most current information. Addresses and telephone numbers of these agencies, as well as of individual experts and research centers, may be found in the Master Resources List.

**Resources**

**For more information on Tay syndrome:** National Organization for Rare Disorders (NORD); Foundation for Ichthyosis and Related Skin Types; National Arthritis and Musculoskeletal and Skin Diseases Information Clearinghouse; International Tremor Foundation.

**For genetic information and genetic counseling referrals:** March of Dimes Birth Defects Foundation; Alliance of Genetic Support Groups.

**References**

Dermatology, 3rd ed.: S.L. Moschella and H.J. Hurley, eds.; W.B. Saunders Company, 1992.

Textbook of Dermatology, 5th ed.: R.H. Champion, et al., eds.; Blackwell Scientific Publications, 1992.

Dermatology, 3rd ed.: O. Braun-Falco, et al.; Springer-Verlag, 1991.

Mendelian Inheritance in Man, 9th ed.: V.A. McKusick; The Johns Hopkins University Press, 1990, p. 1272.

Dermatology in General Medicine: Textbook and Atlas, 3rd ed.: T.B. Fitzpatrick, et al., eds.; McGraw-Hill, 1987.

Genetically Transmitted, Generalized Disorders of Cornification: The Ichthyoses: M.L. Williams, et al.; Dermatol. Clin., January 1987, vol. 5(1), pp. 155–178.

The Tay Syndrome (Congenital Ichthyosis with Trichothiodystrophy): R. Happle, et al.; Eur. J. Pediatr., January 1984, vol. 141(3), pp. 147–152.

# TOXIC EPIDERMAL NECROLYSIS (TEN)

**Description** TEN is characterized by severe epidermal erythema, blisters, and peeling. Onset can occur at any age. The cause is most often a drug reaction.

**Synonyms**

    Acute Toxic Epidermolysis

    Dermatitis Exfoliativa

    Scalded Skin Syndrome

**Signs and Symptoms** The first apparent signs of TEN are intense redness and marked skin tenderness followed by large, easily broken blisters. Slight injury or even touching can cause large sheets of skin to peel. The mucous membranes may also be involved. The condition usually progresses rapidly and within a few days may be severe. Up to 40 percent of cases are fatal. Loss of skin barrier may lead to sepsis; fluid loss may result in dehydration. Usually the skin heals without scarring, but scars resembling those of burns can develop when the skin begins to heal.

**Etiology** The disease is believed to be the result of a drug reaction. Many drugs have been associated, including multiple antibiotics, phenytoin, sulfonamides, and barbiturates.

**Epidemiology** Males and females are affected in equal numbers.

**Related Disorders** See *Epidermolysis Bullosa; Stevens-Johnson Syndrome.*

**Treatment—Standard** Treatment is similar to therapy for severe burns. Contact with peeled skin surface should be minimal. Hospitalization with isolation may be necessary, and ongoing fluid and electrolyte replacement may be needed to correct severe fluid and protein loss. If the disease is caused by a drug reaction, systemic corticosteroids may control the reaction but do not seem to alleviate the skin symptoms. Septicemia and pulmonary infections should be anticipated. Other therapy is symptomatic and supportive.

**Treatment—Investigational** Plasmapheresis may be of benefit in cases caused by a severe reaction to drugs, but the procedure is still investigational. Research is under way in the areas of new wound-healing drugs, antibiotics, and inhibition of blister formation.

Please contact the agencies listed under Resources, below, for the most current information. Addresses and telephone numbers of these agencies, as well as of individual experts and research centers, may be found in the Master Resources List.

**Resources**

**For more information on toxic epidermal necrolysis:** National Organization for Rare Disorders (NORD); NIH/National Arthritis and Musculoskeletal and Skin Diseases Information Clearinghouse; Dystrophic Epidermolysis Bullosa Research Association of America; Dystrophic Epidermolysis Bullosa Research Association (U.K.).

**For information on clinical facilities:** University of Washington School of Medicine, St. Louis, Missouri; Rockefeller University, New York, New York; Children's Hospital, Philadelphia, Pennsylvania; University of Pennsylvania, Philadelphia, Pennsylvania.

**References**

Dermatology, 3rd ed.: S.L. Moschella and H.J. Hurley, eds.; W.B. Saunders Company, 1992.

Textbook of Dermatology, 5th ed.: R.H. Champion, et al., eds.; Blackwell Scientific Publications, 1992.

Dermatology, 3rd ed.: O. Braun-Falco, et al.; Springer-Verlag, 1991.

Dermatology in General Medicine: Textbook and Atlas, 3rd ed.: T.B. Fitzpatrick, et al., eds.; McGraw-Hill, 1987.

Improved Burn Center Survival of Patients with Toxic Epidermal Necrolysis Managed Without Corticosteroids: P.H. Halebian, et al.; Ann. Surg., November 1986, vol. 204(5), pp. 503–512.

Plasmapheresis in Severe Drug-Induced Toxic Epidermal Necrolysis: D. Kamanabroo, et al.; Arch. Dermatol., December 1985, vol. 121(12). pp. 1548–1549.

# URTICARIA PIGMENTOSA

**Description** Urticaria pigmentosa is the name of a cutaneous form of mastocytosis, a disorder of excessive mast cell proliferation. Urticaria pigmentosa is generally benign and self-limiting.

**Synonyms**

Infantile Mastocytosis

**Signs and Symptoms** Reddish-brown, pruritic macules and papules appear on the epidermis overlying dermal collections of mast cells. Lesions may rarely be present in bone or other organs. The skin lesions become urticarial when they are rubbed or exposed to heat. Sometimes lesions are bullous. Other symptoms of mastocytosis include headache, malaise, flushing, abdominal pain, and diarrhea, but these are uncommon in urticaria pigmentosa.

**Etiology** The etiology is not known. The symptoms are those of release of histamine and other vasodilatory substances from the mast cell infiltrates.

**Epidemiology** Onset is generally during the first year of life. Lesions usually disappear by adolescence. Males and females are affected in equal numbers.

**Related Disorders** See ***Mastocytosis,*** in which there is multisystem mast cell infiltration.

**Treatment—Standard** Treatment is symptomatic and supportive. Topical steroids may be useful, as may antihistamines given systemically. Symptomatic urticaria pigmentosa has been treated with oral disodium cromoglycate, cimetidine (sometimes combined with chlorpheniramine or propantheline), and with ketotifen.

**Treatment—Investigational** Please contact the agencies listed under Resources, below, for the most current information. Addresses and telephone numbers of these agencies, as well as of individual experts and research centers, may be found in the Master Resources List.

**Resources**

**For more information on urticaria pigmentosa:** National Organization for Rare Disorders (NORD); Mastocytosis Chronicles; NIH/National Arthritis and Musculoskeletal and Skin Diseases Information Clearinghouse.

**References**

Cecil Textbook of Medicine, 19th ed.: J.B. Wyngaarden, et al., eds.; W.B. Saunders Company, 1992, p. 1456.

Mendelian Inheritance in Man, 10th ed.: V.A. McKusick; The Johns Hopkins University Press, 1992, p. 700.

Nelson Textbook of Pediatrics, 14th ed.: R.E. Behrman, ed.-in-chief; W.B. Saunders Company, 1992, pp. 600, 1662–1663.

Textbook of Dermatology, 5th ed.: R.H. Champion, et al., eds.; Blackwell Scientific Publications, 1992, pp. 2067–2071.

Blistering Disorders in Childhood: L.F. Eichenfield, et al.; Pediatr. Clin. North Am., August 1991, vol. 38(4), pp. 959–976.

Dermatology, 3rd ed.: O. Braun-Falco, et al.; Springer-Verlag, 1991.

Harrison's Principles of Internal Medicine, 12th ed.: J.D. Wilson, et al., eds.: McGraw-Hill, 1991, pp. 332, 335, 1426.

The Skin in Mastocytosis: N.A. Soter; J. Invest. Dermatol., March 1991, vol. 96(3), pp. 32S–38S, discussion 38S–39S.

Urticaria Pigmentosa: Systemic Evaluation and Successful Treatment with Topical Steroids: C. Guzzo, et al.; Arch. Dermatol., February 1991, vol. 127(2) pp. 191–196.

Birth Defects Encyclopedia: M.L. Buyse, ed.-in-chief; Blackwell Scientific Publications, 1990, pp. 1737–1738.

Dictionary of Medical Syndromes, 3rd ed.: S.I. Magalini, et al., eds.; J.B. Lippincott Company, 1990, pp. 629–630.

Histamine Release from Skin Mast Cells and Basophils in Patients with Urticaria Pigmentosa: H. Nolte, et al.; Acta Derm. Venereol., 1990, vol. 70(2), pp. 154–156.

Urticaria Pigmentosa: Histaminuria and Treatment: A.I. Tabar, et al.; Allergol. Immunopathol. (Madr.), March–April 1990, vol. 18(2), pp. 101–103.

Dermatology in General Medicine: Textbook and Atlas, 3rd ed.: T.B. Fitzpatrick, et al., eds.; McGraw-Hill, 1987.

# VITILIGO

**Description** Vitiligo is an acquired disorder characterized by an absence of melanocytes, which results in decreased or absent pigmentation in patches of skin. Vitiliginous patches may be localized or widespread.

**Synonyms**

> White Spot Disease

**Signs and Symptoms** The areas of absent pigmentation appear white under a Wood's light. They are usually sharply demarcated and symmetrical in shape, and typically appear on the face, neck, axillae, elbows, hands, knees, and feet, although they can occur anywhere on the skin. They are common around body orifices. The hair in affected areas may be white. The depigmented lesions burn easily in the sun and should be protected by application of sunscreens.

**Etiology** The cause is unknown. Vitiligo is sometimes familial, although the exact mode of inheritance is not determined. The disorder is 10 to 15 times more common in patients with autoimmune diseases and has been associated with pernicious anemia, Addison disease, hypothyroidism, and alopecia areata. Organ-specific antibodies have recently been detected in patients with vitiligo, indicating that destruction of melanocytes may have an immune basis. The disorder also is associated with head trauma. Vitiligo sometimes is associated with melanoma, and patients should be screened for these malignant tumors.

**Epidemiology** Onset is usually before age 20.

**Treatment—Standard** Small lesions may be camouflaged with cosmetic creams. Topical corticosteroids are sometimes effective for localized patches. Broad-spectrum sunscreens protect against sunburn. For larger areas of involvement, patients may use psoralen photochemotherapy (PUVA), with systemic psoralens administered orally followed by exposure to UV-A from sunlight or an artificial source.

The agent benoquin (SPI Pharmaceuticals, Costa Mesa, CA) is being reintroduced for use as a depigmenting drug in cases of vitiligo.

**Treatment—Investigational** Please contact the agencies listed under Resources, below, for the most current information. Addresses and telephone numbers of these agencies, as well as of individual experts and research centers, may be found in the Master Resources List.

**Resources**

**For more information on vitiligo:** National Organization for Rare Disorders (NORD); National Vitiligo Foundation; Frontier's International Vitiligo Foundation; National Foundation for Vitiligo and Pigment Disorders; NIH/National Arthritis and Musculoskeletal and Skin Diseases Information Clearinghouse.

**References**

Dermatology, 3rd ed.: S.L. Moschella and H.J. Hurley, eds.; W.B. Saunders Company, 1992.

Textbook of Dermatology, 5th ed.: R.H. Champion, et al., eds.; Blackwell Scientific Publications, 1992.

Dermatology, 3rd ed.: O. Braun-Falco, et al.; Springer-Verlag, 1991.

Harrison's Principles of Internal Medicine, 12th ed.: J.D. Wilson, et al., eds.; McGraw-Hill, 1991, pp. 326–328.

Mendelian Inheritance in Man, 9th ed.: V.A. McKusick; The Johns Hopkins University Press, 1990, p. 969.

Cecil Textbook of Medicine, 18th ed.: J.B. Wyngaarden and L.H. Smith, Jr., eds.; W.B. Saunders Company, 1988, pp. 2344–2345.

Dermatology in General Medicine: Textbook and Atlas, 3rd ed.: T.B. Fitzpatrick, et al., eds.; McGraw-Hill, 1987.

# WEBER-CHRISTIAN DISEASE

**Description** Weber-Christian disease is characterized by recurrent febrile episodes with formation of nonsuppurating subcutaneous fat nodules.

**Synonyms**

> Nodular Nonsuppurative Panniculitis
>
> Pfeiffer-Weber-Christian Syndrome

**Signs and Symptoms** Onset of Weber-Christian disease usually is gradual, with nodules appearing in the subcutaneous tissue of the arms, legs, thighs, buttocks, and abdomen. The overlying skin usually is erythematous. Accompanying symptoms may include fever, enlargement of the spleen and lymph nodes, malaise, sore throat, chills, nausea, and anemia, and pain in the joints, muscles, or abdomen. Symptoms may subside spontaneously after days or weeks, but may recur weeks, months, or years later.

**Etiology** The cause is unknown; allergic factors may be involved, or a predisposition of fatty tissue to a granulomatous reaction. Weber-Christian disease must be differentiated from similar nodular lesions associated with diabetes mellitus, systemic lupus erythematosus, subacute bacterial endocarditis, tuberculosis, iodide and bromide therapy, withdrawal from large doses of corticosteroids, and pancreatitis.

**Epidemiology** Weber-Christian disease most often affects adult women, usually between the ages of 20 and 40 years.

**Related Disorders** See *Mesenteritis, Retractile.*

**Treatment—Standard** Treatment is symptomatic and supportive. If the disorder is associated with an underlying condition, treatment of that disorder can alleviate the symptoms of Weber-Christian disease.

**Treatment—Investigational** Treatment with oral cyclophosphamide has shown some promise in preliminary clinical trials. Thalidomide is being tested as a treatment, although this drug must not be taken by pregnant women. Physicians wishing to test thalidomide as a treatment for this disorder may contact Pediatric Pharmaceutical.

Please contact the agencies listed under Resources, below, for the most current information. Addresses and telephone numbers of these agencies, as well as of individual experts and research centers, may be found in the Master Resources List.

**Resources**

**For more information on Weber-Christian disease:** National Organization for Rare Disorders (NORD); NIH/National Arthritis and Musculoskeletal and Skin Diseases Information Clearinghouse; NIH/National Institute of Allergy and Infectious Diseases.

**References**

Dermatology, 3rd ed.: S.L. Moschella and H.J. Hurley, eds.; W.B. Saunders Company, 1992.

Textbook of Dermatology, 5th ed.: R.H. Champion, et al., eds.; Blackwell Scientific Publications, 1992.

Dermatology, 3rd ed.: O. Braun-Falco, et al.; Springer-Verlag, 1991.

Dermatology in General Medicine: Textbook and Atlas, 3rd ed.: T.B. Fitzpatrick, et al., eds.; McGraw-Hill, 1987.

Cyclophosphamide-Induced Remission in Weber-Christian Panniculitis: W. Kirch, et al.; Rheumatol. Int., 1985, 5(5), pp. 239–240.

# WELLS SYNDROME

**Description** Wells syndrome is characterized by raised, red, swollen, and warm areas of skin with associated pain.

**Synonyms**

Eosinophilic Cellulitis

Granulomatous Dermatitis with Eosinophilia

**Signs and Symptoms** The skin develops raised, swollen, red areas on the trunk and limbs. The episodes are usually of rapid onset. Skin blistering has also been known to develop. Often Wells syndrome will recur spontaneously after a period of years, with swelling and redness developing for no apparent reason. An attack may last up to 6 weeks. Large areas of skin may be affected. Microscopic studies reveal characteristic flame figures and an abnormal number of eosinophils in the red and swollen areas of skin, underlying fat, and blood.

**Etiology** Wells syndrome sometimes occurs as an exaggerated response to bites of arthropods (spiders, bees, fleas, ticks, or mites), or it may have other causes, such as surgery, fungal infections, parastic infections, or drugs. There may be an autoimmune basis for the disorder.

**Epidemiology** Wells syndrome affects males and females of all ages in equal numbers.

**Related Disorders** See *Anaphylaxis.*

In **cellulitis,** the skin becomes red, swollen, and painful over a large area. There may be accompanying chills and fever. This disorder can be caused by Group A β-hemolytic streptococci, or in older persons it is sometimes caused by Group G streptococci.

**Contact dermatitis** is an inflammatory reaction in the skin in response to irritants and allergens. It is marked by inflamed skin and, possibly, blisters at the site of contact with an offending agent. If acute, the area may be edematous, crusty, scaly, and exudative. The patient complains of burning pain and, as a rule, pruritus.

**Treatment—Standard** Steroids may be administered. However, the disorder often resolves itself after several weeks. Other treatment is symptomatic and supportive.

**Treatment—Investigational** Please contact the agencies listed under Resources, below, for the most current information. Addresses and telephone numbers of these agencies, as well as of individual experts and research centers, may be found in the Master Resources List.

**Resources**

**For more information on Wells syndrome:** National Organization for Rare Disorders (NORD); NIH/Institute of Allergy and Infectious Diseases.

**References**

Clinical Dermatology, 2nd ed.: T.P. Habif, ed.: C.V. Mosby Company, 1990, pp. 189–194.

Wells Syndrome, Insect Bites, and Eosinophils: J.W. Melski: Dermatol. Clin., April 1990, vol. 8(2), pp. 287–293.

Eosinophilic Infiltration with Flame Figures: A Distinctive Tissue Reaction Seen in Wells Syndrome and Other Diseases: C. Wood, et al.; Am. J. Dermatopathol, June 1986, vol. 8(3), pp. 186–193.

Eosinophilic Cellulitis (Wells Syndrome): G.B. Fisher, et al.; Int. J. Dermatol., March 1985, vol. 24(2), pp. 101–107.

# XERODERMA PIGMENTOSUM

**Description** Xeroderma pigmentosum is a rare skin disorder that begins during early childhood. It is characterized by photosensitivity to sunlight and the early development of hyper- and hypopigmentation in exposed skin. Cutaneous malignancies are common, and patients have numerous basal cell and squamous cell carcinomas as well as melanomas.

**Signs and Symptoms** The first sign of xeroderma pigmentosum is severe infantile photosensitivity followed by extensive freckling in exposed skin. Telangiectasia as well as diffuse hyper- and hypopigmentation appears in the exposed skin.

Malignancies of the skin may occur before age 5, and the face and skin may appear old. Growth retardation, short stature, neurologic dysfunction, and mental retardation may occur in some persons.

Ocular findings include photophobia, excessive lacrimation, keratitis, corneal opacities, and tumors of the eyelid or cornea.

**Etiology** The disorder is transmitted as an autosomal recessive trait. Several forms exist, but each is caused by impaired excisional repair of photo-damaged DNA. Thymine dimer excision is defective in most forms of xeroderma pigmentosum, as is repair of chemically induced DNA damage.

**Epidemiology** Xeroderma pigmentosum affects approximately 1:100,000 persons, and there are an estimated 250,000 cases in the United States. Children of both sexes may be affected as early as the first year of life.

**Related Disorders** See *Malignant Melanoma.*

**Treatment—Standard** Total protection of the skin from sunlight is necessary for patients with xeroderma pigmentosum to prevent the development of additional skin lesions. In some cases surgery has been performed with limited success. Other treatment is symptomatic and supportive.

**Treatment—Investigational** Application of a catalase cream appears to prevent tumors in some children. Ointments containing vitamin A derivatives are also being investigated. Isotretinoin has been shown to reduce the recurrence of tumors, but the drug is very toxic and many patients find the side effects intolerable. T4 endonuclease V.B. liposome encapsulated (T4N5) is an orphan drug being used to prevent the skin cancers and other skin abnormalities of xeroderma pigmentosum. The drug is available from Applied Genetics.

Please contact the agencies listed under Resources, below, for the most current information. Addresses and telephone numbers of these agencies, as well as of individual experts and research centers, may be found in the Master Resources List.

**Resources**

**For more information on xeroderma pigmentosum:** National Organization for Rare Disorders (NORD); Xeroderma Pigmentosum Registry; The Skin Cancer Foundation; NIH/National Cancer Institute Physician Data Query Phoneline; NIH/National Arthritis and Musculoskeletal and Skin Diseases Information Clearinghouse.

**For genetic information and genetic counseling referrals:** March of Dimes Birth Defects Foundation; Alliance of Genetic Support Groups.

**References**

Dermatology, 3rd ed.: S.L. Moschella and H.J. Hurley, eds.; W.B. Saunders Company, 1992.

Textbook of Dermatology, 5th ed.: R.H. Champion, et al., eds.; Blackwell Scientific Publications, 1992.

Dermatology, 3rd ed.: O. Braun-Falco, et al.; Springer-Verlag, 1991.

Dermatology in General Medicine: Textbook and Atlas, 3rd ed.: T.B. Fitzpatrick, et al., eds.; McGraw-Hill, 1987.

Microinjection of Human Cell Extracts Corrects Xeroderma Pigmentosum Defect: A.J. de Jonge, et al.; EMBO J., 1983, vol. 2(5), pp. 637–641.

Skin Signs of Systemic Disease: I.M. Braverman; W.B. Saunders Company, 1981.

Xeroderma Pigmentosum, Defective DNA Repair—and Schistosomiasis?: J. German; Ann. Gen., Paris 1980, vol. 23(2), pp. 69–72.

# 8 | GASTROINTESTINAL DISORDERS
## By William F. Balistreri, M.D.

There are a number of rare disorders that can affect various portions of the gastrointestinal tract, including disorders of the upper and lower intestine, the liver, and the pancreas. The clinical consequences primarily relate to altered digestion and metabolism. These disorders may present with malabsorption and, therefore, failure to thrive or weight loss. Watery diarrhea may be a manifestation of disorders of carbohydrate transport; the degree of severity can range from troublesome to life-threatening. Chronic blood loss from the gastrointestinal tract may be seen in polyposis syndromes.

Disorders that affect the liver may present with mild degrees of unconjugated hyperbilirubinemia that have little consequence (e.g., Gilbert syndrome). However, a severe form of unconjugated hyperbilirubinemia (Crigler-Najjar syndrome) is life-threatening, with relentless accumulation of bilirubin and the development of kernicterus and death without liver transplantation. The presence of conjugated hyperbilirubinemia (cholestasis) is never benign—this always indicates hepatobiliary dysfunction. Cholestasis is the presenting sign of biliary atresia.

Recognition of these rare disorders of the gastrointestinal tract is important, since certain ones are responsive to specific or supportive therapy. Patients with achalasia will be cured with dilatation or surgical myotomy. Persons with Budd-Chiari syndrome can be recognized by the development of hepatomegaly, often with ascites; surgical therapy is required. The recognition of gluten-sensitive enteropathy (celiac sprue) will allow the institution of a gluten-free diet, which will (1) reverse the gut injury; (2) allow for more effective absorption of dietary nutrients; and (3) decrease the potential for malignant degeneration. The malignant potential of the familial polyposis syndromes and Gardner syndrome must also be recognized so that early, aggressive surgery can be performed.

Early detection of biliary atresia is also critical, since the successful establishment of bile flow is dependent upon the age at which surgical drainage is performed. Prompt diagnosis of Hirschsprung disease is also imperative because delayed discovery can result in abdominal distention and poor weight gain, with the potential complication of toxic megacolon with perforation and death. Patients with Caroli disease, plagued by persistent cholangitis with infection of the dilated biliary ductal system, may benefit from early, aggressive antibiotic therapy.

Eosinophilic gastroenteritis is a poorly understood disorder; it may, however, respond to dietary or steroid therapy. Patients with inborn errors of carbohydrate transport, such as glucose-galactose malabsorption and sucrase-isomaltase deficiency, will require restriction of the offending carbohydrate from the diet, thereby diminishing the diarrhea.

Patients with intestinal pseudo-obstruction can present with a lifelong history of constipation, and while no effective therapy has yet been defined, palliative procedures are available.

# GASTROINTESTINAL DISORDERS
*Listings in This Section*

# ACHALASIA

**Description** A motor disorder of the esophagus, achalasia is distinguished by dilation of the esophagus, impaired peristalsis, and failure to relax the lower esophageal sphincter.

**Synonyms**

>Cardiospasm
>Dyssynergia Esophagus
>Esophageal Aperistalsis
>Megaesophagus

**Signs and Symptoms** Onset is gradual. Patients are likely to complain of dysphagia and of chest pain, which may range from transient discomfort to overwhelming agony. Gastric contents may be regurgitated or may enter the tracheobronchial tree. Nighttime regurgitation is reported in approximately one-third of cases. Significant weight loss may occur in untreated cases. A nocturnal cough may also be present.

Pneumonia, pulmonary infections, and strangulation can occur from aspiration of the esophageal contents. Esophageal carcinoma occurs in approximately 5 percent of cases.

Radiology is often useful in diagnosis, as dilation of the esophagus and retention of food, secretions, and barium can be seen. Manometric examination may also be useful. Pharmacologic stimulation and endoscopy are not advised.

**Etiology** The cause of achalasia is not known. The condition may be caused by degeneration of Auerbach's plexus. In some cases, it may be inherited as an autosomal recessive genetic trait.

**Epidemiology** While achalasia affects mainly adults between the ages of 20 and 40, the disorder may occur at any age. Achalasia affects males and females in equal numbers, except in those cases that are thought to be inherited. In familial cases of achalasia, males are twice as likely to be diagnosed with this disorder.

**Treatment—Standard** Treatment is directed at removing the obstruction caused by failure of the lower esophageal sphincter to relax. This may be done pharmacologically, manipulatively, or surgically.

Isosorbide, a long-acting nitrate, or nifedipine, a calcium channel blocker, may provide some relief.

Balloon dilation aimed at the lower esophageal sphincter, effective in about 85 percent of cases, can be complicated by bleeding and perforation. The success rate of Heller myotomy, in which the muscular fibers in the lower esophageal sphincter are cut, is also about 85 percent.

**Treatment—Investigational** Please contact the agencies listed under Resources, below, for the most current information. Addresses and telephone numbers of these agencies, as well as of individual experts and research centers, may be found in the Master Resources List.

**Resources**

**For more information on achalasia:** National Organization for Rare Disorders (NORD); NIH/National Digestive Diseases Information Clearinghouse.

**For genetic information and genetic counseling referrals:** March of Dimes Birth Defects Foundation; Alliance of Genetic Support Groups.

**References**

Achalasia: New Thoughts on an Old Disease: C.M. Farr; J. Clin. Gastroentrol., July 1992, vol. 15(1), pp. 2–4.

Cecil Textbook of Medicine, 19th ed.: J.B. Wyngaarden, et al., eds.; W.B. Saunders Company, 1992, pp. 643–646.

Mendelian Inheritance in Man, 10th ed.: V.A. McKusick; The Johns Hopkins University Press, 1992, pp. 92–94.

Primary Treatment of Esophageal Achalasia: Long-Term Results of Myotomy and/or Fundoplication: L. Bonavina; Arch. Surg., February 1992, vol. 127(2), pp. 222–226.

Harrison's Principles of Internal Medicine, 12th ed.: J.D. Wilson, et al., eds.; McGraw-Hill, 1991, pp. 1224–1225.

Birth Defects Encyclopedia: M.L Buyse, ed.-in-chief; Blackwell Scientific Publications, 1990, p. 641.

# ALAGILLE SYNDROME

**Description** Alagille syndrome, a genetic liver disorder, is characterized by insufficient bile flow due to a congenital paucity of intrahepatic bile ducts.

**Synonyms**

>Arteriohepatic Dysplasia
>Cholestasis with Peripheral Pulmonary Stenosis
>Intrahepatic Bile Duct Paucity
>Syndromatic Hepatic Ductular Hypoplasia

**Signs and Symptoms** Jaundice is usually present at birth. The hepatic malformation is accompanied by other anomalies, including structural abnormalities of the eye, cardiac valve and arterial malformations, and abnormally shaped (butterfly) vertebrae. Facial characteristics include a broad forehead, a straight nose with a bulbous tip, deep-set eyes spaced widely apart, and a pointed jaw. Fingers may be short. Symptoms can range from mild to severe.

**Etiology** The syndrome is thought to be inherited as an autosomal dominant trait.

**Epidemiology** Alagille syndrome is a rare disorder that frequently occurs in more than one person in a family and in many generations of an affected family.

**Related Disorders** See *α-1-Antitrypsin Deficiency; Zellweger Syndrome.*

**Cholestasis-lymphedema syndrome** is a genetic disorder characterized by impaired bile flow and jaundice at birth, which tends to recur throughout life. Hypoplasia of lymph vessels results in edema of the legs, usually at 5 or 6 years of age.

**Byler disease (progressive familial intrahepatic cholestasis)** is an inherited liver disorder with an early onset. It is characterized by loose, foul-smelling stools, jaundice, hepatomegaly, splenomegaly, and short stature.

**Treatment—Standard** Treatment of Alagille syndrome is symptomatic and supportive. Genetic counseling is recommended for patients and their families.

**Treatment—Investigational** Ursodeoxycholic acid is being studied as therapy for patients with Alagille syndrome by William F. Balistreri, M.D., Children's Hospital Medical Center, Cincinnati, OH.

Please contact the agencies listed under Resources, below, for the most current information. Addresses and telephone numbers of these agencies, as well as of individual experts and research centers, may be found in the Master Resources List.

**Resources**

**For more information on Alagille syndrome:** National Organization for Rare Disorders (NORD); Alagille Syndrome Alliance; American Liver Foundation; United Liver Association; Children's Liver Foundation; The Arc (a national organization on mental retardation); NIH/National Digestive Diseases Information Clearinghouse.

**For genetic information and genetic counseling referrals:** March of Dimes Birth Defects Foundation; Alliance of Genetic Support Groups.

**References**

Mendelian Inheritance in Man, 9th ed.: V.A. McKusick; The Johns Hopkins University Press, 1990, p. 187.

Arteriohepatic Dysplasia (Alagille Syndrome): Extreme Variability Among Affected Family Members: S.A. Shulman, et al.; Am. J. Med. Genet.; October 1984, vol. 19(2), pp. 325–332.

Possible Defect in the Bile Secretory Apparatus in Arteriohepatic Dysplasia (Alagille's Syndrome): A Review with Observations on the Ultrastructure of Liver: P. Valencia-Mayoral, et al.; Hepatology, July–August 1984, vol. 4(4), pp. 691–698.

# BILIARY ATRESIA

**Description** The most common form of extrahepatic biliary atresia is the closure of bile ducts near the porta hepatis; distal biliary atresia is much less common.

**Signs and Symptoms** Signs of biliary atresia (jaundice, pale stools, dark urine, and hepatomegaly) usually are not evident until the infant is 2 weeks old. Within 6 to 10 weeks, however, certain features may have developed: irritability (from itchiness), growth delay, and portal hypertension.

Other abnormalities that may be present in children with biliary atresia include renal and cardiac malformations. Asplenia or polysplenia may also be present.

Liver biopsy, laparotomy, and cholangiography are used in diagnosis.

**Etiology** The etiology is unknown.

**Epidemiology** The incidence is 1:10,000 to 1:15,000 live births. Males and females are both affected.

**Related Disorders** See *Hepatitis, Neonatal,* in which the intrahepatic bile ducts are underdeveloped, unlike the extrahepatic abnormality seen in biliary atresia.

**Treatment—Standard** The type of surgical repair performed, including Kasai hepatoportoenterostomy, depends on the type and area of abnormality found. Even with successful surgical intervention, some hepatic dysfunction may remain. The Kasai procedure may be used as an early intermediate procedure to support the child's growth until liver transplantation is feasible.

**Treatment—Investigational** Please contact the agencies listed under Resources, below, for the most current information. Addresses and telephone numbers of these agencies, as well as of individual experts and research centers, may be found in the Master Resources List.

**Resources**

**For more information on biliary atresia:** National Organization for Rare Disorders (NORD); American Liver Foundation; United Liver Association; Children's Liver Foundation; NIH/National Digestive Diseases Information Clearinghouse.

**For genetic information and genetic counseling referrals:** March of Dimes Birth Defects Foundation; Alliance of Genetic Support Groups.

### References

MR Imaging of Biliary Cysts in Children with Biliary Atresia: Clinical Associations and Pathologic Correlation: B.W. Betz, et al.; Am. J. Roentgenol., January 1994, vol. 162(1), pp. 167–171.

Biliary Atresia Splenic Malformation Syndrome: An Etiologic and Prognostic Subgroup: M. Davenport, et al.; Surgery, June 1993, vol. 113(6), pp. 662–668.

Extrahepatic Biliary Atresia and Associated Anomalies: Etiologic Heterogeneity Suggested by Distinctive Patterns of Associations: R. Carmi, et al.; Am. J. Med. Genet., March 15, 1993, vol. 45(6), pp. 683–693.

Imaging in the Pediatric Liver Transplantation: S.J. Westra, et al.; Radiographics, September 1993, vol. 13(5), pp. 1081–1089.

Cecil Textbook of Medicine, 19th ed.: J.B. Wyngaarden, et al., eds.; W.B. Saunders Company, 1992, pp. 790, 799.

The Efficacy of Kasai Operation for Biliary Atresia: A Single Institutional Experience: J.N. Linn, et al.; J. Pediatr. Surg., June 1992, vol. 27(6), pp. 704–706.

Mendelian Inheritance in Man, 10th ed.: V.A. McKusick; The Johns Hopkins University Press, 1992, p. 1251.

Nelson Textbook of Pediatrics, 14th ed.: R.E. Behrman, ed.-in-chief; W.B. Saunders Company, 1992, pp. 1009–1012.

Familial Biliary Atresia in Three Siblings Including Twins: B.M. Smith, et al.; J. Pediatr. Surg., November 1991, vol. 26(1), pp. 1131–1133.

Harrison's Principles of Internal Medicine, 12th ed.: J.D. Wilson, et al., eds.; McGraw-Hill, 1991, p. 1356, 1365.

Neonatal Hepatitis and Extrahepatic Biliary Atresia Associated with Cytomegalovirus Infection in Twins: M.H. Hart, et al.; Am. J. Dis. Child., March 1991, vol. 145(3), pp. 302–305.

Biliary Atresia and Its Complications: A.S. Knisely; Ann. Clin. Lab. Sci., March–April 1990, vol. 29(2), pp. 540–542.

Birth Defects Encyclopedia: M.L Buyse, ed.-in-chief; Blackwell Scientific Publications, 1990, pp. 223–224.

Biliary Atresia: E.R. Howard, et al.; Br. J. Hosp. Med., February 1989, vol. 41(2), pp. 123–124, 128–130.

Gastrointestinal Disease, 4th ed.: M.H. Sleisenger, et al.; W.B. Saunders Company, 1989, pp. 1639–1640.

# BUDD-CHIARI SYNDROME

**Description** Budd-Chiari syndrome is a rare hepatic vascular disorder characterized by abnormal enlargement of the liver due to occlusion of the major hepatic veins. The obstruction usually results from thrombosis or congenital webs that form at the junction of the hepatic veins and the inferior vena cava.

**Synonyms**

      Hepatic Veno-Occlusive Disease

      Rokitansky Disease

**Signs and Symptoms** Abdominal pain is common and usually accompanied by ascites, edema of the legs, and mild jaundice. Hepatomegaly is present. Hemoglobinuria also may be observed. When the obstruction is severe, onset of the disorder can be sudden and acute. The chronic form of Budd-Chiari syndrome is characterized by an insidious onset and less severe pain; liver enlargement occurs gradually. The associated portal hypertension that develops causes impaired liver function and serious liver damage.

Routine biochemical testing is of little diagnostic value. Liver biopsy tests can reveal central cell deterioration, development of fibrous growths, and occlusion of the terminal hepatic veins.

**Etiology** In about 70 percent of cases, the cause of the blockage is due to an underlying disorder. The syndrome can be associated with hypercoagulable states (polycythemia vera or another myeloproliferative disorder; oral contraceptives, or pregnancy), or with a tumor in the inferior vena cava. Other potential causes include exposure to radiation and arsenic, trauma, sepsis, certain chemotherapy drugs, and, in some parts of the world, drinking a beverage made from pyrrolidizine plant alkaloids (bush tea).

**Epidemiology** Males and females are equally affected. Patients between the ages of 20 and 40 years tend to be most susceptible.

**Related Disorders** Lesions of the hepatic artery or of the hepatic venous system may produce symptoms similar to those of Budd-Chiari syndrome.

**Treatment—Standard** Treatment depends on the underlying disorder and the location and extent of the occlusion. Diagnostic procedures such as x-ray, CT scanning, MRI, and ultrasound are useful for this purpose. Liver biopsy reveals changes in cell structure. Therapeutic choices include medical treatment of ascites, angioplasty, shunting, and, in some cases, liver transplantation.

**Treatment—Investigational** Please contact the agencies listed under Resources, below, for the most current information. Addresses and telephone numbers of these agencies, as well as of individual experts and research centers, may be found in the Master Resources List.

**Resources**

**For more information on Budd-Chiari syndrome:** National Organization for Rare Disorders (NORD); American Liver Foundation; United Liver Association; Children's Liver Foundation; NIH/National Digestive Diseases Information Clearinghouse.

**References**

Internal Medicine, 3rd ed.: J.H. Stein, ed.-in-chief; Little, Brown and Company, 1990, pp. 516–517.

Comparison of Ultrasonography, Computed Tomography and 99mTc Liver Scan in Diagnosis of Budd-Chiari Syndrome: S. Gupta, et al.; Gut, March 1987, vol. 38(3), pp. 242–247.

Treatment of the Budd-Chiari Syndrome with Percutaneous Transluminal Angioplasty: Case Report and Review of the Literature: J. Sparano, et al.; Am. J. Med., April 1987, vol. 82(4), pp. 821–828.

Results of Portal Systemic Shunts in Budd-Chiari Syndrome: C. Vons, et al.; Ann. Surg., April 1986, vol. 203(4), pp. 366–370.

# CAROLI DISEASE

**Description** In Caroli disease the intrahepatic bile ducts are characterized by segmental cystic dilatation. Complications often occur and include stone formation, recurrent cholangitis, and hepatic abscesses.

**Synonyms**

Acute Cholangitis

Congenital Dilatation of Intrahepatic Bile Ducts

**Signs and Symptoms** Abdominal pain, sepsis, fever, and jaundice occur in individuals with Caroli disease. Symptoms may manifest in childhood or as late as the 6th decade of life.

**Etiology** This rare disorder is believed to result from abnormal prenatal development of the intrahepatic bile ducts. Caroli disease may be associated with cystic disease of the kidney or other organs.

**Epidemiology** Males are affected by Caroli disease more often than females.

**Related Disorders Benign tumors of the extrahepatic bile ducts,** including papillomas, adenomas, fibroadenomas, adenomyomas, leiomyomas, granular cell myoblastomas, neurinomas, and hamartomas, may occur. Surgical removal of the neoplasm is the appropriate treatment.

**Carcinoma of the extrahepatic bile ducts,** although rare, may occur.

**Helminthiasis of the bile ducts** caused by the parasite *Ascaris lumbricoides* has been reported worldwide. Helminthiasis of the bile ducts caused by the parasite *C. sinensis* occurs almost entirely in the Far East.

**Treatment—Standard** Surgical resection of cysts and removal of stones may be appropriate. Antibiotics and drainage are supportive but are seldom successful treatments. Death may result from gram-negative septicemia.

**Treatment—Investigational** Ursodeoxycholic acid is being studied as a treatment for Caroli disease. Researchers hope that ursodeoxycholic acid will help to reduce the formation of stones in the liver and gallbladder.

Please contact the agencies listed under Resources, below, for the most current information. Addresses and telephone numbers of these agencies, as well as of individual experts and research centers, may be found in the Master Resources List.

**Resources**

**For more information on Caroli disease:** National Organization for Rare Disorders (NORD); NIH/National Digestive Diseases Information Clearinghouse; American Liver Foundation; United Liver Association; Children's Liver Foundation.

**For genetic information and genetic counseling referrals:** March of Dimes Birth Defects Foundation; Alliance of Genetic Support Groups.

**References**

Ursodeoxycholic Acid Treatment of Primary Hepatolithiasis in Caroli's Syndrome: E. Ros, et al.; Lancet, August 1993, vol. 342(8868), p. 404–406.

Internal Medicine, 2nd ed.: J.H. Stein, ed.-in-chief; Little, Brown and Company, 1987, p. 261.

Caroli's Disease: New Diagnostic and Therapeutic Approaches: S. L. Newman, et al.; South. Med. J., December 1986, vol. 79(12), pp. 1587–1590.

Scintigraphic and Radiographic Findings in Caroli's Disease: A.J. Moreno, et al.; Am. J. Gastroenterol., April 1984, vol. 79(4), pp. 299–303.

Successful Treatment of Caroli's Disease by Hepatic Resection: Report of Six Patients: N. Nagasue; Ann. Surg., December 1984, vol. 200(6), pp. 718–723.

# CELIAC SPRUE

**Description** Celiac sprue is an inherited intestinal malabsorption disorder associated with intolerance to gluten.

**Synonyms**

Celiac Disease

Gee-Herter Disease

Gee-Thaysen Disease

Gluten Enteropathy

Huebner-Herter Disease
Nontropical Sprue

**Signs and Symptoms** Symptoms range from severe to mild; celiac sprue can be asymptomatic. Age at onset also varies, with the disease becoming evident in infancy or adulthood.

Affected children from 6 months to 3 years of age may have diarrhea, projectile vomiting, and a bloated abdomen. Growth is retarded. Frequent symptoms in adults include weight loss, chronic fatty diarrhea, abdominal cramping and distention, and myopathy. Food craving, weakness, and fatigue are also common.

In patients with celiac sprue, the intestinal villi are partially or totally absent, and the absorptive surface is flattened or reduced. Symptoms depend on the degree of mucosal damage and the duration of nutrient malabsorption. Vitamin and mineral deficiencies may result in anemia, mucous membrane deterioration, follicular hyperkeratosis, osteomalacia, osteoporosis, decreased blood coagulation, or muscle cramps. Malabsorption of protein, salt, and water can produce dehydration, electrolyte depletion, growth retardation, and edema. Lactose intolerance, peripheral neuropathy, and central nervous system lesions can also occur. Less commonly, dermatitis herpetiformis may be seen. Most patients with dermatitis herpetiformis have some degree of gluten enteropathy, but are only minimally symptomatic.

Difficulty in concentration, decreased mental alertness, and impaired memory may occur. Behavioral changes such as irritability and crankiness may be noted, especially in children. There have even been cases of dementia.
**Etiology** The genetic inheritance is probably dominant with incomplete penetrance. HLA-B8 antigen has been identified in 80 percent of persons with the disease. Typical mucosal abnormalities can appear in healthy siblings of affected persons.
**Epidemiology** Celiac sprue occurs equally in males and females. Although the disorder begins in infancy following exposure to gluten, most commonly it is diagnosed in adulthood.
**Related Disorders** Celiac sprue can be differentiated from **Whipple Disease** and **tropical sprue** by a jejunal biopsy that shows flat or absent villi and by clinical improvement after withdrawal of dietary gluten. People with **Systemic Lupus Erythematosus,** diabetes type I, or **Sjögren Syndrome** have an increased risk of celiac sprue.
**Treatment—Standard** Over 75 percent of patients respond to a gluten-free diet, with symptoms usually improving within weeks. Intestinal histologic improvement may not be evident for months. Appropriate dietary supplementation may be indicated, with fat-soluble vitamins, minerals, and hematinics. Patients who do not respond initially to gluten withdrawal may benefit from limited treatment with oral steroids. Occasionally, antibiotics or pancreatic enzymes are given.
**Treatment—Investigational** Please contact the agencies listed under Resources, below, for the most current information. Addresses and telephone numbers of these agencies, as well as of individual experts and research centers, may be found in the Master Resources List.
**Resources**

**For more information on celiac sprue:** National Organization for Rare Disorders (NORD); Celiac Sprue Association/USA; Gluten Intolerance Group of North America; NIH/National Digestive Diseases Information Clearinghouse; Joseph A. Murray, M.D., Center for Digestive Disease, University of Iowa Hospital and Clinics.

**For genetic information and genetic counseling referrals:** March of Dimes Birth Defects Foundation; Alliance of Genetic Support Groups.
**References**

Cecil Textbook of Medicine, 19th ed.: J.B. Wyngaarden, et al., eds.; W.B. Saunders Company, 1992, pp. 742–743.
Celiac Sprue: J.S. Trier; N. Engl. J. Med., December 12, 1991, vol. 325(24), pp. 1709–1719.
Harrison's Principles of Internal Medicine, 12th ed.: J.D. Wilson, et al., eds.; McGraw-Hill, 1991, pp. 1264–1265.
Nelson Textbook of Pediatrics, 13th ed.: R.E. Behrman, ed.-in-chief; W.B. Saunders Company, 1987, pp. 804–805.

# CRONKHITE-CANADA DISEASE

**Description** Cronkhite-Canada disease is characterized by generalized gastrointestinal polyposis, alopecia, hyperpigmentation, and nail atrophy.
**Synonyms**

Allergic Granulomatous Angiitis
Canada-Cronkhite Disease
Gastrointestinal Polyposis with Ectodermal Changes

**Signs and Symptoms** Polyps composed of dilated cystic glands appear on the walls of the large and small intestines. Alactasia, diarrhea, malabsorption, hypoproteinemia, and intestinal loss of electrolytes occur. Lung involvement, cutaneous lesions, and large ecchymotic plaques may be seen in affected individuals. Approximately 15 percent of affected individuals develop colon cancer.

**Etiology** There is some evidence that this rare disease is hereditary.

**Epidemiology** Middle-aged and elderly women are more frequently affected than men.

**Related Disorders** See *Familial Polyposis; Gardner Syndrome; Peutz-Jeghers Syndrome.*

**Turcot syndrome** is an extremely rare inherited disorder characterized by familial polyposis and tumors of the central nervous system (e.g., medulloblastoma, glioblastoma, or ependymoma). Symptoms may include diarrhea, rectal bleeding, and abdominal discomfort. Neurologic symptoms vary greatly and depend on the type and location of the tumor. Symptoms may include ataxia and impaired speech.

**Treatment—Standard** Medical treatment is not helpful in the management of Cronkhite-Canada disease; surgical removal of polyps or gastric resection may be necessary. Nutritional supplementation or a nutritionally balanced liquid diet may be necessary. Other treatment is symptomatic and supportive.

**Treatment—Investigational** Please contact the agencies listed under Resources, below, for the most current information. Addresses and telephone numbers of these agencies, as well as of individual experts and research centers, may be found in the Master Resources List.

**Resources**

**For more information on Cronkhite-Canada disease:** National Organization for Rare Disorders (NORD); NIH/National Digestive Diseases Information Clearinghouse.

**References**

Complete Remission in Cronkhite-Canada Syndrome: D.M. Russell, et al.; Gastroenterology, July 1993, vol. 85(1), pp. 180–185.

Cronkhite-Canada Syndrome Associated with Colon Cancer: Report of a Case: N. Murai, et al.; Surg. Today, 1993, vol. 23(9), pp. 825–829.

Cecil Textbook of Medicine, 19th ed.: J.B. Wyngaarden, et al., eds.; W.B. Saunders Company, 1992, p. 716.

Mendelian Inheritance in Man, 10th ed.: V.A. McKusick; The Johns Hopkins University Press, 1992, p. 902.

Birth Defects Encyclopedia: M.L Buyse, ed.-in-chief; Blackwell Scientific Publications, 1990, pp. 1400–1401.

Dictionary of Medical Syndromes, 3rd ed.: S.I. Magalini, et al., eds.; J.B. Lippincott Company, 1990, p. 212.

Gastrointestinal Disease, 4th ed.: M.H. Sleisenger, et al.; W.B. Saunders Company, 1989, pp. 489, 1511–1513.

Cronkhite-Canada Syndrome Associated with a Rectal Cancer and Adenomatous Changes in Colonic Polyps: Y. Katayama, et al.; Am. J. Surg. Pathol., January 1985, vol. 9(1), pp. 65–71.

# DUBIN-JOHNSON SYNDROME

**Description** Dubin-Johnson syndrome is a familial chronic form of nonhemolytic jaundice. The presence of a brown, coarsely granular pigment in the centrilobular hepatocytes is pathognomonic of the condition.

**Synonyms**

Chronic Idiopathic Jaundice

Conjugated Hyperbilirubinemia

Hyperbilirubinemia II

**Signs and Symptoms** In individuals affected by Dubin-Johnson syndrome, the liver is deeply pigmented owing to the intracellular presence of a melanin-like substance; otherwise, the organ is histologically normal. Conjugated hyperbilirubinemia occurs, and bile appears in the urine.

**Etiology** The syndrome, probably inherited as an autosomal recessive trait, is thought to result from a defect in the excretion of conjugated bilirubin and certain other organic anions (e.g., sulfobromophthalein) by the liver. Bile salt excretion is not impaired. The cause of pigment deposition in the liver is unknown.

**Epidemiology** Dubin-Johnson syndrome affects males and females in equal numbers. Age at onset of symptoms may be 10 weeks to 56 years. Individuals of Middle Eastern Jewish descent are affected disproportionately to other populations or ethnic groups.

**Related Disorders** See *Primary Biliary Cirrhosis.*

**Rotor syndrome** is a variant of Dubin-Johnson syndrome. Less frequent than Dubin-Johnson, it is also usually mild and involves much the same symptoms. These include occasional pain in the right upper quadrant and mild jaundice. Enlargement of the liver may also occur. The prognosis is generally favorable.

**Treatment—Standard** No treatment may be necessary, although symptomatic and supportive modalities may be appropriate.

**Treatment—Investigational** Please contact the agencies listed under Resources, below, for the most current information. Addresses and telephone numbers of these agencies, as well as of individual experts and research centers, may be found in the Master Resources List.

**Resources**

**For more information on Dubin-Johnson syndrome:** National Organization for Rare Disorders (NORD); American Liver Foundation; United Liver Association; Children's Liver Foundation; NIH/National Digestive Diseases Information Clearinghouse.

**For genetic information and genetic counseling referrals:** March of Dimes Birth Defects Foundation; Alliance of Genetic Support Groups.

**References**
   Mendelian Inheritance in Man, 9th ed.: V.A. McKusick; The Johns Hopkins University Press, 1990, pp. 1253–1254.
   The Metabolic Basis of Inherited Disease, 6th ed.: C.R. Scriver, et al., eds.; McGraw-Hill, 1989, pp. 1391–1408.
   Bile Salt Transport in the Dubin-Johnson Syndrome: J.G. Douglas, et al.; Gut, October 1980, vol. 21(10), pp. 890–893.

# FAMILIAL POLYPOSIS

**Description** Familial polyposis is characterized by initially benign polyps in the mucous lining of the gastrointestinal tract.

**Synonyms**
>   Adenomatous Polyposis of the Colon
>   Intestinal Polyposis I

**Signs and Symptoms** Bleeding and diarrhea are the most common symptoms. Cramping abdominal pain and weight loss may also occur. Chronic rectal bleeding may result in secondary anemia. Untreated patients develop bowel cancer, usually by their late 30s. Some patients are asymptomatic until a malignancy is diagnosed.

   Some affected individuals may also develop desmoids, usually on the neck, head, and upper arms, as well as extracolonic fibromas.

**Etiology** Familial polyposis is inherited through an autosomal dominant gene believed to be on the long arms of chromosome 5 (5q21–q22). The gene may control the manufacture of a cell growth substance.

**Epidemiology** Familial polyposis occurs in 1:5,000 to 1:10,000 individuals and accounts for about 1 percent of colorectal cancers. The greatest incidence of the disorder occurs between ages 20 and 45 years, although diagnosis has been made in teenage patients and in persons older than 45.

**Related Disorders** See *Peutz-Jeghers Syndrome; Gardner Syndrome; Cronkhite-Canada Syndrome.*

   **Turcot syndrome** is an extremely rare inherited disorder characterized by familial polyposis and tumors of the central nervous system (e.g., medulloblastoma, glioblastoma, or ependymoma). Symptoms may include diarrhea, rectal bleeding, and abdominal discomfort. Neurologic symptoms vary greatly and depend on the type and location of the tumor. Symptoms may include ataxia and impaired speech.

**Treatment—Standard** Early diagnosis is important to prevent malignancy. All children and siblings of a patient should undergo lifelong periodic rectal examination from puberty onward. Surgical removal of the colon may prevent cancer. Surgical methods include joining the ileum and rectum and monitoring for rectal polyps, removing the rectum and an ileostomy, removing the lining of the rectum and developing a reservoir from the ileum, and removing the rectum and constructing an internal abdominal pouch with a nipple valve.

**Treatment—Investigational** Please contact the agencies listed under Resources, below, for the most current information. Addresses and telephone numbers of these agencies, as well as of individual experts and research centers, may be found in the Master Resources List.

**Resources**

   **For more information on familial polyposis:** National Organization for Rare Disorders (NORD); Familial Polyposis Registry (for information on national and international familial polyposis and colon cancer registries, please check with NORD); NIH/National Digestive Diseases Information Clearinghouse; American Cancer Society; NIH/National Cancer Institute; United Ostomy Association.

   **For genetic information and genetic counseling referrals:** March of Dimes Birth Defects Foundation; Alliance of Genetic Support Groups.

**References**
   Expression of Hormone Receptors, Cathepsin D, and HER-2/NER Ocoprotein in Normal Colon and Colonic Disease: S. Galandiuk, et al.; Arch. Surg., June 1993, vol. 128(6), pp. 637–642.
   Function of Ileal J Pouch-Anal Anastomosis in Patients with Familial Adenomatous Polyposis: C. Penna, et al.; Br. J. Surg., June 1993, vol. 80(6), pp. 765–767.
   Similar Functional Results After Restorative Proctocolectomy in Patients with Familial Adenomatous Polyposis and Mucosal Ulcerative Colitis: J.J. Tjandra, et al.; Am. J. Surg., March 1993, vol. 165(2), pp. 322–325.
   Cecil Textbook of Medicine, 19th ed.: J.B. Wyngaarden, et al., eds.; W.B. Saunders Company, 1992, pp. 715–716.
   Familial Adenomatous Polyposis: Case Report and Review of Extracolonic Manifestations: K.A. Konsker; Mt. Sinai J. Med., January 1992, vol. 59(1), pp. 85–91.
   Hereditary Colon Cancer Newsletter: Spring 1992, vol. 9(1).
   Mendelian Inheritance in Man, 10th ed.: V.A. McKusick; The Johns Hopkins University Press, 1992, pp. 894–900.
   Overview of Screening and Management of Familial Adenomatous Polyposis: M. Rhodes, et al.; Gut, January 1992, vol. 33(1), pp. 125–131.
   Population Genetics of Colonic Cancer: R.W. Burt, et al.; Cancer, September 1992, vol. 60(6 suppl.), pp. 1719–1722.
   Birth Defects Encyclopedia: M.L Buyse, ed.-in-chief; Blackwell Scientific Publications, 1990, pp. 982–986.
   Dictionary of Medical Syndromes, 3rd ed.: S.I. Magalini, et al., eds.; J.B. Lippincott Company, 1990, p. 465.
   Gastrointestinal Disease, 4th ed.: M.H. Sleisenger, et al.; W.B. Saunders Company, 1989, pp. 1487–1491.

# GARDNER SYNDROME

**Description** Gardner syndrome is a rare variant of familial polyposis of the large bowel, associated with supernumerary teeth, fibrous dysplasia of the skull, osteomas of the skull and mandible, fibromas, and epithelial cysts.

**Synonyms**
>Bone Tumor–Epidermoid Cyst–Polyposis
>Familial Adenomatous Polyposis with Extraintestinal Manifestations
>Intestinal Polyposis III
>Oldfield Syndrome
>Polyposis, Gardner Type
>Polyposis–Osteomatosis–Epidermoid Cyst Syndrome

**Signs and Symptoms** Symptoms generally appear during late childhood or after puberty. Multiple colonic adenomas are accompanied by rectal bleeding, diarrhea or constipation, abdominal pain, and weight loss. Osteomas, soft tissue tumors, and abnormal dentition are evident. Affected individuals have a propensity to develop a variety of extracolonic malignant tumors, and the risk of colon cancer is close to 100 percent. Some patients develop congenital hypertropy of retinal pigment epithelium **(CHRPE).**

**Etiology** The syndrome is inherited as an autosomal dominant trait. The responsible gene has been located on the long arm of chromosome 5 (5q21–22q).

**Epidemiology** Approximately 1:15,000 people in the United States are affected by this disorder, males and females in equal number. Symptoms usually begin at the age of 20 but have been known to appear in infancy or old age.

**Related Disorders** See *Familial Polyposis; Peutz-Jeghers Syndrome; Cronkhite-Canada Disease.*

**Turcot syndrome** is an extremely rare inherited disorder characterized by familial polyposis and tumors of the central nervous system (e.g., medulloblastoma, glioblastoma, or ependymoma). Symptoms may include diarrhea, rectal bleeding, and abdominal discomfort. Neurologic symptoms vary greatly and depend on the type and location of the tumor. Symptoms may include ataxia and impaired speech.

**Treatment—Standard** Cancer prevention is the major goal in Gardner syndrome. Resection of the colon and rectum or ileoproctostomy may be necessary. New polyps must be excised or fulgurated.

**Treatment—Investigational** Researchers are investigating the use of the nonsteroidal anti-inflammatory drug sulindac (Clinoril) in the treatment of intestinal polyps associated with Gardner syndrome.

Please contact the agencies listed under Resources, below, for the most current information. Addresses and telephone numbers of these agencies, as well as of individual experts and research centers, may be found in the Master Resources List.

**Resources**

**For more information on Gardner syndrome:** National Organization for Rare Disorders (NORD); NIH/National Digestive Diseases Information Clearinghouse; Familial Polyposis Registry; United Ostomy Association; American Cancer Society; NIH/National Cancer Institute; NIH/National Cancer Institute Physician Data Query Phoneline.

**For genetic information and genetic counseling referrals:** March of Dimes Birth Defects Foundation; Alliance of Genetic Support Groups.

**References**
Disappearance of Duodenal Polyps in Gardner's Syndrome with Sulindac Therapy: A.L. Parker, et al.; Am. J. Gastroenterol., January 1993, vol. 88(1), pp. 93–94.

Cecil Textbook of Medicine, 19th ed.: J.B. Wyngaarden, et al., eds.; W.B. Saunders Company, 1992, pp. 715–716.

Mendelian Inheritance in Man, 10th ed.: V.A. McKusick; The Johns Hopkins University Press, 1992, p. 897.

Effective Chemotherapy for Abdominal Desmoid Tumor in a Patient with Gardner's Syndrome: Report of a Case: A. Kitamura, et al.; Dis. Colon Rectum, September 1991, vol. 34(9), pp. 822–826.

Extracolonic Manifestations of the Familial Adenomatous Polyposis Syndromes: R.K. Harned, et al.; Am. J. Roentgenol., March 1991, vol. 156(3), pp. 481–485.

Birth Defects Encyclopedia: M.L Buyse, ed.-in-chief; Blackwell Scientific Publications, 1990, pp. 984–985.

Dictionary of Medical Syndromes, 3rd ed.: S.I. Magalini, et al., eds.; J.B. Lippincott Company, 1990, p.337.

Gastrointestinal Disease, 4th ed.: M.H. Sleisenger, et al.; W.B. Saunders Company, 1989, pp. 1504–1507.

The Metabolic Basis of Inherited Disease, 6th ed.: C.R. Scriver, et al., eds.; W.B. Saunders Company, 1989, p. 362.

# GASTRITIS, GIANT HYPERTROPHIC

**Description** Giant hypertrophic gastritis is a chronic disorder distinguished by the presence of large coiled ridges or folds, which may resemble polyps, in the stomach's inner wall. Inflammation may or may not occur.

**Synonyms**

>   Ménétrier Disease
>
>   Protein-Losing Gastroenteropathy

**Signs and Symptoms** The most obvious clinical manifestation is pain or discomfort, accompanied by tenderness, in the upper middle region of the abdomen. Associated symptoms are anorexia, nausea, vomiting, diarrhea, and, in 40 percent of cases, hematemesis. Less frequently, ulcerlike pains are reported following eating.

If protein seeps into the abdominal cavity, hypoproteinuria and edema result. Because the risk of gastric carcinoma may be increased in patients with this condition, periodic examination is necessary.

Biopsy or x-rays, and sometimes endoscopy, are generally necessary for differential diagnosis.

**Etiology** The cause is unknown. There is some indication that in extremely rare cases, the disorder may be inherited as an autosomal dominant genetic trait.

**Epidemiology** The disorder usually affects adults between the ages of 30 and 60 years, though a childhood variety has been described. Men are affected more often than women.

**Related Disorders** See *Gastric Lymphoma, Non-Hodgkin Type; Cronkhite-Canada Syndrome; Amyloidosis.*

**Gastric carcinoma** is often associated with giant hypertrophic gastritis. The 3rd most commonly occurring gastrointestinal cancer in the United States, gastric carcinoma is characterized by a distended stomach, enlarged gastric folds, obstructing lesions, and an ulcerated mass in the stomach. It generally affects men over 50 and persons who consume foods high in salt and nitrates rather than a diet high in vegetables and fresh fruits.

**Treatment—Standard** A high-protein diet, anticholinergic drugs, and acid blockers may correct hypoproteinemia. Gastric resection is rarely necessary.

**Treatment—Investigational** Octreotide may be useful in reducing protein loss associated with giant hypertrophic gastritis.

Please contact the agencies listed under Resources, below, for the most current information. Addresses and telephone numbers of these agencies, as well as of individual experts and research centers, may be found in the Master Resources List.

**Resources**

**For more information on giant hypertrophic gastritis:** National Organization for Rare Disorders (NORD); NIH/National Digestive Diseases Information Clearinghouse.

**References**

Menetrier's Disease: A Form of Hypertrophic Gastropathy or Gastritis?: H.C. Wolfsen, et al.; Gastroenterology, May 1993, vol. 104(5), pp. 1310–1319.

Octreotide Reduces Enteral Protein Losses in Menetrier's Disease: P. Yeaton, et al.; Am. J. Gastroenterol., January 1993, vol. 88(1), pp. 95–98.

Cecil Textbook of Medicine, 19th ed.: J.B. Wyngaarden, et al., eds.; W.B. Saunders Company, 1992, pp. 651–652.

Mendelian Inheritance in Man, 10th ed.: V.A. McKusick; The Johns Hopkins University Press, 1992, p. 412.

Menetrier's Disease: Evolution of Disease Under Histamine-2 Receptor Antagonists: M. Geist; Am. J. Gastroenterol., May 1992, vol. 87(5), pp. 648–650.

Nelson Textbook of Pediatrics, 14th ed.: R.E. Behrman, ed.-in-chief; W.B. Saunders Company, 1992, p. 680.

Hypertrophic Gastropathy with Gastric Adenocarcinoma: Menetrier's Disease and Lymphocytic Gastritis?: J.F. Mosnier; Gut, December 1991, vol. 32(12), pp. 1565–1567.

Dictionary of Medical Syndromes, 3rd ed.: S.I. Magalini, et al., eds.; J.B. Lippincott Company, 1990, pp. 586–587.

Gastrointestinal Disease, 4th ed.: M.H. Sleisenger, et al.; W.B. Saunders Company, 1989, pp. 802–804.

Menetrier's Disease: A Trivalent Gastropathy: T.M. Sundt; Ann. Surg., December 1988, vol. 208(6), pp. 694–701.

Familial Giant Hypertrophic Gastritis (Menetrier's Disease): B. Larsen, et al.; Gut, November 1987, vol. 28(11), pp. 1517–1521.

# GASTROENTERITIS, EOSINOPHILIC (EG)

**Description** This form of gastritis is distinguished by heavy infiltration of eosinophils in the lining of the stomach, small intestine, and/or large intestine. The infiltration generally causes cramping abdominal pain, diarrhea, and vomiting. The disorder is classified into patterns I, II, and III.

**Signs and Symptoms Pattern I** is distinguished by extensive infiltration of eosinophils in the area below the submucosa and muscle wall. It commonly involves the stomach but may affect the small intestine or colon as well. Nausea, vomiting, abdominal pain, and sometimes obstruction are among the symptoms.

In **pattern II,** eosinophilic infiltration occurs mainly in the mucous and submucosal membranes. In children the gastric mucosa is usually involved, while in adults pattern II tends to affect the small intestine. Symptoms include diarrhea, abdominal and back pain, edema, and mild to moderate malabsorption. Laboratory analysis may reveal iron-deficiency anemia, hypoproteinemia, steatorrhea, and other abnormalities.

**Pattern III,** the rarest form of EG, usually involves the subserosal and serosal membranes of the stomach and is characterized by an accumulation of eosinophil-containing fluid in the abdomen. This fluid can infiltrate the serous membrane of the lungs. Chest pain, fever, shortness of breath, and limited motion of the chest wall are among the symptoms.

**Etiology** The precise cause is unknown, but some cases may be the result of hypersensitivity to certain foods or other unknown allergens.

**Epidemiology** Individuals with a history of allergies, eczema, and seasonal asthma are more likely to develop EG, which affects males and females in equal numbers. The disease usually occurs between the ages of 30 and 60.

**Related Disorders** See *Celiac Sprue.*

**Treatment—Standard** Prednisone is usually effective. Eliminating foods that cause an allergic reaction may help some patients. In severe cases, surgery may be required to remove intestinal obstructions. Additional treatment is symptomatic and supportive.

**Treatment—Investigational** Sodium chromoglycate is being investigated.

Please contact the agencies listed under Resources, below, for the most current information. Addresses and telephone numbers of these agencies, as well as of individual experts and research centers, may be found in the Master Resources List.

**Resources**

**For more information on eosinophilic gastroenteritis:** National Organization for Rare Disorders (NORD); NIH/National Digestive Diseases Clearinghouse.

**References**

Cecil Textbook of Medicine, 18th ed.: J.B. Wyngaarden and L.H. Smith, Jr., eds.; W.B. Saunders Company, 1988, p. 807.

Eosinophilic Gastroenteritis: Ultrastructural Evidence for a Selective Release of Eosinophil Major Basic Protein: G. Torpier, et al.; Clin. Exp. Immunol., December 1988, vol. 74(3), pp. 404–408.

Near Fatal Eosinophilic Gastroenteritis Responding to Oral Sodium Chromoglycate: R. Moots, et al.; Gut, September 1988, vol. 29(9), pp. 1282–1285.

Eosinophilic Gastroenteritis Presenting with Biliary and Duodenal Obstruction: M. Rumans, et al.; Am. Gastroenterol., August 1987, vol. 82(8), pp. 775–778.

Internal Medicine, 2nd ed.: J.H. Stein, ed.-in-chief; Little, Brown and Company, 1987, p. 136.

# GILBERT SYNDROME

**Description** One of a benign group of metabolic abnormalities, Gilbert syndrome is a hereditary disorder involving a defect in the clearance of serum bilirubin by the liver. This syndrome is common but innocuous. It is marked by a persistent jaundice, which may fluctuate in severity.

**Synonyms**

Constitutional Liver Dysfunction
Familial Jaundice
Gilbert Disease
Gilbert-Lereboullet Syndrome
Hyperbilirubinemia I
Icterus Intermittens Juvenilis
Meulengracht Disease
Unconjugated Benign Bilirubinemia

**Signs and Symptoms** The onset of Gilbert syndrome is shortly after birth but may not be recognized for many years. A mild jaundice appears at about age 10 and is more common in males than females. There is a general lack of awareness of the jaundice initially. The jaundice may increase with fasting, stress, and exposure to cold. Fatigue, nausea, abdominal pain, and, rarely, diarrhea are common associated symptoms.

The mild jaundice may be especially evident on the face, palms, and plantar surfaces. Formation of pigmented skin thickenings similar to nevi and xanthelasma on eyelids can occur. An increase in pigmentation on exposure to light and heat are other symptoms of this disorder. Bradycardia, hypothermia, neuromuscular hypersensitivity, and migraine headaches may also be present. Enlargement of the liver and spleen are rarely seen.

Symptoms and jaundice become more pronounced following exertion, alcohol intake, and/or infections. A slight reduction of red cell survival is found in 50 percent of patients.

**Etiology** Gilbert syndrome is inherited as an autosomal dominant disease, but a clear genetic pattern is often hard to establish. A misdiagnosis of chronic hepatitis is sometimes made.

A defect in uptake or clearance of unconjugated bilirubin from plasma by the liver is a possible cause of this disorder. Reduced bilirubin uridine diphosphate (UDP) glucuronyl transferase activity could possibly explain hyperbilirubinemia and impaired clearance of pigment, but it is not the only mechanism responsible for the syndrome. Attempts to find a consistent impairment of bilirubin conjugation or decrease of glycuronyl transferase activity have failed.

**Epidemiology** Gilbert syndrome affects both sexes but is more common in males, appearing at about the age of 10 years. The male to female ratio is 4:1.

**Related Disorders** See ***Dubin-Johnson Syndrome.***

**Rotor syndrome** is a variant of Dubin-Johnson syndrome. Less frequent than Dubin-Johnson syndrome, it is also usually mild and involves much the same symptoms. These include occasional pain in the right upper quadrant and mild jaundice. Enlargement of the liver may also occur. The prognosis is generally favorable.

**Crigler-Najjar syndrome** is a congenital nonhemolytic jaundice in infants. This is a very rare disease that can be inherited through both dominant and recessive traits. The dominant type involves a later onset of jaundice and destructive changes in the brain. The recessive form usually involves severe deep jaundice from birth and some changes in the brain function.

**Treatment—Standard** Treatment is unnecessary. If jaundice becomes a cosmetic problem, phenobarbitol, which reduces the bilirubin level, may be prescribed. Careful regulation of the diet is important, as fasting increases hyperbilirubinemia. Prognosis is good since the disease is benign.

**Treatment—Investigational** Please contact the agencies listed under Resources, below, for the most current information. Addresses and telephone numbers of these agencies, as well as of individual experts and research centers, may be found in the Master Resources List.

**Resources**

For more information on Gilbert syndrome: National Organization for Rare Disorders (NORD); American Liver Foundation; United Liver Association; Children's Liver Foundation; NIH/National Digestive Diseases Information Clearinghouse.

For genetic information and genetic counseling referrals: March of Dimes Birth Defects Foundation; Alliance of Genetic Support Groups.

**References**

Mendelian Inheritance In Man, 6th ed.: V.A. McKusick; The Johns Hopkins University Press, 1983, p. 283.

Unconjugated Hyperbilirubinemia: Physiologic Evaluation and Experimental Approaches to Therapy: Berk, P.D., et al.; Ann. Intern. Med., April 1975, vol. 82(4), pp. 552–570.

# GLUCOSE-GALACTOSE MALABSORPTION

**Description** Glucose-galactose malabsorption is a familial disorder of transport produced by deficient intestinal monosaccharidase. The condition is clinically identical to disaccharide intolerance.

**Synonyms**

> Carbohydrate Intolerance
> Complex Carbohydrate Intolerance

**Signs and Symptoms** In children, the inability to digest carbohydrates causes diarrhea and failure to gain weight. In adults the disorder manifests as abdominal distention, nausea, diarrhea, cramps, borborygmus, and flatus.

**Etiology** Glucose-galactose intolerance is inherited as an autosomal recessive trait.

**Epidemiology** No statistics on the epidemiology of this extremely rare disorder are available.

**Related Disorders** See ***Galactosemia, Classic.***

**Lactose intolerance** is a malabsorption syndrome in which deficiency of the intestinal enzyme lactase causes impaired absorption of lactose from the small bowel. The disorder is easily controlled by adherence to a lactose-free diet or administration of oral lactase (e.g., Lactaid).

**Treatment—Standard** Treatment consists of a lactose-free diet with oral calcium supplementation. Fructose (and sometimes sucrose) may be substituted as a source of carbohydrate calories.

**Treatment—Investigational** Please contact the agencies listed under Resources, below, for the most current information. Addresses and telephone numbers of these agencies, as well as of individual experts and research centers, may be found in the Master Resources List.

**Resources**

For more information on glucose-galactose intolerance: National Organization for Rare Disorders (NORD); NIH/National Digestive Diseases Information Clearinghouse.

For genetic information and genetic counseling referrals: March of Dimes Birth Defects Foundation; Alliance of Genetic Support Groups.

**References**

Mendelian Inheritance in Man, 9th ed.: V.A. McKusick; The Johns Hopkins University Press, 1990, pp. 1208–1209.

The Metabolic Basis of Inherited Disease, 6th ed.: C.R. Scriver, et al., eds.; McGraw-Hill, 1989, pp. 2463–2471.

Complex Carbohydrate Intolerance: Diagnostic Pitfalls and Approach to Management: J.D. Loyd-Still, et al.; J. Pediatr., May 1988, vol. 112(5), pp. 709–713.

Glucose-Galactose Malabsorption: Demonstration of Specific Jejunal Brush Membrane Defect: I.W. Booth, et al.; Gut, December 1988, vol. 29(12), pp. 1661–1665.

Internal Medicine, 2nd ed.: J.H. Stein, ed.-in-chief; Little, Brown and Company, 1987, p. 140, 880.

# HEPATIC FIBROSIS, CONGENITAL

**Description** Congenital hepatic fibrosis is a rare congenital disorder that affects both the liver and kidneys. The typical liver abnormalities are hepatomegaly, portal hypertension, and hepatic fibrosis. Many patients with congenital hepatic fibrosis also have polycystic kidney disease. Gastrointestinal bleeding is the main clinical problem in patients with congenital hepatic fibrosis.

**Signs and Symptoms** Congenital hepatic fibrosis usually presents in children, with the obvious symptoms being a swollen abdomen; a firm, slightly enlarged liver; and/or hematemesis due to bleeding in the stomach and intestines.

The main findings in congenital hepatic fibrosis are identified through diagnostic testing. Many of the following signs are present in patients with this disorder: portal hypertension, hepatic fibrosis, nephromegaly, gastrointestinal bleeding, polycystic kidney disease, and splenomegaly. Liver function tests are usually normal. The diagnosis of congenital hepatic fibrosis is confirmed by liver biopsy.

**Etiology** Congenital hepatic fibrosis is thought to be inherited as an autosomal recessive trait.

**Epidemiology** Congenital hepatic fibrosis affects males and females in equal numbers and is normally detected in the first 10 years of life.

**Related Disorders** See *Caroli Disease; Medullary Cystic Disease; Medullary Sponge Kidney; Polycystic Kidney Diseases.*

**Treatment—Standard** Treatment is symptomatic and supportive. To prevent gastrointestinal hemorrhage, portal hypertension may need to be treated surgically. Aspirin and alcohol should be avoided.

Treatment of polycystic kidney disease consists of management of urinary infections and secondary portal hypertension. Kidney function may deteriorate very slowly in some patients. Usually kidney function is normal or only slightly impaired when congenital hepatic fibrosis is found along with polycystic kidney disease in older children. Patients eventually need dialysis in order to remove toxins from the blood. Transplantation of a kidney or liver may be indicated.

Genetic counseling may be of benefit for patients and their families.

**Treatment—Investigational** Please contact the agencies listed under Resources, below, for the most current information. Addresses and telephone numbers of these agencies, as well as of individual experts and research centers, may be found in the Master Resources List.

**Resources**

**For more information on congenital hepatic fibrosis:** National Organization for Rare Disorders (NORD); American Liver Foundation; Children's Liver Foundation; Polycystic Kidney Research Foundation; NIH/National Kidney and Urologic Diseases Information Clearinghouse; National Kidney Foundation; American Kidney Fund; National Association of Patients on Hemodialysis and Transplantation.

**For genetic information and genetic counseling referrals:** March of Dimes Birth Defects Foundation; Alliance of Genetic Support Groups.

**References**

Cecil Textbook of Medicine, 19th ed.: J.B. Wyngaarden, et al., eds.; W.B. Saunders Company, 1992, p. 849.

The Kidney, 4th ed.: B.M. Brenner and F.C. Rector, Jr., eds.; W.B. Saunders Company, 1991, pp. 1670–1672.

Birth Defects Encyclopedia: M.L Buyse, ed.-in-chief; Blackwell Scientific Publications, 1990, pp. 861–862.

Mendelian Inheritance in Man, 9th ed.: V.A. McKusick; The Johns Hopkins University Press, 1990, pp. 1430–1431.

# HIRSCHSPRUNG DISEASE

**Description** Hirschsprung disease is characterized by the absence at birth of myenteric ganglion cells in a distal segment of the large bowel. Peristaltic activity in the involved segment is absent or abnormal, causing continuous spasm, obstruction, and massive hypertrophic dilatation of the normal proximal colon. The aganglionic segment usually remains narrowed, but may dilate passively.

**Synonyms**

Congenital Megacolon

Megacolon, Aganglionic

**Signs and Symptoms** Symptoms of Hirschsprung disease usually appear soon after birth, with constipation, abdominal distention, and vomiting evident in affected neonates. Older infants may become anorexic, lose the physiologic urge to defecate, and have a palpable colon, visible peristalsis, and failure to thrive. The longer the disorder persists untreated, the greater the risk of toxic enterocolitis, which may be fatal.

Diagnosis is made by rectal biopsy of the mucous lining.

**Etiology** It has been suggested that Hirschsprung disease results from a defect in early fetal development caused by maternal hyperthermia. The condition may also be inherited as an autosomal recessive trait (Hirschsprung disease with ulnar polydactyly, polysyndactyly of the big toe, and ventricular septal defect), or as an X-linked disorder (Hirschsprung disease with type D brachydactyly). The gene associated with the disease has been mapped to chromosome 10 (10q11.2). Acquired forms of Hirschsprung disease, or cases of the disease that occur along with other disorders, usually occur as a result of either intestinal nerve or muscular failure or the use of drugs that can cause decreased or cessation of motility in the intestines.

**Epidemiology** Males are affected more often than females. The disorder occurs in approximately 1:5,000 births.

**Related Disorders** Patients with Down syndrome and Waardenburg syndrome may have aganglionic megacolon.

**Treatment—Standard** The initial treatment of Hirschsprung disease in infants is colostomy at a site proximal to the aganglionic segment. Resection of the colon and definitive repair may be deferred until the infant is larger. Prognosis after surgery is generally good, with most infants achieving satisfactory bowel control.

**Treatment—Investigational** Dr. Arvinda Chakekavarti of the University of Pittsburgh is conducting a study on the families of Hirschsprung disease patients. Patients with families having more than one living affected member or those with multiple abnormalities along with Hirschsprung disease (excluding Down syndrome patients) are eligible for the study.

Please contact the agencies listed under Resources, below, for the most current information. Addresses and telephone numbers of these agencies, as well as of individual experts and research centers, may be found in the Master Resources List.

**Resources**

**For more information on Hirschsprung disease:** National Organization for Rare Disorders (NORD); NIH/National Digestive Diseases Information Clearinghouse; American Pseudo-obstruction and Hirschsprung's Disease Society; Pull-Through Network.

**For genetic information and genetic counseling referrals:** March of Dimes Birth Defects Foundation; Alliance of Genetic Support Groups.

**References**

Human Genetics Disorders: The Journal of NIH Research, August 1994, vol. 6(8), pp. 115-134.

Mendelian Inheritance in Man, 9th ed.: V.A. McKusick; The Johns Hopkins University Press, 1990, pp. 1313–1314.

Management of Hirschsprung's Disease in Adolescents: R.R. Ricketts, et al.; Am. Surg., April 1989, vol. 55(4), pp. 219–225.

Hirschsprung's Disease: Identification of Risk Factors for Enterocolitis: D.H. Teitelbaum, et al.; Ann. Surg., March 1988, vol. 207(3), pp. 240–244.

Adult Hirschsprung's Disease: An Experience with the Duhamel-Martin Procedure with Special Reference to Obstructed Patients: N.B. Natsikas, et al.; Dis. Colon Rectum, March 1987, vol. 30(3), pp. 204–206.

Internal Medicine, 2nd ed.: J.H. Stein, ed.-in-chief; Little, Brown and Company, 1987, pp. 7, 125–126, 171.

Segmental Intestinal Muscular Thinning: A Possible Cause of Intestinal Obstruction in the Newborn: J.F. Johnson, et al.; Radiology, December 1987, vol. 165(3), pp. 659–660.

# INTESTINAL PSEUDO-OBSTRUCTION

**Description** Intestinal pseudo-obstruction is characterized by hypomotility of the intestinal walls. The condition resembles a true obstruction, but no evidence of organic obstruction is present at laparotomy.

**Synonyms**

Congenital Short Bowel Syndrome

Hypomotility Disorder

Pseudointestinal Obstruction Syndrome

**Signs and Symptoms** Constipation, colicky pain, vomiting, and weight loss or failure to thrive are characteristic of this condition, which may be present at birth. Central nervous system deterioration, speech disturbances, and neuromuscular symptoms may also occur.

**Etiology** Intestinal pseudo-obstruction may occur as a complication of other disorders, including scleroderma, myxedema, amyloidosis, muscular dystrophy, hypokalemia, chronic renal failure, and diabetes mellitus. The cause of the condition is unknown. An autosomal dominant inheritance has been suggested.

**Epidemiology** Males and females are affected in equal numbers.

**Related Disorders Megacystis microcolon intestinal hypoperistalsis syndrome** is characterized by bowel and bladder dysfunction. Catheterization and anticholinergic drugs may be helpful in management, producing temporary asymptomatic periods. Surgery followed by enteral or parenteral nutrition may, however, be necessary.

**Paralytic ileus** results from paralysis of the bowel wall caused by peritonitis or shock. Symptoms are similar to those of intestinal pseudo-obstruction.

**Acute colonic pseudo-obstruction (Ogilvie syndrome)** is characterized by hypomotility of the colon. Decompression of the enlarged colon is appropriate treatment.

A **tumor, abscess, or other mechanical blockage** may cause intestinal obstruction.

The following disorders may precede the development of intestinal pseudo-obstruction: **Myxedema** is characterized by hypothyroidism accompanied by coarse, dry hair and skin; evidence of intellectual impairment; and numerous other anomalies. Affected individuals have a dull facial expression. The condition may be treated with a variety of thyroid hormone preparations. **Anticholinergic toxicity** and **opiate toxicity** are adverse drug reactions that may produce intestinal pseudo-obstruction. See also ***Amyloidosis; Scleroderma.***

**Treatment—Standard** If intestinal pseudo-obstruction has occurred as a secondary effect of another disorder, treatment of the underlying condition is the goal of therapy. The administration of antibiotics, enteral or parenteral nutrition, and, sometimes, surgical removal of the dilated sections of intestine may help to control malabsorption and diarrhea, improve nutrition, and relieve pain.

**Treatment—Investigational** The orphan drug cisapride, which induces peristalsis in intestinal pseudo-obstruction, is being tested. For more information, contact Paul Hyman, M.D., at Harbor UCLA Medical Center's Pediatric Gastrointestinal Motility Center, or Janssen Pharmaceutica.

Please contact the agencies listed under Resources, below, for the most current information. Addresses and telephone numbers of these agencies, as well as of individual experts and research centers, may be found in the Master Resources List.

**Resources**

**For more information on intestinal pseudo-obstruction:** National Organization for Rare Disorders (NORD); American Pseudo-obstruction and Hirschsprung's Disease Society; NIH/National Digestive Diseases Information Clearinghouse; Frances Harley, M.D., University of Alberta, Canada.

**For information on parenteral or enteral nutrition:** Parent Education Network.

**For genetic information and genetic counseling referrals:** March of Dimes Birth Defects Foundation; Alliance of Genetic Support Groups.

**References**

Chronic Idiopathic Intestinal Pseudo-Obstruction Caused by Visceral Neuropathy Localised in the Left Colon: Report of Two Cases: H. Suzuki, et al.; Jpn. J. Surg., July 1987, vol. 17(4), pp. 302–306.

Chronic Idiopathic Intestinal Pseudo-Obstruction: Clinical and Intestinal Manometric Findings: V. Stanghellini, et al.; Gut, January 1987, vol. 28(1), pp. 5–12.

Familial Intestinal Pseudoobstruction Dominated by a Progressive Neurologic Disease at a Young Age: J. Faber, et al.; Gastroenterology, March 1987, vol. 92(3), pp. 786–790.

Internal Medicine, 2nd ed.: J.H. Stein, ed.-in-chief; Little, Brown and Company, 1987, pp. 1065–1066.

Problems of Trace Elements and Vitamins During Long-Term Parenteral Nutrition: A Case Report of Idiopathic Intestinal Pseudo-Obstruction: H. Kadowski, et al.; JPEN, May–June 1987, vol. 11(3), pp. 322–325.

Familial Visceral Neuropathy with Autosomal Dominant Transmission: E.A. Mayer, et al.; Gastroenterology, December 1986, vol. 91(6), 1528–1535.

# MALLORY-WEISS SYNDROME

**Description** Mallory-Weiss syndrome is characterized by slitlike lacerations of the gastric mucosa, longitudinally placed at or slightly below the esophagogastric junction.

**Synonyms**

Gastroesophageal Laceration-Hemorrhage Syndrome

**Signs and Symptoms** Hematemesis or melena generally follows hours or days of vomiting, retching, or hiccups.

**Etiology** The esophagogastric lacerations of Mallory-Weiss syndrome are usually caused by vomiting, but they may also result from trauma to the chest or abdomen, intense snoring, hiccups, gastritis, or cancer chemotherapy.

**Epidemiology** The disorder was originally described in alcoholics, but it may occur in other situations as described above.

**Related Disorders Boerhaave syndrome** is characterized by esophageal rupture, an emergency situation with a high mortality rate. Mediastinitis and pleural effusion should be treated immediately by surgical repair and drainage.

**Peptic ulcer** is a common disorder that is recurrent and chronic. The goal of treatment is to neutralize or decrease gastric activity.

**Esophageal varices** occur in the azygos and portal veins in individuals with portal hypertension.

**Treatment—Standard** Most episodes of bleeding from Mallory-Weiss syndrome stop spontaneously. However, ligation of the lacerations or an angiographically guided infusion of vasopressin into the left gastric artery may be required.

**Treatment—Investigational** The effectiveness of embolization is being evaluated as a treatment for massive uncontrolled bleeding of the esophagus.

The orphan drug sodium tetradecyl sulfate (Sotradecol) is being used as an experimental treatment for bleeding esophageal varices. For more information contact Elkins-Sinn, in Cherry Hill, New Jersey.

Please contact the agencies listed under Resources, below, for the most current information. Addresses and telephone numbers of these agencies, as well as of individual experts and research centers, may be found in the Master Resources List.

**Resources**

**For more information on Mallory-Weiss syndrome:** National Organization for Rare Disorders (NORD); NIH/National Digestive Diseases Information Clearinghouse.

**References**

Internal Medicine, 3rd ed.: J.H. Stein, ed.-in-chief; Little, Brown and Company, 1990, pp. 310–311.

Percutaneous Transhepatic Embolization of Gastroesophageal Varices: Results in 400 Patients: C.L. Hermine, et al.; April 1989, vol. 152(4), pp. 775–760.

Upper Gastrointestinal Bleeding: J. Lancaster; Prim. Care, March 1988, vol. 15(1), pp. 31–41.

Multipolar Electrocoagulation in the Treatment of Active Upper Gastrointestinal Tract Hemorrhage: A Prospective Controlled Trial: L. Laine; N. Engl. J. Med., June 1987, vol. 316(26), pp. 1613–1617.

Snore-Induced Mallory-Weiss Syndrome: J. Merrill; J. Clin. Gastroenterol., February 1987, vol. 9(1), pp. 88–89.

Mallory-Weiss Syndrome: A Study of 224 Patients: C. Sugawa, et al.; Am. J. Surg., January 1983, vol. 145(1), pp. 30–33.

Mallory-Weiss Tear: A Complication of Cancer Chemotherapy: M. Fishman, et al.; Cancer, December 1983, vol. 52(11), pp. 2031–2032.

# MICROVILLUS INCLUSION DISEASE

**Description** Microvillus inclusion disease is a progressive intestinal disease characterized by chronic, severe, watery diarrhea occurring in infants at or soon after birth.

**Synonyms**

> Congenital Familial Protracted Diarrhea
> Congenital Microvillus Atrophy
> Davidson Disease
> Familial Enteropathy

**Signs and Symptoms** Diarrhea persists after oral feeding. Dehydration, acidosis, growth retardation, and developmental delay may be observed in affected infants.

**Etiology** Microvillus inclusion disease is a congenital defect in the intestinal wall that is inherited as an autosomal recessive trait.

**Epidemiology** Males and females are affected in equal numbers.

**Related Disorders Familial chloride diarrhea** is characterized by profuse watery stools with excessive chloride content. Infants born with this autosomal recessive disorder are often premature.

**Infantile diarrhea with abnormal hair** is a progressive malabsorption syndrome that develops around the 3rd week of life. Affected infants have dark, kinky hair that falls out easily; large, low-set ears; a flat nasal bridge; and a large mouth. The disorder is inherited as an autosomal recessive trait.

**Congenital sodium diarrhea** results from defective sodium exchange in the bowels. This recessive disorder is present at birth.

**Treatment—Standard** Microvillus inclusion disease is treated with intravenous feeding. Genetic counseling is recommended.

**Treatment—Investigational** An analogue of somatostatin being tested for treatment of prolonged diarrhea shows some promise.

Please contact the agencies listed under Resources, below, for the most current information. Addresses and telephone numbers of these agencies, as well as of individual experts and research centers, may be found in the Master Resources List.

**Resources**

**For more information on microvillus inclusion disease:** National Organization for Rare Disorders (NORD); NIH/National Digestive Diseases Information Clearinghouse.

**For genetic information and genetic counseling referrals:** March of Dimes Birth Defects Foundation; Alliance of Genetic Support Groups.

### References

Microvillus Inclusion Disease: An Inherited Defect of Brush-Border Assembly and Differentiation: E. Cutz, et al.; N. Engl. J. Med., March 9, 1989, vol. 320(10), pp. 646–651.

Microvillus Inclusion Disease: Specific Diagnostic Features Shown by Alkaline Phosphatase Histochemistry: B.D. Lake; J. Clin. Pathol., August 1988, vol. 41(8), pp. 880–882.

Biochemical Abnormality in Brush Border Membrane Protein of a Patient with Congenital Microvillus Atrophy: L. Carruthers, et al.; J. Pediatr. Gastroenterol. Nutr., December 1985, vol. 4(6), pp. 902–907.

# PEUTZ-JEGHERS SYNDROME

**Description** Peutz-Jeghers syndrome is a hereditary disorder characterized by polyps on the mucous lining of the intestinal wall and dark discolorations on the skin and mucous membrane surfaces.

**Synonyms**

> Hutchinson-Weber-Peutz Syndrome
> Intestinal Polyposis II
> Intestinal Polyposis–Cutaneous Pigmentation Syndrome
> Jeghers Syndrome
> Melanoplakia–Intestinal Polyposis
> Peutz-Touraine Syndrome

**Signs and Symptoms** Intussusception and bleeding are the most common symptoms. Discrete brown to black macules occur around the lips; inside the mouth on the mucosal lining of the cheeks; on the fingers, palms of the hands, forearms, and toes; and around the naval. Polyps occur most often in the jejunum and ileum but may be present anywhere in the gastrointestinal tract. Severe bleeding can cause anemia and recurrent pain that disappears with massage, physical manipulation, or contorting the body. Intussusception can cause complications, such as intestinal obstruction and gangrene. The polyps are benign hamartomas, but about 50 percent of patients develop intestinal and nonintestinal malignancies, particularly in the pancreas, ovaries, and breast, as adults.

**Etiology** Peutz-Jeghers syndrome is an inherited autosomal dominant trait.

**Epidemiology** Approximately 1:120,000 children in the United States are afflicted with this disorder. Males and females are affected in equal numbers.

**Related Disorders** See *Familial Polyposis; Gardner Syndrome; Cronkhite-Canada Disease.*

**Turcot syndrome** is an extremely rare inherited disorder characterized by familial polyposis and tumors of the central nervous system (e.g., medulloblastoma, glioblastoma, or ependymoma). Symptoms may include diarrhea, rectal bleeding, and abdominal discomfort. Neurologic symptoms vary greatly and depend on the type and location of the tumor. Symptoms may include ataxia and impaired speech.

**Treatment—Standard** Periodic x-rays of the gastrointestinal tract from childhood through adolescence monitor changes in size and number of polyps. Large individual polyps or particularly heavily affected sections of the intestine can be removed surgically. If intestinal gangrene develops, the involved section must be resected.

**Treatment—Investigational** Please contact the agencies listed under Resources, below, for the most current information. Addresses and telephone numbers of these agencies, as well as of individual experts and research centers, may be found in the Master Resources List.

### Resources

**For more information on Peutz-Jeghers syndrome:** National Organization for Rare Disorders (NORD); NIH/National Digestive Diseases Information Clearinghouse; American Cancer Society; NIH/National Cancer Institute Physician Data Query Phoneline.

**For genetic information and genetic counseling referrals:** March of Dimes Birth Defects Foundation; Alliance of Genetic Support Groups.

### References

Cancer in Peutz-Jeghers Syndrome: K. Hizawa, et al.; Cancer, November 1993, vol. 72(9), pp. 2777–2781.

Peutz-Jeghers Syndrome: P.J. Morrison; N. Engl. J. Med., September 1993, vol. 329(11), p. 774.

Cecil Textbook of Medicine, 19th ed.: J.B. Wyngaarden, et al., eds.; W.B. Saunders Company, 1992, pp. 717–718.

Mendelian Inheritance in Man, 10th ed.: V.A. McKusick; The Johns Hopkins University Press, 1992, pp. 899–900.

Nelson Textbook of Pediatrics, 14th ed.: R.E. Behrman, ed.-in-chief; W.B. Saunders Company, 1992, p. 993.

Peutz-Jeghers Syndrome: J.L. Buck, et al.; Radiographics, March 1992, vol. 12(2), pp. 365–378.

The Peutz-Jeghers Syndrome: Case Reports: S. Dorfman, et al.; Invest. Clin., 1991, vol. 32(2), pp. 59–65.

Peutz-Jeghers Syndrome: CT and US Demonstration of Small Bowel Polyps: R.N. Sener, et al.; Gastrointest. Radiol., Winter 1991, vol. 16(1), pp. 21–23.

Birth Defects Encyclopedia: M.L Buyse, ed.-in-chief; Blackwell Scientific Publications, 1990, pp. 983–984.

Dictionary of Medical Syndromes, 3rd ed.: S.I. Magalini, et al., eds.; J.B. Lippincott Company, 1990, p. 685.

Peutz-Jeghers Syndrome: A Call for Intraoperative Enteroscopy: R.G. Panos, et al.; Am. Surg., May 1990, vol. 56(5), pp. 331–333.

Gastrointestinal Disease, 4th ed.: M.H. Sleisenger, et al.; W.B. Saunders Company, 1989, pp. 1508–1510.

Smith's Recognizable Patterns of Human Malformation, 4th ed.: K.L. Jones; W.B. Saunders Company, 1988, p. 462.

# POLYCYSTIC LIVER DISEASE

**Description** Polycystic liver disease is an inherited disorder characterized by multiple cysts in the liver. Abdominal discomfort from swelling of the liver may occur; however, most patients are asymptomatic.

**Signs and Symptoms** Cysts range in diameter from a few millimeters to over 15 cm. Symptoms rarely occur although the liver gradually enlarges as it is replaced by cysts. Abdominal discomfort may occur due to the stretching of the liver. Fever may also occur as a result of infection or bleeding into a cyst. Rarely, jaundice may occur if the bile ducts are compressed by a cyst. Portal hypertension occurs only if the portal vein is compressed by a cyst. Liver function is generally unaffected if the liver has only a few cysts or if the cysts are small.

Fifty percent of patients with polycystic liver disease have cysts in their kidneys as well. Rarely, cystlike lesions occur in the pancreas, lungs, spleen, and other organs.

**Etiology** Polycystic liver disease is inherited as an autosomal dominant trait. Liver cysts may also occur as a result of abnormally developed bile ducts in the fetus.

**Epidemiology** Polycystic liver disease affects males and females in equal numbers. It may occur at any age; however, cysts are less common during childhood.

**Related Disorders** See *Caroli Disease.*

**Solitary cysts of the liver** are most often present in the right part of the liver. They may contain as little as a few milliliters or more than a liter of fluid. Most cysts cause no symptoms. Among patients that do have symptoms, the most common are abdominal discomfort, nausea, and vomiting.

**Echinococcosis** is transmitted by the parasitic tapeworm Echinococcus and results in hepatic cysts. It is most common in central and eastern Europe and rare in the United States. The cyst of *Echinococcus granulosus* is usually solitary, located in the right part of the liver, and causes no symptoms. *Echinococcus multilocularis* may cause many cysts in the liver and may extend beyond it. A few patients may have abdominal pain and a slight swelling. Rupture of a cyst, infection, or an allergic reaction may occur as complications.

**Treatment—Standard** Treatment may not be necessary in many cases. For patients with troublesome symptoms, aspiration of large cysts may be performed. Genetic counseling may be of benefit to patients and their families. Other treatment is symptomatic and supportive.

**Treatment—Investigational** Researchers are investigating unroofing, fenestration, and hepatectomy to treat large, troublesome cysts in polycystic liver disease. Rarely, surgical intervention may be needed to treat portal hypertension when it occurs as a rare complication in polycystic liver disease.

Please contact the agencies listed under Resources, below, for the most current information. Addresses and telephone numbers of these agencies, as well as of individual experts and research centers, may be found in the Master Resources List.

**Resources**

**For more information on polycystic liver disease:** National Organization for Rare Disorders (NORD); American Liver Foundation; United Liver Association; Children's Liver Foundation.

**For genetic information and genetic counseling referrals:** March of Dimes Birth Defects Foundation; Alliance of Genetic Support Groups.

**References**

Massive Hepatomegaly in Adult Polycystic Liver Disease: M.K. Kwok and K.J.Lewin; Am. J. Surg. Pathol., April 1988, vol. 12(4), pp. 321–324.

Therapeutic Dilemmas in Patients with Symptomatic Polycystic Liver Disease: R.H. Turnage, et al.; Am. Surg., June 1988, vol. 54(6), pp. 365–372.

Internal Medicine, 2nd Ed.: J.H. Stein, ed.-in-chief; Little, Brown and Company, 1987, p. 241.

Mendelian Inheritance in Man, 7th ed.: V.A. McKusick; The Johns Hopkins University Press, 1986, p. 608.

# PRIMARY BILIARY CIRRHOSIS

**Description** Primary biliary cirrhosis is a chronic, progressive disease occurring in 4 stages and thought to be related to abnormalities in the immune system. In later stages of the disease, cholestasis of the intrahepatic bile ducts results in jaundice. Excessive amounts of copper accumulate in the liver (but the relationship of these elevated levels to the disease is not understood), and fibrous or granular induration of the soft liver tissue develops.

**Synonyms**

Hanot Cirrhosis

**Signs and Symptoms** Commonly, the patient with primary biliary cirrhosis is a woman of about 50 who complains of persistent, generalized itching; dark urine; pale stools; and jaundice. The disease has 4 symptomatic stages stemming from unrelieved obstruction of the extrahepatic bile ducts.

In **stage I,** hepatomegaly, centrilobular bile stasis, cell degeneration, and focal areas of necrosis occur. Unexplained itching is common and is often worse at night. Increased amounts of melanin pigmentation appear in the skin, and excoriation occurs. Fatigue and unexplained weight loss are common.

In **stage II,** proliferation and dilatation of the portal ducts and ductules are more widespread but less specific. Biopsy shows loss of normal bile ducts and increased numbers of those with irregularly shaped lumens. Fibrous cells infiltrate and spread within the liver. Bile stoppage is limited to portal areas.

In **stage III,** cholestasis of bile acids, bilirubin, copper, and other substances normally excreted into bile cause progressive damage. The medium-sized bile ducts become inflamed and distorted. Over a period of time the itching, jaundice, and hyperpigmentation increase. Xanthomas may be noticeable on the skin and may occur in internal organs. Excessive amounts of lipids and cholesterol are found circulating in the blood. The bile acid concentration in the intestines is inadequate for complete digestion and absorption of triglycerides in the diet. Additionally, normal absorption of vitamins A, D, E, and K as well as calcium may be diminished, and iron-deficiency anemia may develop. Muscle wasting, spider angiomas, palmar erythema, ascites and edema, and, in about 25 percent of patients, the bony tenderness of osteoporosis and osteomalacia occur.

**Stage IV** represents the end-stage of lesion formation, with widespread cirrhosis and regenerative nodules. Jaundice becomes pronounced.

Patients may die within 5 to 10 years of the first appearance of the disease, primarily because of the development of portal hypertension.

**Etiology** The cause is not known. An immunologic relationship is suspected because IgG is present in the sera of 95 percent of patients with primary biliary cirrhosis; however, these circulating antibodies, which react with mitochondrial antibodies, are seldom present in other forms of liver disease. Since 90 percent of those affected with the disease are women over age 50, an endocrine contribution is also suggested.

**Epidemiology** The disease, a rare form of biliary cirrhosis, affects females over 50 years of age in approximately 90 percent of cases.

**Related Disorders Extrahepatic bile duct obstruction** originates outside the liver but may produce symptoms similar to those of primary biliary cirrhosis. **Obstructive biliary cirrhosis** is characterized by fibroid or granular hardening of the soft liver tissue due to bile duct obstruction rather than the deterioration inside the liver that is typical of primary biliary cirrhosis.

**Alcoholic cirrhosis** is characterized by gradual hardening of the soft tissue of the liver, a condition that frequently develops in alcoholics. The early stage is marked by liver enlargement due to fatty infiltration with mild fibrosis. In late stages, normal liver lobes are replaced with small nodules, separated by a framework of fine fibrous tissue strands (hobnail liver).

**Treatment—Standard** Since this is a prolonged, chronic, and incurable disease, treatment is often directed at relieving itching, malabsorption, fluid retention, portal hypertension, and late-stage hepatic insufficiency. Topical menthol lotions, sedation, and cholestyramine relieve itching in almost all patients. Large-volume plasmapheresis may relieve itching in patients who do not respond to drug treatment. A balanced high-calorie diet is adequate, but fat intake may be reduced to below 30 to 40 gm per day if the patient complains of diarrhea. Malabsorption of fat-soluble vitamins may be treated with vitamins K1, A, and D, and with calcium. Iron-deficiency anemia responds to oral iron supplements. Folic acid is recommended for patients taking cholestyramine because the drug may produce a folic acid deficiency. Folic acid and cholestyramine should be taken several hours apart.

In severe cases, liver transplantation may be considered.

**Treatment—Investigational** Several drugs including colchicine, prednisolone, D-penicillamine, azathioprine, ursodeoxycholic acid, cyclosporine A, and chlorambucil are being evaluated for therapy.

The orphan drug Actigall (ursodiol) has been approved for testing in the treatment of primary biliary cirrhosis. Clinical trials have indicated that the drug delays progression of the disease and that the earlier the drug is given, the better the results. The drug is manufactured by Ciba-Geigy Corporation.

The orphan drug Ursofalk (ursodeoxycholic acid) is being tested by the Food and Drug Administration as a treatment of primary biliary cirrhosis. The drug is manufactured by Axcan Pharma.

Please contact the agencies listed under Resources, below, for the most current information. Addresses and telephone numbers of these agencies, as well as of individual experts and research centers, may be found in the Master Resources List.

**Resources**

**For more information on primary biliary cirrhosis:** National Organization for Rare Disorders (NORD); Primary Biliary Cirrhosis Patient Support Network; American Liver Foundation; United Liver Association; Children's Liver Foundation; NIH/National Digestive Diseases Information Clearinghouse.

**References**

Ursodiol for the Long-Term Treatment of Primary Biliary Cirrhosis: R.E. Poupon, et al.; N. Engl. J. Med., May 12, 1994, vol. 330(19), pp. 1342–1347.

Clinical and Statistical Analyses of New and Evolving Therapies for Primary Biliary Cirrhosis: R.H. Wiesner, et al.; Hepatology, May–June 1988, vol. 8(3), pp. 668–676.

Treatment of Pruritis in Primary Biliary Cirrhosis with Rifampin: Results of a Double-Blind, Crossover, Randomized Trial: C.N. Ghent, et al.; Gastroenterology, February 1988, vol. 94(2), pp. 488–493.

Internal Medicine, 2nd ed.: J.H. Stein, ed.-in-chief; Little, Brown and Company, 1987, pp. 1065–1066.

Transplantation of Liver, Heart, and Lungs for Primary Biliary Cirrhosis and Primary Pulmonary Hypertension: J. Wallwork, et al.; Lancet, July 1987, vol. 2(8552), pp. 182–185.

# SUCROSE-ISOMALTOSE MALABSORPTION, CONGENITAL

**Description** Congenital sucrose-isomaltose malabsorption results from an inborn deficiency of the enzyme sucrase-isomaltase. Characteristic symptoms result from the ingestion of table sugar or certain other carbohydrates.

**Synonyms**

> Disaccharide Intolerance I
> Sucrase-α-Dextrinase Deficiency, Congenital

**Signs and Symptoms** Diarrhea is the major symptom. Affected children may be unable to gain weight on a normal diet, since the diarrhea can be severe enough to purge other nutrients before they can be absorbed. Adults may experience abdominal cramps, bloating, and flatus.

**Etiology** The disorder is transmitted through autosomal recessive genes.

**Epidemiology** Congenital sucrose-isomaltose malabsorption affects children from birth, and males and females in equal numbers. Some patients may be only mildly affected; others may have moderate to severe forms of the disorder.

**Related Disorders Lactose intolerance** is a malabsorption syndrome in which deficiency of the intestinal enzyme lactase causes impaired absorption of lactose from the small bowel. The disorder is easily controlled by adherence to a lactose-free diet or administration of oral lactase (e.g., Lactaid).

**Treatment—Standard** Congenital sucrose-isomaltose malabsorption is treated by administering the sucrase-isomaltase enzyme derived from a type of yeast. Symptoms are prevented by avoiding sucrose and sucrose-containing foods.

**Treatment—Investigational** The orphan product Sucrase (yeast derived) is being tested for treatment of congenital sucrose-isomaltose malabsorption under the direction of William R. Treem, M.D., of Hartford Hospital, Hartford, Connecticut.

Please contact the agencies listed under Resources, below, for the most current information. Addresses and telephone numbers of these agencies, as well as of individual experts and research centers, may be found in the Master Resources List.

**Resources**

**For more information on congenital sucrose-isomaltose malabsorption:** National Organization for Rare Disorders (NORD); NIH/National Digestive Diseases Information Clearinghouse; Research Trust for Metabolic Diseases in Children.

**For genetic information and genetic counseling referrals:** March of Dimes Birth Defects Foundation; Alliance of Genetic Support Groups.

**References**

Enzyme-Substitution Therapy with the Yeast Saccharomyces Cerevisiae in Congenital Sucrase-Isomaltase Deficiency: H.K. Harms, et al.; N. Engl. J. Med., May 21, 1987, vol. 316(21), pp. 1306–1309.

The Metabolic Basis of Inherited Disease, 5th ed.: J.B. Stanbury, et al., eds.; McGraw-Hill, 1983, pp. 1731–1733.

# WALDMANN DISEASE

**Description** Waldmann disease is characterized by dilatation of the lymphatics of the intestinal lamina propria. The disorder may be congenital or acquired.

**Synonyms**

> Familial Dysproteinemia
> Familial Hypoproteinemia with Lymphangiectatic Enteropathy
> Hypercatabolic Protein-Losing Enteropathy
> Hypoproteinemia, Idiopathic
> Intestinal Lymphangiectasia
> Lymphangiectatic Protein-Losing Enteropathy
> Neonatal Lymphedema Due to Exudative Enteropathy

**Signs and Symptoms** Gross, often asymmetrical edema, intermittent diarrhea, nausea, vomiting, and abdominal pain occur in children or young adults. Protein-losing enteropathy, steatorrhea, chylous effusions, lymphopenia, and ascites may also be present. Serum albumin, IgA, and IgG are markedly reduced. Diagnosis is made by serial small bowel biopsy.

**Etiology** Waldmann disease may be inherited as an autosomal dominant trait characterized by congenital malformation of the lymphatics. The condition may also be acquired as a secondary effect of tuberculous enteritis, granulomatous enteritis, lymphoma, retroperitoneal fibrosis, pancreatitis, or constrictive pericarditis.

**Epidemiology** Both males and females are affected.

**Related Disorders** See *Hemolytic-Uremic Syndrome; Glucose-Galactose Malabsorption; Intestinal Pseudo-obstruction; Gastritis, Giant Hypertrophic.*

**Lactose intolerance** is a malabsorption syndrome in which deficiency of the intestinal enzyme lactase causes impaired absorption of lactose from the small bowel. The disorder is easily controlled by adherence to a lactose-free diet or administration of oral lactase (e.g., Lactaid).

**Treatment—Standard** Treatment of Waldmann disease is accomplished with a low-fat diet supplemented by medium-chain triglycerides. Sodium restriction and diuretic therapy may be helpful in some patients. Occasionally surgical resection of the involved intestinal segment may be necessary.

**Treatment—Investigational** Please contact the agencies listed under Resources, below, for the most current information. Addresses and telephone numbers of these agencies, as well as of individual experts and research centers, may be found in the Master Resources List.

**Resources**

**For more information on Waldmann disease:** National Organization for Rare Disorders (NORD); National Lymphatic and Venous Diseases Foundation; NIH/National Digestive Diseases Information Clearinghouse.

**For genetic information and genetic counseling referrals:** March of Dimes Birth Defects Foundation; Alliance of Genetic Support Groups.

**References**

Cecil Textbook of Medicine, 19th ed.: J.B. Wyngaarden, et al., eds.; W.B. Saunders Company, 1992, p. 829.
Coeliac Disease and Lymphangiectasia: V.N. Perisic; Arch. Dis. Child., January 1992, vol. 67(1), pp. 134–136.
Mendelian Inheritance in Man, 10th ed.: V.A. McKusick; The Johns Hopkins University Press, 1992, p. 679.
Nelson Textbook of Pediatrics, 14th ed.: R.E. Behrman, ed.-in-chief; W.B. Saunders Company, 1992, p. 982.
Bleeding from Duodenal Lymphangiectasia: V.N. Perisic; Arch. Dis. Child., January 1991, vol. 66(1), pp. 153–154.
Birth Defects Encyclopedia: M.L Buyse, ed.-in-chief; Blackwell Scientific Publications, 1990, pp. 979–981.
Gastrointestinal Disease, 4th ed.: M.H. Sleisenger, et al.; W.B. Saunders Company, 1989, pp. 1951–1952.
Dietary Management of Intestinal Lymphangiectasia Complicated by Short Gut Syndrome: J.M. Thompson, et al.; Human Nutrition and Applied Nutrition, April 1986, vol. 40(2), pp. 136–140.

# WANDERING SPLEEN

**Description Congenital wandering spleen** (pediatric) is a very rare birth defect characterized by the absence or underdevelopment of one or all of the ligaments that hold the spleen in its normal position in the upper left abdomen. The spleen may "wander" into the lower abdomen or pelvis and be mistaken for an unidentified abdominal mass. The symptoms of wandering spleen are typically related to splenomegaly or the abnormal position of the spleen in the abdomen. Enlargement may be due to the torsion of the splenic arteries and veins or an infarct in the spleen. Symptoms of wandering spleen may include abdominal pain and discomfort, nausea, vomiting, fatigue, frequent urination, and/or menstrual abnormalities. **Acquired wandering spleen** may occur during adulthood as a result of accidents or other underlying conditions that may weaken the ligaments that hold the spleen in its normal position (e.g., connective tissue disease or pregnancy).

**Synonyms**

> Displaced Spleen
> Drifting Spleen
> Floating Spleen
> Splenic Ptosis
> Splenoptosis

**Signs and Symptoms** Some children with congenital wandering spleen may be asymptomatic, whereas others may experience acute or chronic abdominal pain. In most cases, episodes of pain may be related to the spontaneous torsion and detorsion of the mobile spleen. Infants with congenital wandering spleen may attempt to relieve pain by stretching. Other symptoms may include a bulging abdominal mass, constipation, bloating, nausea, vomiting, frequent and difficult urination, and/or menstrual problems in women. In some cases, the spleen may lack proper blood supply as a result of torsion of the splenic arteries. In these cases, symptoms may include abdominal pain, splenomegaly, bleeding into the abdomen, fibrosis of the spleen, and/or necrosis of splenic tissue. In severe cases, blood flow into the spleen is diminished, and the spleen may become greatly enlarged as it sequesters blood elements, such as platelets and red blood cells. Resulting symptoms may include fatigue, weakness, blood in the stools, anemia, hematemesis, and/or thrombocytopenia.

The diagnosis of wandering spleen may be suspected when an abdominal mass is present, especially if pain can be relieved by moving the mass toward the upper left quadrant of the abdomen, which is the normal position of the spleen. Wandering spleen may be confirmed by specialized examinations, such as ultrasonography and CT scan, which enable the physician to view the structure, size, and placement of the spleen within the abdomen or pelvis. Doppler studies may demonstrate impaired blood flow in and out of the spleen. In radioisotopic scanning, the level of function of the liver and spleen is studied. Doppler and radioisotopic studies may demonstrate that blood flow to the spleen is compromised as a result of torsion of the splenic artery. These studies may also show that there is functional asplenia or an infarct.

**Etiology** The cause of wandering spleen is not known. Congenital wandering spleen may be the result of a defect in the development of the mesogastrium dorsum that gives rise to the ligaments that normally hold the spleen in the upper left abdomen. Affected children may be missing one or all of these ligaments, or, if present, the ligaments are not positioned properly. Symptoms usually develop as a result of the abnormal position of the spleen in the lower abdomen or because of splenomegaly. Acquired wandering spleen may occur during adulthood because of accident or injury, another underlying disorder (e.g., connective tissue disease), or abnormal laxity of the ligaments caused by pregnancy.

**Epidemiology** Congenital wandering spleen affects more males than females during the first 2 years of life. However, between the ages of 2 and 21 years, this disorder seems to affect males and females in equal numbers. The exact reason for this is not fully understood. Approximately 100 cases of congenital wandering spleen have been reported in the medical literature. About 51 of these cases occurred in children under the age of 10 years.

Acquired wandering spleen usually occurs during adulthood, and it affects females 20 times more frequently than males. This is probably due to the laxity of the splenic ligaments during the childbearing years. Pregnancy is thought to contribute to the laxity, which increases the frequency of acquired wandering spleen among women who have had children.

There are a total of about 450 cases of all forms of wandering spleen documented in the medical literature.

**Related Disorders** Symptoms of the following disorders can be similar to those of wandering spleen: peritonitis, appendicitis, diverticulitis, and cholecystitis. Other common diseases may also have symptoms that are similar to those of wandering spleen. These include pyelonephritis, hiatal hernia, hepatitis, gastric ulcer, gastroenteritis, and pancreatitis. The following disorders may be associated with wandering spleen as secondary characteristics; comparisons are not necessary for a differential diagnosis: thrombocytopenia and prune belly syndrome. Other conditions that have been associated with wandering spleen include the absence or abnormal enlargement of a kidney, infectious mononucleosis, malaria, sickle cell anemia, and Hodgkin disease.

**Treatment—Standard** The treatment of wandering spleen depends on the severity of symptoms and on a complete evaluation to determine the size, location, and functional status of the spleen. Although most treatments are aimed at conserving the spleen and maximizing its function, surgical removal is often considered.

A conservative approach to the treatment of wandering spleen includes the observation of the affected individuals for signs of compromised splenic function or enlargement, and prevention of injury, such as avoidance of contact sports or other activities that might damage the unprotected spleen.

Since most children with congenital wandering spleen will experience episodes of torsion and acute pain, the treatment of choice may be splenopexy to anchor the spleen back in the proper position in the upper left abdomen. In many cases, the spleen can be preserved and the risk of torsion and infarct is reduced. The spleen is placed in mesh (Dexon snood) and sutured in place in the upper left abdomen. This type of surgery may be considered for the treatment of congenital or acquired wandering spleen if there is no evidence of torsion, acute abdominal pain, abnormal enlargement of the spleen, and/or other complications before surgery.

When wandering spleen causes chronic abdominal pain, abnormal enlargement of the spleen, and/or deficiencies of one or more necessary blood elements (e.g., thrombocytopenic hypersplenism), the treatment of choice is usually splenectomy. Acute abdominal pain associated with wandering spleen is considered a surgical emergency and may require immediate splenectomy. Splenopexy has not been a successful treatment for these cases.

The possible complications of splenectomy may include postsplenectomy infection syndrome, which is characterized by overwhelming life-threatening sepsis. People who have had a splenectomy are at higher lifetime risk for serious infections than the general population. Immunizations to boost immunity against *Hemophilus influenzae, Streptococcus Pneumoniae, Neisseria meningitidis,* and other contagious diseases are usually administered before the splenectomy is performed. All people who have had a splenectomy must be observed carefully in case of fever or other symptoms of infection. Antibiotics may be prescribed to help prevent infectious disease, especially in children under the age of 2 years. Prophylactic antibiotic therapy is required for all people who have had a splenectomy whenever they undergo medical or dental procedures.

**Treatment—Investigational** Please contact the agencies listed under Resources, below, for the most current information. Addresses and telephone numbers of these agencies, as well as of individual experts and research centers, may be found in the Master Resources List.

### Resources

**For more information on wandering spleen:** National Organization for Rare Disorders (NORD); NIH/National Institute of Child Health and Human Development; March of Dimes Birth Defects Foundation.

### References

Acute Abdomen Caused by Torsion of the Pedicle in a Wandering Spleen: M. Cainzos, et al.; Hepatogastroenterology, February 1993, vol. 40(1), pp. 78–80.

Splenoptosis (Wandering Spleen): E. Balik, et al.; Eur. J. Pediatr. Surg., June 1993, vol. 3(3), pp. 174–175.

Torsion of Wandering Spleen: The Whorled Appearance of the Splenic Pedicle on CT: L.E. Swischuk, et al.; Pediatr. Radiol., 1993, vol. 23(6), pp. 476–477.

Cecil Textbook of Medicine, 19th ed.: J.B. Wyngaarden, et al., eds.; W.B. Saunders Company, 1992, pp. 978, 982–983.

Nelson Textbook of Pediatrics, 14th ed.: R.E. Behrman, ed.-in-chief; W.B. Saunders Company, 1992, p. 1289.

Pediatric Wandering Spleen: Case Report and Review of Literature: M.L. Rodkey, et al.; Clin. Pediatr., May 1992, vol. 31(5), pp. 289–294.

The Splenic Snood: An Improved Approach for the Management of the Wandering Spleen. S.P. Schmidt, et al.; J. Pediatr. Surg., August 1992, vol. 27(8), pp. 1043–1044.

Wandering Spleen: Anatomic and Radiologic Considerations: K.B. Allen, et al.; South. Med. J. October 1992, vol. 85(10), pp. 976–984.

The Wandering Spleen: Collective Review: M. Buehner, et al.; Obstet. Gynecol., October 1992, vol. 175(4), pp. 373–387.

Elective Splenopexy for Wandering Spleen: J.H. Seashore, et al.; J. Pediatr. Surg., February 1990, vol. 25(2), pp. 270–272.

Chronic Torsion of the Wandering Spleen: W.E. Shiels, et al.; Pediatr. Radiol., 1989, vol. 19(6–7), pp. 465–467.

Pediatric Wandering Spleen—The Case for Splenopexy: Review of 35 Reported Cases in the Literature:. K.B. Allen, et al.; J. Pediatr. Surg., May 1989, vol. 24(5), pp. 432–435.

Wandering Spleen Presenting As an Adnexal Mass: N.M. Aquino, et al.; J. Natl. Med. Assoc., March 1989, vol. 81(3), pp. 331, 334.

Torsion of a Wandering Spleen: S. Franic, et al.; Can. Assoc. Radiol. J., September 1988, vol. 39(3), pp. 232–234.

Acute Urinary Retention As Presenting Symptom of Torsion of a Wandering Spleen: N. Samuel, et al.; Eur. J. Obstet. Gynecol. Reprod. Biol., February 1985, vol. 19(2), pp. 109–111.

Torsion of a Wandering Spleen: M. Witz, et al.; Postgrad. Med. J., February 1985, vol. 61(712), pp. 181–182.

# 9 | INHERITED RENAL AND GENITOURINARY DISORDERS
## By Russell W. Chesney, M.D.

The kidney and genitourinary tract can be afflicted by more than 235 inherited disorders and 75 chromosomal abnormalities resulting in renal defects. Some inherited renal disorders are reasonably common, including diabetic nephropathy or familial nephrolithiasis, which can affect a substantial portion of the population (0.5 to 1.0 percent). But many are quite rare, with an incidence of 1:10,000 to 1:100,000.

Clinical manifestations of these disorders comprise a broad spectrum; e.g., hematuria, proteinuria, hydronephrosis, nephrolithiasis, renal dysplasia, mono- or polycystic kidneys, tubulointerstitial nephritis, and renal medullary disease. Other abnormalities include renal vascular stenosis, aminoaciduria, glycosuria, and various other tubular abnormalities that result in the hyperexcretion of organic solutes or ions. A common final development is renal insufficiency, which leads to the symptom complex called uremia, further known as "end-stage renal disease."

Although it is difficult to generalize about the diversity of genetic renal disorders, the following universal principles concerning inherited renal disease can be identified.

1. More than one child in a family may be affected; a family history should be obtained.
2. The child with hereditary renal disease frequently presents with growth failure.
3. The inherited pattern is usually autosomal recessive, but it may also be autosomal dominant, X-linked recessive, or X-linked dominant.

Inherited renal disease is diagnosed by conventional nephrologic diagnostic procedures, including a history and physical, a family history, urinalysis, renal ultrasonography, pyelography, and percutaneous renal biopsy. The techniques used to diagnose inborn errors of metabolism are also necessary to discern those conditions that include a renal component as part of their systemic involvement. For example, several lysosomal storage diseases include renal abnormalities; thus, lysosomal enzyme activity must be measured and a renal biopsy must be performed to detect changes in the renal tubule or glomerulus. Many renal disorders also influence the serum concentration of electrolytes, blood urea nitrogen, and creatinine. Various acid-base disturbances occur, including metabolic acidosis with a normal anion gap, hyperchloremia (found in proximal or distal renal tubular acidosis), metabolic acidosis with an increased anion gap (found in diabetic nephropathy), and hypokalemic metabolic alkalosis (common in Bartter syndrome). These disorders may also impair several normal functions of the kidney: plasma filtration, so as to reduce glomerular filtration rate; reabsorption by the proximal or distal tubule or collecting duct, resulting in excessive excretion of ions or organic solutes; secretion, which results in retention of excreted substances, such as uric acid; production of kidney-derived hormones, including erythropoietin and 1,25-dihydroxy vitamin $D_3$; concentration and dilution of the final urine, which is observed in nephrogenic diabetes insipidus or sickle cell nephropathy; and the regulation of blood pressure. Uremia results in a fixed osmotic specific gravity.

The child who presents with either acute or chronic oliguric renal failure poses the greatest dilemma. A diagnosis must be made in the face of life-threatening hyperkalemia, volume overload, congestive heart failure, and hypertension. Figure 9.1 offers an approach to such a child. This chart lists only the more common disorders and is not exhaustive. Oliguria has four major causes: obstruction, prerenal azotemia as observed in dehydration, and acute or chronic renal failure. The child with acute renal failure will usually exhibit physical findings that point to the cause of renal failure, such as pyoderma or pharyngitis associated with poststreptococcal glomerulonephritis, or a facial rash and arthralgia associated with systemic lupus erythematosus. The child with chronic renal failure will present with short stature, anemia, anorexia, and hyperpigmentation because of the deposition in skin of nitrogenous waste products not excreted by failing kidneys. Other physical features pointing to chronic renal failure are enlarged kidneys in polycystic kidney disease, lenticonus and deafness in Alport hereditary nephritis, photophobia and hepatomegaly in cystinosis, and polyuria and anemia in medullary cystic disease. Inherited diseases are far more likely to result in chronic rather than acute renal failure.

Therapy is now available for a variety of inherited renal diseases. Cystinuria can be treated with D-penicillamine or α-methylpropinylglycine, which reduces the excretion of relatively insoluble cystine by the formation of more soluble mixed disulfides. The progression toward end-stage renal disease can be slowed by cysteamine in patients with cystinosis. Indomethacin can improve the profound hypokalemia of Bartter syndrome. Tight metabolic control of hyperglycemia will forestall nephropathy in diabetes, although this needs to be proved.

Patients with nephrogenic diabetes insipidus will have a marked reduction in urine volume if placed on a sodium chloride–restricted diet in conjunction with a thiazide diuretic. For children who develop uremia because of an inherited renal disorder, the techniques of hemodialysis and peritoneal dialysis and renal transplantation are successful in reversing uremia.

Renal disease is frequently a component of other inherited disorders, particularly those in which there is systemic involvement. Renal manifestations occur in these conditions for several reasons: (1) Enzymatic abnormalities affecting other organs, such as the brain, retina, or liver, may also be found in the kidney, an active metabolic organ; (2) glomerular or tubular function, which involves complex metabolic or signal-transduction pathways, may be impaired by toxic metabolites as in tyrosinosis or hereditary fructose intolerance; (3) systemic inflammatory conditions, in which mediators of inflammation lead to alterations in glomerular permselectivity, result in alterations in glomerular filtration rate and proteinuria; and (4) lysosomal enzyme damage of glomerular and tubular cells occurs in various lysosomal storage diseases. With the technique of positional cloning, the genes for many obscure familial renal disorders are now being elucidated. Hence, our understanding of renal disease has increased tremendously over the past several years.

### References

Renal Diseases in Children: Clinical Evaluation and Diagnosis: A.Y. Barakat; Springer-Verlag, 1990.

Isolated Renal Tubular Disorders: R.W. Chesney and A.L. Friedman; in Diseases of the Kidney, 6th ed.: R.L. Schrier and C.M. Gottschalk; Little, Brown and Company, 1993, pp. 611–634.

**Figure 9.1   Clinical presentation of oliguric renal failure**

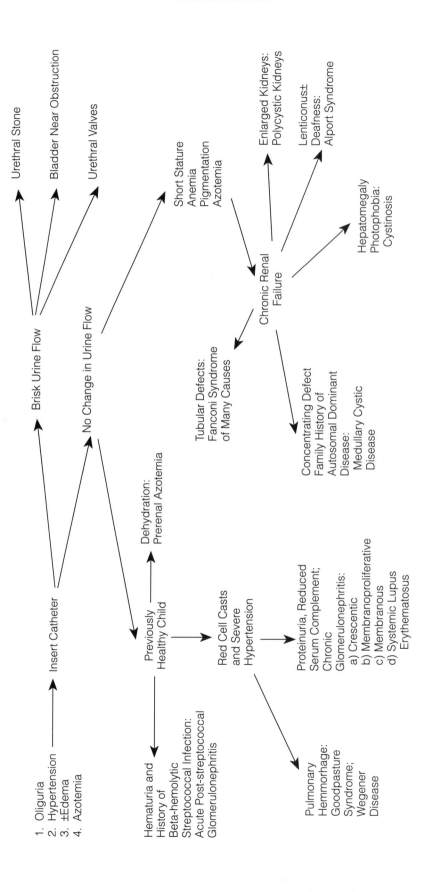

# INHERITED RENAL AND GENITOURINARY DISORDERS
*Listings in This Section*

# ALPORT SYNDROME

**Description** The syndrome encompasses a group of hereditary renal disorders marked by progressive deterioration of the glomerular basement membrane, which in a high proportion of cases leads to chronic renal failure, uremia, and the development of end-stage renal disease **(ESRD).** Uremia and renal failure may cause cardiac disturbances and renal osteodystrophy. In some forms of Alport syndrome, vision and hearing are also impaired.

Alport syndrome is classified according to its mode of inheritance, the age of onset of uremia, and features other than renal abnormalities. Six types of the disorder, designated I–VI, have been described. Juvenile forms are characterized by the development of ESRD before age 31. In adult forms, ESRD occurs after age 31.

**Synonyms**
> Epstein Syndrome (Type V)
> Hereditary Nephritis
> Nephritis and Nerve Deafness, Hereditary
> Nephropathy and Deafness, Hereditary

**Signs and Symptoms** The characteristic renal glomerular basement membrane abnormality probably causes hematuria and proteinuria. When chronic renal failure, uremia, or ESRD develops, other signs and symptoms appear. Symptoms of uremia and chronic renal failure (see below) begin insidiously.

Renal failure may lead to abnormalities of bone formation, calcium and phosphorus metabolism, and conversion of vitamin D to its active metabolite, as well as excessive parathyroid hormone secretion. Hypocalcemia and hyperphosphatemia are characteristic findings.

Ocular abnormalities may occur in the juvenile forms of Alport syndrome. Lenticonus or spherophakia may be noted. Cataracts, retinal macular flecks, or fundus albipunctatus may also be present. Children with Alport syndrome may be myopic.

Acoustic nerve or cochlear deafness also occurs in some forms of the syndrome, with high-tone hearing loss being a prominent feature.

Signs and symptoms of uremia include anorexia, nausea and vomiting, peptic ulcer disease, weakness, fatigue, hypersomnia, lassitude, dry skin, and pruritus. A urine-like breath odor is frequently noted in association with pallor, dyspnea, hypertension, fluid retention, and edema. Nerve conduction defects and attention deficits are common.

**Etiology** Alport syndrome may be inherited as an autosomal dominant or an X-linked dominant trait, or it may occur through gene mutation. An autosomal recessive inheritance has also been reported. The 6 types of Alport syndrome and their modes of inheritance are as follows:

**Type I,** a juvenile form characterized by renal disease with nerve deafness and ocular abnormalities, is an autosomal dominant disorder.

**Type II,** a juvenile form that includes renal disease with nerve deafness and ocular abnormalities, is X-linked dominant.

**Type III,** an adult form that includes renal disease with nerve deafness, is X-linked dominant.

**Type IV,** an adult form that affects only the kidney, is X-linked dominant. No vision or hearing impairment is present.

**Type V** (Epstein syndrome), which includes nerve deafness and thrombocytopathia, is an autosomal dominant disorder. This rare type has not yet been classified as a juvenile or an adult form.

**Type VI,** a juvenile form that includes kidney disease with nerve deafness and ocular abnormalities, is autosomal dominant.

**Epidemiology** Approximately 1:50,000 Americans carries the gene for Alport syndrome, although not all of them develop the syndrome. About 15 to 18 percent of affected newborns have no family history of renal disease. These cases may represent spontaneous gene mutation. The syndrome is more frequent and more severe in men. No racial preponderance or geographic clusters have been noted.

**Related Disorders** See *Fabry Disease; Medullary Cystic Disease.*

See also *Hematuria, Benign Familial*. The abnormalities of the glomerular basement membrane that characterize Alport syndrome are not found in benign familial hematuria, and proteinuria is not a feature.

**Glomerulonephritis** is characterized by inflammatory changes in the glomeruli. Manifestations include hematuria and proteinuria, facial edema, oliguria, and hypertension. Nephrotic syndrome and chronic renal failure may also occur.

**Treatment—Standard** Chronic renal failure caused by Alport syndrome must be treated vigorously. Renal function and certain components in the blood are regularly monitored. Fluid intake and diet, particularly salt and protein content, may be restricted and drugs prescribed. Control of hypertension and prompt and aggressive treatment of urinary tract and ear infections are important to maintain function of either organ.

Dialysis or renal transplantation may be used to treat chronic renal failure and ESRD. Because of the slight or inapparent disease in some female family members, care must be taken in selecting living related kidney donors.

In some cases, successful kidney transplantation has halted the progression of hearing loss. Transplantation of the cornea or removal of the lens may be helpful in patients with visual problems.

Other treatment is symptomatic and supportive. Genetic counseling is indicated for patients and their families.

**Treatment—Investigational** Calcium acetate is a new orphan drug being used in the treatment of hyperphosphatemia in ESRD. It is manufactured by Pharmedic Co.

Please contact the agencies listed under Resources, below, for the most current information. Addresses and telephone numbers of these agencies, as well as of individual experts and research centers, may be found in the Master Resources List.

**Resources**

**For more information on Alport syndrome:** National Organization for Rare Disorders (NORD); Hereditary Nephritis Foundation; Alport Syndrome-Hereditary Nephritis Study; NIH/National Kidney and Urologic Diseases Information Clearinghouse; National Kidney Foundation; American Kidney Fund.

**For genetic information and genetic counseling referrals:** March of Dimes Birth Defects Foundation; Alliance of Genetic Support Groups.

**References**

Internal Medicine, 4th ed.: J.H. Stein, ed.-in-chief; Little, Brown and Company, 1994, pp. 2516, 2750–2751.

Alport Syndrome: M.C. Gregory and C.L. Atkins; *in* Diseases of the Kidney, 5th ed.; Little, Brown and Company, 1993, pp. 571–591.

Mendelian Inheritance in Man, 10th ed.: V.A. McKusick; The Johns Hopkins University Press, 1992, pp. 54–55, 1210, 1784–1785, 1804.

Hereditary Nephropathies: M.C. Gregory, et al.; *in* Textbook of Internal Medicine; Lippincott, 1988, ch. 118.

# EXSTROPHY OF THE BLADDER

**Description** Exstrophy of the bladder is a congenital anomaly characterized by the absence of a portion of the lower abdominal wall and the anterior vesical wall, and eversion of the posterior vesical wall through the opening. Urine is excreted through this opening.

**Synonyms**

Ectopia Vesicae

**Signs and Symptoms** The anomaly results in incontinence. The pubic arch is open, and the ischia are widely separated and connected by a fibrous band. The connection between the ureter and the bladder is constricted, and the ureters are dilated. If the defect is not corrected, ureteral reflux will occur, and pyelonephritis and renal failure are likely to develop.

Diagnosis of the disorder may be made prenatally. Ultrasound studies of the developing fetus can reveal specific features that are characteristic of this abnormality (e.g., protrusion of the bladder wall through the abdomen). Early prenatal diagnosis can lead to surgical intervention shortly after birth.

**Etiology** Exstrophy of the bladder may result from rupture of the fetal bladder or from transposition of the earliest embryologic form of the organ due to a change in position of the vitelline duct.

**Epidemiology** The incidence of the abnormality is 7 times higher in males than in females.

**Related Disorders** More severe than exstrophy of the bladder, **exstrophy of the cloaca sequence** is a rare congenital defect that is obvious at birth. Like exstrophy of the bladder, it is characterized by the absence of a portion of the lower abdominal wall and the anterior vesical wall, and eversion of the posterior vesical wall through the opening. In addition, a portion of intestinal mucosa may also protrude through the abdominal wall. The anus is usually missing or stenotic. Most infants have an omphalocele.

**Treatment—Standard** Treatment consists of primary closure of the exstrophic bladder, often using a segment of colon to form the anterior and superior portion of the bladder wall. Approximately 70 percent of infants are successfully treated with this surgical procedure. An alternative but rarely used procedure to correct the defect is by ureterosigmoidostomy, with or without a colostomy. A third corrective procedure is ileal or colon loop urinary diversion.

Reconstruction of the genitalia, when necessary, is usually begun before the age of 2 years.

The outlook for maintaining normal renal function after surgical correction is relatively good. However, some individuals may experience long-term urinary problems, such as kidney stones, kidney infections, and varying degrees of urinary incontinence. Other treatment is symptomatic and supportive.

**Treatment—Investigational** Please contact the agencies listed under Resources, below, for the most current information. Addresses and telephone numbers of these agencies, as well as of individual experts and research centers, may be found in the Master Resources List.

**Resources**

**For more information on exstrophy of the bladder:** National Organization for Rare Disorders (NORD); National Support Group for Exstrophy of the Bladder; NIH/National Kidney and Urologic Diseases Information Clearinghouse; Simon Foundation; Help for Incontinent People.

**For genetic information and genetic counseling referrals:** March of Dimes Birth Defects Foundation.

**References**

The Failed Exstrophy Closure: Strategy for Management: J.P. Gearhart, et al.; Br. J. Urol., February 1993, vol. 71(2), pp. 217–220.

Cecil Textbook of Medicine, 19th ed.: J.B. Wyngaarden, et al., eds.; W.B. Saunders Company, 1992, p. 614.

Nelson Textbook of Pediatrics, 14th ed.: R.E. Behrman, ed.-in-chief; W.B. Saunders Company, 1992, pp. 1373–1374.

Results of Surgical Treatment in Children with Bladder Exstrophy: A. Csontai, et al.; Br. J. Urol., December 1992, vol. 70(6), pp. 683–685.

Birth Defects Encyclopedia: M.L Buyse, ed.-in-chief; Blackwell Scientific Publications, 1990, pp. 226–227.

Sonographic Findings in the Prenatal Diagnosis of Bladder Exstrophy: R. Jaffe, et al.; Am. J. Obstet. Gynecol., March 1990, vol. 162(3), pp. 675–678.

Closure of the Exstrophic Bladder: An Evaluation of the Factors Leading to Its Success and Its Importance in Urinary Continence: D.A. Husmann, et al.; J. Urol., August 1989, vol. 142(2 pt 2), pp. 522–524, discussion pp. 542–543.

Long-Term Followup of 207 Patients with Bladder Exstrophy: An Evolution in Treatment: J.P. Connor, et al.; J. Urol., September 1989, vol. 142(3), pp. 793–795.

State-of-the-Art Reconstructive Surgery of Bladder Exstrophy at The Johns Hopkins Hospital: J.P. Gearhart, et al.; Am. J. Dis. Child., December 1989, vol. 143(12), pp. 1475–1478.

Smith's Recognizable Patterns of Human Malformation, 4th ed.: K.L. Jones, ed.: W.B. Saunders Company, 1988, pp. 566–567.

# HEMATURIA, BENIGN FAMILIAL

**Description** Benign familial hematuria is a hereditary nonprogressive renal disorder that begins in childhood. It is characterized by episodes of hematuria and scattered thinning of the glomerular basement membrane.

**Synonyms**

> Hematuria, Benign Recurrent
> Hematuria, Essential

**Signs and Symptoms** The hematuria may be macro- or microscopic and is often preceded by a respiratory infection. Little or no proteinuria occurs, and renal function is unaffected. In children, the urine may clear after each episode; in adults, the hematuria may be more persistent.

**Etiology** The cause is unknown. A genetic predisposition transmitted through autosomal dominant genes is suspected. The disorder's frequent appearance after respiratory infections may be significant.

**Epidemiology** Benign familial hematuria occurs more frequently in males than females, and more often in children and young adults.

**Related Disorders** See *IGA Nephropathy; Alport Syndrome.*

**Chronic renal failure** can be a complication of many kidney diseases or a symptom of a variety of diseases and conditions. It occurs gradually when the kidneys can no longer filter waste products from the blood. Polyuria, hematuria, proteinuria, hypertension, and anemia may occur.

**Treatment—Standard** Treatment may not be necessary, or is symptomatic and supportive. Genetic counseling may be helpful.

**Treatment—Investigational** Please contact the agencies listed under Resources, below, for the most current information. Addresses and telephone numbers of these agencies, as well as of individual experts and research centers, may be found in the Master Resources List.

**Resources**

**For more information on benign familial hematuria:** National Organization for Rare Disorders (NORD); National Kidney Foundation; American Kidney Fund; NIH/National Kidney and Urological Diseases Information Clearinghouse.

**For genetic information and genetic counseling referrals:** March of Dimes Birth Defects Foundation; Alliance of Genetic Support Groups.

**References**

Hematuria: C.E. Kashtan; *in* Primer on Kidney Diseases: A. Greenberg, ed.; Academic Press, 1994, ch. 4.

Mendelian Inheritance in Man, 10th ed.: V.A. McKusick; The Johns Hopkins University Press, 1992, pp. 460–461.

Internal Medicine, 3rd ed.: J.H. Stein, ed.-in-chief; Little, Brown and Company, 1990, p. 914.

Establishing the Diagnosis of Benign Familial Hematuria: The Importance of Examining the Urine Sediment of Family Members: S. Blumenthal, et al.; JAMA, April 15, 1988, vol. 259(15), pp. 2263–2266.

Benign Familial Hematuria: N. Yoshikawa, et al.; Arch. Pathol. Lab. Med., August 1988, vol. 112(8), pp. 794–797.

# HEMOLYTIC-UREMIC SYNDROME (HUS)

**Description** HUS is a syndrome of diverse etiologies defined as a microangiopathic hemolytic anemia, thrombocytopenia, and acute kidney failure with hematuria and proteinuria.

**Synonyms**
Gasser Syndrome

**Signs and Symptoms** Onset usually is abrupt; in most cases the first sign is diarrhea, with or without blood in the stool (hematochezia). Other characteristics include vomiting, dehydration, labored breathing, hematemesis, melena, petechiae, hypertension, and seizures. Thrombocytopenia and anemia usually occur. The kidneys are primarily affected, and anuria may be present. The onset of anemia (pallor) and oliguria may occur abruptly during the course of the diarrhea.

Approximately 60 percent of children with HUS develop acute kidney failure, which usually reverses after dialysis. Chronic kidney failure occurs in approximately 10 percent of children, who require lifelong dialysis or transplantation. Kidney involvement is generally more severe in adults, and cortical necrosis may occur.

**Etiology** The cause is unknown. An association with *Escherichia coli* infection is found in 70 percent of cases in North America and 35 percent of cases in the United Kingdom. The *E. coli* strains associated with HUS (O157:_; O157:H7; O111; O25:H11; and others) produce verocytotoxins similar to the toxins produced by *Shigella dysenteriae*. HUS usually appears abruptly in children 3 to 10 days after an episode of gastroenteritis or viral upper respiratory tract infections. In adults, it most commonly affects women and is often associated with pregnancy or the use of birth control pills.

**Epidemiology** The syndrome occurs rarely, and most frequently in children under the age of 4 years, and in pregnant or postpartum women. It is occasionally seen in older children and nonpregnant adults. Some areas of the world (e.g., Argentina) have a much higher incidence than North America, but the west coast of the United States appears to be an endemic region.

**Related Disorders** See ***Purpura, Thrombotic Thrombocytopenic.***

**Treatment—Standard** Infants and children recover more easily than adults. Dialysis may be necessary for children and postpartum women. Fresh frozen plasma transfusions may be used. The orphan drug erythropoetin **(EPO)**, used in the treatment of anemia related to kidney dialysis, should not be prescribed.

**Treatment—Investigational** Plasmapheresis may be beneficial in severe cases, but is still under investigation to analyze side effects and effectiveness.

Please contact the agencies listed under Resources, below, for the most current information. Addresses and telephone numbers of these agencies, as well as of individual experts and research centers, may be found in the Master Resources List.

**Resources**

**For more information on hemolytic-uremic syndrome:** National Organization for Rare Disorders (NORD); NIH/National Kidney and Urologic Diseases Information Clearinghouse; National Kidney Foundation; American Kidney Fund.

**References**

Internal Medicine, 4th ed.: J.H. Stein, ed.-in-chief; Little, Brown and Company, 1994, pp. 802, 869, 2727.

Hemolytic-Uremic Syndrome Associated with an Infection by Verotoxin-Producing *Escherichia coli* 0111 in a Woman on Oral Contraceptives: K.O. Stenger, et al.; Clin. Nephrol., March 1989; vol. 29(3), pp. 153–158.

Cytoxin-Producing *Escherichia coli* and the Hemolytic-Uremic Syndrome: T.G. Cleary; Pediatr. Clin. North Am., June 1988, vol. 35(5), pp. 485–501.

Illnesses Associated with *Escherichia coli* 0157:H7 Infections. A Broad Clinical Spectrum: P.M. Griffin, et al.; Ann. Intern. Med., November 1, 1988, vol. 109(9), pp. 705–712.

# HEPATORENAL SYNDROME

**Description** Hepatorenal syndrome develops as a result of severe liver disease; the kidneys appear normal. The disorder is seen in 2 forms, one milder than the other.

**Signs and Symptoms** Unique circulatory abnormalities occur in hepatorenal syndrome. Cardiac output is increased. The arteries of the systemic circulation widen. The renal arteries narrow, causing a decrease in renal blood flow.

The more severe form of the syndrome is characterized by ascites, jaundice, and rapidly progressive renal failure, with oliguria and azotemia and, in some cases, proteinuria and hematuria. The jaundice may be accompanied by dark urine and an enlarged and tender liver. Anorexia, fever, fatigue, and weakness may be present. Hepatic or portosystemic encephalopathy may develop, possibly causing changes in mental acuity, personality changes, inappropriate behavior, depression, and sleep disturbances.

In the 2nd form of the syndrome, jaundice is milder, renal failure advances less rapidly, and hepatic encephalopathy does not occur.

**Etiology** Reported causes of the syndrome include hepatitis, advanced cirrhosis, obstructive jaundice, liver cancer, and tumors of the bile ducts. In many cases a precipitating factor can be identified, such as an infection or gastrointestinal bleeding.

**Epidemiology** The syndrome occurs equally in males and females with severe liver disease.

**Related Disorders** Most cases of acute renal failure are distinguished from hepatorenal syndrome by underlying renal abnormalities, such as renovascular disease; glomerular disturbances associated with infections, Goodpasture syndrome, polycystic kidney disease, or Wegener granulomatosis; acute interstitial nephritis, commonly related to drugs or infections; intratubular obstruction; or acute tubular necrosis. (See *Goodpasture Syndrome; Polycystic Kidney Diseases; Wegener Granulomatosis.)*

**Treatment—Standard** Treatment is primarily directed toward correcting the characteristic circulatory disturbances. Three methods have been used: head-out water immersion (immersion of the body in water, leaving the head out, which redistributes the blood from the arms and legs to the trunk); paracentesis; and peritoneovenous shunting.

Other treatment is symptomatic and supportive.

**Treatment—Investigational** Liver transplantation has been used for patients who do not respond to other therapies.

The effectiveness of transfusion with fresh frozen plasma and the use of lumbar sympathectomy in treating the acute renal failure are being evaluated. The therapeutic roles of drugs such as atrial natriuretic peptide, calcium channel blockers, prostaglandins, and the liver hormone glomerulopressin are under investigation.

Please contact the agencies listed under Resources, below, for the most current information. Addresses and telephone numbers of these agencies, as well as of individual experts and research centers, may be found in the Master Resources List.

**Resources**

**For more information on hepatorenal syndrome:** National Organization for Rare Disorders (NORD); American Liver Foundation; Children's Liver Foundation; NIH/National Kidney and Urologic Diseases Information Clearinghouse.

**References**

The Hepatorenal Syndrome: P.S. Kellerman and S.L. Linas; AKF Nephrology Letter, November 1988, vol. 5(4), pp. 47–54.

Pathophysiology of the Hepatorenal Syndrome and Potential for Therapy: M. Levy; Am. J. Cardiol., December 14, 1987, vol. 60(17), pp. 66I–72I.

# IgA Nephropathy

**Description** IgA nephropathy occurs during childhood and young adulthood. Hematuria related to IgA nephropathy usually occurs after a viral infection of the upper respiratory or gastrointestinal tract.

**Synonyms**

Berger Disease
Idiopathic Renal Hematuria
Mesangial IgA Nephropathy

**Signs and Symptoms** The first recognizable sign of IgA nephropathy is hematuria due to acute nephritis or glomerulonephritis. There is often mild proteinuria with slowly progressive renal changes. Loin pain may occur, but hypertension or edema is unusual during the initial phase of the disease.

IgA nephropathy may progress slowly for several decades and can result in progressive renal failure in 35 percent of cases.

**Etiology** A postinfectious process is suspected as the cause of IgA nephropathy. An immune association is postulated because of an increase in the immunoglobulin IgA factor, but the mechanisms leading to glomerular immune deposit formation are unclear.

**Epidemiology** IgA nephropathy affects males 2 or 3 times more often than females and usually occurs between the ages of 15 and 35. It is one of the leading causes of acute nephritis in young people in the United States, Europe, and Japan. The incidence is significantly higher in American Indians than in any other ethnic group studied, and it is more prevalent in whites than in blacks. A study showed an annual occurrence rate of approximately 94:100,000 young men tested upon induction into the military.

**Related Disorders** See *Purpura, Schoenlein-Henoch; Systemic Lupus Erythematosus.*

**Treatment—Standard** No specific treatment for IgA nephropathy has been shown to be effective for all patients. Some have responded to oral steroid therapy, especially in the early stages of the disease. Long-term remission of symptoms has been achieved with the use of cyclophosphamide, even after therapy was withdrawn. Kidney transplantation has been successful for many persons.

**Treatment—Investigational** Cyclosporin may be an effective treatment for certain patients with relapsing IgA nephropathy. However, if the drug is discontinued, most patients will relapse.

Please contact the organizations listed under Resources, below, for the most current information. Addresses and telephone numbers of these agencies, as well as of individual experts and research centers, may be found in the Master Resources List.

**Resources**

**For more information on IgA nephropathy:** National Organization for Rare Disorders (NORD); IgA Nephropathy Support Network; American Kidney Fund; National Kidney Foundation; NIH/National Kidney and Urologic Diseases Information Clearinghouse.

**References**

Cyclosporin in the Treatment of Steroid-Responsive and Steroid-Resistant Nephrotic Syndrome in Adults: E. Maher, et al.; Nephrol. Dial. Transplant., 1988, vol. 3(6).

IgA Nephropathy, the Most Common Glomerulonephritis Worldwide: A Neglected Disease in the United States?: Am. J. Med., January 1988, vol. 84(1), pp. 129–132.

Proteinuria in IgA Nephropathy: K. Neelakantappa, et al.; Kidney Int., March 1988, vol. 33(3), pp. 716–721.

Steroid Therapy in IgA Nephropathy: A Retrospective Study in Heavy Proteinuric Cases: Y. Kobayaski, et al.; Nephron, 1988, vol. 48(1), pp. 12–17.

Tonsillar Distribution of IgA and IgG Immunocytes and Production of IgA Subclasses and J Chain in Tonsillitis Vary with the Presence or Absence of IgA Nephropathy: J. Nagy, et al.; Scand. J. Immunol., April 1988, vol. 27(4), pp. 393–399.

# INTERSTITIAL CYSTITIS

**Description** Interstitial cystitis is a slowly progressive inflammatory disease of the bladder characterized by pressure and pain above the pubic area along with increased frequency and urgency of urination. This occurs because of chronic inflammation of the lining of the bladder and swelling of the interior walls of the bladder. Affected individuals urinate frequently because of a smaller than normal bladder capacity. In a small percentage of cases, people with interstitial cystitis also have scarring and ulcerations on the membranes that line the bladder. Interstitial cystitis typically affects young and middle-aged women.

**Synonyms**

>Hunner Ulcer or Syndrome
>Panmural Fibrosis
>Submucosal Cystitis
>Submucosal Ulcer of the Bladder

**Signs and Symptoms** The major symptoms of interstitial cystitis include the urgent need for frequent urination and the ability to eliminate only small amounts of urine at one time. The symptoms are the same as those caused by common bladder infections, but in interstitial cystitis there is usually no infection and the symptoms are not relieved by antibiotic treatment. The symptoms occur both during the day and at night. People with this disorder may urinate as many as 50 to 60 times during the day and 20 to 30 times during the night. Sleep deprivation may lead to fatigue, anxiety, and/or depression.

Most people with interstitial cystitis experience pain and pressure above the pubic area, which slowly disappears after urination. Pain may also occur in the pelvic area, the genitals, and around the rectum. If immediate urination is delayed, the pain may be extreme. Other symptoms may include hematuria, dysuria, painful sexual intercourse, and sometimes incontinence.

The symptoms of interstitial cystitis are usually slowly progressive and may become more severe over the course of months or years. However, the symptoms seem to plateau after about 5 years in most people.

A common complication of interstitial cystitis is repeated infection of the urinary tract following the use of medical instruments in examination or treatment procedures. If the ureter becomes narrower than normal, some affected individuals may experience hydronephrosis, possibly leading to kidney damage.

Cystoscopy usually reveals abnormally thick bladder walls, areas of inflammation, areas of bleeding, and fibrosis within the mucosal lining of the bladder. Inflammatory changes include the replacement of muscle by fibrous tissue, an abnormally thin and patchy mucosal layer, an increase in the number of blood vessels, and degeneration of the blood vessels around the bladder.

Mast cells may be present within the mucosal lining of the bladder of some people with interstitial cystitis. Measurement of urinary volume typically reveals a decrease in the amount of urine that is passed during each urination. A biopsy of the bladder to rule out the possibility of carcinoma in situ is recommended.

**Etiology** The exact cause of interstitial cystitis is not known. Some studies suggest that it may be an autoimmune disease of the bladder's connective tissue. Many people with interstitial cystitis have a strong history of allergies, but few report having had infections of the urinary tract. Some research suggests that interstitial cystitis may be associated with abnormalities of the thin, protective mucosal lining of the walls of the bladder (glycosaminoglycan or GAG layer). Defects in this lining may lead to the development of chronic inflammation or ulceration. Other studies are investigating the role of glycosaminoglycan uronates. There is some evidence that certain uronates may be deficient in some people with interstitial cystitis.

**Epidemiology** Interstitial cystitis affects females 10 times more frequently than males. Some cases have also been diagnosed in children. The symptoms of this disorder usually begin between 20 and 50 years of age, but the average onset is about 40 years of age. There may be as many as 450,000 cases of interstitial cystitis in the United States, but many of these patients are undiagnosed or misdiagnosed.

**Related Disorders** See *Reiter Syndrome.*

**Cystitis** is a common inflammatory bladder disease characterized by painful and frequent urination. Pain and pressure may be present in the pelvic and genital area, and there may be hematuria. Acute cystitis may occur because of a bacterial infection of the lower urinary tract, radiation therapy, or treatment with certain immunosuppressant drugs (e.g., cyclophosphamide). In radiation-induced cystitis, cysts may form in the interior walls of the bladder.

**Cystitis colli (cystanchenitis)** is an acute inflammatory condition of the neck of the bladder. The symptoms are similar to those of interstitial cystitis and may include painful and frequent urination accompanied by pain in the pelvic area.

**Cancer of the bladder (carcinoma in situ)** is characterized by malignant growths on the bladder walls that may destroy the mucosal lining. Symptoms may include pain and pressure in the pelvis and genitals accompanied by frequent and painful urination. Blood may be present in the urine.

**Endometriosis** is a common gynecologic condition that is characterized by the inability to shed the tissue that normally lines the uterus before menstruation. This excess tissue may sometimes spread to other areas of the body, including the bladder and lungs. Symptoms may include lower back pain, pain in the thighs, repeated miscarriages, and/or infertility. When endometrial tissue spreads to the bladder, the symptoms can be similar to those of interstitial cystitis, including frequent and painful urination.

**Prostatitis** is a common infection of the prostate gland. Acute bacterial prostatitis is characterized by chills, high fever, low back pain, and/or painful joints. Other symptoms may include the frequent urge to urinate, accompanied by difficult and painful urination. Acute cystitis usually accompanies acute prostatitis. Males with chronic bacterial prostatitis experience frequency and urgency of urination, pain and burning sensations during urination, and excessive urination at night.

**Treatment—Standard** Treatment is palliative, not curative. Approximately 30 percent of people with interstitial cystitis experience short-term relief from hydraulic distention. Repeated bladder distentions may be done to try to increase the urinary capacity of the bladder. Another procedure, instillation of dimethyl sulfoxide (**DMSO**) into the bladder, provides some relief. Other drugs that may be used instead of DMSO include cortisone acetate, silver nitrate, and oxychlorosene sodium (Clorpactin). Electrofulguration may temporarily relieve some symptoms of interstitial cystitis and allow ulcerations to heal.

Glucocorticoids may be administered orally. Anticholinergic drugs, such as propantheline bromide or oxybutinyn chloride, may also relieve symptoms of interstitial cystitis. Other oral medications may include nonsteroidal anti-inflammatory drugs (e.g., benzydamine), antispasmodic drugs, antihistamines, muscle relaxants, or heparin. Antidepressant drugs, such as anitriptylin or doxepin, may be also be administered. These drugs may help relieve pain and help some patients to sleep for longer periods of time. Some people with interstitial cystitis may improve when alcohol, caffeine, artificial sweeteners, citrus fruits, and/or tomatoes are eliminated from the diet.

When the urogenital pain associated with interstitial cystitis is severe, a transcutaneous electrical nerve stimulator, or TENS unit, may be used to alter nerve transmissions to the bladder and help to block pain impulses. Other severely affected individuals may have pain medications administered via lumbar epidural block.

When the symptoms of interstitial cystitis do not respond to bladder lavage or drug therapy, surgery may be performed to increase the size of the bladder. In one surgical procedure known as ileocystoplasty or sigmoidoplasty/uretosigmoidostomy, the size of the bladder is increased using tissue from the intestine. In extremely severe cases, a cystectomy may have to be performed to shift urine flow into the small or large intestine.

**Treatment—Investigational** In a small preliminary study of people with severe interstitial cystitis who had not responded to conventional therapies, 5 patients were treated with laser therapy (neodymium-YAG laser) on the interior walls of the bladder. In 4 of these patients, severe bladder pain and frequent urination stopped within several days after therapy. Bladder capacity was found to be increased, and complications from laser treatment were low. Fifteen months after treatment, these patients had no recurrence of severe symptoms, although some had mild urinary frequency. Larger long-term studies are needed to determine the safety and effectiveness of laser therapy for the possible treatment of severe interstitial cystitis.

A 5-year research program began in 1987 at the University of Pennsylvania to develop a comprehensive database on people with interstitial cystitis and to examine possible causes of the disorder. This research focused on the GAG layer, which acts as a protective lining in the bladder. If defective, the GAG layer might allow the penetration of substances in the urine that could cause interstitial cystitis. Researchers are also exploring substances in the urine that might irritate the bladder wall. Possible hormonal, immunologic, and infectious causes of interstitial cystitis are also being investigated.

The orphan drug sodium pentosan polysulphate (Elmiron) is an oral medication that may help to restore the GAG layer. In some studies, approximately 40 to 60 percent of people with interstitial cystitis showed some improvement while on this medication. Larger studies of Elmiron are currently under way to determine the long-term safety and effectiveness of this drug for the treatment of interstitial cystitis. For more information contact Baker Cummins Pharmaceuticals.

Studies are under way to determine the effectiveness of combining certain drugs for the treatment of interstitial cystitis. In one study the bladder is "washed" with a long acting anesthetic known as marcaine combined with hydrocortisone, heparin, and sodium bicarbonate. More studies are needed to determine the long-term safety and effectiveness of these drugs for the treatment of interstitial cystitis.

Although antihistamine drugs do not seem to be an effective treatment for interstitial cystitis, research is under way to determine the effects of the antihistamine atarax (Vistaril). More study is required before antihistamines can be recommended for the treatment of interstitial cystitis.

A research project at the Tufts New England Medical Center is exploring the role of mast cells in interstitial cystitis. The drug nalmefene, which is believed to inhibit mast cell activity, and the orphan drug nifedipine are being tested for the treatment of interstitial cystitis.

Please contact the agencies listed under Resources, below, for the most current information. Addresses and telephone numbers of these agencies, as well as of individual experts and research centers, may be found in the Master Resources List.

### Resources

**For more information on interstitial cystitis:** National Organization for Rare Disorders (NORD); Interstitial Cystitis Association of America; NIH/National Kidney and Urologic Diseases Information Clearinghouse.

### References

Lumbar Epidural Blockage for Management of Pain in Interstitial Cystitis: P.P. Irwin, et al.; Br. J. Urol., April 1993, vol. 71(4), pp. 413–416.

The Natural History of Interstitial Cystitis: A Survey of 374 Patients: J.A. Koziol, et al.; J. Urol., March 1993, vol. 149(3), pp. 465–469.

Urinary Glycosaminoglycan Excretion As a Laboratory Marker in the Diagnosis of Interstitial Cystitis: R.E. Hurst, et al.; J. Urol., January 1993, vol. 149(1), pp. 31–35.

Cecil Textbook of Medicine, 19th ed.: J.B. Wyngaarden, et al., eds.; W.B. Saunders Company, 1992, pp. 593–594.

Interstitial Cystitis: A Bladder Disease Finds Legitimacy: V. Ratner, et al.; J. Women's Health, Spring 1992, vol. 1(1), pp. 63–68.

Characteristics of Mast Cells in Normal Bladder, Bacterial Cystitis and Interstitial Cystitis: T.J. Christmas, et al.; Br. J. Urol., November 1991, vol. 68(5), pp. 473–478.

Problems in the Surgical Treatment of Interstitial Cystitis: D.E. Nurse, et al.; Br. J. Urol., August 1991, vol. 68(2), pp. 153–154.

Dictionary of Medical Syndromes, 3rd ed.: S.I. Magalini, et al., eds.; J.B. Lippincott Company, 1990, pp. 223–224.

Successful Treatment of Interstitial Cystitis with Sodium Pentosanpolysulfate: C.L. Parsons, et al.; J. Urol., July 1983, vol. 130(1), pp. 51–53.

General Urology, 10th ed.: D. Smith, ed.; Lange Medical Publications, 1981, pp. 470–84.

The Treatment of Interstitial Cystitis by Cystolysis with Observations on Cystoplasty: A Review After 7 Years: P.H. Worth; Br. J. Urol., June 1980, vol. 52(3), p. 32.

# LOKEN-SENIOR SYNDROME

**Description** Loken-Senior syndrome is an inherited disorder characterized by nephronophthisis, with or without medullary cystic disease, and by progressive eye disease. Typically, this disorder becomes apparent during the first year of life.

### Synonyms

Nephronophthisis-Associated Ocular Anomalies, Familial Juvenile
Renal Dysplasia–Blindness, Hereditary
Renal Dysplasia–Retinal Aplasia, Loken-Senior Type
Renal-Retinal Dystrophy, Familial
Renal-Retinal Syndrome
Senior-Loken Syndrome

**Signs and Symptoms** Kidney problems typically develop very gradually, with much time elapsing before symptoms become apparent. Progressive kidney failure occurs as a result of tubular degeneration. This can cause uremia and chronic interstitial nephritis. Eventually the patient may have symptoms such as nausea, vomiting, weight loss, fatigue, anemia, and ultimately kidney failure. Progressive atrophy of the retina also occurs, resembling the retinal atrophy either of Leber congenital amaurosis or of retinitis pigmentosa.

**Etiology** Loken-Senior syndrome is inherited as an autosomal recessive trait.

**Epidemiology** Loken-Senior syndrome affects males and females in equal numbers. There have been more than 150 cases of this disorder reported in the medical literature.

**Related Disorders** See *Leber Congenital Amaurosis; Retinitis Pigmentosa; Medullary Cystic Disease; Polycystic Kidney Disease.*

**Treatment—Standard** Patients with uremia need close monitoring. Diet must be carefully controlled. An increase of calories in the diet should be coupled with a reduction in the total content of dietary protein. Sufficient carbohydrates and fats should be consumed to provide energy and prevent the body from metabolizing its own proteins. Kidney failure may need to be managed with hemodialysis. Kidney transplantation is sometimes indicated. When the retinal atrophy in Loken-Senior syndrome resembles that of retinitis pigmentosa, the patient may benefit from various visual aids. Genetic counseling may be of benefit for patients and their families.

**Treatment—Investigational** Researchers at the Cullen Eye Institute of the Baylor College of Medicine in Houston, TX, and the Hospital For Sick Children in Toronto, Canada, are studying a group of inherited retinal disorders including Leber congenital amaurosis. Families with at least two affected members whose parents are both living are needed to participate in the program. For information, please contact Richard A. Lewis, M.D., at the Cullen Eye Institute, and Maria A. Musarella, M.D., at the Hospital For Sick Children.

Please contact the agencies listed under Resources, below, for the most current information. Addresses and telephone numbers of these agencies, as well as of individual experts and research centers, may be found in the Master Resources List.

**Resources**

**For more information on Loken-Senior syndrome:** National Organization for Rare Disorders (NORD); National Kidney Foundation; American Kidney Fund; NIH/National Kidney and Urologic Diseases Information Clearinghouse; National Association of Patients on Hemodialysis and Transplantation; NIH/National Eye Institute; Foundation Fighting Blindness; National Association for Parents of the Visually Impaired; National Association for the Visually Handicapped.

**For genetic information and genetic counseling referrals:** March of Dimes Birth Defects Foundation; Alliance of Genetic Support Groups.

**References**

Mendelian Inheritance in Man, 10th ed.: V.A. McKusick; The Johns Hopkins University Press, 1992, pp. 1675–1676.

Birth Defects Encyclopedia: M.L Buyse, ed.-in-chief; Blackwell Scientific Publications, 1990, p. 1463.

Senior-Loken Syndrome (Familial Renal-Retinal Dystrophy) and Coats' Disease: J.S. Schuman, et al.; Am. J. Ophthalmol., December 15, 1985, vol. 100(6), pp. 822–827.

Senior-Loken Syndrome: Nephronophthisis and Tapeto-Retinal Degeneration: J.P. Fillastre, et al.; Clin. Nephrol., January 1976, vol. 5(1), pp. 14–19.

# MEDULLARY CYSTIC DISEASE

**Description** Medullary cystic disease is a genetic nephropathy that usually appears in children or young adults (**familial juvenile nephronopthisis**) and progresses gradually to the onset of uremia, either in childhood or adulthood. It is the 2nd most common cause of chronic kidney failure in childhood. Other affected individuals may not experience any symptoms until adulthood (**adult-onset medullary cystic disease**). A third variant of the disease is characterized by retinal degeneration (**renal-retinal dysplasia**).

**Synonyms**

Adult-Onset Medullary Cystic Disease

Familial Juvenile Nephronophthisis

Renal-Retinal Dysplasia

**Signs and Symptoms** The initial manifestation is often a severe polyuria and sodium wasting. Metabolic acidosis with or without hyperchloremia may be present. Other symptoms include polydipsia, general weakness, pallor, and incontinence, particularly at night (noctural enuresis). Affected children frequently have growth retardation and signs of bone disease. Many patients compensate so well during the development of the disorder that medullary cystic disease goes unrecognized until uremia develops. Anemia may be an early clue to medullary cystic disease.

Laboratory findings are similar to those in chronic renal failure, although proteinuria is not evident. Intravenous urography reveals small kidneys; medullary cysts may be seen with ultrasonography or arteriography.

A subset of patients with renal-retinal dysplasia experience visual impairment caused by degenerative changes in the retina and are difficult to fit for corrective glasses. Unusual amounts of pigment may also accumulate in the retina, causing inflammation. Further visual impairment may be caused by retinitis pigmentosa.

**Etiology** Familial juvenile nephronopthisis is inherited as an autosomal recessive genetic trait. The gene that causes this form of the disease is thought to be located on the short arm of chromosome 2 (2p24). Adult-onset medullary cystic disease is inherited as an autosomal dominant genetic trait.

**Epidemiology** Fifty percent of cases are diagnosed in childhood, 20 percent not until adulthood. In some cases, onset has occurred as late as the 7th decade. The juvenile form of the disease is thought to occur in 1:50,000 children in the United States.

**Related Disorders** See *Medullary Sponge Kidney; Polycystic Kidney Diseases; Loken-Senior Syndrome.*

**Treatment—Standard** The polyuria is resistant to vasopressin. Treatment consists of management of uremia when it occurs. Diet is monitored. An increase in caloric intake should be accompanied by a reduction in total dietary protein. Sufficient carbohydrates and fats should be consumed to provide energy and prevent the body from metabolizing its own proteins. In severe cases, kidney transplantation may be considered. Recurrence of the disease has not been noted in people undergoing transplantation. Genetic counseling is recommended for patients and their families. Other treatment is symptomatic and supportive.

**Treatment—Investigational** Please contact the agencies listed under Resources, below, for the most current information. Addresses and telephone numbers of these agencies, as well as of individual experts and research centers, may be found in the Master Resources List.

**Resources**

For more information on medullary cystic disease: National Organization for Rare Disorders (NORD); NIH/National Kidney and Urologic Diseases Information Clearinghouse; National Kidney Foundation; American Kidney Fund.

For genetic information and genetic counseling referrals: March of Dimes Birth Defects Foundation; Alliance of Genetic Support Groups.

**References**

Online Mendelian Inheritance in Man (OMIM): V.A. McKusick; The Johns Hopkins University, last edit date 6/8/94, entry number 25610.

Cecil Textbook of Medicine, 19th ed.: J.B. Wyngaarden, et al., eds.; W.B. Saunders Company, 1992, p. 612.

Mendelian Inheritance in Man, 10th ed.: V.A. McKusick; The Johns Hopkins University Press, 1992, pp. 888, 1582–1583.

Nelson Textbook of Pediatrics, 14th ed.: R.E. Behrman, ed.-in-chief; W.B. Saunders Company, 1992, p. 1346.

Harrison's Principles of Internal Medicine, 12th ed.: J.D. Wilson, et al., eds.; McGraw-Hill, 1991, p. 1198.

The Kidney, 4th ed.: B.M. Brenner and F.C. Rector, Jr., eds.: W.B. Saunders Company, 1991, pp. 1675–1676.

Birth Defects Encyclopedia: M.L Buyse, ed.-in-chief; Blackwell Scientific Publications, 1990, pp. 1008–1009.

Dictionary of Medical Syndromes, 3rd ed.: S.I. Magalini, et al., eds.; J.B. Lippincott Company, 1990, p. 628.

Renal Medullary Cystic Disease: Findings at Urography and Ultrasonography: A. Olsen, et al.; Acta Radiol., September–October 1988, vol. 29(5), pp. 527–529.

Combined Tubular Dysfunction in Medullary Cystic Disease: A. Chagnac, et al.; Arch. Intern. Med., May 1986, vol. 146(5), pp. 1007–1009.

# MEDULLARY SPONGE KIDNEY

**Description** Medullary sponge kidney is a hereditary congenital defect occurring in one or both kidneys and characterized by marked dilatation of the collecting tubules, which may be associated with nephrolithiasis and hematuria.

**Synonyms**

> Sponge Kidney
> Tubular Ectasia

**Signs and Symptoms** Urinary tract infections often are the first sign of the underlying abnormality.

Nephrolithiasis with renal colic, loin pain, and the excretion of small stones is a prominent feature of medullary sponge kidney. The stones, which form in the dilated portions of the collecting tubules, consist of calcium oxalate, calcium phosphate, and other calcium salts. About 13 percent of all patients who develop renal calculi have medullary sponge kidney. The disorder seldom progresses to end-stage renal failure, although reduced glomerular filtration rates have been observed.

The most common functional abnormalities include the loss of urinary concentrating capacity and metabolic acidosis secondary to renal tubular acidosis.

**Etiology** The disorder is inherited in an autosomal dominant pattern. A possible relationship between hyperparathyroidism and medullary sponge kidney has been proposed. Medullary sponge kidney is also found in individuals with the Beckwith-Wiedemann syndrome (see *Beckwith-Wiedemann Syndrome).*

**Epidemiology** The incidence is higher in males than in females. Although symptoms may begin at any age, they usually develop during adolescence or in adults between the ages of 30 and 50.

**Treatment—Standard** Patients should take in sufficient fluids in order to excrete about 2 liters of urine daily. Those with hypercalciuria may benefit from long-term therapy with thiazide diuretics as well as a high fluid intake. For patients with calcium urolithiasis and normal calcium excretion, oral phosphate therapy may be useful. A low-calcium diet may prevent stone formation. Yearly urinalysis and urine culture are advisable.

Many patients with medullary sponge kidney have recurrent urinary tract infections and should probably receive prophylactic antibiotics.

**Treatment—Investigational** The orphan drugs calcium acetate (Braintree Laboratories) and calcium carbonate (R&D Laboratories) are being investigated for the treatment of hyperphosphatemia associated with end-stage renal disease, which can occur as a rare complication in some people with medullary sponge kidney.

Please contact the agencies listed under Resources, below, for the most current information. Addresses and telephone numbers of these agencies, as well as of individual experts and research centers, may be found in the Master Resources List.

**Resources**

**For more information on medullary sponge kidney:** National Organization for Rare Disorders (NORD); NIH/National Kidney and Urologic Diseases Information Clearinghouse; National Kidney Foundation.

**References**

Experience Using Extracorporeal Shock-Wave Lithotripsy to Treat Urinary Calculi in Problem Kidneys: W.C. Chen, et al.; Urol. Int., 1993, vol. 51(1), pp. 32–38.

Prophylactic Role of Extracorporeal Shock Wave Lithotripsy in the Management of Nephrocalcinosis: H. Vandeursen, et al.; Br. J. Urol., April 1993, vol. 71(4), pp. 392–395.

Cecil Textbook of Medicine, 19th ed.: J.B. Wyngaarden, et al., eds.; W.B. Saunders Company, 1992, p. 612.

Nelson Textbook of Pediatrics, 14th ed.: R.E. Behrman, ed.-in-chief; W.B. Saunders Company, 1992, p. 1346.

Harrison's Principles of Internal Medicine, 12th ed.: J.D. Wilson, et al., eds.; McGraw-Hill, 1991, pp. 1197–1198.

The Kidney, 4th ed.: B.M. Brenner and F.C. Rector, Jr., eds.: W.B. Saunders Company, 1991, pp. 1676–1679.

Medullary Sponge Kidney on Axial Computed Tomography: Comparison with Excretory Urography: J.M. Ginalski, et al.; Eur. J. Radiol., March–April 1991, vol. 12(2), pp. 104–107.

Birth Defects Encyclopedia: M.L Buyse, ed.-in-chief; Blackwell Scientific Publications, 1990, p. 1008.

Dictionary of Medical Syndromes, 3rd ed.: S.I. Magalini, et al., eds.; J.B. Lippincott Company, 1990, p. 150.

Does Medullary Sponge Kidney Cause Nephrolithiasis?: J.M. Ginalski, et al.; Am. J. Roentgenol., August 1990, vol. 155(2), pp. 299–302.

# POLYCYSTIC KIDNEY DISEASES (PKD)

**Description** The presence of bilateral renal cysts characterizes these inherited diseases. Renal cystic enlargement over time results in encroachment on normal renal tissue, with loss of renal function. The enlargement of renal tissue also stretches renal vasculature and results in hypertension.

Infantile and adult forms of PKD exist.

**Signs and Symptoms** Onset of the infantile form is soon after birth. The abdomen is enlarged, and the kidneys are palpable. Dehydration and emaciation are frequently noted. Fibrosis of the liver associated with hypertension and splenomegaly often occurs in infants and children with PKD.

In the adult form, symptoms usually develop in the 30s and result from cystic pressure; they include lumbar pain, hematuria, and colic. Hypertension may be present. Splenomegaly is often found, and hepatic cysts occur in about one-third of cases. There is also a high associated incidence of intracranial aneurysms. Most patients with severe cystic kidneys develop end-stage renal failure and require dialysis.

**Etiology** The infantile form is an autosomal recessive disorder. The adult form, which is autosomal dominant, has been found to be caused by more than one defective gene. The defective genes are located on chromosome 16 and are so closely linked on the short arm of the chromosome that they are usually inherited together, although this is not the case in about 5 percent of affected persons. These variations may account for clinical differences in patients with PKD.

**Epidemiology** Approximately 500,000 persons in the United States are affected. The disorder accounts for 8 to 10 percent of cases of end-stage renal disease.

**Related Disorders** See *Medullary Cystic Disease; Medullary Sponge Kidney.*

**Glomerular cystic disease** is similar to PKD, but the liver and spleen are unaffected.

**Treatment—Standard** Treatment consists of management of urinary infections and secondary hypertension. When uremia occurs, it is managed by an increase in caloric intake combined with a reduction in total dietary protein. Sufficient carbohydrates and fat must be provided to meet energy requirements.

With dialysis, a normal hematocrit can be achieved. Renal transplantation is sometimes indicated, but the use of parental and sibling donors may be impractical because of the familial nature of the disease. Genetic counseling is recommended for affected families.

Magnetic resonance angiography may be used for screening of intracranial aneurysms in patients with autosomal dominant PKD.

**Treatment—Investigational** The orphan drug calcium acetate (Pharmedic Company) is being used in the treatment of hyperphosphatemia in end-stage renal disease.

Research on autosomal recessive polycystic kidney disease is being pursued by Lisa M. Guay-Woodford, M.D., Norman D. Rosenblum, M.D., Kathy L. Jabs, M.D., William E. Harmon, M.D., and E. William Harris, Jr., M.D., Ph.D., at Children's Hospital in Boston.

Clinical trials are under way to study intracranial aneurysms in autosomal dominant polycystic disease. Please contact William D. Kaehny, M.D., at the University of Colorado Health Science Center.

Taxol is being tested on mice for treatment of PKD. It is thought that taxol may delay the progression of PKD in humans and prevent or delay kidney transplantation or dialysis.

Please contact the agencies listed under Resources, below, for the most current information. Addresses and telephone numbers of these agencies, as well as of individual experts and research centers, may be found in the Master Resources List.

### Resources

**For more information on polycystic kidney diseases:** National Organization for Rare Disorders (NORD); Polycystic Kidney Research Foundation; NIH/National Kidney and Urologic Diseases Information Clearinghouse; American Kidney Fund; National Kidney Foundation; National Association of Patients on Hemodialysis and Transplantation.

**For genetic information and genetic counseling referrals:** March of Dimes Birth Defects Foundation; Alliance of Genetic Support Groups.

### References

Cecil Textbook of Medicine, 19th ed.: J.B. Wyngaarden, et al., eds.; W.B. Saunders Company, 1992, pp. 142, 480, 609–611.

The Diagnosis and Prognosis of Autosomal Dominant Polycystic Kidney Disease: P.S. Parfrey, et al.; N. Engl. J. Med., October 18, 1990, vol. 323(16), pp. 1085–1090.

# RENAL AGENESIS, BILATERAL

**Description** The failure of both kidneys to develop in utero results in oligohydramnios. The lack of amniotic fluid may cause compression of the fetus and further fetal malformations. Bilateral renal agenesis is more common in infants with a parent who has a renal anomaly, particularly unilateral renal agenesis. Studies have shown that unilateral and bilateral renal agenesis may be genetically related.

**Synonyms**

Hereditary Renal Adysplasia

Urogenital Adysplasia, Hereditary

**Signs and Symptoms** Premature labor, breech delivery, and a disproportionately low birth weight are often associated with bilateral renal agenesis.

A typical facies includes ocular hypertelorism, a "parrot-beak" nose, a receding chin, and large, low-set ears deficient in cartilage (the so-called **Potter facies).** Other characteristics may include excess and dehydrated skin, prominent epicanthal folds, the facial expression of an older infant, and deformities of the hands and feet. The uterus and upper vagina may be absent in females; males may lack the seminal vesicles and spermatic duct. Gastrointestinal anomalies include the absence of a rectum, esophagus, and duodenum. Other abnormalities that may occur are the presence of only one umbilical artery and major deformities of the lower trunk and lower limbs. Pulmonary hypoplasia and pneumothorax are common associated findings.

**Etiology** The disorder has an autosomal dominant mode of inheritance.

**Epidemiology** Bilateral renal agenesis occurs more frequently in males than in females. It is a very rare disorder.

**Related Disorders** See *Sirenomelia Sequence; Fraser Syndrome; Branchio-Oto-Renal Syndrome.*

**Oligohydramnios sequence (Potter syndrome)** is characterized by an insufficient level of amniotic fluid, which may be due to the absence of fetal urinary output or to chronic leakage of fluid from the amniotic sac.

**Cat-eye syndrome (coloboma of iris-anal atresia syndrome)** is a genetic disorder that is marked by a fissure in the iris and the absence of an anal opening. Associated abnormalities may include renal agenesis.

**MURCS association (Müllerian duct, renal, and cervical vertebral defects)** is a rare disorder characterized by malformation of the vertebrae and absence of a vagina and kidneys.

**Rokitansky sequence** is a disorder in which the vagina and uterus are incompletely formed.

**Treatment—Standard** Treatment is symptomatic and supportive for patients with this disorder. Most children will die of renal insufficiency.

**Treatment—Investigational** Please contact the agencies listed under Resources, below, for the most current information. Addresses and telephone numbers of these agencies, as well as of individual experts and research centers, may be found in the Master Resources List.

### Resources

**For more information on bilateral renal agenesis:** National Organization for Rare Disorders (NORD); American Kidney Fund; National Kidney Foundation; NIH/National Institute of Diabetes, Digestive and Kidney Diseases.

**For genetic information and genetic counseling referrals:** March of Dimes Birth Defects Foundation; Alliance of Genetic Support Groups.

**References**

Mendelian Inheritance in Man, 10th ed.: V.A. McKusick; The Johns Hopkins University Press, 1992, pp. 1131–1132.

Smith's Recognizable Patterns of Human Malformation, 4th ed.: K.L. Jones; W.B. Saunders Company, 1988, pp. 572–573.

# RENAL GLYCOSURIA

**Description** Renal glycosuria is a rare metabolic disorder in which abnormal amounts of glucose are excreted into the urine when the blood glucose levels are normal or low. There are 2 types: primary and congenital.

**Synonyms**

> Diabetes, True Renal
> Glucosuria

**Signs and Symptoms Primary renal glycosuria** occurs without any apparent functional or structural abnormalities of the kidney. It tends to occur in pregnant women and almost always disappears after childbirth.

**Congenital renal glycosuria** is a rare inherited disorder characterized by the inability of the intestines to absorb glucose and by an excessive amount of glucose in the urine. Since glycosuria is the primary symptom of this disorder, a fasting blood glucose test and a glucose oxidase test must be performed to differentiate renal glycosuria from diabetes mellitus.

**Etiology** The cause is probably a defect in the renal glucose transport protein. Renal glycosuria is recognized as a metabolic disorder and is believed to be inherited as an autosomal recessive trait. Because some patients eventually develop diabetes mellitus, some believe the disorder may precede the onset of diabetes, but this has not been proved.

**Epidemiology** Males and females are equally affected. The incidence in women is higher during pregnancy, with the glycosuria subsiding after delivery. Some patients with severe renal failure also have renal glycosuria.

**Related Disorders** See *Cystinosis; Rickets, Hypophosphatemic.*

**Treatment—Standard** Treatment may not be necessary. Since an excessive loss of glucose can occur with this disorder, fasting should be avoided; theoretically it could lead to hypoglycemia. Severe diarrhea in infants with renal glycosuria must be treated to avoid dehydration. Genetic counseling may be beneficial. Other treatment is symptomatic and supportive.

**Treatment—Investigational** Please contact the agencies listed under Resources, below, for the most current information. Addresses and telephone numbers of these agencies, as well as of individual experts and research centers, may be found in the Master Resources List.

**Resources**

**For more information on renal glycosuria:** National Organization for Rare Disorders (NORD); American Kidney Fund; National Kidney Foundation; NIH/National Digestive Diseases Information Clearinghouse.

**For genetic information and genetic counseling referrals:** March of Dimes Birth Defects Foundation; Alliance of Genetic Support Groups.

**References**

The Metabolic and Molecular Base of Inherited Disease, 7th ed.: C.R. Scriver, et al., eds.; McGraw-Hill, 1995, ch. 116.

Internal Medicine, 4th ed.: J.H. Stein, ed.-in-chief; Little, Brown and Company, 1994, pp. 2753–2754.

Mendelian Inheritance in Man, 10th ed.: V.A. McKusick; The Johns Hopkins University Press, 1992, p. 1422.

Complete Absence of Tubular Glucose Reabsorption: A New Type of Renal Glucosuria: B.S. Oemar et al.; Clin. Nephrol., March 1987, vol. 27(3), pp. 156–160.

# RICKETS, HYPOPHOSPHATEMIC

**Description** Hypophosphatemic rickets is a rare genetic form of rickets characterized by a renal tubular defect in transport of phosphate and altered renal metabolism of vitamin D. Additionally, intestinal absorption of calcium and phosphate is decreased, which compounds hypophosphatemia and leads to osteomalacia. Major manifestations include skeletal changes and retarded growth.

**Synonyms**

> Familial Hypophosphatemic (Vitamin D–Resistant) Rickets
> Hereditary Type II Hypophosphatemia

Phosphate Diabetes
X-Linked Hypophosphatemia
X-Linked Vitamin D–Resistant Rickets

**Signs and Symptoms** Signs and symptoms are usually first noticed after 12 to 18 months of age. Dental problems may develop, such as delayed eruption of teeth, or caries and abscesses, especially of the dental pulp. Skeletal abnormalities include softening or thinning of bones, fractures, and abnormal bony extensions at the site of muscular attachments. Other characteristics include weakness, intermittent muscle cramps, a waddling walk due to abnormalities in the hip joint, pain in the knees, knock-knees or bowlegs, diminished growth (especially of the legs), and abnormal skull or rib development.

The symptoms and signs range from mild to severe. Some patients may have no noticeable symptoms, while others have pain and stiffness of the back, hips, and shoulders, possibly limiting mobility. Very rarely, some hair loss may occur. One rare acquired form of this disorder may be associated with a benign tumor that secretes a phosphaturic substance.

**Etiology** The most common form of hypophosphatemic rickets is inherited as an X-linked dominant trait. Symptoms are caused by altered metabolism of phosphorus, calcium, and vitamin D, although the exact mechanism for this is unclear. One important factor in the pathogenesis of this disease is impaired reabsorption of phosphorus by the renal proximal tubules, with resultant hypophosphatemia. Because of the hypophosphatemia, mineralization of bone is impaired.

**Epidemiology** The disorder occurs in males and females in equal numbers, but is usually more severe in males. Asymptomatic hypophosphatemic adult carriers are always females.

**Related Disorders** Rickets occurs in several forms, either acquired or inherited, all of which are characterized by weakening of bones due to abnormal calcium metabolism as well as possible decreases in magnesium or phosphorus levels.

**Rickets** is due to vitamin D deficiency resulting in deficient calcification of osteoid. This condition can develop at any age and can be successfully treated with high doses of vitamin D.

**Pseudo–vitamin D–deficiency rickets (vitamin D–dependent rickets, type I)** is characterized by more severe skeletal changes and weakness than those of hypophosphatemic rickets, and onset is earlier. This disorder is caused by abnormal vitamin D metabolism and is inherited as an autosomal recessive trait. Serum calcium levels are decreased, although phosphate levels may be normal or only slightly decreased. Aminoaciduria occurs because of a proximal tubule abnormality. Intermittent muscle cramps are due to hypocalcemia. Convulsions and abnormalities of the spine and pelvis may also develop.

**Osteomalacia** is characterized by gradual softening and bending of the bones. Pain may occur in varying degrees of severity. Softening is due to defective calcification of bone, resulting from vitamin D deficiency or renal dysfunction. Osteomalacia is more common in women than in men, and often develops during pregnancy. It can exist alone or in association with other disorders, such as hypophosphatemic rickets.

**Fanconi syndrome** is characterized by renal proximal tubular dysfunction and bone abnormalities similar to those of hypophosphatemic rickets. Excess amounts of phosphate, amino acids, bicarbonate, glucose, and uric acid are excreted in the urine. This rare disorder is thought to be inherited in an autosomal recessive pattern. Bone abnormalities include rickets in children and osteomalacia in adults. Fanconi syndrome may be associated with a variety of inherited metabolic disorders. See *Cystinosis; Lowe Syndrome; Fructose Intolerance, Hereditary; Wilson Disease; Galactosemia, Classic.* Other associated disorders include a form of tyrosinemia and a glycogen storage disorder.

**Treatment—Standard** Hypophosphatemic rickets is treated with both oral phosphate and vitamin D, usually in the form of calcitriol. The dosage of calcitriol is gradually increased until bone healing occurs. This treatment must be carefully monitored to prevent hypercalciuria and nephrocalcinosis. Vitamin D alone reduces renal loss of phosphate but does not affect the patient's growth rate, the intestinal absorption of phosphate, or renal function. Phosphate alone may improve intestinal absorption of calcium and phosphate as well as enhance bone healing, but these effects may not be sustained without concomitant administration of vitamin D.

Covering teeth with chrome crowns may be effective in preventing spontaneous dental abscesses. Genetic counseling may benefit patients and their families. Those rare cases of hypophosphatemic rickets that are caused by bone tumors can be treated through surgical removal of the tumor, whenever feasible.

**Treatment—Investigational** Bone growth abnormalities associated with hypophosphatemic rickets can be surgically corrected in an attempt to prevent further shortening or deformities of affected arms or legs. However, this should not be attempted before hypophosphatemia has been corrected with phosphate and calcitriol therapy.

In a study carried out with Australian children having X-linked hypophosphatemic rickets using the enzyme calcitriol (1,25-dihydroxy vitamin $D_3$) and phosphate, a slight increase in height was noted. Nephrocalcinosis also occurred. Conservative use of calcitriol and careful observation of patients to guard against serious kidney damage are recommended. Treatment should be discontinued when growth has stopped.

The orphan drug Osteo-D (secalciferol, manufactured by Lemon Company) is being tested for treatment of hypophosphatemic rickets.

Studies are also being conducted to determine the optimal dosage of 24,25-dihydroxy vitamin D, a vitamin D metabolite. In some cases, this drug may be used as an adjunct to standard treatment along with phosphates and vitamin D. For more information, contact Kate Holbrook at Yale University School of Medicine.

Please contact the agencies listed under Resources, below, for the most current information. Addresses and telephone numbers of these agencies, as well as of individual experts and research centers, may be found in the Master Resources List.

### Resources

**For more information on hypophosphatemic rickets:** National Organization for Rare Disorders (NORD); NIH/National Institute of Diabetes, Digestive and Kidney Diseases Information Clearinghouse.

**For genetic information and genetic counseling referrals:** March of Dimes Birth Defects Foundation; Alliance of Genetic Support Groups.

### References

Tibial Bowing Exacerbated by Partial Premature Epiphyseal Closure in Sex-Linked Hypophosphatemic Rickets: W.H. McAlister, et al.; Radiology, February 1987, vol. 162(2), pp. 461–463.

Early Diagnosis and Early Treatment of Hypophosphatemic Vitamin D–Resistant Rickets: E. Schaumberger, et al.; Klin. Pediatr., January–February 1986, vol. 198(1), pp. 44–48.

Prophylactic Dental Treatment for a Patient with Vitamin D–Resistant Rickets: Report of Case: G.H. Breen; J. Dent. Child., January–February 1986, vol. 53(1), pp. 38–43.

# 10 ENDOCRINE DISORDERS

*By Thomas P. Foley, Jr., M.D.,*
*and David N. Finegold, M.D.*

During the past few decades, there have been dramatic advances in the science of endocrinology, leading to better understanding of the impact of genetic and environmental factors upon inherited endocrine disorders as well as of the pathophysiologic processes that disrupt endocrine function. The contributions of these discoveries to diagnostic and therapeutic potentials are extraordinary and have made endocrinology a discipline in which diagnoses can be made with precision and appropriate, safe treatment prescribed.

The classic definition of endocrinology—the integration and communication between endocrine tissues, which release chemical signals into the circulation that act on distant target tissues—is too limited. The definition now needs to incorporate local mediators via autocrine and paracrine mechanisms that modify action by amplification or inhibition and tissue growth factors and regulatory peptides that function independently. Increasing amalgamation of other systems with the endocrine system has led to new fields of study, such as psychoneuroendocrinology, immunopathoendocrinology, and reproductive endocrinology.

Molecular biology, coupled with new immunologic and biochemical approaches, has provided a profound influence and new insights into the study and classification of endocrine disorders. It is now possible to diagnose patients with rare disorders who were previously assigned the term *an experiment in nature,* to identify the inherent problem at the level of the responsible gene, and to study the problem in terms of deletion or mutation for the transcription of the hormones themselves, hormonal receptors, or postreceptor functions. Transgenic animals can be produced, bred, and studied to further delineate results of hormonal excesses or transcription of genes with single point mutations. Through these types of studies, mechanisms of both inherited and acquired endocrine diseases can be examined in exquisite detail at the cellular and molecular levels, and therapeutic strategies more appropriately designed for these diseases.

Endocrine disorders themselves are common in the practices of internal medicine and pediatrics. Some, such as hypogonadism and acquired hypothyroidism, may be readily treated by skilled medical practitioners. Others have vague symptomatology leading to a delay in appropriate diagnosis or, especially in young children, rapid onset of catastrophic proportions requiring immediate appropriate diagnosis and treatment. Medical practitioners, therefore, must continually consider the possibility of an underlying endocrine cause for commonly observed symptoms such as loss of energy, nausea, diarrhea, and changes in skin turgor, pigmentation, and texture, as well as for infertility, sexual ambiguity, loss of libido, and amenorrhea. Because of the subtlety and variation in clinical presentation for many of the conditions described in this section, prompt consultation with an appropriate specialist in adult or pediatric endocrinology needs to be obtained.

If an endocrine cause is found and promptly treated, preservation of good health can be expected. Especially in the very young pediatric age group, unrecognized endocrine disorders, such as adverse changes in serum electrolyte and fluid balance, alterations in calcium and phosphorus relationships, elevation or depression in blood glucose level, and elevation or depression in thyroid hormone level, can lead to irreparable health hazards and mental and psychomotor retardation.

Therefore, as our wealth of knowledge rapidly expands, diagnostic methods become more sophisticated and precise, and therapeutic possibilities through hormonal and synthetic analogue therapies become more available, the practitioner needs to be aware of the symptoms of uncommon diseases as well as the consultants (specialists, disease-focused self-help groups, or governmental agencies) through whom important, pertinent information can be acquired. In addition, these rare conditions deserve not only study as medical curiosities but also full support from insurance companies and the pharmaceutical industry to furnish the hormones and medications required to provide the potential of total replacement therapies and restoration of optimal health for a lifetime. A better understanding of the etiology and pathogenesis of endocrine disorders, improved diagnostic techniques, and an expanded number of therapeutic modalities can only improve health care for the unfortunate few who are afflicted with these diseases.

# ENDOCRINE DISORDERS
*Listings in This Section*

# ACHARD-THIERS SYNDROME

**Description** Achard-Thiers syndrome is caused by hyperadrenocorticism, which results in diabetes and virilization.

**Synonyms**

> Adenoma-Associated Virilism of Older Women
>
> Diabetic Bearded-Woman Syndrome

**Signs and Symptoms** The major symptoms of Achard-Thiers syndrome are typically those associated with classical diabetes, including hyperglycemia and glucosuria, associated with polyuria, polydipsia, hunger, and weight loss.

The excessive production of adrenocortical androgens results in hirsutism, a deepening of the voice, acne, clitoromegaly, and/or a reduction in the size of the breasts. Patients present with enlarged face and trunk but slender arms and legs. If untreated, some women develop hypertension, heart disease, and hyperadrenocorticism.

Achard-Thiers syndrome is also associated with anomalies of the adrenal glands and ovaries. Abnormal changes in the pancreas result in impaired production of insulin, abnormal carbohydrate metabolism, and diabetes.

**Etiology** Adenomas are the usual cause of the enlargement and hypersecretion of the adrenal cortex in Achard-Thiers syndrome.

**Epidemiology** Achard-Thiers syndrome affects postmenopausal women.

**Related Disorders Acquired adrenogenital syndrome** is a rare endocrine disorder caused by a tumor in the adrenal glands that results in overproduction of androgens or late-onset congenital adrenal hyperplasia. In an adult female, the symptoms may include hirsutism, alopecia, acne, deepening voice, and abnormally large muscles.

**Diabetes** is a complex endocrine disease in which the body produces too little insulin or is not able to use insulin properly. In both type I (insulin-dependent) and type II (noninsulin-dependent) forms, symptoms include polyuria, polydipsia, constant hunger, and unexplained weight loss. Long-term complications may affect the nervous system, heart, kidneys, and eyes.

**Treatment—Standard** The standard treatment for Achard-Thiers syndrome includes the surgical removal of portions of the adrenal gland, especially if a tumor is present. Diabetes is managed by diet and/or insulin or other medications.

**Treatment—Investigational** Please contact the agencies listed under Resources, below, for the most current information. Addresses and telephone numbers of these agencies, as well as of individual experts and research centers, may be found in the Master Resources List.

**Resources**

**For more information on Achard-Thiers syndrome:** National Organization for Rare Disorders (NORD); National Adrenal Diseases Foundation; NIH/National Institute of Diabetes, Digestive and Kidney Diseases; American Diabetes Association National Service Center.

**References**

Cecil Textbook of Medicine, 19th ed.: J.B. Wyngaarden, et al., eds.; W.B. Saunders Company, 1992, pp. 1387–1388.

Textbook of Endocrinology, 8th ed.: J.D. Wilson and D.W. Foster, eds.; W.B. Saunders Company, 1992, pp. 720–721, 1140.

Dictionary of Medical Syndromes, 3rd ed.: S.I. Magalini, et al., eds.; J.B. Lippincott Company, 1990, p. 6.

Adrenal Androgens in Insulin-Dependent Diabetes Mellitus: M. Small; Diabetes Res., June 1989, vol. 11(2), pp. 93–95.

Characterization of Hyperandrogenism with Insulin-Resistant Diabetes Type A: M. Gibson, et al.; Fertil. Steril., May 1980, vol. 33(5), pp. 501–505.

# ACROMEGALY

**Description** Acromegaly is an insidious disorder of growth hormone excess that manifests itself in abnormal enlargement of bones of the extremities and head, especially the frontal bone and jaws, and thickening of soft tissues, including those of the heart.

**Synonyms**

> Marie Disease

**Signs and Symptoms** Symptoms are slowly progressive after puberty, becoming prominent in middle age. Facial features coarsen with the growth of soft tissues and cartilage. Facial bones are prominent, the jaw protrudes, and overbite leads to wide separation of the teeth. The voice usually deepens and sounds husky. Osseous overgrowth and cartilage hypertrophy lead to osteoarthritis; kyphoscoliosis may occur. Enlargement of the hands and feet is gradual. Compression of the spinal nerve root may lead to functional abnormalities and pain. Darkening of the skin and hirsutism may be apparent. Cardiomegaly (which may lead to congestive heart failure), hepatomegaly, splenomegaly, and renal enlargement may occur. At times there is enlargement of the thyroid and adrenal glands.

Approximately 25 percent of patients are hypertensive. Pituitary enlargement can produce headache, visual abnormalities, and hormonal imbalances. Since excessive growth hormone (**GH**) is antagonistic to the action of insulin, 50 percent of patients have elevated glucose levels. The metabolic rate may quicken, and the activity of the sweat and sebaceous glands may increase.

At a late stage, myopathy and peripheral neuropathy may develop. Visual impairment may progress, even to blindness. If untreated, 25 percent of patients have glycosuria, polydipsia, and polyphagia.

**Etiology** Hypersecretion of GH is most often due to a pituitary adenoma involving the somatotrophic cells of the anterior lobe; less often, ineffective control of these cells by the hypothalamus is responsible. GH-secreting tumors may sometimes be due to overstimulation by the hypothalamus.

An exogenous cause of acromegaly in otherwise normal children is prolonged, excessive therapy with human growth hormone (**HGH**).

**Epidemiology** Acromegaly affects males and females in equal numbers.

**Related Disorders Gigantism** or **giantism,** also caused by hypersecretion of GH, occurs prepubertally. It is associated with enlarged soft tissues and late epiphyseal closure, which produces excessive growth during childhood; height may exceed 7 or 8 feet. Onset of hypopituitarism later in the course may result in myopathy and hypogonadism. Sexual development may be normal, or it may be affected by associated hypogonadism. In some cases, peripheral neuropathy may develop.

The hereditary **multiple endocrine neoplasia (MEN) syndrome I (Wermer syndrome; polyendocrine adenomatosis)** has the hallmarks of excessive growth and multiple tumors or endocrine hypersecretion. The patient may have diarrhea and abdominal pain. A child may have hypoglycemia, and an adult, peptic ulcers. At times, epileptic seizures occur.

**Acromegaloidism** is thought to be caused by the excessive production of insulin-like growth factor I (**IGF-1**) and by insulin resistance. The symptoms are similar to those of acromegaly: coarse facial features; a deep, hoarse voice; enlargement of the hands and feet; and hirsutism. Other symptoms may include hypoglycemia, excessive sweating, headaches, and visual disturbances. GH levels, however, are normal.

See *Marfan Syndrome; McCune-Albright Syndrome; Sotos Syndrome.*

**Treatment—Standard** The usual treatment of acromegaly is surgical excision of a pituitary adenoma or partial or total surgical removal of the pituitary gland, perhaps supplemented by irradiation. If the entire gland is removed, lifelong hormonal replacement therapy is essential. GH suppressors, including estrogen, medroxyprogesterone, chlorpromazine, and somatostatin (the latter must be given parenterally), have had only limited success. In mild cases or in elderly patients, dopamine agonists such as bromocryptine have been used adjunctively.

**Treatment—Investigational** Treatment of acromegaly is now possible with the somatostatin analogue (Sandostatin). This medication significantly lowers the mean plasma GH concentrations and, when given preoperatively, causes significant shrinkage of invasive pituitary macroadenomas, with improved surgical remission rates. Treatment with somatostatin analogue is available in many medical centers in the United States.

Please contact the agencies listed under Resources, below, for the most current information. Addresses and telephone numbers of these agencies, as well as of individual experts and research centers, may be found in the Master Resources List.

**Resources**

**For more information on acromegaly:** National Organization for Rare Disorders (NORD); NIH/National Arthritis and Musculoskeletal and Skin Diseases Information Clearinghouse.

**References**

Cecil Textbook of Medicine, 19th ed.: J.B. Wyngaarden, et al., eds.; W.B. Saunders Company, 1992, pp. 1234–1236.

Textbook of Endocrinology, 8th ed.: J.D. Wilson and D.W. Foster, eds.; W.B. Saunders Company, 1992, pp. 268–290.

Acromegaly: S. Melmed; N. Engl. J. Med., April 1990, vol. 322(14), pp. 966–977.

Somatostatin Proves Effective in Treating Resistant Acromegaly: A.J. Clark; Res. Resource Rep., April 1988, pp. 5–7.

Acromegalic Heart Disease: Influence of Treatment of the Acromegaly on the Heart: R.P. Hayward, et al.; Q.J. Med., January 1987, vol. 62(237), pp. 41–58.

Acromegaly: J.D. Nabarro; Clin. Endocrinol. (Oxf.), April 1987, vol. 26(4), pp. 481–512.

Somatomedin–C Levels in Treated and Untreated Patients with Acromegaly: F. Roelfsema, et al.; Clin. Endocrinol. (Oxf.), February 1987, vol. 26(2), pp. 137–144.

The Pathogenesis of Acromegaly: Clinical and Immunocytochemical Analysis in 75 Patients: E.R. Laws, Jr., et al.; J. Neurosurg., July 1985, vol. 63(1), pp. 35–38.

Plasma Insulin-Like Growth Factor-I/Somatomedin-C in Acromegaly: Correlation with the Degree of Growth Hormone Hypersecretion: A.L. Barkan, et al.; J. Clin. Endocrinol. Metab., vol. 67(1) pp. 69–73.

Preoperative Treatment of Acromegaly with Long-Acting Somatostatin Analog SMS 201-995: Shrinkage of Invasive Pituitary Macroadenomas and Improved Surgical Remission Rate: A.L. Barkan, et al.; J. Clin. Endocrinol. Metab., vol. 67(5), pp. 1040–1047.

Treatment of Acromegaly with the Long-Acting Somatostatin Analog SMS 201-995: A.L. Barkan, et al.; J. Clin. Endocrinol. Metab., vol. 66(1), pp. 16–23.

# ACTH DEFICIENCY

**Description** Decreased or absent adrenocorticotropic hormone (**ACTH**) and abnormally low levels of cortisol and steroid hormones mark this disorder.

**Synonyms**

Adrenocorticotropic Hormone Deficiency, Isolated

**Signs and Symptoms** ACTH deficiency usually manifests during adulthood; a few cases in children have been identified. The patient may experience weight loss, anorexia, muscle weakness, nausea, vomiting, and hypotension. As a rule, hypoglycemia, hyponatremia, and hyperkalemia are present. Blood tests may show no detectable level of ACTH, and cortisol levels may be subnormal. Urinary free cortisol concentrations are low, as are plasma androgen levels. Although the male distribution of body hair is usually normal, females have sparse pubic and axillary hair. Decreased skin pigmentation is the norm, but in some it may be normal or even increased. Emotionally, patients may range from being depressed to exhibiting frank psychosis.

**Etiology** ACTH deficiency is idiopathic; hypothalamic or pituitary abnormalities have been suggested. The symptoms are a reflection of understimulation of the adrenal cortex by ACTH, which results in insufficient hormone secretion.

**Epidemiology** Males and females are affected in equal numbers. Symptoms usually become apparent in adulthood, but laboratory tests can reveal ACTH deficiency in asymptomatic infants.

**Related Disorders** See *Adrenal Hyperplasia, Congenital; Addison Disease.*

**Secondary adrenal insufficiency** stems from insufficient production or release of ACTH. Causes range from prolonged corticosteroid therapy, adenomas, and granulomas of the pituitary gland to postpartum pituitary necrosis.

**Treatment—Standard** Replacement with cortisone constitutes therapy. Replacement enables patients to lead a normal life, with the exception that they require increased doses of cortisone replacement therapy in the presence of moderate and severe stress.

**Treatment—Investigational** Please contact the agencies listed under Resources, below, for the most current information. Addresses and telephone numbers of these agencies, as well as of individual experts and research centers, may be found in the Master Resources List.

**Resources**

**For more information on ACTH deficiency:** National Organization for Rare Disorders (NORD); National Adrenal Diseases Foundation; NIH/National Digestive Diseases Information Clearinghouse.

**References**

Internal Medicine, 2nd ed.: J.H. Stein, et al., eds.; Little, Brown and Company, 1987, p. 1899.

# ADDISON DISEASE

**Description** Addison disease is the result of chronic, usually progressive hypofunction of the adrenal cortex. Deficiencies of cortisol and aldosterone lead to hypoglycemia, hypotension, and electrolyte imbalance (low sodium and chloride, and high potassium levels). The imbalance causes increased water excretion, followed by hypotension and dehydration. Major characteristics are fatigability, gastrointestinal discomfort, light-headedness, syncope, and an increase in skin pigmentation.

**Synonyms**

Adrenal Hypoplasia

Adrenocortical Hypofunction

Adrenocortical Insufficiency

Chronic Adrenocortical Insufficiency

Glucocorticoid Resistance Syndrome

Primary Adrenal Insufficiency

Primary Failure Adrenocortical Insufficiency

**Signs and Symptoms** Weakness, fatigue, anorexia, increased water excretion, hypotension, and darkened pigmentation of scars, skin folds, and mucous membranes are early symptoms and signs. In addition, there may be black freckles over the head and shoulder areas. Neonates present in profound shock and hypoglycemic within the first hour of life. This presentation is shared by all disorders that cause hypoglucocorticoidism and mineralocorticoid deficiency.

Later developments are nausea, dehydration from vomiting and diarrhea, dizziness, cold intolerance, syncopal attacks, apathy, mental confusion, fever, abdominal pain, and hypoglycemia. Adrenal crisis may occur, signaled by a marked sudden loss of strength; severe abdominal, lower back, or leg pain; and/or renal failure.

**Etiology** Autoimmune-mediated atrophy accounts for about three-quarters of cases; the rest are due to partial destruction of the gland by such factors as tuberculosis, tumor, or amyloidosis. Acute infection, trauma, surgery, or sodium loss through heavy sweating can trigger adrenal crisis.

In rare cases, Addison disease is thought to be inherited as an X-linked genetic trait (**X-linked Addison disease**). **Congenital Addison disease** is thought to be inherited as an **autosomal dominant genetic trait.** Symptoms typically begin during childhood or adolescence.

**Epidemiology** Males and females are affected in equal numbers, at a rate of approximately 4:100,000. Onset may occur at any age.

**Related Disorders** See *ACTH Deficiency; Adrenoleukodystrophy; Amyloidosis; Adrenal Hyperplasia, Congenital; Cushing Syndrome; Schmidt Syndrome.*

**Treatment—Standard** In chronic adrenal insufficiency, replacement therapy consists of hydrocortisone and 9-α-fluorohydrocortisone, taken with meals. To avert adrenal crisis during infection, trauma, surgery, and other stress, the patient must increase the oral dosage or administer hydrocortisone by injection. Adrenal crisis demands *immediate* intravenous administration of high-dose hydrocortisone succinate or phosphate and fluid and electrolyte (normal saline) replacement; a short-term course of a vasopressor may be indicated to maintain blood pressure. Patients should carry a card or wear a tag stating that they have Addison disease.

**Treatment—Investigational**

Please contact the agencies listed under Resources, below, for the most current information. Addresses and telephone numbers of these agencies, as well as of individual experts and research centers, may be found in the Master Resources List.

**Resources**

**For more information on Addison disease:** National Organization for Rare Disorders (NORD); National Adrenal Diseases Foundation; NIH/National Digestive Diseases Information Clearinghouse.

**References**

Cecil Textbook of Medicine, 19th ed.: J.B. Wyngaarden, et al., eds.; W.B. Saunders Company, 1992, pp. 1340, 1460–1461.

Mendelian Inheritance in Man, 10th ed.: V.A. McKusick; The Johns Hopkins University Press, 1992, pp. 36, 1772–1773.

Harrison's Principles of Internal Medicine, 12th ed.: J.D. Wilson, et al., eds.; McGraw-Hill, 1991, pp. 1729–1731.

Delayed Diagnosis of Addison's Disease: J.R. Paterson, et al.; Ann. Clin. Biochem., July 1990, vol. 27(4), pp. 378–381.

Schmidt's Syndrome: A Rare Cause of Puberty Menorrhagia: J.B. Sharma, et al.; Int. J. Gynaecol. Obstet., December 1990, vol. 33(4), pp. 373–375.

Hyperkalaemic Periodic Paralysis: A Rare Presentation of Addison's Disease: J.M. Sowden, et al.; Postgrad. Med. J., April 1989, vol. 65(762), pp. 238–48.

Textbook of Endocrine Physiology: J.E. Griffin and S.R. Ojeda, eds.; Oxford University Press, 1988, pp. 258–259.

# ADRENAL HYPERPLASIA, CONGENITAL (CAH)

**Description** CAH comprises a group of disorders resulting from defective synthesis of adrenal corticosteroids secondary to mutations in the genes regulating the enzymes of corticoid biosynthesis. Lack of glucocorticoids, especially cortisol, causes various metabolic problems. The response to low levels of cortisol is increased production of corticotropin (**ACTH**). Lack of mineralocorticoids, primarily aldosterone, causes sodium and water losses, which in some cases can be fatal. The various forms of CAH represent defects in the different stages of corticosteroid synthesis, usually hydroxylation reactions at certain positions on the original cholesterol molecule.

CAH can result from congenital lipoid hyperplasia (adrenal insufficiency with male pseudohermaphroditism; steroid acute regulatory [**StAR**] protein deficiency); 3-β-hydroxysteroid dehydrogenase (**HSD**) deficiency; 17-α-hydroxylase deficiency with 17-20-lyase deficiency; 17-β-hydroxysteroid deficiency (17-ketosteroid reductase deficiency); 21-hydroxylase deficiency; 17-20-desmolase deficiency; 11-β-hydroxylase deficiency; and corticosterone methyloxidase deficiency, types I, II.

**Synonyms**

Adrenogenital Syndrome

**Signs and Symptoms** The phenotype of the inborn errors of steroid biosynthesis is highly variable. In several forms of CAH in which adrenomegaly produces abnormally large amounts of androgens, abnormalities of sexual development may be the most conspicuous consequence, particularly masculinization of the external genitalia in females. Deficiencies of glucocorticoids occur in some cases despite the adrenal hypertrophy, causing symptoms of Addison disease. These include weakness, nausea, vomiting, anorexia, irritability, depression, hyperpigmentation of the skin, hypotension, inability to tolerate cold, and inability to respond physiologically to stress; even patients who produce adequate corticosteroids under normal conditions usually cannot meet the increased requirement. Life-threatening addisonian crisis can then occur. A deficiency of aldosterone can lead to sodium depletion, dehydration, and circulatory collapse.

**21-Hydroxylase deficiency** accounts for 95 percent of the cases of CAH. It causes pseudohermaphroditism in females, but male infants appear normal. Females are born with abnormalities of the external genitalia that range from mild clitoromegaly to fusion of the labia so that the infant appears to have a phallus with undescended testes. Internally, the female reproductive organs are present; however, labial fold fusion may seal off the vagina from the exterior. These children are often raised as boys until the small size of the phallus becomes apparent at about age 4. Very rarely, genetic females live their lives as males. Untreated females do not menstruate and are infertile. Physical growth may initially be rapid, but retardation occurs fairly soon, and adult stature is short. Untreated affected females may have psychological problems. Newborn screening programs can identify the disease within the first week of life to prevent acute adrenal insufficiency, shock, and possibly death during the first month of life.

Beginning at age 3 or 4, males exhibit pseudoprecocious puberty. High levels of androgens suppress hormones required for normal puberty, testicular development, and spermatogenesis. Since the disorder is not initially apparent in boys, there is risk of an unanticipated, potentially fatal gluco- or mineralocorticoid deficiency crisis.

About one-third of patients with 21-hydroxylase deficiency also have a deficiency of aldosterone, which results in natriuresis, dehydration, hypovolemia, and hypotension. Symptoms develop 5 to 10 days after birth and include lethargy, vomiting, diarrhea, and circulatory collapse. Untreated, the disorder is rapidly fatal.

In **congenital lipoid hyperplasia (adrenal cortex male pseudohermaphroditism; StAR protein deficiency),** the most prominent feature is male pseudohermaphroditism. The disorder is characterized by failure of the external male genitalia to masculinize, and by hypospadias. There is accompanying impaired androgen action. This form of CAH can be life-threatening to infants.

**3-β-Hydroxysteroid dehydrogenase deficiency** occurs early in the synthetic chain of reactions required to produce adrenal corticosteroid hormones. Androgens, glucocorticoids, and mineralocorticoids are not synthesized. Hypospadias and ambiguous external genitalia are common in male infants. Virilization of females is not noticeable or does not occur at all. Salt loss is a frequent cause of adrenal crisis. Infants usually survive no more than a few hours unless diagnosed and treated rapidly. A few patients with incomplete forms of this defect have been described. These fail to be symptomatic until later in childhood (mild clitoromegaly, acne, and advanced maturation of the skeleton) or until adulthood. The late-onset form is characterized by menstrual irregularity and hirsutism.

**17-Hydroxylase deficiency** deprives genetic males of androgens during fetal development. As a consequence, they are born with female external genitalia; if cryptorchidism occurs, testicular malignancy may occur later in life. Other characteristics are amenorrhea, hypertension, hypokalemia, and the failure to develop secondary sexual traits.

**17-20-Desmolase deficiency** results in genetic males having female or ambiguous external genitalia. The adrenal glands are normal in size, and production of gluco- and mineralocorticoids is adequate.

**11-β-Hydroxylase deficiency** causes virilization in females and precocious puberty in males. Both males and females have hypertension and short stature.

**17-α-Hydroxylase deficiency** usually goes undetected until adolescence when there is a lack of secondary sexual development in males and females. Genetic males have female external genitalia. Females fail to menstruate or develop breasts. There is no production of androgens by the testes, and the ovaries fail to produce estrogen. Low levels of blood potassium and hypertension are other important characteristics of the disorder.

Symptoms of **nonclassical adrenal hyperplasia (NAH)** include infertility, premature sexual development, severe acne, excessive facial hair in women, and short stature in men. Symptoms of NAH are all caused by excess androgen at or before birth. The term *NAH* is no longer helpful since mutational analysis may be performed for this class of disorders.

**Etiology** Most adrenal hyperplasias are inherited as autosomal recessive disorders, and in most a gene mutation can be identified. Gene localizations are as follows: 21-hydroxylase deficiency, 6p21.3 (HLA region); 11-β-hydroxylase deficiency, 8q21; 3-β-HSD deficiency, 1p13.1; lipoid adrenal hyperplasia (StAR protein deficiency), not localized. However, in 17-β-HSD, the disorder may also be inherited as an X-linked recessive trait.

**Epidemiology** The most common form of CAH, 21-hydroxylase deficiency, is estimated to affect between 1:5,000 and 1:15,000 persons in the United States and Europe. In the Yupik Eskimo, however, the incidence of the salt-wasting form of CAH may be as high as 1:282. Other forms of CAH are much rarer.

Milder mutations resulting in adrenal hyperplasia affect approximately 1:30 Ashkenazic Jews, 1:40 Hispanics, 1:50 Yugoslavians, and 1:300 Italians.

**Related Disorders** Virilization of female fetuses and children, or accelerated sexual maturity in males, may also result from androgen-producing tumors or maternal ingestion of androgenic substances. The congenital absence of gonads and the development of cryptorchidism can also result in abnormal sexual development.

See *Turner Syndrome; Addison Disease; Hermaphroditism; Klinefelter Syndrome.*

**Treatment—Standard** Diagnosis and genetic sex determination are possible during the first trimester of pregnancy to prevent unexpected circulatory crises in the neonate and to permit maternal dexamethasone therapy to suppress fetal androgen secretion that could prevent any surgical modification of the external genitalia. After the first trimester, diagnosis again can be established by measuring estriol levels in the amniotic fluid. Oral corticosteroid therapy corrects the endocrine deficiency and must continue throughout life. Glucocorticoids are replaced orally with hydrocortisone or cortisol, cortisone acetate by injections, and prednisone for adults. Mineralocorticoid deficiency is corrected with 9-$\alpha$-fluorohydrocortisone therapy and intravenous therapy with physiologic saline; both are necessary to maintain proper sodium and water balance. Treated girls menstruate regularly and may have normal pregnancies. In boys, androgen suppression permits normal puberty, testicular development, and the production of viable sperm.

A decrease in androgen secretion may cause some regression of enlarged genital structures, but in many cases (especially when therapy begins late), surgical reconstruction of the external genitalia of girls is necessary.

Once identified, individuals with mutations resulting in a mild phenotype for adrenal hyperplasia can also be treated with cortisol orally to reverse most of the symptoms, including infertility.

Genetic counseling is beneficial for patients and their families.

**Treatment—Investigational** Intrauterine treatment of female fetuses affected with **21-hydroxylase deficiency** has been started during early pregnancy with dexamethasone and continued until birth. This treatment suppresses the adrenal glands, and the external sex organs are normal at birth. The mother must be closely monitored for side effects. Further study is needed to determine the long-term safety and effectiveness of this treatment.

Please contact the agencies listed under Resources, below, for the most current information. Addresses and telephone numbers of these agencies, as well as of individual experts and research centers, may be found in the Master Resources List.

**Resources**

**For more information on congenital adrenal hyperplasia:** National Organization for Rare Diseases (NORD); Magic Foundation for Children's Growth, Congenital Adrenal Hyperplasia Division; National Adrenal Diseases Foundation; Congenital Adrenal Hyperplasia Support Association; NIH/National Institute of Child Health and Human Development; Research Trust for Metabolic Diseases in Children.

**For genetic information and genetic counseling referrals:** March of Dimes Birth Defects Foundation; Alliance of Genetic Support Groups.

**References**

Role of Steroidogenic Acute Regulatory Protein in Adrenal and Gonadal Steroidogenesis: D. Lin, et al.; Science, 1995, vol. 267, pp. 1828–1851.

Cecil Textbook of Medicine, 19th ed.: J.B. Wyngaarden, et al., eds.; W.B. Saunders Company, 1992, pp. 1331–1333, 1377.

Genetic Disorders of Adrenal Hormone Synthesis: M.I. Rice; Hormone Res., 1992, vol. 37(suppl. 3), pp. 22–33.

Maternal Side Effects of Prenatal Dexamethasone Therapy for Fetal Congenital Adrenal Hyperplasia: S. Pang, et al.; J. Clin. Endocrinol. Metab., July 1992, vol. 75(1), pp. 249–253.

Mendelian Inheritance in Man, 10th ed.: V.A. McKusick; The Johns Hopkins University Press, 1992, pp. 1188–1193.

Nelson Textbook of Pediatrics, 14th ed.: R.E. Behrman, ed.-in-chief; W.B. Saunders Company, 1992, pp. 1444–1449.

Textbook of Endocrinology, 8th ed.: J.D. Wilson and D.W. Foster, eds.; W.B. Saunders Company, 1992, pp. 565–570.

Congenital Adrenal Hyperplasias: W.L. Miller; Endocrinol. Metab. Clin. North Am., 1991, vol. 20(4), pp. 721–749.

Birth Defects Encyclopedia: M.L. Buyse, ed.-in-chief; Blackwell Scientific Publications, 1990, pp. 1595–1599, 1602–1604.

Clinical Pediatric Endocrinology: S.A. Kaplan; W.B. Saunders Company, 1990, pp. 185–194.

Dictionary of Medical Syndromes, 3rd ed.: S.I. Magalini, et al., eds.; J.B. Lippincott Company, 1990, pp. 18–21.

Prenatal Treatment of Congenital Adrenal Hyperplasia Resulting from 21-Hydroxylase Deficiency: R. David, et al.; J. Pediatr., November 1984, vol. 105(5), pp. 799–803.

Recent Advances in 21-Hydroxylase Deficiency: M.I. New, et al.; Ann. Rev. Med., 1984, vol. 35, pp. 649–663.

The Adrenal Cortex: Physiological Function and Disease; Vol. XVIII, Major Problems in Internal Medicine: D.H. Nelson; W.B. Saunders Company, 1980, pp. 177–197.

Congenital Adrenal Hyperplasia: M.I. New and L.S. Levine; in Monographs on Endocrinology, vol. 26, Springer-Verlag, 1984.

Diurnal Variation in Blood 17-Hydroxyprogesterone Concentrations in Untreated Congenital Adrenal Hyperplasia: J. Slonim; Arch. Dis. Child., vol. 59(8), pp. 743–747.

# AHUMADA–DEL CASTILLO SYNDROME

**Description** Ahumada–del Castillo syndrome represents a dysfunction of the pituitary-hypothalamic axis. It is one of a group of disorders affecting women and is not correlated with pregnancy.

**Synonyms**

Amenorrhea-Galactorrhea Syndrome
Amenorrhea–Galactorrhea–FSH Decrease Syndrome
Argonz–del Castillo Syndrome
Galactorrhea-Amenorrhea Without Pregnancy
Nonpuerperal Galactorrhea-Amenorrhea

**Signs and Symptoms** Symptoms consist of galactorrhea and amenorrhea. The breasts and nipples are of normal size and appearance, as are the secondary sexual characteristics.

Laboratory tests reveal elevated levels of prolactin and low gonadotropin secretion.

**Etiology** The underlying abnormality is unknown. Evidence suggests that small tumors in the pituitary-hypothalamic region are sometimes responsible. The tumors are frequently microscopic and difficult to detect.

Rarer causes of galactorrhea-amenorrhea syndromes are hypothyroidism, chronic use of dopamine-antagonistic drugs such as chlorpromazine, and discontinuance of oral contraceptive agents.

**Epidemiology** Ahumada–del Castillo is a rare endocrinopathy that affects females only. Symptoms usually begin during adulthood.

**Related Disorders** Galactorrhea-amenorrhea syndromes include ***Chiari-Frommel Syndrome,*** which is correlated with pregnancy, and ***Forbes-Albright Syndrome,*** which is associated with demonstrable tumors in the sella turcica.

**Treatment—Standard** Drugs such as bromocriptine and lergotrile mesilate lower prolactin levels, thereby stopping abnormal milk secretion and often restoring menstrual function. Small tumors may in some cases be excised; others may respond to irradiation. When another underlying disorder is the cause, the galactorrhea-amenorrhea syndrome resolves upon successful treatment of the disorder.

**Treatment—Investigational** In a small study of pergolide, prolactin levels were lowered. Longer-term studies are needed to determine pergolide's safety and effectiveness.

Please contact the agencies listed under Resources, below, for the most current information. Addresses and telephone numbers of these agencies, as well as of individual experts and research centers, may be found in the Master Resources List.

**Resources**

**For more information on Ahumada–del Castillo syndrome:** National Organization for Rare Disorders (NORD); NIH/National Institute of Child Health and Human Development; Resolve.

**References**

Cecil Textbook of Medicine, 19th ed.: J.B. Wyngaarden, et al., eds.; W.B. Saunders Company, 1992, pp. 1365–1366.

A Comparison of the Efficacy and Safety of Pergolide and Bromocriptine in the Treatment of Hyperprolactinemia: S.W. Lamberts, et al.; J. Clin. Endocrinol. Metab., March 1991, vol. 723, pp. 635–641.

Dictionary of Medical Syndromes, 3rd ed.: S.I. Magalini, et al., eds.; J.B. Lippincott Company, 1990, p. 44.

Hyperprolactinemia and Female Infertility: E.E. Jones; J. Reprod. Med., February 1989, vol. 34(2), pp. 117–126.

Novak's Textbook of Gynecology, 11th ed.: H. Jones III, et al., eds.; Williams and Wilkins, 1988, pp. 351–357.

Hyperprolactinemia in Nonpregnant Women Due to Pituitary Tumors: L.G. Tolstoi; Life Sci., June 1986, vol. 38(22), pp. 1981–1989.

# ALSTROM SYNDROME

**Description** Alstrom syndrome is a genetic disorder with visual and hearing impairments beginning as early as infancy. Diabetes mellitus and obesity are also associated with this disorder. Acanthosis nigricans, hyperuricemia, and hyperlipidemia have also been reported in patients with Alstrom syndrome.

**Signs and Symptoms** Retinitis pigmentosa, with loss of central vision, occurs before the age of 1 year, and functional blindness is common by adolescence. Nystagmus may be present, and cataracts may develop during early adulthood. Glaucoma, a dislocated lens, and other eye abnormalities have been reported

Gradual loss of hearing (nerve deafness) occurs in childhood and by adolescence has developed into clinical deafness. Childhood obesity is common, and insulin-dependent diabetes mellitus or glucose intolerance may develop in early adulthood. Chronic nephropathy may be present and may result in renal failure.

Acanthosis nigricans, alopecia of the scalp, and/or aminoaciduria may be present. Hypogonadism, which can result in delayed puberty, may also occur. Secondary sexual characteristics may develop normally.

**Etiology** Alstrom syndrome is inherited as an autosomal recessive trait.

**Epidemiology** More males than females are affected. Approximately 20 cases have been reported.

**Related Disorders** See ***Bardet-Biedl Syndrome; Choroideremia; Usher Syndrome.***

**Hallgren syndrome** is characterized by deafness at birth accompanied by progressive visual impairment, including nystagmus and cataracts. Other symptoms may include delayed development, vestibulocerebellar ataxia, mental deficiency, and psychosis.

The following disorders may be associated with Alstrom syndrome as secondary characteristics. They are not necessary for a differential diagnosis:

**Insulin-dependent diabetes mellitus** is a common disorder that affects females and males approximately equally. Although it is idiopathic, genetic factors seem to play a role. The onset is marked by polyuria, extreme thirst, constant hunger, and unexplained weight loss.

See also ***Retinitis Pigmentosa.***

**Treatment—Standard** An electroretinogram **(ERG)** may be used to detect abnormalities in the retina, and an electrooculogram **(EOG)** may be used to measure retinal function. In cases where cataracts significantly impair vision, surgery is indicated. Whether or not surgery helps to improve vision often depends on how far the retinal changes have advanced.

To make the maximum use of their remaining vision, those with Alstrom syndrome can use such optical aids as Corning and NOIR glasses, the Fresnel Prising telescope, microscopes, and night vision devices. Nonoptical aids include the Apollo Laser, Visualtek closed-circuit television, the Wide Angle Mobility Light, paper guides, large-print typewriters, adjustable stands, reading machines, and talking computers.

There is no treatment for nerve deafness. Hearing aids may help to maximize use of remaining hearing, and speech therapy may enhance the ability of a child to communicate orally. In the case of deafness associated with Alstrom syndrome, teaching a child sign language may not be an option as vision loss is a feature of this disorder. Therefore, educational methods and options should be chosen carefully.

Strict dietary measures and exercise programs may help to control obesity, as well as aid in the management of diabetes mellitus and glucose intolerance associated with Alstrom syndrome. In most of the diagnosed cases of Alstrom syndrome, diabetes was controlled by diet and exercise alone. However, it was necessary in some cases to treat the diabetes with insulin.

If insulin therapy should become necessary for diabetes associated with Alstrom syndrome, a daily routine of insulin injection, controlled diet, exercise to burn off glucose, and testing for blood sugar level is vital in achieving and maintaining good blood sugar control. Insulin must be given by injection, usually 2 or more times each day. Portable pumps have been developed that administer insulin continuously. The management of diabetes may reduce the risk of kidney failure and the need for dialysis.

Genetic counseling may be of benefit for patients and their families. Other treatment is symptomatic and supportive.

**Treatment—Investigational** Dr. Jan Marshall at Jackson Laboratory in Bar Harbor, Maine, is studying blood samples from affected individuals and their families in order to identify the gene that causes Alstrom syndrome.

The orphan drug Cronnassial (Fida Pharmaceutical) is under investigation for treatment of some symptoms of retinitis pigmentosa, but its effectiveness in individuals with Alstrom syndrome is unproved.

Please contact the agencies listed under Resources, below, for the most current information. Addresses and telephone numbers of these agencies, as well as of individual experts and research centers, may be found in the Master Resources List.

**Resources**

**For more information on Alstrom syndrome:** National Organization for Rare Disorders (NORD); NIH/National Eye Institute; Foundation Fighting Blindness; National Association for the Visually Handicapped; NIH/National Institute of Deafness and Other Communication Disorders; National Information Center on Deafness; American Society for Deaf Children; American Diabetes Association; Juvenile Diabetes Foundation International

**For genetic information and genetic counseling referrals:** March of Dimes Birth Defects Foundation; Alliance of Genetic Support Groups

**References**

Longitudinal Study of the Early Electroretinographic Changes in Alstrom's Syndrome: F. Tremblay, et al.; Am. J. Ophthalmol. May 1993, vol. 115(5), pp. 657–665.

Mendelian Inheritance in Man, 10th ed.: V.A. McKusick; The Johns Hopkins University Press, 1992, pp. 1210–11.

Nelson Textbook of Pediatrics, 14th ed.: R.E. Behrman, ed.-in-chief; W.B. Saunders Company, 1992, p. 1585.

Birth Defects Encyclopedia: M.L. Buyse, ed.-in-chief; Blackwell Scientific Publications, 1990, pp. 93–94.

Dictionary of Medical Syndromes, 3rd ed.: S.I. Magalini, et al., eds.; J.B. Lippincott Company, 1990, pp. 41–42.

A Patient with Features of Both Bardet-Biedl and Alstrom Syndromes: C. Hauser, et al.; Eur. J. Pediatr., August 1990, vol. 149(11), pp. 783–785.

Ophthalmologic and Systemic Manifestations of Alstrom's Disease: R.H. Millay, et al.; Am. J. Ophthalmol., October 1986, vol. 202(4), pp. 482–490.

# ASHERMAN SYNDROME

**Description** Asherman syndrome is the result of intrauterine adhesions.

**Synonyms**

Intrauterine Synechiae

Uterine Synechiae

**Signs and Symptoms** Amenorrhea and infertility commonly occur. Endometritis often precedes this syndrome.

**Etiology** Dilation and curettage **(D&C),** sporadic endometritis, and endometritis caused by tuberculosis are possible causes.

**Epidemiology** Asherman syndrome affects females only.

**Related Disorders** See *Primary Amenorrhea; Stein-Leventhal Syndrome.*

In **secondary amenorrhea**, menstruation ceases as a result of D&C or acute endometritis.

**Endometriosis** is caused by an inability of the uterus to shed accumulated tissue prior to menstruation. Excess tissue can spread as far as the lungs, although it usually attaches to the bowels or intestines. Symptoms are pain in the lower back, in the thighs, or during the menstrual cycle.

**Pelvic inflammatory disease (PID)** is an infection of the fallopian tubes, cervix, uterus, or ovaries. It occurs most often in young women who are sexually active. PID is transmitted by sexual intercourse, childbirth, or abortion. Neisseria gonorrhoeae is the cause in 40 to 60 percent of patients.

**Treatment—Standard** A hysteroscope can confirm the diagnosis of Asherman syndrome. A D&C is performed to separate the adhesions, and an intrauterine contraceptive device (**IUD**) is inserted. Antibiotics are prescribed. Hormonal therapy is also used to encourage menstruation.

**Treatment—Investigational** The adhesions due to Asherman syndrome have been vaporized with an Nd-YAG laser, which causes minimal injury to the tissue. Although laser surgery is common, its use in the removal of uterine tissue is relatively new.

Please contact the agencies listed under Resources, below, for the most current information. Addresses and telephone numbers of these agencies, as well as of individual experts and research centers, may be found in the Master Resources List.

**Resources**

**For more information on Asherman syndrome:** National Organization for Rare Disorders (NORD); National Women's Health Network; NIH/National Institute of Child Health and Human Development.

**References**

Cecil Textbook of Medicine, 19th ed.: J.B. Wyngaarden, et al., eds.; W.B. Saunders Company, 1992, pp. 1435–1436.

Spontaneous Uterine Rupture During Pregnancy After Treatment of Asherman Syndrome: J.L. Deaton, et al.; Am. J. Obstet. Gynecol., May 1989, vol. 160 (5 pt. 1), pp. 1053–1054.

Treatment of Minimal and Moderate Intrauterine Adhesions (Asherman Syndrome): B. Ismajovich, et al.; J. Reprod. Med., October 1985, vol. 30(10), pp. 769–772.

Asherman Syndrome: A Comparison of Therapeutic Methods: J.S. Sanfilippo, et al.; J. Reprod. Med., June 1982, vol. 27(6), pp. 328–330.

# BARTTER SYNDROME

**Description** Bartter syndrome is a rare disorder of renal metabolism.

**Synonyms**

> Aldosteronism with Normal Blood Pressure
> Hyperaldosteronism with Hypokalemic Alkalosis
> Hyperaldosteronism Without Hypertension
> Juxtaglomerular Hyperplasia

**Signs and Symptoms** The majority of symptoms reflect a large urinary loss of potassium due to hypersecretion of renin. The patient may experience polydipsia, polyuria, mental retardation, weakness, short stature, and cramps in the muscles of the extremities.

**Etiology** The syndrome is thought to be inherited as an autosomal recessive trait. Investigations suggest the involvement of 2 renal dysfunctions: increased prostaglandin synthesis or a defect in chloride reabsorption.

**Epidemiology** Bartter syndrome affects males and females in equal numbers. While more frequent in children than in adults, it can occur at any age.

**Related Disorders** **Renal tubular acidosis** is a disorder in which renal secretion of hydrogen and reabsorption of bicarbonate are deficient. Sequelae may be chronic metabolic acidosis and potassium depletion, osteomalacia, or rickets.

See *Anemia, Fanconi.*

**Treatment—Standard** Counteraction of potassium loss is usually achieved with albumin and aldosterone antagonists. Other drug therapy may employ aspirin, indomethacin plus spironolactone, or triamterene. Otherwise, treatment is symptomatic and supportive. Patients and their families may benefit from genetic counseling.

**Treatment—Investigational** Enalapril has raised serum potassium levels in trials dealing with patients with this disorder.

Please contact the agencies listed under Resources, below, for the most current information. Addresses and telephone numbers of these agencies, as well as of individual experts and research centers, may be found in the Master Resources List.

**Resources**

**For more information on Bartter syndrome:** National Organization for Rare Disorders (NORD); National Kidney Foundation; American Kidney Fund; The Arc (a national organization on mental retardation); NIH/National Digestive Diseases Information Clearinghouse.

**For genetic information and genetic counseling referrals:** March of Dimes Birth Defects Foundation; Alliance of Genetic Support Groups.

**References**

Mendelian Inheritance in Man, 9th ed.: V.A. McKusick; The Johns Hopkins University Press, 1990, pp. 1061, 1267–1268.

The Juxtaglomerular Apparatus in Bartter's Syndrome and Related Tubulopathies: An Immunocytochemical and Electron Microscopic Study: R. Raugner, et al.; Virchows Arch. [A], 1988, vol. 412(5), pp. 459–470.

Total Body Potassium in Bartter's Syndrome Before and During Treatment with Enalapril: A. van de Stolpe, et al.; Nephron 1987, vol. 45(2), pp. 122–125.

Renal Tubular Reabsorption of Chloride in Bartter's Syndrome and Other Conditions with Hypokalemia: J.A. Rodriguez-Portales, et al.; Clin. Nephrol., December 1986, vol. 26(6), pp. 269–272.

# CARCINOID SYNDROME

**Description** Carcinoid syndrome is a rare malignant disease affecting the small bowel, stomach, and/or pancreas. Slow-growing tumors can metastasize to the liver, lungs, and ovary.

**Synonyms**

Carcinoid Tumor

Endocrine Tumors

Malignant Carcinoid Syndrome

Metastatic Carcinoid Tumor

**Signs and Symptoms** Initially asymptomatic, patients usually do not exhibit signs of carcinoid syndrome until the tumor has had years to grow. It is most often characterized by flushing, wheezing, and diarrhea, which can be debilitating. The diarrhea may be severe enough to cause life-threatening dehydration and electrolyte imbalance. Abdominal pain, blockage of hepatic arteries, and excessive urinary peptide excretion may be present. Congestive heart failure may occur, associated with right-sided valvular cardiac disease. A **carcinoid crisis** may develop rarely, with life-threatening hypotension.

**Etiology** Carcinoid syndrome is idiopathic. It has been suggested that the tumors develop from endocrine cells in the gastrointestinal tract, usually the ileum, the gonads, the bronchi, or the pancreas.

**Epidemiology** The incidence of carcinoid tumors is approximately 8:100,000. Males and females of all ages are equally affected. It may be that prevalence is greater than suspected because of lack of diagnosis; not all patients have the initial triad of flushing, wheezing, and diarrhea.

**Related Disorders** See *Cushing Syndrome; Zollinger-Ellison Syndrome.*

**Pancreatic cholera (vipoma)** is characterized by watery diarrhea, hypokalemia, and acidosis. In most cases the disorder is due to a non-B islet cell pancreatic tumor that secretes vasoactive intestinal polypeptide (**VIP**) and peptide histidine isoleucine. The episodes of diarrhea in association with profound loss of potassium, hypochlorhydria, and metabolic acidosis can be life-threatening.

**Treatment—Standard** Therapy may involve the use of doxorubicin, 5-fluorouracil, dacarbazine, dactinomycin, or cisplatin. It may also employ a combination of drugs for malignant carcinoid tumors including streptozocin and 5-fluorouracil or streptozocin and cyclophosphamide. Other drug therapy may include parachlorophenylalanine, cyproheptadine, tamoxifen, and interferon. Surgical removal of the tumors has proved successful in some patients, as has hepatic artery ligation or occlusion.

A somatostatin analogue has proved effective in blocking flushing and relieving diarrhea and wheezing; symptoms usually improve within a few days. This drug has also been successful in the prophylaxis of carcinoid crisis and as an adjunct for patients undergoing surgery or starting chemotherapy.

**Treatment—Investigational** Please contact the agencies listed under Resources, below, for the most current information. Addresses and telephone numbers of these agencies, as well as of individual experts and research centers, may be found in the Master Resources List.

**Resources**

**For more information on carcinoid syndrome:** National Organization for Rare Disorders (NORD); American Cancer Society; NIH/National Cancer Institute Physician Data Query Phoneline.

**References**

Advances in Diagnostic and Treatment Methods in Carcinoids: B. Hyde; Res. Resources Rept., 1989, vol. 13(1), pp. 1–4.

The Carcinoid Syndrome: A Treatable Malignant Disease: L. Kvols; Oncology, 1988, vol. 2(2), pp. 33–39.

Carcinoid Crisis During Anesthesia: Successful Treatment with a Somatostain Analogue: H.M. Marsh, et al.; Anesthesiology, 1987, vol. 66(1), pp. 89–91.

Effect of Somatostatin Analog on Water and Electrolyte Transport and Transit Time in Human Small Bowel: M. Duano, et al.; Dig. Dis. Sci., 1987, vol. 32(10), pp. 1092–1096.

Vipoma Syndrome: H.S. Mekhuian, et al.; Semin. Oncol., September 1987, vol. 14(3), pp. 282–289.

Treatment of the Malignant Carcinoid Syndrome: L. Kvols, et al.; N. Engl. J. Med., September 11, 1986, vol. 315(11), pp. 663–666.

Vipoma Syndrome: Effect of a Synthetic Somatostatin Analogue: W.C. Santangelo, et al.; Scand. J. Gastroenterol., 1986, vol. 21(119), pp. 187–190.

Effect of a Long-Acting Somatostatin Analogue in a Patient with Pancreatic Cholera: P.N. Maton, et al.; N. Engl. J. Med., January 3, 1985, vol. 312, pp. 17–21.

# CHIARI-FROMMEL SYNDROME

**Description** Chiari-Frommel syndrome is a postpartum endocrine disorder in which lactation, anovulation, and amenorrhea persist long after childbirth. The absence of normal hormonal cycles may eventually lead to uterine atrophy. Some cases resolve spontaneously, with return of normal hormone levels and reproductive function.

**Synonyms**

Chiari I Syndrome
Frommel-Chiari Syndrome
Lactation-Uterus Atrophy
Postpartum Galactorrhea-Amenorrhea Syndrome

**Signs and Symptoms** The pregnancy preceding the onset of Chiari-Frommel syndrome is typically normal, and childbirth and initial lactation are uneventful. However, normal menses and ovulation do not resume, and persistent discharge from the nipples occurs, sometimes lasting for years. Other clinical findings include emotional lability, headache, backache, abdominal pain, visual deficits, occasionally obesity, and, in long-standing cases, uterine atrophy. Laboratory findings include high levels of prolactin and low urinary levels of estrogen and gonadotropins.

**Etiology** The cause of the abnormality of the hypothalamic-pituitary axis underlying Chiari-Frommel syndrome is not known. Most cases are attributable to pituitary tumors. Tiny hypothalamic lesions may also be involved. An association with oral contraceptive use has been suggested.

**Epidemiology** Chiari-Frommel Syndrome affects postpartum females.

**Related Disorders** See *Ahumada–del Castillo Syndrome; Forbes-Albright Syndrome.*

**Treatment—Standard** Medical and surgical therapy may be used to treat Chiari-Frommel syndrome. Large pituitary tumors causing the disorder may be removed surgically, but excision of small tumors may not be feasible. Bromocriptine is prescribed to reduce prolactin levels and restore ovulatory cycles.

**Treatment—Investigational** Please contact the agencies listed under Resources, below, for the most current information. Addresses and telephone numbers of these agencies, as well as of individual experts and research centers, may be found in the Master Resources List.

**Resources**

**For more information on Chiari-Frommel syndrome:** National Organization for Rare Disorders (NORD); NIH/National Institute of Child Health and Human Development; Resolve.

**References**

Cecil Textbook of Medicine, 19th ed.: J.B. Wyngaarden, et al., eds.; W.B. Saunders Company, 1992, pp. 1365–1366.

Mendelian Inheritance in Man, 10th ed.: V.A. McKusick; The Johns Hopkins University Press, 1992, p. 62.

Textbook of Endocrinology, 8th ed.: J.D. Wilson and D.W. Foster, eds.; W.B. Saunders Company, 1992, p. 959.

Dictionary of Medical Syndromes, 3rd ed.: S.I. Magalini, et al., eds.; J.B. Lippincott Company, 1990, p. 44.

Novak's Textbook of Gynecology, 11th ed.: H. Jones III, et al. eds.; Williams and Wilkins, 1988, pp. 351–356.

Hyperprolactinemia Anemorrhea and Galactorrhea: M.C. Koppelman; Ann. Int. Med., 1984, vol. 10, pp. 115–121.

# CONN SYNDROME

**Description** Conn syndrome is a rare metabolic endocrine disorder characterized by oversecretion of aldosterone, causing hypervolemia, hypernatremia, and hypokalemic alkalosis. Aldosterone causes transfer of sodium in exchange for potassium and hydrogen in the kidneys, in the salivary and sweat glands, and in the cells of the mucous membranes of the intestines. The renin-angiotensin mechanism and, to a lesser extent, the adrenocorticotropin hormone (**ACTH**) regulate aldosterone secretion. The sodium and water retention resulting from increased aldosterone secretion not only causes hypervolemia but also reduces renin secretion.

## Synonyms

> Aldosteronism, Primary
> Glucocorticoid Suppressible Hyperaldosteronism
> Hyperaldosteronism, Primary

**Signs and Symptoms** Hypernatremia, hypervolemia, and hypokalemic alkalosis can cause periods of weakness, unusual sensations such as tingling and warmness, a transient paralysis, and muscle spasms. Hypertension is expected, and polyuria and polydipsia often occur.

**Etiology** The most frequent cause is a unilateral adenoma of the adrenal cortex glomerulosa cells. The origin of the tumor is unknown. Less commonly an adrenal carcinoma or hyperplasia underlies Conn syndrome. Glucocorticoid suppressible hyperaldosteronism is the result of an anti-Lepore-type fusion of the CYP 11B2 and CYP 11B1 genes.

**Related Disorders Secondary aldosteronism** is characterized by increased adrenal cortex production of aldosterone resulting from stimuli exogenous to the adrenal glands, probably the result of excessive secretion of renin secondary to constriction of the renal vessels. The disorder is similar to Conn syndrome and related to hypertension and disorders with fluid retention and/or edema, such as congestive heart failure and cirrhosis with ascites. This syndrome also occurs as a symptom of other renal disorders, but unlike Conn syndrome, it is marked by decreased sodium levels and increased plasma-renin activity.

See *Bartter Syndrome.*

**Treatment—Standard** A search for adenoma in both adrenal glands is essential, although there is most often a unilateral lesion. Therapy consists of removal of the tumor. Among the choices for follow-up drug therapy are mitotane, spironolactone, or hydrochlorothiazide.

**Treatment—Investigational** Please contact the agencies listed under Resources, below, for the most current information. Addresses and telephone numbers of these agencies, as well as of individual experts and research centers, may be found in the Master Resources List.

## Resources

**For more information on Conn syndrome:** National Organization for Rare Disorders (NORD); National Adrenal Diseases Foundation; NIH/National Digestive Diseases Information Clearinghouse; NIH/National Heart, Lung and Blood Institute Information Center.

## References

Mutations in the CYP 11B1 (11-Beta-Hydroxylase) and CYP 11B2 (Aldosterone Synthase) Genes Causing CMOII Deficiency, 11-Beta-Hydroxylase Deficiency, and Glucocorticoid Suppressible Hyperaldosteronism: L. Pascoe, et al.; Am. J. Hum. Genet., 1992, vol. 51(suppl.), p. A28.

Clinical Implications of Primary Aldosteronism with Resistant Hypertension: E.L. Bravo, et al.; Hypertension, 1988, vol. 11(2 pt. 2), pp. 1207–1211.

Isolated Clinical Syndrome of Primary Aldosteronism in Four Patients with Adrenocortical Carcinoma: D. Farge, et al.; Amer. J. Med., 1987, vol. 83(4), pp. 635–640.

Pure Primary Hyperaldosteronism Due to Adrenal Cortical Carcinoma: D.J. Greathouse, et al.; Amer. J. Med., 1984, vol. 76(6), pp. 1132–1136.

Aging and Aldosterone: R. Hegstad, et al.; Amer. J. Med., 1983, vol. 74(3), pp. 442–448.

# CUSHING SYNDROME

**Description** Cushing syndrome consists of myriad clinical abnormalities that are the result of hypersecretion of corticosteroids by the adrenal cortex.

## Synonyms

> Adrenal Cortex Adenoma
> Adrenal Hyperfunction Resulting from Pituitary ACTH Excess
> Adrenal Neoplasm
> Cushing's III
> Ectopic Adrenocorticotropic Hormone (ACTH) Syndrome

**Signs and Symptoms** Excessive weight gain produces fat deposits in the face, causing a rounded shape, and in the supraclavicular and dorsal cervical areas. The trunk is obese, but the arms and legs remain slender. The face is reddened, and the skin is thin, fragile, and slow to heal. Weakened connective tissue causes reddish-blue stretch marks on the arms, breasts, axillae, abdomen, buttocks, and thighs. Children and adolescents experience weight gain, growth retardation, and hypertension.

In women, hirsutism affects the face, neck, chest, abdomen, and thighs; menstrual disorders are common. In men, fertility is often decreased and the sex drive diminished or absent.

Hypertension occurs in 85 percent of patients. Osteoporosis, hyperglycemia, severe weakness and fatigue, and psychiatric disturbances may also be present.

**Etiology** Cushing syndrome is caused by excessive secretion of cortisol, often due to hormone-secreting benign adrenal or pituitary tumors. Seventy percent of cases in adults are due to a pituitary tumor or hyperplasia from hypothalamic corticotropin-releasing factor **(CRF)** secretion, resulting in **Cushing disease.** Extremely rare in children, **ectopic ACTH syndrome** is caused in 17 percent of adult cases by hormone-secreting malignant tumors, such as oat cell carcinomas of the lung. About 13 percent of adult cases are due to benign adrenal adenomas.

A rare, idiopathic adrenal response to gastric inhibitory peptides **(GIPS)** may increase cortisol levels.

An exogenous cause of elevated cortisol levels is corticosteroid therapy (e.g., prednisone), which results in Cushing syndrome.

**Epidemiology** Cushing syndrome affects 5 times more women than men. Onset is most common at ages 30 to 40; women who have just given birth are at higher risk.

**Related Disorders** See *Addison Disease.*

**Cushing disease** is characterized by hypersecretion of ACTH as a result of adrenal hyperplasia. It is a major cause of symptoms associated with Cushing syndrome.

**Treatment—Standard** Pituitary tumors may be removed by transphenoidal adenomectomy, with a success rate of over 80 percent. After surgery, the expected drop in the production of ACTH can be temporarily compensated with hydrocortisone. Therapy usually lasts for less than 1 year. If the patient is not a candidate for surgery or surgery proves unsuccessful, irradiation of the pituitary gland for 6 weeks is indicated. The rate of improvement is 40 to 50 percent for adults and 80 percent for children.

Mitotane alone or in combination with irradiation is used to inhibit cortisol production and speed recovery. Aminoglutethimide, metyrapone, or ketoconazole also controls the production of cortisol.

Trilostane (Modrastane) has been approved for treatment of Cushing syndrome.

The destruction of ACTH-secreting tumor cells is essential to reverse the effects of ectopic ACTH syndrome. Surgery, radiation, chemotherapy, or immunotherapy, in conjunction with the administration of mitotane, may be indicated.

If cortisol levels are elevated because of corticosteroid therapy, the dosage should be reduced until the symptoms are under control, or therapy should be changed to once every other day if the therapeutic effect can be retained.

**Treatment—Investigational** A glucocorticoid antagonist, RU 486, is undergoing clinical trials in the treatment of Cushing syndrome.

George P. Chrousos, M.D., at the Developmental Endocrinology Branch, National Institutes of Health, is studying patients with Cushing syndrome.

Research is underway to determine the effectiveness of octreotide (Sandostatin) in shrinking corticotropin-secreting adenomas.

Bilateral femoral catheterization to reach the inferior petrosal sinuses followed by sampling after stimulation with corticotropin-releasing hormone is under investigation for evaluating patients with Cushing syndrome. For more information, contact Karen Elkind-Hirsch, Ph.D., at Methodist Hospital, Houston, Texas.

David N. Orth, M.D., at Vanderbilt University, Nashville, Tennessee, is conducting clinical trials to study the diagnosis and treatment of Cushing syndrome.

Hormonal evaluation of patients with Cushing syndrome is being conducted by Roy E. Weiss, M.D., Ph.D., at the University of Chicago.

Please contact the agencies listed under Resources, below, for the most current information. Addresses and telephone numbers of these agencies, as well as of individual experts and research centers, may be found in the Master Resources List.

**Resources**

**For more information on Cushing syndrome:** National Organization for Rare Disorders (NORD); National Cushing Syndrome Association; National Adrenal Diseases Foundation; Cushing Support and Research Foundation; Brain and Pituitary Foundation of America.

**References**

Cushing Syndrome in Children and Adolescents: M.A. Magiakou, et al.; N. Engl. J. Med., September 1994, vol. 331(10), pp. 629–635.

Bronchial Carcinoid Tumors: D.G. Davila, et al.; Mayo Clin. Proc., August 1993, vol. 68(8), pp. 795–803.

Paraendocrine Syndromes: S.T. Pierce; Curr. Opin. Oncol., July 1993, vol. 5(4), pp. 639–645.

The Pathology of Cushing's Disease: K. Kovacs; J. Steroid Biochem. Mol. Biol., April 1993, vol. 45(1–3), pp. 179–182.

Unpredictable Hypersecretion of Cortisol in Cushing's Disease: Detection by Daily Salivary Cortisol Measurements: A.R. Hermus, et al.; Acta Endocrinol., May 1993, vol. 128(5), pp. 428–432.

Bilateral Adrenocortical Adenomas Causing Cushing's Syndrome: Report of Two Cases with Enzyme Histochemical and Ultrastructural Studies and a Review of the Literature: M. Aiba, et al.; Arch. Pathol. Lab. Med., February 1992, vol. 116(2), pp. 146–150.

Cecil Textbook of Medicine, 19th ed.: J.B. Wyngaarden, et al., eds.; W.B. Saunders Company, 1992, pp. 1284–1288.

Endocrinopathies of Hyperfunction: Cushing's Syndrome and Aldosteronism: J. Gumowski, et al.; AACN Clin. Issues Crit. Care Nurs., May 1992, vol. 3(2), pp. 331–349.

Food-Dependent Cushing's Syndrome Mediated by Aberrant Adrenal Sensitivity to Gastric Inhibitory Polypeptide: Y. Reznik, et al.; N. Engl. J. Med., October 1992, vol. 327(14), pp. 981–986.

Gastric Inhibitory Polypeptide-Dependent Cortisol Hypersecretion: A New Case History: A. LaCroix, et al.; N. Engl. J. Med., October 1992, vol. 327(14), pp. 974–980.

Nelson Textbook of Pediatrics, 14th ed. R.E. Behrman, ed.-in-chief; W.B. Saunders Company, 1992, pp. 1448–1450.

Neuroendocrinology: Clinical and Experimental: M.F. Scanlon; Curr. Opin. Neurol. Neurosurg., June 1992, vol. 5(3), pp. 379–382.

Potential Indications for Octreotide in Endocrinology: K. von Werder, et al.; Metabolism, September 1992, vol. 41(9 suppl. 2), pp. 91–98.

The Role of Octreotide (Sandostatin) in Nongrowth Hormone-, Nonthyroid Stimulating Hormone-, and Nonprolactin-Secreting Adenomas: A. Warner; Metabolism, September 1992, vol. 41(9 suppl. 2), pp. 59–61.

Textbook of Endocrinology, 8th ed.: J.D. Wilson and D.W. Foster, eds.; W.B. Saunders Company, 1992, pp. 536–562.

ACTH-Producing Pituitary Tumors: J.R. Grua, et al.; Endocrinol. Metab. Clin. North Am., June 1991, vol. 29(2), pp. 319–362.

Dictionary of Medical Syndromes, 3rd ed.: S.I. Magalini, et al., eds.; J.B. Lippincott Company, 1990, pp. 217–218.

Internal Medicine, 2nd ed.: J.H. Stein, ed.-in-chief; Little, Brown and Company, 1987, pp. 1947–1951.

# DENYS-DRASH SYNDROME

**Description** Denys-Drash syndrome is characterized by the combination of abnormal kidney function, malignant renal neoplasm in children, and pseudohermaphroditism.

**Synonyms**

Drash Syndrome

Nephropathy–Pseudohermaphroditism–Wilms Tumor

Pseudohermaphroditism–Nephron Disorder–Wilms Tumor

Wilms Tumor and Pseudohermaphroditism

Wilms Tumor–Pseuodohermaphroditism–Glomerulopathy

Wilms Tumor–Pseudohermaphroditism–Nephropathy

**Signs and Symptoms** Major symptoms of the complete form of Denys-Drash syndrome are abnormal kidney function, nephroblastoma, and pseudohermaphroditism. The incomplete form of Denys-Drash syndrome combines abnormal kidney function with either pseudohermaphroditism or nephroblastoma.

Some patients with Denys-Drash syndrome may develop malignancies of the testes or ovaries, abnormalities of the reproductive and urinary systems, vesicoureteral reflux, and hydronephrosis.

**Etiology** Denys-Drash syndrome is a result of mutations in the Wilms tumor suppressor (**WT1**) gene. The mutations exert a dominant negative effect.

**Epidemiology** One hundred fifty cases have been reported in the medical literature.

**Related Disorders** See *Wilms Tumor; Adrenal Hyperplasia, Congenital; Klinefelter Syndrome; Reifenstein Syndrome*

**17-β-Hydroxysteroid dehydrogenase deficiency** (also known as **17-ketosteroid reductase deficiency**) causes impairment in the production of steroids. Male pseudohermaphroditism is present, and there is no enlargement of the adrenal gland. This disorder is inherited as either an autosomal recessive or an X-linked trait.

**Treatment—Standard** Patients with progressive kidney disease can be maintained on dialysis. Some patients may choose to undergo transplant surgery.

Removal of the ovaries or testes may be recommended to avoid malignancy.

Genetic counseling may be of benefit for patients and their families.

Other treatment is symptomatic and supportive.

**Treatment—Investigational** Please contact the agencies listed under Resources, below, for the most current information. Addresses and telephone numbers of these agencies, as well as of individual experts and research centers, may be found in the Master Resources List.

**Resources**

**For more information on Denys-Drash syndrome:** National Organization for Rare Disorders (NORD); National Kidney Foundation; American Kidney Fund; American Cancer Society; NIH/National Institute of Child Health and Human Development.

**For genetic information and genetic counseling referrals:** March of Dimes Birth Defects Foundation; Alliance of Genetic Support Groups.

**References**

The Denys-Drash Syndrome: R.F. Mueller; J. Med. Genet., 1994, vol. 31, pp. 471–477.

A Case Report of Drash Syndrome in a 46,XX Female: T.L. Melocoton, et al.; Am. J. Kidney Dis., October 1991, vol. 18(4), pp. 503–508.

Birth Defects Encyclopedia: M.L. Buyse, ed.-in-chief; Blackwell Scientific Publications, 1990, pp. 1780–1781.

Mendelian Inheritance in Man, 9th ed.: V.A. McKusick; The Johns Hopkins University Press, 1990, p. 984.

A Report of 4 Patients with Drash Syndrome and a Review of the Literature: J.C. Jensen, et al.; J. Urol. May 1989, vol. 141(5), pp. 174–176.

The Drash Syndrome Revisited: Diagnosis and Follow-Up: A.L. Friedman, et al.; Am. J. Med. Genet., 1987, vol. 3(suppl.), pp. 293–296.

# DERCUM DISEASE

**Description** Dercum disease is characterized by subcutaneous lipomas that exert pressure on nerves, causing extreme pain and weakness.

**Synonyms**
> Adiposa Dolorosa
> Juxta-articular Adiposis Dolorosa

**Signs and Symptoms** Painful, irregularly shaped, soft fatty tissue deposits occur most frequently in the trunk, forearms, knees, and thighs. These deposits may spontaneously resolve, leaving hardened tissue or pendulous folds of skin. In some cases, severe asthenia is present. Some patients may experience depression, but it is not known whether depression is a symptom of the disorder or a response to the pain of chronic illness.

**Etiology** Dercum disease is autosomal dominant.

**Epidemiology** Dercum disease usually affects obese females age 45 to 60. It has been recorded in more than one member of the same family and has been known to affect persons of normal weight. Cases of men affected by Dercum disease have been reported in the literature.

**Related Disorders** Symptoms of Dercum disease are similar to those of arthritis.

**Treatment—Standard** Treatment is directed primarily at easing painful episodes. Surgical excision of fatty tissue deposits around joints may temporarily relieve symptoms; recurrence is common. Intravenous infusions of lidocaine bring temporary relief, but periodic infusions may be necessary to sustain the effect. Mexiletine, taken orally, may also eliminate pain for variable periods. Psychotherapy may help patients cope with long-term intense pain. Other treatment is symptomatic and supportive.

**Treatment—Investigational** Please contact the agencies listed under Resources, below, for the most current information. Addresses and telephone numbers of these agencies, as well as of individual experts and research centers, may be found in the Master Resources List.

**Resources**

   **For more information on Dercum disease:** National Organization for Rare Disorders (NORD); NIH/National Digestive Diseases Information Clearinghouse; American Chronic Pain Association; National Pain Outreach Association.

**References**

Mendelian Inheritance in Man, 9th ed.: V.A. McKusick; The Johns Hopkins University Press, 1990, p. 31.

Dercum Disease (Adiposa Dolorosa): Treatment of Severe Pain with Intravenous Lidocaine: P. Petersen, et al.; Pain, 1987, vol. 28(1), pp. 77–80.

A Case of Adiposis Dolorosa: Lipid Metabolism and Hormone Secretion: A. Taniguchi, et al.; Int. J. Obes., 1986, vol. 10(4), pp. 277–281.

Dercum Disease (Adiposa Dolorosa): A Case Report and Review of the Literature: T.J. Bonatus, et al.; Clin. Orthop., 1986, vol. 205, pp. 251–253.

# DIABETES INSIPIDUS (DI)

**Description** DI, a disorder of the neurohypophyseal system, is characterized by the excretion of large amounts of urine of low specific gravity, by dehydration, and by polydipsia. The more common neurohypophyseal DI or central DI, which can be inherited, acquired, or idiopathic, is due to a deficiency of antidiuretic hormone (**ADH;** vasopressin). The rarer congenital nephrogenic diabetes insipidus (**NDI**) is caused by failure of the renal tubules to respond to ADH, preventing reabsorption of water.

**Synonyms**
> Vasopressin-Sensitive Diabetes Insipidus (Central or Neurogenic Diabetes Insipidus)
> Vasopressin-Resistant Diabetes Insipidus (Nephrogenic Diabetes Insipidus)

**Signs and Symptoms** Onset of all types of DI may be abrupt and may occur at any age. From 3 to 30 liters of fluid may be ingested and excreted per day. Some patients may experience nocturia and fever. Loss of consciousness is the result of insufficient retention of fluids. Poor weight gain in children or weight loss may be evident because the need for excessive fluid intake prevents adequate caloric intake.

In central or neurogenic DI, polydipsia and polyuria vary in severity among patients. Symptoms may also include weakness, fatigue, and dryness of the mouth and skin. Other physical symptoms and signs are usually those of the underlying disorder.

In nephrogenic DI, infants develop polydipsia and polyuria. Since infants cannot communicate thirst, severe dehydration with hypernatremia, fever, vomiting, or convulsions should signal the possibility of NDI. Mental retardation may result.

**Etiology** Central or neurogenic DI can be inherited (X-linked forms as well as autosomal dominant forms) as the result of mutations in the arginine vasopressin gene (**ARVP**), acquired (the result of hypophysectomy, trauma, malignancy, histiocytosis, granuloma, vascular abnormalities, infection), or idiopathic. The idiopathic form affects approximately 50 percent of patients with DI. It is essential to perform imaging studies of the brain in any patient with neurogenic DI.

Nephrogenic DI may occur as an X-linked recessive trait. The defective gene is on the long arm of the X chromosome (Xq28). Other cases are inherited as an autosomal dominant trait. Another defective gene (aquaporin-2), which causes nephrogenic DI, is localized to chromosome 12q12–13. Nephrogenic DI may also be acquired as the result of drug toxicity.

**Epidemiology** The inherited forms of diabetes insipidus usually affect males. Females can be carriers.

**Related Disorders Diabetes mellitus (insulin dependent)** is a more common disorder in which insulin replacement is required. Environmental factors may play a role in determining which predisposed people acquire the deficiency. Females and males are equally affected. Polydipsia and polyuria are the most obvious symptoms and the only symptoms in common with DI.

**Treatment—Standard** Eradication of a lesion may be indicated in some cases. The most effective control of neurogenic DI is obtained with the commercially available, long-acting synthetic ADH analogue desmopressin acetate (**DDAVP**), which appears to enhance antidiuretic activity with minimal adverse effects on the vascular system or smooth muscles. DDAVP may be insufflated with a spray dispenser or blown high into the nasal passages with an tube insufflator. In many patients, nasal irritation may be a drawback to this form of treatment.

Thiazide diuretics are effective for treating the polyuria in patients with both neurogenic and nephrogenic DI.

DDAVP is of little use in chronic treatment of nephrogenic DI. Chlorpropamide, used to treat hyperglycemia in diabetes mellitus, is effective in reducing polyuria in neurogenic DI patients. However, hypoglycemia is a significant adverse reaction to chlorpropamide therapy. Clofibrate and carbamazepine also have been used successfully. Partial or total substitutions for clofibrate or carbamazepine can be made. Some patients may benefit from the use of one of these agents in combination with a diuretic.

A laboratory test is available to determine if DI is the inherited form of nephrogenic DI and to identify women who may be carriers.

**Treatment—Investigational** Research in treating DI is ongoing. Prostaglandin synthesis inhibitors under investigation have not shown uniform effectiveness. Use of hydrochlorothiazide-amiloride in the treatment of congenital NDI has indicated that treatment with both of these compounds may possibly be more effective than hydrochlorothiazide alone and can be a satisfactory alternative to the hydrochlorothiazide-prostaglandin synthetase inhibitor combination in the treatment of NDI.

Gary L. Robertson, M.D., at Northwestern Memorial Hospital in Chicago, is studying the genetic basis of neurogenic DI.

Robert S. Wildin, M.D., at the University of Texas, Galveston, is studying genetic mutations in the renal vasopressin receptor to learn more about its function in congenital NDI.

Please contact the agencies listed under Resources, below, for the most current information. Addresses and telephone numbers of these agencies, as well as of individual experts and research centers, may be found in the Master Resources List.

**Resources**

**For more information on diabetes insipidus:** National Organization for Rare Diseases (NORD); American Diabetes Association; NIH/National Diabetes Information Clearinghouse; Diabetes Insipidus and Related Disorders Network; The Arc (a national organization on mental retardation).

**For genetic information and genetic counseling referrals:** March of Dimes Birth Defects Foundation; Alliance of Genetic Support Groups.

**References**

Treatment of Nephrogenic Diabetes Insipidus with Prostaglandin Synthesis-Inhibitors: S. Libber, et al., eds.; J. Pediatr., February 1986, vol. 108(2), pp. 305–311.

Hydrochlorothiazide-Amiloride in the Treatment of Congenital Nephrogenic Diabetes Insipidus: V. Alon and J.C. Chan; Am. J. Nephrol., 1985, vol. 5(1), pp. 9–13.

# FORBES-ALBRIGHT SYNDROME

**Description** Forbes-Albright syndrome is one of a group of disorders associated with hypersecretion of prolactin by the pituitary.

**Synonyms**

      Galactorrhea-Amenorrhea Syndrome

      Nonpuerperal Amenorrhea-Galactorrhea

      Nonpuerperal Galactorrhea

**Signs and Symptoms** Onset of galactorrhea and amenorrhea in women and of galactorrhea and other changes in men usually occurs between the ages of 20 and 40. Women with galactorrhea and amenorrhea have breasts and nipples of normal size and appearance, but the pattern of body hair may change and libido may decrease. Obesity and exceptionally oily skin are characteristics in some patients.

Men may have gynecomastia and galactorrhea. Even in the absence of galactorrhea, men may experience a lessening of libido and impotence, and a decrease in sperm.

High levels of prolactin and low concentrations of gonadotropins, e.g., follicle-stimulating hormone (**FSH**), are typical findings.

**Etiology** The primary cause of the syndrome is a hormone-secreting pituitary tumor or, at times, a tumor in the hypothalamus. Also to blame may be hypothyroidism, chronic use of dopamine antagonists (e.g., chlorpromazine), and discontinuation of oral contraceptives.

**Epidemiology** Forbes-Albright syndrome occurs predominantly in females and is rare in males.

**Related Disorders** See *Chiari-Frommel Syndrome; Ahumada–del Castillo Syndrome.*

**Treatment—Standard** Surgical removal of the neoplasm is usually curative. For smaller or inoperable tumors, irradiation or treatment with bromocriptine or lergotrile mesilate is indicated. These drugs lower prolactin levels, thereby preventing abnormal lactation, and often produce normal menses.

**Treatment—Investigational** Please contact the agencies listed under Resources, below, for the most current information. Addresses and telephone numbers of these agencies, as well as of individual experts and research centers, may be found in the Master Resources List.

**Resources**

  **For more information on Forbes-Albright syndrome:** National Organization for Rare Disorders (NORD); NIH/National Institute of Child Health and Human Development.

**References**

Assessment and Management of Galactorrhea: D.S. Edge, et al.; Nurse Pract., June 1993, vol. 18(6), pp. 35–36, 38, 43–44.

Textbook of Endocrinology, 8th ed.: J.D. Wilson and D.W. Foster, eds.; W.B. Saunders Company, 1992, pp. 958–959.

Cecil Textbook of Medicine, 19th ed.: J.B. Wyngaarden, et al., eds.; W.B. Saunders Company, 1992, pp. 1365–1368.

Dictionary of Medical Syndromes, 3rd ed.: S.I. Magalini, et al., eds.; J.B. Lippincott Company, 1990, p. 44.

Novak's Textbook of Gynecology, 11th ed.: H. Jones III, et al., eds.; Williams and Wilkins, 1988, pp. 351–357.

# FRÖLICH SYNDROME

**Description** Frölich syndrome is characterized by delayed puberty, small testes, and obesity; it primarily affects males. In recent years, Frölich syndrome has referred exclusively to such features in boys who have lesions in the hypothalamus. Teenagers with this disorder must be differentiated from those who simply have a familial trait of slower-than-normal growth or **Prader-Willi syndrome.**

**Synonyms**

      Adiposogenital Dystrophy

      Babinski-Frölich Syndrome

      Dystrophia Adiposogenitalis

      Hypothalamic Infantilism-Obesity

      Launois-Cleret Syndrome

      Sexual Infantilism

**Signs and Symptoms** Obesity accompanies delayed puberty and secondary sexual characteristics. Body growth may also be slow, and patients often remain short in stature. Fingernails are often malformed or undersized. Headaches are common. Some patients may have mental retardation, visual disturbances, and, rarely, diabetes mellitus.

**Etiology** In some cases the anterior pituitary fails to secrete the hormones necessary for puberty because of a lesion, usually caused by a tumor or inflammation resulting from an infection, such as tuberculosis or encephalitis. In the remaining cases, Frölich syndrome is due to lesions in the hypothalamus, which produces substances that stimulate the pituitary and is believed to regulate the appetite.

**Epidemiology** More males than females are affected.

**Related Disorders Hypogonadotropic hypogonadism** is a disorder of the development of the region of the hypothalamus that regulates the production of gonadotropins.

See ***Borjeson Syndrome; Bardet-Biedl Syndrome; Prader-Willi Syndrome.***

**Treatment—Standard** Hormonal replacement therapy is indicated, but hypothalamic tumors should be removed if possible. The patient's appetite makes it difficult to achieve weight control.

**Treatment—Investigational** Please contact the agencies listed under Resources, below, for the most current information. Addresses and telephone numbers of these agencies, as well as of individual experts and research centers, may be found in the Master Resources List.

**Resources**

**For more information on Frölich syndrome:** National Organization for Rare Disorders (NORD); NIH/National Institute of Neurological Disorders and Stroke; Human Growth Foundation; Short Stature Foundation; Magic Foundation for Children's Growth; The Arc (a national organization on mental retardation).

**References**

Textbook of Endocrinology, 8th ed.: J.D. Wilson and D.W. Foster, eds.; W.B. Saunders Company, 1992, pp. 192–193.

Dictionary of Medical Syndromes, 3rd ed.: S.I. Magalini, et al., eds.; J.B. Lippincott Company, 1990, pp. 18–21.

# GRAVES DISEASE

**Description** Hyperthyroidism, goiter, exophthalmos, tachycardia, and dermopathy are the major characteristics of Graves disease.

**Synonyms**

Basedow Disease

Exophthalmic Goiter

Parry Disease

Thyrotoxicosis

**Signs and Symptoms** The major features of Graves disease do not necessarily occur together and often run courses independent of each other. There may be periods of remission. The diffusely enlarged goiter may be asymmetric, with an enlarged pyramidal lobe. Ten to 15 percent of adults may not have goiter at diagnosis. Besides exophthalmos, the other often characteristic ocular findings include inflammation and conjunctival edema; ophthalmoplegia may occur in the more severe cases. Diplopia and photophobia may also be present. The dermopathy, though rare, most often presents as erythematous, pruritic swelling over the pretibial area.

Other findings include hyperactivity, tachycardia, gynecomastia, and, less often, clubbing of the fingers and toes.

**Etiology** The cause of Graves disease is unknown, and inheritance is unclear. The pathogenesis is autoimmune-mediated by thyrotropin **(TSH)** receptor antibodies, also known as thyroid-stimulating immunoglobulins class $G_1$.

**Epidemiology** Graves disease can occur at any age but is most common in the 20s and 30s. Females are affected more often than males. A 1987 survey of 924 hyperthyroid patients from 17 thyroid centers in 6 European countries indicated that 60 percent of hyperthyroid adults and more than 90 percent of hyperthyroid children have Graves disease.

**Related Disorders** See ***Hashimoto Disease.***

**Treatment—Standard** Antithyroid drugs are preferred initially by many physicians, since ablative procedures more often produce hypothyroidism. Antithyroid drugs (e.g., propylthiouracil and methimazole) are also preferred for children, teenagers, and pregnant women. These drugs, however, seem to result in fewer lasting remissions. Thyroxine in conjuction with antithyroid drug therapy may be helpful to further control hormone release.

Radioactive iodine ablative therapy is preferred by many centers, especially in patients above age 40, because of its effectiveness in treating thyrotoxicosis without the possible complications of surgical procedures. The hypothyroidism that ensues must be anticipated and treated.

Surgery is usually reserved for patients refractory to other therapies. Lifelong follow-up is indicated postthyroidectomy.

Initial symptomatic control of thyrotoxicosis is achieved with β-adrenergic blocking agents that are continued until antithyroid drug therapy has rendered the patient euthyroid.

Genetic counseling may benefit those patients and their families with a strong familial history. Other treatment is symptomatic and supportive.

**Treatment—Investigational** Please contact the agencies listed under Resources, below, for the most current information. Addresses and telephone numbers of these agencies, as well as of individual experts and research centers, may be found in the Master Resources List.

**Resources**

   **For more information on Graves disease:** National Organization for Rare Disorders (NORD); American Autoimmune-Related Diseases Association; Graves Disease Foundation; National Graves Disease Foundation; Thyroid Foundation of America; Paget Foundation; NIH/National Digestive Diseases Information Clearinghouse.

   **For genetic information and genetic counseling referrals:** March of Dimes Birth Defects Foundation; Alliance of Genetic Support Groups.

**References**

Administration of Thyroxine in Treated Graves' Disease: Effects on the Level of Antibodies to Thyroid-Stimulation Hormone Receptors and on the Risk of Reoccurrence of Hyperthyroidism: K. Hashizume, et al., N. Engl. J. Med., April 1991, vol. 324, pp. 947–953.

Treatment for Graves' Disease: Telling the Thyroid to Rest: P.W. Ladenson, N. Engl. J. Med., April 1991, vol. 324, pp. 989–1000.

Internal Medicine, 3rd ed.: J.H. Stein, ed.-in-chief; Little, Brown and Company, 1990, pp. 2174–2178.

Mendelian Inheritance in Man, 9th ed.: V.A. McKusick; The Johns Hopkins University Press, 1990, pp. 1509–1510.

Graves Disease: Manifestations and Therapeutic Options: K.F. McFarland, et al.; Postgrad. Med., 1988, vol. 83(4), pp. 275–282.

High Serum Progesterone in Hyperthyroid Men with Graves Disease: K. Nomura, et al.; J. Clin. Endocrinol. Metab., 1988, vol. 66(1), pp. 230–232.

Graves Disease Associated with Histologic Hashimoto's Thyroiditis: S.A. Falk, et al.; Otolaryngol. Head Neck Surg., 1985, vol. 93(1), pp. 86–91.

# GROWTH HORMONE DEFICIENCY (GHD)

**Description** A sufficient quantity of growth hormone **(GH),** manufactured in the pituitary, is required during infancy and childhood to maintain normal linear growth and normalize sexual maturity. Growth hormone deficiency causes an absence or delay of lengthening and widening of the skeletal bones inappropriate to the chronological age of the child.

   There are several types of GHD: IA, IB, IIB, and III.

**Signs and Symptoms** Growth increments are the most important criteria in the diagnosis of GHD. Normal levels of growth usually follow a pattern, and if growth during a recorded 6- to 12-month period is within those levels, it is unlikely that a growth disorder exists.

   Growth in the first 6 months of life is usually 16 to 17 cm, and in the second 6 months, about 8 cm. During the 2nd year, 10 or more cm are normal. Growth in the 3rd year should equal 8 cm or more, and in the 4th year, 7 cm. In the years between ages 4 and 10, an average of 5 or 6 cm is normal. Ten percent deviation in these norms is the standard in assessing a growth abnormality. If a child falls below the 10 percent deviation in growth, he or she should then be tested for abnormally low levels of growth hormone.

   The infant with GHD is usually of normal weight and length at birth. During the newborn period, the infant may become hypoglycemic. Micropenis may be present in males. Signs and symptoms common to children with GHD are abnormal rates of development of facial bones, slow tooth eruption, delayed skeletal development, fine hair, and poor nail growth. They may also experience truncal obesity, a high-pitched voice, and delayed closure of the fontanelles.

   **GHD IA** is characterized by prenatal growth retardation. The infant usually has a normal response to administration of GH at first, then develops antibodies to the hormone. The child is small in relation to his or her siblings and becomes a very short adult.

   **GHD IB** is similar to IA, but some growth hormone is present at birth. The child may respond to treatment with GH.

   **GHD IIB** is similar to IB, but with a different inheritance.

   **GHD III** is similar to the above, but also with a different inheritance.

   Laboratory testing is necessary before a diagnosis of GHD is made, because growth and maturity delays can be caused by a wide variety of factors, including normal genetic influences.

**Etiology** The growth hormone gene is located on the long arm of chromosome 17. In some children, GHD is of unknown origin; in others, it may be inherited or familial. GHD IA and IB are inherited as autosomal recessive traits. GHD IIB inheritance is autosomal dominant. GHD III is inherited through X-linked transmission, affecting only males. GHD may occur after damage to the hypothalamus and/or pituitary from tumors, cysts, inflammation, trauma, and developmental abnormalities. Mutations in the growth hormone gene **(GH1)** and pituitary transcription factor **(PIT1),** a protein important in regulating genes controlling pituitary development and expression of the genes for growth hormone, thyroid hormone, and prolactin, have been found in patients with GHD.

**Epidemiology** For all forms of inherited GHD, except GHD III, males and females are affected equally. Growth hormone deficiency is rarely seen in association with other disorders, such as Down syndrome, CHARGE association, cystic fibrosis, chronic renal failure, and Turner syndrome. There may be approximately 15,000 to 20,000 children in the United States with pituitary dwarfism caused by GHD.

**Related Disorders** See *Turner Syndrome; Down Syndrome; CHARGE Association; Cystic Fibrosis; Growth Hormone Insensitivity Syndrome.*

**Treatment—Standard** Confirming GHD in a child with growth retardation is most important. Tests used include GH stimulation by insulin-arginine, exercise, glucagon, clonidine, or L-dopa. Estrogen or testosterone and propranolol are added to enhance the GH response to the stimulation tests. When a diagnosis of GHD can be made, treatment can then be instituted. Short children whose levels of growth hormone have not been tested or are tested and found to be normal should not be treated with human growth hormone **(HGH).** Commercially available, biotechnology engineered HGH is very expensive, and many health insurance companies will not reimburse for the product unless laboratory tests confirm GHD. Moreover, adverse effects of HGH on healthy short children without GHD have not been adequately assessed.

Recombinant HGH is available worldwide as an injection. Children with GHD are usually started on a dose of recombinant HGH based on body weight as soon as the condition is recognized. The dosage gradually increases with the increase in body weight to its highest during puberty, and discontinued by approximately age 17.

**Treatment—Investigational** Please contact the agencies listed under Resources, below, for the most current information. Addresses and telephone numbers of these agencies, as well as of individual experts and research centers, may be found in the Master Resources List.

**Resources**

**For more information on growth hormone deficiency:** National Organization for Rare Disorders (NORD); Magic Foundation for Children's Growth; Human Growth Foundation; Short Stature Foundation; Little People of America; NIH/National Institute of Child Health and Human Development.

**For genetic information and genetic counseling referrals:** March of Dimes Birth Defects Foundation; Alliance of Genetic Support Groups.

**References**

Biosynthetic Human Growth Hormone in the Treatment of Growth Hormone Deficiency: J.H. Holcombe, et al.; Acta Paediatr. Scand. Suppl., 1990, vol. 367, pp. 44–48.

Clinical Pediatric Endocrinology: S.A. Kaplan; W.B. Saunders Company, 1990, pp. 1–56.

Growth Hormone for Short Stature Not Due to Classic Growth Hormone Deficiency: J.F. Cara, et al.; Pediatr. Clin. North Am., December, 1990, vol. 37(6), pp. 1229–1254.

Growth Hormone Therapy: L. Shulman, et al.; Am. Fam. Physician, May 1990, vol. 41(5), pp. 1541–1546.

Mendelian Inheritance in Man, 9th ed.: V.A. McKusick; The Johns Hopkins University Press, 1990, pp. 377–380, 887–888, 1426–1427.

Urinary Growth Hormone Excretion As a Screening Test for Growth Hormone Deficiency: J.M. Walker, et al.; Arch. Dis. Child, January 1990, vol. 65(1), pp. 89–92.

Cecil Textbook of Medicine, 18th ed.: J.B. Wyngaarden and L.H. Smith, Jr., eds.; W.B. Saunders Company, 1988, pp. 1290–1297, 2205.

Smith's Recognizable Patterns of Human Malformation, 4th ed.: K.L. Jones; W.B. Saunders Company, 1988, pp. 614–618, 762–763.

Diagnostic Recognition of Genetic Disease: W.L. Nyhan, et al.; Lea and Febiger, 1987, pp. 706–709, 712, 718.

# GROWTH HORMONE INSENSITIVITY SYNDROME (GHIS)

**Description** GHIS, a genetic disorder, is the result of growth hormone **(GH)** receptor or post-GH receptor mutations.

**Synonyms**

> Growth Hormone Binding Protein
> Growth Hormone Receptor
> Growth Hormone Receptor Deficiency
> Laron-Type Dwarfism
> Pituitary Dwarfism II

**Signs and Symptoms** Proportionate severe short stature is evident at birth or soon after. Delayed tooth eruption, a disproportion between the growth of the head and jaw, a saddle nose, and deep-set eyes are characteristic. Elevated levels of GH indicate the inability of patients to use the GHs they produce. Hypoglycemia is common. Sexual maturation in boys occurs at about age 22 and in girls at 16 to 19 years of age. Hands and feet are smaller than normal. Obesity and a high-pitched voice may also be present.

**Etiology** GHIS is inherited as an autosomal recessive genetic disorder. The gene is localized to chromosome 5p13.1–p12. The defect in this gene causes GH receptor defects that interfere with GH binding and signal transduction. The disorder may differ from family to family.

**Epidemiology** Six females to every 2 males are effected. Although first recognized in Mediterranean peoples and in those of Middle Eastern Jewish ancestry, GHIS may occur in any ethnic group and is especially prevalent in regions of Ecuador.

**Related Disorders** See *Coffin-Siris Syndrome; Cockayne Syndrome.*

**Treatment—Standard** Insulin-like growth factor 1, manufactured by several pharmaceutical companies, has been shown to increase linear growth. It is associated with very few dose-related side effects. Replacement therapy with exogenous human growth hormone **(HGH)** is not effective because the body cannot utilize it. Hypoglycemia must be treated to prevent further complications. Other treatment is symptomatic and supportive.

Genetic counseling is indicated for patients and their families.

**Treatment—Investigational** Please contact the agencies listed under Resources, below, for the most current information. Addresses and telephone numbers of these agencies, as well as of individual experts and research centers, may be found in the Master Resources List.

**Resources**

**For more information on growth hormone insensitivity syndrome:** National Organization for Rare Disorders (NORD); Magic Foundation for Children's Growth; Human Growth Foundation; Short Stature Foundation; Little People of America; NIH/National Institute of Child Health and Human Development.

**For genetic information and genetic counseling referrals:** March of Dimes Birth Defects Foundation; Alliance of Genetic Support Groups.

**References**

Mendelian Inheritance in Man, 9th ed.: V.A. McKusick; The Johns Hopkins University Press, 1990, pp. 1426–1427.

Characterization of the Human Growth Hormone Receptor Gene and Demonstration of a Partial Gene Deletion in Two Patients with Laron-Type Dwarfism: P.J. Godowski, et al.; Proc. Nat. Acad. Sci. USA, October 1989, vol. 86(20), pp. 8083–8087.

Laron Dwarfism and Mutations of the Growth Hormone Receptor Gene: S. Amelm, et al.; N. Engl. J. Med., October 1989, vol. 321(15), pp. 1426–1427.

Puberty in Laron-Type Dwarfism: Z. Laron, et al.; Eur. J. Pediatr., June 1980, vol. 134 (1), pp. 79–83.

# HASHIMOTO DISEASE

**Description** Hashimoto disease is a major cause of hypothyroidism and goiter. In its progression it can totally destroy the thyroid gland, but usually the patient has an enlarged thyroid gland with normal or mildly abnormal thyroid function tests.

**Synonyms**

Chronic Lymphocytic Thyroiditis
Hashimoto Syndrome
Hashimoto Thyroiditis
Lymphadenoid Goiter
Struma Lymphomatosa

**Signs and Symptoms** The main characteristic is a painless goiter, which on palpation feels firm and either smooth or nodular. Thyroid function studies initially are normal if the disease process has not yet affected the secretion of thyroid hormone.

**Etiology** The cause is unknown. The disease is the prototype of an autoimmune association. There may be a familial predisposition to the disorder, but the precise factors determining its development in certain individuals are not understood. The diagnosis is established by the presence of antibodies in serum to thyroglobulin and/or thyroid peroxidase.

**Epidemiology** Men and women of any age can develop the syndrome, but it occurs most often in women between the ages of 30 and 50. Patients with such chromosomal disorders as Turner syndrome, Down syndrome, and Klinefelter syndrome are at greater risk.

**Related Disorders** See *Graves Disease.*

**Subacute thyroiditis,** a fairly common inflammation of the thyroid, usually manifests about 2 weeks after a respiratory viral infection. Considerable pain and tenderness in the thyroid area accompany difficulty in swallowing. The radioiodine uptake is low, and the erythrocyte sedimentation rate is elevated. Most patients obtain relief from an analgesic or an anti-inflammatory drug, and in time the thyroid levels become normal.

**Riedel thyroiditis,** the result of fibrous tissue formation in the thyroidal area, is very rare and occurs exclusively in adults beyond the 4th decade of life. The thyroid is enlarged, hard, and fixed, but nontender. Hypothyroidism results from progressive destruction of the gland.

**Hypothyroidism** may be congenital or acquired, and occurs alone or in conjuction with other diseases. Major symptoms include goiter, dull facial expression, puffiness around the eyes, drooping eyelids, thinning hair, fatigue, and weight gain. Mental functioning may be affected.

**Treatment—Standard** Upon replacement with synthetic thyroid hormone, the goiter usually will shrink significantly, usually within 2 to 4 weeks. Lifetime replacement therapy is necessary.

**Treatment—Investigational** Please contact the agencies listed under Resources, below, for the most current information. Addresses and telephone numbers of these agencies, as well as of individual experts and research centers, may be found in the Master Resources List.

**Resources**

**For more information on Hashimoto disease:** National Organization for Rare Disorders (NORD); Thyroid Foundation of America; NIH/National Digestive Diseases Information Clearinghouse.

**For genetic information and genetic counseling referrals:** March of Dimes Birth Defects Foundation; Alliance of Genetic Support Groups.

**References**

Harrison's Principles of Internal Medicine, 12th ed.: J.D. Wilson, et al.; McGraw-Hill, 1991, pp. 1711–1712.
Internal Medicine, 3rd ed.: J.H. Stein, ed.-in-chief; Little, Brown and Company, 1990, pp. 2179–2180.
Mendelian Inheritance in Man, 8th ed.: V.A. McKusick; The Johns Hopkins University Press, 1986, p. 296.

# HERMAPHRODITISM, TRUE

**Description** True hermaphroditism is characterized by the presence of both male and female gonadal tissue in the same gonad or on opposite sides in the same individual.

**Synonyms**

Hermaphroditism

**Signs and Symptoms** The external genitalia are often morphologically ambiguous. Approximately 15 percent of those affected have a normal penis, and 5 percent have normal female external genitalia.

Internally, the most common presentation is an ovary and a testis. An ovotestis along with a normal ovary is also common, accompanied by the fallopian tube and in 90 percent of cases a uterus. The epididymis is present in approximately one-third of affected individuals. If a penis is present, hypospadias and cryptorchidism may occur. Tumors of the ovaries or testes are present in approximately 2 percent of reported cases.

At puberty, approximately one-half of those children who have not had sexual reassignment surgery will menstruate. A child born with a penis and raised as a male without undergoing a hysterectomy may experience menstruation as cyclical periods of hematuria. Gynecomastia occurs in approximately 80 percent of affected males. Pregnancy and childbirth are possible after surgical removal of the testes or testicular tissue and correction of the external genitalia. Individuals with testicular tissue may have fertile sperm.

**Etiology** True hermaphroditism is an error in embryologic development. It may be inherited as an autosomal recessive trait, although an autosomal dominant inheritance may occur.

Although born with the correct number of chromosomes, approximately two-thirds of patients show abnormalities of their sex chromosomes. A Y chromosome may be translocated to either an X chromosome or to an autosome. Abnormalities may also arise from hyper- or hyposecretion of hormones during the first trimester of fetal development.

**Epidemiology** The incidence in the United States is unknown, but the disorder probably occurs in less than 1:50,000 individuals.

**Related Disorders** See *Klinefelter Syndrome; Turner Syndrome*

**Female pseudohermaphroditism** occurs when a genetically female embryo is exposed to hypersecretion of androgens or when an infant overproduces these hormones. The internal female genitalia are normal, while the external genitalia are male or ambiguous. Clitoromegaly and a common outlet for the urethra and vagina may be present. Other symptoms as adolescents and adults include absence of breast development, hirsutism, virilization, amenorrhea, obesity, a short and thick neck, and protruding abdomen accompanied by thin arms and legs.

**Male pseudohermaphroditism** is a genetic disorder characterized by defective development of external male genitalia. The testes are usually normal. However, other external genitalia may be female.

**Treatment—Standard** To avoid gender confusion later in life, patients should be assigned a sexual identity as soon as possible. Criteria should be based on the appearance of the external genitalia, the formation of the internal genitalia, and the ease in which reconstruction can be carried out along one sexual line or the other.

A clitoral reduction on sex-assigned females is usually completed as early as possible to facilitate sexual identification. Vaginal reconstruction is usually delayed until puberty to avoid vaginal stenosis. In sex-assigned males, hypospadias is usually surgically corrected before the age of 2 or 3.

When an ovotestis and a uterus are present, the ovotestis and any male internal structures are usually removed, and feminizing surgery of the external genitalia is performed. If two ovotestes are present and there is a clear line of demarcation between the 2 types of tissue, the testicular portion is usually removed and the external genitalia surgically feminized. In both cases, the child is raised as female.

If a testis is present on one side and an ovotestis on the other, the testis is usually brought into the scrotum only if the external genitalia can be surgically reconstructed and the child raised as male.

If an ovary is present on one side and a testis on the other, sexual assignment is usually decided by evaluation of the appearance and function of the external genitalia. Appropriate surgical correction is then performed.

Genetic counseling may be of benefit for patients and their families.

**Treatment—Investigational** Please contact the agencies listed under Resources, below, for the most current information. Addresses and telephone numbers of these agencies, as well as of individual experts and research centers, may be found in the Master Resources List.

**Resources**

**For more information on true hermaphroditism:** National Organization for Rare Disorders (NORD); Dr. John Mahoney, Professor, Pediatrics and Psychology; NIH/National Institute of Child Health and Human Development.

**For genetic information and genetic counseling referrals:** March of Dimes Birth Defects Foundation; Alliance of Genetic Support Groups.

**References**

True Hermaphroditism with Bilateral Ovotestis: A Case Report: M. Bergmann, et al.; Int. J. Androl., April 1989, vol. 12(2), pp. 139–147.
Early Gender Assignment in True Hermaphroditism: F.I. Luks, et al.; J. Pediatr. Surg., December 1988, vol. 23(12), pp. 1122–1126.
True Hermaphroditism: Diagnosis and Surgical Treatment: S. Guaschino, et al.; Clin. Exp. Obstet. Gynecol., 1988, vol. 15(3), pp. 74–79.
Mendelian Inheritance in Man, 8th ed.: V.A. McKusick; The Johns Hopkins University Press, 1986, pp. 984–985.

# HYPOPHOSPHATASIA

**Description** A genetic metabolic bone disorder, hypophosphatasia is a manifestation of bony demineralization and lack of calcium deposit in the osteoid and in the cartilage of the long bones in early years. The disorder causes rachitic changes. There are 4 subdivisions: infantile (neonatal); childhood; adult; and pseudohypophosphatasia.

**Synonyms**

Hypercalciuric Rickets

Hypophosphatemic Rickets with Hypercalciuria, Hereditary

**Signs and Symptoms** In hypophosphatasia, rachitic radiographic abnormalities, a low serum alkaline phosphatase, and urinary excretion of phosphoethanolamine are diagnostic.

**Infantile hypophosphatasia** is the most frequently encountered form of the abnormality. As a rule, onset is before age 6 months, but diagnosis prenatally is possible. Demineralization is often accompanied by increased intracranial pressure, which may cause exophthalmos. Hypercalcemia and hypercalciuria may be present; calcium in the renal tubules may cause renal failure. Weakening and bending of the bones is usual, giving a picture of rickets. Significant bone abnormalities may develop.

Onset of **childhood hypophosphatasia** is generally after age 6 months and consists of loss of newly erupted teeth, increased proneness to infection, and retarded growth. X-rays may reveal abnormalities in the epiphyses and the shafts of the long bones.

**Adult hypophosphatasia** is rare. The patient has a history of early loss of baby teeth and rachitic symptoms as a child. Early in adulthood, the patient's permanent teeth often loosen and fall out or require extraction. The bones are less dense than they should be, and the patient is apt to be fracture-prone.

In **pseudohypophosphatasia,** the serum alkaline phosphatase is normal, whereas the other manifestations of hypophosphatasia are present.

**Etiology** With the exception of pseudohypophosphatase, a lack of alkaline phosphatase is responsible for the signs and symptoms of hypophosphatase. The infantile, childhood, and adult forms are hereditary; the infantile and childhood types are autosomal recessive, and the adult form is autosomal dominant. Alkaline phosphatase **(ALP1),** the gene responsible for the disorder, regulates the expression of the alkaline phosphatase protein.

**Epidemiology** All forms of hypophosphatasia affect males and females in equal numbers.

**Related Disorders** The hallmark of all types of rickets, either hereditary or acquired, is weakening of the bones as a result of faulty calcium metabolism and impaired bone mineralization. When a dietary lack of vitamin D is responsible, a supplement is curative if given before completion of bone development.

In **osteomalacia,** pain of varying severity accompanies softening and bending of the bones. The bones lack calcium either because of inadequate vitamin D or a renal disorder. Osteoamalacia is more common among women than men, and onset often coincides with pregnancy. Osteomalacia can be a separate entity but may also occur with other disorders, as in hypophosphatemic rickets.

**Pseudo–vitamin D–deficiency rickets (vitamin D–dependent rickets, type I)** usually starts in early infancy and causes significant skeletal changes (such as bending of the bones) and weakness. Episodic muscle cramping, convulsions, and spinal and pelvic abnormalities may occur. Inherited abnormal vitamin D-dependent metabolism is responsible. The disorder is autosomal recessive. The serum calcium is very low; the serum phosphate is only slightly below normal or normal. Renal dysfunction causes excessive excretion of amino acids.

See *Rickets, Vitamin D–Deficiency; Osteogenesis Imperfecta; Paget Disease of Bone; Rickets, Hypophosphatemic.*

**Treatment—Standard** Ultrasonography combined with alkaline phosphatase assay and x-ray of the fetus can make the diagnosis of hypophosphatasia prenatally in severe cases.

Vitamin D and its metabolites should be avoided in hypophosphatasia. A long-term course of oral phosphate supplements may be effective in some patients. Other treatment is symptomatic and supportive. Genetic counseling is indicated for patients' families.

**Treatment—Investigational** A few patients with severe cases of infantile hypophosphatasia have received transfusions of alkaline phosphatase–rich plasma to supplement the lack of alkaline phosphatase.

Please contact the agencies listed under Resources, below, for the most current information. Addresses and telephone numbers of these agencies, as well as of individual experts and research centers, may be found in the Master Resources List.

**Resources**

**For more information on hypophosphatasia:** National Organization for Rare Disorders (NORD); NIH/National Arthritis and Musculoskeletal and Skin Diseases Information Clearinghouse; Research Trust for Metabolic Diseases in Children; Michael P. Whyte, M.D., Shriners' Hospital for Crippled Children, St. Louis, Missouri.

**For genetic information and genetic counseling referrals:** March of Dimes Birth Defects Foundation; Alliance of Genetic Support Groups.

**References**

The Metabolic Basis of Inherited Disease, 6th ed.: C.R. Scriver, et al., eds.; McGraw-Hill, 1989, pp. 2845–2856.

Enzyme Replacement Therapy for Infantile Hypophosphatasia Attempted by Intravenous Infusions of Alkaline Phosphatase-Rich Paget Plasma: Results in Three Additional Patients: M.P. Whyte, et al.; J. Pediatr., December 1984, vol. 105(6), pp. 926–933.

Infantile Hypophosphatasia: Enzyme Replacement Therapy by Intravenous Infusion of Alkaline Phosphatase-Rich Plasma from Patients with Paget Bone Disease: M.P. Whyte, et al.; J. Pediatr., September 1982, vol. 101(3), pp. 379–386.

Infantile Hypophosphatasia Diagnosed at 4 Months and Surviving at 2 Years: A. Albeggiani, et al.; Helv. Paediatr. Acta, 1982, vol. 37(1), pp. 49–58.

# KALLMANN SYNDROME

**Description** Kallmann syndrome is an inherited disorder characterized by hypogonadism and anosmia.

**Synonyms**

Hypogonadism with Anosmia

Hypogonadotropic Hypogonadism and Anosmia

**Signs and Symptoms** Delayed puberty is characteristic. Anosmia is common. Other symptoms include color blindness, cleft lip or palate, hearing loss, renal agenesis, abnormal development of secondary sex characteristics, and infertility.

In more severe forms, mental retardation and abnormalities of the skeleton, such as syndactyly, a short 4th finger, or craniofacial asymmetry, may occur.

Females may experience estrogen deficiency, dyspareunia, osteoporosis, and hot flashes. Males may have absence of palpable testes (cryptorchidism) and micropenis.

In a very rare form of the disorder, patients exhibit spastic paraplegia.

**Etiology** The abnormal development of the rhinencephalon interferes with communication between the hypothalamus and the pituitary, causing the hyposecretion of luteinizing hormone (**LH**) and of follicle-stimulating hormone (**FSH**).

Kallmann Syndrome can be inherited as an autosomal dominant, autosomal recessive, or X-linked recessive disorder. The X-linked form is thought to be caused by a deletion on the short arm of the X chromosome at the location of the KALIG-1 gene.

**Epidemiology** This disorder affects 1:10,000 males and 1:50,000 females.

**Related Disorders** See *Klinefelter Syndrome; Noonan Syndrome; Turner Syndrome.*

**Treatment—Standard** Treatment with luteinizing hormone-releasing hormone (**LHRH**) is indicated to stimulate secondary sex characteristics and sexual function.

Fertility in both sexes may be obtained with gonadotropin-releasing hormone (**GnRH**) therapy and in some cases a combination of GnRH and spermatogenesis.

The production of sex cells may be achieved with repeated injections of human chorionic gonadotropin (**HCG**) in males, and human menopausal gonadotropin (**HMG**) in females.

Genetic counseling may be of benefit for patients and their families.

Other treatment is symptomatic and supportive.

**Treatment—Investigational** Please contact the agencies listed under Resources, below, for the most current information. Addresses and telephone numbers of these agencies, as well as of individual experts and research centers, may be found in the Master Resources List.

**Resources**

**For more information on Kallmann syndrome:** National Organization for Rare Disorders (NORD); American Cleft Palate Cranial Facial Association; The Arc (a national organization on mental retardation); NIH/National Institute of Child Health and Human Development.

**For genetic information and genetic counseling referrals:** March of Dimes Birth Defects Foundation; Alliance of Genetic Support Groups.

**References**

Cecil Textbook of Medicine, 19th ed.: J.B. Wyngaarden, et al., eds.; W.B. Saunders Company, 1992, pp. 1416–1417.

Birth Defects Encyclopedia: M.L. Buyse, ed.-in-chief; Blackwell Scientific Publications, 1990, p. 1000.

Mendelian Inheritance in Man, 9th ed.: V.A. McKusick, ed.; The Johns Hopkins University Press, 1990, pp. 546, 1283, 1660.

Principles of Neurology, 4th ed.: R.D. Adams and M. Victor, eds.; McGraw-Hill, 1989, p. 185.

Internal Medicine, 2nd ed.: Jay H. Stein, ed.-in-chief; Little, Brown and Company, 1987, pp. 1985–1986.

Ophthalmic Midline Dysgenesis in Kallmann Syndrome: M.J. Jaffe, et al.; Ophthalmic Paediatr. Genet., November 1987, vol. 8(3), pp. 171–174.

# LIPODYSTROPHY

**Description** The lipodystrophies, a cluster of rare inherited or acquired metabolic disorders, are associated with defects in adipose tissue that cause total or partial loss of body fat, irregularities of carbohydrate and lipid metabolism, marked endogenous insulin resistance, and a malfunctioning immune system. Systemic involvement occurs in varying degrees.

The disorders are categorized into 3 forms: **total lipodystrophy** (congenital and acquired forms); **partial lipodystrophy** (acquired and familial forms, and lipoatrophic diabetes mellitus); and **localized lipodystrophy** (including mesenteric, membranous, and centrifugal forms). Categorization is made on the basis of anatomic distribution of the lipodystrophy.

**Synonyms**

Acquired Lipodystrophy

Acquired Partial Lipodystrophy (Cephalothoracic Lipodystrophy)

Barraquer-Simons Disease

Centrifugal Lipodystrophy

Familial Lipodystrophy of Limbs and Lower Trunk (Reverse Partial Lipodystrophy; Kobberling-Dunnigan Syndrome; Lipoatrophic Diabetes Mellitus)

Hollaender-Simons Disease

Insulin Lipodystrophy

Leprechaunism

Membranous Lipodystrophy

Mesenteric Lipodystrophy

Nasu Lipodystrophy

Partial Lipodystrophy

Progressive Lipodystrophy

Seip Syndrome (Berardinelli Syndrome; Congenital Lipoatrophic Diabetes)

Simons Syndrome

Unilateral Partial Lipodystrophy

**Signs and Symptoms Total lipodystrophy,** major body-wide loss of adipose tissue, is associated with abnormal carbohydrate and lipid metabolism.

Congenital total lipodystrophy is characterized by a severe loss of subcutaneous fat in the face, trunk, and limbs. The muscles and bones stand out because of the lack of subcutaneous fat. Acanthosis nigricans may appear in the skin folds, particularly in the axillae, usually at onset of puberty. Hirsutism and skin thickening may occur. Hepatomegaly, mild-to-moderate hypertension, renal disease, and genital hypertrophy are often seen. Mental retardation may occur. Symptoms may be delayed until diabetes mellitus manifests, usually at puberty. Insulin resistance, hyperglycemia, and hypertriglyceridemia are characteristic.

When acquired, total lipodystrophy usually has its onset during childhood or adulthood, with loss of adipose tissue in the same pattern as that of the inherited form. Associated abnormalities are also similar, except that liver involvement may be more severe in acquired total lipodystrophy.

**Partial lipodystrophy** may also be hereditary or acquired. In the inherited form the trunk and limbs are most often the sites of lipoatrophy. The muscle prominence, renal disease, and hepatomegaly of total lipodystrophy are not present. Genital enlargement and a mild acanthosis nigricans may occur. Insulin resistance, hyperglycemia, and hypertriglyceridemia are characteristic. Onset is most often at puberty but may occur in middle age.

The acquired form (cephalothoracic progressive lipodystrophy) is the most frequently encountered type of lipodystrophy. It may often occur after another illness. The face, upper trunk, and upper limbs are affected. Renal disease is moderately severe, and insulin resistance, hyperglycemia, and hypertriglyceridemia are characteristic. Muscle prominence and hypertension are not present. Hepatomegaly, genital hypertrophy, and acanthosis nigricans are rare. Associated abnormalities include central nervous system dysfunction, menstrual disorders, ovarian abnormalities, and hypogonadism. Symptoms include coldness of affected sites, abdominal discomfort, diarrhea, headaches, nervousness, and fatigue.

Lipoatrophic diabetes mellitus, which is linked to partial lipodystrophy, may accompany either the inherited or the acquired form. The familial form is characterized by lipoatrophy of the trunk and limbs, sparing the face and neck. Acanthosis nigricans and genital hypertrophy are commonly present, but hepatic and renal involvement are not. Onset usually is at puberty but may occur in middle age.

The acquired form of lipoatrophic diabetes mellitus may be generalized as well as partial. Acanthosis nigricans, hyperlipidemia, and hepatosplenomegaly are present. Consequently, lipoatrophic diabetes mellitus may be mistaken for total lipodystrophy if the pattern of lost fat tissue is generalized. Acquired lipoatrophic diabetes mellitus may occur in childhood or early adulthood; as a rule, it begins during adolescence or in the early adult years.

Partial lipodystrophy associated with developmental abnormalities is hereditary. The areas involved are the face and buttocks. A nonprogressive disease with onset during infancy or early childhood, its characteristics are visual problems **(Rieger anomaly),** short stature, underdevelopment of the midface, hypotrichosis, and insulin-dependent diabetes. Dental malformations are also present.

**Localized lipodystrophies** have readily identifiable hallmarks: multiple lesions that are small, well-defined atrophic areas. A frequent association is lymphocytic panniculitis. The disorder may occur in various forms, including mesenteric, membranous, and centrifugal lipodystrophy.

Mesenteric lipodystrophy is characterized by small intestinal adipose tissue.

Membranous lipodystrophy is characterized by bilateral multiple cystic bone lesions that precede neuropsychiatric symptoms, including dementia, seizures, and ataxia. Additionally, the ocular lens may be affected.

Centrifugal lipodystrophy is a rare localized disorder identified by a small indentation in the skin that enlarges to become a circle. Severe atrophied subcutaneous adipose tissue causes the depression in the skin.

**Etiology** Congenital total lipodystrophy is inherited as an autosomal recessive trait; the acquired form is sporadic.

Acquired partial lipodystrophy is usually sporadic. The inherited form is autosomal dominant, although X-linked dominant inheritance has been reported.

Localized lipodystrophy may or may not be associated with an inflammatory mechanism. Forms may also occur secondary to events such as insulin injection and diphtheria/pertussis/tetanus **(DPT)** vaccine.

**Epidemiology** Males and females are equally affected in congenital total lipodystrophy; in the other forms, females are affected more often than males.

**Related Disorders** See *Adrenal Hyperplasia, Congenital; Cushing Syndrome; Diencephalic Syndrome.*

**Treatment—Standard** No drugs are specific for the lipodystrophies. Extended courses of pimozide, a dopamine receptor–blocking drug, have been ineffective. Diet has some benefit in metabolic disorders; small frequent feedings and partial substitution of medium-chain triglycerides for polyunsaturated fats appear practical. Implants of monolithic silicon rubber as replacement of lost soft facial tissue have been successful. Dentures may be cosmetically beneficial for some patients. Long-term treatment is usually confined to associated systemic disorders, such as renal or endocrine dysfunction.

For the patient with a genetic form of lipodystrophy, genetic counseling is recommended. Other treatment is symptomatic and supportive.

**Treatment—Investigational** Late stages of some cases of lipodystrophy with severe renal disease may necessitate a transplant. This experimental procedure is recommended only in patients who are refractory to more conventional treatment.

Abhimanyu Garg, M.D., at the University of Texas Southwestern Medical Center, is studying pathogenic mechanisms and genetic defects associated with the lipodystrophies.

Please contact the agencies listed under Resources, below, for the most current information. Addresses and telephone numbers of these agencies, as well as of individual experts and research centers, may be found in the Master Resources List.

**Resources**

**For more information on lipodystrophy:** National Organization for Rare Disorders (NORD); National Lipid Diseases Foundation; NIH/National Digestive Diseases Information Clearinghouse; American Diabetes Association; The Arc (a national organization on mental retardation); Research Trust for Metabolic Diseases in Children; International Tremor Foundation.

**For genetic information and genetic counseling referrals:** March of Dimes Birth Defects Foundation; Alliance of Genetic Support Groups.

### References

Mendelian Inheritance in Man, 9th ed.: V.A. McKusick; The Johns Hopkins University Press, 1990, pp. 574–575, 1475, 1662.

Familial Partial Lipodystrophy: Two Types of an X-Linked Dominant Syndrome, Lethal in the Hemizygous State: J. Kobberling, et al.; J. Med. Genet., vol. 23(2), pp. 120–127.

Lipolysis: Pitfalls and Problems in a Series of 1,246 Procedures: S. Cohen; Aesthetic Plast. Surg., vol. 9(3), pp. 209–214.

Membranous Lipodystrophy (Nasu Disease): Clinical and Neuropathological Study of a Case: M. Minagawa, et al.; Clin. Neuropathol., vol. 4(1), pp. 38–45.

Ultrastructural Abnormalities of the Liver in Total Lipodystrophy: A. Klar, et al.; Arch. Pathol. Lab. Med., vol. 111(2), pp. 197–199.

# McCune-Albright Syndrome

**Description** McCune-Albright syndrome is a multisystem disorder in which there is polyostotic fibrous dysplasia.

**Synonyms**

> Albright Syndrome
> Fibrous Dysplasia, Monostotic
> Fibrous Dysplasia, Polyostotic
> Fuller-Albright Syndrome
> Osteitis Fibrosa Disseminata
> Precocious Puberty with Polyostotic Fibrous Dysplasia and Abnormal Pigmentation

**Signs and Symptoms** Infants present characteristic skin pigmentations. Abnormal growth of fibrous bone tissue may be increasingly painful and crippling. Any bone may be invaded, but the lesions most often occur in the extremities, pelvis, ribs, and the base of the skull. The patient is fracture-prone. Shortening of the limbs and other osseous deformities may develop. Patchy pigmentation with large, irregular café au lait spots may appear. Premature puberty may manifest as early as age 3 months and is more common in females than males. While menses occur early, it may be years before the breasts develop and axillary hair appears. Fertility in young patients is very rare, but in adults with McCune-Albright syndrome it is normal. Acromegaly or gigantism may result from pituitary hypersecretion of growth hormone **(GH).** Pituitary hyperfunction may coincide with Cushing syndrome. Hyperthyroidism, hypercorticism, and pheochromocytoma may also occur.

**Etiology** McCune-Albright syndrome is typically caused by mutations in the guanine nucleotide-binding protein gene **(GNAS1).** Symptoms vary because of postzygotic somatic cell mutation mosaicism. GNAS1 is located at chromosome 20q13.2–13.3

**Albright hereditary osteodystrophy** and some hormone-secreting tumors may be the result of mutations of this gene. Accelerated ovarian function due to hyperthyroidism or premature activation of the hypothalamic-pituitary-ovarian axis may explain the early puberty in females with the syndrome.

**Epidemiology** McCune-Albright syndrome affects more females than males at a ratio of 3:2. Approximately 50 percent of patients, usually females, experience early puberty. Hundreds of cases have been described in the medical literature in the United States since Albright first recognized the disorder in 1937.

**Related Disorders** See *Acromegaly; Cushing Syndrome; Neurofibromatosis.*

**Gigantism,** also caused by hypersecretion of GH, occurs before puberty. It is associated with enlarged soft tissues and late epiphyseal closure, which produces excessive growth during childhood; height may reach 7 or 8 feet. Onset of hypopituitarism later in the course may result in myopathy and hypogonadism. Sexual development may be normal, or it may be affected by associated hypogonadism. In some cases peripheral neuropathy may develop.

**Treatment—Standard** X-rays reveal areas of fibrous growth that replace normal bone tissue. Blood tests reveal elevated levels of serum alkaline phosphatase. Treatment is symptomatic and supportive. Depending on age, severity of symptoms, and size of the lesion, orthopedic procedures may be indicated. Calcitonin may be effective in treating chronic bone pain and high levels of serum alkaline phosphatase. In some severe cases, radioiodine ablation or thyroidectomy may be indicated to control persistent hyperthyroidism. LHRH analogues may be helpful in cases of precocious puberty, especially for females.

**Treatment—Investigational** Trials of the aromatase inhibitor testolactone, which blocks the synthesis of estrogens, are ongoing in the treatment of premature puberty in females with McCune-Albright syndrome. Cortical bone grafting has been investigated for treating fibrous dysplasia.

Please contact the agencies listed under Resources, below, for the most current information. Addresses and telephone numbers of these agencies, as well as of individual experts and research centers, may be found in the Master Resources List.

**Resources**

**For more information on McCune-Albright syndrome:** National Organization for Rare Disorders (NORD);

NIH/National Arthritis and Musculoskeletal and Skin Diseases Information Clearinghouse; International Center for Skeletal Dysplasia; McCune-Albright Syndrome Division of The Magic Foundation.

**For genetic information and genetic counseling referrals:** March of Dimes Birth Defects Foundation; Alliance of Genetic Support Groups.

### References

Mendelian Inheritance in Man, 10th ed.: V.A. McKusick; The Johns Hopkins University Press, 1992, pp. 449–450.

Nelson Textbook of Pediatrics, 14th ed.: R.E. Behrman, ed.-in-chief; W.B. Saunders Company, 1992, pp. 1411–1412.

Textbook of Endocrinology, 8th ed.: J.D. Wilson and D.W. Foster, eds.; W.B. Saunders Company, 1992, pp. 1200–1203, 1510.

Activating Mutations of the Stimulatory G Protein in the McCune-Albright Syndrome: L.S. Weinstein, et al.; N. Engl. J. Med., December 12, 1991, vol. 325(24), pp. 1688–1695.

Harrison's Principles of Internal Medicine, 12th ed.: J.D. Wilson, et al.; McGraw-Hill, 1991, pp. 1945–1947.

The McCune-Albright Syndrome: The Whys and Wherefores of Abnormal Signal Transduction: M. A. Levine; N. Engl. J. Med., December 12, 1991, vol. 325(24), pp. 1688–1695.

Birth Defects Encyclopedia: M.L. Buyse, ed.-in-chief; Blackwell Scientific Publications, 1990, pp. 739–740.

Cecil Textbook of Medicine, 19th ed.: J.B. Wyngaarden, et al., eds.; W.B. Saunders Company, 1992, pp. 1358, 1388, 1435.

Dictionary of Medical Syndromes, 3rd ed.: S.I. Magalini, et al., eds.; J.B. Lippincott Company, 1990, pp. 558–559.

Smith's Recognizable Patterns of Human Malformation, 4th ed.: K.L. Jones; W.B. Saunders Company, 1988, p. 454.

Neurofibromatosis and Albright's Syndrome: V.M. Ricciardi; Dermatol. Clin., January 1987, vol. 5(1), pp. 193–203.

Fibrous Dysplasia of the Femoral Neck. Treatment by Cortical Bone Grafting: W.F. Enneking, et al.; J. Bone Joint Surg. Am., December 1986, vol. 68(9), pp. 1415–1422.

Treatment of Precocious Puberty in the McCune-Albright Syndrome with the Aromatase Inhibitor Testolactone: J.D. Malley, et al.; N. Engl. J. Med., October 1986, vol. 315(18), pp. 1115–1119.

# NELSON SYNDROME

**Description** Nelson syndrome is marked by abnormal hormone secretion and an enlarged pituitary gland.

**Synonyms**

Pituitary Tumor After Adrenalectomy

**Signs and Symptoms** Symptoms are hyperpigmentation, headaches, visual field disturbances, and, in females, amenorrhea. The pituitary gland is enlarged, leading to the headaches and visual symptoms. Laboratory tests reveal elevated levels of ACTH and β-melanocyte–stimulating hormone (**β-MSH**).

**Etiology** Nelson syndrome can develop following bilateral adrenalectomy as treatment for Cushing syndrome. Growth of a preexisting or an occult pituitary tumor may also be responsible.

**Epidemiology** Nelson syndrome occurs in approximately 5 to 10 percent of patients following bilateral adrenalectomy. In contrast, tumor-induced Nelson syndrome is rare. Males and females are affected in equal numbers.

**Treatment—Standard** Irradiation is used to impair abnormal pituitary growth. If the gland presses on an adjacent area of brain and is symptomatic, surgical removal is indicated. Microsurgical removal of ACTH adenomas, using the transphenoidal approach, is an appropriate treatment for Nelson syndrome.

**Treatment—Investigational** One study found that bromocriptine (a dopamine agonist) and cyproheptadine (a serotonin antagonist) caused a significant drop in plasma ACTH levels stimulated by corticotropin-releasing factor (**CRF**). After a longer course of cyproheptadine, however, plasma ACTH levels were again elevated. Consequently, the usefulness of the drug appears limited.

Please contact the agencies listed under Resources, below, for the most current information. Addresses and telephone numbers of these agencies, as well as of individual experts and research centers, may be found in the Master Resources List.

**Resources**

**For more information on Nelson syndrome:** National Organization for Rare Disorders (NORD); NIH/National Institute of Neurological Disorders and Stroke.

### References

Trans-Sphenoidal Microsurgical Treatment of Nelson's Syndrome: T. Fukushima; Neurosurg. Rev., 1985, vol. 8(3–4), pp. 185–194.

Effects of Bromocriptine and Cyproheptadine on Basal and Corticotropin-Releasing Factor (CRF)-Induced ACTH Release in a Patient with Nelson's Syndrome: Y. Hirata, et al.; Endocrinol. Jpn., October 1984, vol. 31(5), pp. 619–626.

# PRECOCIOUS PUBERTY

**Description** True precocious puberty is the result of premature initiation of the function of the hypothalamic-pituitary axis. Premature release of the luteinizing hormone-releasing hormone (**LHRH**) by the hypothalamus triggers secretion of the pituitary gonadatropin hormones. As a consequence, the gonads function at an inappropriately early age. Precocious puberty per se has many subdivisions: isosexual, heterosexual, gonadotropin-dependent (true precocious puberty), gonadotropin-independent, male-limited (familial testotoxicosis), cerebral, central, and idiopathic.

## Synonyms

 Familial Testotoxicosis
 Gonadotropin-Independent Familial Sexual Precocity
 Pubertas Praecox

**Signs and Symptoms** In females the breasts start to develop before age 8, or menarche occurs before age 10, and growth is rapid. In males, onset as manifest by testicular enlargement is before age 10; boys grow facial, axillary, and pubic hair; growth, including that of the penis, accelerates; the voice deepens; and behavior becomes aggressive. Puberty may take place before age 3 in some children.

Children with precocious puberty are taller than their peers. Since osseous maturity is usually hastened in precocious puberty, closure of the epiphyses occurs prematurely and patients may be short in stature in adulthood.

In **isosexual precocious puberty,** feminizing signs appear in girls, masculinization in boys.

**Heterosexual precocious puberty** causes signs of virilization in girls and feminization in boys.

**Cerebral precocious puberty** differs in cause but mimics true precocious puberty.

**Central precocious puberty** is attended by changes that concern the central nervous system.

**Gonadotropin-dependent precocious puberty** is marked by high gonadotropin levels in girls. Girls with McCune-Albright syndrome may have this type of precocious puberty.

**Gonadotropin-independent precocious puberty** usually affects boys who have low levels of gonadotropin. Girls with McCune-Albright syndrome may have this form of precocious puberty.

**Idiopathic precocious puberty** is associated with EEG irregularities in girls. The cause of the unusual brain waves is unclear.

**Etiology** Usually precocious puberty is idiopathic. In some instances, it is due to an endocrine disorder. **Cerebral precocious puberty** is associated with a brain abnormality. **Male-limited precocious puberty (familial testotoxicosis)** has been demonstrated to be caused by a gain of function mutation of LHRH. This results in hypersensitivity to circulating levels of LH. This is a sex-limited dominant trait.

Among the uncommon underlying disorders in girls are hypothalamic neoplasm, neurofibromatosis, congenital brain lesions, postinfectious encephalitis, hydrocephalus, and craniopharyngiomas. Very rare causes are oral contraceptives, other estrogen-containing drugs, or meat with a high estrogen content. Primary hypothyroidism and McCune-Albright syndrome often accompany precocious puberty.

Other considerations are hormone-secreting ovarian or adrenal neoplasms. Possibly the most frequently seen sex steroid-secreting tumors among girls with precocious puberty are estrogen-secreting ovarian granulosa-thecal cell tumors. Some girls may have benign ovarian cysts.

**Epidemiology** The incidence of precocious puberty in girls is approximately twice that in boys. Approximately 80 percent of the cases in girls are idiopathic, but disease underlies 60 percent of the cases in boys.

**Related Disorders** See *McCune-Albright Syndrome; Adrenal Hyperplasia, Congenital; Neurofibromatosis.*

**Pseudo-precocious puberty** is associated with high steroid concentrations. Such levels are present because of cortocosteroid therapy, hormone-producing tumors (usually ovarian or testicular), or adrenal disorders that cause hormonal hypersecretion. Sexual development and maturity may appear normal, but ovulation or spermatogenesis may not occur because of gonadal immaturity.

**Adrenogenital syndrome** comprises a group of conditions due to adrenocortical hyperplasia or glandular malignancy. Virilization of women or precocious puberty in boys are hallmarks. Hypersecretion of adrenocortical androgenic steroids is present.

**Treatment—Standard** Therapy depends upon the cause of precocious puberty. Glucocorticoid suppression of ACTH is indicated for girls with **heterosexual precocious puberty** due to congenital adrenal hyperplasia. Girls with **precocious puberty** and **McCune-Albright syndrome** respond to the aromatase-inhibitor testolactone, a blocker of estrogen synthesis. Some hypothalamic lesions and ovarian tumors or cysts can be excised. Once identified, exogenous hormones can be eliminated. Replacement therapy with levothyroxine is indicated for girls with **precocious puberty caused by primary hypothyroidism,** in whom closure of the epiphyses is late.

The orphan drug Supprelin (histrelin acetate), manufactured by Ortho, has been approved for treatment of precocious puberty. It minimizes sex changes in boys and girls and slows accelerated bone maturation. It is given once a day subcutaneously. The orphan drug leuprolide acetate (Lupron Injection), manufactured by Tap Pharmaceuticals, has been approved for treatment of central precocious puberty.

**Male-limited precocious puberty** has been treated with ketoconizole. Genetic counseling is recommended for families of patients with male-limited precocious puberty and other hereditary types of this disorder.

**Treatment—Investigational** A course of at least 6 months of a combination of spironolactone and testolactone has been used experimentally in males with **isosexual precocious puberty.** These patients have abnormally rapid growth, and the goal of drug therapy is to restore the rates of growth and maturation to normal prepubertal levels.

For girls with **gonadotropin-dependent precocious puberty,** intranasal administration of the hormone-suppressing drug nafarelin acetate may be useful.

For children with **central precocious puberty,** an orphan drug, deslorelin (Somagard), manufactured by Roberts Laboratories, is available.

Please contact the agencies listed under Resources, below, for the most current information. Addresses and telephone numbers of these agencies, as well as of individual experts and research centers, may be found in the Master Resources List.

**Resources**

**For more information on precocious puberty:** National Organization for Rare Disorders (NORD); National Adrenal Diseases Foundation; NIH/National Institute of Child Health and Human Development; Brain and Pituitary Foundation of America.

**For genetic information and genetic counseling referrals:** March of Dimes Birth Defects Foundation; Alliance of Genetic Support Groups.

**References**

The Treatment of Familial Male Precocious Puberty with Spironolactone and Testolactone: L. Laue, et al.; N. Engl. J. Med., February 23, 1989, vol. 320(8), pp. 496–502.

CT of Cerebral Abnormalities in Precocious Puberty: K.G. Rieth, et al.; AJR, June 1987, vol. 148(6), pp. 1231–1238.

Intranasal Nafarelin: An LH-RH Analogue Treatment of Gonadotropin-Precocious Puberty: T.H. Lin, et al.; J. Pediatr., December 1986, vol. 109(6), pp. 954–958.

Treatment of Precocious Puberty in the McCune-Albright Syndrome with the Aromatase Inhibitor Testolactone: P.P. Feuillan, et al.; N. Engl. J. Med., October 30, 1986, vol. 315(18), pp. 1115–1119.

# REIFENSTEIN SYNDROME

**Description** Reifenstein syndrome (partial androgen insensitivity) is a hereditary form of male pseudohermaphroditism.

**Synonyms**

Androgen Insensitivity Syndrome, Partial
Familial Incomplete Male Pseudohermaphroditism, Type I
Gilbert-Dreyfus Syndrome
Incomplete Testicular Feminization
Lubs Syndrome
Rosewater Syndrome

**Signs and Symptoms** Genetically the patient is male and has testicular tissue, but the external genitalia are ambiguous. The severity of androgen insensitivity determines how this syndrome presents itself. In the least severe cases, the only symptom may be few or no sperm. More severe cases may result in hypogonadism, hypospadias, seminiferous tubular sclerosis, cryptorchidism, and gynecomastia. Leydig cell hyperplasia may lead to impotence later in life. The degree of feminization at puberty is not as marked as in other forms of pseudohermaphroditism. Facial and chest hair may be sparse or missing, and the voice may have a high pitch.

**Etiology** Reifenstein syndrome is inherited as an X-linked recessive disorder. The weight of evidence suggests that this disorder is a result of mutations in the androgen receptor **(AR)** gene.

**Epidemiology** The disorder occurs only in males, but females are carriers. There have been many reports of multiple males in a family inheriting the syndrome.

**Related Disorders** See *Klinefelter Syndrome.*

**Male pseudohermaphroditism** is a genetic disorder in which the individual has testes but possesses both female and male sexual characteristics. If never treated, the body type is usually female and the male characteristics are not apparent until puberty.

**17-β-Hydroxysteroid dehydrogenase deficiency** (also known as **17-ketosteroid reductase deficiency**) is inherited as either an autosomal recessive or X-linked recessive gene and causes impairment in the production of steroids. Male pseudohermaphroditism is present, and there is no enlargement of the adrenal gland.

**17-α-Hydroxylase deficiency** (also known as **17-hydroxylation deficiency**) usually goes undetected until adolescence. The adrenal gland and testes fail to produce androgens, while the ovaries produce no estrogens. Because males are not exposed to androgens during fetal development, they are born with female external genitalia, although testes are buried within the abdominal cavity. Characteristic are hypertension, hypokalemia, and failure to menstruate or to develop such secondary sexual traits as breasts or body hair.

**3-β-Hydroxysteroid dehydrogenase deficiency** occurs early in the chain of reactions required to produce adrenal corticosteroids. Androgens, glucocorticoids, and mineralocorticoids fail to synthesize, and untreated infants with the complete defect usually survive no more than a few hours. Boys are born with female or ambiguous external genitalia. Virilization of females is not as noticeable or does not occur at all. A few patients with incomplete forms of this disorder are not symptomatic until later in childhood or until adulthood; females may have mild clitoromegaly, acne, hirsutism, and advanced maturation of the skeleton.

**Treatment—Standard** Patients with more severe defects and every male with androgen unresponsiveness should be raised as females, undergo corrective surgery prepubertally, and use estrogen therapy at puberty.

Genetic counseling may be of benefit for patients and their families.

**Treatment—Investigational** Please contact the agencies listed under Resources, below, for the most current information. Addresses and telephone numbers of these agencies, as well as of individual experts and research centers, may be found in the Master Resources List.

**Resources**

**For more information on Reifenstein syndrome:** National Organization for Rare Disorders (NORD); John Mahoney, M.D., Johns Hopkins University; NIH/National Institute of Child Health and Human Development; Finding Our Own Ways.

**For genetic information and genetic counseling referrals:** March of Dimes Birth Defects Foundation; Alliance of Genetic Support Groups.

**References**

The Metabolic Basis of Inherited Disease, 6th ed.: C.R. Scriver, et al., eds.; McGraw Hill, 1989, pp. 1931–1932.

Cecil Textbook of Medicine, 18th ed.: J.B. Wyngaarden and L.H. Smith, Jr., eds.; W.B. Saunders Company, 1988, pp. 1399–1400, 1418.

Clinical and Endocrinological Characterization of Two Subjects with Reifenstein Syndrome Associated with Qualitative Abnormalities of the Androgen Receptor: H.U. Schweikert, et al.; Human Res., 1987, vol. 25(2), pp. 72–79.

Mendelian Inheritance in Man, 8th ed.: V.A. McKusick; The Johns Hopkins University Press, 1986, p. 1711.

# RICKETS, VITAMIN D–DEFICIENCY

**Description** Vitamin D–deficiency rickets, which appears during infancy and childhood, is characterized primarily by bone disease and retarded growth. Vitamin D is needed for the metabolism of calcium and phosphorus and deposition of calcium and phosphate in the bone matrix.

**Synonyms**

Nutritional Rickets

Rickets

**Signs and Symptoms** Symptoms include restlessness and lack of sleep. Growth is slowed, and there is a delay in crawling, sitting, or walking. The skull is thin at the top and back (craniotabes); there is bossing; and fontanelle closure is delayed. Beading occurs where the ribs and their cartilages join (rachitic rosary).

If the disorder is not treated, the ends of the long bones may become enlarged and the legs may become bowed. Muscles can become weak and the chest may become deformed because of the pull of the diaphragm on the ribs weakened by rickets (Harrison groove). Abnormal development and decay of teeth may also occur.

In more severe, untreated cases of this disorder, the bones may become fragile, and fractures easily occur. Convulsions, muscle twitching, and tetany spasms of the wrist and ankle joints may also be present. Occasionally, when recurrent, severe hypocalcemia is present because of the lack of vitamin D, mental retardation may develop.

**Etiology** The vitamin deficiency can be caused by poor nutrition, a lack of exposure to the sun, or intestinal malabsorption syndromes.

**Epidemiology** Males and females are affected in equal numbers. Babies of nursing mothers themselves deficient in vitamin D can be affected.

The disorder is rare in the United States but not uncommon in certain areas of the world. However, in the United States, children who are dark-skinned and living in cloudy northern cities, as well as children on restricted diets due to cultural or religious beliefs, are more likely to develop vitamin D–deficiency rickets.

In areas of the world where cultural habits curtail exposure to sun, or the amount of sun in a day or season is otherwise limited, the disorder tends to be more prevalent. Northern Yemen and Kuwait are areas of prevalence. Rickets is also more common in regions of Asia where there is not only limited exposure to the sun, but also low intake of meat due to a vegetarian diet.

**Related Disorders** See *Lowe Syndrome; Rickets, Hypophosphatemic.*

**Fanconi syndrome** is a rare disorder characterized by kidney dysfunction and bone abnormalities similar to those of vitamin D–deficiency rickets. Excess amounts of phosphate, amino acids (usually bicarbonate), glucose, and uric acid are eliminated in the urine. Bone symptoms include rickets in children and osteomalacia in adults. Fanconi syndrome is thought to be inherited through recessive genes. The syndrome may be associated with a variety of inherited metabolic disorders (see *Cystinosis; Fructose Intolerance, Hereditary; Galactosemia; Tyrosinemia I; Wilson Disease*). Glycogen storage disorders are also associated.

**Infantile scurvy** is caused by a lack of vitamin C in the diet. Symptoms include anemia, irritability, anorexia, weakness, failure to gain weight, oral lesions, loosening of the teeth, and bleeding under the tissue layer covering the bones. Scurvy is treated with large amounts of vitamin C.

**Osteomalacia** is the adult presentation of rickets and is characterized by a gradual softening and bending of the bones. Pain may be present in varying degrees of severity. Softening occurs because solid bones have failed to calcify as a result of a kidney dysfunction or the lack of vitamin D. The disorder is more common in females than males, and often begins during pregnancy. It can exist alone or in association with other disorders.

**Pseudo–vitamin D–deficiency rickets (vitamin D–dependent rickets, type I)** is characterized by more severe skeletal changes and weakness than those of hypophosphatemic rickets. The disorder is inherited as an autosomal recessive trait and is caused by impaired 1-hydroxylation of 25-hydroxy vitamin D. This type of rickets often begins earlier than hypophosphatemic rickets. Hypocalcemia is severe, and there is aminoaciduria. Intermittent muscle cramps and convulsions may occur. Abnormalities of the spine and pelvis may also develop. **Type II** is an unknown, postreceptor abnormality of 1,25-dihydroxy vitamin D.

**Treatment—Standard** The disorder can be prevented by providing a normal balanced diet to infants and children, assuming that they are exposed to adequate amounts of sun.

Treatment is accomplished with doses of vitamin D given daily until the bone disease is cured. The dose can then be reduced to the daily recommended requirement.

In more severe cases when cramps, convulsions, muscle twitching, and tetany of the ankle and wrist joints are present, treatment with vitamin D is supplemented with intravenous calcium salts.

**Treatment—Investigational** Please contact the agencies listed under Resources, below, for the most current information. Addresses and telephone numbers of these agencies, as well as of individual experts and research centers, may be found in the Master Resources List.

**Resources**

**For more information on vitamin D–deficiency rickets:** National Organization for Rare Disorders (NORD); NIH/National Institute Digestive Diseases Information Clearinghouse.

**References**

Internal Medicine, 2nd ed.: J.H. Stein, ed.-in-chief; Little, Brown and Company, 1987, pp. 2106–2112.

Nutritional Rickets: K.W. Feldman, et al.; Am. Fam. Physicians, November 1990, vol. 42(5), pp. 1311–1318.

High Prevalence of Rickets in Infants on Macrobiotic Diets: P.C. Dagnelie, et al.; Am. J. Clin. Nutr., February 1990, vol. 51(2), pp. 202–208.

Nutritional Rickets in San Diego: I. Hayward, et al.; Am. J. Dis. Child, October 1987, vol. 141(10), pp. 1060–1062.

Vitamin D Deficiency Rickets: D.M. Kruger, et al.; Clin. Orthop., November 1987, vol. 224, pp. 277–283.

Photosynthesis of Vitamin D in the Skin: Effect of Environmental and Lifestyle Variables: M.F. Holick; Fed. Proc., April 1987, vol. 46(5), pp. 1876–1882.

The Importance of Limited Exposure to Ultraviolet Radiation and Dietary Factors in the Etiology of Asian Rickets: A Risk-Factor Model: J.B. Henderson, et al.; Q. J. Med., May 1987, vol. 63(241), pp. 413–425.

High Levels of Childhood Rickets in Rural North Yemen: P. Underwood, et al.; Soc. Sci. Med., 1987, vol. 24(1), pp. 37–41.

Vitamin D–Deficiency Rickets in Kuwait: The Prevalence of a Preventable Disease: M.M. Lubani, et al.; Ann. Trop. Paediatr., September 1989, vol. 9(3), pp. 134–139.

Osteomalacia of the Mother: Rickets of the Newborn: W. Park, et al.; Eur. J. Pediatr., May 1987, vol. 146(3), pp. 292–293.

# SCHMIDT SYNDROME

**Description** Schmidt syndrome is defined as the association of Addison disease and primary hypothyroidism. Other endocrine and non-endocrine deficiencies may occur, such as insulin-dependent diabetes mellitus and failure of the gonads, parathyroids, and autoimmune-type abnormalities. Most cases are sporadic. Increased risk for autoimmune disease is known, but the inheritance is uncertain.

**Synonyms**

Multiple Endocrine Deficiency Syndrome, Type II

**Signs and Symptoms** Symptoms of Schmidt syndrome are *Addison Disease* and primary hypothyroidism.

Because of the varied manifestations associated with glandular deficiencies, there are many signs and symptoms of Schmidt syndrome, in addition to Addison disease and primary hypothyroidism: chronic candidiasis of mucosal surfaces, skin, and nails; thymoma; thymic dysplasia; hyperthyroidism; diabetes mellitus type I; adrenal failure; pernicious anemia; cataracts; keratoconjunctivitis; band keratopathy; pancreatic insufficiency; chronic hepatitis; vitiligo; cirrhosis; and alopecia.

Gonadal failure causes an absence of secondary sex characteristics or regression of preexisting secondary sex characteristics in association with elevated gonadotropins.

**Etiology** Schmidt syndrome is idiopathic. An autoimmune basis has been demonstrated, and it has been found to be familial in some cases. It may be inherited as an autosomal dominant or autosomal recessive trait.

**Epidemiology** Schmidt syndrome affects females approximately 4 times more than males. This disorder usually becomes apparent at about age 30.

**Related Disorders** See *APECED Syndrome.*

**Treatment—Standard** Each disorder in Schmidt syndrome is treated separately.

**Diabetes mellitus** is treated with daily insulin injections, a controlled diet, exercise to burn off glucose, and testing for blood sugar level. Urine testing for ketonuria is recommended during illness, and blood for hemoglobin A1 or A1C is tested quarterly to assess glucose control.

**Hypothyroidism** is treated with levothyroxine, a synthetic thyroid hormone. Thyroid function is monitored annually to ensure adequacy of therapy.

**Hypoadrenalism** is treated with replacement cortisol and Florinef (9-α-fludrocortisone).

**Pernicious anemia** is treated with vitamin B12.

**Gonadal failure** is treated with hormones.

Genetic counseling may be of benefit for patients and their families who have the inherited form of Schmidt syndrome.

**Treatment—Investigational** Genetic factors have been shown to be associated with diabetes, which could lead to prevention of the disorder in genetically susceptible persons. In related studies, insulin-producing beta cells were infected and destroyed by common viruses, the preface to vaccine development. Pancreas transplantation has had limited success, primarily due to problems with rejection. Insulin pumps for unstable diabetes have been successful for many patients.

Please contact the agencies listed under Resources, below, for the most current information. Addresses and telephone numbers of these agencies, as well as of individual experts and research centers, may be found in the Master Resources List.

**Resources**

**For more information on Schmidt syndrome:** National Organization for Rare Disorders (NORD); National Adrenal Diseases Foundation; Thyroid Foundation of America; American Diabetes Association; Juvenile Diabetes Foundation International; National Foundation for Vitiligo and Pigment Disorders; Celiac Sprue Association/USA; Myasthenia Gravis Foundation; NIH/National Digestive Diseases Information Clearinghouse.

**For genetic information and genetic counseling referrals:** March of Dimes Birth Defects Foundation; Alliance of Genetic Support Groups.

**References**

Cecil Textbook of Medicine, 19th ed.: J.B. Wyngaarden, et al., eds.; W.B. Saunders Company, 1992, pp. 1460–1461.

Mendelian Inheritance in Man, 9th ed.: V.A. McKusick, ed.; The Johns Hopkins University Press, 1990, p. 1472.

Schmidt Syndrome: A Rare Case of Puberty Menorrhagia: J.B. Sharma, et al.; Int. J. Gynaecol., December 1990, vol. 33(4), pp. 373–375.

Myasthenia Gravis and Schmidt Syndrome: J.K. McAlpine, et al.; Postgrad. Med. J., October 1988, vol. 64(756), pp. 787–788.

# SHEEHAN SYNDROME

**Description** Sheehan syndrome is characterized by hypopituitarism associated with profound blood loss during and after childbirth, and consequent postpartum collapse.

**Synonyms**

> Postpartum Hypopituitarism
> Postpartum Panhypopituitarism
> Postpartum Pituitary Necrosis
> Simmond Disease

**Signs and Symptoms** The varying manifestations of Sheehan syndrome depend on the degree of hypopituitarism. The signs and symptoms correlate with the extent of the deficiency of prolactin, gonadotropins, thyroid-stimulating hormone **(TSH),** adrenocorticotropin **(ACTH),** and growth hormone **(GH).**

The full-blown condition is associated with evidence of deficient gonadotropins: postpartum failure of lactation, amenorrhea, absence of regrowth of pubic hair, and slowly vanishing axillary hair. Breasts and genitalia atrophy.

The hallmarks of hypothyroidism, triggered by deficient TSH, usually appear gradually; myxedema, for example, may not become apparent for years or decades.

Hypoglycemia may develop in association with GH and ACTH deficiency, causing a lack of cortisol; GH deficiency is associated with increased insulin sensitivity, some loss of muscle strength, and mild anemia.

ACTH deficiency's manifestations are chronic hypotension with fainting and proneness to infection, even from cuts and abrasions. These features usually become apparent weeks or months postpartum.

**Etiology** Severe arteriolar spasm in the vessels supplying the hypothalamus, occurring in shock, is considered to be the cause of Sheehan syndrome. Spasm leads to anterior pituitary ischemia. The amount of cellular damage correlates with the severity and duration of arteriolar spasm.

**Epidemiology** Sheehan syndrome affects women with postpartum hemorrhage and circulatory collapse.

**Treatment—Standard** Hormonal replacement therapy (i.e., ovarian, thyroid, and adrenocortical hormones) is indicated. Mild, partial ACTH deficiency may not require continuing cortisol replacement therapy except as emergency therapy during times of stress.

**Treatment—Investigational** Please contact the agencies listed under Resources, below, for the most current information. Addresses and telephone numbers of these agencies, as well as of individual experts and research centers, may be found in the Master Resources List.

**Resources**

**For more information on Sheehan syndrome:** National Organization for Rare Disorders (NORD); NIH/National Digestive Diseases Information Clearinghouse.

# STEIN-LEVENTHAL SYNDROME

**Description** Stein-Leventhal syndrome is characterized by amenorrhea or abnormal menses, hirsutism, obesity, and infertility.

**Synonyms**

> Bilateral Polycystic Ovarian Syndrome
> Ovarian Hyperthecosis
> Polycystic Bilateral Ovarian Syndrome
> Sclerocystic Ovarian Disease

**Signs and Symptoms** Initial symptoms usually occur soon after puberty and before age 20. If the menses have been normal, they become irregular and gradually lessen over several months until they stop. Sometimes heavy flow intervenes during stretches of amenorrhea.

Infertility or the growth of facial hair often brings the patient to the physician's office. Signs of virilization include voice changes and male-pattern hirsutism. Obesity is often present. The ovaries become polycystic and may increase in size. Frequently the uterus is undersized. The patient is anovulatory.

**Etiology** The cause of Stein-Leventhal syndrome is unclear. It is often inherited as an autosomal dominant genetic trait. Some women may have a genetic predisposition to the disorder. The susceptibility gene is located on chromosome 6 (human leukocyte antigen **[HLA]**). Generally, the irregularities are attributed to the hypothalamic-pituitary-ovarian axis. Occasionally, an androgen-producing ovarian tumor is responsible.

**Epidemiology** Stein-Leventhal syndrome occurs in young women.

**Related Disorders** See *Primary Amenorrhea; Ahumada–del Castillo Syndrome; Forbes-Albright Syndrome.*

**Mullerian aplasia** is characterized by the absence at birth of the uterus and vagina in a female with normal ovarian function and normal external genitalia. Secondary sexual characteristics are normal. The initial symptom is usually amenorrhea.

**Treatment—Standard** Diagnosis of Stein-Leventhal syndrome is confirmed by amenorrhea and the presence of high levels of testosterone in the blood. For the woman who desires pregnancy, clomiphene will often produce ovulation and normal menstruation. Pregnancy occurs in about 50 percent of treated patients. If clomiphene does not produce the desired effects, human chorionic gonadotropin accompanied by follicle-stimulating hormone (**FSH**) is a 2nd choice. If neither treatment is effective, ovarian wedge resection, or removal of the cystic portions of the ovaries, can be performed. Recurrence is common, however.

Treatment with low-dosage oral contraceptives or long-acting progestins, such as medroxyprogesterone, is indicated even when pregnancy is not a goal; it is important to suppress ovarian hormone production. Otherwise, irregular bleeding may be distressing. Furthermore, endometrial changes can trigger the development of premalignant or malignant disorders. Ovarian hormone production can be fully suppressed with low-dosage oral contraceptives or long-acting progestins, such as medroxyprogesterone.

**Treatment—Investigational** David Ehrmann, M.D., at the University of Chicago Medical Center, is studying the effectiveness of Flutamide in controlling hair growth.

Please contact the agencies listed under Resources, below, for the most current information. Addresses and telephone numbers of these agencies, as well as of individual experts and research centers, may be found in the Master Resources List.

**Resources**

**For more information on Stein-Leventhal syndrome:** National Organization for Rare Disorders (NORD); NIH/National Institute of Child Health and Human Development; Resolve; National Women's Health Network.

**References**

Ovulation Induction with Low-Dose Follicle-Stimulating Hormone in Women with the Polycystic Ovary Syndrome: O. Dale, et al.; Acta. Obstet. Gynecol. Scand., January 1993, vol. 72(1), pp. 43–46.

Cecil Textbook of Medicine, 19th ed.: J.B. Wyngaarden, et al., eds.; W.B. Saunders Company, 1992, pp. 1367, 1369.

Increased Risk for Polycystic Ovary Syndrome Associated with Human Leukocyte Antigen DQA1*0501: C. Ober; Am. J. Obstet. Gynecol., December 1992, vol. 167(6), pp. 1803–1806.

Mendelian Inheritance in Man, 10th ed.: V.A. McKusick; The Johns Hopkins University Press, 1992, pp. 1037–1038.

Textbook of Endocrinology, 8th ed.: J.D. Wilson and D.W. Foster, eds.; W.B. Saunders Company, 1992, pp. 768–769.

Which Hormone Tests for the Diagnosis of Polycystic Ovary Syndrome?: S. Robinson, et al.; Br. J. Obstet. Gynaecol., March 1992, vol. 99(3), pp. 232–238.

Novak's Textbook of Gynecology, 11th ed.: H. Jones III, et al., eds.; Williams and Wilkins, 1988, pp. 104, 369–371.

# ZOLLINGER-ELLISON SYNDROME

**Description** Zollinger-Ellison syndrome is associated with refractory peptic ulcers, marked gastric hyperacidity, and, usually, small gastrin-secreting tumors (gastrinomas). Benign or malignant tumors develop most often in the pancreas but are also found in the stomach, duodenum, mesentery, spleen, or the abdominal lymph nodes.

**Synonyms**

> Gastrinoma
> Multiple Endocrine Neoplasia, Type I
> Pancreatic Ulcerogenic Tumor Syndrome
> Partial Multiple Endocrine Adenomatosis

**Signs and Symptoms** Exquisite pain from ulcers in the stomach, duodenum, jejunum, and/or esophagus is likely, and diarrhea and steatorrhea are often present. The ulcers may be refractory to any type of treatment for years, during which time the serum potassium remains low. Life-threatening complications, such as obstruction, perforations, and bleeding may occur. About 40 percent of patients have tumors, and approximately 50 percent of these are malignant.

**Etiology** Since 1982, 2 forms of Zollinger-Ellison syndrome have been recognized: sporadic and autosomal dominant; there may be other as yet unidentified forms. Onset of the sporadic type is usually in the mature years. The autosomal dominant type is a symptom of **multiple endocrine adenomatosis.** The cause of the tumors associated with Zollinger-Ellison syndrome is unknown. The symptoms are caused by excessive secretion of gastrin.

**Epidemiology** Onset of Zollinger-Ellison syndrome may be during the childhood years, but the time of diagnosis is most often between ages 20 to 70. Males and females are affected in equal numbers.

**Related Disorders** Endocrinopathy, such as **hyperparathyroidism** and **adrenal** or **pituitary adenomas** may be associated with the **multiple endocrine neoplasia (MEN) syndrome I (Wermer syndrome; polyendocrine adenomatosis).**

**Duodenal ulcers** have a high incidence. Their development may stem from a familial proneness, or a course of corticosteroids may be the trigger. Other potential factors are cirrhosis of the liver, chronic pancreatitis, cystic fibrosis, or pulmonary emphysema.

See *Cushing Syndrome.*

**Treatment—Standard** Control of gastric acid secretion with antacids and drugs such as cimetidine and ranitidine, with or without anticholinergic agents, has replaced gastrectomy as treatment for most patients. Higher-than-routine doses are often required. In 1989, omeprazole was approved for the treatment of Zollinger-Ellison syndrome and other severe gastric conditions. The rate of efficacy is rising, an effect of the success of imaging procedures that pinpoint the tumor site. Surgical removal in conjunction with chemotherapy may be beneficial for some patients. Genetic counseling may be helpful.

**Treatment—Investigational** New diagnostic tests are being developed, such as transhepatic pancreatic vein catheterization supplemented by the determination of local hormone gradients. This may permit preoperative location of even the smallest tumors; the current success rate for tumor surgery is 20 percent. Severing the vagus nerve is under investigation to interrupt the stimulation of acid-secreting tissue. Patients who require very high doses of standard drugs may be candidates for this surgery.

Please contact the agencies listed under Resources, below, for the most current information. Addresses and telephone numbers of these agencies, as well as of individual experts and research centers, may be found in the Master Resources List.

**Resources**

**For more information on Zollinger-Ellison syndrome:** National Organization for Rare Disorders (NORD); NIH/National Digestive Diseases Information Clearinghouse.

**For genetic information and genetic counseling referrals:** March of Dimes Birth Defects Foundation; Alliance of Genetic Support Groups.

**References**

Current Management of Zollinger-Ellison Syndrome: R.T. Jensen, et al.; Drugs, August 1986, vol. 32(2), pp. 188–196.

Diagnosis and Curative Therapy in Zollinger-Ellison Syndrome: W.H. Hacki; Schweiz. Med. Wochenschr., April 1985, vol. 115(17), pp. 575–581.

Zollinger-Ellison Syndrome: H.D. Becker; Wien. Klin. Wochenschr., February 1984, vol. 96(4), pp. 138–144.

# 11 ARTHRITIS AND CONNECTIVE TISSUE DISEASES
## By Marc C. Hochberg, M.D., M.P.H., and Raymond H. Flores, M.D.

Arthritis and other diseases of the musculoskeletal system, including the diffuse connective tissue diseases, constitute the most common cause of disability in the adult civilian population of the United States. They are the leading cause of mobility limitation and the second leading cause of activity limitation among adults ages 18 and above. It is recognized that over 100 diseases can cause arthritis. An overview of the classification of the rheumatic diseases, as suggested by the Arthritis Foundation, is listed in Table 11.1.

Diseases associated with arthritis generally present in one of three major fashions: 1) arthritis alone; 2) arthritis as the dominant clinical finding but with extra-articular lesions; or 3) arthritis as one part of a diffuse multisystem disease. The individual conditions covered in this chapter were selected as representing four major groups of "less common" arthritis and musculoskeletal diseases: the seronegative spondyloarthropathies, to be distinguished from rheumatoid arthritis (Table 11.2); the diffuse connective tissue diseases (Table 11.3); the vasculitides and related syndromes (Table 11.4); and miscellaneous orthopedic conditions producing localized musculoskeletal pain and dysfunction.

The first step in evaluating the patient who presents with a musculoskeletal or rheumatic complaint is conducting a thorough history and physical examination. Most of the rheumatic diseases are more common in women than men, except for ankylosing spondylitis, Reiter syndrome, gout, and polyarteritis nodosa. The age of the patient also provides diagnostic clues. Occurrence of the rheumatic diseases can largely be subdivided into those affecting children and adolescents; those affecting young patients (between 18 and 40 years), such as ankylosing spondylitis, Reiter syndrome,

---

**Table 11.1    Classification of the rheumatic diseases**

    I. Diffuse connective tissue diseases
   II. Seronegative spondyloarthropathies
  III. Osteoarthritis
  IV. Infectious arthritis
   V. Arthritis associated with metabolic and/or endocrine disorders
  VI. Neoplasms of bones and joints
 VII. Arthritis associated with neurovascular disorders
VIII. Primary bone and cartilage disorders
  IX. Nonarticular rheumatism
   X. Miscellaneous conditions

Modified from Primer on the Rheumatic Diseases, 10th ed.: H.R. Schumacher, Jr., J.H. Klippel, and W.J. Koopman, eds.; Arthritis Foundation, 1993. Used with permission.

**Table 11.2  Classification of seronegative spondyloarthropathies**

Ankylosing spondylitis
Reiter syndrome
Psoriatic arthritis
Arthritis associated with inflammatory bowel disease

gonococcal arthritis, and systemic lupus erythematosus; those affecting middle-aged patients (between 40 and 65 years), such as gout, rheumatoid arthritis, and the diffuse connective tissue diseases; and those affecting elderly patients (65 years and older), such as polymyalgia rheumatica, giant cell arteritis, osteoarthritis, and pseudogout (calcium pyrophospate dihydrate crystal deposition disease).

It is important to identify the type and pattern of joint involvement: whether 1) the arthritis is inflammatory (accompanied by warmth, erythema, and soft tissue swelling) or noninflammatory; 2) the course has been episodic or persistent; 3) the number of joints involved is oligoarticular (fewer than five joints) or polyarticular (five or more joints); 4) the pattern of involvement has been migratory or additive; 5) the distribution of involvement is bilateral and symmetric or asymmetric; and 6) the axial skeleton, including the sacroiliac joints, is involved or uninvolved.

After a detailed review of the musculoskeletal symptoms and signs, the presence of extra-articular features and systemic manifestations must be determined. In particular, a thorough examination of the skin, eyes, blood vessels, and cardiopulmonary systems should be performed to evaluate for evidence of multisystem involvement. The absence of such manifestations would suggest that the patient has a primarily arthritic disease; in contrast, the dominance of such manifestations would suggest the presence of a multisystem disease, particularly a diffuse connective tissue disease or systemic vasculitis.

Laboratory testing usually serves to confirm the clinical diagnosis arrived at by the above process. In patients with arthritis, sampling of synovial fluid may be diagnostic in the presence of infection or microcrystalline disease (either gout or pseudogout), and may be helpful in distinguishing inflammatory from noninflammatory causes of arthritis. Routine hematologic tests are usually nonspecific; however, elevation of the erythrocyte sedimentation rate (**ESR**) indicates the presence of a systemic inflammatory process. In patients with an ESR above 100 mm/hr, the physician should consider the diagnoses of polymyalgia rheumatica and/or giant cell arteritis, when appropriate, or conduct a further evaluation for abnormal serum proteins (multiple myeloma, macroglobulinemia), occult infection, and occult malignancy.

Serologic testing is often performed in patients with arthritis and musculoskeletal diseases. Positive tests for rheumatoid factor and antinuclear antibodies are highly sensitive for the diagnosis of rheumatoid arthritis and the presence of a diffuse connective tissue disease, respectively. However, it must be noted that both rheumatoid factor and antinuclear antibodies are present in up to 5 percent of normals, and up to 15 percent of elderly patients aged 65 and above. Therefore,

**Table 11.3  Classification of diffuse connective tissue diseases**

Rheumatoid arthritis
Juvenile arthritis
Systemic lupus erythematosus
Scleroderma (systemic sclerosis)
Polymyositis/dermatomyositis
Sjögren syndrome
Diffuse fasciitis with or without eosinophilia
Overlap syndromes
Systemic necrotizing vasculitis

**Table 11.4    Classification of systemic vasculitides**

Polyarteritis nodosa
Allergic granulomatosis
Wegener granulomatosis
Giant cell arteritis
Takayasu arteritis
Kawasaki syndrome
Behçet syndrome
Buerger disease
Relapsing polychondritis
Hypersensitivity angiitis

the presence of these autoantibodies alone does not make a diagnosis; the diagnosis rests on the clinical presentation, which is confirmed by results of serologic testing.

In patients suspected of having a diffuse connective tissue disease, it is appropriate to characterize the positive test for antinuclear antibodies by obtaining tests for antibodies to double-stranded deoxyribonucleic acid **(DNA),** and extractable nuclear antigens, including nuclear ribonucleoprotein **(nRNP),** Sm, Ro, La, and in individuals suspected of having scleroderma, Scl-70. The presence of antibodies to double-stranded DNA and/or Sm is highly specific for a diagnosis of systemic lupus erythematosus. The presence of antibodies to nRNP is seen in patients with several connective tissue diseases, including systemic lupus erythematosus, scleroderma, and the overlap syndrome, mixed connective tissue disease. The presence of antibodies to Ro and La is seen in patients with systemic lupus erythematosus and Sjögren syndrome. Tests for anticentromere antibody should be performed in patients with Raynaud phenomenon. It is important that these tests be performed in reliable clinical laboratories; "false positive" tests can result in incorrect diagnostic labeling and inappropriate therapies.

Finally, because the diseases discussed in this chapter are rare, it is entirely appropriate for the primary care physician to seek consultation with a specialist, usually a rheumatologist, for a diagnostic evaluation, including recommendations for medical management. Listings of rheumatologists by geographic area are available through the local chapters of the Arthritis Foundation and the American College of Rheumatology. In instances of rare orthopedic conditions producing localized musculoskeletal pain and dysfunction, consultation with an orthopedic surgeon is appropriate. It is hoped that increased awareness of the rare musculoskeletal and connective tissue diseases by the primary care physician, coupled with timely referral for subspecialty consultation, will lead to improved diagnosis, management, and outcomes for patients with these conditions.

In addition to using this resource, readers are encouraged to obtain their individual copies of the *Primer on the Rheumatic Diseases* through their local chapters of the Arthritis Foundation; this soft-cover volume provides a concise yet thorough description of the rheumatic diseases, focusing on clinical presentation, diagnosis, and management. Additional patient education materials are also readily available through local chapters of the Arthritis Foundation.

# ARTHRITIS AND CONNECTIVE TISSUE DISEASES
*Listings in This Section*

# AMYLOIDOSIS

**Description** Amyloidosis is the term applied to a group of metabolic disorders in which the fibrillar protein amyloid accumulates in tissue, to the extent that the function of affected organs is impaired. The accumulation may be localized, general, or systemic. Various imperfect systems are used for classifying amyloidosis. The most widely used is based on the chemistry of the fibrils.

The most common form of amyloidosis is **AL** or light-chain-related (**primary** amyloidosis). This form of the disease may occur independently of other disease, or in the presence of multiple myeloma. The tongue, thyroid gland, intestinal tract, liver, and spleen are typically affected. Cardiac involvement may result in congestive heart failure.

**AA** amyloidosis (**secondary** amyloidosis) is most often discovered during the course of chronic inflammatory disease, such as rheumatoid arthritis, chronic infections (such as osteomyelitis), and familial Mediterranean fever. Kidneys, liver, and spleen are commonly impaired by AA amyloidosis, but the adrenal glands, lymph nodes, and vascular system may be affected as well. In addition, the skin inflammation that occurs with recurrent injections seems to induce AA amyloidosis. Nephrotic syndrome and renal failure cause the most fatalities in this category. AA amyloidosis is reported in approximately 1 percent of cases of chronic inflammatory disease in the United States.

The amyloidosis of **aging** is observed in the heart, and, sometimes, the pancreas and brain.

**Hemodialysis-associated** amyloidosis is seen in patients who have experienced long-term hemodialysis.

**Familial** amyloidosis is found in a series of genetically transmitted diseases that typically affect the kidney, heart, skin, and other areas of the body.

**Signs and Symptoms** Manifestations are nonspecific. Generally, involved organs become rubbery and firm, with a waxy appearance. Often they are enlarged. Biopsy is necessary for diagnosis.

Kidneys: The nephrotic syndrome is usually accompanied by proteinuria, which worsens as the disease progresses and may finally result in renal failure. The kidney becomes small, pale, and hard. Renal tubular defects, renal vein thrombosis, and hypertension may also be noted. Amyloid may accumulate in other parts of the urogenital system, such as the bladder or ureter.

Liver and spleen: Hepato- and splenomegaly are the most notable signs. The function of the liver is significantly affected only late in the course of the disease, although elevated alkaline phosphatase and other liver function abnormalities may be detected earlier. Occurrence in the spleen increases the risk of traumatic rupture.

Heart: Cardiac involvement occurs frequently and is reflected in cardiomegaly, arrhythmias, murmurs, electrocardiogram abnormalities, and, particularly, congestive failure. Nodular deposits of amyloid may be present on pericardial and endocardial surfaces, and valvular lesions may be noted.

Gastrointestinal system: Symptoms may be similar to those of gastric carcinoma and frequently develop in association with chronic diseases, including tuberculosis and granulomatous ileitis. Amyloid accumulation in the GI tract may cause motility abnormalities in the esophagus and small and large intestines. Malabsorption, ulceration, bleeding, gastric atony, pseudo-obstruction, protein loss, and diarrhea may also be noted. Infiltration of the tongue may cause macroglossia.

Skin: Microscopic or macroscopic dermal involvement occurs in at least half of primary and secondary amyloidosis cases, and in all cases of amyloid neuropathy. Waxy-looking papules appear on the face and neck; in axillary, anal, and inguinal regions; and in mucosal areas such as the ear canal or tongue. Areas of swelling, purpura, alopecia, glossitis, and xerostomia are also found.

Nervous system: Neurologic manifestations often appear in hereditary amyloidoses, and those associated with multiple myeloma. Peripheral neuropathy may be present, as well as hypohidrosis, postural hypotension, Adie syndrome (tonic pupil), hoarseness, sphincter dysfunction, and an increase in the concentration of cerebrospinal fluid protein.

Respiratory system: Pulmonary symptoms often parallel cardiac symptoms. Air passages and ducts may be obstructed by accumulations of amyloid in the nasal sinuses, larynx, and trachea.

Other: Amyloid arthropathy, which occurs in 6 to 15 percent of multiple myeloma cases, may involve articular cartilage or the synovial membrane and fluid. Symptoms are similar to those of rheumatoid arthritis. Amyloid deposits in muscle tissue may cause pseudomyopathy. Results of hematologic involvement may include fibrinogenopenia, increased fibrinolysis, and deficiency of certain clotting factors.

**Etiology** Little is known about the etiology, although it appears that the various forms of amyloidosis result from different causes. Secondary amyloidosis apparently results from excessive antigenic stimuli that accompany chronic inflammatory or infectious disease. Hereditary amyloidosis is thought to be autosomal dominant, except when associated with familial Mediterranean fever, which seems to be autosomal recessive.

**Epidemiology** Amyloidosis affects males and females equally. AA amyloidosis (secondary amyloidosis) occurs in 3 to 5 percent of cases of rheumatoid arthritis. In the United States, approximately 1:100,000 to 1:1,000,000 people are carriers of the defective gene that causes hereditary amyloidosis. A high percentage of patients with familial Mediterranean fever develop systemic amyloidosis.

**Treatment—Standard** No uniformly effective treatment has been found to cure the disease or reverse amyloid deposition. In secondary amyloidosis, treatment of the underlying disorder may control the disease adequately, if begun in time. In addition, chronic colchicine therapy appears to improve survival. Patients with AL amyloidosis, whether they have myeloma or not, may benefit from myeloma-like protocols.

Patients with cardiac involvement may experience increased sensitivity to digitalis drugs, which should therefore be used only with extreme caution.

In cases with severe renal involvement, dialysis or kidney transplantation may be necessary. Transplantation has been successful for several patients. It is thought, however, that amyloidosis will eventually recur in the transplanted kidney.

Localized amyloid tumors may be surgically removed, generally without further complications or recurrence.

The most successful treatment has been the preventive use of colchicine in patients with familial Mediterranean fever.

Genetic counseling may be of benefit for patients and their families with hereditary forms of amyloidosis.

**Treatment—Investigational** α-Interferon is being evaluated as a treatment, and trials are being conducted using colchicine in patients with AL and AA amyloidosis. Two different chemotherapy programs are under investigation by researchers at the Mayo Clinic (Morie A. Gertz, M.D.) as treatment for primary systemic amyloidosis. A combination of colchicine, melphalan, and prednisone is being studied (Martha Skinner, M.D., and Alan S. Cohen, M.D., at Boston University School of Medicine) to determine their long-term safety and effectiveness in amyloidosis patients.

Please contact the agencies listed under Resources, below, for the most current information. Addresses and telephone numbers of these agencies, as well as of individual experts and research centers, may be found in the Master Resources List.

**Resources**

**For more information on amyloidosis:** National Organization for Rare Disorders (NORD); NIH/National Arthritis and Musculoskeletal and Skin Diseases Information Clearinghouse; Merrill Benson, M.D., Indiana University.

**For genetic information and genetic counseling referrals:** March of Dimes Birth Defects Foundation; Alliance of Genetic Support Groups.

**References**

Mendelian Inheritance in Man, 10th ed.: V.A. McKusick; The Johns Hopkins University Press, 1992, pp. 66, 1214–1215, 1786.
Amyloidosis: A.S. Cohen, et al.; Curr. Opin. Rheumatol., February 1991, vol. 3(1), pp. 125–138.
Amyloid and Amyloidoses: R. Kisilevsky; Mod. Pathol., July 1991, vol. 4(4), pp. 514–518.
Birth Defects Encyclopedia: M.L. Buyse, ed.-in-chief; Blackwell Scientific Publications, 1990, pp. 99–109.
Arthritis and Allied Conditions, 11th ed.: D.J. McCarty; Lea and Febiger, 1989, pp. 1273–1293.
The Metabolic Basis of Inherited Disease, 6th ed.: C.R. Scriver, et al., eds.; McGraw-Hill, 1989, pp. 2439–2460.
Cecil Textbook of Medicine, 18th ed.: J.B. Wyngaarden and L.H. Smith, Jr., eds.; W.B. Saunders Company, 1988, pp. 359–360, 1198–1203.

# ANKYLOSING SPONDYLITIS

**Description** Ankylosing spondylitis is an inflammatory arthritis affecting the sacroiliac joints, spine, and paraspinal structures.

**Synonyms**

Bekhterev-Strümpell Syndrome
Marie-Strümpell Disease
Spondyloarthritis

**Signs and Symptoms** Back pain and postures assumed in response to the arthritic vertebrae are frequent features. The pain often is worst after periods of rest and at night, is associated with morning stiffness and gel phenomenon, and improves with exercise and use of heat.

Muscle spasm early in the course of the disease and ankylosis as the disease progresses may prevent normal flexion of the spine during bending. Advanced disease may cause immobility of the entire spine, resulting in a straight "poker spine." X-rays show sacroiliitis and may also show spinal involvement with syndesmophyte formation and fusion of apophyseal joints.

Symptoms involving peripheral joints, including hips and shoulders, are the first to appear in 20 percent of cases. Neck movement may become limited.

About one-third of patients develop iritis. Respiratory capacity may be decreased as a result of the fixed position of the chest cage due to costovertebral joint involvement. Neurologic complications include incontinence and absence of ankle jerks due to compression of the cauda equina. In fewer than 10 percent of cases, the heart is involved, causing heart block, arrhythmias, and/or aortic insufficiency after long-standing disease.

**Etiology** Although the cause of ankylosing spondylitis is unknown, familial clustering and the association with HLA-B27 strongly indicate a genetic basis. Evidence suggests that the disease occurs when a genetically predisposed person is affected by a bacterium, virus, or other environmental factor, not yet identified.

This disorder is also suspected of being an autoimmune disease.

Some cases of ankylosing spondylitis may be inherited as an autosomal dominant genetic trait. The symptoms are produced more readily in males and may be related to the presence of the HLA-B27 antigen. The gene is located on the short arm of chromosome 6.

**Epidemiology** Ankylosing spondylitis usually begins between the ages of 20 and 40. The disorder occurs more often among whites than blacks and is at least 3 times more common in men than in women, who usually experience milder symptoms.

**Related Disorders** See *Psoriatic Arthritis; Reiter Syndrome.*

**Rheumatoid arthritis** is a chronic, often progressive form of arthritis resulting in destruction of diarthrodial joints. Symmetrical inflammation, pain, swelling, and decreased mobility are symptoms. The disease is most common among females and those of middle age. The course of the disease is highly variable and may include episodes of remission.

**Infectious arthritis** is the result of tissue invasion by bacteria, virus, or fungi. Symptoms include fever and chills, accompanied by intense inflammation of the joint(s). Within hours or days, affected joint(s) become painful, swollen, red, and stiff. Rapid onset may indicate bacterium as the cause. Viral or fungal agents cause a slower progression of the disease.

**Osteoarthritis** is the most common form of arthritis. Characteristics include degeneration of articular cartilage and hypertrophy of the tissue surrounding the joints. The exact cause is unknown, but biochemical, genetic, metabolic, and endocrine factors have been implicated. Stress may aggravate the condition. Symptoms include joint pain after exercise, stiffness, tenderness, and swelling. Walking may be difficult because of knee, hip, or spine involvement.

**Treatment—Standard** Diagnosis of ankylosing spondylitis can be confirmed through clinical evaluation and x-rays that demonstrate sacroileitis and apophyseal fusion. Most patients respond well to medications given to reduce pain and inflammation, combined with exercises to improve posture and strengthen muscle groups to counteract potential deformity. This is particularly true for patients who contract ankylosing spondylitis early in life and for whom treatment begins early in the course of the disease.

Nonsteroidal anti-inflammatory drugs are effective in treating patients. Narcotics and systemic corticosteroid are to be avoided.

Exercises should emphasize back movements, especially extension, straightening of the thoracic vertebrae, and deep breathing. The patient should get ample rest, sleeping on his or her back on a firm mattress with a flat pillow or none at all. Some persons benefit from back braces. Swimming is an excellent exercise.

Therapeutic measures usually eliminate the need for surgery to straighten the spine.

**Treatment—Investigational** Please contact the agencies listed under Resources, below, for the most current information. Addresses and telephone numbers of these agencies, as well as of individual experts and research centers, may be found in the Master Resources List.

**Resources**

**For more information on ankylosing spondylitis:** National Organization for Rare Disorders (NORD); Ankylosing Spondylitis Association; Arthritis Foundation; NIH/National Arthritis and Musculoskeletal and Skin Diseases Information Clearinghouse.

**For genetic information and genetic counseling referrals:** March of Dimes Birth Defects Foundation; Alliance of Genetic Support Groups.

**References**

Ankylosing Spondylitis: I. Haslock; Baillieres Clin. Rheumatol., February 1993, vol. 7(1), pp. 99–115.

Ankylosing Spondylitis: A Common Cause of Low Back Pain: A. Escalante; Postgrad. Med., July 1993, vol. 94(1), pp. 153–160, 166.

Management of the Patient with Rheumatic Diseases Going to Surgery: R. Sorokin; Med. Clin. North Am., March 1993, vol. 77(2), pp. 453–464.

Cecil Textbook of Medicine, 19th ed.: J.B. Wyngaarden, et al., eds.; W.B. Saunders Company, 1992, pp. 1516–1518.

HLA Molecules in Autoimmune Diseases: W.E. Braun; Clin. Biochem., June 1992, vol. 25(3), pp. 187–191.

Infection and the Immunopathogenesis of Seronegative Spondyloarthropathies: A. Keat; Curr. Opin. Rheumatol., August 1992, vol. 4(4), pp. 494–499.

Infection as a Cause of Reactive Arthritis, Ankylosing Spondylitis, and Rheumatic Fever: L.W. Moreland, et al.; Curr. Opin. Rheumatol., August 1992, vol. 4(4), pp. 534–542.

Mendelian Inheritance in Man, 10th ed.: V.A. McKusick; The Johns Hopkins University Press, 1992, p. 82.

Nelson Textbook of Pediatrics, 14th ed.: R.E. Behrman, ed.-in-chief; W.B. Saunders Company, 1992, pp. 621–622.

Radiographic Evaluation of the Degenerative Cervical Spine: K.A. Rahim, et al.; Orthop. Clin. North Am., July 1992, vol. 23(3), pp. 395–403.

Therapy for the Seronegative Spondyloarthropathies: J. Buxhaum; Curr. Opin. Rheumatol., August 1992, vol. 4(4), pp. 500–506.

Harrison's Principles of Internal Medicine, 12th ed.: J.D. Wilson, et al., eds.; McGraw-Hill, 1991, pp. 1451–1453.

Birth Defects Encyclopedia: M.L. Buyse, ed.-in-chief; Blackwell Scientific Publications, 1990, pp. 146–147.

Dictionary of Medical Syndromes, 3rd ed.: S.I. Magalini, et al., eds.; J.B. Lippincott Company, 1990, p. 53.

Arthritis and Allied Conditions, 11th ed.: D.J. McCarty; Lea and Febiger, 1989, pp. 934–943.

# ARTERITIS, GIANT CELL

**Description** Giant cell arteritis is part of a generalized vascular disorder displaying granulomatous inflammation. The chronic inflammation is so frequently confined to the aortic arch branches, principally the temporal arteries, that it is designated as a distinct entity. The disorder is a panarteritis; the greatest changes show focal necrosis and granulomatous inflammation with giant cells. Any of the large elastic arteries are susceptible. Venous involvement is extremely rare.

**Synonyms**

> Cranial Arteritis
>
> Granulomatous Arteritis
>
> Temporal Arteritis

**Signs and Symptoms** Onset may be either acute or gradual, with flu-like symptoms such as low-grade fever, muscle pain, mild anemia, and severe stiffness. A few patients experience respiratory tract symptoms, including cough, sore throat, and hoarseness. Such manifestations may direct attention away from the underlying arteritis.

Headache is a common and early symptom. Severe throbbing and boring or stabbing temporal pain is often accompanied by redness, swelling, tenderness, pulsations, and knotting of the temporal artery. The scalp may be tender.

Frequent involvement of the internal carotid system results in ophthalmic and retinal vessel disease. Half the patients have visual symptoms, but only 10 percent experience visual loss. Early diagnosis and treatment are important in preventing permanent visual loss. The process may involve other vessels, such as the coronary, carotid, subclavian, pulmonary, renal, and mesenteric arteries. The disorder has serious complications, including a potential for cerebral vascular accident, coronary artery occlusion, and arterial insufficiency of the extremities, as well as blindness. Aortic aneurysm formation with or without dissection may be a late complication. Angiograms show smooth, tapered arterial occlusions or stenosis.

Polymyalgia rheumatica involving the neck, shoulder, and hip girdle musculature, accompanied by synovitis, especially of the knees, is common.

**Etiology** The cause is unknown. A genetic predisposition has been suggested. The immune system has been implicated in recent data, but a causal relationship has not been established. Familial cases have been reported, and research indicates that some people may have a genetic predisposition to the disease.

**Epidemiology** Incidence is approximately 24:100,000 persons aged 50 and above. The disease develops from age 50 to 90, with average onset at about 70 years. Women are affected twice as often as men. Whites are affected more often than blacks or other ethnic/racial groups.

**Related Disorders** See *Polymyalgia Rheumatica; Polymyositis; Takayasu Arteritis.*

**Vasculitis** is an inflammation of the veins, arteries, and/or capillaries. This disorder may occur alone or in conjunction with allergic and rheumatic diseases. Symptoms include blood clots, weakened vessel walls, muscle pain, joint pain, fever, weight loss, loss of appetite, abdominal pain, and shortness of breath. Localized symptoms are dependent on the type and size of vessel involved, as well as on the distribution of vessels affected. Various vasculitic (arteritic) syndromes have been described.

**Treatment—Standard** Diagnosis is confirmed by a complete clinical evaluation, blood tests, and temporal artery biopsy. Treatment should begin immediately in order to avoid serious complications, such as stroke and blindness. High doses of corticosteroids (60 to 80 mg/day) control initial local and systemic symptoms. Prednisone may be given in large doses until symptoms cease and laboratory findings (elevated erythrocyte sedimentation rate) return to normal. This process usually lasts for 2 to 4 weeks. Initial therapy is followed by giving a gradually reduced dosage (about 10 percent per month) for 2 years or longer to prevent recurrence. The disease is monitored by checking the sedimentation rate. A rise in the rate along with arteritic or polymyalgia symptoms heralds a return of the illness.

**Treatment—Investigational** For patients unable to tolerate high doses of corticosteroid, other drugs such as azathioprine, methotrexate, and dapsone are being studied.

Please contact the agencies listed under Resources, below, for the most current information. Addresses and telephone numbers of these agencies, as well as of individual experts and research centers, may be found in the Master Resources List.

## Resources

**For more information on giant cell arteritis:** National Organization for Rare Disorders (NORD); NIH/National Heart, Lung and Blood Institute.

## References

Giant Cell Arteritis: Epidemiology and Treatment: E. Nordboerg, et al.; Drugs Aging, February 1994, vol. 4(2), pp. 135–144.

Familial Giant Cell Arteritis: Report of an HLA-Typed Sibling Pair and a Review of the Literature: R. Wernick, et al.; Clin. Exp. Rheumatol., January–February 1994, vol. 12(1), pp. 63–66.

The Clinical and Laboratory Course of Polymyalgia Rheumatica/Giant Cell Arteritis After the First Two Months of Treatment: V. Kyle, et al.; Ann. Rheum. Dis., December 1993, vol. 52(12), pp. 847–850.

The Diagnosis and Management of Arteritis: N.D. Karanjia, et al.; J. R. Soc. Med., May 1993, vol. 86(5), pp. 267–270.

Diagnosis and Management of Temporal Arteritis: A Review and Case Report: T. Grosvenor, et al.; Optom. Vis. Sci., September 1993, vol. 70(9), pp. 771–777.

Fluorescein Angiography in the Diagnosis of Giant Cell Arteritis: R.M. Siatkowski, et al.; Am. J. Ophthalmol., January 1993, vol. 115(1), pp. 57–63.

Cecil Textbook of Medicine, 19th ed.: J.B. Wyngaarden, et al., eds.; W.B. Saunders Company, 1992, pp. 1544–1547.

Giant Cell Arteritis: E. Nordboerg, et al.; Curr. Opin. Rheumatol., February 1992, vol. 4(1), pp. 23–30.

Giant Cell Arteritis and Polymyalgia Rheumatica: A.G. DiBartolomeo, et al.; Postgrad. Med., February 1, 1992, vol. 91(2), pp. 107–109, 112.

Mendelian Inheritance in Man, 10th ed.: V.A. McKusick; The Johns Hopkins University Press, 1992, pp. 1066–1067.

Presenting Features and Outcomes in Patients Undergoing Temporal Artery Biopsy: A Review of 98 Patients: W.L. Chmelewski, et al.; Arch. Intern. Med., August 1992, vol. 152(8), pp. 1690–1695.

Temporal Arteritis: A Form of Systemic Panarteritis: A. Sendino, et al.; Ann. Rheum. Dis., September 1992, vol. 51(9), pp. 1082–1084.

Harrison's Principles of Internal Medicine, 12th ed.: J.D. Wilson, et al., eds.; McGraw-Hill, 1991, pp. 1461–1462.

Dictionary of Medical Syndromes, 3rd ed.: S.I. Magalini, et al., eds.; J.B. Lippincott Company, 1990, pp. 423–424.

Textbook of Rheumatology, 3rd ed.: W.N. Kelley, et al.; W.B. Saunders Company, 1989, pp. 1200–1208.

# ARTERITIS, TAKAYASU

**Description** Takayasu arteritis is an inflammation of the large elastic arteries and the aorta. The disorder is a progressive polyarteritis resulting in the reduction of blood flow to the head and arms, and loss of the major pulses. Irregular segmental stenosis of the large arteries and aortic regurgitation are also likely to be part of the clinical picture.

## Synonyms

Aortic Arch Syndrome
Brachiocephalic Ischemia
Martorell Syndrome
Occlusive Thromboaortopathy
Pulseless Disease
Young Female Arteritis

**Signs and Symptoms** Prodromes mimic acute febrile illness with systemic manifestations of fever, anorexia, malaise, myalgias, and arthralgias. Progressive obstructive arterial disease and arterial stenosis follow the acute period of the disease (pulseless phase). When the aorta and carotid arteries are involved, the patient experiences lightheadedness, dizziness, and syncope, which is probably the result of cerebral ischemia. Carotid and superficial temporal pulses may be lost. Most patients develop cardiac and cerebral insufficiencies. There may be episodes of blindness, dim vision, and frank stroke. Symptoms of brachial involvement include extremity weakness and claudication, cool skin, and the absence of radial pulses. Blood pressure may be imperceptible. Raynaud phenomenon is occasionally observed. Additional signs include systolic murmurs, erythema nodosum, fever, atrophy of facial muscles and soft tissues, and premature cataracts. Prognosis is more favorable when the disease progresses slowly and the patient has the opportunity to develop adequate collateral or secondary circulation.

**Etiology** The cause is unclear. Certain evidence (e.g., elevated globulins levels, the presence in serum of antiaorta antibodies) suggests an immunologic process and possibly an autoimmune association, not contradicted by the familial and racial incidence associations as discussed below. Studies have shown increased frequency in Asians with HLA-Bw52, and increased frequency in North Americans with HLA-DR4. An infectious etiology has not been proved. Some people may be genetically predisposed to the disease.

**Epidemiology** The disease is common in Japan and occurs throughout the Orient. It has been seen in India and is reported to occur frequently in South America. Females are primarily affected (80 to 90 percent of cases), generally between 10 and 30 years of age.

**Related Disorders** See *Arteritis, Giant Cell; Polymyalgia Rheumatica.*

**Polyarteritis nodosa** is a rare inflammatory systemic disease characterized by nodules along the small and medium-sized arteries. Initial symptoms include fever, chills, fatigue, and weight loss. In addition, abdominal pain, peripheral neuropathy, skin eruptions, arthralgia, and/or general myalgia are common. It may cause ischemia to various organs as well as blood clots.

**Treatment—Standard** Thoracic and abdominal aortography are required to diagnose and evaluate the extent of Takayasu arteritis. Treatment should begin as soon as diagnosis is suspected, in order to avoid serious complications such as arterial occlusion and blindness. High doses of corticosteroids control initial local and systemic symptoms. Prednisone may be given in large doses until symptoms cease and laboratory findings return to normal. This process usually lasts 2 to 4 weeks. Initial therapy is followed by giving a gradually reduced dosage (about 10 percent/month) for 2 years or longer to prevent recurrence. The disease is monitored by checking the sedimentation rate. A rise in the rate along with recurrence of symptoms heralds a return of the illness. Cytotoxic therapy may be useful in individuals with refractory disease.

Reconstructive vascular surgery may be helpful in selected patients with inactive disease. Heparin may be given to those patients who experience ischemia.

**Treatment—Investigational** Two surgical procedures are under investigation for the treatment of Takayasu arteritis. In the first, percutaneous transluminal balloon angioplasty is used to widen arteries. In the other, coronary artery bypass grafting is used. Patients with short areas of narrowed arteries achieve greater relief than those with long areas of constriction.

Please contact the agencies listed under Resources, below, for the most current information. Addresses and telephone numbers of these agencies, as well as of individual experts and research centers, may be found in the Master Resources List.

**Resources**

**For more information on Takayasu arteritis:** National Organization for Rare Disorders (NORD); NIH/National Heart, Lung and Blood Institute.

**References**

Immunopathogenesis, Diagnosis, and Treatment of Giant Cell Arteritis, Temporal Arteritis, Polymyalgia Rheumatica, and Takayasu's Arteritis: D.B. Hellman; Curr. Opin. Rheumatol., January 1993, vol. 5(1), pp. 25–32.

Balloon Angioplasty of the Aorta in Takayasu's Arteritis: Initial and Long-Term Results: S. Tyagi, et al.; Am. Heart J., October 1992, vol. 124(4), pp. 876–882.

Cecil Textbook of Medicine, 19th ed.: J.B. Wyngaarden, et al., eds.; W.B. Saunders Company, 1992, pp. 2157.

Mendelian Inheritance in Man, 10th ed.: V.A. McKusick; The Johns Hopkins University Press, 1992, pp. 1222.

Pathological Studies on Takayasu's Arteritis: M. Hotchi; Heart Vessels, 1992, vol. 7(suppl.), pp. 11–17.

Pulmonary Artery Disease in Takayasu's Arteritis: Angiographic Findings: I. Yamada, et al.; AJR Am. J. Roentgenol., August 1992, vol. 159(2), pp. 263–269.

Revascularization for Coronary Ostial Stenosis in Takayasu's Disease with Calcified Aorta: M. Tanaka, et al.; Ann. Thorac. Surg., May 1992, vol. 53(3), pp. 894–895.

Takayasu's Arteritis and Atherosclerosis: P.G. Jorens, et al.; J. Cardiovasc. Surg., May–June 1991, vol. 32(3), pp. 373–375.

Textbook of Rheumatology, 3rd ed.: W.N. Kelley, et al.; W.B. Saunders Company, 1989, pp. 1190–1192.

Heart Disease, 3rd ed.: E. Braunwald; W.B. Saunders Company, 1988, pp. 1563–1565.

Pulmonary Diseases and Disorders, 2nd ed.: A.P. Fishman; McGraw-Hill, 1988, pp. 1143–1145.

# BEALS SYNDROME

**Description** Beals syndrome is an inherited disorder in which the joints bend but cannot straighten.

**Synonyms**

Arachnodactyly, Contractural Beals Type

Beals-Hecht Syndrome

Contractural Arachnodactyly, Congenital

Contractures, Multiple with Arachnodactyly

Ear Anomalies–Contractures–Dysplasia of Bone with Kyphoscoliosis

**Signs and Symptoms** Contractures of the joints of the fingers, hips, knees, ankles, and elbows are typical. Improvement is often gradual and spontaneous. Occasionally the knee and hand contractures persist, but physical therapy tends to improve the condition. Also common are "crumpled" ears and arachnodactyly.

Other symptoms include kyphoscoliosis, which may be present during infancy or progress with age; pectus carinatum; pectus excavatum; keratoconus; a delay in motor development due to the contractures; myopia; taller than normal height; and mitral valve prolapse.

**Etiology** Beals syndrome is inherited as an autosomal dominant trait with variable expression.

**Epidemiology** Males and females are affected in equal numbers. Approximately 20 affected families as well as many isolated cases have been reported.

**Related Disorders** See ***Arthrogryposis Multiplex Congenita; Marfan Syndrome.*** See also ***Keratoconus*** and ***Mitral Valve Prolapse Syndrome,*** disorders that occur in conjunction with Beals syndrome.

**Treatment—Standard** Patients with Beals syndrome can improve mobility of joints by undergoing physical therapy. Keratoconus can usually be corrected with glasses or contact lenses.

Although surgery is not usually recommended for patients with mitral valve prolapse, in rare cases replacement of the affected valve is indicated. The use of oral contraceptives by women with mitral valve prolapse is not recommended, and antibiotics should be prescribed before minor or major surgery to avoid infection.

Plastic surgery may be performed to correct the ears.

Genetic counseling may be of benefit for patients and their families.

**Treatment—Investigational** Drugs such as β-blockers and moricizene (Ethmozine) may alleviate many of the heart rhythm abnormalities associated with mitral valve prolapse. Other symptoms such as palpitations, dizziness, and fainting spells may also respond to these drugs.

Please contact the agencies listed under Resources, below, for the most current information.

**Resources**

**For more information on Beals syndrome:** National Organization for Rare Disorders (NORD); Coalition of Heritable Disorders of Connective Tissue; NIH/National Arthritis and Musculoskeletal and Skin Diseases Information Clearinghouse.

**For genetic information and genetic counseling referrals:** March of Dimes Birth Defects Foundation; Alliance of Genetic Support Groups.

**References**

Birth Defects Encyclopedia: M.L. Buyse, ed.-in-chief; Blackwell Scientific Publications, 1990, p. 174.

Mendelian Inheritance in Man, 9th ed.: V.A. McKusick; The Johns Hopkins University Press, 1990, p. 225.

Smith's Recognizable Patterns of Human Malformation, 4th ed.: K.L. Jones; W.B. Saunders Company, 1988, p. 424.

# BEHÇET SYNDROME

**Description** Behçet syndrome is a chronic relapsing inflammatory disorder marked by eye inflammation, oral and genital ulcers, and certain other skin lesions, as well as varying multisystem involvement including the joints, blood vessels, central nervous system, and gastrointestinal tract.

**Signs and Symptoms** The most frequent initial sign is aphthous stomatitis; the lesions heal in a few days to a month but recur. Similar genital lesions recur less frequently.

Ocular symptoms include posterior uveitis, iridocyclitis, a transient hypopyon iritis, and chorioretinitis. Although the ocular lesions may resolve, chronic recurrence of the inflammation may result in partial loss of vision or complete blindness after 4 to 8 years.

Cutaneous hypersensitivity is seen in most Behçet patients, with a pustule and erythema developing within 24 hours at the site of a pinprick into sterile skin (pathergy). The skin lesions typically resemble erythema nodosum, most commonly over the lower legs.

At least 50 percent of patients develop arthralgia or a polyarthritis before, during, or after the onset of Behçet syndrome. The arthritis usually affects large joints, ranges from mild to severe in nature, and occasionally becomes chronic. Joint damage is rarely present.

Vascular involvement includes thrombophlebitis of the large veins and arterial occlusion and aneurysm. Rarely, pulmonary embolism occurs.

The lesions of aphthous stomatitis may be found elsewhere in the gastrointestinal tract. Symptoms vary from mild abdominal discomfort to ulcerative colitis or regional enteritis and malabsorption problems.

The central nervous system becomes involved in about 10 percent of patients. Central nervous system symptoms are first seen on the average of 16 months after the initial onset of Behçet syndrome symptoms. Recurrent attacks of meningoencephalitis or meningitis result in neurologic damage, with such manifestations as ocular and pseudobulbar palsies and cerebellar ataxia.

**Etiology** The cause of Behçet syndrome is unclear. Genetic predisposition, autoimmune mechanisms, and viral infection are under consideration.

**Epidemiology** Seen most frequently in the Middle East and Asia, especially Japan, the syndrome occurs twice as often in men between 20 and 30 years of age than in women, and is a leading cause of blindness. However, in the United States and Australia it is more prevalent in women than in men and less severe. In the United States about 15,000 persons may be affected.

**Related Disorders** See *Reiter Syndrome; Stevens-Johnson Syndrome.*

**Treatment—Standard** Attacks often remit spontaneously. Topical corticosteroids may relieve the pain of oral lesions, and lidocaine mouthwash also will alleviate pain. Chronic therapy with colchicine is effective in preventing recurrent attacks of oral and genital ulcers. Joint, skin, and mucosal inflammation may be reduced with high-dose oral glucocorticoids, but there is some question as to their use in posterior uveitis. Chlorambucil has been successful in treating uveitis and meningoencephalitis, but the possible toxic effects of this drug must be considered in its use.

**Treatment—Investigational** A study of 96 Japanese patients reported in The Lancet, May 20, 1989, indicates that cyclosporine treatment for oral ulcers, skin lesions, and optic inflammation may be beneficial. Additional studies in the United States, Israel, and Japan also suggest that the use of cyclosporine may lessen or prevent the occurrence of uveitis. Side effects of cyclosporine include nephrotoxicity; it also has been reported that disease activity resumes quickly when the drug is stopped.

Azathioprine as well as chlorambucil (mentioned above) has been used to control the symptoms of eye disease in persons with Behçet syndrome. Further research is needed.

Thalidomide, an orphan drug, is being tested for its effectiveness in treatment; this drug, however, should not be used in pregnant women because of its known ability to cause severe birth defects. Physicians wishing to inquire about testing thalidomide should contact the Andrulis Research Corporation. Thalidomide is also available in England under special license from Penn Pharmaceuticals of Tredegar, South Wales.

Transfer factor is under investigation as a possible treatment for Behçet syndrome.

Please contact the agencies listed under Resources, below, for the most current information. Addresses and telephone numbers of these agencies, as well as of individual experts and research centers, may be found in the Master Resources List.

**Resources**

**For more information on Behçet syndrome:** National Organization for Rare Disorders (NORD); American Behçet's Disease Association; Arthritis Foundation; J.D. O'Duffy, M.D., Mayo Clinic Behçet's Clinic; NIH/National Arthritis and Musculoskeletal and Skin Diseases Information Clearinghouse; .

**References**

HLA Antigen Familial Study in Complete Behçet's Syndrome Affecting Three Sisters: J.S. Villaneuva; An. Rheum. Dis., February 1993, vol. 52(2), pp. 155–157.

Miscellaneous Vasculitic Syndromes Including Behçet's Disease and Central Nervous System Vasculitis: N.B. Allen; Curr. Opin. Rheumatol., January 1993, vol. 5(1), pp. 51–56.

Cecil Textbook of Medicine, 19th ed.: J.B. Wyngaarden, et al., eds.; W.B. Saunders Company, 1992, p. 1550.

Low Dose Cyclosporin A Versus Pulsed Cyclophosphamide in Behçet's Syndrome: A Single Masked Trial: Y. Ozyazgan; Br. J. Ophthalmol., April 1992, vol. 76(4), pp. 241–243.

Mendelian Inheritance in Man, 10th ed.: V.A. McKusick; The Johns Hopkins University Press, 1992, pp. 142–143.

Nelson Textbook of Pediatrics, 14th ed.: R.E. Behrman, ed.-in-chief; W.B. Saunders Company, 1992, pp. 636–637.

The Repetitive Vascular Catastrophes of Behçet's Disease: A Case Report with Review of the Literature: A. Sherif, et al.; Ann. Vasc. Surg., January 1992, vol. 6(1), pp. 85–89.

Medical and Surgical Treatment of Seronegative Spondyloarthropathi: F. Kozin; Curr. Opin. Rheumatol., August 1991, vol. 3(4), pp. 592–596.

Ophthalmology. Principles and Concepts, 7th ed.: Frank W. Newell; Mosby Year Book, 1991, pp. 300, 334–335.

Systemic Lupus Erythematosus, Dermatomyositis, Scleroderma, Vasculopathies, and Other Connective Tissue Disorders in Children: L.B. Tucker; Curr. Opin. Rheumatol., October 1991, vol. 3(5), pp. 844–853.

Clinical Ophthalmology, 2nd ed.: J.J. Kanski, ed.; Butterworth-Heinemann, 1990, pp. 148–150.

Cyclosporine in Behçet's Disease Resistant to Conventional Therapy: Laura E. Caspers-Velu, et al.; Ann. Ophthalmol., 1989.

Principles of Neurology, 4th ed.: R.D. Adams and M. Victor, eds.; McGraw-Hill, 1989, pp. 375, 560.

Textbook of Rheumatology, 3rd ed.: W.N. Kelley, et al.; W.B. Saunders Company, 1989, pp. 1209–1214.

# BUERGER DISEASE

**Description** Buerger disease is an occlusive and inflammatory disorder affecting the peripheral blood vessels. The clinical and pathologic manifestations are severe pain, Raynaud phenomenon, venous thrombosis, and ulcerations.

**Synonyms**

    Occlusive Peripheral Vascular Disease
    Thromboangiitis Obliterans

**Signs and Symptoms** Intermediate and small-sized arteries and veins are affected, with chronic inflammation and thrombosis. Major vessels are only occasionally involved.

Coldness in the extremities is usually the first complaint, and pain in the affected areas is nearly intolerable. Digital ulcers may be present, as may hyperhidrosis. Red and tender raised areas abruptly appear in the skin near the valves of superficial veins, resolve gradually over several weeks, and reappear. Remissions and exacerbations up to a month long are typical, with occluded areas eventually outstripping collateral circulation, resulting in ischemia.

In advanced Buerger disease there may be gangrene and intermittent claudications that mimic arteriosclerosis obliterans.

**Etiology** The cause is unknown; however, cigarette smoke seems to be primarily associated. Repeated blunt injury to the hand or fingers may contribute to the development of the disease.

**Epidemiology** Males are affected more often than females in a ratio of 75:1. The greatest incidence is between 20 and 45 years of age, and in men who smoke and are of Jewish or Oriental heritage.

**Related Disorders** See *Arteritis, Giant Cell; Arteritis, Takayasu; Polyarteritis Nodosa; Wegener Granulomatosis.*

**Treatment—Standard** Discontinuing the use of nicotine relieves vasoconstriction and improves circulation. Skin ulcerations should be treated immediately. Calcium channel blockers, pentoxifylline, thromboxane inhibitors, and epoprostenol may relieve symptoms. Surgery has been used to treat the pain but does not change the course.

**Treatment—Investigational** Preganglionic sympathectomy is recommended by some when vasospasm is excessive in advancing thromboangiitis obliterans, but not in mild cases or when gangrene is widespread. Surgical intervention is still under debate.

Revascularization combined with pharmacologic therapy using heparin, urokinase, and PGE1, is being investigated as a means to enhance circulation.

Please contact the agencies listed under Resources, below, for the most current information. Addresses and telephone numbers of these agencies, as well as of individual experts and research centers, may be found in the Master Resources List.

**Resources**

**For more information on Buerger disease:** National Organization for Rare Disorders (NORD); NIH/National Heart, Lung and Blood Institute.

**References**

Buerger's Disease (Thromboangiitis Obliterans): J.W. Joyce; Rheum. Dis. Clin. North Am., 1990, vol. 16, pp. 463–470.

Fate of the Ischemic Limb in Buerger's Disease: T. Ohta, et al.; Br. J. Surg., March 1988, vol. 75(3), pp. 259–262.

Thromboangiitis Obliterans (Buerger's Disease) of the Temporal Arteries: J.T. Lie, et al.; Hum. Path., May 1988, vol. 19(5), pp. 598–602.

Thromboangiitis Obliterans (Buerger's Disease) in a Saphenous Vein Arterial Graft: J.T. Lie; Hum. Path., April 1987, vol. 18(4), pp. 402–404.

# DE BARSEY SYNDROME

**Description** De Barsey syndrome is an inherited disorder whose major features relate to systemic connective tissue anomalies of the skin, muscles, eyes, ears, small joints, long bones, and forehead.

**Synonyms**

Corneal Clouding–Cutis Laxa–Mental Retardation
Cutis Laxa–Growth Deficiency Syndrome
De Barsy–Moens–Diercks Syndrome
Progeroid Syndrome of De Barsey

**Signs and Symptoms** The major characteristic is cutis laxa on areas where the skin is normally loose. Especially noticeable on the face, this disorder gives the patient a mournful or aged appearance. Other symptoms include athetosis; hypotonia; large, prominent ears; cloudy cornea of the eye; frontal bossing; unusual flexibility of the small joints; and short stature.

Infrequently, symptoms may include a partially transparent vein pattern, mental retardation, dislocated joints at birth, cataracts, sparse hair, and thin lips.

**Etiology** De Barsey syndrome is inherited as an autosomal recessive trait.

**Epidemiology** Of the approximately 25 cases reported, males were affected slightly more often than females.

**Related Disorders** See *Cutis Laxa; Ehlers-Danlos Syndrome; Hutchinson-Gilford Syndrome; Pseudoxanthoma Elasticum.*

**Treatment—Standard** Genetic counseling may be of benefit for patients and their families. Other treatment is symptomatic and supportive.

**Treatment—Investigational** Please contact the agencies listed under Resources, below, for the most current information. Addresses and telephone numbers of these agencies, as well as of individual experts and research centers, may be found in the Master Resources List.

**Resources**

**For more information on De Barsey syndrome:** National Organization for Rare Disorders (NORD); NIH/National Arthritis and Musculoskeletal and Skin Diseases Information Clearinghouse; The Arc (a national organization on mental retardation).

**For genetic information and genetic counseling referrals:** March of Dimes Birth Defects Foundation; Alliance of Genetic Support Groups.

**References**

Birth Defects Encyclopedia: M.L. Buyse, ed.-in-chief; Blackwell Scientific Publications, 1990, p. 476.

Mendelian Inheritance in Man, 9th ed.: V.A. McKusick; The Johns Hopkins University Press, 1990, p. 1118.

Syndrome of Congenital Cutis Laxa with Ligamentous Laxity and Delayed Development: Report of a Brother and Sister from Turkey: G. Ogur et al.; Am. J. Med. Genet., September 1990, vol. 37(1), pp. 6–9.

Congenital Cutis Laxa with Retardation of Growth and Development: M.A. Patton et al.; J. Med. Genet., September 1987, vol. 24(9), pp. 556–561.

# DUPUYTREN CONTRACTURE

**Description** Dupuytren contracture commonly involves an abnormal fibrotic process of the palmar fascia that results in flexor contracture of the fingers, pain, and loss of function. Rarely, the feet are affected.

**Signs and Symptoms** Abnormal contractile connective tissues consisting of nodules and bands form in the palmar fascia. Initially, nodular thickening and dimpling of the skin are seen. Further growth of nodules and thickening of fascial cords develop, resulting in contracture. The disorder is usually bilateral, affecting the ring finger most often. Pain may be felt in the fingers and palm. Eventually the contractures may become disabling.

**Etiology** An autosomal dominant inheritance with variable penetrance has been suggested. Dupuytren contracture seems to be associated with several diseases, including Peyronie disease, diabetes mellitus, epilepsy, alcoholism, and rheumatoid arthritis. Injury to the hand has been reported to be a precipitating factor.

**Epidemiology** Adult white males are primarily affected, especially northern Europeans. The disorder is rarely seen in children and does not occur in persons of pure African and Asian heritage. Men afflicted with Peyronie disease may also have Dupuytren contracture.

**Related Disorders** Interphalangeal nodules of new growth of fibrous tissue may occur. They are most likely genetic in origin.

**Treatment—Standard** Pain is treated with analgesics, local heat, and corticosteroid injections into the lesion. Physical therapy is useful for preventing atrophy of the unused hand and forearm muscles. Surgical intervention has been recommended, even early intervention to prevent deformity, but procedures are complicated by such factors as neurovascular involvement within the fibrotic mass, and recurrence of contractures due to remaining abnormal connective tissue bands.

Genetic counseling may be beneficial to some patients and their families.

**Treatment—Investigational** Please contact the agencies listed under Resources, below, for the most current information. Addresses and telephone numbers of these agencies, as well as of individual experts and research centers, may be found in the Master Resources List.

**Resources**

**For more information on Dupuytren contracture:** National Organization for Rare Disorders (NORD); NIH/National Arthritis and Musculoskeletal and Skin Diseases Information Clearinghouse.

**For genetic information and genetic counseling referrals:** March of Dimes Birth Defects Foundation; Alliance of Genetic Support Groups.

**References**

Mendelian Inheritance in Man, 9th ed.: V.A. McKusick; The Johns Hopkins University Press, 1990, pp. 272–273.

Arthritis and Allied Conditions, 11th ed.: D.J. McCarty; Lea and Febiger, 1989, pp. 1475–1477.

Cytogenetic Studies in Dupuytren's Contracture: D.H. Wurster-Hill, et al.; Am. J. Hum. Genet., September 1988, vol. 43(3), pp. 285–292.

Dupuytren's Contracture, Alcohol Consumption, and Chronic Liver Disease: P. Attali, et al.; Arch. Int. Med., June 1987, vol. 146(6), pp. 1065–1067.

Dupuytren's Disease in Blacks: M.V. Makhlouf, et al.; Ann. Plast. Surg., October 1987, vol. 19(4), pp. 334–336.

Salvage of Severe Recurrent Dupuytren's Contracture on the Ring and Small Fingers: H.K. Watson, et al.; J. Hand Surg., March 1987, vol. 12(2), pp. 287–289.

# EHLERS-DANLOS SYNDROMES (EDS)

**Description** EDS comprise a diverse group of inherited systemic connective tissue disorders whose major features relate to the joints and the skin. The various forms are labeled I through X to XI, depending on the categorization.

**Synonyms**

Arthrochalasis Multiplex Congenita

Cutis Hyperelastica

India Rubber Skin

Meekeren-Ehlers-Danlos Syndrome

Van Meekeren I Syndrome

**Signs and Symptoms** The clinical picture varies considerably. Characteristics in general include hyperelastic, fragile skin, hyperextensibility of joints with frequent luxations, a tendency toward bleeding and bruising, soft pseudotumors, calcified cysts and atrophic scars, and visceral anomalies. Intelligence is usually normal. Facial characteristics may be normal in appearance or may include widely spaced eyes with epicanthal folds, a broad nasal bridge, and "lop" ears.

Most striking is the soft, velvety skin that can be pulled away from underlying structures and will then return to its original position. Although hyperelastic, the skin is abnormally fragile, which is reflected in easily formed hematomas and soft pseudotumors. Minor trauma may cause gaping wounds and be difficult to suture, and surgical complications may also arise because of deep-tissue frailty. The elbows, knees, shins, and other bony prominences may have paper-thin, red-brown shiny scars. Legs and forearms may have subcutaneous nodules that move and often calcify. "India rubber men" or "human pretzels" display the abnormal positioning of joint hyperextensibility.

Ocular symptoms include strabismus, which occurs frequently; a blue membrane around the sclera; perforation of the globe; diminished cornea; and myopia with associated glaucoma.

Other characteristics include gastrointestinal hernias and diverticula, and synovial effusion. Premature birth can occur as a result of maternal tissue extensibility and fetal membrane fragility. Congenital hip dislocations and clubfeet are due to the loose-jointedness.

Diagnosis usually can be confirmed by the presence of 2 or more of the following cardinal features: cutaneous hyperelasticity, joint hyperextensibility, easy bruising, atrophic scars and pseudotumors, and calcified subcutaneous cysts.

**Etiology** Ehlers-Danlos syndromes are inherited as autosomal dominant, autosomal recessive, or X-linked recessive traits.

**Epidemiology** The syndromes are most prevalent among white persons of European ancestry but may occur in dark-skinned individuals. Men and women are equally affected. Joint and skin symptoms most often are seen at an early age, but in some cases are not evident until adulthood.

**Treatment—Standard** Treatment is essentially supportive. Care should be taken to avoid lacerations and trauma to the joints. Homeostasis must be maintained during surgical procedures, and any time suturing is required, tissue tension should be minimized. Careful obstetric supervision must be observed during pregnancy and delivery to prevent premature birth and hemorrhaging.

**Treatment—Investigational** Researchers at the Washington State University Department of Veterinary Microbiology and Pathology have identified cats and dogs with certain types of Ehlers-Danlos syndrome, and are studying the biochemical defects that cause the syndrome.

Genetic linkage studies are under way to determine if Ehlers-Danlos X-linked and Menkes syndrome, both of which display problems with copper metabolism, are located on the same gene. Affected families who want to participate in the studies should contact Dr. Yang (510-596-6916) or Dr. Packman (415-476-4337).

Please contact the agencies listed under Resources, below, for the most current information. Addresses and telephone numbers of these agencies, as well as of individual experts and research centers, may be found in the Master Resources List.

**Resources**

**For more information on Ehlers-Danlos syndrome:** National Organization for Rare Disorders (NORD); Ehlers-Danlos National Foundation; NIH/National Arthritis and Musculoskeletal and Skin Diseases Information Clearinghouse.

**References**

Mendelian Inheritance in Man, 9th ed.: V.A. McKusick; The Johns Hopkins University Press, 1990, pp. 283–287, 1158–1161, 1589.

Arthritis and Allied Conditions, 11th ed.: D.J. McCarty; Lea and Febiger, 1989, pp. 1337–1340.

Textbook of Rheumatology, 3rd ed.: W.N. Kelley, et al.; W.B. Saunders Company, 1989, pp. 1698–1703.

Cecil Textbook of Medicine, 18th ed.: J.B. Wyngaarden and L.H. Smith, Jr., eds.; W.B. Saunders Company, 1988, pp. 1178–1180.

# EOSINOPHILIC FASCIITIS

**Description** Eosinophilic fasciitis is characterized by inflammation and loss of elasticity in the fascial tissues of the hands, arms, legs, and feet.

**Synonyms**

Diffuse Fasciitis with Eosinophilia

Eosinophilic Syndrome

Shulman Syndrome

**Signs and Symptoms** Pain, swelling, and inflammation of the skin, which can assume an orange-peel (peau d'orange) appearance, are some early manifestations. The arms and forearms are affected more often than the thighs and legs. Trunk involvement occurs in approximately 50 percent of reported cases, but the face is usually spared. Arm and leg movements gradually become restricted. Tenosynovitis often leads to contractures of the fingers and to carpal tunnel syndrome. Fatigue, weight loss, myalgia, and arthritis may also occur. Strenuous physical activity may intensify symptoms.

An association with serious hematologic disorders, such as aplastic anemia, hemolytic anemia, and thrombocytopenia, has been noted in approximately 10 percent of patients. Rarely, cardiac involvement and Sjögren syndrome have been described.

Diagnosis is made by full-thickness biopsy of the affected skin, deep enough to include adjacent muscle fibers. Thickened and inflamed fascia are characteristic. Peripheral eosinophilia is seen in 80 to 90 percent of patients, particularly early in the course of the disease.

**Etiology** The exact cause of eosinophilic fasciitis is unknown. An attack commonly follows strenuous physical activity. Some scientists believe that it may be a variant of scleroderma. Others believe it to be an autoimmune disease.

**Epidemiology** Eosinophilic fasciitis occurs most frequently in white males 40 to 60 years old. Onset is preceded in about 50 percent of cases by unusual physical exertion.

**Related Disorders** See *Scleroderma.*

**Carpal tunnel syndrome** is a common disorder caused by compression of the median nerve in one or both wrists. It is characterized by numbness, tingling, burning, and pain in the hand and wrist. The feeling that the hand has "gone to sleep" is common.

**Treatment—Standard** Many patients respond favorably to corticosteroid therapy, especially prednisone, which may be required for 2 months or longer. Cimetidine may be used as an alternative. The most dramatic response to corticosteroids occurs early in the course of the disease. Spontaneous and sometimes complete remission may occur following an interval of 2 to 5 years. Corticosteroid therapy may not be completely successful, and recurrence of the disorder has been observed after discontinuation of therapy. Unfavorable responses to corticosteroid therapy usually indicate the presence of another disorder, such as aplastic anemia, thrombocytopenia, hemolytic anemia, or Hodgkin disease. Physical therapy is important in the prevention and treatment of limb stiffness and contractures.

**Treatment—Investigational** Please contact the agencies listed under Resources, below, for the most current information. Addresses and telephone numbers of these agencies, as well as of individual experts and research centers, may be found in the Master Resources List.

**Resources**

**For more information on eosinophilic fasciitis:** National Organization for Rare Disorders (NORD); NIH/National Arthritis and Musculoskeletal and Skin Diseases Information Clearinghouse; Centers for Disease Control.

**References**

Eosinophilic Fasciitis in a Pair of Siblings: G.T. Thomson, et al.; Arthritis Rheum., January 1989, vol. 32(1), pp. 96–99.

Cecil Textbook of Medicine, 18th ed.: J.B. Wyngaarden and L.H. Smith, Jr., eds.; W.B. Saunders Company, 1988, p. 2021.

Eosinophilic Faciitis: Clinical Spectrum and Therapeutic Response in 52 Cases: S. Lakhanpal, et al.; Semin. Arthritis Rheum., May 1988, vol. 17(4), pp. 221–231.

Internal Medicine, 2nd ed.: J.H. Stein, ed.-in-chief; Little, Brown and Company, 1987, pp. 1294–1296.

# FAMILIAL MEDITERRANEAN FEVER (FMF)

**Description** The salient features of FMF are recurrent attacks of fever accompanied by self-limiting peritonitis, pleuritis, and, sometimes, arthritis.

**Synonyms**

  Armenian Syndrome
  Benign Paroxysmal Peritonitis
  Familial Paroxysmal Polyserositis
  Periodic Amyloid Syndrome
  Periodic Peritonitis Syndrome
  Recurrent Polyserositis
  Reimann Periodic Disease
  Reimann Syndrome
  Siegel-Cattan-Mamou Syndrome

**Signs and Symptoms** Symptoms of recurrent FMF attacks typically include fever and polyserositis, which causes severe abdominal and pleuritic pain. The abdominal pain may mimic appendicitis. The abdominal attacks generally last up to 24 hours but may continue for 4 days. Almost three-quarters of patients have attacks of arthritis that are exquisitely painful and accompanied by some swelling and by limitation of motion. They usually end within 7 days, with joint function restored, but can continue for several weeks or months. There may be painful, erythematous, and swollen skin lesions on the lower legs. Some patients experience depression and other psychological difficulties.

*Amyloidosis* occurs in almost half of those patients who are Sephardic Jews, but less often in those of other cultures. Amyloid nephropathy may be fatal. Intestinal obstruction and meningitis may be complications.

**Etiology** The disease is inherited as an autosomal recessive trait. In non-Ashkenazic Jews, the gene responsible is located on the short arm of chromosome 16. The exact biochemical or structural defect is unknown. An inborn metabolic error or an endocrine defect is suspected.

**Epidemiology** The disease generally begins in childhood or in the teen years and continues intermittently throughout life. Males are affected more often than females, and the majority of those affected have their origins in the Mediterranean Sea region and include Sephardic and Iraqi Jews, Turks, Levantine Arabs, and Armenians. Approximately half of those affected with FMF have no known family history of the disease.

**Related Disorders** *Amyloidosis* is associated with FMF as a secondary characteristic and is not necessary for diagnosis.

**Treatment—Standard** Although the reason is not understood, colchicine seems to prevent attacks of FMF as well as amyloidosis. If an attack is ongoing, large doses of colchicine will halt the symptoms. Corticosteroids have not proved effective. Narcotics should be used judiciously because the intense pain necessitates large doses.

If the kidneys are involved by amyloidosis, renal dialysis or transplantation may be necessary.

**Treatment—Investigational** Please contact the agencies listed under Resources, below, for the most current information. Addresses and telephone numbers of these agencies, as well as of individual experts and research centers, may be found in the Master Resources List.

**Resources**

**For more information on familial Mediterranean fever:** National Organization for Rare Disorders (NORD); NIH/National Institute of Digestive Diseases Information Clearinghouse.

**For genetic information and genetic counseling referrals:** March of Dimes Birth Defects Foundation; Alliance of Genetic Support Groups.

**References**

Familial Mediterranean Fever (FMF) in Moroccan Jews: Demonstration of a Founder Effect by Extended Haplogype Analysis: I. Aksentijevich, et al.; Am. J. Hum. Genet., September 1993, vol. 53(3), pp. 644–651.

Case Report: Severe Pyoderma Associated with Familial Mediterranean Fever: Favorable Response to Colchicine in Three Patients: G. Lugassy, et al.; Am. J. Med. Sci., July 1992, vol. 304(1), pp. 29–31.

Cecil Textbook of Medicine, 19th ed.: J.B. Wyngaarden, et al., eds.; W.B. Saunders Company, 1992, pp. 1140–1141.

Mendelian Inheritance in Man, 10th ed.: V.A. McKusick; The Johns Hopkins University Press, 1992, pp. 1518–1520.

Twin Studies in Familial Mediterranean Fever: M. Shohat, et al.; Am. J. Med. Genet., September 1992, vol. 44(2), pp. 179–182.

Birth Defects Encyclopedia: M.L. Buyse, ed.-in-chief; Blackwell Scientific Publications, 1990, p. 733.

Dictionary of Medical Syndromes, 3rd ed.: S.I. Magalini, et al., eds.; J.B. Lippincott Company, 1990, pp. 813–814.

Arthritis and Allied Conditions, 11th ed.: D.J. McCarty; Lea and Febiger, 1989, pp. 995–998.

# FELTY SYNDROME

**Description** Felty syndrome is an unusual complication of rheumatoid arthritis (**RA**) in which patients have splenomegaly and granulocytopenia. The syndrome occurs in approximately 1 percent of patients with RA.

**Synonyms**

Splenomegaly with Rheumatoid Arthritis

**Signs and Symptoms** Characteristics include leukopenia associated with recurrent infections; thrombocytopenia; splenomegaly; and a yellowish-brown skin discoloration over the lower extremities. Leg ulcers, stomatitis, anemia, vasculitis, swelling of lymph nodes, and fever also may occur.

**Etiology** The cause of the granulocytopenia in patients with Felty syndrome is not clear at this time. It is believed to be multifactorial, involving antigranulocyte antibodies and/or other unknown immunologic disturbance. The granulocytopenia is associated with frequent infections, most commonly involving the skin and respiratory tract.

**Epidemiology** The syndrome seems to occur mostly in middle-aged and elderly women, although it has been reported in men as well.

**Related Disorders Rheumatoid arthritis** usually occurs in middle-aged and older persons, mostly women, but can also affect children. It is characterized by pain, stiffness, swelling, and joint deformities. The hands, wrists, knees, feet, ankles, and shoulders are most commonly affected. Felty syndrome occurs in about 1 percent of patients with RA.

**Treatment—Standard** Splenectomy for serious or recurrent infections arising from Felty syndrome is successful in about half of all patients. Other therapies are those used for RA, such as anti-inflammatory drugs, including gold, penicillamine, or methotrexate. Anemia associated with Felty syndrome can be treated with blood transfusions or erythropoietin. The prognosis is generally uncertain and depends on several variables, including the general health of the patient and the combination of symptoms occurring in a patient. Patients with Felty syndrome have an increased risk of developing non-Hodgkin lymphoma.

**Treatment—Investigational** Lithium has been used experimentally to treat Felty syndrome. Preliminary studies appear positive.

Please contact the agencies listed under Resources, below, for the most current information. Addresses and telephone numbers of these agencies, as well as of individual experts and research centers, may be found in the Master Resources List.

**Resources**

**For more information on Felty syndrome:** National Organization for Rare Disorders (NORD); Arthritis Foundation; NIH/National Arthritis and Musculoskeletal and Skin Diseases Information Clearinghouse.

**References**

Lithium Carbonate Therapy in Severe Felty's Syndrome: M.J. Mant, et al.; Arch. Intern. Med., 1986, vol. 146, pp. 277–280.
Felty's Syndrome in a Child: A.M. Rosenberg, et al.; J. Rheumatol., December 1984, vol. 11(6), pp. 835–837.


# FORESTIER DISEASE

**Description** Forestier disease is one of the many forms of osteoarthritis in which bone spurs occur along the spine without breakdown of spinal discs.

**Synonyms**

> Diffuse Idiopathic Skeletal Hyperostosis (DISH)
> Spinal Diffuse Idiopathic Skeletal Hyperostosis
> Vertebral Ankylosing Hyperostosis

**Signs and Symptoms** Bony overgrowth, or "spurs," develop in the thoracic and lumbar regions of the spine. Stiffness, mild discomfort, and limitation of motion may result. Other sites include tendon osseous junctions of peripheral joints. Patients may feel pain in the affected area(s), and nerve compression or entrapment may cause irritation. Uncommonly, diffuse idiopathic skeletal hyperostosis may cause dysphagia or dysphonia related to compression by large, bulky spurs.

**Etiology** The exact cause of Forestier disease is unknown. Aging, trauma, or playing sports may cause the bony overgrowths to occur. Disorders that involve disturbances in cartilage metabolism, such as diabetes mellitus, acromegaly, or certain inherited connective tissue disorders, may be associated (see *Acromegaly*).

**Epidemiology** Forestier disease is a common subtype of osteoarthritis. It generally affects men and women over the age of 50.

**Related Disorders** See *Ankylosing Spondylitis.*

**Osteoarthritis** is a common degenerative joint disease characterized by loss of cartilage, deformities of bones and joints, and thickening of the surrounding ligaments and membranes at the joint margins with areas of bony outgrowths (osteophytes or spurs). Osteoarthritis develops when cartilage repair does not keep pace with cartilage degeneration. It may occur as a result of trauma to the bone, aging, obesity, or other underlying diseases that cause damage to the joint or its cartilage, such as congenital dislocation of the hip or rheumatoid arthritis.

**Spondylosis** is osteoarthritis of the spine. It is usually associated with deterioration of the spinal disks in between the vertebrae; this does not occur in Forestier disease.

**Rheumatoid arthritis** is characterized by anorexia; fatigue; painful, inflamed, and deformed joints; and early morning stiffness chiefly in the hands, knees, feet, jaw, and cervical spine. Once affected, a patient's joints remain painful or uncomfortable for weeks, months, or even years.

**Treatment—Standard** Testing includes imaging techniques such as x-rays and CT scans. Treatment may include nonsteroidal anti-inflammatory drugs. Surgery to correct deformities may be indicated. Other treatment is symptomatic and supportive.

**Treatment—Investigational** Please contact the agencies listed under Resources, below, for the most current information. Addresses and telephone numbers of these agencies, as well as of individual experts and research centers, may be found in the Master Resources List.

**Resources**

**For more information on Forestier disease:** National Organization for Rare Disorders (NORD); NIH/National Arthritis and Musculoskeletal and Skin Diseases Information Clearinghouse; Arthritis Foundation; Ankylosing Spondylitis Association; Coalition of Heritable Disorders of Connective Tissue.

**References**

Diffuse Idiopathic Skeletal Hyperostosis Causing Acute Thoracic Myelopathy: A Case Report and Discussion: A. Reisner, et al.; Neurosurgery, March 1990, vol. 26(3), pp. 507–511.

Diffuse Idiopathic Skeletal Hyperostosis (DISH) of the Spine: A Cause of Back Pain? A Controlled Study: P. Schlapbach, et al.; Br. J. Rheumatol. August 1989, vol. 28(4), pp. 299–303.

Dysphagia Due to Diffuse Idiopathic Skeletal Hyperostosis: W. J. Shergy, et al.; Am. Fam. Physician., April 1989, vol. 39(4), pp. 149–152.

Cecil Textbook of Medicine, 18th ed.: J.B. Wyngaarden and L.H. Smith, Jr., eds.; W.B. Saunders Company, 1988, pp. 2039–2041.

Dysphonia Caused by Forestier's Disease: I. Gay and J. Elidan; Ann. Otol. Rhinol. Laryngol., May–June 1988, vol. 97(3 pt. 1), pp. 275–276.

Diffuse Idiopathic Skeletal Hyperostosis with Dysphagia: A Review: E. Eviatar and M. Harell; J. Laryngol. Otol., June 1987, vol. 101(6), pp. 627–632.

Radiographic, Clinical, and Histopathologic Evaluation with Surgical Treatment of Forestier's Disease: J. G. Barsamian, et al.; Oral Surg. Oral Med. Oral Pathol., February 1985, vol. 59(2), pp. 136–141.

# GORHAM DISEASE

**Description** Gorham disease is a bone disorder characterized by bone loss associated with angiomatous proliferation.

**Synonyms**

Disappearing Bone Disease
Gorham-Stout Syndrome
Gorham Syndrome
Idiopathic Massive Osteolysis
Massive Gorham Osteolysis
Massive Osteolysis
Morbus Gorham-Stout Disease
Progressive Massive Osteolysis
Vanishing Bone Disease

**Signs and Symptoms** Bone loss may occur in such places as the hand, arm, shoulder, ribs, hemipelvis, or femur. When the lower jaw, upper jaw, tooth sockets, or other bones in the head or neck are affected, possible symptoms are pain, loose teeth, fractures, facial deformity, and recurrent meningitis. Fibrous tissue appears in areas of bone loss. Fractures promote the progression of the disease, and angiomas cause swelling. Some patients experience chylous pleural effusion in conjunction with Gorham disease.

**Etiology** Gorham disease is idiopathic.

**Epidemiology** Males are affected slightly more often than females in all the age groups.

**Related Disorders** See *Osteonecrosis; Gaucher Disease; Kienboeck Disease.*

**Treatment—Standard** Testing for Gorham disease includes x-rays and CT scans. Diagnosis can be made by biopsy. Gorham disease may be treated with radiation, surgery, bone grafting, and drugs. Pleural effusion may be treated by draining. Other treatment is symptomatic and supportive.

**Treatment—Investigational** Please contact the agencies listed under Resources, below, for the most current information. Addresses and telephone numbers of these agencies, as well as of individual experts and research centers, may be found in the Master Resources List.

**Resources**

**For more information on Gorham disease:** National Organization for Rare Disorders (NORD); NIH/National Arthritis and Musculoskeletal and Skin Diseases Information Clearinghouse.

**References**

Radiotherapy of Morbus Gorham-Stout: The Biological Value of Low Irradiation Dose: L. Handl-Zeller, et al.; Br. J. Radiol., March 1990, vol. 63(747), pp. 206–208.

A 20-Year Follow-up Study of a Case of Surgically Treated Massive Osteolysis: S. Turra, et al.; Clin. Orthop., January 1990, vol. 250, pp. 297–302.

Gorham Disease Affecting the Maxillofacial Skeleton: Y. Anavi, et al.; Head Neck, November–December 1989, vol. 11(6), pp. 550–557.

Massive Osteolysis of the Femur (Gorham Disease): A Case Report and Review of the Literature: A.A. Mendez, et al.; J. Pediatr. Orthop. September–October 1989, vol. 9(5), pp. 604–608.

Cecil Textbook of Medicine, 18th ed.: J.B. Wyngaarden and L.H. Smith, Jr., eds.; W.B. Saunders Company, 1988, pp. 1474–1475.

Cytochemical Localization of Alkaline and Acid Phosphatase in Human Vanishing Bone Disease: G.R. Dickson, et al.; Histochemistry, 1987, vol. 87(6), pp. 569–572.

"Disappearing Bone Disease" in the Hand;. R.S. Carneiro, et al.; J. Hand Surg. [Am.], July 1987, vol. 12(4), pp. 629–634.

Gorham's Syndrome: A Case Report and Review of the Literature: N.D. Choma, et al.; Am. J. Med., December 1987, vol. 83(6), pp. 1151–1156.

Massive Gorham Osteolysis of the Right Hemipelvis Complicated by Chylothorax: Report of a Case in a 9-Year-Old Boy Successfully Treated by Pleurodesis: N. Hejgaard, et al.; J. Pediatr. Orthop., January–February 1987, vol. 7(1), pp. 96–99.

# HAJDU-CHENEY SYNDROME

**Description** Hajdu-Cheney syndrome is a disorder of the connective tissue. The most distinctive features are ulcerating lesions on the palms of the hands and soles of the feet accompanied by acro-osteolysis. Abnormal development appears in the bones, joints, and teeth. A decrease in bone mass and changes in the skull and jawbone are also features of this syndrome.

**Synonyms**

      Acro-Osteolysis with Osteoporosis and Changes in Skull and Mandible

      Arthro-Dento-Osteodysplasia

      Cheney Syndrome

**Signs and Symptoms** The main symptoms include acro-osteolysis; wormian bones; a small, recessed mandible; osteoporosis; a thick depression in the back of the head; persistent open joint between the bones of the cranium; loose joints; and early loss of teeth. Other features are short stature (usually due to collapse of the spinal column); small or missing frontal sinus; unequal growth of the long bones that may cause dislocations, bowing, or outward twisting of the knees; dislocation of the patella; high, narrow palate; hernia; projecting ears; a deep voice; distinctive facial features (a short neck, thick eyebrows, coarse hair, low-set ears); hearing loss; and syndactyly.

**Etiology** The majority of cases are idiopathic. Multiple cases in one family are thought to be inherited as an autosomal dominant trait.

**Epidemiology** Of the 30 reported cases in the United States and western and central Europe, males and females were affected in equal numbers.

**Related Disorders** See *Gaucher Disease; Gorham Disease; Kienboeck Disease; Legg-Calvé-Perthes Syndrome; Osteonecrosis.*

**Treatment—Standard** Patients with Hajdu-Cheney syndrome should have regular neurologic checkups in order to detect any complications due to bone abnormalities. Hearing and sight should be checked after confirmation of diagnosis. Occupational and physical therapy may be helpful in preventing developmental delay and in improving proper muscle and skeletal function. Surgery and bone grafting may be indicated for patients with severe tissue destruction. Genetic counseling may be of benefit for patients and their families. Other treatment is symptomatic and supportive.

**Treatment—Investigational** Please contact the agencies listed under Resources, below, for the most current information. Addresses and telephone numbers of these agencies, as well as of individual experts and research centers, may be found in the Master Resources List.

**Resources**

    **For more information on Hajdu-Cheney syndrome:** National Organization for Rare Disorders (NORD); Coalition of Heritable Disorders of Connective Tissue; NIH/National Arthritis and Musculoskeletal and Skin Diseases Information Clearinghouse.

    **For genetic information and genetic counseling referrals:** March of Dimes Birth Defects Foundation; Alliance of Genetic Support Groups.

**References**

    Birth Defects Encyclopedia: M.L. Buyse, ed.-in-chief; Blackwell Scientific Publications, 1990, pp. 827–829.

    Cervical Instability As an Unusual Manifestation of Hajdu-Cheney Syndrome of Acroosteolysis: D. Herscovici, Jr., et al.; Clin. Orthop., June 1990, vol. 255, pp. 111–116.

    High Turnover Osteoporosis in Acro-Osteolysis (Hajdu-Cheney Syndrome): V. Nunziata, et al.; J. Endocrinol. Invest., March 1990, vol. 13(3), pp. 251–255.

    Mendelian Inheritance in Man, 9th ed.: V.A. McKusick; The Johns Hopkins University Press, 1990, pp. 17–18.

    A 20-Year Follow-up Study of a Case of Surgically Treated Massive Osteolysis: S. Turra, et al.; Clin. Orthop., January 1990, vol. 250, pp. 297–302.

# KAWASAKI SYNDROME

**Description** Kawasaki syndrome is a childhood illness characterized by fever, lymphadenopathy, rash, polyarteritis, and vasculitis.

**Synonyms**

      Mucocutaneous Lymph Node Syndrome

**Signs and Symptoms** The fever typically begins abruptly and lasts for about 2 weeks but may be sustained over 1 month. Other symptoms occurring in the first 5 days of Kawasaki disease include bilateral conjunctivitis, stomatitis, cervical adenopathy, and rash. The palms of the hands and soles of the feet become erythematous, and in about 7 days after onset the hands and feet are edematous; after a few more days, the ends of the fingers and toes are desquamative. A painful arthritis may occur at this time, usually symmetric and involving large and small joints. Thrombocytosis may develop about 10 days after onset of fever and not disappear for several weeks.

Cardiac complications occur in about one-third to one-half of cases and include aneurysms, myocarditis, coronary vasculitis, pericardial effusions, arrhythmias, and, rarely, congestive heart failure and valvular disease.

Other complications include diarrhea, vomiting, hepatitis, gallbladder disease, cough, depression, and seizures.

**Etiology** The exact cause of Kawasaki syndrome is not fully understood. Research is under way to determine if the disease is caused by staphylococcus or streptococcus bacteria or by special toxins released by them.

Recent research suggests that the syndrome may be caused by a retrovirus. The virus has not yet been identified, but antibodies to retroviruses have been found in the white blood cells of Kawasaki patients.

**Epidemiology** The disease is seen predominantly in children under the age of 5. Extremely rare occurrences have been reported in patients in their 20s. There is a slight prevalence of males over females, with serious complications found more often in males. Kawasaki syndrome has been reported throughout the world.

**Related Disorders** See *Hand-Foot-Mouth Syndrome.*

**Treatment—Standard** Early high-dose intravenous gamma globulin along with low-dose aspirin may reduce the development of coronary artery complications and will reduce fever and inflammation of the respiratory tract mucous membranes, central nervous system, joints, and skin. Treatment with corticosteroids is not recommended.

The duration of aspirin therapy for prevention of coronary aneurysm is relative to the disease course and usually lasts over a period of several months. With the onset of an aneurysm, aspirin therapy is continued as an anticoagulant, and bypass surgery may be indicated.

Close long-term follow-up is essential. Frequent electrocardiogram evaluation is recommended. Two-dimensional echocardiography with appropriate coronary angiography is suggested if coronary aneurysm is suspected.

**Treatment—Investigational** The benefits of a single high dose of intravenous immune globulin with aspirin as compared to several low doses are being studied for initial treatment of Kawasaki syndrome.

Current researchers of the disease include Jane W. Newburger, M.D., of the Children's Hospital in Boston, Massachusetts, and Drs. Fred Rosen and James Gamble at the Harvard Medical School.

Please contact the agencies listed under Resources, below, for the most current information. Addresses and telephone numbers of these agencies, as well as of individual experts and research centers, may be found in the Master Resources List.

**Resources**

**For more information on Kawasaki syndrome:** National Organization for Rare Disorders (NORD); NIH/National Institute of Allergy and Infectious Diseases; Centers for Disease Control.

**References**

Adult Coronary Aneurysms Related to Kawasaki Disease: B. Albat, et al., J. Cardiovasc Surg., February 1994, vol. 35(1), pp. 57–60.

Guidelines for Long-Term Management of Patients with Kawasaki Disease: Report from the Committee on Rheumatic Fever, Endocarditis, and Kawasaki Disease, Council on Cardiovascular Disease in the Young, American Heart Association: A.S. Dajani, et al.; Circulation, February 1994, vol. 89(2), pp. 916–922.

Long-Term Outcome of Myocardial Revascularization in Patients with Kawasaki Coronary Artery Disease: A Multicenter Cooperative Study: S. Kitamura, et al.; J. Thorac Cardiovasc. Surg., March 1994, vol. 107(3), pp. 663–673, discussion 673–674.

Management of Kawasaki Disease in the British Isles: R. Dhilon, et al.; Arch Dis. Child, December 1993, vol. 69(6), pp. 631–636, discussion 637–638.

Biologically Active Extracellular Products of Oral Viridans Streptococci and the Aetiology of Kawasaki Disease: H. Ohkuni, et al.; J. Med. Microbiol., November 1993, vol. 39(5), pp. 352–362.

Kawasaki Disease: D.Y. Leung; Curr. Opin. Rheumatol., January 1993, vol. 5(1), pp. 41–50.

Kawasaki Disease: S. Nadel; Curr. Opin. Pediatr., February 1993, vol. 5(1), pp. 29–34.

Kawasaki Disease and Its Cardiac Sequelai: R.P. Sundel, et al.; Hosp. Pract., November 1993, vol. 28(11), pp. 51–54, 57–60, 64–66.

Kawasaki Disease: Early Presentation to the Otolaryngologist: M.A. Seichshnaydre, et al.; Otolaryngol. Head Neck Surg., April 1993, vol. 108(4), pp. 344–347.

Toxic Shock Syndrome Toxin-Secreting Staphylococcus Aureus in Kawasaki Syndrome: D.Y.M. Leung, et al.; Lancet, December 1993, vol. 342(8884), pp. 1385–1388.

Cecil Textbook of Medicine, 19th ed.: J.B. Wyngaarden, et al., eds.; W.B. Saunders Company, 1992, pp. 981, 2301.

Effect of High Doses of Intravenously Administered Immune Globulin on Natural Killer Cell Activity in Peripheral Blood: R.W. Finberg, et al.; J. Pediatr., March 1992, vol. 120(3), pp. 376–380.

Infectious Diseases: S.L. Gorbach, ed.; W.B. Saunders Company, 1992, pp. 1370–1374.

Nelson Textbook of Pediatrics, 14th ed.: R.E. Behrman, ed.-in-chief; W.B. Saunders Company, 1992, pp. 629–631.

Harrison's Principles of Internal Medicine, 12th ed.: J.D. Wilson, et al., eds.; McGraw-Hill, 1991, pp. 1462–1463.

Dictionary of Medical Syndromes, 3rd ed.: S.I. Magalini, et al., eds.; J.B. Lippincott Company, 1990, p. 491.

Kawasaki Syndrome: D.W. Wortmann and A.M. Nelson; Rheum. Dis. Clin. North Am., 1990, vol. 16, pp. 363–375.

The Heart, 3rd ed.: E. Braunwald; W.B. Saunders Company, 1988, pp. 1014–1016.

# KIENBOECK DISEASE

**Description** In Kienboeck disease, derangements of the lunate bone, acquired during inflammation or injury, occur that may limit the extent of motion in the wrist.

**Synonyms**
     Lunatomalacia

**Signs and Symptoms** Degenerative changes in the lunate result in softening, deterioration, fragmentation, or compression of the affected bone. Symptoms are recurrent tenderness and pain, and thickening, swelling, and stiffness of the soft tissues overlying the lunate. Range of motion in the wrist usually is compromised. Formation of new bone will resolve the disorder.

Diagnostic procedures include arthroscopy, CT scan, and radiography.

**Etiology** Kienboeck disease is caused by inflammation or injury to the wrist.

**Epidemiology** Onset is usually in childhood, and females are affected more often than males.

**Related Disorders.**

**Carpal tunnel syndrome,** a peripheral nerve entrapment neuropathy, results from compression of the median nerve as it passes through the carpal tunnel at the wrist. Pain, numbness, and paresthesias in the wrist and areas of the hand supplied by the median nerve are characteristic. With timely treatment, the prognosis in most cases is favorable.

**Juvenile osteoporosis** is a porous or atrophic condition of the bony tissue that may cause fractures or pain in various bones, including the wrist. Onset is before or during puberty, with spontaneous remission occurring within several years. The cause is unknown.

**Sudeck atrophy,** or posttraumatic osteoporosis, is acute atrophy of bone tissue following a seemingly minor injury, such as a sprain. Bones in the wrists and ankles are the most frequently affected.

**Treatment—Standard** Surgical intervention for Kienboeck disease may be necessary. Inflammation may require the use of drugs. Other treatment is symptomatic and supportive.

**Treatment—Investigational** Please contact the agencies listed under Resources, below, for the most current information. Addresses and telephone numbers of these agencies, as well as of individual experts and research centers, may be found in the Master Resources List.

**Resources**

**For more information on Kienboeck disease:** National Organization for Rare Disorders (NORD); NIH/National Arthritis and Musculoskeletal and Skin Diseases Information Clearinghouse.

**References**

Excision of the Lunate in Kienboeck's Disease: Results After Long-Term Follow-Up: H. Kawai, et al.; J. Bone Joint Surg. Br., March 1988, vol. 70(2), pp. 287–292.

Ulna-Minus Variance and Kienboeck's Disease: P.A. Nathan, et al.; J. Hand Surg., September 1987, vol. 12(5), pp. 777–778.

# KÖHLER DISEASE

**Description** Köhler disease is a foot disorder in which progressive degeneration of the navicular bone causes pain and swelling of the foot.

**Synonyms**
     Navicular Osteochondrosis

**Signs and Symptoms** The affected foot is swollen and particularly tender along the length of the arch. Walking and other weight-bearing activities cause further discomfort and a limp. The bone eventually regenerates and heals itself.

**Etiology** The cause is unknown. The disease is apparently not hereditary or caused by injury.

**Epidemiology** Males are affected more often than females. The disease usually occurs in children between the ages of 3 and 5.

**Related Disorders** See *Tarsal Tunnel Syndrome; Erythromelalgia.*

**Burning feet syndrome (Gopalan syndrome)** is marked by burning, aching pain and cramps in the soles of the feet and sometimes palms of the hands. A deficiency of a B vitamin is suspected.

**Freiberg disease** (see also *Osteonecrosis),* characterized by foot pain that is exacerbated by weight-bearing or walking, is caused by progressive osteonecrosis of the head of the 2nd metatarsal. Treatment may require surgery.

**Treatment—Standard** Diagnosis of Köhler disease can be made by x-ray. Recovery is aided by avoiding weight-bearing on the affected foot, or supporting the weight-bearing with short-leg plaster casts or specially designed shoes. Recovery usually occurs in less than 1 year, rarely taking more than 2 years. Patients permanently regain full function of the foot.

**Treatment—Investigational** Please contact the agencies listed under Resources, below, for the most current information. Addresses and telephone numbers of these agencies, as well as of individual experts and research centers, may be found in the Master Resources List.

**Resources**

**For more information on Köhler disease:** National Organization for Rare Disorders (NORD); NIH/National Arthritis and Musculoskeletal and Skin Diseases Information Clearinghouse.

**References**

Dorsiflexion Osteotomy in Freiberg's Disease: P. Kinnard and R. Lirette; Foot Ankle Int., April 1989, vol. 9(5), pp. 226–231.

Freiberg's Infraction of the Second Metatarsal Head with Formation of Multiple Loose Bodies: G. Scartozzi, et al.; J. Foot Surg., May–June 1989, vol. 28(3), pp. 195–199.

Köhler's Osteochondrosis of the Tarsal Navicular: Case Report with Twenty-Eight Year Follow-Up: K.M. Devine and R.E. Van Demark, Sr.; S.D.J. Med., September 1989, vol. 42(9), pp. 5–6.

Köhler's Disease of the Tarsal Navicular: Long-Term Follow-up of Twelve Cases: E. Ippolito, et al.; J. Ped. Orth., August 1984, vol. 4(4), pp. 416–417.

Köhler's Disease of the Tarsal Navicular: G.A. Williams and H.R. Cowell; Clin. Orth., July–August 1981, vol. 158, pp. 53–58.

# LEGG-CALVÉ-PERTHES SYNDROME

**Description** Legg-Calvé-Perthes syndrome affects the hip joint, with abnormalities in bone growth during the early years that may result in permanent deformity of the hip joint in young adulthood.

**Synonyms**

Coxa Plana

Slipped Capital Femoral Epiphysis

**Signs and Symptoms** Without warning, mild aching in the hip may occur, followed by inability to move the affected leg normally. Hip pain may increase in intensity and muscle spasms develop. The bone may shorten enough to cause an obvious limp. Osteonecrosis of the femoral head may be seen in persons with Legg-Calvé-Perthes syndrome.

**Etiology** The syndrome is thought to be inherited as an autosomal dominant trait. Damage to the early developing hip joint bone is caused by reduced vascular supply to the femur.

**Epidemiology** Onset of the disorder is between 6 and 12 years of age. Males are affected more often than females.

**Related Disorders Juvenile (rheumatoid) arthritis** may have symptoms similar to Legg-Calvé-Perthes syndrome.

**Treatment—Standard** Anti-inflammatory medication and analgesics are the primary choices for patient management. Non-weight-bearing with crutch walking may be necessary for several months. Additional treatment is symptomatic and supportive.

**Treatment—Investigational** Please contact the agencies listed under Resources, below, for the most current information. Addresses and telephone numbers of these agencies, as well as of individual experts and research centers, may be found in the Master Resources List.

**Resources**

**For more information on Legg-Calvé-Perthes syndrome:** National Organization for Rare Disorders (NORD); Arthritis Foundation; NIH/National Arthritis, Musculoskeletal and Skin Diseases Information Clearinghouse.

**For genetic information and genetic counseling referrals:** March of Dimes Birth Defects Foundation; Alliance of Genetic Support Groups.

**References**

Mendelian Inheritance in Man, 9th ed.: V.A. McKusick; The Johns Hopkins University Press, 1990, pp. 563–564.

Legg-Calvé-Perthes Disease in a Family: Genetic or Environmental: M. O'Sullivan, et al.; Clin. Orth., October 1985, vol. 199, pp. 179–181.

Lesions of the Femoral Neck in Legg-Perthes Disease: F.N. Silverman, AJR, June 1985, vol. 144(6), pp. 1249–1254.

Long-Term Follow-up of Legg-Calvé-Perthes Disease: M.P. McAndrew, et al.; J. Bone Joint Surg. Am., July 1984, vol. 66(6), pp. 860–869.

# MARDEN-WALKER SYNDROME

**Description** Marden-Walker syndrome is a connective tissue disorder that is inherited as an autosomal recessive trait.

**Synonyms**

Connective Tissue Disorder, Marden-Walker Type

**Signs and Symptoms** Droopy eyelids, a flat nasal bridge, low-set ears, an abnormal jaw, and a fixed facial position are characteristic. Other features include curvature of the spine causing a hunchback, joint contractures, a cleft or high-arched palate, growth delay, and slow muscle movement.

In addition, a small head circumference, heart abnormalities, irregular sexual and urinary systems, a decrease in bone mass, pectus carinatum or pectus excavatum, a preauricular tag, abnormally small eyes, a short neck, a small mouth, and a low hairline may appear.

The following have all been associated with Marden-Walker syndrome: duodenal bands, pyloric stenosis, loss of appetite, failure of the body to absorb nutrients adequately, stomach pain, and weight loss caused by pancreatic insufficiency.

**Etiology** Marden-Walker syndrome is inherited as an autosomal recessive trait.

**Epidemiology** Of the 20 cases reported, males were affected more often than females.

**Related Disorders** See *Cerebro-Oculo-Facio-Skeletal Syndrome.*

**Arthrogryposis multiplex congenita** is a congenital disease characterized by reduced mobility of multiple joints at birth due to proliferation of fibrous tissue. Joint motion of all limbs is limited.

**Schwartz-Jampel syndrome** is characterized by the inability of muscles to relax after contracting (myotonia). Typical are abnormal bone formation and abnormalities of the face and eyes. Other anomalies include short stature, low birth weight, short neck, pectus carinatum, curvature of the spine causing a hunchback, and joint contractures.

**Treatment—Standard** Genetic counseling may be of benefit for patients and their families. Other treatment is symptomatic and supportive.

**Treatment—Investigational** Please contact the agencies listed under Resources, below, for the most current information. Addresses and telephone numbers of these agencies, as well as of individual experts and research centers, may be found in the Master Resources List.

**Resources**

**For more information on Marden-Walker syndrome:** National Organization for Rare Disorders (NORD); Coalition of Heritable Disorders of Connective Tissue; American Cleft Palate Cranial Facial Association; NIH/National Arthritis and Musculoskeletal and Skin Diseases Information Clearinghouse;

**For genetic information and genetic counseling referrals:** March of Dimes Birth Defects Foundation; Alliance of Genetic Support Groups.

**References**

Congenital Myopathy with Oculo-Facial Abnormalities (Marden-Walker Syndrome): N. Linder, et al.; Am. J. Med. Genet., June 1991, vol. 39(4), pp. 377–379.

Birth Defects Encyclopedia: M.L. Buyse, ed.-in-chief; Blackwell Scientific Publications, 1990, pp. 1103–1104.

Expanded Spectrum of Findings in Marden-Walker Syndrome: G.P. Pineda, et al.; Am. J. Med. Genet., August 1990, vol. 36(4), pp. 495–499.

Mendelian Inheritance in Man, 9th ed.: V.A. McKusick; The Johns Hopkins University Press, 1990, p. 1309.

A 26-Month-Old Child with Marden-Walker Syndrome and Pyloric Stenosis: D. Gossage, et al.; Am. J. Med. Genet., April 1987, vol. 26(4), pp. 915–919.

# METATROPHIC DYSPLASIA I

**Description** Metatrophic dysplasia I is characterized by extremely small stature with short arms and legs. Other features include a narrow thorax, short ribs, and kyphoscoliosis, which develops into short trunk dwarfism.

**Synonyms**

> Chondrodystrophy, Hyperplastic
> Dwarfism, Metatrophic
> Metatrophic Dwarfism Syndrome
> Metatrophic Dysplasia

**Signs and Symptoms** Abnormal skeletal development includes short ribs; short, deformed arms and legs; kyphoscoliosis; and extremely short stature. A long, narrow thorax; bulging joints with limited mobility of the knees and hips; and unusually increased extension of the finger joints are typical. An unusually long torso and ensuing short trunk dwarfism due to curvature of the spine are apparent early. Kyphosis is typical.

X-rays show growth insufficiency of the vertebral column, with flattening of vertebrae and often growth insufficiency at the hip and shoulder joints. A hump at the end of the spine is also apparent.

**Etiology** Metatrophic dysplasia I can be inherited as an autosomal dominant or autosomal recessive trait.

**Epidemiology** Males and females are affected in equal numbers.

**Related Disorders** See *Kniest Dysplasia; Morquio Syndrome.*

**Treatment—Standard** Treatment is symptomatic and supportive. When partial dislocation of the cervical vertebrae is present, the joint can be fused together to prevent damage to the cervical part of the spinal cord.

Genetic counseling may be of benefit for patients and their families.

**Treatment—Investigational** Please contact the agencies listed under Resources, below, for the most current information. Addresses and telephone numbers of these agencies, as well as of individual experts and research centers, may be found in the Master Resources List.

**Resources**

   **For more information on metatrophic dysplasia I:** National Organization for Rare Disorders (NORD); Metatrophic Dysplasia Hotline; Magic Foundation for Children's Growth; Human Growth Foundation; NIH/National Institute of Child Health and Human Development; Parents of Dwarfed Children.

   **For genetic information and genetic counseling referrals:** March of Dimes Birth Defects Foundation; Alliance of Genetic Support Groups.

**References**

Birth Defects Encyclopedia: M.L. Buyse, ed.-in-chief; Blackwell Scientific Publications, 1990, pp. 1135–1136.

Mendelian Inheritance in Man, 9th ed.: V.A. McKusick; The Johns Hopkins University Press, 1990, p. 1323.

Odontoid Hypoplasia with Vertebral Cervical Subluxation and Ventriculomegaly in Metatrophic Dysplasia: M. Shohat, et al.; J. Pediatr., February 1989, vol. 114(2), pp. 239–243.

Smith's Recognizable Patterns of Human Malformation, 4th ed.: K.L. Jones; W.B. Saunders Company, 1988, p. 318.

# MIXED CONNECTIVE TISSUE DISEASE (MCTD)

**Description** The signs and symptoms of MCTD overlap those of systemic lupus erythematosus **(SLE),** scleroderma, and polymyositis. Salient features are sequential manifestations of symptoms and high titers of antibodies to a ribonuclease-sensitive extractable nuclear antigen (anti-RNP antibodies).

**Signs and Symptoms** Early signs and symptoms include fever of unknown origin, Raynaud phenomenon, edematous hands, fatigue, and nondeforming arthritis.

   The overlapping features develop sequentially over several years. Arthritis occurs in almost every case of MCTD but rarely results in deformities similar to those seen in rheumatoid arthritis. Muscle pain occurs commonly, and an inflammatory myopathy may be present that is indistinguishable clinically and histologically from polymyositis. Skin changes also are universal and include those of SLE, including malar rash and discoid plaques, as well as those of scleroderma. In addition, mucosal ulcerations in the mouth and sicca symptoms may be present.

   Pulmonary and cardiac involvement includes pulmonary hypertension and an associated pericarditis, both of which can be asymptomatic for years. Involvement of the gastrointestinal tract includes esophageal and bowel dysmotility. Renal involvement in patients with MCTD is rare; its occurrence indicates the presence of another primary connective tissue disease, especially SLE. Hematologic disorders, including anemia and leukopenia, may develop. Neurologic complications, only seen in about 10 percent of patients, include trigeminal neuropathy.

**Etiology** The cause is not known; however, an immunologic association is well documented. All patients have high titers of antibodies to nuclear RNP, resulting in a positive test for antinuclear antibodies in a speckled pattern. Patients lack antibodies to double-stranded DNA and the Sm antigen.

**Epidemiology** Onset is known to be from 4 to 80 years; however, most patients are in their late 30s. Nearly all patients are women. The disease is not associated with any specific geographic area.

**Related Disorders** MCTD overlaps a multitude of other illnesses. See *Raynaud Disease and Phenomenon; Systemic Lupus Erythematosus; Scleroderma; Polymyositis; Dermatomyositis.*

**Treatment—Standard** Many symptoms of MCTD respond in some degree to corticosteroids. Mild forms may be helped by nonsteroidal anti-inflammatory drugs, antimalarials, or low doses of corticosteroids.

**Treatment—Investigational** Please contact the agencies listed under Resources, below, for the most current information. Addresses and telephone numbers of these agencies, as well as of individual experts and research centers, may be found in the Master Resources List.

**Resources**

   **For more information on mixed connective tissue disease:** National Organization for Rare Disorders (NORD); Arthritis Foundation; American Autoimmune Related Diseases Association; Coalition of Heritable Disorders of Connective Tissue; United Scleroderma Foundation; Scleroderma Information Exchange; Scleroderma Research Foundation; Sjögren Syndrome Foundation; Lupus Foundation of America; Systemic Lupus Erythematosus Foundation; NIH/National Arthritis and Musculoskeletal and Skin Diseases Information Clearinghouse.

**References**

Textbook of Rheumatology, 3rd ed.: W.N. Kelley, et al.; W.B. Saunders Company, 1989, pp. 1148–1165.

# OLLIER DISEASE

**Description** Ollier disease is a skeletal dysplasia usually of childhood onset, affecting the long bones and cartilage in joints of the arms and legs.

**Synonyms**

   Multiple Cartilaginous Enchondroses

**Signs and Symptoms** Onset during childhood is gradual. Involvement may be either uni- or bilateral.

The head and upper body are normal. If just one leg is affected, the patient may limp; if the disease is bilateral, short stature may result. Deformities may develop in the wrists and ankles. Dislocation of the elbows or other joints with resulting fractures may occur.

The abnormal growth of bone and cartilage eventually stops. Rare associations with chondrosarcoma and ovarian juvenile granulosa cell tumor have been reported.

**Etiology** The cause is unknown. Overgrowth of cartilaginous cells in some skeletal and joint areas may result in cortex thinning and distortion of growth in the metaphyses.

**Epidemiology** Males and females are equally affected.

**Related Disorders** See *Maffucci Syndrome,* an autosomal dominant congenital disorder in which hemangiomas as well as enchondromas are present.

**Exostosis,** an epiphyseal growth abnormality inherited as a dominant trait, is an extremely rare condition, occurring chiefly among natives of Micronesia. Although usually symptom-free, the patient may experience pain because of pressure from benign exostoses. The disorder is most frequent and severe in males.

**Treatment—Standard** Surgical extension of the affected limb has been helpful, as has prosthetic joint replacement when appropriate. Fractures routinely heal without unusual complications.

**Treatment—Investigational** Please contact the agencies listed under Resources, below, for the most current information. Addresses and telephone numbers of these agencies, as well as of individual experts and research centers, may be found in the Master Resources List.

**Resources**

**For more information on Ollier disease:** National Organization for Rare Disorders (NORD); NIH/National Institute of Diabetes, Digestive and Kidney Diseases.

**References**

Treatment of Multiple Enchrondromatosis (Ollier's Disease) of the Hand: J.F. Fatti, et al.; Orthopedics, April 1986, vol. 9(4), pp. 512–518.

Multiple Chondrosarcomas in Dyschondroplasia (Ollier's Disease): S.R. Cannon, et al.; Cancer, February 15, 1985, vol. 55(4), pp. 836–840.

Ollier's Disease: An Assessment of Angular Deformity, Shortening, and Pathological Fracture in Twenty-One Patients: F. Shapiro; J. Bone Surg. Am., January 1982, vol. 64-A(1), pp. 95–103.

# OSGOOD-SCHLATTER DISEASE

**Description** Osgood-Schlatter disease is a nonprogressive, self-limited, inflammatory condition associated with abnormal bone and cartilage formation in the tibial tubercle.

**Synonyms**

Osteochondrosis, Tibial Tubercle

**Signs and Symptoms** The typical symptoms, swelling accompanied by tenderness and pain, worsen with increased exercise or stretching. The disease is bilateral in about one-half of patients. Osgood-Schlatter disease runs a limited course (weeks to months), and the affected area will usually regenerate. Long-term effects are uncommon, although tibial fractures and joint pain have been documented years after the initial diagnosis of the disease.

**Etiology** The cause is unknown. Precipitating factors may include traumatic injury, chronic irritation, and misuse of immature bone or of the quadriceps.

**Epidemiology** Adolescent males who are athletically active are the most frequently affected.

**Treatment—Standard** Treatment consists initially of immobilization of the affected leg with a cast. If this is not adequate, complete bed rest is necessary. Surgery for grafting or removal of debris has been required in some cases. Any other treatment is supportive and symptomatic.

**Treatment—Investigational** Please contact the agencies listed under Resources, below, for the most current information. Addresses and telephone numbers of these agencies, as well as of individual experts and research centers, may be found in the Master Resources List.

**Resources**

**For more information on Osgood-Schlatter disease:** National Organization for Rare Disorders (NORD); NIH/National Arthritis and Musculoskeletal and Skin Diseases Information Clearinghouse; Arthritis Foundation.

**References**

Avulsion Fracture of the Tibial Tuberosity in Late Adolescence: P. Nimityongskul, et al.; J. Trauma, April 1988, vol. 28(4), pp. 505–509.

Management of Sports Injuries in Children and Adolescents: C. Stanitski; Orth. Clin. N. Amer., October 1988, vol. 19(4), pp. 689–698.

The Sequelae of Osgood-Schlatter's Disease in Adults: J. Hogh, et al.; Int. Orth., 1988, vol. 12(3), pp. 213–215.

Tibial Sequestrectomy in the Management of Osgood-Schlatter Disease: I. Trail; J. Ped. Orth., September–October 1988, vol. 8(5), pp. 554–557.

# OSTEONECROSIS

**Description** Osteonecrosis, a slowly progressive disorder of bone destruction, is most often due to inadequate blood supply to a bone. Most commonly affected are the ends of long bones, such as the femoral heads and condyles and humeral heads. This produces pain in the hips, knees, and shoulders, respectively.

**Synonyms**

Avascular Necrosis of Bone

Ischemic Necrosis of Bone

**Signs and Symptoms** Pain usually occurs when standing, walking, or lifting, becoming more intense when pressure is exerted on the bones or joints. The pain may progress, eventually occurring while at rest or even disturbing sleep. Other symptoms include muscle spasms, joint stiffness, and limitation of range of motion.

**Etiology** Conditions that affect the vascular supply to bone can cause osteonecrosis. Trauma that results in dislocation or fracture of the neck of the femur is a common cause. Certain drugs (e.g., glucocorticoids), radiation, and chemotherapy can also adversely affect the blood supply to bone, as can kidney transplantation, sickle cell disease, and alcoholism, all of which can be associated with osteonecrosis.

**Epidemiology** Osteonecrosis can occur at any age, but is most prevalent in persons between 30 and 60 years. Males are affected more by osteonecrosis of the hip; females, of the knee. The disease is also more common in persons with rheumatic diseases, especially those treated with glucocorticoids (e.g., rheumatoid arthritis, systemic lupus erythematosus), other patients treated with steroids (e.g., asthmatics), alcoholics, diabetics, and skin divers who have experienced "the bends."

**Related Disorders** Osteonecrosis may be produced by a wide variety of diseases, disorders, and traumatic situations. See *Legg-Calvé-Perthes Syndrome; Gaucher Disease; Polycythemia Vera; Osteopetrosis; Systemic Lupus Erythematosus.*

**Sickle cell disease** refers to several disorders in which sickle-, or crescent-, shaped erythrocytes in the peripheral blood become rigid and lodge in capillaries. Pain results from the ensuing disruption in the flow of oxygen to tissue and organs.

**Caisson disease (decompression sickness; "the bends"),** caused by the formation of nitrogen bubbles in the tissues and blood, occurs from a very rapid reduction of air pressure after rising quickly from deep water with high atmospheric pressure, to normal air pressure. Caisson disease is characterized by painful joints, osteonecrosis, chest tightness, giddiness, abdominal pain, vomiting, and visual difficulties. Convulsions and paralysis may also occur.

The **osteopetroses** are a group of rare inherited disorders marked by increased bone density, brittleness of bone, and, in some cases, skeletal abnormalities.

**Treatment—Standard** Diagnosis of the underlying cause is the primary basis for establishing treatment. X-rays are useful in diagnosing osteonecrosis and determining the extent of bone damage. However, when x-rays are normal in early disease, bone scans and magnetic resonance imaging may reveal the diagnosis.

Limiting weight-bearing activities, standing, and walking, and avoiding alcohol may help the recovery process. Pain is relieved with aspirin or other nonsteroidal anti-inflammatory medications. Core decompression may help relieve pain in early osteonecrosis. Joint replacement surgery may be necessary when there is a fracture or when the bone has collapsed.

Bones damaged by osteonecrosis will usually undergo progressive remodeling with the development of secondary osteoarthritis of the contiguous joint. Surgical management, either core decompression or joint arthroplasty, is often required.

**Treatment—Investigational** Please contact the agencies listed under Resources, below, for the most current information. Addresses and telephone numbers of these agencies, as well as of individual experts and research centers, may be found in the Master Resources List.

**Resources**

**For more information on osteonecrosis:** National Organization for Rare Disorders (NORD); Arthritis Foundation; NIH/National Arthritis, Musculoskeletal and Skin Diseases Information Clearinghouse.

**References**

Ischemic Necrosis of Bone: T.M. Zizic and D. Hungerford; *in* Harris, et al.: Textbook of Rheumatology, 3rd ed., W.B. Saunders Company, 1990.

Cecil Textbook of Medicine, 18th ed.: J.B. Wyngaarden and L.H. Smith, Jr., eds.; W. B. Saunders Company, 1988. p. 1517.

Influence of Alcohol Intake, Cigarette Smoking, and Occupational Status on Idiopathic Osteonecrosis of the Femoral Head: K. Matsuo, et al.; Clin. Orth., September 1988, vol. 234, pp. 115–123.

Osteonecrosis of the Femoral Head:. Pathogenesis and Long-Term Results of Treatment: M. Meyers; Clin. Orth., June 1988, vol. 231, pp. 51–61.

Osteonecrosis of the Hip in the Sickle Cell Diseases: Treatment and Complications: G. Hanker, et al.; J. Bone Surg. Am., April 1988, vol. 70(4), pp. 499–506.

# PAGET DISEASE OF BONE

**Description** Paget disease of bone is a chronic, slowly progressive skeletal condition of abnormally rapid bone destruction and reformation in which the new bone is structurally abnormal, dense, and fragile. The areas most frequently affected are the spine, skull, pelvis, thighs, and lower legs.

**Synonyms**

>   Corticalis Deformans
>   Hyperostosis Corticalis Deformans
>   Osteitis Deformans

**Signs and Symptoms** Early symptoms include bone pain, joint pain (especially back, hips, and knees), and headache. Physical signs include enlargement and bowing of the thighs (femurs) and lower legs (tibias), and frontal bossing with enlargement of the skull.

As the disease progresses, other signs and symptoms may appear: further bowing of the affected limb, a waddling gait, muscle and sensory disturbances, and hearing loss. High-output congestive heart failure may occur. Osteogenic sarcoma is a rare complication.

Most cases are asymptomatic and mild, and can be identified on pelvic x-rays. When symptoms occur, they are often vague and hard to distinguish from those of many other diseases, including lumbar spine disease and osteoarthritis.

Differential diagnosis includes normal serum calcium and phosphorous and elevated serum alkaline phosphatase as compared with other osteitis conditions that usually do not have the elevated serum alkaline phosphatase, and the characteristic lesions of the occiput and femur on x-ray.

**Etiology** The disease may be hereditary, but the actual cause has not been confirmed. Recent research implicates a slow virus. Pain is caused by direct bone involvement, osteoarthritis due to abnormal joint restructuring, and nerve root impingement.

**Epidemiology** Persons between 50 and 70 years of age are most frequently affected, although young adults have been diagnosed with the disease. Males are affected more often than females. Because so many cases are mild and go undiagnosed and untreated, the estimate of 3 million cases in the United States is considered below the actual incidence. Paget disease of bone is more prevalent in those with western European heritage.

**Related Disorders** See *Engelmann Disease; Hypophosphatasia; Spinal Stenosis; Hyperostosis Frontalis Interna.*

**Treatment—Standard** Treatment is symptomatic and focuses on relieving pain and preventing deformity, fractures, and loss of mobility.

Diphosphonates are effective and are given intermittently for periods not exceeding 6 months, with observation of the alkaline phosphatase level. In patients who do not respond to diphosphonates, calcitonin is often used (see below, under Treatment—Investigational).

**Treatment—Investigational** There is ongoing research in the areas of bone tissue; the effect of Paget disease on collagen synthesis; the action of calcitonin, parathyroid, and other hormone secretions; and the assessment of bone regeneration.

For research on using calcitonin in patients who have side effects or are resistant to diphosphonates, please contact Roy D. Altman, M.D., at the University of Miami School of Medicine.

For research studying etiology of the disease, and clinical studies on possible viral causes, please contact Robert Canfield, M.D., Ethel Siris, M.D., and Thomas Jacobs, M.D., at Columbia Presbyterian Hospital.

Please contact the agencies listed under Resources, below, for the most current information. Addresses and telephone numbers of these agencies, as well as of individual experts and research centers, may be found in the Master Resources List.

**Resources**

For more information on **Paget disease of bone:** National Organization for Rare Disorders (NORD); Paget's Foundation; NIH/National Arthritis and Musculoskeletal and Skin Diseases Information Clearinghouse.

For **genetic information and genetic counseling referrals:** March of Dimes Birth Defects Foundation; Alliance of Genetic Support Groups.

**References**

Cecil Textbook of Medicine, 19th ed.: J.B. Wyngaarden, et al., eds.; W.B. Saunders Company, 1992, pp. 1431–1433.
Mendelian Inheritance in Man, 9th ed.: V.A. McKusick; The Johns Hopkins University Press, 1990, p. 703.
Paget's Disease of Bone: R.L. Merkow, et al.; Orthop. Clin. North Am., January 1990, vol. 21(1), pp. 171–189.
Textbook of Rheumatology, 3rd ed.: W.N. Kelley, et al.; W.B. Saunders Company, 1989, pp. 1742–1743.

# Polyarteritis Nodosa (PAN)

**Description** PAN is an inflammatory necrotizing systemic vascular disease characterized by nodules along the length of small and medium-sized arteries. In varying degrees, the lesions involve most of the arteries throughout the body and are segmental. The clinical picture is polymorphic, with many manifestations seemingly unrelated.

**Synonyms**

> Necrotizing Angiitis
> Periarteritis
> Periarteritis Nodosa
> Polyarteritis

**Signs and Symptoms** Initial symptoms and signs include fever, chills, fatigue, and weight loss. Systemic manifestations include abdominal pain, combined motor and sensory peripheral neuropathy, skin lesions, arthritis, muscle pain, and testicular pain. Gastrointestinal bleeding may occur.

The inflammatory vascular process causes arterial constriction resulting in tissue ischemia, thrombosis, occasional aneurysms, and an increased potential for arterial rupture. The kidneys are most often involved, and hypertension is common. Disease severity ranges from mild to rapidly fatal. The course is usually acute; most deaths due to vasculitis occur within 1 year of onset.

Diagnosis is confirmed by either biopsy or visceral angiography demonstrating aneurysms.

**Etiology** There is no one apparent cause, and the majority of patients have no predisposing event or circumstance. The disorder has been observed in drug abusers, particularly those using amphetamines, and in hepatitis-B patients. Research suggests that polyarteritis nodosa is an autoimmune disease possibly initially triggered by a viral infection.

**Epidemiology** Most often polyarteritis nodosa affects men between 40 and 60 years of age, but it has been seen in every age group. Approximately 1:100,000 persons is affected, with males having the disease 2 to 3 times more frequently than females.

**Related Disorders** The clinical symptoms of polyarteritis may be produced by a wide variety of related disorders, requiring a comprehensive process of differential diagnosis. See *Churg-Strauss Syndrome; Arteritis, Giant Cell; Arteritis, Takayasu; Wegener Granulomatosis.*

**Cogan syndrome** is a very rare polyarteritis-like disorder characterized by interstitial keratitis, vertigo, tinnitus, and hearing loss. In addition, systemic symptoms such as congestive heart failure, intestinal hemorrhage, splenomegaly, hypertension, and muscle and bone abnormalities may occur. If corticosteroid drug therapy is begun early, it can result in clearing of inflamed eyes and in hearing recovery. Cogan syndrome can occur at any age and affects men and women equally.

**Treatment—Standard** Primary treatment consists of high-dose corticosteroids (60 to 80 mg/day) such as prednisone for the relief of inflammation and immunosuppression. Cyclophosphamide in doses of 1 to 2 mg/kg/day has also been found to be effective. If indicated, aggressive treatment for hypertension should be part of the management program. Surgery is required where gastrointestinal problems, such as infarction of bowel, perforation, and bleeding, indicate such intervention. Additional treatment is supportive and symptomatic.

**Treatment—Investigational** Plasmapheresis may be of benefit in some cases of polyarteritis nodosa, but its safety and efficacy are still under investigation.

The National Institute of Allergy and Infectious Diseases is conducting a study on a treatment for polyarteritis nodosa. Participants must be at least 14 years old and have had a recent onset of the illness.

Please contact the agencies listed under Resources, below, for the most current information. Addresses and telephone numbers of these agencies, as well as of individual experts and research centers, may be found in the Master Resources List.

**Resources**

**For more information on polyarteritis nodosa:** National Organization for Rare Disorders (NORD); NIH/National Institute for Allergy and Infectious Diseases.

**References**

Textbook of Rheumatology, 3rd ed.: W.N. Kelley, et al.; W.B. Saunders Company, 1989, pp. 1172–1179.

Clinical Findings and Prognosis of Polyarteritis Nodosa and Churg-Strauss Angiitis: A Study in 165 Patients: L. Guillevin, et al.; British J. of Rheum., August 1988, vol. 27(4), pp. 258–264.

Pulmonary Diseases and Disorders, 2nd ed.: A.P. Fishman; McGraw-Hill, 1988, pp. 1127–1128.

Internal Medicine, 2nd ed.: J.H. Stein, ed.-in-chief; Little, Brown and Company, 1987, pp. 856, 857, 1282–1284.

# POLYMYALGIA RHEUMATICA

**Description** Polymyalgia rheumatica is marked by muscular pain and stiffness and generalized symptoms that include fatigue and fever. The disorder is comparatively benign and exquisitely responsive to treatment, and rarely results in permanent muscle weakness or atrophy.

**Synonyms**
> Anarthritic Syndrome
> Anarthritic Rheumatoid Disease

**Signs and Symptoms** Onset is typically abrupt, with pain and stiffness in the neck, shoulders, upper arms, lower back, hips, and thighs. Distal extremities usually are not affected. The stiffness and pain are bilateral and are most severe in the morning and after long periods of rest and inactivity. Muscle tenderness and weakness may occur, but examination of the muscles usually does not reveal any abnormality. Low-grade fever, anorexia, weight loss, fatigue, malaise, and depression may be among the initial symptoms. A peripheral rheumatoid-like arthritis occurs in about one-third of patients.

The sedimentation rate is markedly elevated, often above 100 mm/hr using the Westergren method. Also increased are serum albumin, globulins, and fibrinogen. A nonhemolytic anemia may be present. The disease has remissions and exacerbations; however, permanent disability, even after months or years of disease, is unusual.

**Etiology** The cause is not known. An immunologic association and genetic predisposition have been suggested.

**Epidemiology** Prevalence is about 50:100,000 persons aged 50 or older.

**Related Disorders** Polymyalgia rheumatica and giant cell arteritis occur in the same patient population, and often both are present in the same individual. See *Arteritis, Giant Cell; Polymyositis/Dermatomyositis.*

**Treatment—Standard** Nonsteroidal anti-inflammatory drugs may be used for patients without vascular symptoms or signs. If those are not effective, low to moderate doses of prednisone up to 20 mg/day are used. In patients with cranial symptoms suggestive of giant cell arteritis, high-dose corticosteroids, particularly prednisone, are given. Rapid improvement in symptoms of polymyalgia rheumatica usually results within a few days after beginning prednisone. After symptoms resolve, a gradual reduction in dosage for maintenance at a rate of 10 percent per month over several months is begun. Occasionally, patients require treatment for several years. Side effects of prednisone must be carefully monitored, with further reduction in dosage or even discontinuation if side effects persist.

**Treatment—Investigational** Please contact the agencies listed under Resources, below, for the most current information. Addresses and telephone numbers of these agencies, as well as of individual experts and research centers, may be found in the Master Resources List.

**Resources**

**For more information on polymyalgia rheumatica:** National Organization for Rare Disorders (NORD); Arthritis Foundation; NIH/National Arthritis and Musculoskeletal and Skin Diseases Information Clearinghouse.

**References**

Textbook of Rheumatology, 3rd ed.: W.N. Kelley, et al.; W.B. Saunders Company, 1989, pp. 1200–1208.

# POLYMYOSITIS/DERMATOMYOSITIS

**Description** **Polymyositis** is marked by inflammatory and degenerative changes in the muscle fibers and the supporting collagen connective tissue, resulting in muscle weakness.

**Dermatomyositis** is identical to polymyositis, but with the addition of a characteristic rash.

In childhood, dermatomyositis is more common than polymyositis alone.

**Signs and Symptoms** Typically, muscle weakness has an insidious onset, occurring primarily in the neck, trunk, and proximal extremities. The hands, feet, and facial muscles usually escape involvement. Eventually, it becomes difficult for the patient to rise from a sitting position, climb stairs, lift objects, or reach overhead. Late in the chronic stage, muscle atrophy and contractures of the extremities may develop. Occasionally, joint pain and tenderness are present. In about one-third of patients, the polyarthralgia may be accompanied by swelling and other signs of nondeforming arthritis.

Interstitial pneumonitis, manifested by dyspnea and coughing, may be an early symptom. Raynaud phenomenon is usually limited to the fingers and does not always occur. Numb and shiny red areas around and under the nailbeds may also appear.

Gastrointestinal involvement is essentially confined to the upper esophagus; the pharynx is involved as well. Dysphagia is a common symptom and may result in aspiration pneumonia. Abdominal symptoms, most often seen in children with juvenile dermatomyositis, include melena and hematemesis arising from gastrointestinal ulcerations.

Cardiac irregularities evident on electrocardiogram have been reported, as has acute renal failure due to excess myoglobin in the urine during rhabdomyolysis. Associated malignancy, usually carcinoma, occurs in about 15 percent of patients aged 45 and over with new-onset polymyositis.

In **dermatomyositis,** cutaneous lesions may appear before muscle involvement. There may be periorbital edema, a patchy facial erythema, and erythematous dermatitis over the extensor surfaces of the joints, particularly the hands (Gottron papules). The lesions usually fade completely, leaving a brownish pigmentation, atrophy, or vitiligo. In some patients, cutaneous changes are similar to scleroderma, especially the distribution of subcutaneous calcification seen in children. Particularly in untreated patients, the calcinosis universalis tends to be more comprehensive than in scleroderma.

**Etiology** The cause is not known. Immunologic mechanisms and a genetic influence have been suggested. Injectable bovine collagen has been implicated in the onset of a dermatomyositis-like syndrome. Viral infections and toxoplasmosis have also been implicated.

**Epidemiology** Polymyositis and dermatomyositis may appear at any age, although 60 percent of cases occur between the ages of 30 and 60. Females are affected twice as often as males.

Childhood dermatomyositis occurs most often between 5 and 15 years of age. Dermatomyositis in adults aged 45 and above is more commonly associated with malignancy than is polymyositis.

**Related Disorders** See *Scleroderma; Systemic Lupus Erythematosus.*

**Treatment—Standard** Initial treatment is with high-dose corticosteroids such as prednisone. Muscle enzyme activity (i.e., creatine phosphokinase levels) is measured to gauge treatment effectiveness. Generally, the enzymes return to normal ranges within 6 to 12 weeks, followed by increased muscular strength. At that time, corticosteroid dosage can be gradually reduced. However, in some cases of adult polymyositis, there is either a poor response to prednisone or a need for indefinitely prolonged treatment with prednisone. In such instances, the immunosuppressive drugs methotrexate and azathioprine have been beneficial for those failing to respond to corticosteroids.

Surgical intervention is required if gastrointestinal perforation occurs.

In patients with dermatomyositis, antimalarials (e.g., hydroxychloroquine) may be helpful for control of skin rash.

**Treatment—Investigational** At the NIH, cyclophosphamide in combination with mesna is being tested in severely afflicted patients who are unresponsive to steroid therapy. Other investigational protocols involve the use of cyclosporine. Efficacy has not yet been determined for either of these approaches.

The orphan product intravenous immune globulin (Immuno Clinic Research Corp.) has been approved for treatment of polymyositis/dermatomyositis. Its long-term efficacy and safety have yet to be proved, however.

Frederick W. Miller, M.D., and Lisa G. Rider, M.D., at the National Institutes of Health, are studying the genetic factors responsible for certain connective tissue diseases, including polymyositis and dermatomyositis.

Paul Poltz at the National Institute of Arthritis and Musculoskeletal and Skin Diseases is studying the natural history and pathogenesis of polymyositis, dermatomyositis, and other idiopathic inflammatory myopathies.

Please contact the agencies listed under Resources, below, for the most current information. Addresses and telephone numbers of these agencies, as well as of individual experts and research centers, may be found in the Master Resources List.

**Resources**

**For more information on polymyositis/dermatomyositis:** National Organization for Rare Disorders (NORD); NIH/National Arthritis and Musculoskeletal and Skin Diseases Information Clearinghouse; Arthritis Foundation; National Support Group for Myositis; Dermatomyositis and Polymyositis Support Group.

**References**

A Controlled Trial of High-Dose Intravenous Immune Globulin Infusions As Treatment for Dermatomyositis: M.C. Dalakas, et al.; N. Engl. J. Med., December 1993, vol. 329(27), pp. 1993–2000.

Arthritis and Allied Conditions, 11th ed.: D.J. McCarty; Lea and Febiger, 1989, pp. 1092–1117.

Textbook of Rheumatology, 3rd ed.: W.N. Kelley, et al.; W.B. Saunders Company, 1989, pp. 1265–1273, 1274–1275.

Cecil Textbook of Medicine, 18th ed.: J.B. Wyngaarden and L.H. Smith, Jr., eds.; W.B. Saunders Company, 1988, pp. 1978, 2341.

# PSEUDOGOUT

**Description** Pseudogout is characterized by deposits of calcium pyrophosphate dihydrate (**CPPD**) crystals in one or more joints, causing symptoms and signs that mimic gout and other arthritides.

**Synonyms**

Articular Chondrocalcinosis

Calcium Pyrophosphate Dihydrate Crystal Deposition Disease

**Signs and Symptoms** Acute attacks of pseudogout involve swelling, stiffness, warmth, and pain, usually in one joint, most often the knee. Episodes last from 1 day to several weeks and can subside without treatment. They can be severe but are usually not as disabling or painful as gout itself.

A milder, chronic form of pseudogout produces symptoms similar to those of the acute episode but less painful.
**Etiology** The cause of the crystal deposition is unknown. There is evidence that some cases of pseudogout are familial. Associations seem to exist with certain metabolic conditions, such as hyperparathyroidism, familial hypocalciuric hypercalcemia, and hemochromatosis, and with surgery or other trauma as well as aging.
**Epidemiology** Pseudogout appears in mature adults. Some studies indicate a greater prevalence in women; other studies indicate a greater prevalence in men. Asymptomatic articular calcinosis is common in persons over age 50. A familial pattern of incidence has been observed in several countries.
**Related Disorders Gout** is a recurrent acute arthritis that results from deposition of monosodium urate crystals in persons with hyperuricemia. In most cases, gout is responsive to drugs and diet therapy.
**Treatment—Standard** There is at present no known way to prevent the formation of CPPD crystals or to satisfactorily remove existing ones.

Acute attacks of pseudogout are treated in several ways. The excess fluid and CPPD crystals are drained from the affected joint. If only one joint is involved, a corticosteroid may be injected locally. Colchicine is effective for treating pseudogout as well as true gout. Aspirin and other nonsteroidal anti-inflammatory drugs may be used. Chronic colchicine therapy may decrease the frequency and severity of future attacks.

During an attack, the affected joint may need rest and protection with splints or canes. Once the episode subsides, or in the milder chronic form, rest should be balanced with carefully monitored appropriate exercise.

Surgical intervention and repair may be needed in rare cases of severe joint damage, pain, instability, or immobility, owing to the development of secondary osteoarthritis.
**Treatment—Investigational** Please contact the agencies listed under Resources, below, for the most current information. Addresses and telephone numbers of these agencies, as well as of individual experts and research centers, may be found in the Master Resources List.
**Resources**

**For more information on pseudogout:** National Organization for Rare Disorders (NORD); Arthritis Foundation; NIH/National Arthritis and Musculoskeletal and Skin Diseases Information Clearinghouse.
**References**

Primer on the Rheumatic Diseases, 10th ed.: H.R. Schumacher, Jr., ed.; Arthritis Foundation, 1993, pp. 219–222.
Arthritis and Allied Conditions, 11th ed.: D.J. McCarty; Lea and Febiger, 1989, pp. 1711–1731.
Cecil Textbook of Medicine, 18th ed.: J.B. Wyngaarden and L.H. Smith, Jr., eds.; W.B. Saunders Company, 1988, p. 2037.

# PSORIATIC ARTHRITIS

**Description** Psoriatic arthritis is an arthritic condition that is associated with psoriasis of the skin and/or nails and a negative test for rheumatoid factor **(RF)**.
**Synonyms**

Arthropathic Psoriasis
Psoriatic Spondyloarthritis
**Signs and Symptoms** The characteristic symptoms are inflammation of the joints and surrounding tissues accompanied by psoriasis of the nails and psoriatic plaques on the scalp, elbows, knees, and lower spine. The psoriasis usually precedes joint involvement (80 percent of cases); in 20 percent of cases, the joint involvement appears first.

The psoriasis is seen as erythematous, silvery-gray, sharply demarcated spots or plaques that usually appear on the scalp, behind the ears, on the elbows and knees, and on the skin over the sacrum.

The joints most commonly affected are the distal interphalangeal **(DIP)** joints of the hands and feet, as well as the wrists, knees, and ankles. Rheumatoid nodules are not present. Exacerbations and remissions tend to occur, as in patients with rheumatoid arthritis **(RA)**; however, progression to chronic arthritis and severe deformities is less common than in patients with RA.

There are 5 clinical subtypes of psoriatic arthritis: 1) "classical," with involvement limited to the DIP joints of the hands and feet; 2) an asymmetric oligoarthritis usually involving knees, ankles, wrists, and feet; 3) a symmetric polyarthritis resembling RA; 4) an axial arthritis (ankylosing spondylitis) usually involving sacroiliac joints and lumbar and cervical spine; and 5) arthritis mutilans.

X-rays show DIP joint involvement. Destruction of large and small joints may occur with joint fusion. Laboratory findings reveal the presence of HLA-B27 antigen in the blood of most patients with psoriatic arthritis with axial involvement.

Patients with inflammatory polyarthritis testing negative for rheumatoid factor should be examined for undetected or minimal psoriasis.
**Etiology** The cause is unknown.

**Epidemiology** Between 5 and 8 percent of patients with psoriasis have psoriatic arthritis. The disorder is more common in women and usually first appears between the ages of 20 and 30 years. However, onset can occur at any age.

**Related Disorders** The clinical symptoms of psoriatic arthritis are similar to a variety of diseases and syndromes.

**Rheumatoid arthritis (RA)** is characterized by symmetric joint inflammation. The skin is usually not involved.

**Acute gouty arthritis** attacks are accompanied by great pain; the big toe is a frequent site. The disorder usually is self-limiting and lasts, untreated, about 1 to 2 weeks.

See ***Reiter Syndrome.***

**Treatment—Standard** Treatment is similar to that of RA (including rest, joint protection, appropriate exercises), but with some significant differences. All patients should be treated with nonsteroidal anti-inflammatory drugs (NSAIDs). The most effective NSAIDs for patients with psoriatic arthritis include diclofenac, sulindac, tolmetin, and indomethacin.

The cutaneous lesions of psoriatic arthritis are treated as for psoriasis.

Use of antimalarial medications is generally discouraged.

For severely affected patients, folic acid antagonists and immunosuppressive drugs, particularly methotrexate, have been effective in relieving psoriatic lesions and joint inflammation in patients; *meticulous care should be exercised in the use of methotrexate because of its potential toxicity.* Physical and occupational therapy, tailored for the individual patient, should be encouraged. Patients who fail to respond to NSAIDs alone should be referred to a rheumatologist for further treatment.

**Treatment—Investigational** Please contact the agencies listed under Resources, below, for the most current information. Addresses and telephone numbers of these agencies, as well as of individual experts and research centers, may be found in the Master Resources List.

**Resources**

**For more information on psoriatic arthritis:** National Organization for Rare Disorders (NORD); National Psoriasis Foundation; Psoriasis Research Association; Arthritis Foundation; NIH/National Arthritis and Musculoskeletal and Skin Diseases Information Clearinghouse.

**References**

Arthritis and Allied Conditions, 11th ed.: D.J. McCarty; Lea and Febiger, 1989, pp. 954–971.

Cecil Textbook of Medicine, 18th ed.: J.B. Wyngaarden and L.H. Smith, Jr., eds.; W.B. Saunders Company, 1988, p. 2327.

# RAYNAUD DISEASE AND PHENOMENON

**Description Raynaud disease,** characterized by episodes of vasospasm in the fingers and skin, is considered to be the benign primary form of **Raynaud phenomenon,** which occurs in association with systemic disorders.

**Synonyms**

Raynaud Syndrome

Symmetric Asphyxia

**Signs and Symptoms** Usually sequential phases of pallor, cyanosis, and rubor are seen, but a dramatic stark white pallor of the affected fingers and toes may be the only element of the triad to occur. The initial pallor may be the result of vasospasm of the digital arteries or arterioles; cyanosis is probably due to stasis in affected venules and capillaries; and after a time, ranging from minutes to hours, hyperemia causes a striking rubor.

Initially, only 1 or 2 fingertips may be involved. As the disorder progresses, all the fingers in their entirety, except the thumbs, may be affected. Symptoms vary and may include feelings of numbness or cold, severe aching or pain, tingling or throbbing, a sensation of tightness, pins and needles, and severe paresthesias. Over an extended period of time, trophic changes may occur, and severe cases may develop fingertip ulcerations or gangrene. Sometimes progression is more rapid.

The possibility of associated disease should be explored, e.g., systemic lupus erythematosus, systemic sclerosis, and other connective tissue diseases. Differential diagnosis should rule out other causes of digital ischemia such as frostbite, vibration-induced trauma, atherosclerotic or Buerger disease, and cervical rib syndrome. Unilateral symptoms are likely to be a different entity. If patients present with single limb involvement, structural arterial disease of that limb should be investigated.

**Etiology** The cause is uncertain. There is discussion as to whether sympathetic nervous system hyperactivity or local arterial abnormalities are the explanation for the clinical findings. Genetic inheritance has not been ruled out. Precipitating factors include stress and exposure to cold.

**Epidemiology** Women, especially those 30 years and older, are affected 5 times more often than men. Recent studies suggest that up to 5 percent of women may have Raynaud disease.

**Related Disorders** Raynaud phenomenon may be an early presenting symptom of several diseases and disorders. See ***Scleroderma; Systemic Lupus Erythematosus; Sjögren Syndrome; Mixed Connective Tissue Disease;***

***Polymyositis/Dermatomyositis.*** Digital pain is also seen in Fabry disease and carpal tunnel syndrome (see ***Fabry Disease).*** Other associated conditions include some categories of vasculitis, neurogenic lesions, drug intoxications with ergot and methysergide, dysproteinemias, myxedema, and primary pulmonary hypertension.

**Unilateral episodic vasoconstriction of the fingers** may result from frostbite and structural abnormalities of the arteries.

**Posttraumatic vasospasm of the fingers** may result in symptoms of Raynaud disease. Possible causes include white vibratory finger syndrome.

**Treatment—Standard** Basic management includes avoidance of exposure to cold and of other vasoconstrictive factors, such as smoking and certain drugs. An α-adrenoceptor blocker (e.g., prazosin), a calcium blocker (e.g., nifedipine), or phenobarbital, in addition to phenoxybenzamine, guanethidine, pentoxifylline, dipyridamole, methyldopa, reserpine, topical nitroglycerin, and low-dose aspirin, may be beneficial. Biofeedback has been useful in some instances.

Any underlying disorder of Raynaud phenomenon must be diagnosed and treated. Sympathectomy is generally more effective for patients with Raynaud disease who do not respond to other therapies than for those with Raynaud phenomenon.

**Treatment—Investigational** Ketanserin, a serotonin antagonist manufactured by Janssen Pharmaceutica, is being investigated for digital vascular symptoms of Raynaud disease.

An orphan drug, Iloprost, manufactured by Berlex Laboratories, is being studied for the treatment of Raynaud phenomenon with digital ulcers when it occurs with scleroderma.

Captopril and nifedipine (Bristol-Myers Squibb) and thymoxamine (Parke-Davis) are being tested for treating Raynaud disease.

Please contact the agencies listed under Resources, below, for the most current information. Addresses and telephone numbers of these agencies, as well as of individual experts and research centers, may be found in the Master Resources List.

**Resources**

**For more information on Raynaud disease and phenomenon:** National Organization for Rare Disorders (NORD); NIH/National Heart, Lung, and Blood Institute; Raynaud's Association Trust; Raynaud's Scleroderma Association; Scleroderma Information Exchange; American Heart Association.

**References**

The Diagnostic Puzzle and Management Challenge of Raynaud's Syndrome: E. Davis; Nurse Pract., March 1993, vol. 18(32), pp. 18, 21–22, 25.

Managing Raynaud's Phenomenon: A Practical Approach: A.C. Adee; Am. Fam. Physician, March 1993, vol. 47(4), pp. 823–829.

Raynaud's Syndrome: An Enigma after 130 Years: T.J. Cleophas, et al.; Angiology, March 1993, vol. 44(3), pp. 196–209.

Cecil Textbook of Medicine, 19th ed.: J.B. Wyngaarden, et al., eds.; W.B. Saunders Company, 1992, pp. 355–358.

The Many Faces of Scleroderma: J.D. Smiley; Am. J. Med. Sci., November 1992, vol. 304(5), pp. 319–333.

Mendelian Inheritance in Man, 10th ed.: V.A. McKusick; The Johns Hopkins University Press, 1992, p. 967.

Raynaud's Phenomemon: E.V. Lally; Curr. Opin. Rheumatol., December 1992, vol. 4(6), pp. 825–836.

Treatment of Systemic Sclerosis: F.M. Wigley; Curr. Opin. Rheumatol., December 1992, vol. 4(6), pp. 878–886.

Internal Medicine, 3rd ed.: J.H. Stein, ed.-in-chief; Little, Brown and Company, 1990, p. 223.

Principles of Neurology: R.D. Adams and M. Victor, eds.; McGraw-Hill, 1989, pp. 176–178.

# REITER SYNDROME

**Description** Reiter syndrome (one form of **reactive arthritis**) is characterized by a triad of arthritis, nongonococcal urethritis, and conjunctivitis, and by lesions of the skin and mucosal surfaces. An enteric initiating component has been recognized in some patients. Symptoms may not appear simultaneously; they may alternate; and there may be spontaneous remissions and recurrences.

**Synonyms**

> Arthritis Urethritica
> Blennorrheal Idiopathic Arthritis
> Feissinger-Leroy-Reiter Syndrome
> Polyarthritis Enterica
> Ruhr Syndrome
> Urethro-Oculo-Articular Syndrome
> Venereal Arthritis
> Waelsch Syndrome

**Signs and Symptoms** Although the initial symptoms are urethritis or enteritis, with arthritis and other symptoms appearing 4 days to 4 weeks later, the patient may not request help from the physician until the arthritis appears. The initial symptoms may be revealed only after some questioning, either because the patient did not make the connection or was embarrassed.

The initial urethritis may be painful, and a purulent discharge and hematuria may be present. Cultures of the genitourinary discharge do not reveal *Neisseria gonorrhoeae* but may demonstrate *Chlamydia* organisms. The enteric organisms involved are discussed below.

Arthritis usually begins abruptly, affects more than one joint, and is asymmetric. Joints of the legs and feet are involved most often; small joints of the hands are almost never affected. Joints are warm, red, swollen, and painful. Although episodes of arthritis usually last at least 2 to 4 months, symptoms may begin to subside within 2 to 6 weeks. Remission in the setting of treatment often occurs within the first year, but some attacks last several years. In such cases, the involved joints may be permanently damaged.

Extra-articular musculoskeletal findings include tendinitis (often involving the Achilles tendon), plantar fasciitis resulting in pain at the bottom of the heel, dactylitis (sausage toes), and a diffuse enthesitis involving insertions of tendons to bone. Ankylosing spondylitis develops in 10 to 20 percent of patients with sacroiliac and lumbar spine involvement.

Conjunctivitis is most often mild and bilateral, lasting a few days; however, it often recurs. Occasionally, the uvea also becomes inflamed (uveitis or iritis), with symptoms of photophobia; glaucoma, cataracts, and blindness may rarely develop in severe cases (approximately 5 percent).

Mucocutaneous vesicular lesions develop on the glans penis, palmar surfaces, and soles of the feet, and in the mouth, urethra, and bladder. They become eroded and erythematous but cause little pain and resolve quickly. The lesions of **keratoderma blennorrhagica,** found on the hands, arms, and trunk, are scaly and crusty and resemble pustular psoriasis, eventually peeling off. The fingernails also become brittle, thick, and opaque.

Rarely, patients develop cardiac abnormalities, including an incompetent aortic valve and cardiac conduction defects.

Laboratory findings include anemia, elevated levels of white blood cells in the blood and synovial fluids, and an elevated erythrocyte sedimentation rate. Tests for rheumatoid factor are negative. HLA-B27 is found in two-thirds to three-quarters of patients.

**Etiology** The precipitating event for sexually acquired Reiter syndrome is urethritis from *Chlamydia trachomatis* or *Ureaplasma urealyticum.* Infectious agents causing enteric reactive arthritis include *Shigella flexneri,* salmonella, yersinia, and campylobacter. The HLA-B27 antigen is a predisposing factor. Recently, Reiter syndrome has been recognized to occur in men with symptomatic HIV infection and AIDS, probably because of their increased risk of exposure to the above organisms.

**Epidemiology** Sexually acquired Reiter syndrome is seen almost exclusively in males between 20 to 40 years of age. Enteric reactive arthritis is seen equally in males and females, and occasionally in children.

**Related Disorders** Reiter syndrome may be mimicked by arthritis with coexistent gonorrheal urethritis. **Behçet Syndrome** has symptoms of oral and genital lesions, uveitis, and arthritis, but they are distinctly different from those of Reiter syndrome.

**Treatment—Standard** Treatment is symptomatic. Nonsteroidal anti-inflammatory drugs (NSAIDs) such as indomethacin, diclofenac, tolmetin, sulindac, or phenylbutazone usually relieve the arthritis. In severe cases, folic acid antagonists such as methotrexate may relieve joint inflammation. *Methotrexate must be used with caution because of its potential toxicity.* Physical therapy may be useful during recovery from arthritis.

Urethritis should be treated with tetracycline. An appropriate antibiotic can be used to treat enteric pathogens. Severe, recurring conjunctivitis may require drops containing steroids.

**Treatment—Investigational** Please contact the agencies listed under Resources, below, for the most current information. Addresses and telephone numbers of these agencies, as well as of individual experts and research centers, may be found in the Master Resources List.

**Resources**

For more information on Reiter syndrome: National Organization for Rare Disorders (NORD); Arthritis Foundation; NIH/National Arthritis and Musculoskeletal and Skin Diseases Information Clearinghouse; Centers for Disease Control.

**References**

Rheumatologic Disease and Associated Ocular Manifestations: B.P. Mahoney, et al.; J. Am. Optom. Assoc., June 1993, vol. 64(6), pp. 403–415.

Cecil Textbook of Medicine, 19th ed.: J.B. Wyngaarden, et al., eds.; W.B. Saunders Company, 1992, pp. 1518–1519.

HLA-B27 and Clinical Features in Reiter's Syndrome: T. Tuncer; Clin. Rheumatol., June 1992, vol. 11(2), pp. 239–242.

Oculocutaneous Manifestations Observed in Multisystem Disorders: J.P. Callen, et al.; Dermatol. Clin., October 1992, vol. 10(4), pp. 709–716.

Anterior Uveitis and Hypopyon: L.P. D'Alessandro, et al.; Am. J. Ophthalmol., September 1991, vol. 112(3), pp. 317–321.

Infection As a Cause of Arthritis: L.W. Moreland; Curr. Opin. Rheumatol., August 1991, vol. 3(4), pp. 639–649.

Ophthalmology: Principles and Concepts, 7th ed.: Frank W. Newell; Mosby Year Book, 1991, pp. 300, 334–335.

Birth Defects Encyclopedia: M.L. Buyse, ed.-in-chief; Blackwell Scientific Publications, 1990, pp. 146–147.

Clinical Ophthalmology, 2nd ed.: J.J. Kanski, ed.; Butterworth-Heinemann, 1990, p. 143.

Dictionary of Medical Syndromes, 3rd ed.: S.I. Magalini, et al., eds.; J.B. Lippincott Company, 1990, p. 755.

Arthritis and Allied Conditions, 11th ed.: D.J. McCarty; Lea and Febiger, 1989, pp. 944–953.

# RELAPSING POLYCHRONDRITIS

**Description** Relapsing polychondritis is a clinical syndrome characterized by inflammation and degeneration of the body's cartilaginous framework. Included are the nose, ears, joints, and the laryngotracheobronchial tree. Occasionally, the aortic valve is affected.

**Synonyms**

> Generalized or Systemic Chondromalacia
> Meyenburg-Altherz-Vehlinger Syndrome
> Relapsing Perichondritis
> Von Meyenburg Disease

**Signs and Symptoms** The course is marked by exacerbations and remissions. Fever and leukocytosis may be present. Episcleritis is a common symptom.

In one or both ears, pain, tenderness, and swelling of the cartilage may occur suddenly and then spread to the fleshy portion of the outer ear. Cartilaginous destruction may follow recurrences, leaving the ears with a drooping appearance. Middle ear inflammation is likely to lead to eustachian tube obstruction, and recurrent attacks may cause hearing loss. Attacks vary in severity and in duration, lasting from days to weeks.

Joint involvement may range from mild arthralgia to severe synovitis.

Two-thirds of patients develop nasal chondritis. Again, recurrent episodes may lead to cartilage destruction and collapse of the nasal bridge, resulting in nasal congestion and a saddle-nose deformity.

Collapse of the tracheal or bronchial wall may lead to speech difficulties, respiratory complications, and even death. In rare instances, heart valve abnormalities and kidney inflammation and dysfunction develop.

**Etiology** The cause is unknown; an immunologic mechanism is suspected.

**Epidemiology** The illness occurs equally in both sexes, usually from 40 to 60 years of age. All races are affected, but the syndrome predominantly affects whites.

**Related Disorders** See *Wegener Granulomatosis.*

**Treatment—Standard** Treatment usually is with nonsteroidal anti-inflammatory drugs (NSAIDs), dapsone, and corticosteroids. In severe cases, azathioprine, cyclophosphamide, and 6-mercaptopurine have been found to be useful immunosuppressants. The most severe cases may require heart valve replacement or a tracheostomy.

**Treatment—Investigational** Some cases may remit after use of the immunosuppressant cyclosporine-A. Continued research is necessary to fully evaluate the safety and effectiveness of this treatment.

Please contact the agencies listed under Resources, below, for the most current information. Addresses and telephone numbers of these agencies, as well as of individual experts and research centers, may be found in the Master Resources List.

**Resources**

**For more information on relapsing polychrondritis:** National Organization for Rare Disorders (NORD); Arthritis Foundation; NIH/National Institute of Arthritis, Musculoskeletal and Skin Diseases Information Clearinghouse; Polychrondritis and Rheumatoid Arthritis Clinic, Beth Israel Hospital.

**References**

Textbook of Rheumatology, 3rd ed.: W.N. Kelley, et al.; W.B. Saunders Company, 1989, pp. 1513–1521.

Cardiac Involvement in Relapsing Polychondritis: A. Balsa-Criado, et al.; J. Int. Cardiol., March 1987, vol. 14(3), pp. 381–383.

Internal Medicine, 2nd ed.: J.H. Stein, ed.-in-chief; Little, Brown and Company, 1987, pp. 631, 664, 1311.

Pulmonary Function in Relapsing Polychondritis: W.S. Krell, et al.; Am. Rev. Respir. Dis., June 1986, vol. 133(6), pp. 1120–1123.

Relapsing Polychondritis: Survival and Predictive Role of Early Disease Manifestations: C.J. Michet, et al.; Ann. Int. Med., January 1986, vol. 104(1), pp. 74–78.

# RETROPERITONEAL FIBROSIS

**Description** Retroperitoneal fibrosis is a disorder in which fibrotic tissue forms behind the peritoneum, causing ureteral obstruction.

**Synonyms**

> Idiopathic Retroperitoneal Fibrosis
> Ormond Disease

**Signs and Symptoms** Vague pain in the lower back or abdomen is the most common symptom. Other symptoms include loss of appetite, weight loss, fever, nausea, and anemia. Impaired movement of a limb may occur intermittently, and jaundice may be present. Occasionally, bleeding in the stomach and intestine occurs. About 10 percent of patients have difficulty urinating. A palpable mass can be felt in the rectum or abdomen in about 15 percent of patients. In some patients the inferior vena cava may be encased by the fibrous tissue, but this rarely causes obstruction.

Complications include hypertension and blood vessel blockage, and tissue growth may become malignant in rare cases.

**Etiology** The exact cause of retroperitoneal fibrosis is not known in about two-thirds of patients. Methysergide, which is used in the treatment and prevention of migraine headaches, may be the cause in 12 percent of cases. Malignant tumors are the cause in 8 percent of patients. Trauma and surgery are possible factors.

**Epidemiology** Males are affected twice as often as females. Seventy percent of patients are 50 to 70 years old. Children are rarely affected.

**Related Disorders** See *Carcinoid Syndrome; Scleroderma.*

**Vasculitis** is an inflammation of the veins, arteries, and/or capillaries. This disorder may occur alone or in conjunction with allergic and rheumatic diseases. Symptoms include blood clots, weakened vessel walls, muscle pain, joint pain, fever, weight loss, loss of appetite, abdominal pain, and shortness of breath. Localized symptoms are dependent on the type and size of vessel involved, as well as on the distribution of vessels affected. Various vasculitic (arteritic) syndromes have been described.

**Treatment—Standard** Treatment of retroperitoneal fibrosis depends on the location and extent of the tissue growth. Surgery is often successful in freeing a constricted organ. Steroid drug therapy may be used along with surgery, or in patients who are at high risk for surgery. In some cases, this disorder subsides spontaneously.

**Treatment—Investigational** Azathioprine has proved effective in a few cases, and progesterone has been used in Latin America. More research is needed to determine the safety and effectiveness of these drugs.

Please contact the agencies listed under Resources, below, for the most current information. Addresses and telephone numbers of these agencies, as well as of individual experts and research centers, may be found in the Master Resources List.

**Resources**

**For more information on retroperitoneal fibrosis:** National Organization for Rare Disorders (NORD); National Kidney Foundation; NIH/National Digestive Diseases Information Clearinghouse.

**References**

Cecil Textbook of Medicine, 19th ed.: J.B. Wyngaarden, et al., eds.; W.B. Saunders Company, 1992, p. 273.

Idiopathic Retroperitoneal Fibrosis: An Update: P.M. Higgins, et al.; Dig. Dis., 1990, vol. 8(4), pp. 206–222.

Idiopathic Retroperitoneal Fibrosis: Is Serum Alkaline Phosphatase a Marker of Disease Activity?: I.G. Barrison, et al.; Postgrad. Med. J., March 1988, vol. 64(749), pp. 239–241.

Non-Operative Management of Retroperitoneal Fibrosis: P.M. Higgins, et al.; Br. J. Surgery, June 1988, vol. 75(6), pp. 573–577.

Internal Medicine, 2nd ed.: J.H. Stein, et al., eds.; Little, Brown and Company, 1987, pp. 455–456.

# SCLERODERMA

**Description** Scleroderma is a connective tissue disorder characterized by skin thickening, Raynaud phenomenon, and a spectrum of systemic disorders.

**Synonyms**

CREST Syndrome

Dermatosclerosis

Systemic Sclerosis

**Signs and Symptoms** Clinical manifestations in early stages vary considerably, and the classical cutaneous lesions may appear later. Arthralgia, morning stiffness, fatigue, and weight loss are common features. Raynaud phenomenon is an early and frequent complaint (see **CREST syndrome,** below).

Leathery indurations of the skin are widespread and symmetrical, succeeded by atrophy and pigmentation. **Morphea,** a localized form of scleroderma, is seen usually between ages 20 and 50 and begins with an inflammatory stage. Firm, hard, oval-shaped plaques that have ivory centers and are encircled by a violet ring on the trunk, face, and extremities follow the first stage. Many patients improve spontaneously. Generalized morphea is more rare and serious and involves the dermis but not the internal organs. **Linear scleroderma** appears as a bandlike thickening of skin on the arm or leg. It is most likely to be unilateral but may be bilateral. Generally surfacing in young children, the first sign is failure of one limb to grow as rapidly as its counterpart. The band may extend from the hip to heel or shoulder to hand, and have a loss of deep tissue.

Systemic manifestations of scleroderma (systemic sclerosis) encompass a wide range of disturbances, including inflammatory myopathy (see *Polymyositis/Dermatomyositis);* edema of the fingers and hands; and microvascular, pulmonary (progressive interstitial fibrotic lung disease), renal (rapidly progressive renal failure), cardiovascular (myocardial accelerated hypertension), gastrointestinal (esophageal and colonic dysmotility), and immunologic abnormalities.

**CREST syndrome** is an acronym for (**C**)alcinosis, (**R**)aynaud phenomenon, (**E**)sophageal dysfunction, (**S**)clerodactyly, and (**T**)elangiectasia. Calcium salts accumulate subcutaneously and in many organs. Raynaud phenomenon affects symmetrical digits and may lead to digital ulcers and autoamputation. Dysfunction of the lower esophagus results in acid reflux and esophageal scarring; strictures may occur. Loss of peristalsis in the small intestine causes malabsorption and increased bacterial growth. Sclerodactyly results in decreased function of the fingers and toes. Telangiectasias, while not debilitating, are unsightly. Patients with the CREST syndrome are at increased risk of developing pulmonary hypertension.

**Etiology** The cause is unknown. The immune and vascular systems and connective tissue metabolism are known to play some part in the disease process.

**Epidemiology** It is estimated that between 50,000 and 100,000 persons are presently affected with scleroderma in the United States. The disease is 3 to 4 times more common in women than men. All ages are susceptible, but onset is highest in midlife.

**Related Disorders** See *Mixed Connective Tissue Disease; Raynaud Disease and Phenomenon; Systemic Lupus Erythematosus; Polymyositis/Dermatomyositis.*

**Treatment—Standard** Treatment is supportive and symptomatic. Fibrosis of the skin and internal organs may be treated with D-penicillamine and colchicine. Other skin care includes lubricating creams and antibiotic ointments for ulcerations. If Raynaud phenomenon is present, nifedipine, reserpine, guanethidine, phenoxybenzamine, nicotinic acid, diltiazem, verapamil, and/or prazosin may be useful. Rarely, calcinosis requires surgical intervention. For arthralgia or arthritis, nonsteroidal anti-inflammatory agents are generally given, although some patients may require low-dose corticosteroids.

Symptomatic management of pulmonary hypertension involves supplemental oxygen. The treatment of choice for renal involvement and hypertension is captopril and enalapril. Nifedipine and dipyridamole may be tried when myocardial perfusion abnormalities are present. Nonsteroidal anti-inflammatory drugs and corticosteroids are used to treat the symptoms of pericarditis.

When the esophagus and gastrointestinal tract are inflamed or ulcerated, the treatment of choice is $H_2$ blockers, such as cimetidine or ranitidine; omeprazole may also be used. Cisapride, newly released, may be helpful as well. Metoclopramide has been found to be beneficial for dysmotility. Acid reflux can be partially controlled by dietary measures. Several small and frequent meals per day lighten the work of the gastrointestinal system. Sitting upright for at least 2 hours after eating aids digestion.

Good oral hygiene is important because gum disease is common in scleroderma. Some patients experience excessive dryness of the mouth and eyes, or *Sjögren Syndrome.*

**Treatment—Investigational** Several experimental treatments are currently being evaluated. Early steps in the cellular synthesis of excess collagen have been blocked by retinoids for some types of scleroderma. Recombinant γ-interferon has been shown to inhibit oversynthesis of collagen. Ketanserin, a serotonin antagonist, may be successful for treating Raynaud phenomenon. Cyclosporine has potential in the treatment of dermatologic disorders, including those seen in collagen vascular diseases. Chlorambucil and photophoresis are also being evaluated for effectiveness. Dimethyl sulfoxide has been used experimentally to treat scleroderma. The efficacy and safety of xomazyme COS and photophoresis are under investigation, and octreotide acetate (manufactured by Sandoz) is undergoing trials to increase motility and to relieve abdominal symptoms. The orphan drug Iloprost is being studied for treating Raynaud phenomenon when accompanied by scleroderma. Gary W. Hunninghake, M.D., and Barbara White, M.D., at the University of Iowa Hospitals and Clinics, are conducting clinical trials to study bronchoalveolar lavage in interstitial lung disease associated with scleroderma.

Please contact the agencies listed under Resources, below, for the most current information. Addresses and telephone numbers of these agencies, as well as of individual experts and research centers, may be found in the Master Resources List.

**Resources**

**For more information on scleroderma:** National Organization for Rare Disorders (NORD); United Scleroderma Foundation; Scleroderma Research Foundation; Scleroderma Information Exchange; NIH/National Arthritis and Musculoskeletal and Skin Diseases Information Clearinghouse.

**References**

Cecil Textbook of Medicine, 19th ed.: J.B. Wyngaarden, et al., eds.; W.B. Saunders Company, 1992, pp. 1530–1535.

Extracorporeal Photochemotherapy Induces the Production of Tumor Necrosis Factor-Alpha by Monocytes: Implications for the Treatment of Cutaneous T-Cell Lymphomas and Systemic Sclerosis: B.R. Vowels; J. Invest. Dermatol., May 1992, vol. 98(5), pp. 686–692.

Genetic and Environmental Factors in Systemic Sclerosis: R.I. Fox; Curr. Opin. Rheumatol., December 1992, vol. 4(6), pp. 857–861.

The Many Faces of Scleroderma: J.D. Smiley; Am. J. Med. Sci., November 1992, vol. 304(5), pp. 319–333.

Mendelian Inheritance in Man, 10th ed.: V.A. McKusick; The Johns Hopkins University Press, 1992, p. 1006.

Treatment of Systemic Sclerosis: F.M. Wigley; Curr. Opin. Rheumatol., December 1992, vol. 4(6), pp. 878–886.

Epidemiology of Scleroderma: A.J. Silman, Curr. Opin. Rheumatol., December 1991, vol. 3(6), pp. 967–972.

Treatment of Systemic Sclerosis: T.A. Medsger; Ann. Rheum. Dis., November 1991, vol. 50(4), pp. 877–886.

Treatment of Systemic Sclerosis: V. Steen; Curr. Opin. Rheumatol., December 1991, vol. 3(6), pp. 979–985.

Use of Angiotensin-Converting-Enzyme Inhibitors in the Management of Renal Disease: J.P. Asher; Clin. Pharm., January 1991, vol. 10(10), pp. 25–31.

Birth Defects Encyclopedia: M.L. Buyse, ed.-in-chief; Blackwell Scientific Publications, 1990, pp. 1515–1516.

Arthritis and Allied Conditions, 11th ed.: D.J. McCarty; Lea and Febiger, 1989, pp. 460–461, 1142–1144.

Textbook of Rheumatology, 3rd ed.: W.N. Kelley, et al.; W.B. Saunders Company, 1989, pp. 1215–1244.

Treatment of Autoimmune Disease with Extracorporeal Photochemotherapy: Progressive Systemic Sclerosis: A.H. Rook; Yale J. Biol. Med., November–December 1989, vol. 62(6), pp. 639–645.

# SJÖGREN SYNDROME (SJS)

**Description** Sjögren syndrome, an autoimmune disorder characterized by degeneration of the mucus-secreting glands (exocrine glands), particularly the lacrimal and salivary glands, is also associated with rheumatic disorders such as rheumatoid arthritis.

**Synonyms**

> Autoimmune Exocrinopathy
> Dacryosialoadenopathia Atrophicans
> Gougerot-Houwer-Sjogren
> Keratoconjuctivitis Sicca
> Secreto-Inhibitor-Xerodermatostenosis
> Sicca Syndrome

**Signs and Symptoms Primary SjS** is characterized solely by keratoconjunctivitis sicca and xerostomia. In **secondary SjS,** keratoconjunctivitis sicca and/or xerostomia occur in the setting of a connective tissue disease, most often rheumatoid arthritis **(RA).**

Most patients with Sjögren syndrome have primary SjS. The onset of symptoms is insidious. Decreased production of saliva and consequent dry mouth make chewing and swallowing food difficult. The lack of saliva causes particles of food to stick to the cheeks, gums, and throat. Teeth decay easily, leading to dental caries, gingivitis, and pyorrhea.

As the lacrimal glands atrophy, tears decrease, causing keratoconjunctivitis sicca and leaving the patient with a feeling of grittiness and burning in the eyes. The eyelids may stick together.

Dryness may extend to the skin and to the mucous membranes of the nose, throat, and vagina.

Patients with primary SjS may have extraglandular (systemic) disease as well, affecting lungs, kidneys, blood vessels (vasculitis), and muscles. Patients may experience arthritis, rash (palpable purpura on the lower extremities, photosensitive dermatitis on the face, arms, and other sun-exposed areas), fever, and neurologic involvement. The latter may involve seizures, psychosis, dementia, and strokelike syndromes. Primary SjS may occasionally terminate in a lymphoid malignancy. Patients with systemic disease usually have positive blood tests for antinuclear antibodies and antibodies to Ro and La antigens.

A number of tests are available for the diagnosis of SjS: 1) eye examination, including Schirmer's test (measurement of tear production) and rose bengal staining (looking for keratitis); 2) measurement of either unstimulated or stimulated saliva production; 3) examination of cells from the lip (minor salivary gland biopsy) to determine whether lymphocytes are present in the salivary glands; and 4) blood tests, including ANA (antinuclear antibody) and anti-Ro and anti-La antibodies.

All patients suspected of having SjS should be examined by an ophthalmologist. Patients with SjS who have positive blood tests for anti-Ro antibodies should be evaluated by a rheumatologist for evidence of extraglandular involvement.

**Etiology** The cause is unknown. Sjögren syndrome is an autoimmune disorder that is known to have a genetic predisposition (HLA-DR3) and often occurs in patients with rheumatoid arthritis, systemic lupus erythematosus, and other connective tissue diseases.

**Epidemiology** The syndrome affects 9 females to every male. Ninety percent of persons with the disorder are postmenopausal women, although symptoms may be apparent at an earlier age. Recent data suggest that men with symptomatic HIV infection may develop a syndrome similar to Sjögren syndrome.

**Related Disorders** See *Keratomalacia; Ligneous Conjunctivitis; Systemic Lupus Erythematosus.*

**Rheumatoid arthritis (RA),** an inflammatory autoimmune disorder of unknown etiology, is characterized by morning stiffness and polyarthritis (chiefly the hands, wrists, knees, feet, shoulders, and hips). Once affected, a joint may remain painful and swollen for weeks, months, and even years. About 25 percent of RA patients also have secondary SjS.

**Mikulicz disease** is a benign chronic disorder of the parotid and lacrimal glands. Symptoms include dryness of the mouth, difficulty swallowing, and tooth decay. Blurred vision and the absence of or a decrease in tears may be evident.

**Treatment—Standard** Treatment depends on symptoms. No specific therapy, however, presently restores glandular secretion.

Ocular symptoms may be relieved by the use of artificial tears and lubricating creams at bedtime.

For oral symptoms, artificial saliva can be used to wet the mouth. Patients may benefit from chewing sugarless gum or using sugarless hard candies.

Systemic medication such as corticosteroids and hydroxychloroquine and other immunosuppressive agents are occasionally needed for certain complications (the extraglandular features described above).

All patients should be routinely checked by ophthalmologists and dentists. Patients with extraglandular features should be under the care of rheumatologists.

**Treatment—Investigational** The National Institute of Dental Research is conducting studies on several drugs for treatment of SjS. For more information, please contact Alice Macynski, R.N.

Bromhexine is an orphan drug being tested as a treatment for mild to moderate keratoconjunctivitis sicca. It is manufactured by Boehringer Ingelheim Pharmaceuticals.

Cyclosporine and OcuNex ophthalmic solution are being studied in the treatment for severe dry eyes. The drug Pilocarpine (salagen tablets) is being tested for the treatment of dry mouth.

Please contact the agencies listed under Resources, below, for the most current information. Addresses and telephone numbers of these agencies, as well as of individual experts and research centers, may be found in the Master Resources List.

**Resources**

**For more information on Sjögren syndrome:** National Organization for Rare Disorders (NORD); Sjögren Syndrome Foundation; National Sjögren's Syndrome Association; Arthritis Foundation; American Autoimmune-Related Diseases Association; NIH/National Institute of Dental Research; NIH/National Arthritis and Musculoskeletal and Skin Diseases Information Clearinghouse.

**References**

Mendelian Inheritance in Man, 9th ed.: V.A. McKusick; The Johns Hopkins University Press, 1990, pp. 1477–1478.

Primary Sjögren's Syndrome in Men: Clinical Serologic and Immunogenetic Features: R. Molina, et al.; Am. J. Med., January 1986, vol. 80(1), pp. 23–31.

Treatment of Primary Sjögren's Syndrome with Hydrochloroquine: R.I. Fox, et al.; Am. J. Med., October 1988, vol. 85(4A), pp. 62–67.

Molecular Characterization of a Major Auto-Antibody Associated Cross-Reactive Idiotype in Sjögren's Syndrome: T.J. Kipps, et al.; J. Immunol., June 1989, vol. 142(12), pp. 4261–4268.

# SYSTEMIC LUPUS ERYTHEMATOSUS (SLE)

**Description** SLE is a multisystem inflammatory disease of connective tissue involving immunologically mediated tissue injury. Many abnormalities are associated.

**Synonyms**

Disseminated Lupus Erythematosus

**Signs and Symptoms** Fatigue is an early and frequent feature. Other constitutional symptoms include fever, swollen glands, anorexia, weight loss, headaches, alopecia, and edema.

Arthritis, arthralgia, and myalgia occur in over 90 percent of patients, in some cases preceding the onset of systemic disease by months or years. The arthritis is often migratory, occurs most often in the knees and finger and wrist joints, and is symmetric. Joint involvement is usually nonerosive.

Dermatologic manifestations occur in over 80 percent of patients. Photosensitive lesions include both annular, discoid lesions and bullae. The classic erythematous butterfly rash across the bridge of the nose and cheeks appears in about 50 percent of patients, often lasting hours or days. Lesions of the mucous membranes occur in about 35 percent of patients.

Vascular involvement includes telangiectasia, Raynaud phenomenon, and vasculitis. Pulmonary involvement includes pleurisy, cough, and pneumonitis. Cardiovascular abnormalities include pericarditis, myocarditis, and coronary artery disease. Hematologic abnormalities include anemia, leukopenia, lymphocytopenia, and thrombocytopenia in addition to the lymphadenopathy often seen early in the disease.

Renal abnormalities associated with SLE include proteinuria, interstitial nephritis, and diffuse proliferative and membranous glomerulonephritis. Neuropsychiatric symptoms include depression, anxiety, psychosis, seizures, stroke, neuropathy, and meningitis.

Tentative diagnosis can be made if 4 of the following criteria are present (using the ARA Revised Criteria for the Classification of SLE): arthritis involving 2 or more joints; malar rash; discoid rash; oral or nasal ulcers; photosensitivity; pleuritis or pericarditis; positive LE cell test, presence of anti-DNA or anti-Sm, or a chronic false-positive serologic test for syphilis; proteinuria over 0.5 gm/day, cellular casts in the urine; seizures or psychosis; hemolytic anemia, leukopenia, lymphopenia, or thrombocytopenia; and an abnormal antinuclear antibody titer.

The SLE patient may experience exacerbations (flares) of symptoms, which can be triggered by such factors as stress, infections, and exposure to sunlight.

**Etiology** The cause is still unknown. Immunologic, genetic, environmental, hormonal, and infectious factors have all been implicated.

SLE-like symptoms have also been induced by some drugs, including hydralazine, procainamide, isoniazid, methyldopa, and chlorpromazine.

**Epidemiology** Ninety percent of SLE cases occur in women, at any age, although the peak incidence is between 15 and 55 years. Black women are affected 3 times as often as white women, and the disorder also is commonly seen in Chinese women. Estimates of the prevalence in the United States vary considerably; however, most reliable estimates are about 50:100,000.

**Related Disorders** See *Scleroderma; Polymyositis/Dermatomyositis; Mixed Connective Tissue Disease; Polyarteritis Nodosa; Sjögren Syndrome; Raynaud Disease and Phenomenon; Purpura, Thrombotic Thrombocytopenic.*

**Treatment—Standard** Symptoms such as joint pain and fever commonly respond to aspirin or other nonsteroidal anti-inflammatory agents. Antimalarial drugs (hydroxychloroquine and chloroquine) treat skin lesions and joint pain effectively, although side effects such as visual disturbances and nausea may occur during prolonged treatment. Standard treatment for more severe manifestations of SLE is corticosteroid therapy; in particular, high dosages of prednisone or its equivalent. Initial treatment and maintenance dosages vary according to organ system involvement, response, side effects, and duration of use. Corticosteroid creams and lotions effectively control rashes and skin irritation but should be used with caution on the face and in the presence of skin infection. Since infections are a leading cause of death in SLE patients, their management should be aggressive. Oral contraceptives should be avoided.

**Treatment—Investigational** Although immunosuppressive treatment has been in use for several years, it is still considered experimental. It is thought that suppression of the immune system will also suppress the formation of harmful immune complexes appearing to cause widespread organ and tissue destruction. Unfortunately, such therapy increases the risk of infections. Drugs used with the corticosteroids are cyclophosphamide or azathioprine.

Other investigational management includes the use of corticosteroids via intravenous bolus ("pulse steroids"), and attempts to physically remove the immune complexes from the circulation by plasmapheresis or lymphoplasmapheresis.

Researchers studying cyclophosphamide, also used in the therapy of some malignancies, are treating patients with lupus nephritis as well as some severe cases of CNS lupus that do not respond to steroids, with intravenous boluses of cyclophosphamide given at 4-week intervals. Side effects and long-term efficacy are still under investigation.

Other experimental treatments under investigation include intravenous immune globulin; a monoclonal antibody (sponsored by Medclone) for immunization against lupus nephritis; and an orphan product dehydroepiandrosterone (**DHEA**) (manufactured by Genelabs Technologies) to treat SLE and steroid-dependent SLE patients.

Please contact the agencies listed under Resources, below, for the most current information. Addresses and telephone numbers of these agencies, as well as of individual experts and research centers, may be found in the Master Resources List.

**Resources**

**For more information on systemic lupus erythematosus:** National Organization for Rare Disorders (NORD); Lupus Foundation of America; Systemic Lupus Erythematosus Foundation; American Lupus Society; NIH/National Arthritis and Musculoskeletal and Skin Diseases Information Clearinghouse; American Autoimmune-Related Diseases Association.

**References**

Medical Progress. Systemic Lupus Erythematosus: J.A. Mills; N. Engl. J. Med., June 1994, vol. 330(26), pp. 1871–1879.

Arthritis and Rheumatism: M. Reichlin, et al.; Arthritis Rheum., April 1992, vol. 35(4), pp. 457–464.

Cecil Textbook of Medicine, 19th ed.: J.B. Wyngaarden, et al., eds.; W.B. Saunders Company, 1992, pp. 1522–1530.

Mendelian Inheritance in Man, 10th ed.: V.A. McKusick; The Johns Hopkins University Press, 1992, pp. 675–676.

Systemic Lupus Erythematosus: M.C. Hochberg; Rheum. Dis. Clin. North Am., August 1991, vol. 16(3), pp. 617–639.

Systemic Lupus Erythematosus: D.S. Pisetsky; Curr. Opin. Immunol., December 1991, vol. 3(6), pp. 917–923.

Treatment of Systemic Lupus Erythematosus: M.L. Miller; Curr. Opin. Rheumatol., October 1991, vol. 3(5), pp. 803–808.

Arthritis and Allied Conditions, 11th ed.: D.J. McCarty; Lea and Febiger, 1989, pp. 1022–1079.

Textbook of Rheumatology, 3rd ed.: W.N. Kelley, et al.; W.B. Saunders Company, 1989, pp. 1101–1146.

# TIETZE SYNDROME

**Description** Tietze syndrome affects the upper costal cartilages, usually the 2nd, with tenderness, pain, and swelling.

**Synonyms**
>Chondropathia Tuberosa
>Costochondritis

**Signs and Symptoms** Pain, tenderness, and fusiform or spindle-shaped swelling occur in 1 or more of the 4 upper ribs. The tenderness and swelling are localized. The pain may have a sudden or gradual onset and may be mild or severe, dull or sharp, gripping, or neuralgic in nature. Sudden coughing or deep breathing accentuates the pain, and often precedes the swelling. The pain typically diminishes after a few weeks or months, but the swelling may persist.

**Etiology** The cause is unknown.

**Epidemiology** The syndrome usually affects older children and young adults. Males and females are affected in equal numbers.

**Related Disorders Benign and malignant tumors** and **angina pectoris** may mimic this syndrome.

**Spinal root lesions or compression** may cause chest pain similar to that seen in Tietze syndrome. The pain develops after sudden movement of the body such as straining, coughing, sneezing, or laughing.

**Chest wall pain** is a broad term given to several conditions characterized by noncardiac anterior chest wall pain. A dull, aching pain results as a result of straining, poor posture, or inflammation or infiltration of the chest muscles, ligaments, or cartilage. Chest wall pain may also arise from irritation of a nerve root in the upper spine or neck, or a fractured rib. Tietze syndrome is included in this group of ailments.

**Costal chondritis (costochondritis),** inflammation of rib cartilage, is characterized by pain, sometimes radiating, in the chest wall that may be similar to that of Tietze syndrome. However, the swelling seen in Tietze is absent.

**Treatment—Standard** Treatment consists of local heat and anti-inflammatory or analgesic medication. Usually the pain subsides after a few weeks or months. Swelling may remain for a longer period of time.

**Treatment—Investigational** Please contact the agencies listed under Resources, below, for the most current information. Addresses and telephone numbers of these agencies, as well as of individual experts and research centers, may be found in the Master Resources List.

**Resources**

**For more information on Tietze syndrome:** National Organization for Rare Disorders (NORD); NIH/National Arthritis, Musculoskeletal and Skin Diseases Information Clearinghouse.

**References**

Internal Medicine, 2nd ed.: J.H. Stein, ed.-in-chief; Little, Brown and Company, 1987, p. 610.

Clinical Experience of Drug Treatments for Mastalgia: J.K. Pye, et al.; Lancet, August 1985, vol. 2(8451), pp. 373–377.

Musculoskeletal Chest Wall Pain: A.G. Fam, et al.; J. Can. Med. Assoc., September 1, 1985, vol. 133(5), pp. 379–389.

# 12 OPHTHALMOLOGIC DISORDERS
### By Richard Alan Lewis, M.D., M.S.

The evaluation of anyone, especially a child, with a visual disability or a developmental abnormality of the visual system must depend heavily on the diligence, the prudence, and the accuracy of the complete ophthalmologic evaluation. Unfortunately, some ophthalmologists focus intently on the eyes and ocular adnexa and disregard other obvious facial and cranial defects and other systemic dysmorphic features. Nonetheless, the ophthalmologist provides key information to the thorough evaluation of a dysmorphic individual, including a unique knowledge and analysis of visual embryology, of ocular and systemic pathology, of the natural history and prognosis of visual disorders, and of the burden of ocular diseases.

Both primary physicians and specialists in a multidisciplinary clinic who must evaluate, diagnose, and manage children with craniofacial defects involving the visual system should befriend an ophthalmologist, perhaps a pediatric ophthalmologist, who has demonstrated devotion to thoroughness and accuracy and who is willing to explore the patient's immediate and extended family members for variable signs of hereditary disorders. Since many heritable diseases occur with predictable mendelian patterns of inheritance, ophthalmologists must also acknowledge that their responsibility often extends beyond the individual patient and that they are obligated to search for other affected family members and to educate individuals at risk for the disorder or for bearing affected offspring.

As in all other realms of human genetics, the primary obligation of the ophthalmologist and primary physician is to establish a diagnosis. That diagnosis must be specific rather than symptomatic. A clinical diagnosis of "nystagmus" is not acceptable, since numerous defects in the development and organization of the central nervous system, the optic nerve, or the retina, let alone defects in the anterior segment of the globe, can result in nystagmus. Nystagmus is a sign, not a unique diagnosis. Similarly, the primary physician should advise the ophthalmologist about other dysmorphic features with which visual handicaps appear to be associated, especially other defects in the embryogenesis or morphology of the central nervous system.

As in other genetic disease, the evaluation of the proband may involve recovery of previously written records of the patient's evaluation; copies of personal or family photographs, albums, or paintings; prior neuroimaging studies, fundus photographs, and fluorescein angiograms; and the records of electrodiagnostic studies, color-vision tests, and other psychophysiologic investigations, before new investigations are planned. Usually, the recovery of reports is *not* adequate, since, for example, neuroradiologists may attend cranial defects or anomalies of brain structure and ignore aberrations in the anterior visual pathways, orbit, or globes. The verbal report of a previously "normal computed tomography **(CT)** scan" may change dramatically when one finds that the actual films demonstrate only normal intracranial contents and that no views record the anterior visual pathways, chiasm and pituitary, and orbits. Additional studies, reconstructions, or, preferably, magnetic resonance imaging **(MRI)** scans, may be necessary to complete the diagnostic assessment.

The ascertainment and personal examination of at-risk relatives may also prove extremely important. Those examinations may include siblings (for recessive disorders) or both parents (for dominant or X-linked ones) for discovery of minor manifestations. Physicians may recover photographs to look for variable facial features, previous CT or MRI scans, pathology slides, and other biochemical or chromosomal studies. For example, the evaluation of children with congenital cataracts mandates the thorough examination of both parents for minor manifestations of autosomal dominant cataracts with variable expressivity. Similarly, biomicroscopy of the lens of the adolescent or preadolescent for features of Steinert myotonic dystrophy *without* examination of both parents may lead to highly erroneous conclusions. Lastly, some X-linked disorders have distinctive carrier states in the mothers of new, "isolated" males; the clarification of the carrier status changes an isolated event to one with a definable recurrence risk. To counsel an adult in the reproductive age group about a childhood disorder, it may be necessary to recover documents to establish a historical diagnosis that the parents retain by memory. For example, I once counseled a 21-year-old young woman who was a survivor of unilateral retinoblastoma. Recovery and review of the original histopathology slides established a diagnosis of persistent hyperplastic primary vitreous **(PHPV)** and showed no evidence of intraocular neoplasm. Nonetheless, the parents had believed firmly for 20 years that the enucleated eye had contained a malignant embryonal tumor. The recurrence risk for PHPV is extremely low, whereas the recurrence risk for retinoblastoma depends substantially on other clinical and genetic parameters!

The investigation of the family history must be meticulous. That family history should ascertain the parentage and may investigate consanguinity, incest, and nonpaternity. Even in the absence of known consanguinity by descent, the geographic origin of the parents, particularly if not born in the United States, or the geographic proximity of their places of birth may imply consanguinity from a geographic isolate, even if language differences, lack of records, and verbal history fail to establish it.

The absence of a family history of a specific disorder does not exclude the possibility of affected individuals. In the presence of a disease that can be transmitted as an autosomal dominant trait, recall and examination of both parents are mandatory to exclude minimal manifestations. A child with profound colobomatous microphthalmia and "no family history" may have a minimally affected parent with anterior stromal hypoplasia in the characteristic inferior nasal meridian of one iris or a minor choroidal coloboma at the equator of one ocular fundus that is detectable only by biomicroscopy or indirect ophthalmoscopy performed by a careful and comprehensive ophthalmologist. Omission of this step in the evaluation of the affected child has led to inappropriate counseling of recurrence risks and the subsequent birth of another, occasionally even more severely affected, offspring.

Ancillary diagnostic studies may include chromosomal analysis, biochemical tests, molecular studies, audiometry, ultrasound of the orbit or globe, and neuroimaging. High resolution chromosomal analysis may be appropriate in any high-risk multisystem disorder. For ophthalmologists, the two key indications are unexplained mental retardation with ocular findings that seem not necessarily associated, and any multisystem anomalies where the eye and the central nervous system are involved simultaneously. Of course, chromosomal analysis is mandatory in known embryonal malignancies, such as retinoblastoma or aniridia–Wilms tumor.

The primary physician should engage the ophthalmologist in the assessment of contiguous gene syndromes, when one disease of a known single gene inheritance is associated with other unexplained features or diseases. The recent association of choroideremia with microcephaly, severe neurosensory hearing impairment, short stature, obesity, and developmental delay may lead to discovery of a visible or molecular deletion on chromosome Xq21. A number of contiguous gene syndromes involve the ocular system. WAGR syndrome (Wilms tumor, aniridia, genitourinary anomalies, mental retardation) occurs as a result of a deletion of chromosome 11p13. Retinoblastoma may be a hallmark of the associative deletion at chromosome 13q14, along with microcephaly, broad nose, short neck, short thumb and great toe, and ear pits. Retinitis pigmentosa has been noted in a deletion of Xp21, in association with Duchenne muscular dystrophy, chronic granulomatous disease, and the McLeod red cell phenotype. The simultaneous occurrence of a recognizable "single gene" ocular disease with two or more other recognizable genetic events should lead the ophthalmologist to contemplate the explanation of a contiguous deletion and to seek the appropriate chromosomal or molecular confirmation. Chromosomal analysis may also be important when individuals with a female appearance present with X-linked traits, such as color blindness, which classically afflict "only" males. Examples of Turner syndrome with color-vision deficiency or testicular feminization with color-vision deficiency have been recorded.

Still, one may need to explain the isolated case, the infant, child, or even adolescent who is the only individual in the family afflicted with an apparent genetic disorder. The primary physician and the ophthalmologist should consider the possibility that this individual represents the new mutation, the first individual in the family to have the disease. For example, nearly one-half of individuals with classical neurofibromatosis, NF 1, are the first individuals afflicted with the disorder in their families. Once the mutation has occurred, however, the recurrence risk for offspring and subsequent generations of this individual follows a classical autosomal dominant pattern. If a new mutation for an autosomal dominant is considered, the physicians should inquire about the paternal age at the time the child was born. There is an increasing risk of new mutation, single gene, autosomal dominant disorders in the offspring of older-age-group fathers. The possibility that a person is the only affected individual in the family with a disorder would raise the prospect that the disorder is recessive and thus is determined by the coincident inheritance of a recessive gene from each (normal-appearing) carrier parent. A search for parental consanguinity—the classic features of a common geographic, religious, family, or (maiden) surname background—would be appropriate.

Sometimes the isolated case does not represent a genetic or inherited disorder, but rather a somatic mutation. There is reasonable evidence that segmental neurofibromatosis (and perhaps even unilateral retinoblastoma) is not strictly speaking a germinal mutation, but rather a postzygotic somatic event. Are the physicians certain that the biological parents are accurately identified? Rarely, parents will adopt a child and never admit in the child's presence that he or she has been adopted until well after the recognition of a heritable disorder later. Nonpenetrance or minimal expressivity of either a dominant or an X-linked trait can be resolved by diligent investigation of parents and other relatives or of an obligate carrier mother. Lastly, a child may be an isolated case of an apparently genetic disorder because the diagnosis is not correct. Drugs, prenatal infections, and other environmental insults can create dysmorphisms that distantly resemble genetic disease. For example, congenitally deaf, nonverbal children with pigmentary retinopathy may have Usher syndrome type I, or they may have congenital rubella syndrome.

Most especially, the ophthalmologist must remain informed about the evolution of gene mapping and its implications for mutational diagnosis, carrier detection, premorbid ascertainment, and prenatal diagnosis. The identification of suitable families for research provides an invaluable resource for all humankind. There is no substitute for the DNA in a simple blood sample!

The ophthalmologist must be sensitive to these vagaries and must be willing to extend his search beyond the affected patient to the immediate family, including siblings and both parents. Information that the ophthalmologist can provide in these situations will amplify tremendously the abilities of the primary physicians to sort a clinical problem and to establish a firm diagnosis as the basis for counseling the individual and the family about recurrence risks, natural history and outcomes, and reproductive choices.

# OPHTHALMOLOGIC DISORDERS
*Listings in This Section*

# ANIRIDIA (AN)

**Description** Aniridia, a genetic disorder of vision and ocular structure, is characterized by partial or nearly complete agenesis of the iris in one or both eyes. Four forms **(AN-I, AN-II, AN-III, AN-IV)** have been characterized and their signs distinguished. AN-IV, the **WAGR syndrome,** consists of (**W**)ilms tumor, (**A**)niridia, (**G**)enitourinary anomalies, and mental (**R**)etardation.

**Synonyms**

Irideremia

**Signs and Symptoms** Vision is preserved in some mild cases. **AN-I** is marked by variable expression of the disorder. Hypoplasia of the iris is rarely unilateral. In **AN-II,** abnormalities of the iris may occur alone or in combination with other disorders such as cataracts, glaucoma, nystagmus, corneal pannus, and underdevelopment of the fovea.

A 3rd type of aniridia, **AN-III,** is associated with mental retardation. The 4th type, **AN-IV (WAGR syndrome),** occurs with Wilms tumor and genitourinary abnormalities. In most cases there is also delayed mental development. The ocular abnormalities may include congenital cataracts, nystagmus, and ptosis. Other abnormalities such as micrognathia, growth deficiency, and microcephaly may be present.

**Etiology** AN-I has been assigned to chromosome 2 and is transmitted as an autosomal dominant trait. AN-II results from defects on chromosome 11 in the gene homologous to the PAX6 gene in mouse. It is inherited as an autosomal dominant trait, although some cases appear to be genetic mutations. An autosomal recessive inheritance is suspected in AN-III. WAGR syndrome always results from a contiguous deletion of chromosome 11p13.

**Epidemiology** All types of aniridia affect males and females in equal numbers. The incidence is approximately 1:100,000 to 1:200,000 live births in the United States.

**Related Disorders** See *WAGR Syndrome; Rieger Syndrome.*

In **iridogoniodysgenesis,** a genetic eye structure disorder in newborns, the defect is underdevelopment of the stroma of the iris.

**Dominant juvenile-onset open-angle glaucoma,** which must be distinguished from autosomal recessive primary congenital glaucoma, has onset of symptoms delayed until childhood or adolescence. Other cases may represent an early onset of some other complex forms of glaucoma. Dominant juvenile-onset open-angle glaucoma has been mapped to chromosome 1q, but the causative gene has not been isolated.

**Treatment—Standard** Treatment is usually directed toward improvement of useful vision. If there is a refractive error, a patient may benefit from corrective lenses. Drugs may be helpful in control of glaucoma, but frequently surgery will be needed. Surgery may be necessary for cataracts. Genetic counseling is recommended for all patients, regardless of the type of aniridia. Patients with AN-IV should be evaluated with karyotype for the deletion that raises the risk of developing Wilms tumor; abdominal sonogram, CT scan, or laparotomy with renal biopsy may be necessary. Other treatment is symptomatic and supportive.

**Treatment—Investigational** Please contact the agencies listed under Resources, below, for the most current information. Addresses and telephone numbers of these agencies, as well as of individual experts and research centers, may be found in the Master Resources List.

**Resources**

**For more information on aniridia:** National Organization for Rare Disorders (NORD); NIH/National Eye Institute; Vision Foundation; National Association for Parents of the Visually Impaired; National Association for the Visually Handicapped; The Arc (a national organization on mental retardation).

**For genetic information and genetic counseling referrals:** March of Dimes Birth Defects Foundation; Alliance of Genetic Support Groups.

**References**

Mendelian Inheritance in Man, 11th ed.: V.A. McKusick; The Johns Hopkins University Press, 1994, pp. 109–111.

Genomic Structure, Evolutionary Conservation and Aniridia Mutations in the Human PAX6 Gene: T. Glaser, et al.; Nat. Genet., 1992, vol. 2, pp. 232–239.

Resolution of the Two Loci for Autosomal Dominant Aniridia, AN1 and AN2, to a Single Locus on Chromosome 11p13: L.A. Lyons, et al.; Genomics, 1992, vol. 13, pp. 925–930.

Suppression of Tumorigenicity in Wilms Tumor by the p15.5–p14 Region of Chromosome 11: S.F. Dowdy, et al.; Science, 1991, vol. 254, pp. 293–295.

11p13 Deletion, Wilms' Tumour, and Aniridia: Unusual Genetic, Non-Ocular and Ocular Features of Three Cases: V. Jotterand, et al.; Br. J. Ophthalmol., 1990, vol. 74, pp. 568–570.

Two Anonymous DNA Segments Distinguish the Wilms' Tumor and Aniridia Loci: L.M. Davis, et al.; Science, August 1988, vol. 241, pp. 840–842.

Familial Isolated Aniridia Associated with a Translocation Involving Chromosomes 11 and 22 [t (11;22) (p13;q12.2)]: J.W. Moore, et al.; Hum. Genet., April 1986, vol. 72(4), pp. 297–302.

Wilms' Tumor Detection in Patients with Sporadic Aniridia: Successful Use of Ultrasound: A.L. Friedman; Am. J. Dis. Child, February 1986, vol. 140(2), pp. 173–174.

Wilms' Tumor with Aniridia/Iris Dysplasia and Apparently Normal Chromosomes: V.M. Riccardi, et al.; J. Pediatr., April 1982, vol. 100(4), pp. 574–577.

Autosomal Dominant Aniridia: Probable Linkage to Acid Phosphatase Locus on Chromosome 2: R.E. Ferrell, et al.; Proc. Natl. Acad. Sci. USA, March 1980, vol. 77(3), pp. 1580–1582.

# BLEPHAROPHIMOSIS, PTOSIS, EPICANTHUS INVERSUS SYNDROME (BPES)

**Description** BPES is a disorder characterized by eyelids that are abnormally narrow horizontally (blepharophimosis), a vertical fold of skin from the lower eyelid up either side of the nose (epicanthus inversus), and drooping of the upper eyelids (ptosis or blepharoptosis). Two types of the syndrome are thought to occur. **Type I** BPES also involves female infertility, is inherited as an autosomal dominant genetic trait, and is transmitted by affected males to their offspring. Premature ovarian failure, the cause of which is unknown, usually prevents females from reproducing. **Type II** BPES is also transmitted as an autosomal dominant genetic trait. Males and females can transmit the disorder to their offspring; it is not associated with female infertility.

**Synonyms**
> Blepharophimosis, Epicanthus Inversus, and Ptosis
> Blepharophimosis, Epicanthus Inversus, and Ptosis Syndrome

**Signs and Symptoms** In addition to the major symptoms of BPES (blepharophimosis, ptosis, epicanthus inversus), the eyelid fold may also be absent. Other findings include telecanthus, a low bridge of the nose, incomplete development or cupping of the external ears, and, more rarely, microphthalmos, a high-arched palate, displaced tear ducts, and infertility in females.

**Etiology** Both forms of BPES are inherited as autosomal dominant traits. Recent findings suggest that the defective gene may be found on the long arm (q) of chromosome 3.

**Epidemiology** BPES affects males slightly more often than females, especially in those type I families where limited reproduction of females reduces the relative number of affected female births.

**Related Disorders** See *Waardenburg Syndrome.*

**Treatment–Standard** Eye surgery may be performed to reduce the epicanthus inversus and to repair blepharophimosis and ptosis. Genetic counseling may be of benefit for patients and their families. Other treatment is symptomatic and supportive.

**Treatment—Investigational** Please contact the agencies listed under Resources, below, for the most current information. Addresses and telephone numbers of these agencies, as well as of individual experts and research centers, may be found in the Master Resources List.

**Resources**

For more information on blepharophimosis, ptosis, epicanthus inversus syndrome: National Organization for Rare Disorders (NORD); NIH/National Institute of Child Health and Human Development; National Craniofacial Foundation; FACES—National Association for the Craniofacially Handicapped; Society for the Rehabilitation of the Facially Disfigured; Forward Face; Children's Craniofacial Association; Craniofacial Family Association; AboutFace.

For genetic information and genetic counseling referrals: March of Dimes Birth Defects Foundation; Alliance of Genetic Support Groups.

**References**

Mendelian Inheritance in Man, 11th ed.: V.A. McKusick; The Johns Hopkins University Press, 1994, pp. 196–197.

Birth Defects Encyclopedia: M.L. Buyse, ed.-in-chief; Blackwell Scientific Publications, 1990, pp. 228–229.

Parental Age in Blepharophimosis, Ptosis, Epicanthus Inversus, Telecanthus Complex: W.H. Finley, et al.; Am. J. Med. Genet., August 1990, vol. 36(4), pp. 414–417.

Blepharophimosis and Its Association with Female Infertility: C.A. Jones, et al.; Br. J. Ophthalmol., 1984, vol. 68, pp. 533–534.

Additional Findings in the Syndrome of Blepharoptosis, Blepharophimosis, Epicanthus Inversus, and Telecanthus: R. Kohn; J. Pediatr. Ophthalmol. Strabismus, May–June 1983, vol. 20(3), pp. 98–100.

The Blepharophimosis, Ptosis, and Epicanthus Inversus Syndrome: Delineation of Two Types: J. Zlotogora, et al.; Am. J. Hum. Genet., September 1983, vol. 35(5), pp. 1020–1027.

Blepharophimosis, Ptosis, Epicanthus Inversus, and Primary Amenorrhea, a Dominant Trait: P.L. Townes, et al.; Arch. Ophthalmol., 1979, vol. 97, pp. 1664–1666.

# BROWN SYNDROME

**Description** This congenital or acquired disorder is manifested by an inability to raise the adducted eye above the horizontal plane and is due to an abnormality of the tendon sheath of the superior oblique muscle that mechanically limits eye elevation.

**Synonyms**

> Superior Oblique Tendon Sheath Syndrome
> Tendon Sheath Adherence, Superior Oblique

**Signs and Symptoms** The hallmark feature of Brown syndrome is limited vertical movement in the affected eye, with adduction or abduction restricted or totally absent. Other signs include squinting, ptosis, palpebral fissure, strabismus, and backward head tilt. No imbalance in the lower field or overaction of the ipsilateral superior oblique muscle occurs. Fusion and stereopsis are good at near. Corrected visual acuity is normal. Hypotropia is present in the affected eye in the primary position, and elevation in the nasal field is absent or severely limited. Limitation of elevation decreases as the involved eye is abducted, with full elevation occurring upon completed abduction. Upon adduction of the affected eye, "downshoot" of depression of that eye occurs and the palpebral fissure widens. Temporal excursions of the involved eye are normal. One eye is usually affected, but the disorder may be bilateral in approximately 10 percent of cases.

**Etiology** The disorder is due to a shortened or restricted tendon sheath of the superior oblique muscle, a thickening of the sheath that restricts its passage through the trochlea, or an abnormal insertion of the tendon. Congenital Brown syndrome may very rarely be inherited as an autosomal dominant trait, but it is usually an isolated trait. Acquired Brown syndrome may result from surgical or nonsurgical trauma (as following a superior oblique muscle tuck) or from trochlear inflammation due to an underlying inflammatory disorder, such as lupus or rheumatoid arthritis.

**Epidemiology** The disorder is slightly more common among females than males.

**Related Disorders** See *Duane Syndrome.*

**Treatment—Standard** Usually nothing is done. Alignment of the eyes may improve with age. Surgery is indicated only if there is a need to improve an unsightly compensatory head posture when the patient adopts binocular fusion. For those patients requiring surgery, the most common revision is tenectomy of the superior oblique muscle. If Brown syndrome is a result of lupus or rheumatoid arthritis, treatment of the underlying disease may moderate the symptoms.

**Treatment—Investigational** Please contact the agencies listed under Resources, below, for the most current information. Addresses and telephone numbers of these agencies, as well as of individual experts and research centers, may be found in the Master Resources List.

**Resources**

> **For more information on Brown syndrome:** National Organization for Rare Disorders (NORD).

**References**

Brown's Syndrome: A Longitudinal Long-Term Study of Spontaneous Course: E. Gregerson, et al.; Acta Ophthalmol., June 1993, vol. 71(3), pp. 371–376.

Natural History of Presumed Congenital Brown Syndrome: T.J. Kaban, et al.; Arch. Ophthalmol., July 1993, vol. 111(7), pp. 943–946.

Acute-Onset Brown's Syndrome Associated with Pansinusitis: R.A. Saunders, et al.; Arch. Ophthalmol., January 1990, vol. 108(1), pp. 58–60.

Birth Defects Encyclopedia: M.L. Buyse, ed.-in-chief; Blackwell Scientific Publications, 1990, p. 249.

Brown's Syndrome: An Unusual Ocular Complication of Rheumatoid Arthritis: C. Cooper, et al.; Ann. Rheum. Dis., March 1990, vol. 49(3), pp. 188–189.

Simultaneous Superior Oblique Sheathectomy and Inferior Oblique Tuck in Congenital Brown's Syndrome: S. Veronneau-Troutman; Ann. Ophthalmol., November 1990, vol. 22(11), pp. 406–413.

# CHOROIDEREMIA

**Description** Choroideremia is an X-linked disorder of night vision characterized by a characteristic ophthalmoscopic appearance of extensive peripheral atrophy of the retinal pigment epithelium and choriocapillaris and relative preservation of the inner retina and optic disk tissue until late in the disease.

**Synonyms**

> Choroidal Sclerosis
> Progressive Choroidal Atrophy
> Progressive Tapetochoroidal Dystrophy

# ATLAS OF VISUAL DIAGNOSIS

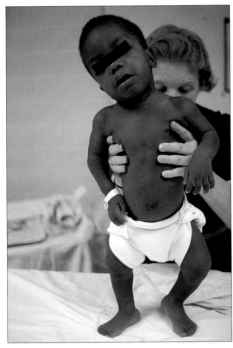

Achondroplasia (see p. 8)

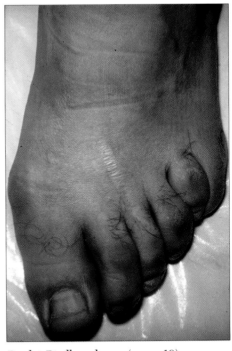

Bardet-Biedl syndrome (see p. 19)

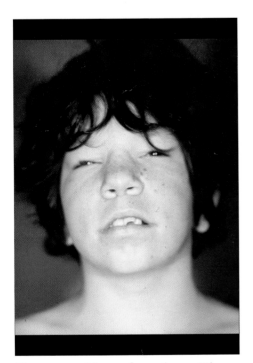

Chromosome 18p- syndrome (see p. 39)

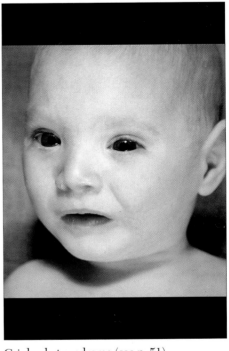

Cri du chat syndrome (see p. 51)

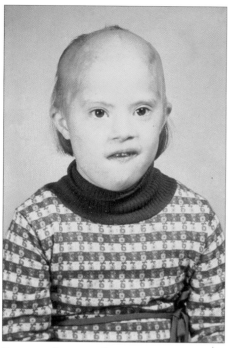

Down syndrome with alopecia (see p. 57)

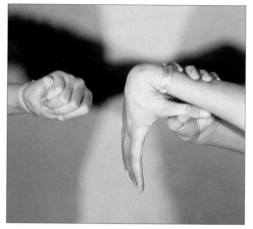

Marfan syndrome (see p. 98)

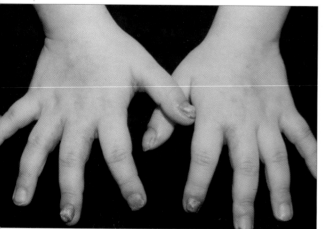

Moniliasis secondary to hypoparathyroidism
(see DiGeorge syndrome, p. 56)

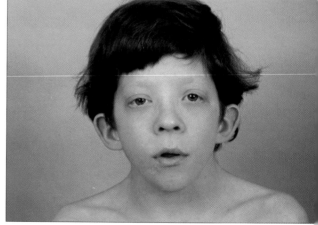

Noonan syndrome (see p. 110)

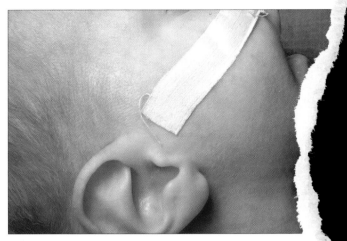

Trisomy 18 syndrome (see p. 153)

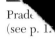

Prad
(see p. 1.

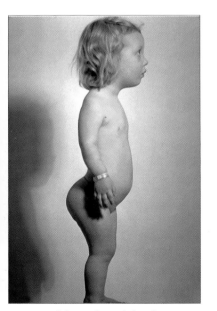

Spondyloepiphyseal dysplasia
(see pp. 140, 141)

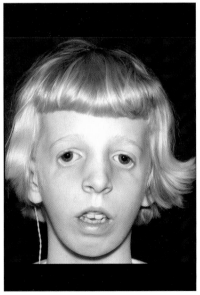

Treacher Collins syndrome
(see p. 147)

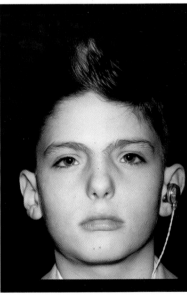

Waardenburg syndrome (see p. 158)

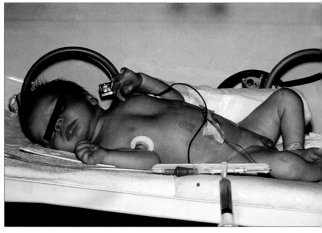

Catastrophically ill newborn with citrullinemia (see p. 187).
This degree of hypotonia is typical of hyperammonemia.

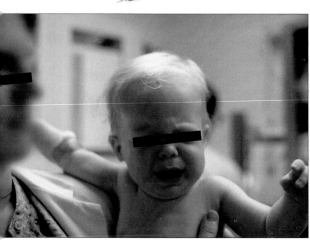

Nephropathic cystinosis (see p. 188)

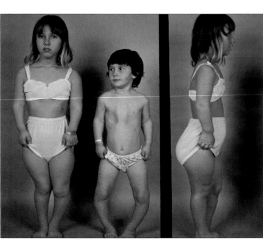

Hypophosphatemic rickets (see p. 704)

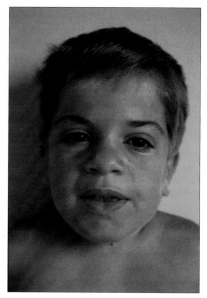

Hunter syndrome (see p. 201)

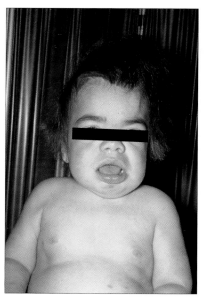

Hurler syndrome (see p. 202)

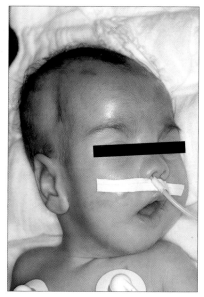

Zellweger syndrome (see p. 248)

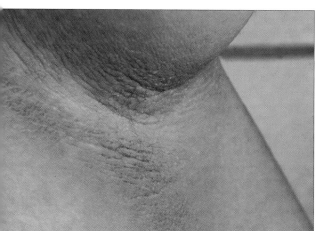

Acanthosis nigricans (see p. 606)

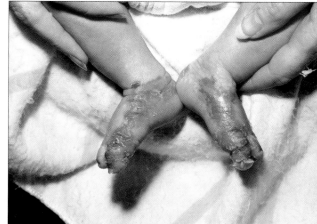

Acrodermatitis enteropathica (see p. 608)

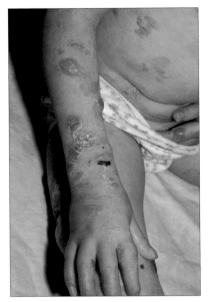

Epidermolysis bullosa simplex
(see p. 621)

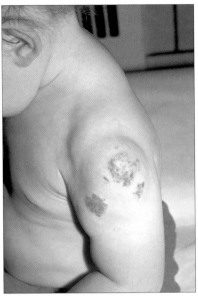

Mixed hemangioma. The deep
(cavernous) component is skin-colored
and the superficial (capillary) component is red. (see p. 613)

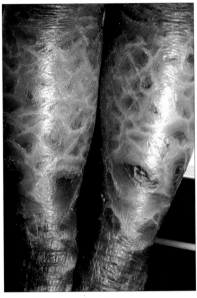

Lamellar recessive ichthyosis
(see p. 640)

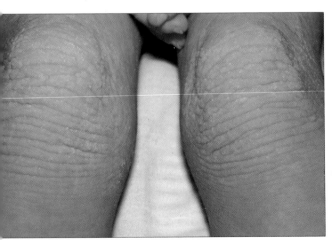

Epidermolytic hyperkeratosis (see p. 623)

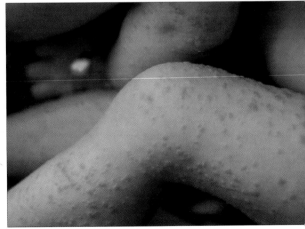

Gianotti-Crosti syndrome (see p. 629)

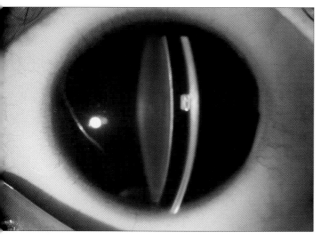

Aniridia (see p. 792)

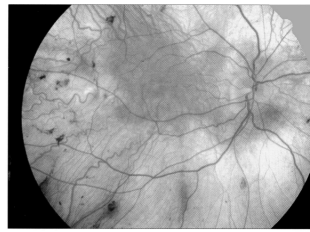

Choroideremia (see p. 794)

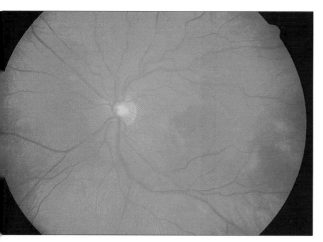

Serpiginious choroiditis (see p. 795)

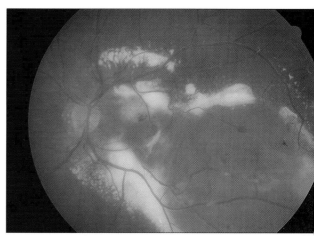

Coats disease (see p. 796)

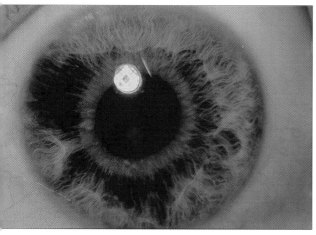

Essential iris atrophy (see p. 803)

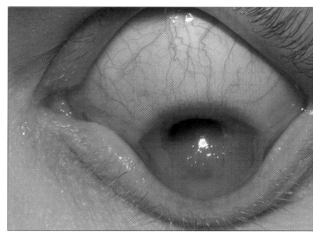

Keratoconus with acute hydrops (see p. 804)

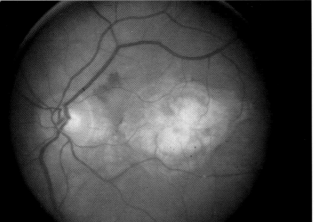

Disciform macular degeneration (see p. 808)

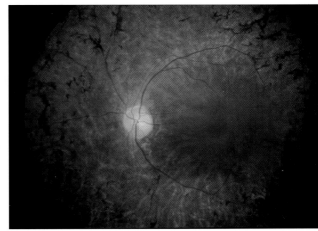

Retinitis pigmentosa (see p. 811)

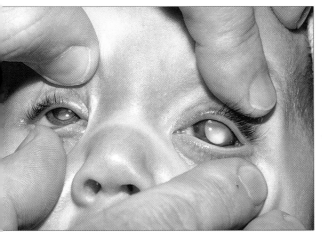

Bilateral retinoblastoma (see p. 812)

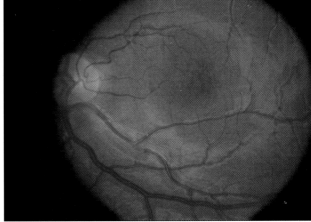

Juvenile X-linked retinoschisis (see p. 818)

**Signs and Symptoms** Night blindness, usually occurring in childhood, is often the first noticeable symptom. Degeneration of the vessels of the choroid and functional damage to the retina occur later in life and usually lead to progressive peripheral vision field loss and eventual blindness.

Prenatal diagnosis by linkage and by mutational analysis is feasible.

**Etiology** The X-linked trait has been mapped to Xq21, isolated, and cloned.

**Epidemiology** Usually males are affected; females are carriers. Occasionally, however, older females may present severe manifestations of the carrier state and be symptomatic. In the Salla area of northern Finland, an unusually high concentration of cases has occurred, affecting 1:40 persons.

**Related Disorders** See *Retinitis Pigmentosa.*

**Gyrate atrophy of the choroid and retina** is an autosomal recessive disorder characterized by a peripheral circular-patterned degeneration of the choroid and retina, and by hyperornithinemia caused by defects in ornithine aminotransferase.

**Treatment—Standard** Treatment is supportive. Organizations providing services to sight-impaired individuals may be helpful. Genetic counseling is recommended.

**Treatment—Investigational** Please contact the agencies listed under Resources, below, for the most current information. Addresses and telephone numbers of these agencies, as well as of individual experts and research centers, may be found in the Master Resources List.

**Resources**

**For more information on choroideremia:** National Organization for Rare Disorders (NORD); NIH/National Eye Institute; Foundation Fighting Blindness; Texas Association for Retinitis Pigmentosa; National Federation of the Blind; American Council of the Blind; American Foundation for the Blind; Vision Foundation; Council of Families with Visual Impairment; National Association for Parents of the Visually Impaired; National Association for the Visually Handicapped; National Library Service for the Blind and Physically Handicapped.

**For genetic information and genetic counseling referrals:** March of Dimes Birth Defects Foundation; Alliance of Genetic Support Groups.

**References**

Mendelian Inheritance in Man, 11th ed.: V.A. McKusick; The Johns Hopkins University Press, 1994, pp. 2326–2329.

Retinal Degeneration in Choroideremia: Deficiency of Rab Geranylgeranyl Transferase: M.C. Seabra, et al.; Science, 1993, vol. 259, pp. 377–381.

Isolation of a Candidate Gene for Choroideremia: D.E. Merry, et al.; Proc. Natl. Acad. Sci. USA, 1992, vol. 89, pp. 2135–2139.

Choroideremia and Deafness with Stapes Fixation: A Contiguous Gene Deletion Syndrome in Xq21: D.E. Merry, et al.; Am. J. Hum. Genet., vol. 45, 1989, pp. 530–540.

Multipoint Linkage Analysis of Loci in the Proximal Long Arm of the Human X Chromosome: Application of Mapping the Choroideremia Locus: J.G. Lesko, et al.; Am. J. Hum. Genet., April 1987, vol. 40(4), pp. 303–311.

Choroideremia-Locus Maps Between DXS3 and DXS11 on Xq: A. Gal, et al.; Hum. Genet., June 1986, vol. 73(2), pp. 123–126.

Mapping X-Linked Ophthalmic Diseases: Provisional Assignment of the Locus for Choroideremia to Xq13–q24: R.A. Lewis, et al.; Ophthalmology, 1985, vol. 92, pp. 800–806.

Choroideremia: A Clinical, Electron Microscopic, and Biochemical Report: M.M. Rodrigues, et al.; Ophthalmology, 1984, vol. 91, pp. 873–883.

# CHOROIDITIS, SERPIGINOUS

**Description** Serpiginous choroiditis is a rare chronic eye disorder characterized by recurrent, progressive, irregularly shaped (serpiginous) lesions involving the retinal pigment epithelium and the choriocapillaris, typically involving both eyes.

**Synonyms**

Geographic Choroiditis
Geographic Helicoid Serpiginous Choroidopathy
Helicoid Choroiditis

**Signs and Symptoms** Lesions usually begin at the back of the eye near the optic disk and may then extend in any direction along the eye layers. Lesions may also begin at other locations and spread toward the optic disk. The disorder has 2 stages: an acute stage, during which lesions develop and/or spread, and a chronic stage, during which the disease does not progress but inactive lesions are associated with scarring, atrophy, and/or clumping of pigment. Recurrences usually start in scar tissue left by old lesions. Symptoms of serpiginous choroiditis appear only if the macula is damaged. A sudden painless decrease in central or paracentral vision in one eye may be the first noticeable sign of disease. Blurred central vision and/or positive scotomas are characteristic symptoms. Both eyes are commonly affected, although the 2nd eye may not develop lesions for weeks to years after the 1st eye. Peripheral vision remains normal in most cases. A subretinal neovascular membrane may grow from the choriocapillaris and cause vision distortion and/or blurring in some people with serpiginous choroiditis. If a neovascular membrane affects the macular region of the retina, central vision loss may occur.

**Etiology** The exact cause of serpiginous choroiditis is not known. It has been suggested that an abnormal immune response may cause localized vasculitis of the eye, leading to the development of serpiginous choroiditis. A few affected individuals have been reported to have had chronic exposure to an unusual variety of chemicals, but the relationship between this exposure and the development of serpiginous choroiditis is highly speculative at this time.

**Epidemiology** Serpiginous choroiditis affects males and females in equal numbers. Symptoms usually appear during the early to middle adult years.

**Related Disorders** See *Epitheliopathy, Acute Posterior Multifocal Placoid Pigment, Macular Degeneration.*

**Posterior uveitis** is an eye disorder characterized by inflammation of the uvea. The sclera, cornea, and retina may also be affected. Posterior uveitis affects the rear hemisphere of the eye, while anterior uveitis and intermediate uveitis affect areas of the front hemisphere. Scars left by posterior uveitis on the eye membranes may cause impaired vision. Major symptoms include blurred vision, metamorphopsia, and floating black spots in the visual field. If the foveal area is affected, central vision loss may occur. Onset may be sudden or gradual, depending on the cause of the disorder. In many cases, this disorder occurs as a complication of toxoplasmosis or other infections. In other cases, the cause cannot be determined.

**Tuberculous uveitis** is a very rare type of inflammation of the uvea and may be difficult to differentiate from other types of uveitis. Tuberculous uveitis is characterized by a long, chronic course and by involvement of the choroid and the retina of the eye. Symptoms may appear suddenly and may include blurred vision, metamorphopsia, floating black spots in the visual field, and/or impaired central vision. Diagnosis may be made by indirect evidence, which may include a lack of response to steroid therapy, positive test results for tuberculosis, and/or the ruling out of other causes for the uveitis. In some cases, tentative therapy for tuberculosis (i.e., the antimycobacterial drug Isoniazid) may be administered to determine if the uveitis responds. If the treatment is effective, tuberculous uveitis is the probable diagnosis.

**Treatment—Standard** Periodic clinical examinations are recommended for people with serpiginous choroiditis to monitor the status of the disease and allow early detection of neovascular membrane development. Krypton or argon laser treatments may arrest the progress of neovascular membranes associated with serpiginous choroiditis. Vision aids and/or specialized equipment (i.e., closed circuit television) may help to offset ultimate vision impairment associated with serpiginous choroiditis. Other treatment is symptomatic and supportive.

**Treatment—Investigational** Some people with serpiginous choroiditis have been treated with the following medications: the immunosuppressive agent cyclosporine-A, triple agent immunosuppressive therapy (azathioprine, cyclosporine, and prednisone in combination), and/or the antiglaucoma agent acetazolamide. Success rates have varied, and further studies are needed to determine the long-term safety and effectiveness of these drugs in the treatment of serpiginous choroiditis.

Please contact the agencies listed under Resources, below, for the most current information. Addresses and telephone numbers of these agencies, as well as of individual experts and research centers, may be found in the Master Resources List.

**Resources** For more information on **serpiginous choroiditis:** National Organization for Rare Disorders (NORD); NIH/National Eye Institute; Vision Foundation; National Association for the Visually Handicapped.

**References**

Treatment of Cystoid Macular Edema with Acetazolamide in a Patient with Serpiginous Choroidopathy: R.L. Steinmentz, et al.; Retina, 1991, vol. 11, pp. 412–415.

Triple Agent Immunosuppression in Serpiginous Choroiditis: P.L. Hooper, et al.; Ophthalmology, June 1991, vol. 98(6), pp. 944–951, discussion pp. 951–952.

Cyclosporine-A in the Treatment of Serpiginous Choroiditis: A.G. Secchi, et al.; Int. Ophthalmol., October 1990, vol. 14(5–6), pp. 395–399.

Experience in the Differential Diagnosis of Peripapillary "Geographic" Choroid Disease and Tuberculous Chorioretinitis: E.I. Ustinova, et al.; Vestn. Oftalmol., November–December 1990, vol. 106(6), pp. 43–46.

Macular Serpiginous Choroiditis: A.M. Mansour, et al.; Retina, 1988, vol. 8, pp. 125–131.

The Late Stage of Serpiginous (Geographic) Choroiditis: I.H. Chisholm, et al.; Am. J. Ophthalmol., 1976, vol. 82, pp. 343–351.

# COATS DISEASE

**Description** Coats disease is a rare eye disorder that usually presents during the first 10 years of life. This disorder is characterized by a white or yellowish area of exudate in the macular area or peripheral retina associated with telangiectatic malformations of retinal blood vessels. Loss of vision and retinal detachment may occur. Coats disease is found usually in one eye only and progresses slowly if untreated. Rare bilateral cases affect one eye far more severely than the other.

**Synonyms**

Exudative Retinitis

**Signs and Symptoms** The main signs of Coats disease are retinal telangiectasia, yellow fundus reflex, and strabismus. Early Coats disease is characterized by large yellowish areas within the retina as well as beneath it. There will also be dilated telangiectatic blood vessels in the peripheral retina, well away from the exudation.

In the majority of cases, this disorder progresses for many years. Eventually, detachment of the retina, the development of a retrolental mass, secondary cataract, rubeosis iridis, secondary uveitis, secondary glaucoma, and shrinking of the eyeball may also occur with this disorder.

Rarely, a similar vascular anomaly has been reported in some families with Landouzy-Dejerine muscular dystrophy.

**Etiology** The specific cause of Coats disease is not known. It is presumed to be a nongenetic, nonhereditary anomaly in the embryologic development of retinal blood vessels.

**Epidemiology** Coats disease affects males more often than females. This disorder usually occurs during childhood, but may, in milder forms, be identified in adults in the 3rd and 4th decades.

**Treatment—Standard** Coats disease may be treated with both photocoagulation and cryotherapy to destroy the areas of telangiectatic blood vessels. If massive exudation has pooled in the macular area, obliteration of the source of the leakage (i.e., the abnormal blood vessels) will not necessarily ensure the recovery of central vision after the exudate resorbs.

**Treatment—Investigational** Please contact the agencies listed under Resources, below, for the most current information. Addresses and telephone numbers of these agencies, as well as of individual experts and research centers, may be found in the Master Resources List.

**Resources**

**For more information on Coats disease:** National Organization for Rare Disorders (NORD); Foundation Fighting Blindness; National Federation of the Blind; American Council of the Blind; American Foundation for the Blind; National Association for Parents of the Visually Impaired; National Association for the Visually Handicapped; Council of Families with Visual Impairment; NIH/National Eye Institute.

**References**

Coats'-Type Retinitis Pigmentosa: J.A. Khan, et al.; Surv. Ophthalmol., March–April 1988, vol. 32(5), pp. 317–332.

Metamorphosis of Retinal Exudation Following Argon Laser Photocoagulation of Retinal Telangiectasia: A.F. Cruess, et al.; Retina, 1983, vol. 3, pp. 261–264.

Coats' Disease: Evaluation of Management: M.E. Ridley, et al.; Ophthalmology, 1982, vol. 89, pp. 1381–1387.

Coats' Disease: I. Egerer, et al.; Arch. Ophthalmol., 1974, vol. 92, pp. 109–112.

# CONE DYSTROPHY

**Description** Cone dystrophy is a rare disorder of the eye that is usually inherited. However, there have been numerous reports of isolated cases appearing in a previously unaffected family. The cone cells and rod cells in the retina of the eye deteriorate, causing impaired vision. This disorder normally occurs during the 1st to 3rd decades of life.

**Synonyms**

Combined Cone-Rod Degeneration

Cone-Rod Degeneration, Progressive

Cone-Rod Dystrophy

Retinal Cone Degeneration

Retinal Cone Dystrophy

Retinal Cone-Rod Dystrophy

**Signs and Symptoms** Symptoms of Cone dystrophy may include impaired central vision, faulty color vision (usually red-green or blue-yellow defects), day blindness, and nystagmus. Some patients may have lesions in the middle of the retina known as bull's-eye macular lesions, and there may be a lack of color in the optic disk.

When Cone dystrophy is associated with an X-linked inheritance, there may be a golden yellow sheen throughout the retina, and the patient may become blind because of dark spots in the visual field. This X-linked form of the disorder occurs only in males. Female carriers of the gene occasionally show extremely mild features of the disorder.

**Etiology** Cone dystrophy may occur as an isolated event, or it may be caused by X-linked recessive, autosomal dominant, or autosomal recessive inheritance. Autosomal dominant inheritance with later (post-adolescence) onset is the most common.

**Epidemiology** Cone dystrophy affects males and females equally when there is an autosomal dominant or autosomal recessive inheritance. Males and females are equally affected when the disorder occurs as an isolated event.

However, when Cone dystrophy is inherited as an X-linked disorder, it affects only males, although female carriers can show mild symptoms. The X-linked form of the disorder is the rarest.

**Related Disorders** See *Macular Degeneration; Retinitis Pigmentosa.*

**Stargardt disease/fundus flavimaculatus** is an autosomal recessive disorder with onset between 6 and 15 years. It is characterized by a central "bull's-eye" macular dystrophy and loss of central vision to at least 20/200. A fluorescein angiogram will show a dark or "silent" choroid, distinguishing it from Cone dystrophy.

**Oguchi disease** is also known as hereditary night blindness and may be associated with vitamin A deficiency. This nonprogressive disorder occurs predominantly in Japan and usually begins in infancy. The main symptom of this disorder is limited vision in dim light. Characteristic retinal findings differ in the light-adapted retina compared with the dark-adapted retina.

**Treatment—Standard** Routine care from an ophthalmologist is required. Visual aids may help as vision decreases. Eyeglasses such as Corning 550 CPF are used to protect the eye from excess light. Genetic counseling may be of benefit for patients and their families. Other treatment is symptomatic and supportive.

**Treatment—Investigational** Please contact the agencies listed under Resources, below, for the most current information. Addresses and telephone numbers of these agencies, as well as of individual experts and research centers, may be found in the Master Resources List.

**Resources**

For more information on **Cone dystrophy:** National Organization for Rare Disorders (NORD); Foundation Fighting Blindness; Association for Macular Diseases; NIH/National Eye Institute.

For **genetic information and genetic counseling referrals:** March of Dimes Birth Defects Foundation; Alliance of Genetic Support Groups.

**References**

Mendelian Inheritance in Man, 11th ed.: V.A. McKusick; The Johns Hopkins University Press, 1994, pp. 1298–1299, 2337–2338.

Birth Defects Encyclopedia: M.L. Buyse, ed.-in-chief; Blackwell Scientific Publications, 1990, pp. 1475–1476.

Autosomal Dominantly Inherited Macular Dystrophy with Preferential Short-Wavelength Sensitive Cone Involvement: G.H. Bresnick, et al.; Am. J. Ophthalmol., 1989, vol. 108(3), pp. 265–276.

Hereditary Macular Dystrophy Without Visible Fundus Abnormality: Y. Miyake, et al.; Am. J. Ophthalmol., 1989, vol. 108, pp. 292–299.

Progressive Peripheral Cone Dysfunction: K.G. Noble, et al.; Am. J. Ophthalmol., 1988, vol. 106(5), pp. 557–560.

# CONJUNCTIVITIS, LIGNEOUS

**Description** Ligneous conjunctivitis is a bilateral membranous conjunctivitis seen in childhood and is occasionally associated with lesions of other mucous membranes, including the trachea and vagina.

**Signs and Symptoms** The symptoms of ligneous conjunctivitis are redness of the conjunctiva, persistent tearing that evolves slowly, the growth of pseudomembranes on the tarsal conjunctiva, and lesions of the mucous membranes that develop into tough, thick, firm, knotty masses replacing the normal mucous membranes. The changes in the mucous membranes have a woodlike (ligneous) consistency. These features are typically bilateral. Some patients with this disorder may also have ligneous lesions and inflammation of the mucous membranes in the larynx, vocal chords, nose, gingiva, trachea, bronchi, vagina, and/or cervix.

Ligneous conjunctivitis resolves spontaneously in some patients. Tracheobronchitis (and secondary pneumonia) and airway obstruction due to recurrent growth of ligneous membranes sometimes occur.

**Etiology** Although the exact cause of ligneous conjunctivitis is not known, it may be an autoimmune disease. Multiple cases of this disorder have occurred within the same family, suggesting an autosomal recessive trait.

**Epidemiology** Ligneous conjunctivitis appears to affect females more commonly than males. This disorder usually appears during childhood.

**Related Disorders** See *Sjögren Syndrome; Keratoconjunctivitis, Vernal.*

**Conjunctivitis** is a common group of disorders caused by an infection of the conjunctiva from bacteria or viruses. The eye becomes red and irritated with a sandy or burning feeling. The disease may be associated with a cold, sore throat, or other viral illness and is most common in children. Viral conjunctivitis is highly contagious.

**Treatment—Standard** Treatment of ligneous conjunctivitis is not universally successful. The topical use of hyaluronidase and chymotrypsin, either before or without removal of the affected pseudomembranes, has been successful in some patients. Repeated surgical stripping of the affected membranes may not influence recurrence, unless the area is also treated with topical lubricants and/or cromolyn. Frequent treatment with topical cyclosporine has completely resolved the membranous problems in some patients and slowed recurrences in others.

Surgical stripping of the affected membranes in the trachea is best accomplished when anesthesia is given with a mask. This procedure eliminates the problem of membranes' becoming dislodged and obstructing the airways. Other treatment is symptomatic and supportive.

**Treatment—Investigational** Please contact the agencies listed under Resources, below, for the most current information. Addresses and telephone numbers of these agencies, as well as of individual experts and research centers, may be found in the Master Resources List.

**Resources**

**For more information on ligneous conjunctivitis:** National Organization for Rare Disorders (NORD); NIH/National Eye Institute.

**For genetic information and genetic counseling referrals:** March of Dimes Birth Defects Foundation; Alliance of Genetic Support Groups.

**References**

Immunohistologic Findings and Results of Treatment with Cyclosporine in Ligneous Conjunctivitis: E.J. Holland, et al.; Am. J. Ophthalmol., February 1989, vol. 107, pp. 160–166.

Ligneous Conjunctivitis: A Clinicopathologic Study of 17 Cases: A.A. Hidayat, et al.; Ophthalmology, August 1987, vol. 94(8), pp. 949–959.

Ligneous Tracheobronchitis: An Unusual Case of Airway Obstruction: M.F. Babcock, et al.; Anesthesiology, November 1987, vol. 67(5), pp. 819–821.

Ligneous Conjunctivitis: An Autosomal Recessive Disorder: J.B. Bateman, et al.; J. Pediatr. Ophthalmol. Strabismus, May–June 1986, vol. 23(3), pp. 137–140.

# DUANE SYNDROME

**Description** Duane syndrome is a congenital ocular disorder characterized by impaired horizontal motility.

**Synonyms**

>DR Syndrome
>Duane Retraction Syndrome
>Eye Retraction Syndrome
>Retraction Syndrome
>Stilling-Turk-Duane Syndrome

**Signs and Symptoms** The syndrome is usually unilateral and most commonly involves the left eye. In 10 percent of patients, the syndrome is bilateral. Features include a defect in horizontal motility and retraction of the globe on attempted adduction, and minimal to substantial face turn to the side of the affected eye. Fusion typically is good. Visual acuity is normal, and the involved globe is otherwise healthy. The disorder is congenital and stationary. The majority of people with Duane syndrome have straight eyes in the primary position.

**Duane syndrome type I** affects adduction. On attempted adduction, the affected eye displays retraction of the globe with narrowing of the palpebral fissure and minimal restriction on versions and forced duction.

**Duane syndrome type II** affects abduction. On attempted abduction, the fissure is widened but abduction does not occur or is limited to a few degrees past midline.

**Duane syndrome type III** affects both adduction and abduction.

Many researchers deem the subtype classification unhelpful.

**Etiology** The syndrome may be supranuclear in origin or may occur when horizontal rotators (one or both) are replaced with inelastic bands of fibrous tissue. Extremely rare examples of families with purported dominant transmission have been reported. Electromyography overwhelmingly supports the hypothesis of paradoxic innervation, that is, that the disorder is caused by co-contraction of both lateral and medial rectus muscles alone or in combination with abnormality of extraocular muscle. Presumably, the nuclear/supranuclear embryologic defect leads to secondary muscle changes later and thus the positive traction test and gradual esodeviation later in life.

**Epidemiology** Females are affected more frequently than males.

**Related Disorders** See *Brown Syndrome.*

Duane syndrome may occur in association with Klippel-Feil syndrome (see *Klippel-Feil Syndrome)* and with Wildervanck syndrome (see *Wildervanck Syndrome).* Epibulbar dermoids, preauricular skin tags, and Goldenhar syndrome may rarely be associated with Duane syndrome (see *Goldenhar Syndrome).*

**Strabismus** is a common eye condition in which the eyes are not aligned properly.

**Treatment—Standard** In mild case in which vision is not impaired, treatment is usually unnecessary. If face turning or orbit retraction is severe, maximal recession or a Z-tenotomy of the medial rectus in the involved eye may be performed.

**Treatment—Investigational** Please contact the agencies listed under Resources, below, for the most current information. Addresses and telephone numbers of these agencies, as well as of individual experts and research centers, may be found in the Master Resources List.

**Resources**

**For more information on Duane syndrome:** National Organization for Rare Disorders (NORD); NIH/National Eye Institute.

**For genetic information and genetic counseling referrals:** March of Dimes Birth Defects Foundation; Alliance of Genetic Support Groups.

### References

Mendelian Inheritance in Man, 11th ed.: V.A. McKusick; The Johns Hopkins University Press, 1994, p. 437.

Online Mendelian Inheritance in Man: V.A. McKusick; The Johns Hopkins University Press, last edit date June 27, 1994, entry number 126800.

Duane's Retraction Syndrome: P.A. DeRespinis, et al.; Surv. Ophthalmol., November–December 1993, vol. 38(3), pp. 257–288.

Medial Rectus Electromyographic Abnormalities in Duane Syndrome: N. Saad, et al.; J. J. Pediatr. Ophthalmol. Strabismus, March–April 1993, vol. 30(3), pp. 88–91.

Electrooculography and Discriminant Analysis in Duane's Syndrome and Sixth-Cranial-Nerve Palsy: M.C. Yang, et al.; Graefes Arch. Clin. Exp. Ophthalmol., 1991, vol. 229(1), pp. 52–56.

A Magnetic Resonance Imaging Study of the Upshoot-Downshoot Phenomenon of Duane's Retractions Syndrome: J.N. Bloom, et al.; Am. J. Ophthalmol., May 15, 1991, vol. 111(5), pp. 548–554.

Ophthalmology: Principles and Concepts, 7th ed.: F.W. Newell; Mosby Year Book, 1991, pp. 394, 397–398.

Bilateral Duane Syndrome Associated with Hypogonadotropic Hypogonadism and Anosmia (Kallman Syndrome): M. Cordonnier, et al.; Bull. Soc. Belge. Ophtalmol., 1990, vol. 239, pp. 29–35.

The Treatment of Duane Syndrome by an Inversion of the Right Lateral Muscle: C.V. Gobin, et al.; Bull. Soc. Belge. Ophtalmol., 1989, vol. 232, pp. 77–85.

# EALES DISEASE

**Description** Eales disease is a rare vision disorder that appears as an inflammation and white haze around the outercoat of the veins in the retina.

### Synonyms

    Idiopathic Peripheral Periphlebitis

    Eales Retinopathy

**Signs and Symptoms** Eales disease usually presents itself with blurred vision resulting from vitreous hemorrhage. At the onset of the disorder, the small peripheral veins of the retina show inflammatory cuffing. As the disease progresses, the inflammation around the veins extends further posteriorly. Eales disease may also be associated with peripheral retinal neovascularization in areas of vaso-obliteration.

The more advanced cases of Eales disease are characterized by a noninflammatory occlusive vasculopathy and extensive hemorrhages into the retina. Vitreous hemorrhages also occur, usually from neovascularization. In rare cases, the retina may become detached, from either retinal tears or traction. Rubeosis iridis may occur, and there may be loss of vision and damage to the optic disk resulting from neovascular glaucoma.

**Etiology** The cause of Eales disease is not known. The disorder seems to occur spontaneously, with no precipitating factors such as injury, infection, heredity, etc.

**Epidemiology** The disorder is most prevalent among young males and typically affects both eyes.

**Related Disorders Arteriosclerotic retinopathy** is a noninflammatory condition characterized by hemorrhages into the retina and vitreous, impaired oxygenation of the retina, and hardening of the arterial walls.

**Treatment—Standard** Treatment of Eales disease is symptomatic and supportive. Laser sectoral or panretinal photocoagulation may eliminate the ischemia of the retina caused by obliteration of blood vessels and slow down excessive formation of new blood vessels. Vitreous hemorrhages and detachment of the retina may be managed through pars plana vitrectomy and conventional retinal detachment procedures.

**Treatment—Investigational** Please contact the agencies listed under Resources, below, for the most current information. Addresses and telephone numbers of these agencies, as well as of individual experts and research centers, may be found in the Master Resources List.

### Resources

**For more information on Eales disease:** National Organization for Rare Disorders (NORD); NIH/National Eye Institute.

### References

The Evaluation of Patients with Eales' Disease: W.A. Renie, et al.; Retina, 1983, vol. 3, pp. 243–248.

# EPITHELIOPATHY, ACUTE POSTERIOR MULTIFOCAL PLACOID PIGMENT

**Description** Acute posterior multifocal placoid pigment epitheliopathy, a rare, acquired ocular disorder, is characterized by a sudden loss of vision and a cluster of inflammatory patches in the outer retina and retinal pigment epithelium.

**Signs and Symptoms** A rapid but temporary loss of vision that often subsides without treatment is characteristic. Multiple yellow-white placoid lesions appear in the posterior pole of the retina in each eye. After resolution of the plaques, pigment alterations are usually permanent. The vision loss may be permanent if the plaques occur sub-foveally, but more than 90 percent of patients recover 20/30 or better visual acuity within a few months of onset. Recurrences have been reported but are quite uncommon, especially after 1 year beyond the initial episode.

**Etiology** A viral etiology is suspected, but none has been isolated.

**Epidemiology** Males and females are affected in equal numbers. The disorder is rare in children under 15 years of age.

**Related Disorders** **Multifocal evanescent white dot syndrome (MEWDS)** and **acute retinal pigment epitheliitis** may be confused. These and other disorders share the common denominators of abnormal choroidal perfusion and focal retinal pigment epithelial infarction.

**Serpigenous choroiditis** has a similar appearance in the retina, but bilaterality is almost universal, and recurrences, at unpredictable intervals until the fovea is destroyed, are expected. See ***Choroiditis, Serpigenous.***

**Treatment—Standard** Treatment is minimal, symptomatic, and supportive. Rarely, anterior uveitis may require temporary suppression with topical corticosteroids and mydriatics.

**Treatment—Investigational** Please contact the agencies listed under Resources, below, for the most current information. Addresses and telephone numbers of these agencies, as well as of individual experts and research centers, may be found in the Master Resources List.

**Resources**

**For more information on acute posterior multifocal placoid pigment epitheliopathy:** National Organization for Rare Disorders (NORD); NIH/National Eye Institute.

**References**

Acute Posterior Multifocal Placoid Pigment Epitheliopathy: An Indocyanine Green Angiographic Study: R.S. Dhaliwal, et al.; Retina, 1993, vol. 13, pp. 317–325.

Long-Term Visual Function in Acute Posterior Multifocal Placoid Pigment Epitheliopathy: M.D. Wolf, et al.; Arch. Ophthalmol., 1991, vol. 109, pp. 800–803.

Long-Term Follow-up of Acute Multifocal Posterior Placoid Pigment Epitheliopathy: D.F. Williams and W.F. Mieler; Br. J. Ophthalmol., December 1989, vol. 73(12), pp. 985–990.

Acute Posterior Multifocal Placoid Pigment Epitheliopathy and Cerebral Vasculitis: C.A. Wilson, et al.; Arch. Ophthalmol., June 1988, vol. 106, pp. 796–800.

Acute Posterior Multifocal Placoid Pigment Epitheliopathy: T. Autzen, et al.; Acta Ophthalmol., June 1986, vol. 64(3), pp. 267–270.

# IRIDOCORNEAL ENDOTHELIAL (ICE) SYNDROMES

## CHANDLER SYNDROME

**Description** Chandler syndrome is a very rare eye disorder characterized by endothelial proliferation, corneal edema, glaucoma, and, less commonly, iris atrophy. The disorder may result in vision loss.

**Synonyms**

ICE Syndrome, Chandler Type
Iridocorneal Endothelial (ICE) Syndrome, Chandler Type
Dystrophia Endothelialis Cornea
Iris Atrophy with Corneal Edema and Glaucoma

**Signs and Symptoms** Chandler syndrome, essential iris atrophy, and Cogan-Reese syndrome are variants in the spectrum of iridocorneal endothelial **(ICE)** syndromes whose symptoms often overlap. Chandler syndrome may cause blurred vision, ocular pain and swelling, and eventual loss of vision. Usually only one eye is affected; however, the other eye may eventually become involved.

**Etiology** The exact cause of Chandler syndrome is not known.

**Epidemiology** Chandler syndrome affects middle-aged females more often than males.

**Related Disorders** See ***Cogan-Reese Syndrome; Essential Iris Atrophy.***

**Treatment—Standard** Treatment usually involves the use of eye drops to control the glaucoma and edema. Pilocarpine and β-blockers are drugs used for this purpose. If these methods are unsuccessful, surgery may be indicated.

**Treatment—Investigational** Please contact the agencies listed under Resources, below, for the most current information. Addresses and telephone numbers of these agencies, as well as of individual experts and research centers, may be found in the Master Resources List.

**Resources**
**For more information on Chandler syndrome:** National Organization for Rare Disorders (NORD); NIH/National Eye Institute; National Society to Prevent Blindness.

**References**
Ophthalmology: Principles and Concepts, 7th Ed.: F.W. Newell; Mosby Year Book, 1991, pp. 275–76.
Pathogenesis of Chandler's Syndrome, Essential Iris Atrophy and the Cogan-Reese Syndrome (Part I): Alterations of the Corneal Endothelium: J.A. Alvarado, et al.; Invest. Ophthalmol. Vis. Sci., June 1986, vol. 27(6), pp. 853–872.
Pathogenesis of Chandler's Syndrome, Essential Iris Atrophy and the Cogan-Reese Syndrome (Part II): Estimated Age at Disease Onset: J.A. Alvarado, et al.; Invest. Ophthalmol. Vis. Sci., June 1986, vol. 27(6), pp. 873–882.

# COGAN-REESE SYNDROME

**Description** Cogan-Reese syndrome is an extremely rare eye disorder characterized by a matted or smudged appearance to the surface of the iris, the development of nodular iris nevi, peripheral anterior synechiae, and/or glaucoma. Secondary glaucoma may lead to vision loss. This disorder is usually unilateral and progresses slowly.

**Synonyms**
>ICE Syndrome, Cogan-Reese Type
>Iridocorneal Endothelial (ICE) Syndrome, Cogan-Reese Type
>Iris Nevus Syndrome
>Iris Naevus Syndrome

**Signs and Symptoms** Cogan-Reese syndrome, essential iris atrophy, and Chandler syndrome are variants in the spectrum of iridocorneal endothelial (**ICE**) syndromes whose features often overlap. The development of Cogan-Reese syndrome is gradual and may be preceded by symptoms of essential iris atrophy and/or Chandler syndrome. The matted appearance of the iris and development of nodules on the iris distinguish Cogan-Reese syndrome from the other 2 ICE syndromes.

Other features of Cogan-Reese syndrome may include corneal edema and/or abnormalities in the corneal endothelium. Glaucoma may occur, leading to vision loss. Ectropion uveae often occur in patients with Cogan-Reese syndrome. A transparent membrane may appear across the surface of the iris.

**Etiology** The cause of Cogan-Reese syndrome is not known.

**Epidemiology** Cogan-Reese syndrome predominantly affects young and middle-aged females.

**Related Disorders** See *Chandler Syndrome; Essential Iris Atrophy.*

**Axenfeld anomaly** is characterized by displacement of Schwalbe's line, iris processes, and peripheral anterior synechiae. It is considered to be an inherited defect, while the ICE syndromes are thought to be acquired disorders.

**Rieger anomaly** is characterized by attachment of portions of the iris to the cornea, a distorted pupil, peripheral corneal opacification, hypoplasia, and/or secondary glaucoma. When Rieger anomaly occurs in association with dental abnormalities and facial malformations, it is referred to as Rieger syndrome. Like Axenfeld anomaly, Rieger anomaly is considered to be an inherited, developmental defect; Rieger syndrome transmits as an autosomal dominant trait. See *Rieger Syndrome.*

Whether Axenfeld and Rieger anomalies are separate disorders, or whether they occur together as the **Axenfeld-Rieger syndrome,** continues to be debated.

**Treatment—Standard** Treatment of Cogan-Reese syndrome is usually directed to the secondary glaucoma. Various medicines may be used to control the glaucoma and corneal edema. If these methods are unsuccessful, surgery may be indicated. Trabeculectomy and penetrating keratoplasty have been used to treat Cogan-Reese syndrome.

**Treatment—Investigational** Please contact the agencies listed under Resources, below, for the most current information. Addresses and telephone numbers of these agencies, as well as of individual experts and research centers, may be found in the Master Resources List.

**Resources**
**For more information on Cogan-Reese syndrome:** National Organization for Rare Disorders (NORD); NIH/National Eye Institute; National Society to Prevent Blindness; National Association for the Visually Handicapped; Foundation for Glaucoma Research.

**References**
Prognosis for Penetrating Keratoplasty in Iridocorneal Endothelial Syndrome: P.C. Chang, et al.; Refract. Corneal Surg., March–April 1993, vol. 9(2) pp. 129–132.
Glaucoma and the Iridocorneal Endothelial Syndrome: H.C. Laganowski, et al.; Arch. Ophthalmol., March 1992, vol. 110(3), pp. 346–350.
Ophthalmology: Principles and Concepts, 7th Ed.: F.W. Newell; Mosby Year Book, 1991, pp. 275–276.
A Comparison of the Clinical Variations of the Iridocorneal Endothelial Syndrome: M.C. Wilson, et al.; Arch. Ophthalmol., October 1989, vol. 107(10), pp. 1465–1468.

# ESSENTIAL IRIS ATROPHY

**Description** Essential iris atrophy is a slowly progressive eye disorder characterized by a displaced and/or distorted pupil, patchy areas of thinning and atrophy on the iris, and/or holes in the iris. Usually only one eye is affected. Peripheral anterior synechiae and/or abnormalities in the cornea may lead to secondary glaucoma and vision loss.

**Synonyms**

> Progressive Essential Iris Atrophy
> ICE Syndrome, Essential Iris Atrophy Type
> Iridocorneal Endothelial (ICE) Syndrome, Essential Iris Atrophy Type

**Signs and Symptoms** Essential iris atrophy, Chandler syndrome, and Cogan-Reese syndrome are variants in the spectrum of iridocorneal endothelial (**ICE**) syndromes whose features often overlap. Ectropion uveae often occur in patients with essential iris atrophy. The onset of this disorder is gradual, and the changes in the shape and placement of the pupil are usually noticed before any change in vision occurs. Degeneration and holes in the iris may develop over a period of several years.

Other features of essential iris atrophy may include peripheral anterior synechiae, corneal edema, and/or abnormalities in the corneal endothelium. These changes may lead to glaucoma and vision loss.

**Etiology** The cause of essential iris atrophy is not known. Most researchers suggest that the primary disorder is proliferation and degeneration of the corneal endothelium, with the impact on the iris as a secondary or associated disorder. However, inflammation (uveitis) also occurs with this disease.

**Epidemiology** Essential iris atrophy predominantly affects young and middle-aged females.

**Related Disorders** See *Chandler Syndrome; Cogan-Reese Syndrome.*

**Treatment—Standard** Treatment of essential iris atrophy is usually directed to the secondary glaucoma. Eye drops may be used to control the glaucoma and corneal edema. If these methods are unsuccessful, surgery may be indicated. Trabeculectomy and penetrating keratoplasty have been used to treat essential iris atrophy.

**Treatment—Investigational** Please contact the agencies listed under Resources, below, for the most current information. Addresses and telephone numbers of these agencies, as well as of individual experts and research centers, may be found in the Master Resources List.

**Resources**

**For more information on essential iris atrophy:** National Organization for Rare Disorders (NORD); NIH/National Eye Institute; National Society to Prevent Blindness; National Association for the Visually Handicapped; Foundation for Glaucoma Research.

**References**

Prognosis for Penetrating Keratoplasty in Iridocorneal Endothelial Syndrome: P.C. Chang, et al.; Refract. Corneal Surg., March–April 1993, vol. 9(2), pp. 129–132.

Glaucoma and the Iridocorneal Endothelial Syndrome: H.C. Laganowski, et al.; Arch. Ophthalmol., March 1992, vol. 110(3), pp. 346–350.

Ophthalmology: Principles and Concepts, 7th Ed.: F.W. Newell; Mosby Year Book, 1991, pp. 275–276.

Clinical Ophthalmology, 2nd ed.: J.J. Kanski, ed.; Butterworth-Heinemann, 1990, p. 222.

A Comparison of the Clinical Variations of the Iridocorneal Endothelial Syndrome: M.C. Wilson, et al.; Arch. Ophthalmol., October 1989, vol. 107(10), pp. 1465–1468.

# KERATOCONJUNCTIVITIS, VERNAL

**Description** A noncontagious manifestation of a seasonal allergy, vernal conjunctivitis is a seasonally recurrent bilateral inflammation that usually affects susceptible individuals in the spring or during warm weather.

**Synonyms**

> Seasonal Conjunctivitis
> Spring Ophthalmia

**Signs and Symptoms** Bilateral conjunctival inflammation occurs, causing redness and perhaps blurred vision; cobblestone-like changes appear in the upper and occasionally lower palpebral conjunctiva. The eyes become sensitive to light, and itching is intense. Gelatinous nodules may develop at the limbus. Principal symptoms include tearing, discomfort in bright light, burning, foreign body sensation, and intolerance to contact lens wear.

**Etiology** Vernal keratoconjunctivitis is thought to be an ocular hypersensitivity or allergic reaction to airborne allergens.

**Epidemiology** Males and females are affected equally.

**Related Disorders Conjunctivitis (pink eye)** is a highly contagious viral (and rarely, bacterial) infection of the outer lining of the eye and inner lining of the eyelids. The eyes become red, irritated, and burning; scratchiness, as if caused by sand, occurs. A cold or sore throat may precede the infection, which is most common in children. Sticky mucus in the eye may cause the eyelids to stick together.

**Treatment—Standard** Treatment is symptomatic and supportive. It is essential to identify and treat any causative allergy. Discontinuation of contact lenses may moderate symptoms. Prognosis for ultimate recovery is excellent.

The orphan drug lodoxamide tromethamine (Alomide Ophthalmic Solution—Alcon Laboratories) has been approved for the treatment of vernal keratoconjunctivitis. Other topical astringents, with or without topical and systemic antihistamines, may provide relief.

**Treatment—Investigational** The use of cromolyn sodium in the treatment of ocular allergies such as vernal keratoconjunctivitis is being studied. The orphan drug levocabastine (Iolab Pharmaceuticals) is being used investigationally in the treatment of vernal keratoconjunctivitis.

Please contact the agencies listed under Resources, below, for the most current information. Addresses and telephone numbers of these agencies, as well as of individual experts and research centers, may be found in the Master Resources List.

**Resources**

**For more information on vernal keratoconjunctivitis:** National Organization for Rare Disorders (NORD); NIH/National Eye Institute; NIH/National Institute of Allergy and Infectious Diseases.

**References**

Ocular Allergy and Mast Cell Stabilizers: M.R. Allansmith, et al.; Surv. Ophthalmol., January–February, 1986, vol. 30(4), pp. 229–244.

Vernal Keratoconjunctivitis: New Corneal Findings in Fraternal Twins: W.N. Rosenthal, et al.; Cornea, 1984–1985, vol. 3(4), pp. 288–290.

# KERATOCONUS

**Description** Keratoconus is a change (steepening or ectasia) in the curved transparent outer layer of collagenous tissue constituting the cornea. The resulting cone-shaped cornea causes substantial problems with refraction of light. The disorder progresses slowly and occurs most commonly as an isolated (and asymmetrically bilateral) disease.

**Synonyms**

Conical Cornea

Congenital Keratoconus

**Signs and Symptoms** Inherited forms of this abnormality usually begin after puberty. Symptoms may be unilateral initially and may later become bilateral. Patients frequently need a change in prescription for eyeglasses; astigmatism is common, caused by the progressive ectasia of the cornea. In keratoconus posticus circumscriptus, mental and physical retardation can occur.

**Etiology** The causes are unknown. Both autosomal dominant and recessive inheritances have been suggested.

**Epidemiology** Keratoconus occurs in females slightly more often than males. Onset is more frequent in adolescence than adulthood. One long-term study in the United States indicated a prevalence of 54.5 diagnosed cases of keratoconus per 100,000 population, with unilateral involvement in 41 percent at diagnosis and bilateral disease in 59 percent.

**Related Disorders** Keratoconus may occur alone or in conjunction with other disorders, including some forms of Leber congenital amaurosis, Noonan syndrome, Down syndrome, Ehlers-Danlos syndrome (rarely), aniridia, osteogenesis imperfecta, and atopy (often with eye rubbing).

**Treatment—Standard** Treatment of the visual defect may involve the use of hard contact lenses as a temporary measure. The only "cure" is corneal transplant (penetrating keratoplasty or epikeratoplasty). In some cases, progression may slow enough to obviate treatment. Genetic counseling may be of benefit for patients with an inherited form of keratoconus.

**Treatment—Investigational** Please contact the agencies listed under Resources, below, for the most current information. Addresses and telephone numbers of these agencies, as well as of individual experts and research centers, may be found in the Master Resources List.

**Resources**

**For more information on keratoconus:** National Organization for Rare Disorders (NORD); NIH/National Eye Institute; Eye Bank Association of America; Vision Foundation; National Association for the Visually Handicapped.

**For genetic information and genetic counseling referrals:** March of Dimes Birth Defects Foundation; Alliance of Genetic Support Groups.

**References**

Mendelian Inheritance in Man, 11th ed.: V.A. McKusick; The Johns Hopkins University Press, 1994, pp. 844, 1947.

Prognostic Factors for the Progression of Keratoconus: S.T. Tuft, et al.; Ophthalmology, 1994, vol. 101, pp. 439–447.

Is Keratoconus Genetic?: D.S. Jacobs, et al.; Int. Ophthalmol. Clin., 1993, vol. 33, pp. 249–260.

Long-Term Comparison of Epikeratoplasty and Penetrating Keratoplasty for Keratoconus: R.F. Steinert, et al.; Arch. Ophthalmol., April 1988, vol. 106(4), pp. 493–496.

Clinical and Epidemiological Features of Keratoconus, Genetic and External Factors in the Pathogenesis of the Disease: A. Ihalainen, Acta Ophthalmol., 1986, vol. 178 (suppl.), pp. 1–64.

A 48-Year Clinical and Epidemiologic Study of Keratoconus: R.H. Kennedy, et al.; Am. J. Ophthalmol., March 15, 1986, vol. 101(3), pp. 267–273.

# KERATOMALACIA

**Description** Keratomalacia is an eye disease caused by vitamin A deficiency. Drying and ulceration of the cornea occur as a result of severe malnutrition and especially vitamin A deficiency. Liquefaction and melting of the cornea of both eyes occur in the end-stage of the disease.

**Synonyms**
> Xerotic Keratitis
> Xerophthalmia

**Signs and Symptoms** Vitamin A deficiency may interfere with the eye's ability to adapt to the dark, resulting in night blindness. It may also negatively affect tear production, leading to xerosis of the conjunctiva and the cornea. This may result in a sensation of grittiness in the eyes and photophobia. Shiny, pearly spots of triangular-shaped tissue (Bitôt spots) may appear on the conjunctiva adjacent to the cornea. The cornea may become hazy and gradually dissolve, leading to rupture of the eyeball with extrusion of the eye's contents.

In vitamin A deficiency, cells in the lung, gastrointestinal tract, and urinary tract may be keratinized. The senses of taste and smell may be defective, and there may be a thickening of the skin. Individuals with keratomalacia may develop anemia and an increased susceptibility to infection. Growth retardation is a common symptom in children deprived of vitamin A early in life, especially before bone growth plates have matured.

**Etiology** Keratomalacia is most commonly caused by prolonged dietary deprivation of sources of vitamin A. It occurs most frequently in areas such as Southeast Asia, where rice is the staple. (Rice does not contain the necessary dietary pigment carotene, which the body converts to vitamin A.)

A secondary cause of keratomalacia may be the body's inadequate conversion of carotene to vitamin A. Keratomalacia may also be caused by an interference with absorption, storage, or transport of vitamin A. Interference with absorption or storage of vitamin A may be associated with digestive diseases (sprue), cystic fibrosis, surgery of the pancreas or the small intestine (duodenal bypass), obstruction of the small intestine, obstruction of the bile ducts, chronic diarrhea due to giardiasis, and cirrhosis of the liver (especially in nutritionally deprived chronic alcoholic addiction).

In the United States, vitamin A deficiency in adults is most likely to be secondary to severe malabsorption of the vitamin, or to eating disorders such as anorexia nervosa.

**Epidemiology** Keratomalacia affects males and females in equal numbers. Keratomalacia is very rare in North America and Western Europe, but is a leading cause of blindness in Southeast Asia, India, parts of Africa, and Central and South America, affecting poorly nourished children and adults.

**Related Disorders** See *Sjögren Syndrome; Keratoconus.*

**Interstitial keratitis** is a disorder characterized by chronic inflammation of the deep layers of the cornea. It rarely occurs in the United States. Symptoms may include photophobia, ocular pain, excess lacrimation, and a gradual loss of vision. Interstitial keratitis most commonly affects children and is a late complication of congenital syphilis.

**Treatment—Standard** When treating individuals with keratomalacia, the cause of the deficiency must be corrected. When dietary deficiency of vitamin A is the cause, vitamin A supplements must be administered, often parenterally. However, vitamin A can cause birth defects if given in high doses to pregnant women, so care must be taken in treating women of childbearing years. In general, individuals with keratomalacia respond rapidly to vitamin A replacement therapy if the case is treated early. Dry eyes may be managed with artificial tears. If eye complications have progressed to blindness, little can be done to restore vision. In mild cases of night blindness, improvement is often shown following the systemic administration of vitamin A. More advanced cases may require higher parenteral doses daily for several months. Large doses of vitamin A should be monitored to prevent possible overdose and hepatotoxicity.

If keratomalacia is caused by an interference of absorption, storage, or transport of vitamin A, the underlying disorder must be identified and treated.

**Treatment—Investigational** Please contact the agencies listed under Resources, below, for the most current information. Addresses and telephone numbers of these agencies, as well as of individual experts and research centers, may be found in the Master Resources List.

**Resources**

**For more information on keratomalacia:** National Organization for Rare Disorders (NORD); NIH/National Eye Institute; National Society to Prevent Blindness; Vision Foundation.

### References

Impression Cytology: A Practical Index of Vitamin A Status: G. Natadisastra, et al.; Am. J. Clin. Nutr., September 1988, vol. 48(5), pp. 426–429.

Vitamin A Fortified Monosodium Glutamate and Health, Growth, and Survival of Children: A Controlled Field Trial: Muhilal, et al.; Am. J. Clin. Nutr., November 1988, vol. 48(5), pp. 1271–1276.

Nutritional Blindness: Xerophthalmia and Keratomalacia: A. Sommer; Oxford University Press, 1982.

# LEBER CONGENITAL AMAUROSIS

**Description** Leber congenital amaurosis is a hereditary disorder of the retina that is present at birth. It is characterized by blindness at birth, roving eye movements, pupils that react poorly to light and dilate widely in the dark, a variety of visible changes in the retinas of both eyes, and a nonrecordable electroretinogram from early life.

**Synonyms**

> Congenital Retinal Blindness
> Congenital Retinitis Pigmentosa
> Leber Amaurosis
> Leber Congenital Tapetoretinal Degeneration or Dysplasia
> Congenital Absence of the Rods and Cones

**Signs and Symptoms** In Leber congenital amaurosis, children are born apparently with an absence of light-gathering cells (rods and cones) of the retina. A lack of visual attentiveness at and shortly after birth is the first sign of the disease. Often the eyes are deeply set in childhood, and the child will rub the eyes allegedly to stimulate the retina to produce light (oculodigital stimulation). Absence or reduction of the electrical activity (by the electroretinogram) of the retina is always observed and is necessary for diagnosis.

Some families will have one or more additional features: cataracts evolving in the first 2 decades of life, keratoconus, neurosensory hearing impairment, mental retardation, underdevelopment of the balance centers (cerebellum), and some distinctive behavioral mannerisms or stereotypies. Anomalies of brain stem may be associated with Joubert syndrome. Asphyxiating thoracic dystrophy may occur in Jeune syndrome. Kidney problems occur in Senior syndrome.

**Etiology** Leber congenital amaurosis is a group of disorders nearly always inherited as recessive traits. Rarely, families with dominant transmission have been reported. Leber congenital amaurosis can be seen as part of systemic disorders (e.g., neurologic dysfunction, kidney disease, and, rarely, chromosomal imbalance). It is estimated that 10 or more different genes may be responsible for the same disease appearance.

**Epidemiology** Leber congenital amaurosis, as a recessive disorder, affects males and females in equal numbers.

**Related Disorders** See *Retinitis Pigmentosa; Macular Degeneration.*

**Flecked retina syndromes** are characterized by reduced vision and impaired night vision in some cases. The area behind the retinal vessels appears marked with white or yellow flecks. These flecks are distantly similar to those found in some persons with Leber congenital amaurosis. The retinal and choroidal vessels are usually not affected by these genetic disorders, but rather the retina and the pigment epithelium.

**Oguchi disease** is also known as hereditary night blindness and may be associated with vitamin A deficiency. This nonprogressive disorder occurs predominantly in Japan and usually begins in infancy. The main symptom is limited vision in dim light, but patients often have normal color perception and/or clearness of central vision. It may take between 2 and 8 hours for the eyes of affected individuals to adapt to darkness. The retina appears gray or golden in color, and the retinal vessels stand out with clarity. The optic disk is normal.

**Treatment—Standard** Treatment of Leber congenital amaurosis is symptomatic and supportive. Standard procedures, such as genetic counseling and services that benefit the sight impaired, can be helpful.

**Treatment—Investigational** Researchers at the Cullen Eye Institute of the Baylor College of Medicine in Houston, TX, and The Hospital for Sick Children in Toronto, Canada, are studying a group of inherited retinal disorders including Leber congenital amaurosis. Families with at least 2 affected members whose parents are both living are needed to participate in the program. In Toronto, isolated cases are also being studied by DNA methods. For more information, please contact Richard A. Lewis, M.D., at the Cullen Eye Institute, and Maria A. Musarella, M.D., at the Hospital for Sick Children.

Please contact the agencies listed under Resources, below, for the most current information. Addresses and telephone numbers of these agencies, as well as of individual experts and research centers, may be found in the Master Resources List.

**Resources**

**For more information on Leber congenital amaurosis:** National Organization for Rare Disorders (NORD); NIH/National Eye Institute; Foundation Fighting Blindness; National Association for Parents of the Visually Impaired;

National Association for the Visually Handicapped; American Council of the Blind; American Foundation for the Blind; Council of Families with Visual Impairment; Richard A. Lewis, M.D., Cullen Eye Institute; Maria A. Musarella, M.D., Hospital for Sick Children.

**For genetic information and genetic counseling referrals:** March of Dimes Birth Defects Foundation; Alliance of Genetic Support Groups.

### References

The Natural History of Leber's Congenital Amaurosis: Age-Related Findings in 35 Patients: K.L. Heher, et al.; Ophthalmology, 1992, vol. 99, pp. 241–245.

Clinical Spectrum of Leber's Congenital Amaurosis in the Second to Fourth Decades of Life: D. Smith, et al.; Ophthalmology, 1990, vol. 97, pp. 1156–1161.

Leber's Congenital Amaurosis: Is Mental Retardation a Frequent Associated Defect?: B. Nickel, et al.; Arch. Ophthalmol., July 1982, vol. 100(7), pp. 1089–1092.

Leber's Congenital Amaurosis: K. Mizuno, et al.; Am. J. Ophthalmol., January 1977, vol. 83(1), pp. 32–42.

# LEBER HEREDITARY OPTIC NEUROPATHY (LHON)

**Description** Leber hereditary optic neuropathy is characterized by an abrupt loss of vision, first in one eye, then in the other, usually beginning typically in the middle of the 2nd decade and the 3rd decade, but occasionally as late as the 5th decade, and occurring predominantly in males.

**Synonyms**

> Leber Optic Atrophy
> Hereditary Optic Neuroretinopathy

**Signs and Symptoms** The first symptom is sudden, painless loss of central vision and narrowing of the peripheral field, typically in healthy young men. Involvement of the optic nerve follows, causing severely reduced vision or blindness. The disorder may mimic papillitis, acute optic neuritis, or anterior ischemic optic neuritis. Sometimes heart abnormalities, especially conduction defects, may also occur.

**Etiology** Leber hereditary optic neuropathy is caused by mutations in mitochondrial DNA. The disorder is strictly maternally inherited and passes only through women. Molecular diagnosis may now confirm the clinical diagnosis 100 percent of the time. Definitive molecular diagnosis can obviate expensive, duplicate, invasive investigations and spare potentially harmful therapy.

**Epidemiology** Leber hereditary optic neuropathy affects males more often than females.

**Related Disorders** See *Retinitis Pigmentosa; Papillitis.*

**Treatment—Standard** The pathophysiology of the enzyme defects has yet to yield the development of rational therapy or prevention of the disorder. Services that benefit the sight impaired may be helpful to LHON patients. Genetic counseling may be of benefit for patients and their families. Other treatment is symptomatic and supportive.

**Treatment—Investigational** Family and mutational analysis of mitochondrial defects is available through the laboratories of Douglas C. Wallace, Ph.D., Biochemistry Department, Emory University School of Medicine, Atlanta, GA.

Please contact the agencies listed under Resources, below, for the most current information. Addresses and telephone numbers of these agencies, as well as of individual experts and research centers, may be found in the Master Resources List.

### Resources

**For more information on Leber hereditary optic neuropathy:** National Organization for Rare Disorders (NORD); NIH/National Eye Institute; National Federation of the Blind; American Council of the Blind; American Foundation for the Blind; Vision Foundation; Council of Families with Visual Impairment; Guiding Eyes for the Blind; National Association for Parents of the Visually Impaired; National Association for the Visually Handicapped; National Library Service for the Blind and Physically Handicapped.

**For genetic information and genetic counseling referrals:** March of Dimes Birth Defects Foundation; Alliance of Genetic Support Groups.

### References

Mendelian Inheritance in Man, 11th ed.: V.A. McKusick; The Johns Hopkins University Press, 1994, pp. 2587–2592.

Leber Hereditary Optic Neuroretinopathy: E.K. Nikoskelainen, Curr. Opin. Ophthalmol., 1991, vol. 2, pp. 531–537.

A Mitochondrial DNA Mutation As a Cause of Leber's Hereditary Optic Neuropathy: G. Singh, et al.; N. Engl. J. Med., 1989, vol. 320, pp. 1300–1305.

Mitochondrial DNA Mutation Associated with Leber's Hereditary Optic Neuropathy: D.C. Wallace, et al.; Science, 1988, vol. 242, pp. 1427–1430.

# MACULAR DEGENERATION

**Description** Macular degeneration is the descriptive term for many forms of deterioration of the central area of vision (macula) from a previous state of normalcy. Subtypes of the disorder include Stargardt disease and fundus flavimaculatus (occurring in juveniles); and disciform macular degeneration (termed senile macular degeneration or age-related macular degeneration, and, previously, Kuhnt-Junius disease).

**Synonyms**

Age-Related Macular Degeneration

Juvenile Macular Degeneration

**Signs and Symptoms** Central vision is impaired or absent; peripheral vision is normal. Distortion of vision and central scotoma are associated with the disorder. The condition may progress to a central or scarred stage and then become static.

**Etiology** There are genetic, environmental (including drug-related and toxic), and age-related causes. Age-related macular degeneration has no clearly detectable genetic pattern, although occurrence in siblings, identical twins, and multiple-birth siblings has been reported.

Juvenile forms, including Stargardt disease and fundus flavimaculatus, are usually autosomal recessive.

**Epidemiology** Onset of juvenile macular dystrophy (Stargardt disease; fundus flavimaculatus) is between ages 6 and 15. Age-related macular degeneration is most common after the 6th decade.

**Treatment—Standard** Monitoring of the disorder is indicated. Genetic counseling may be helpful for those with clearly defined variants (e.g., Stargardt disease); examination of siblings is essential.

**Treatment—Investigational** Laser treatment may be useful in early stages of age-related disciform disease.

Inherited retinal diseases, including Stargardt disease and fundus flavimaculatus, are being studied at the Cullen Eye Institute of the Baylor College of Medicine in Houston, Texas. Families with at least 2 affected members and both parents living are needed to participate in this program.

Please contact the agencies listed under Resources, below, for the most current information. Addresses and telephone numbers of these agencies, as well as of individual experts and research centers, may be found in the Master Resources List.

**Resources**

**For more information on macular degeneration:** National Organization for Rare Disorders (NORD); American Foundation for the Blind; Foundation Fighting Blindness; NIH/National Eye Institute; National Association for the Visually Handicapped; Vision Foundation; American Council for the Blind.

**References**

Bilateral Macular Drusen in Age-Related Macular Degeneration: Prognosis and Risk Factors: F.G. Holz, et al.; Ophthalmology, 1994, vol. 101, pp. 1522–1528.

Evaluation of Argon Green vs. Krypton Red Laser for Photocoagulation of Subfoveal Choroidal Neovascularization in the Macular Photocoagulation Study: Macular Photocoagulation Study Group; Arch. Ophthalmol., 1994, vol. 112, pp. 1176–1184.

Laser Photocoagulation for Juxtafoveal Choroidal Neovascularization: Five-Year Results from Randomized Clinical Trials: Macular Photocoagulation Study Group; Arch. Ophthalmol., 1994, vol. 112; pp. 500–509.

Five-Year Follow-up of Fellow Eyes of Patients with Age-Related Macular Degeneration and Unilateral Extrafoveal Choroidal Neovascularization: Macular Photocoagulation Study Group; Arch. Ophthalmol., 1993, vol. 111, pp. 1189–1199.

Risk Factors for Neovascular Age-Related Macular Degeneration: Eye Disease Case-Control Study Group; Arch. Ophthalmol., 1992, vol. 110, pp. 1701–1708.

Argon Laser Photocoagulation for Neovascular Maculopathy: Macular Photocoagulation Study Group; Arch. Ophthalmol., May 1986, vol. 104, pp. 694–701.

Recurrent Choroidal Neovascularization After Argon Laser Photocoagulation for Neovascular Maculopathy: Macular Photocoagulation Study Group; Arch. Ophthalmol., April 1986, vol. 104, pp. 503–512.

Risk Factors in Age-Related Maculopathy Complicated by Choroidal Neovascularization: M.S. Blumenkranz, et al.; Ophthal., May 1986, vol. 93, pp. 552–558.

A Vision Impairment of the Later Years: Macular Degeneration: I.R. Dickman; Distributed as a public service by the American Foundation for the Blind, Public Affairs Pamphlet No. 610.

# NORRIE DISEASE

**Description** Norrie disease is an X-linked hereditary disorder characterized by bilateral blindness at birth.

**Synonyms**

Anderson-Warburg Syndrome

Atrophia Bulborum Hereditaria

Fetal Iritis Syndrome

Oligophrenia-Microphthalmos
Whitnall-Norman Syndrome

**Signs and Symptoms** Males are born blind or become blind very early in life; vitreous hemorrhages and fibro-proliferative and neovascular membranes cover the retina, scar, contract, and create tractional retinal detachments in both eyes. Secondarily, lens opacities and atrophy of the iris may be found in early infancy. Cataracts develop followed by phthisis bulbi. Typical findings are a small anterior chamber and a pupil without light reflex; the iris tends to adhere abnormally to the dense white cataract. By age 5 years, the lens is usually cataractous. By age 10 years, phthisis bulbi becomes apparent.

Mental retardation occurs in more than 50 percent of affected patients, becoming apparent in the first 2 years of life. A progressive neurosensory hearing loss may not be evident until about age 20 years. Diabetes has occurred in some patients. Nonocular symptoms and signs range from the milder (normal intelligence, normal growth, mild hearing loss) to profound mental retardation, short stature, and deafness.

**Etiology** The disease is inherited as an X-linked trait, mapped to Xp11.3–21.1. The candidate gene has been cloned, and mutational analysis is feasible. Prenatal diagnosis has been achieved.

**Epidemiology** The disease affects only males. Carrier females have no phenotypic features.

**Related Disorders** See *Trisomy 13 Syndrome; Usher Syndrome; Retinitis Pigmentosa.*

**Retinal dysplasia** is a hereditary disorder in which an elevated retinal fold arises from the optic disk, covering the macular area and widening toward the temporal fundus. This encroachment may cause blindness.

Other related disorders include **familial exudative vitreoretinopathy** and **retinopathy of prematurity.**

**Treatment—Standard** Surgical reattachment of the retina has been attempted but is never successful. Agencies that provide services for vision- and hearing-impaired individuals may be of benefit, as may genetic counseling.

**Treatment—Investigational** Please contact the agencies listed under Resources, below, for the most current information. Addresses and telephone numbers of these agencies, as well as of individual experts and research centers, may be found in the Master Resources List.

**Resources**

**For more information on Norrie disease:** National Organization for Rare Disorders (NORD); Norrie Disease Association; NIH/National Eye Institute; American Council of the Blind; American Foundation for the Blind; National Association for Parents of the Visually Impaired; National Federation of the Blind.

**For braille or recorded publications:** National Library Service for the Blind and Physically Handicapped; Foundation Fighting Blindness; National Association for the Visually Handicapped; National Association for Parents of the Visually Impaired; Council of Families with Visual Impairment; American Humane Association (for trained hearing dogs); Deafness Research Foundation; National Information Center on Deafness; National Association of the Deaf; American Society for Deaf Children; The Arc (a national organization on mental retardation).

**For genetic information and genetic counseling referrals:** March of Dimes Birth Defects Foundation; Alliance of Genetic Support Groups.

**References**

Mendelian Inheritance in Man, 11th ed.: V.A. McKusick; The Johns Hopkins University Press, 1994, pp. 2493–2495.

Isolation of a Candidate Gene for Norrie Disease by Positional Cloning: W. Berger, et al.; Nat. Genet., 1992, vol. 1, pp. 199–208.

The Norrie Disease Gene Maps to a 150 KB Region on Chromosome Xp11.3.: K.B. Sims, et al.; Hum. Mol. Genet., April 1992, vol. 1(2), pp. 83–89.

Norrie Disease Is Caused by Mutation in an Extracellular Protein Resembling C-Terminal Globular Domain of Mucins: A. Meindl, et al.; Nat. Genet., 1992, vol. 2, pp. 139–143.

Norrie Disease Caused by a Gene Deletion Allowing Carrier Detection and Prenatal Diagnosis: A. de la Chapelle, et al.; Clin. Genet., October 1985, vol. 28(4), pp. 317–320.

# PAPILLITIS

**Description** Papillitis, a progressive inflammation of all or part of the optic nerve, can cause loss of vision. The disorder is usually unilateral but may be bilateral, depending on the etiology.

**Synonyms**

Optic Neuritis

**Signs and Symptoms** The primary symptom is a rapid loss of vision, which can occur within 1 to 2 days of onset and last for months. Movement of the involved eye increases pain, which is characteristically present, especially deep behind the eye in the orbit. Recovery may be spontaneous, but permanent loss of vision is possible if the underlying causes remain undiagnosed and consequently untreated.

An elderly patient with giant cell arteritis may have headaches and fatigue as well as unilateral loss of vision caused by arteritis. In some cases, the other eye may become involved.

**Etiology** In young people, a viral illness or other inflammatory disease may precede development of papillitis. It may be part of a demyelinating process accompanying multiple sclerosis or be due to an occlusive disease affecting the ophthalmic or ciliary vessels, such as giant cell arteritis. Papillitis may occur during meningitis or after syphilis. Metastasis of a tumor to the optic nerve may simulate some forms of optic neuritis. In some cases, there may be no apparent cause.

**Epidemiology** The disease is equally likely to occur in males and females and at any age.

**Related Disorders** See *Arteritis, Giant Cell; Multiple Sclerosis.*

**Retrobulbar neuritis,** an inflammation of the portion of the optic nerve that lies behind the eyeball, is usually unilateral and is characterized by pain on movement of the eye, headache, and a rapid and progressive loss of vision. Retrobulbar neuritis can be associated with multiple sclerosis or viral or infectious diseases; in most cases there is no apparent cause. Imaging studies with contrast of the brain and analysis of spinal fluid are requisite.

**Treatment—Standard** If spontaneous remission does not occur, the disease is usually treated with prednisone or methylprednisolone. A major national collaborative trial (the Optic Neuritis Treatment Trial—ONTT) concluded in 1992 that oral prednisone (1 mg/kg/day) is not only ineffective in speeding recovery or in improving visual outcome after optic neuritis, but increases the patient's risk for future attacks in either the affected or the fellow eye. Thus, there appears to be no role for oral prednisone therapy alone in standard doses for treatment of initial episodes of optic neuritis.

**Treatment—Investigational** Please contact the agencies listed under Resources, below, for the most current information. Addresses and telephone numbers of these agencies, as well as of individual experts and research centers, may be found in the Master Resources List.

**Resources**

**For more information on papillitis:** National Organization for Rare Disorders (NORD); NIH/National Eye Institute.

**References**

Corticosteroids and Optic Neuritis: D.H. Silberberg; N. Engl. J. Med., December 1993, vol. 329(24), pp. 1808–1810.

The Effect of Corticosteroids for Acute Optic Neuritis on the Subsequent Development of Multiple Sclerosis: R.W. Beck, et al.; N. Engl. J. Med., December 1993, vol. 329(24), pp. 1764–1769.

The Optic Neuritis Treatment Trial: Implications for Clinical Practice (Editorial): R.W. Beck; Arch. Ophthalmol., 1992, vol. 110, pp. 331–332.

Optic Neuritis in Children and Its Relationship to Multiple Sclerosis: A Clinical Study in 21 Children: R. Riikonen, et al.; Dev. Med. Child Neurol., June 1988, vol. 30(3), pp. 349–359.

Recovery After Optic Neuritis in Childhood: A. Kriss, et al.; J. Neurosurg. Psychiatry, October 1988, vol. 51(10), pp. 1253–1258.

Causes and Workup of Optic Neuropathy: J.A. McCrary III *in* Walsh and Hoyt's Clinical Neuro-Ophthalmology, vol. 1, 4th ed.: N.R. Miller, ed.; Williams and Wilkins, 1982, pp. 213–328.

# PERIPHERAL UVEITIS (PARS PLANITIS)

**Description** Peripheral uveitis is a vision disorder characterized by inflammation of the peripheral retina and pars plana due to infiltration by cells that produce a snowbank of debris in the vitreous humor and peripheral retina. Severity is greater when symptoms begin in the 1st decade of life, and less when onset is in the 2nd to 4th decades. (The term *pars planitis* is a grammatically incorrect Latin derivative.)

**Synonyms**

Chronic Cyclitis

Pars Planitis

Peripheral Retinal Inflammation

**Signs and Symptoms** Typical of the condition is unilateral or bilateral blurred vision. Intraocular inflammation, particularly vitreitis, mild retinal vasculitis (periphlebitis), and macular edema, can occur. Glaucoma, cataract, phthisis, or other eye complications may develop. With bilateral peripheral uveitis, the involvement of each eye may differ in severity.

**Etiology** The cause is unknown; autoimmune and genetic mechanisms have been suggested. Symptoms and signs are the result of inflammation of the peripheral retina and/or pars plana.

**Epidemiology** The more severe early-onset form of the disorder occurs in about 10 percent of cases. Males and females are affected in equal numbers.

**Related Disorders Cystoid macular edema** may be a complication of peripheral uveitis. It is characterized by edema of the central retina as a result of abnormal leakage of fluid from capillaries.

**Treatment—Standard** The usual therapy is a course of corticosteroids to reduce inflammation. Surgery may be recommended in refractory cases. Diathermy or cryotherapy may be used to seal blood vessels and stop leakage or to treat secondary peripheral retinal neovascularization and vitreous hemorrhage.

**Treatment—Investigational** Please contact the agencies listed under Resources, below, for the most current information. Addresses and telephone numbers of these agencies, as well as of individual experts and research centers, may be found in the Master Resources List.

**Resources**

**For more information on peripheral uveitis (pars planitis):** National Organization for Rare Disorders (NORD); NIH/National Eye Institute.

**References**

Long-Term Visual Outcome and Complications Associated with Pars Planitis: S.M. Malinowski, et al.; Ophthalmology, 1993, vol. 100, pp. 818–825.

Pars Planitis in a Father and Son: K.U. Duinkerke-Eerola, et al.; Ophthalmic Paediatr. Genet., 1990, vol. 11, pp. 305–308.

The Enigma of Pars Planitis (Editorial): T.M. Aaberg; Am. J. Ophthalmol., June 1987, pp. 828–829.

The Significance of the Pars Plana Exudate in Pars Planitis: D.E. Henderly, et al.; Am. J. Ophthalmol., May 1987, vol. 103(5), pp. 669–671.

Pars Planitis in Identical Twins: B.H. Doft; Retina, 1983, vol. 3, pp. 32–33.

Familial Pars Planitis: J.J. Augsburger, et al.; Ann. Ophthalmol., 1981, vol. 13, pp. 553–557.

# RETINITIS PIGMENTOSA (RP)

**Description** Retinitis pigmentosa is the description for a large group of hereditary progressive retinal disorders that begin well after birth with loss of dim-light or night vision, progressive loss of peripheral vision, and classic features of pigmentary retinal deterioration.

**Signs and Symptoms** Night blindness is an early symptom, with onset between ages 10 and 40 (depending on the type of RP present), slowly followed by tunnel vision. The rate and extent of progression are widely variable, even within a family.

**Etiology** More than one-half of cases are isolated, but RP may be recessive, autosomal dominant, or X-linked. At least 50 systemic disorders show some type of retinal involvement similar to RP. Two different X-linked forms of RP, distinguishable by different ophthalmoscopic carrier features in the ocular fundus, have been mapped (in 1984 and 1985) to the short arm of the X chromosome.

In 1989, mutations of the rhodopsin locus on chromosome 3q were shown to be associated with 20 percent of families of autosomal dominant RP. Other genes for dominant retinitis pigmentosa have been mapped to chromosome 6p (peripherin), 4p, 7p, 7q, 8, 17p, and 19q. Scientists have also found recessive genes that cause disorders similar to RP in mice, and it is hoped that this knowledge will lead to benefits for patients with rapidly progressive recessive RP. Phenotypes of RP occur in association with neurodevelopmental delay and ataxia (NARP syndrome), and specific mutations in the mitochondrial DNA.

**Epidemiology** The prevalence of RP is between 1:5,000 and 1:7,000.

**Treatment—Standard** At-risk relatives should be examined to determine the pattern of inheritance, the basis for diagnosis, prognosis, and genetic counseling.

No cure for RP is available. When cataracts significantly interfere with vision, surgical removal may be advisable. Whether surgery improves vision often depends on the extent of retinal damage and the proximity of the constricted visual field to the center of fixation in the fovea.

Optical, nonoptical, and electronic vision aids allow individuals to make the maximum use of their remaining vision.

**Treatment—Investigational** Researchers at the Cullen Eye Institute of the Baylor College of Medicine in Houston, Texas, are studying recessively inherited retinal diseases, including recessive RP. Families with at least 2 affected siblings and both parents living are needed to participate in this program. Families wishing to participate in other genetic studies may contact the Foundation Fighting Blindness.

Please contact the agencies listed under Resources, below, for the most current information. Addresses and telephone numbers of these agencies, as well as of individual experts and research centers, may be found in the Master Resources List.

**Resources**

**For more information on retinitis pigmentosa:** National Organization for Rare Disorders (NORD); Foundation Fighting Blindness; Texas Association for Retinitis Pigmentosa; NIH/National Eye Institute.

**For service organizations for the blind:** American Council of the Blind; American Foundation for the Blind; American Printing House for the Blind; National Association for Parents of the Visually Impaired; National Association for the Visually Handicapped; National Federation of the Blind; National Library Service for the Blind and Physically Handicapped; Recording for the Blind; Council of Families with Visual Impairment; Foundation Fighting Blindness.

**For genetic information and genetic counseling referrals:** March of Dimes Birth Defects Foundation; Alliance of Genetic Support Groups.

## References

Mendelian Inheritance in Man, 11th ed.: V.A. McKusick; The Johns Hopkins University Press, 1994, pp. 1299–1301, 2176–2177, 2522–2525.

On the Molecular Genetics of Retinitis Pigmentosa: P. Humphries, et al.; Science, 1992, vol. 256, pp. 804–813.

Retinal Genetics: A Nullifying Effect for Rhodopsin: R.R. McInnes, et al.; Nat. Genet., 1992, vol. 1, pp. 155–157.

Mutations in the Human Retinal Degeneration Slow Gene in Autosomal Dominant Retinitis Pigmentosa: K. Kajiwara, et al.; Nature, 1991, vol. 354, pp. 480–483.

Birth Defects Encyclopedia: M.L. Buyse, ed.-in-chief; Blackwell Scientific Publications, 1990, pp. 1485–1486.

Linkage to D3S47 (C17) in One Large Autosomal Dominant Retinitis Pigmentosa Family and Exclusion in Another: Confirmation of Genetic Heterogeneity: D.H. Lester, et al.; Am. J. Hum. Genet., 1990, vol. 47, pp. 536–541.

Mutations Within the Rhodopsin Gene in Patients with Autosomal Dominant Retinitis Pigmentosa: T.P. Dryja, et al.; N. Engl. J. Med., 1990, vol. 323, pp. 1302–1307.

Cecil Textbook of Medicine, 18th ed.: J.B. Wyngaarden and L.H. Smith, Jr., eds.; W.B. Saunders Company, 1988, pp. 2236, 2292–2293.

Retinitis Pigmentosa: R.A. Pagon; Surv. Ophthalmol., November–December 1988, vol. 33(3), pp. 137–177.

Prevalence of Retinitis Pigmentosa in Maine: C.H. Bunker, et al.; Am. J. Ophthalmol., 1984, vol. 97, pp. 357–365.

# RETINOBLASTOMA

**Description** Retinoblastoma is a pediatric malignant tumor, often bilateral, that develops in the nerve cell layers (retina) and seems to originate from primitive photoreceptors.

**Signs and Symptoms** Retinoblastoma may occur unilaterally or bilaterally. Unilateral retinoblastoma is usually diagnosed between 1 and 3 years of age (average 23 months); bilateral involvement, by about 8 to 12 months. Unilateral retinoblastoma is typically unifocal; bilateral disease usually has multiple tumor foci in each eye. A cat's-eye reflex in the pupil is often the first sign. Strabismus related to loss of vision, glaucoma, and ocular inflammation also are indicative. On examination, the tumor is yellow to white and varies in size. Calcifications within the tumors are seen in three-quarters of cases. Two to 4 percent of cases occur as **trilateral retinoblastoma,** in which the disease occurs in both eyes and is coupled with neoplasia of the pineal gland.

Other malformations have been reported in patients with a chromosomal contiguous deletion syndrome of 13q, including microcephaly, mental retardation, broad nasal bridge, short thumbs and great toes, ear pits, and short neck.

**Etiology** Most retinoblastomas appear as isolated defects, but about 30 to 40 percent behave as an autosomal dominant trait with variable expressivity. However, both copies of the retinoblastoma gene must be defective, constitutionally or in the eye, for the neoplasm to develop. The retinoblastoma gene, located at chromosome 13q14, has been identified and cloned, and procedures have been developed that in some cases can predict the risk of hereditary retinoblastoma. The retinoblastoma gene product is a nuclear phosphoprotein widely expressed in human tissues and differentially phosphorylated at different stages of the cell growth cycle.

**Epidemiology** The incidence of retinoblastoma is about 1:15,000 live births worldwide. It is the most common form of ocular malignancy in children. Survivors of retinoblastoma appear to be prone to osteosarcoma, because the same gene is involved in both disorders. Other malignancies (e.g., small-cell lung cancer and breast cancer) also occur with greater frequency than the general population risk, with a total lifetime risk of 15 to 30 percent.

**Treatment—Standard** Unilateral retinoblastoma is usually managed by enucleation of the eye. In instances of extremely small tumors, radiation may be tried. With bilateral retinoblastoma, the more involved eye often is enucleated and the other eye treated by photocoagulation, cryotherapy, radiation, and possibly chemotherapy. Often a combination of these treatments is used. Reexamination is usually required at 1- to 2-month intervals. Radiologic surveys for bony metastases and studies of spinal fluid and bone marrow for malignant cells may be done until all viable tumor is destroyed. Examination of siblings and other family members is indicated. Both fresh tumor samples and white blood cells should be submitted at the time of enucleation for mutational analysis to facilitate genetic counseling.

**Treatment—Investigational** Please contact the agencies listed under Resources, below, for the most current information. Addresses and telephone numbers of these agencies, as well as of individual experts and research centers, may be found in the Master Resources List.

**Resources**

**For more information on retinoblastoma:** National Organization for Rare Disorders (NORD); NIH/National Eye Institute; American Cancer Society; NIH/National Cancer Institute Physician Data Query Phoneline.

**For more information on gene mutational analysis:** Brenda Gallie, M.D., Eye Research Institute of Canada, Hospital for Sick Children, Toronto, Ontario (mutational analysis and prenatal diagnosis); Thaddeus P. Dryja, M.D., Massachusetts Eye and Ear Infirmary, Boston, Massachusetts (mutational analysis only).

**For genetic information and genetic counseling referrals:** March of Dimes Birth Defects Foundation; Alliance of Genetic Support Groups.

**References**

The Genetics of Retinoblastoma, Revisited: A. Naumova, et al.; Am. J. Hum. Genet., 1994, vol. 54, pp. 264–273.

The Incidence of Retinoblastoma in the United States: 1974 Through 1985: A. Tamboli, et al.; Arch. Ophthalmol., January 1990, vol. 108, pp. 128–132.

Oncogenic Point Mutations in the Human Retinoblastoma Gene: Their Application to Genetic Counseling: D.W. Yandell, et al.; N. Engl. J. Med., 1989, vol. 321, pp. 1689–1695.

Parental Origin of Mutations of the Retinoblastoma Gene: T.P. Dryja, et al.; Nature, June 15, 1989, vol. 339, pp. 556–558.

Incidence of Second Neoplasms in Patients with Bilateral Retinoblastoma: J.D. Roarty, et al.; Ophthalmology, November 1988, vol. 95, pp. 1583–1587.

Expression of Recessive Alleles by Chromosomal Mechanism in Retinoblastoma: W.K. Cavenee, et al.; Nature, 1983, vol. 305, pp. 779–784.

# SENILE RETINOSCHISIS

**Description** Retinoschisis, the splitting of the retina into 2 layers, in its various forms (typical, juvenile, senile) can be inherited or acquired. The adult, or senile, disorder is characterized by a slow, progressive loss of parts of the far peripheral field of vision corresponding to the areas of the retina that have become split, typically in the inferior temporal quadrants of the retinas.

**Synonyms**
> Giant Cyst of the Retina
> Peripheral Cystoid Retinal Degeneration

**Signs and Symptoms** In typical retinoschisis (Blessig cysts, Iwanoff cysts, peripheral cystoid degeneration of the retina), splitting of the retina frequently occurs bilaterally and symmetrically, usually inferotemporally. The visual field is impaired correspondingly if the cystlike schisis cavities expand substantially. The lesion is a thin, transparent, veil-like, domed membrane that contains the retinal blood vessels (inner wall) and often opacities. The progression of splitting and loss of vision often ceases for many years; in some cases, however, progression may be more rapid, and rarely central vision may be threatened.

Senile retinoschisis is similar to typical retinoschisis but usually occurs in older patients, often without symptoms. It is bilateral in 90 percent of cases. Coalescence of peripheral sacs (Blessig cysts, Iwanoff cysts) may produce symptoms. In the early stage, the cystic space is spanned by thin gray fibers that gradually break, allowing the inner and outer leaves of the retina to separate and form an elevated cyst. In the senile form, the split may extend around the retinal perimeter; it does not usually progress to the back of the retina, and it may remain unchanged for many years.

**Etiology** Senile, or adult, retinoschisis is not considered hereditary.

**Epidemiology** Typical retinoschisis usually occurs in hyperopic young males. Senile retinoschisis usually affects persons in the 5th, 6th, or 7th decades. It affects males and females in equal numbers.

**Related Disorders** See *X-Linked Juvenile Retinoschisis; Macular Degeneration.*

**Treatment—Standard** Typical and senile retinoschisis usually do not require medical treatment. Photocoagulation or cryotherapy can close off the damaged area of the retina if large inner and outer retinal breaks occur or if retinal detachment ensues. Genetic counseling is recommended.

**Treatment—Investigational** Please contact the agencies listed under Resources, below, for the most current information. Addresses and telephone numbers of these agencies, as well as of individual experts and research centers, may be found in the Master Resources List.

**Resources**

**For more information on senile retinoschisis:** National Organization for Rare Disorders (NORD); NIH/National Eye Institute; National Association for the Parents of the Visually Impaired; National Association for the Visually Handicapped; Foundation Fighting Blindness; American Foundation for the Blind; American Council of the Blind; Council of Families with Visual Impairment.

**References**

Long-Term Natural History Study of Senile Retinoschisis with Implications for Management: N.E. Byer; Ophthalmology, September 1986, vol. 93, pp. 1127–1137.

Degenerative Retinoschisis with Giant Outer Layer Breaks and Retinal Detachment: J.M. Sulonen, et al.; Am. J. Ophthalmol., February 1985, vol. 99(2), pp. 114–121.

Argon Laser Treatment of Senile Retinoschisis: Y. Yassur, et al.; Brit. J. Ophthalmol., 1983, vol. 67, pp. 381–384.

Typical and Reticular Degenerative Retinoschisis: B.R. Straatsma and R.Y. Foos; Am. J. Ophthalmol., 1973, vol. 75, pp. 551–575.

# TOLOSA-HUNT SYNDROME

**Description** Tolosa-Hunt syndrome is a spectrum of idiopathic inflammation that may involve the superior orbital fissure or cavernous sinus and presents as painful ophthalmoplegia. The syndrome is characterized by severe, usually unilateral, headaches that often precede the ophthalmoplegia.

**Synonyms**

> Ophthalmoplegia, Painful
> Ophthalmoplegia Syndrome

**Signs and Symptoms** Characteristic features include steady, boring pain in the trigeminal distribution, partial or total ophthalmoplegia with or without pupil involvement, variable vision loss due to an optic neuropathy, proptosis, and a dramatic response to steroid therapy.

Neuroimaging may show a focal or poorly circumscribed mass usually enhanced with contrast and occasionally bony erosion in the sellar or parasellar areas. Neuroimaging, spinal fluid analysis, arteriogram, and laboratory studies to exclude vasculitis, syphilis, sarcoidosis, and tuberculosis are requisite. Nonetheless, Tolosa-Hunt syndrome is a diagnosis of exclusion.

**Etiology** The syndrome is thought to be due to an abnormal autoimmune response coupled with an inflammation in the cavernous sinus and superior orbital fissure.

**Epidemiology** The syndrome occurs equally in males and females. The average age of onset is 41, although the disorder may occur at any age.

**Related Disorders** In **orbital cellulitis,** there is inflammation of the tissues of the orbit. Symptoms include extreme pain, impaired eye movement, edema, fever, and malaise. Possible complications include impaired vision, retinal venous abnormalities, and inflammation of the entire orbital area.

**Cavernous sinus thrombosis** is usually caused by infection and clotting in the vessels behind the eyeballs. It can be a complication of orbital cellulitis or an infection of facial skin. Signs and symptoms include edema, exophthalmos, fever, headache, and possibly convulsions. Prompt treatment with antibiotics, intravenous fluids, occasional anticoagulants, and bed rest is recommended.

**Migraine headaches** are usually unilateral. Patients may have a genetic (dominant) predisposition. Often associated with these painful attacks are irritability, nausea, vomiting, constipation or diarrhea, and photosensitivity. Constriction of the cranial arteries may precede migraine headaches in some patients. Fever and ophthalmoplegia are not part of the symptom complex of migraine.

**Treatment—Standard** A short course of corticosteroids relieves the pain associated with Tolosa-Hunt syndrome dramatically. Pain usually subsides in untreated cases within 15 to 20 days. With drug treatment, pain may abate within 24 to 72 hours, although attacks may recur at any time, on the same or contralateral side.

**Treatment—Investigational** Please contact the agencies listed under Resources, below, for the most current information. Addresses and telephone numbers of these agencies, as well as of individual experts and research centers, may be found in the Master Resources List.

**Resources**

**For more information on Tolosa-Hunt syndrome:** National Organization for Rare Disorders (NORD); NIH/National Institute of Neurological Disorders and Stroke; National Migraine Foundation.

**References**

Is Tolosa-Hunt Syndrome a Limited Form of Wegener's Granulomatosis?: C. Montecucco, et al.; Br. J. Rheumatol., 1993, vol. 32, pp. 640–641.

A New Etiology for Visual Impairment and Chronic Headache: The Tolosa-Hunt Syndrome May Be Only One Manifestation of Venous Vasculitis: J. Hannerz, et al., Cephalalgia, March 1986, vol. 6(1), pp. 59–63.

Steroid Responsive Ophthalmoplegia in a Child: Diagnostic Considerations: R.S. Kandt, et al., Arch. Neurol., June 1985, vol. 42(6), pp. 589–591.

Transient Unilateral Oculomotor Paralysis: E. Kattner, et al., Monatsschr. Kinderheilkd., March 1985, vol. 133(3), pp. 175–177.

The Tolosa-Hunt Syndrome: L.B. Kline; Surv. Ophthalmol., 1982, vol. 27, pp. 79–95.

Tolosa-Hunt Syndrome and Antinuclear Factor: R. Lesser, et al.; Am. J. Ophthalmol., 1974, vol. 77, pp. 732–734.

# USHER SYNDROMES

**Description** The Usher syndromes encompass a group of recessively inherited disorders characterized by night blindness and vision loss similar to that seen in retinitis pigmentosa, in association with congenital neurosensory deafness. These syndromes are considered to be separate from other forms of retinitis pigmentosa. They occur in at least 4 forms and are distinguished by age at onset, severity of symptoms, and chromosomal location.

**Synonyms**
> Hereditary Deafness and Retinitis Pigmentosa
> Retinitis Pigmentosa and Congenital Deafness

**Signs and Symptoms** Usher syndrome type I (USH1) is characterized by complete neurosensory deafness at birth, night-vision problems (nyctalopia) beginning before the age of 10, and progressive loss of peripheral vision beginning before the age of 20. Other syndrome features include unintelligible speech (due to absent hearing at birth), pigmentary retinopathy, nonrecordable electroretinogram, and nonresponsive or hyporesponsive vestibular reflexes. Depending on age of ascertainment, central visual acuity is variable (20/20 to about 20/200); blindness may occur from age 20 to 35.

Usher syndrome type II (USH2) is characterized by moderate to severe neurosensory deafness at birth and the onset of retinitis pigmentosa in the late teens or early 20s. Other features include intelligible but abnormal ("nasal" or "blunted") speech, nyctalopia beginning in the early teens to early 20s, pigmentary retinopathy, mild to moderate visual field loss, a subnormal to nonrecordable electroretinogram, and usually normal vestibular responses. Central visual acuity has the same variability as in USH1, but onset of central loss is later. Hearing declines at about 10 dB/decade.

Usher syndrome type III (USH3) usually begins in puberty with progressive hearing loss. Retinitis pigmentosa begins much later in life.

Usher syndrome type IV (USH4) predominantly affects males. An extremely rare and much debated form of Usher syndrome, USH4 is also characterized by hearing loss and progressive vision disturbances.

**Etiology** The inheritance for USH1, USH2, and USH3 is autosomal recessive. USH4 is thought to be inherited as an X-linked recessive trait. In general, severity of symptoms is symmetrical in affected individuals within a family. USH1C in the Acadian population maps to chromosome 11p; USH1B in the North American population maps to chromosome 11q. A French isolate with a similar phenotype called USH1A maps to chromosome 14q32. The gene for USH2 has been mapped to chromosome 1q41. USH3 has been mapped to chromosome 3q. These same markers do not show linkage for USH1.

The exact reason for the hearing and vision loss in the Usher syndromes is not well understood.

**Epidemiology** The prevalence of the Usher syndromes is approximately 5:100,000 to 10:100,000. The prevalence for USH1 has been found to be higher in persons of French Canadian ancestry in Canada, Louisiana, and east Texas; in persons of Jewish descent in Berlin, Germany; in Argentinians of Spanish descent; and in Nigerians.

**Related Disorders** See *Retinitis Pigmentosa; Alstrom Syndrome.*

**Hallgren syndrome (Graefe-Sjögren syndrome)** is characterized by deafness at birth accompanied by progressive visual impairment, including nystagmus and cataracts. Other symptoms include psychomotor retardation, vestibulocerebellar ataxia, mental deficiency, and psychosis.

**Treatment—Standard** Treatment of the Usher syndromes is symptomatic and supportive. Counseling services to individuals with hearing and vision loss can be helpful; genetic counseling is recommended for patients and families. Surgery to remove cataracts in conjunction with intraocular lens implantation may improve vision in proper candidates.

Early identification of an Usher syndrome in a deaf child is essential. Educational methods and options should be explored carefully during school years. Sign language may be a useful communication skill. However, should vision become severely impaired, tactile sign language may be a useful means of communication.

**Treatment—Investigational** The ongoing investigation of chromosome markers is expected to result in improved gene carrier detection and the ability to provide prenatal testing. Isolation of the genes for the Usher syndromes is being approached by the Center for Hereditary Communication Disorders, Boys Town National Research Hospital, Omaha, Nebraska.

Please contact the agencies listed under Resources, below, for the most current information. Addresses and telephone numbers of these agencies, as well as of individual experts and research centers, may be found in the Master Resources List.

**Resources**

**For more information on the Usher syndromes:** National Organization for Rare Disorders (NORD); National Federation of the Blind; American Council of the Blind; American Foundation for the Blind; Foundation Fighting Blindness; NIH/National Eye Institute; Alexander Graham Bell Association for the Deaf; American Humane Association (for trained hearing dogs); Deafness Research Foundation; National Information Center on Deafness; American Society for Deaf Children; NIH/National Institute on Deafness and Other Communication Disorders.

**For genetic information and genetic counseling referrals:** March of Dimes Birth Defects Foundation; Alliance of Genetic Support Groups.

**References**
Assignment of an Usher Syndrome Type III (USH3) Gene to Chromosome 3q: E-M. Sankila, et al.; Hum. Mol. Genet., 1995, vol. 4, pp. 93–98.

Mendelian Inheritance in Man, 11th ed.: V.A. McKusick; The Johns Hopkins University Press, 1994, pp. 2251–2254.

A Gene for Usher Syndrome Type I (USH1A) Maps to Chromosome 14q: J. Kaplan, et al.; Genomics, 1992, vol. 14, pp. 979–987.

Linkage of Usher Syndrome Type I Gene (USH1B) to the Long Arm of Chromosome 11: W.J. Kimberling, et al.; Genomics, 1992, vol. 14, pp. 988–994.

Localization of Two Genes for Usher Syndrome Type I to Chromosome 11: R.J.H. Smith, et al.; Genomics, 1992, vol. 14, pp. 995–1002.

Localization of Usher Syndrome Type II to Chromosome 1q: W.J. Kimberling, et al.; Genomics, 1990, vol. 7, pp. 245–249.

Mapping Recessive Ophthalmic Diseases: Linkage of the Locus for Usher Syndrome Type II to a DNA Marker on Chromosome 1q: R.A. Lewis, et al.; Genomics, 1990, vol. 7, pp. 250–256.

Usher's Syndrome: CNS Defects Determined by Computed Tomography: T.A. Bloom, et al.; Retina, 1983, vol. 3, pp. 108–113.

Usher's Syndrome, Ophthalmic and Neuro-Otologic Findings Suggesting Genetic Heterogenicity: G.A. Fishman, et al.; Arch. Ophthalmol., September 1983, vol. 101(9), pp. 1367–74.

# WAGR Syndrome

**Description** WAGR syndrome is a rare contiguous gene deletion syndrome in which there is a predisposition to several distinct disorders. The acronym WAGR stands for (**W**)ilms tumor, (**A**)niridia, (**G**)enitourinary anomalies, and mental (**R**)etardation. A combination of 2 or more of these symptoms must be present for an individual to be diagnosed with WAGR syndrome. The clinical picture varies, depending upon the combination of symptoms present. The only feature that has been present in all documented cases of WAGR syndrome, with only one known exception, is aniridia. Mental retardation, Wilms tumor, and/or gonadoblastoma may or may not be present in affected individuals.

**Synonyms**

Wilms Tumor–Aniridia–Gonadoblastoma–Mental Retardation Syndrome

Wilms Tumor–Aniridia–Genitourinary Anomalies–Mental Retardation Syndrome

WAGR Complex

**Signs and Symptoms** The specific symptoms that occur depend upon the combination of disorders present.

**Wilms tumor** occurs in approximately 90 percent of all cases of WAGR syndrome. The onset of Wilms tumor occurs mainly in children under the age of 7, with most cases developing between the ages of 1 and 4. In the early stages of Wilms tumor, there are usually no symptoms. The first signs of the disease may include hematuria, low-grade fever, loss of appetite, pallor, weight loss, fatigue and lethargy, and swelling of the abdomen. In the later stages, slight pain may occur intermittently, or pain may be sudden and sharp. Abdominal swelling is the most common symptom and usually leads to detection of the tumor.

In infants with **aniridia** that is associated with WAGR syndrome, the iris of one or both eyes fails to develop normally before birth. This results in the partial or complete absence of the iris. Aniridia is, with only one known exception, the sole feature that has been present in all documented cases of WAGR syndrome. In almost all cases, aniridia may occur in combination with cataract, corneal pannus formation, nystagmus, and/or partial or complete loss of vision due to glaucoma.

In the medical literature, the letter *G* in the acronym WAGR refers to genitourinary abnormalities, ambiguous genitalia, or gonadoblastoma. **Gonadoblastoma** occurs exclusively in people with gonadal dysgenesis, as is the case in some infants with WAGR syndrome. Although gonadoblastoma is not always manifested in WAGR syndrome, it is important to be aware of the genetic predisposition for this potentially serious disorder so that appropriate steps can be taken. Recently it has become clear that a 2nd locus at 11p15 is associated with Beckwith-Wiedemann syndrome, since loss of heterozygosity in Wilms tumor tissue is confined to 11p15.5 in more than half of all cases. More than half of the tumors seen in Beckwith-Wiedemann syndrome are Wilms tumors. Other genitourinary and reproductive abnormalities may be present in children with WAGR syndrome. In males, these may include ambiguous genitalia, cryptorchidism, and hypospadias.

**Mental retardation** is common in children with WAGR syndrome. However, the severity of the retardation varies greatly from case to case, ranging from severe to mild. Some children with WAGR syndrome may have near normal intelligence.

In rare cases, other symptoms associated with WAGR syndrome may include hemihypertrophy, growth retardation, and/or congenital heart abnormalities.

The disorders associated with WAGR may appear together or in a variety of combinations. In the medical literature, these various groupings may be referred to as distinct disorders, including **aniridia–Wilms tumor association (AWTA), aniridia–ambiguous genitalia–mental retardation (AGR triad),** or **aniridia–Wilms tumor–gonadoblastoma.**

**Etiology** WAGR syndrome is the result of defects in several adjacent genes that occur for unknown reasons. The majority of cases are caused by a deletion of part of the short arm of one of the chromosomes in pair 11. The deletion occurs during early embryonic development and is most commonly paternal in origin. The size and the nature of the deletion on the short arm of chromosome 11 may vary from case to case. However, at least part of band 13 on chromosome 11 is always deleted (del 11p13). The nature and size of the deletion determines which symptoms associated with WAGR syndrome the affected child will have.

In approximately 10 percent of documented cases of WAGR syndrome, one of the parents has a balanced translocation. In these cases, the balanced parental translocation may result in an autosomal dominant mode of inheritance. The features associated with WAGR syndrome may not be manifested in all such cases. When the characteristics associated with WAGR syndrome are expressed, the extent of that expression may vary greatly from case to case, ranging from mild to severe.

**Epidemiology** WAGR syndrome is thought to affect males more frequently than females. However, because some affected individuals have ambiguous external genitalia; incorrect gender identification may occur unless a karyotype is performed.

**Related Disorders** See ***Drash Syndrome; Fraser Syndrome; Aniridia.***

**Treatment—Standard** WAGR syndrome can be diagnosed at birth, based upon a clinical evaluation, characteristic physical findings, and high-resolution karyotyping. In many cases, partial or complete aniridia may be the only physical feature associated with WAGR syndrome that is obvious at birth. In other cases, genitourinary abnormalities may also be apparent.

If a child is the first in the family to have aniridia, chromosomal studies are necessary to determine whether the child has a genetic predisposition for all the disorders associated with WAGR syndrome. Reduced catalase activity has been present in the majority of children with WAGR syndrome because of the proximity of the catalase gene locus to the contiguous deletion. Therefore, if catalase activity is diminished in a child with aniridia, the child should be regularly monitored for the development of Wilms tumor and gonadoblastoma.

Treatment of WAGR syndrome is directed toward the specific symptoms that are apparent in each individual.

**Wilms tumor:** Wilms tumor seems to be caused by loss of function of a zinc finger protein on 11p13. Wilms tumor can often be treated successfully depending on the stage of the tumor at detection and the age and general health of the child. Treatment programs that combine modern surgical techniques (including kidney removal), radiation therapy, and chemotherapy have brought dramatic progress in treating this disease. The chemotherapy regimen currently preferred consists of the drugs dactinomycin and vincristine, which may be combined with doxorubicin. Cyclophosphamide may also be used with this drug regimen to treat tumors that have not responded to the first line of chemotherapy. Other regimens sometimes used to treat Wilms tumor include a combination of the drugs cisplatin and etoposide or a regimen that combines ifosfamide and mesna.

**Aniridia:** The treatment of aniridia is usually directed at improving vision. Drugs or surgery may be helpful for glaucoma and/or cataracts. Contact lenses may have limited benefit. Aniridia is caused by a loss of function of the PAX6 gene.

**Gonadoblastoma and Genitourinary Abnormalities:** Children with aniridia and a genetic predisposition to the other disorders associated with WAGR syndrome should be regularly evaluated to detect abnormal development of the ovaries (streak gonads) or testes. Gonadectomy may be indicated to prevent the occurrence of gonadoblastoma. In cases when gonadoblastoma is actually present, surgery to remove the affected gonad(s) is performed. If one gonad is cancer-free, it still may be removed, since it may be at risk for developing gonadoblastoma. Individuals who have had both gonads removed are given hormone treatment. Because hormone therapy may cause secondary uterine cancer to develop, the uterus (if one is present) may be surgically removed when the gonadectomy is performed initially.

In males with WAGR syndrome, cryptorchidism may be present. If a testis does not properly descend into the scrotum on its own before the child is 1 year of age, hormone treatment may be given. If this treatment is not successful, orchiopexy may be performed. Males with cryptorchidism may also have hypospadias. When hypospadias is identified in infants, routine circumcision soon after birth should not be performed. The foreskin can be essential in aiding surgical repair later in life. Surgical correction is performed as necessary for cosmetic, reproductive, and/or psychological purposes and/or to correct problems with urination. Surgical correction is usually performed before the child is 1 year of age. For individuals with ambiguous genitalia, surgery may be performed to correct some abnormalities, and hormone treatment may be instituted.

**Mental Retardation:** Clinical evaluation should be conducted early in development and on a continuing basis to help determine the presence and extent of mental retardation. Such evaluation can help ensure that appropriate steps are taken to help affected individuals reach their highest potential.

Genetic counseling is important for individuals with WAGR syndrome and for their families. Chromosomal studies are necessary to determine if a balanced translocation is present in one parent. Other treatment is symptomatic and supportive.

**Treatment—Investigational** The National Wilms Tumor Study (**NWTS**) was conducted by a national consortium of hospitals and clinics for the purpose of carrying out controlled clinical trials of new treatments for Wilms tumor. Treatment standards for Wilms tumor patients in the United States are based on this study.

Please contact the agencies listed under Resources, below, for the most current information. Addresses and telephone numbers of these agencies, as well as of individual experts and research centers, may be found in the Master Resources List.

### Resources

**For more information on WAGR syndrome:** National Organization for Rare Disorders (NORD).

**For more information on Wilms tumor:** National Kidney Foundation; American Kidney Fund.

**For more information on Wilms tumor and gonadoblastoma:** American Cancer Society; NIH/National Cancer Institute; NIH/National Cancer Institute Physician Data Query Phoneline; Candlelighters Childhood Cancer Foundation.

**For more information on aniridia, cataracts, and glaucoma:** NIH/National Eye Institute; National Eye Research Foundation; Foundation for Glaucoma Research.

**For more information on genitourinary abnormalities and mental retardation:** NIH/National Institute of Child Health and Human Development.

**For more information on mental retardation:** The Arc (a national organization on mental retardation).

**For genetic information and genetic counseling referrals:** March of Dimes Birth Defects Foundation; Alliance of Genetic Support Groups.

### References

Mendelian Inheritance in Man, 11th ed.: V.A. McKusick; The Johns Hopkins University Press, 1994, pp. 1549–1552.

Online Mendelian Inheritance in Man (OMIM): V.A. McKusick, ed.; The Johns Hopkins University, last edit 7/18/94, Entry Number 194072; last edit 6/1/94, Entry Number 137357; last edit 7/26/94, Entry Number 194080; last edit 5/2/94, Entry Number 136680.

The Distal Region of 11p13 and Associated Genetic Diseases: M. Mannens, et al.; Genomics, 1991, vol. 11, pp. 284–293.

Smallest Region of Overlap in Wilms Tumor Deletions Uniquely Implicates an 11p13 Zinc Finger Gene As the Disease Locus: C.C.T. Ton, et al.; Genomics, 1991, vol. 10, pp. 293–297.

Birth Defects Encyclopedia: M.L. Buyse, ed.-in-chief; Blackwell Scientific Publications, 1990, pp. 361–362.

Complete Physical Map of the WAGR Region of 11p13 Localizes a Candidate Wilms' Tumor Gene: E.A. Rose, et al.; Cell, February 9, 1990, vol. 60(3), pp. 495–508.

Parental Origin of De Novo Constitutional Deletions of Chromosomal Band 11p13: V. Huff, et al.; Am. J. Hum. Genet., 1990, vol. 47, pp. 155–160.

# X-LINKED JUVENILE RETINOSCHISIS (RS)

**Description** X-linked juvenile retinoschisis is a genetic disorder present at birth. RS is due to splitting of the retina, which in turn causes slow, progressive loss of parts of the peripheral fields of vision corresponding to the areas of the retina that have split. Often, RS is associated with the development of retinal cysts. Central visual acuity is invariably impaired by a characteristic retinoschisis of the central fovea of the retina.

### Synonyms

Juvenile Retinoschisis

X-Linked Retinoschisis

**Signs and Symptoms** The retinal split often extends back over the macula and may affect the fovea. In the early stages, the retinal areas that are splitting often exhibit large holes in the inner layer between blood vessels. If breaks develop in both the front and the back layers of the schisis cavity, a true retinal detachment may occur, causing loss of parts of the field of vision. A scotoma with a sharp edge in the area of the schisis appears in the patient's visual field. An electroretinogram shows B-waves that are significantly lower than normal but not obliterated. Cystic macular degeneration, which causes additional loss of vision, always accompanies RS.

Symptoms include reduced central vision (20/40 to 20/200), detachment of all or part of the retina, and occasionally complete retinal atrophy with retinal pigment epithelial degeneration. The patient may develop cysts in the macula and other areas of the retina. The cysts lead to splitting of the retina into retinoschisis "pockets." Bleeding within the schisis cavity or into the vitreous, with or without retinal detachment, may occur.

**Etiology** The disorder is inherited as an X-linked trait. Carrier detection by ophthalmoscopy is not feasible.

**Epidemiology** The disease affects males. The gene appears to be more common in Finland than in other areas of Europe and North America. Populations with high frequency of consanguinity may include affected females, who are invariably more severely afflicted than age-matched affected males. Problems with vision are usually mild up until the age of 40 or 50, after which central vision may slowly worsen.

**Related Disorders** See ***Macular Degeneration.***

**Familial foveal retinoschisis** is another type of juvenile retinoschisis. It involves splitting of tissue only within the retinal fovea. The foveal disease is similar to X-linked juvenile retinoschisis, but the disorder occurs as an autosomal recessive trait.

**Best disease** is a dominant hereditary vision disorder that usually affects the macular region in both eyes. Changes in the macular region, as well as in other areas of the eye, may be noted before visual impairment occurs. The macular area may show a yellow mass resembling the yolk of an egg. With age, the yellow material is absorbed, and a central atrophic scar or occasional disciform scar may develop.

**Treatment—Standard** Genetic counseling may be of benefit for patients and their families. Other treatment is symptomatic and supportive.

**Treatment—Investigational** Gene linkage investigations directed at isolating the responsible gene are being conducted by Paul Sieving, M.D., Ph.D., at the University of Michigan Medical Center.

Please contact the agencies listed under Resources, below, for the most current information. Addresses and telephone numbers of these agencies, as well as of individual experts and research centers, may be found in the Master Resources List.

### Resources

**For more information on X-linked juvenile retinoschisis:** National Organization for Rare Disorders (NORD); NIH/National Eye Institute; Association for Macular Diseases.

**For genetic information and genetic counseling referrals:** March of Dimes Birth Defects Foundation.

### References

Mendelian Inheritance in Man, 11th ed.: V.A. McKusick; The Johns Hopkins University Press, 1994, pp. 2177, 2525–2526.

Refined Localization of the Gene Causing X-Linked Retinoschisis: T. Alitalo, et al.; Genomics, 1991, vol. 9, pp. 505–510.

Linkage Relationship of X-Linked Juvenile Retinoschisis with Xp22.1–p22.3 Probes: P.A. Sieving, et al.; Am. J. Hum. Genet., 1990, vol. 47, pp. 616–621.

Familial Foveal Retinoschisis: R.A. Lewis, et al.; Arch. Ophthalmol., 1977, vol. 95, pp. 1190–1196.

Visual Acuity in 183 Cases of X-Chromosomal Retinoschisis: H. Forsius, et al.; Canad. J. Ophthalmol., 1973, vol. 8, pp. 385–393.

# 13 | ENVIRONMENTAL/TOXIC DISORDERS
## By Robert H. Gray, Ph.D.

The Persian Gulf War has left us with some interesting, inexplicable medical problems. U.S. military personnel returning from Operation Desert Storm and Desert Shield in the Persian Gulf are reporting symptoms of unexpected illnesses. The incidence and possible etiology of the problems encountered in veterans, along with the need for additional data to understand these problems, are discussed in a summary of findings on the Persian Gulf War *(The Persian Gulf Experience and Health,* The National Institutes of Health, Technology Assessment Workshop, April 1994, pp. 1–28). The developing methodology employed for this cohort to obtain a better understanding of the causes of the Persian Gulf War syndrome may be applicable to the study of other rare diseases encountered in various situations.

Under the conditions existing during the Persian Gulf War, it was inevitable that a series of health problems would be encountered and attributed to various infectious agents and to exposure to pesticides, solvents, or particulates resulting in neurologic, respiratory, gastrointestinal, endocrine, or dermatologic abnormalities. However, many of the symptoms being reported among veterans cannot be attributed to common sources and are classified as *unexpected illnesses.* These unexpected illnesses are defined as "previously unrecognized and unanticipated symptom complexes or illnesses that do not fit the traditional diagnostic categories."

In an effort to determine the etiology of these unexpected illnesses, a Persian Gulf War Registry was established to facilitate the collection and analysis of symptoms and other health-related data. By the end of 1994, nearly 35,000 veterans were listed in this registry. Less than 20 percent of the registrants were identified as having the unexpected illnesses. Can the reported symptoms be attributed to stress? It is recognized that the stress levels among military personnel stationed in the Persian Gulf were high. Estimates of fatalities in a full-scale 15-day war could have approached 50,000 of the 500,000 active-duty troops that were deployed to the Persian Gulf region. Detectors in the region on many occasions indicated the presence of chemical weapons and the need to administer drugs designated as pretreatment for nerve gas. However, despite the high stress levels, it is believed that the military personnel were prepared and that stress is not the basis of the unexpected medical problems.

The spectrum of complaints from veterans of the Persian Gulf War includes the following: aching joints, skin rashes, bone pain, weakness, shakiness, headache, dizziness, memory loss, hair loss, chronic fatigue, decreased salivary secretion, gastrointestinal problems (including bleeding), and bleeding gums. Some of the biological, chemical, and physical agents to which veterans were exposed are listed below:

**Leishmaniasis:** Parasite identification was observed in 31 subjects. The infected individuals may be a subset of a larger group diagnosed with visceral leishmaniasis, a condition not usually detected by standard diagnostic tests (bone marrow, skin tests, and serology). Further study on the etiology of leishmaniasis is under way.

**Petroleum vapors, solvents, and smoke:** Many forms of petroleum were sources of human inhalation and dermal exposures. Oil well fires produced a large variety of carbonaceous particulates with metal and partially combusted hydrocarbons. Kerosene and diesel fuel were used for heating. Petroleum products and fuel oil were used widely as dust suppressants. Fumes from petroleum products such as benzene, toluene, xylene can exceed 1 ppm and result in cognitive dysfunction, fatigue, and light-headedness.

**Sand dust:** Sand dust is a common problem in desert regions, resulting from wind or mechanical dispersion from heavy equipment used in the military activities.

**Depleted uranium:** Uranium, in an aerosol form, from impacts and burning metal was reported in localized areas. Uranium exposure induces kidney damage, and aerosolized particulates can accumulate in the lung. Experts feel that the uranium exposure is not the cause of the unexplained illnesses.

**Pyridostigmine bromide (nerve gas pretreatment):** This compound was made available to all and self-administered in tablets (30 mg each) when commanding officers felt that an attack was imminent. In some cases, the drug was administered every 8 hours for up to 1 week or until orders were given to discontinue the treatment. This drug has been used for the treatment of myasthenia gravis at doses up to 6,000 mg/day for life without serious side effects.

**Pesticides:** Several pesticides were used in the Persian Gulf region for vector-borne and rodent-disease prevention. Common pesticides included chlorpyrifos, malathion, lindane, pyrethroids, and several others. The acute adverse effects of exposure to these compounds include headache, dizziness, weakness, blurred vision, nausea, cramps, and pulmonary edema. Acute doses can produce polyneuropathy. No neuropathy has been reported among the examined Persian Gulf War veterans.

**Chemical agent resistant coatings (CARCs):** CARCs were applied to vehicles and equipment shipped to the Persian Gulf region. Toluene diisocyanate is a component of CARCs and can lead to lung sensitization and asthma.

**Biological and chemical warfare agents:** The exposure of military personnel to biological and chemical warfare agents remains controversial. Czech troops reported the detection of sarin and mustard gas. The U.S. Department of Defense reported that there was no evidence to support US military personnel exposure to these agents. However, the report of a special panel set up to investigate the use of biological and chemical warfare was not provided. Therefore, until it can be conclusively determined that chemical and biological warfare agents were not used in the war, the possibility remains that symptoms of unexplained illness could have resulted from their use.

**Vaccines:** Persian Gulf War personnel were vaccinated against two agents of biological warfare, anthrax and botulinum toxin, as well as with other common vaccines. All of the vaccines administered have been used on a wide scale and have not been reported to show long-term adverse effects.

In future studies, symptom prevalence for the cohort (700,000 in this case) needs to be determined through questionnaires or other screening methods. Predeployment health status needs to be established for the cohort as a baseline for these studies. Symptom prevalence of other populations, including military personnel deployed to other locations, needs to be compared with that of the Persian Gulf War veterans. Further research is needed to determine the effect of the stressors of deployment and combat on the symptoms reported. If the effects of stress are understood, then education and training programs prior to deployment and combat could be designed to reduce the stress related to deployment and combat. The role of visceral leishmaniasis in symptoms of Persian Gulf War veterans needs further investigation, which may result in improved diagnostic protocols for this disease.

Rare toxic disorders in humans can occur following exposures to a large spectrum of occupational or environmental toxic agents. The origin of toxic agents may be chemical, physical, or biological. Symptoms produced by such exposures are not always easily traced to the source of the problem. Exposure to some occupational agents is characterized by a latent interval between exposure and onset of the clinical symptoms. Latent periods are highly variable but can be up to 20 years or longer. In addition, the combination of exposures to multiple toxic compounds may mask or alter the expected symptoms once the suspected agent is identified. Enumeration of a comprehensive list of toxic agents or conditions that produce toxic responses in humans is beyond the scope of this chapter. Here, the focus is on selected rare disorders resulting from occupational and environmental exposures.

In this chapter, selected rare toxic/environmental disorders of chemical, physical, or biological origin are described. Exposures of occupational origin include poisoning by selected heavy metals (beryllium, aluminum, antimony, arsenic, cadmium, chromium, cobalt, copper, gold, lead, lithium, manganese, mercury, molybdenum, silver, vanadium, and zinc). Formaldehyde exposure is included as a different type of a toxic chemical. Radiation exposure is discussed as an example of a toxic physical agent. Two environmental disorders—acute mountain sickness (altitude sickness) and an unusual toxin of biological origin (ciguatera fish)—are described.

Care should be exercised while investigating and diagnosing symptoms associated with rare toxic/environmental disorders. The investigation and diagnosis of such disorders require that the physician exhibit extensive "peripheral vision" regarding the characterization of the symptoms being investigated. An acute awareness of the environment in which the patient has been living requires thorough scrutiny. A profile of the patient's workplace, home living conditions, associations with friends and co-workers, leisure time activities, social habits, and general health can be helpful in narrowing the range of suspected problems. The patient's occupational health history should be carefully examined and documented to identify suspected toxic agent exposures and the lengths of such exposures. If occupational exposures are suspected, attempts should be made to document the route (oral, dermal, inhalation, etc.) of exposure, the estimated concentration of the toxin, and the duration of the exposure.

The following patient information may be useful in making a clinical diagnosis.

Comprehensive occupational history including jobs held and their durations.

Is the patient aware of exposure to suspected toxic agents (solvents, dust, etc.)? If so, what are the agents, when did the exposure take place, and what was its duration?

How long have the current symptoms been evident? Have the symptoms appeared and then disappeared?

Was protective equipment recommended in the patient's job? If so, was the equipment used?

Have the patient's co-workers experienced similar symptoms? If so, how many and how long?

Are there known sources of pollution (air or water), with potential harmful health effects near the patient's residence?

Have other members of the patient's family or those living near the patient exhibited similar symptoms? If so, when were the symptoms first observed and how long did they last?

Have there been any new construction or renovation projects initiated, or any new or seasonal maintenance procedures performed in the workplace or at home involving new materials, such as plywood, carpets, or solvents, or recent applications of pesticides or herbicides? In the past, have solvents, pesticides, or herbicides been stored for extended periods near current living areas or working areas? Have there been any recent ventilation or air conditioning system modifications?

What is the smoking history of the patient? If the patient is a smoker, for how many years? How many packs per day? If the patient has quit smoking, how long ago?

Has the patient's diet changed within the last week?

As more is learned about a suspected toxic agent exposure, answers to these questions and to others should aid in eliminating some types of agents and bring one closer to identifying the causal toxic agent. Attempts have been made during the preparation of this chapter to incorporate recent findings from medical literature on the toxic agents covered. New information is, however, continually becoming available. For example, information on radiation sickness is appearing slowly from the aftermath of the Chernobyl accident in 1986. International agencies, such as the World Health Organization, are now initiating studies on the long-term health effects of radiation from the accident. The latter will provide new data in the future on the short- and long-term effects of radiation exposure. Additional information on other rare forms of toxic/environmental disorders can be obtained from state or local health agencies, local poison control centers (e.g., hospitals or clinics), the National Institute for Environmental Health Science, the Centers for Disease Control, the Agency for Toxic Substances Disease Registry, and the Food and Drug Administration.

# ENVIRONMENTAL / TOXIC DISORDERS
*Listings in This Section*

# ACUTE MOUNTAIN SICKNESS

**Description** Acute mountain sickness is a syndrome that may occur in some unacclimated persons who ascend rapidly to altitudes higher than 7,000 to 9,000 feet (2,200 to 2,743 meters).

**Synonyms**

> High-Altitude Illness
> Mareo
> Mountain Sickness
> Puna
> Soroche

**Signs and Symptoms** The syndrome may occur during the first 8 to 24 hours after a person reaches a high altitude. The severity and duration of symptoms vary with the rate of climbing and the ascent height, as well as with the individual's susceptibility. Headache, fatigue, difficulty sleeping, anorexia, nausea, and vomiting may occur, as well as rales, retinal bleeding, and peripheral edema. Oliguria, ataxia, tachycardia, and impaired thinking may also result.

**Etiology** Symptoms occur because of the decrease in available oxygen to the tissues at high altitudes. Decompression-inducible platelet aggregation (**DIPA**) leading to vascular occlusion has been suggested as an etiologic factor in acute mountain sickness.

**Epidemiology** Acute mountain sickness affects males and females in equal numbers. Susceptible persons include those who require more than the normal amount of oxygen, or those who are particularly intolerant of decreased oxygen levels. Individuals who urinate infrequently appear to be particularly susceptible.

**Related Disorders Subacute infantile mountain sickness** is a severe disorder of infants that may occur when they are born at low altitudes and then taken to higher elevations. Thickening of the pulmonary arteries and enlargement of the cavities of the heart have been seen with this disorder.

**High-altitude pulmonary edema** is a severe complication of acute mountain sickness caused by the development of hypoxia at altitudes greater than 9,000 feet. Findings include headaches, vomiting, dyspnea, coughing, rales, tachycardia, and cyanosis. Retinal bleeding, papilledema, problems of memory and orientation, and loss of consciousness may also occur.

**High-altitude cerebral edema,** also a severe consequence of acute mountain sickness, is characterized by headaches, diplopia, visual and auditory hallucinations, loss of consciousness, and ataxia.

**Treatment—Standard** Prompt descent is the most successful treatment for acute mountain sickness. For mild cases, rest coupled with light activity, frequent small meals, no alcohol, and acetaminophen for headache may be the only supportive care needed. For more severe cases, dexamethasone can be used for its anti-inflammatory properties, and acetazolamide for edema, although care should be taken to replace fluids in dehydrated patients.

To prevent acute mountain sickness, a slow, staged ascent, remaining 2 to 5 days at a middle altitude, or prophylactic use of dexamethasone or acetazolamide may be recommended.

**Treatment—Investigational** Researchers are further investigating oxygen therapy and the combination of dexamethasone and acetazolamide for the treatment of acute mountain sickness.

Please contact the agencies listed under Resources, below, for the most current information. Addresses and telephone numbers of these agencies, as well as of individual experts and research centers, may be found in the Master Resources List.

**Resources**

**For more information on acute mountain sickness:** National Organization for Rare Disorders (NORD); NIH/National Institute of Environmental Health Sciences.

**References**

Chronic Mountain Sickness and Chronic Lower Respiratory Tract Disorders: F. Leon-Velarde, et al.; Chest, 1994, vol. 106(1), pp. 151–157.

Acute Mountain Sickness at Moderate Altitudes (Letter): G. Roeggla, et al.; Ann. Intern. Med., 1993, vol. 119(7 pt. 1), p. 633, discussion pp. 633–634.

Acute Mountain Sickness in Children at 2835 Meters: M.K. Theis, et al.; Am. J. Dis. Child., 1993, vol. 147(2), pp. 143–145.

Treatment of Acute Mountain Sickness by Simulated Descent: A Randomised Controlled Trial: P. Bartsch, et al.; BMJ, 1993, vol. 306(6885), pp. 1098–1101.

Acetazolamide in the Treatment of Acute Mountain Sickness: Clinical Efficacy and Effect on Gas Exchange: C.K. Grissom, et al.; Ann. Intern. Med., 1992, vol. 116(6), pp. 461–465.

Current Prevention and Management of Acute Mountain Sickness: F.J. Bia; Yale J. Biol. Med., 1992, vol. 65(4), pp. 337–341.

Acute Mountain Sickness: A Vascular Occlusive Disease: M. Murayama; Medical Hypotheses, March 1990, vol. 31(3), pp. 189–195.

Current Concepts: Acute Mountain Sickness: T.S. Johnson, et al.; N. Engl. J. Med., September 29, 1988, vol. 319(13), pp. 841–845.

High Altitude Cerebral Oedema: C. Clarke; Int. J. Sports Med., April 1988, vol. 9(2), pp. 170–174.

Clinical Features of Patients with High-Altitude Pulmonary Edema in Japan: T. Kobayashi et al.; Chest, November 1987, vol. 92(5), pp. 814–821.

# BERYLLIOSIS

**Description** Berylliosis, the result of inhalation of beryllium dust or fumes, may affect the lungs, skin, eyes, or blood. It can occur acutely or after long-term exposure. Some cases may be delayed as long as 20 years after exposure.

Beryllium is used in the refining of precious metals, in structural materials in the spacecraft industry, in supersonic jets, and in certain components of the space shuttle. Reclaiming beryllium from discarded electronic components and other materials is a separate industry. Beryllium smelter workers may be exposed to high levels of the metal as it is crushed, milled, screened, and melted. Even though the workers are required to wear respirators, contamination may occur, and if dust on their clothes is brought home, other members of their families may develop the condition.

**Synonyms**

> Beryllium Granulomatosis
> Beryllium Pneumonosis
> Beryllium Poisoning

**Signs and Symptoms** Acute berylliosis primarily affects the respiratory system. Chronic exposure is characterized by the formation of pulmonary granulomas, nodular accumulations, or inflammatory cells. Coughing, which is dry at first, later becomes violent and exhausting. Dyspnea and hemoptysis, weight loss, chest pain, and fatigue may develop.

An allergic reaction to beryllium can be manifested as an erythematous, vesicular rash on the face, neck, arms, or hands. Lymphadenopathy may be noted near the affected skin areas.

With prolonged exposure, berylliosis may become chronic. Cyanosis, accompanied by fever and weight loss, may develop, as well as orthopnea. Fingernails may become clubbed, and corneal lesions may be found. It is difficult to distinguish chronic beryllium disease from miliary tuberculosis and sarcoidosis, although central nervous system or salivary gland involvement is more typical of sarcoidosis.

Research indicates that the peripheral blood lymphocyte transformation test may be used to identify berylliosis in its early stages.

**Etiology** Researchers believe that the symptoms of berylliosis are caused by the processes of cell-mediated immunity, including the release of lymphocytes and lymphokines. Beryllium-specific T cells are thought to be involved.

**Epidemiology** Persons at risk for developing berylliosis include those employed in the aerospace, aviation, or nuclear weapons and power industries; those involved in beryllium mining and processing; and those exposed to fluorescent lamp manufacture between 1943 and 1955. In some cases, the families of these employees also may have been exposed, particularly anyone who launders the worker's clothes. Persons living in the vicinity of beryllium refineries have also been affected.

**Related Disorders** See *Alveolitis, Extrinsic Allergic.*

**Treatment—Standard** The source of exposure to beryllium fumes or dust should be removed. In single-exposure acute cases, treatment is symptomatic since the effects are short-term and usually reversible. In chronic cases, corticosteroid therapy may be helpful if begun early in the course of the disease. Bronchoalveolar lavage may be useful in chronic cases, both to confirm the diagnosis and to help remove inorganic particles from the lungs.

**Treatment—Investigational** Long-term intermittent chelation with EDTA is being evaluated.

Please contact the agencies listed under Resources, below, for the most current information. Addresses and telephone numbers of these agencies, as well as of individual experts and research centers, may be found in the Master Resources List.

**Resources**

For more information on berylliosis: National Organization for Rare Disorders (NORD); American Lung Association; NIH/National Institute of Allergy and Infectious Diseases; Centers for Disease Control; NIH/National Institute of Environmental Health Sciences.

**References**

Chronic Beryllium Disease: From the Workplace to Cellular Immunology, Molecular Immunogenetics, and Back: K. Kreiss, et al.; Clin. Immunol. Immunopathol., 1994, vol. 71(2), pp. 123–129.

Beryllium Disease Screening in the Ceramics Industry: Blood Lymphocyte Test Performance and Exposure-Disease Relations: K. Kreiss, et al.; J. Occup. Med., 1993, vol. 35(3), pp. 267–274.

Early Pulmonary Physiologic Abnormalities in Beryllium Disease: G.P. Pappas and L.S. Newman; Am. Rev. Respir. Dis., 1993, vol. 148(3), pp. 661–666.

Epidemiology of Beryllium Sensitization and Disease in Nuclear Workers: K. Kreiss, et al.; Am. Rev. Respir. Dis., 1993, vol. 148(4 pt. 1), pp. 985–991.

A Mortality Study of Workers at Seven Beryllium Processing Plants: E. Ward, et al.; Am . J. Ind. Med., 1992, vol. 22(6), pp. 885–904.

Internal Medicine, 3rd ed.: J.H. Stein, ed.-in-chief; Little, Brown and Company, 1990, p. 706.

Screening Blood Test Identifies Subclinical Beryllium Disease: K. Kreiss, et al.; J. Occup. Med., July 1989, vol. 31(7), pp. 603–608.

Chronic Beryllium Disease: Diagnosis, Radiographic Findings, and Correlation with Pulmonary Function Tests: J.M. Aronchick, et al.; Radiology, June 1987, vol. 163(3), pp. 677–682.

Chronic Beryllium Disease in a Precious Metal Refinery: Clinical Epidemiologic and Immunologic Evidence for Continuing Risk from Exposure to Low Level Beryllium Fumes: M.R. Cullen, et al.; Am. Rev. Respir. Dis., January 1987, vol. 135(1), pp. 201–208.

Mitogenic Effect of Beryllium Sulfate on Mouse B Lymphocytes but Not T Lymphocytes in Vitro: L.S. Newmann and P.A. Campbell; Int. Arch. Allergy Appl. Immunol., 1987, vol. 84(3), pp. 223–227.

Transmission of Occupational Disease to Family Contacts: B. Knishkowy, et al.; Am. J. Ind. Med., 1986, vol. 9(6), pp. 543–550.

# CIGUATERA FISH POISONING

**Description** Gastrointestinal, neurologic, and muscular symptoms occur after ingestion of certain tropical and subtropical fish contaminated with ciguatoxins. More than 400 species of fish have been implicated, including many that are otherwise considered edible, such as snapper, sea bass, and perch. The disease has been occurring more frequently in the United States during the past few years.

**Synonyms**

> Ciguatera Poisoning Syndrome
> Fish Poisoning
> Ichthyosarcotoxism

**Signs and Symptoms** Symptoms of acute ciguatera poisoning may begin as soon as 30 minutes after exposure. Typical initial findings include itching, tingling, and numbness of the lips, tongue, hands, and feet. Other symptoms that also may occur during the first 6 to 17 hours are abdominal cramps, nausea, vomiting, diarrhea, and pruritus. Chills, weakness, restlessness, dizziness, wheezing, myalgias, and arthralgias may develop. Acute symptoms generally resolve within a few days, but disabling neurologic symptoms may continue for several months. In severe cases, there may be rapid progression to dyspnea and muscular paralysis. Death may occur within 24 hours from respiratory arrest or convulsions.

**Etiology** Ciguatera fish poisoning is caused by toxins contained in tropical fish at certain times of the year. Recent reports indicate a ciguatera poisoning syndrome in farm-raised salmon. There is no test for the detection of the toxin, and no known method of cooking the fish can eradicate the toxin.

**Epidemiology** Incidence of ciguatera fish poisoning is highest in tropical countries, particularly those in the Pacific and the Caribbean.

The presence of ciguatoxin has been reported in both semen (producing symptoms in females after sexual intercourse) and breast milk.

**Related Disorders Tetraodon poisoning** results from eating puffer fish that contain the tetraodon toxin. Symptoms are similar to those of ciguatera poisoning, but mortality may be as high as 50 percent. **Scombroid poisoning** is caused by a toxin formed during bacterial decay of fish, and is usually associated with inadequate refrigeration. Symptoms generally begin soon after ingestion and resemble those of a histamine reaction, with flushing, dizziness, urticaria, nausea, and vomiting.

**Treatment—Standard** Gastric lavage should be instituted as soon as possible, and the effects of persistent nausea and vomiting must be treated. Appropriate measures for shock, convulsions, or respiratory failure should begin promptly if these developments occur.

**Treatment—Investigational** Successful treatment of acute ciguatera poisoning with an intravenous infusion of mannitol has recently been reported.

Please contact the agencies listed under Resources, below, for the most current information. Addresses and telephone numbers of these agencies, as well as of individual experts and research centers, may be found in the Master Resources List.

**Resources**

**For more information on ciguatera fish poisoning:** National Organization for Rare Disorders (NORD); Centers for Disease Control.

**For immediate help:** Contact the local poison control center listed in the telephone directory.

**References**

The Ciguatera Poisoning Syndrome from Farm-Raised Salmon: M.J. DiNubile and Y. Hokama; Ann. Intern. Med., 1995, vol. 122(2), pp. 113–114.

Ciguatera Fish Poisoning: W.R. Lange; Am. Fam. Physician, 1994, vol. 50(3), pp. 579–584.

Evolution of Methods for Assessing Ciguatera Toxins in Fish: D.L. Park; Rev. Environ. Contam. Toxicol., 1994, vol. 136, pp. 1–20.

The First Reported Case of Human Ciguatera Possibly Due to a Farm-Cultured Salmon: J.S. Ebesu, et al.; Toxicon, 1994, vol. 32(10), pp. 1282–1286.

Food Safety: Epidemiology of Ciguatera Poisoning: Wkly. Epidemiol. Rec., 1994, vol. 69(49), pp. 365–367.

Ciguatera: A.E. Swift, et al.; J. Toxicol. Clin Toxicol., 1993, vol. 31(1), pp. 1–29.

Ciguatera on Kauai: Investigation of Factors Associated with Severity of Illness: A.R. Katz, et al.; Am. J. Trop. Meg. Hyg., October 1993, vol. 49(4), pp. 448–454.

Coma Due to Ciguatra Poisoning in Rhode Island: D.J. DeFusco, et al.; Am. J. Med., August 1993, vol. 95(2), pp. 240–243.

Study of Factors That Influence the Clinical Response to Ciguatera Fish Poisoning: P. Glaziou, et al.; Toxicon, September 1993, vol. 31(9), pp. 1151–1154.

Cecil Textbook of Medicine, 19th ed.: J.B. Wyngaarden, et al., eds.; W.B. Saunders Company, 1992, pp. 732–733.

Clinical Experience with I.V. Mannitol in the Treatment of Ciguatera: D.G. Blythe, et al.; Bull. Soc. Pathol. Exot., 1992, vol. 85(5 pt. 2), pp. 425–426.

Infectious Diseases: S.L. Gorbach, ed.; W.B. Saunders Company, 1992, pp. 634–635.

Nelson Textbook of Pediatrics, 14th ed.: R.E. Behrman, ed.-in-chief; W.B. Saunders Company, 1992, pp. 1772–1773.

Orthostatic Hypotension in Ciguatera Fish Poisoning: R.J. Geller, et al.; Arch. Intern. Med., October 1992, vol. 152(10), pp. 2131–2133.

Travel and Ciguatera Fish Poisoning: W.R. Lange, et al.; Arch. Intern. Med., October 1992, vol. 152(10), pp. 2049–2053.

Mother's Milk Turns Toxic Following Fish Feast (Letter): D.G. Blythe and D.P. de Sylva; JAMA, October 24–31, 1990, vol. 264(16), p. 2074.

Can Ciguatera Be a Sexually Transmitted Disease?: W.R. Lange, et al.; J. Toxicol. Clin. Toxicol., 1989, vol. 27(3), pp. 193–197.

Ciguatera and Mannitol: Experience with a New Treatment Regimen: J.H. Pearn, et al.; Med. J. Aust., July 17, 1989, vol. 151(2), pp. 77–80.

Successful Treatment of Ciguatera Fish Poisoning with Intravenous Mannitol: N.A. Palafox, et al.; JAMA, May 13, 1988, vol. 259(18), pp. 2740–2742.

# EOSINOPHILIA-MYALGIA SYNDROME

**Description** Eosinophilia-myalgia syndrome is a disorder associated with the oral use of large doses of L-tryptophan (also known as tryptophan), a dietary supplement once available in health food stores. It is a disease of abrupt onset causing severe, disabling, chronic muscle pain; skin symptoms; and other neurotoxic reactions. It can be diagnosed by finding unusually high levels of eosinophils in the blood.

**Synonyms**

> L-Tryptophan Disease
> Eosinophilic Myalgia
> Tryptophan Syndrome

**Signs and Symptoms** Eosinophilia-myalgia syndrome occurs weeks, months, or even years after the oral use of L-tryptophan. The primary symptoms are severe muscle pain and weakness. There may also be associated ulcers of the mouth or other mucous membranes. Sore throat, dyspnea, swollen liver and abdomen, abdominal pain, and fever may also be present. Skin abnormalities resemble scleroderma and include swelling and tightening of the skin, painful itching, and pitting and edema along with peau d'orange skin of the legs. The dermatologic symptoms usually start in the extremities (usually the legs), with the upper body becoming involved later, if at all. Long-term sensorimotor polyneuropathy is evident in 61 percent of patients.

**Etiology** Eosinophilia-myalgia syndrome is caused by the ingestion of oral L-tryptophan. L-Tryptophan that has been contaminated in the manufacturing process with 1-1-ethylidenebis (ETB) causes even more severe symptoms. L-Tryptophan is an essential amino acid present in very small quantities in most foods. However, when purchased as a health food, it is often ingested in unusually high doses, exceeding levels found in the normal diet. The drug was formerly available at health food stores without prescription as a dietary supplement. Although there was no proof of effectiveness, many patients used it to treat depression, premenstrual syndrome, and insomnia. In 1990, the FDA banned L-tryptophan, and it can no longer be purchased in the United States.

**Epidemiology** Eosinophilia-myalgia syndrome affects males and females in equal numbers. According to the Centers for Disease Control, 1,269 cases were reported to them as of February, 1990. Some patients have died.

**Related Disorders** See *Scleroderma; Eosinophilic Fascitis.*

Trichinosis is a disease caused by eating undercooked pork containing *Trichinella spiralis.* Symptoms include eosinophilia, myalgia, circumorbital edema, and fever.

Toxic oil syndrome is associated with the ingestion of contaminated cooking oil. An epidemic of toxic oil syndrome swept Spain during the summer of 1981 and affected over 20,000 persons. Its initial features are fever and pneumonitis, followed by gastrointestinal dysfunction, severe eosinophilia, and severe myalgia.

**Treatment—Standard** Treatment consists of high doses of glucocorticoids to reduce the amount of circulating eosinophils. This treatment, however, does not usually relieve the other symptoms.

**Treatment—Investigational** Please contact the agencies listed under Resources, below, for the most current information. Addresses and telephone numbers of these agencies, as well as of individual experts and research centers, may be found in the Master Resources List.

**Resources**

**For more information on eosinophilia-myalgia syndrome:** National Organization for Rare Disorders

(NORD); NIH/National Arthritis and Musculoskeletal and Skin Diseases; Centers for Disease Control; United Scleroderma Foundation.

### References

Axonal Neuropathy in Eosinophilia-Myalgia Syndrome: S.M. Burns, et al.; Muscle Nerve, 1994, vol. 17(3), pp. 293–298.

Eosinophilic Hepatitis: A New Feature of the Clinical Spectrum of the Eosinophilia-Myalgia Syndrome: P. Martinez-Osuna, et al.; Clin. Rheumatol., 1994, vol. 13(3), pp. 528–532.

The Evolving Spectrum of Eosinophilia Myalgia Syndrome: L.D. Kaufman; Rheum. Dis. Clin. North Am., 1994, vol. 20(4), pp. 973–994.

Acute Encephalopathy Associated with the Eosinophilia-Myalgia Syndrome: J.C. Adair, et al.; Neurology, 1992, vol. 42(2), pp. 461–462.

The Eosinophilia-Myalgia Syndrome and Tryptophan: E.A. Belongia, et al.; Annu. Rev. Nutr., 1992, vol. 12, pp. 235–256.

Pulmonary Manifestations of the Eosinophilia-Myalgia Syndrome Associated with Tryptophan Ingestion: A.C. Campagna, et al.; Chest, 1992, vol. 101(5), pp. 1274–1281.

Review of L-Tryptophan and Eosinophilia-Myalgia Syndrome: J.B. Roufs; J. Am. Diet. Assoc.; 1992, vol. 92(7), pp. 844–850.

Association of the Eosinophilia-Myalgia Syndrome with the Ingestion of Tryptophan: P.A. Hertzman, et al.; N. Engl. J. Med., March 29, 1990, vol. 322(13), pp. 869–873.

Interim Guidance on the Eosinophilia-Myalgia Syndrome (Editorial): Ann. Intern. Med., January 15, 1990, vol. 112( 2).

Scleroderma, Fasciitis, and Eosinophilia Associated with the Ingestion of Tryptophan: R.M. Silver, et al.; N. Engl. J. Med., March 29, 1990, vol. 322(13), pp. 874–881.

Tryptophan-Induced Eosinophilia-Myalgia Syndrome (Editorial): N. Engl. J. Med., March 29, 1990, vol. 322(13), pp. 926–928.

# FORMALDEHYDE POISONING

**Description** Formaldehyde poisoning, which results from breathing the fumes of formaldehyde, can occur while a person is working directly with the chemical, using equipment cleaned with it, or handling materials made from it.

**Synonyms**

> Formaldehyde Exposure
> Formaldehyde Toxicity
> Formalin Intoxication
> Formalin Toxicity

**Signs and Symptoms** Findings are varied. Eye, nose, and throat irritation; headaches; and dermal injury may occur. If formaldehyde is swallowed, it will burn the esophagus and stomach. Acute hemolysis occurs when patients undergo dialysis on machines cleaned with formaldehyde. In extreme cases, formaldehyde poisoning may result in hypotension, arrhythmias, irregular breathing, restlessness, unconsciousness, and coma.

Formaldehyde exposure in mainstream tobacco smoke is suspected of increasing the risk of cancer in smokers. Other recent studies have implicated formaldehyde as a possible human carcinogen; the results do not appear definitive as yet.

**Etiology** Causes are varied and include the handling of products made with formaldehyde, such as chip board and foam insulation; accidental ingestion of formaldehyde; or breathing the vapors given off by the chemical itself. Poisoning may also occur when the chemical is being administered as formalin-soaked packs for cysts, or when formalin is used as a cleaning agent for hospital equipment and is not completely removed.

**Epidemiology** Males and females are affected in equal numbers and in many industrial settings. In occupational settings, poisoning has occurred even with appropriate air filtering equipment. Formaldehyde is also a component of mainstream cigarette smoke, and it may contribute to carcinogenesis among smokers.

**Treatment—Standard** Treatment primarily consists of identification of the source and removal of the chemical from the occupational, domestic, or general environment. Other treatment is symptomatic and supportive.

**Treatment—Investigational** Please contact the agencies listed under Resources, below, for the most current information. Addresses and telephone numbers of these agencies, as well as of individual experts and research centers, may be found in the Master Resources List.

**Resources**

**For more information on formaldehyde poisoning:** National Organization for Rare Disorders (NORD); American Academy of Environmental Medicine; NIH/National Institute of Environmental Health Sciences.

### References

When Disaster Strikes, Is Your Lab Prepared?: K. Miara-Rezutek, et al.; MLO Med. Lab. Obs., January 1995, vol. 27(1), pp. 24–27.

Extrusion of Endodontic Filling Material into the Insertions of the Mylohyoid Muscle: A Case Report: A. Alantar, et al.; Oral Surg. Oral Med. Oral Pathol., November 1994, vol. 78(5), pp. 646–649.

Formaldehyde Exposure, Acute Pulmonary Response, and Exposure Control Options in a Gross Anatomy Laboratory: F. Akbar-Khanzadeh, et al.; Am. J. Ind. Med., July 1994, vol. 26(1), pp. 61–75.

Mortality from Respiratory Cancers (Including Lung Cancer) Among Workers Employed in Formaldehyde Industries: T.D. Sterling and J.J. Weinkam; Am. J. Ind. Med., April 1994, vol. 25(4), pp. 593–602, discussion pp. 603–606.

New Trends in Occupational and Environmental Diseases: The Role of the Occupational Hygienist in Recognizing Lung Diseases: G. Franco; Monaldi Arch. Chest. Dis., June 1994, vol. 49(3), pp. 239–242.

Respiratory Consequences of Exposure to Wood Dust and Formaldehyde of Workers Manufacturing Oriented Strand Board: F.A. Herbert, et al.; Arch. Environ. Health, November 1994, vol. 49(6), pp. 465–470.

Use of Biological Markers in Risk Assessment: A. McMillan, et al.; Risk Anal., October 1994, vol. 14(5), pp. 807–813.

Sources of Pollutants in Indoor Air: H.U. Wanner; IARC Sci. Publ., 1993, vol. 109, pp. 19–30.

Allergy to Formaldehyde and Ethylene-Oxide: J. Bousquet and F.B. Michel; Clin. Rev. Allergy, September 1991, vol. 9(3—4), pp. 357–370.

Formaldehyde Exposure and Health Status In Households: I. Broder, et al.; Environ. Health Perspect., November 1991, vol. 95, pp. 101–104.

Indoor Air Pollutants: A Literature Review: T.F. Cooke; Rev. Environ. Health, 1991, vol. 9(3), pp. 137–160.

Oral Toxicity of Formaldehyde and Its Derivatives: P. Restani and C.L. Galli; Crit. Rev. Toxicol., 1991, vol. 21(5), pp. 315–328.

Clinical and Immunologic Evaluation of 37 Workers Exposed to Gaseous Formaldehyde: L.C. Grammer, et al.; J. Allergy Clin. Immunol., August 1990, vol. 86(2), pp. 177–181.

Mortality from Lung Cancer Among Workers Employed in Formaldehyde Industries: A. Blair, et al.; Am. J. Ind. Med., 1990, vol. 17(6), pp. 683–699.

Quantitative Cancer Risk Estimation for Formaldehyde: T.B. Starr; Risk Analysis, March 1990, vol. 10(1), pp. 85–91.

Cancer Risks Due to Occupational Exposure to Formaldehyde: Results of a Multi-Site Case-Control Study in Montreal: M. Gerin, et al.; Int. J. Cancer, July 15, 1989, vol. 44(1), pp. 53–58.

Formaldehyde: AMA Council on Scientific Affairs; Conn. Med., April 1989, vol. 53(4), pp. 229–235.

Formaldehyde: Council on Scientific Affairs; JAMA, February 24, 1989, vol. 261(8), pp. 1183–1187.

Formaldehyde Exposures from Tobacco Smoke: A Review: T. Godish; Am. J. Public Health, August 1989, vol. 79(8), pp. 1044–1045.

Formaldehyde-Related Health Complaints of Residents Living in Mobile and Conventional Homes: I.M. Ritchie, et al.; Am. J. Public Health, March 1987, vol. 77(3), pp. 323–328.

Formaldehyde-Induced Corrosive Gastric Cicatrization: Case Report: R. Kochhar, et al.; Hum. Toxicol., December 1986, vol. 5(6), pp. 381–382.

Acute Intravascular Hemolysis Due to Accidental Formalin Intoxication During Hemodialysis: K.K. Pun, et al.; Clin. Nephrol., March 1984, vol. 21(3), pp. 188–190.

Formalin Toxicity in Hydatid Liver Disease: A.R. Aggarwal, et al.; Anaesthesia, July 1983, vol. 38(7), pp. 662–665.

# HEAVY METAL POISONING

**Description** Heavy metal poisoning today is generally caused by industrial exposure, although environmental exposure to toxins (e.g., aluminum, arsenic, cadmium, lead, mercury) still occurs. Depending on the type and duration of exposure, the injury may be pulmonary, neurologic, cutaneous, or gastrointestinal.

One particular syndrome, **metal fume fever,** results when a volatilized heavy metal is inhaled. This is an acute, flulike illness characterized by abrupt onset of fever, shaking chills, headache, and cough. Treatment is supportive; the illness is usually brief and self-limited. Occasionally there may be sequelae, however, such as pulmonary edema.

**Signs, Symptoms, and Treatment** Signs and symptoms of heavy metal poisoning vary according to the type of metal overexposure involved.

**Aluminum** containers used in the manufacture and processing of some foods, cosmetics, and medicines, and also aluminum used for water purification, can cause poisoning. Aluminum phosphide, used as a grain preservative, has been associated with serious cardiac disturbances. Workers exposed to aluminum ore suffer inhalation injury that may lead to pulmonary changes, including emphysema. Aluminum poisoning also occurs among patients with chronic renal failure undergoing dialysis, leading to encephalopathy and osteomalacia. Deferoxamine mesylate has been used as a chelating agent, with improved symptoms and bone histology; ocular, auditory, and infectious adverse effects have been reported.

**Antimony** is used for hardening lead and in the manufacture of batteries and cables, as a fire retardant in mattresses, and as therapy for cutaneous and mucosal leishmaniasis. Antimony may cause pulmonary injury and skin cancer, especially in individuals who smoke. Cardiac arrhythmias have also been seen following antimony exposure. Antimony has been suggested as a contributing factor in sudden infant death syndrome. Chelation therapy with dimercaprol is recommended.

**Arsenic** is used in the manufacture of pesticides and in other industrial settings, and also may be found in common substances such as insecticides, and, rarely, in environmental situations such as private wells. Overexposure may cause gastrointestinal disturbances, hypertension, headache, drowsiness, confusion, delirium, seizures, and death. In cases of chronic poisoning, hyperkeratosis of the palms of the hands, weakness, muscle aches, chills, fever, and anemia may develop, as well as cognitive impairment and apparent psychological disturbances. Exposure to arsenic also is associated with an increased risk of cutaneous, tracheal, bladder, and bronchogenic carcinoma, and hepatic hemangiosarcoma. Chelation therapy with dimercaprol or D-penicillamine is recommended. Arsenical neuropathy does not respond well to chelation.

**Beryllium** (see **Berylliosis**).

**Cadmium** is used for many items, including electroplating, storage batteries, vapor lamps, and in some solders. Cadmium is also present in fertilizers and sewage sludge. Overexposure may cause hypertension, emphysema, fatigue, headache, vomiting, anemia, anosmia, renal dysfunction, and osteopenia. There also appears to be an association with prostatic cancer and neuropsychological impairment among cadmium workers. Dimercaprol is contraindicated for chelation therapy. Recent studies on new compounds, such as dithiocarbamate derivatives, give promise of development of useful and safe therapeutic chelating agents.

**Chromium** is used in the manufacture of cars, glass, pottery, and linoleum. Acute exposure is associated with contact dermatitis, gastroenteritis, shock, and toxic nephritis. Chronic exposure can cause perforation of the nasal septum. Overexposure to chromium also is associated with an incidence of respiratory tract cancer 15 to 20 times that found in the general population. Chelation therapy with calcium disodium edetate or dimercaprol is recommended.

**Cobalt,** used in making jet engines, and in other occupations such as diamond polishing, may be associated with gastrointestinal disturbances, tinnitus, neuropathy, respiratory diseases and bronchial hyperreactivity, thyroid dysfunction, cardiomyopathy, and nephrotoxicity. Chelation therapy with dimercaprol is recommended.

**Copper,** used in the manufacture of electrical wires, may cause metal fume disease, gastrointestinal and neurologic disturbances, hepatic *(Wilson Disease)* and renal failure, emphysema, and, it is suggested, hypertension in blacks. Chelation with dimercaprol and possibly D-penicillamine is recommended.

**Gold** is widely used in treatment of rheumatoid arthritis, *Sjögren Syndrome,* and nondisseminated lupus erythematosus. Overexposure to gold may cause dermatitis, headache, vomiting, bone marrow depression, the nephrotic syndrome, jaundice, cholestasis, pneumonitis, gastrointestinal bleeding, and ocular chrysiasis. Gold therapy is usually discontinued when such symptoms occur. Chelation therapy with dimercaprol is recommended.

**Lead** production workers, battery plant workers, welders, and solderers may be overexposed to lead if proper precautions are not taken. Environmental exposure, such as from paint and leaded gasoline, and leaching from certain imported dishware, is becoming less common but still exists. Lead exposure from dust and from lead pipe water mains remain important sources in the environment for young children. Lead levels in the blood of 10 to 15 µg/dL in newborns and very young infants are associated with cognitive and behavioral defects. Lead poisoning may cause miscarriage, birth defects, hearing and eye-hand coordination defects, anemia, abdominal pain ("lead colic"), decreased male fertility, decreased muscular strength and endurance, nephrotoxicity, peripheral neuropathy with wrist drop, hostility, depression, and anxiety. There also may be cognitive and behavioral changes. Chelation therapy with dimercaprol and calcium disodium edetate is recommended.

**Lithium** is widely used in therapeutic management of psychiatric disorders, but also is found in some industrial applications. Overexposure generally occurs during therapeutic usage, when blood levels of the drug increase.

Central nervous system effects include hand tremor, parkinsonism, and memory impairment. Severe gastroenteritis may occur, and arrhythmias, hypotension, the nephrotic syndrome, and renal failure may develop. Nystagmus, carpal tunnel syndrome, a Creutzfeldt-Jakob–like syndrome, and fetal polyhydramnios have been reported.

**Manganese** is used as a purifying agent in the production of several metals. Acute exposure can cause metal fume fever. Chronic exposure among miners has been described as causing hepatic dysfunction and psychiatric disturbances that resemble schizophrenia and neurologic disturbances that resemble parkinsonism. An association between prostatic cancer and manganese exposure has been suggested.

**Mercury** exposure occurs most commonly among dental and chemical workers. Exposure to this metal also may occur from its presence in dental filling amalgam and in some latex paints, and from the ingestion of seafood with high mercury levels. Pulmonary effects may include dyspnea, coughing, and chest pain. In severe cases, interstitial pneumonitis and pulmonary edema may develop. Mercury poisoning also may lead to behavioral and neurologic changes, gastrointestinal disturbances, nephrotoxicity, dehydration, and shock. Mercury pigmentation and possible neuropsychiatric symptoms were reported in an Australian case in which an over-the-counter mercury-containing cosmetic cream was used. Chelation therapy with dimercaprol or D-penicillamine is recommended.

**Molybdenum** is used in the hardening of steel. Overexposure may cause copper depletion, liver and kidney damage, weight loss, and central nervous system changes.

**Silver** exposure may be dental-related or may include working in the manufacture of precious metal powders or chemicals, such as silver nitrate. Overexposure may cause fume fever, gastroenteritis, and argyria. Chelation is ineffective.

**Vanadium** exposure in the workplace includes the manufacture of vanadium pentoxide from magnetite ore. Overexposure may result in metal fume fever, anorexia, throat pain, nasal irritation, and acute bronchitis. Psychiatric disturbances and renal dysfunction have also been noted. A further characteristic finding is a greenish-black discoloration of the tongue. Chelation therapy with calcium disodium edetate is recommended.

**Zinc** is found in paints, enamels, wood preservatives, and rodenticides. Cutaneous reactions have been reported. Inhalation overexposure may lead to metal fume fever, gastrointestinal disturbances, and liver dysfunction. Chelation therapy with edetic acid or dimercaprol is recommended.

**Etiology** Heavy metal poisoning is a result of overexposure from industrial sites, polluted air or water, or contaminated food or cookware.

**Epidemiology** Industrial workers, members of their families, and others living near industrial sites are most commonly exposed to heavy metals.

**Related Disorders** See *Anemia, Fanconi; Wilson Disease.*

**Treatment—Standard** Occupational exposure to heavy metals requires careful prevention through the use of masks and protective clothing.

Treatment consists of various chelating agents as noted above. Gastric lavage is used to remove ingested materials. In the case of inhalation injury, the patient should be removed from the contaminated environment and respiration supported. Bronchodilators may be needed. In case of cerebral edema, treatment with mannitol and corticosteroid drugs, along with intracranial monitoring, is required. If kidney failure develops, hemodialysis may be needed. Treatment is otherwise symptomatic and supportive.

**Treatment—Investigational** Newer chelating agents are being investigated, such as dimercaptosuccinic acid for arsenic exposure, and dithiocarbamate derivatives for cadmium toxicity.

Please contact the agencies listed under Resources, below, for the most current information. Addresses and telephone numbers of these agencies, as well as of individual experts and research centers, may be found in the Master Resources List.

**Resources**

**For more information on heavy metal poisoning:** National Organization for Rare Disorders (NORD); NIH/National Institute of Environmental Health Sciences; Food and Drug Administration.

**References**

The Metal in Our Mettle: R.W. Miller, FDA Consumer; December 1988–January 1989, pp. 24–27.

**Aluminum:**

Treatment of Aluminium Intoxication: A New Scheme for Desferrioxamine Administration: W.G. Douthat, et al.; Nephrol. Dial. Transplant., 1994, vol. 9(10), pp. 1431–1434.

Aluminium and Infants: K. Simmer; J. Paediatr. Child Health, 1993, vol. 29(2), pp. 80–81.

Toxic Effects of Aluminium on Nerve Cells and Synaptic Transmission: H. Meiri, et al.; Prog. Neurobiol., 1993, vol. 40(1), pp. 89–121.

Aluminium Intoxication in Renal Disease: D.N. Kerr, et al.; Ciba Found. Symp., 1992, vol. 169, pp. 123–135, discussion pp. 135–141.

Aluminum Toxicity in Childhood: A. Sedman; Pediatr. Nephrol., 1992, vol. 6(4), pp. 383–393.

Biomedical Aspects of Aluminium: C. Schlatter; Med. Lav., 1992, vol. 83(5), pp. 470–474.

Aluminum Toxicity and Alzheimer's Disease: Is There a Connection?: R.C. Handy; Postgrad. Med., October 1990, vol. 88(5), pp. 239–240.

Aspects of Aluminum Toxicity: C.D. Hewitt, et al.; Clin. Lab. Med., June 1990, vol. 10(2), pp. 403–422.

Deferoxamine for Aluminum Toxicity in Dialysis Patients: P. Hernandez and C.A. Johnson; ANNA J., June 1990, vol. 17(3), pp. 224–228.

Aluminum and Chronic Renal Failure: Sources, Absorption, Transport, and Toxicity: M.R. Wills and J. Savory; Crit. Rev. Clin. Lab. Sci., 1989, vol. 27(1), pp. 59–107.

Aluminum Toxicity in Mammals: A Minireview: J.B. Cannata and J.L. Domingo; Vet. Hum. Toxicol., December 1989, vol. 31(6), pp. 577–583.

Complexation of Labile Metal Ions and Effect on Toxicity: A.E. Martell; Biol. Trace Elem. Res., July–September 1989, vol. 21, pp. 295–303.

Cardiovascular Complications of Aluminum Phosphide Poisoning: S.N. Khosla, et al.; Angiology, April 1988, vol. 39(4), pp. 355–359.

**Antimony:**

Clinical Healing of Antimony-Resistant Cutaneous or Mucocutaneous Leishmaniasis Following the Combined Administration of Interferon-Gamma and Pentavalent Antimonial Compounds: E. Falcoff, et al.; Trans. R. Soc. Trop. Med. Hyg., 1994, vol. 88(1), pp. 95–97.

Cross-Resistance Between Cisplatin and Antimony in a Human Ovarian Carcinoma Cell Line in Vitro (Meeting Abstract): P. Naredi, et al.; Proc. Annu. Meet. Am. Assoc. Cancer Res., 1994, vol. 35, p. A2010 1994.

Sudden Infant Death Syndrome: A Possible Primary Cause: B.A. Richardson; J. Forensic Sci. Soc., 1994, vol. 34(3), pp. 199–204.

Survey of Antimony Workers: Mortality 1961–1992: D. Jones; Occup. Environ. Med., 1994, vol. 51(11), pp. 772–776.

Treatment of Cutaneous Leishmaniasis: A.B. Koff and T. Rosen; J. Am. Acad. Dermatol., 1994, vol. 31(5 pt. 1), pp. 693–708, quiz pp. 708–710.

Dermatitis in Workers Exposed to Antimony in a Melting Process: G.P. White, Jr., et al.; J. Occup. Med., 1993, vol. 35(4), pp. 392–395.

Oral Antimony Intoxications in Man: L.F. Lauwers, et al.; Crit. Care Med., March 1990, vol. 18(3), pp. 324–326.

Severe Arthralgia, Not Related to Dose, Associated with Pentavalent Antimonial Therapy for Mucosal Leishmaniasis: C. Castro, et al.; Trans. R. Soc. Trop. Med. Hyg., 1990, vol. 84(3), p. 362.

**Arsenic:**

Increased Prevalence of Hypertension and Long-Term Arsenic Exposure: C.J. Chen, et al.; Hypertension, 1995, vol. 25(1), pp. 53–60.

Multiple Risk Factors Associated with Arsenic-Induced Skin Cancer: Effects of Chronic Liver Disease and Malnutritional Status: Y.M. Hsueh, et al.; Br. J. Cancer, 1995, vol. 71(1), pp. 109–114.

Arsenic in Drinking Water and Mortality from Vascular Disease: An Ecologic Analysis in 30 Counties in the United States: R.R. Engel and A.H. Smith; Arch. Environ. Health, 1994, vol. 49(5), pp. 418–427.

Differential Cytotoxic Effects of Arsenic on Human and Animal Cells: T.C. Lee and I.C. Ho; Environ. Health Perspect., 1994, vol. 102(suppl. 3), pp. 101–105.

Testing for Arsenic: T.P. Moyer; Mayo Clin. Proc., 1993, vol. 68(12), pp. 1210–1211.

Arsenic Ingestion and Internal Cancers: A Review [See Comments]: M.N. Bates, et al.; Am. J. Epidemiol., 1992, vol. 135(5), pp. 462–476.

An Ecologic Study of Skin Cancer and Environmental Arsenic Exposure: O. Wong, et al.; Int. Arch. Occup. Environ. Health, 1992, vol. 64(4), pp. 235–241.

Ingested Arsenic, Keratoses, and Bladder Cancer: J. Cuzick, et al.; Am. J. Epidemiol., 1992, vol. 136(4), pp. 417–421.

Acute Arsenic Intoxication: J.P. Campbell and J.A. Alvarez; Am. Fam. Physician, December 1989, vol. 40(6), pp. 93–97.

Acute Arsenic Intoxication from Environmental Arsenic Exposure: A. Franzblau and R. Lilis; Arch. Environ. Health, November–December 1989, vol. 44(6), pp. 385–390.

Acute Arsenic Toxicity—An Opaque Poison: J.R. Gray, et al.; Can. Assoc. Radiol. J., August 1989, vol. 40(4), pp. 226–227.

Acute Lead Arsenate Poisoning: G.A. Tallis; Aust. N. Z. J. Med., December 1989, vol. 19(6), pp. 730–732.

Arsenic-Induced Skin Toxicity: R.L. Shannon and D.S. Strayer; Hum. Toxicol., March 1989, vol. 8(2), pp. 99–104.

Encephalopathy: An Uncommon Manifestation of Workplace Arsenic Poisoning?: W.E. Morton and G.A. Caron; Am. J. Ind. Med., 1989, vol. 15(1), pp. 1–5.

Hematologic Effects of Heavy Metal Poisoning: Q.S. Ringenberg, et al.; South. Med. J., September 1988, vol. 81(9), pp. 1132–1139.

**Cadmium:**

Cadmium and Hypertension: S.K. Bakshi, et al.; J. Assoc. Physicians India, 1994, vol. 42(6), pp. 449–450.

Cadmium and Prostate Cancer: M.P. Waalkes and S. Rehm; J. Toxicol. Environ. Health, 1994, vol. 43(3), pp. 251–269.

Beryllium, Cadmium, Mercury, and Exposures in the Glass Manufacturing Industry: Working Group Views and Expert Opinions, Lyon, France, February 9–16, 1993: IARC Monogr. Eval. Carcinog. Risks Hum., 1993, vol. 58, pp. 1–415.

Biomonitoring Exposure to Metal Compounds with Carcinogenic Properties: A. Leonard and A. Bernard; Environ. Health Perspect., 1993, vol. 101(suppl. 3), pp. 127–133.

Renal Tubular Function After Reduction of Environmental Cadmium Exposure: A Ten-Year Follow-Up: K. Iwata, et al.; Arch. Environ. Health, 1993, vol. 48(3), pp. 157–163.

Cadmium As an Environmental Hazard: C.G. Elinder; IARC Sci. Publ., 1992, vol. 118, pp. 123–132.

Cadmium in the Human Environment: Toxicity and Carcinogenicity: Symposium Proceedings, Gargnano, Italy, September 1991. IARC Sci. Publ., 1992, vol. 118, pp. 1–464.

Occupational Exposure to Cadmium and Lung Function: G. Cortona, et al.; IARC Sci. Publ., 1992, vol. 118, pp. 205–210.

Toxicological Principles of Metal Carcinogenesis with Special Emphasis on Cadmium: M.P. Waalkes, et al.; Crit. Rev. Toxicol., 1992, vol. 22(3–4), pp. 175–201.

A Quantitative Study of Iliac Bone Histopathology on 62 Cases with Itai-Itai Disease: M. Noda and M. Kitagawa; Calcif. Tissue Int., August 1990, vol. 47(2), pp. 66–74.

The Search for Chelate Antagonists for Chronic Cadmium Intoxication: M.M. Jones and M.G. Cherian; Toxicology, May 14, 1990, vol. 62(1), pp. 1–25.

Neuropsychological Effects of Occupational Exposure to Cadmium: R.P. Hart, et al.; J. Clin. Exp. Neuropsychol., December 1989, vol. 11(6), pp. 933–943.

Progress of Renal Dysfunction in Inhabitants Environmentally Exposed to Cadmium: T. Kido, et al.; Arch. Environ. Health, May–June 1988, vol. 43(3), pp. 213–217.

**Chromium:**

Nasal Septum Lesions Caused by Chromium Exposure Among Chromium Electroplating Workers: S.C. Lin, et al.; Am. J. Ind. Med., 1994, vol. 26(2), pp. 221–228.

A Study of Chromium Induced Allergic Contact Dermatitis with 54 Volunteers: Implications for Environmental Risk Assessment: J. Nethercott, et al.; Occup. Environ. Med., 1994, vol. 51(6), pp. 371–380.

Biomonitoring Exposure to Metal Compounds with Carcinogenic Properties: A. Leonard and A. Bernard.; Environ. Health Perspect., 1993, vol. 101(suppl. 3), pp. 127–133.

Nickel, Cobalt and Chromium in Consumer Products: A Role in Allergic Contact Dermatitis? D.A. Basketter, et al.; Contact Dermatitis, 1993, vol. 28(1), pp. 15–25.

An Alternative to the USEPA's Proposed Inhalation Reference Concentrations for Hexavalent and Trivalent Chromium: B.L. Finley, et al.; Regul. Toxicol. Pharmacol., 1992, vol. 16(2), pp. 161–176.

Sex Hormones and Semen Quality in Welders Exposed to Hexavalent Chromium: J.P. Bonde and E. Ernst; Hum. Exp. Toxicol., 1992, vol. 11(4), pp. 259–263.

Environmentally Related Diseases of the Urinary Tract: R.A. Goyer; Med. Clin. N. Am., March 1990, vol. 74(2), pp. 377–389.

CT Findings of the Nose and Paranasal Sinuses in Chromium Intoxication: M.J. Kim, et al.; Yonsei Med. J., September 1989, vol. 30(3), pp. 305–309.

Review of Occupational Epidemiology of Chromium Chemicals and Respiratory Cancer: R.B. Hayes; Sci. Total Environ., June 1, 1988, vol. 71(3), pp. 331–339.

**Cobalt:**

Assessment of Risks in Occupational Cobalt Exposures: G. Nordberg; Sci. Total Environ., 1994, vol. 150(1–3), pp. 201–207.

Bronchoalveolar Lavage and Its Role in Diagnosing Cobalt Lung Disease: G. Michetti, et al.; Sci. Total Environ., 1994, vol. 150(1–3), pp. 173–178.

Does Occupational Cobalt Exposure Determine Early Renal Changes?: I. Franchini, et al.; Sci. Total Environ., 1994, vol. 150(1–3), pp. 149–152.

Health Risks Associated with Cobalt Exposure: An Overview: R. Lauwerys and D. Lison; Sci. Total Environ., 1994, vol. 150(1–3), pp. 1–6.

Epidemiological Survey of Workers Exposed to Cobalt Oxides, Cobalt Salts, and Cobalt Metal: B. Swennen, et al.; Br. J. Ind. Med., 1993, vol. 50(9), pp. 835–842.

A Study of Chromium, Nickel and Cobalt Hypersensitivity: A. Arikan and Y. Kulak; J. Marmara Univ. Dent. Fac., 1992, vol. 1(3), pp. 223–229.

Hard Metal Asthma: Cross Immunological and Respiratory Reactivity Between Cobalt and Nickel?: T. Shirakawa, et al.; Thorax, April 1990, vol. 45(4), pp. 267–271.

Rapidly Fatal Progression of Cobalt Lung in a Diamond Polisher: B. Nemery, et al.; Am. Rev. Respir. Dis., May 1990, vol. 141(5 pt. 1), pp. 1373–1378.

The Respiratory Effects of Cobalt: D.W. Cugell, et al.; Arch. Intern. Med., January 1990, vol. 150(1), pp. 177–183.

Evaluation of Right and Left Ventricular Function in Hard Metal Workers: S.F. Horowitz, et al.; Br. J. Ind. Med., November 1988, vol. 45(11), pp. 742–746.

**Copper:**

Mortality from Lung Cancer Among Copper Miners: R. Chen, et al.; Br. J. Ind. Med., 1993, vol. 50(6), pp. 505–509.

The Interaction of Motor, Memory, and Emotional Dysfunction in Wilson's Disease: A. Medalia, et al.; Biol. Psychiatry, 1992, vol. 31(8), pp. 823–826.

Occupational Exposure to Chromium, Copper and Arsenic During Work with Impregnated Wood In Joinery Shops: O. Nygren, et al.; Ann. Occup. Hyg., 1992, vol. 36(5), pp. 509–517.

Cadmium Fume Inhalation and Emphysema [in copper-cadmium alloy manufacturing]: A.G. Davison, et al.; Lancet, March 26, 1988, vol. 1(8587), pp. 663–667.

Hypertension: Heavy Metals, Useful Cations and Melanin As a Possible Repository: C.C. Pfeiffer and R.J. Mailloux; Med. Hypotheses, June 1988, vol. 26(2), pp. 125–130.

**Gold:**

Disease-Modifying Antirheumatic Drugs, Including Methotrexate, Sulfasalazine, Gold, Antimalarials, and Penicillamine: L. Girgis, et al.; Curr. Opin. Rheumatol., 1994, vol. 6(3), pp. 252–261.

Gold Dermatitis: C.G. Webster and J.W. Burnett; Cutis, 1994, vol. 54(1), pp. 25–28.

High Frequency of Contact Allergy to Gold Sodium Thiosulfate: An Indication of Gold Allergy?: B. Bjorkner, et al.; Contact Dermatitis, 1994, vol. 30(3), pp. 144–151.

Kidney Disorders Induced by Non-Steroidal Anti-Inflammatory Agents and Immunomodulators: M. Wakashin and Y. Wakashin; Nippon Naika Gakkai Zasshi, 1994, vol. 83(10), pp. 1747–1751.

Side Effects Induced by Gold Drugs: A Graft-Versus-Host-Like Disease: J. Verwilghen, et al.; J. Lab. Clin. Med., 1994, vol. 123(5), pp. 777–780.

Cholestasis and Pneumonitis Induced by Gold Therapy: J.M. Farre, et al.; Clin. Rheumatol., December 1989, vol. 8(4), pp. 538–540.

Cutaneous Reactions to Drugs Used for Rheumatologic Disorders: D.E. Roth, et al.; Med. Clin. N. Am., September 1989, vol. 73(5), pp. 1275–1298.

Leucopenia in Rheumatoid Arthritis: Relationship to Gold or Sulphasalazine Therapy: R.S. Amos and D. E. Bax; Br. J. Rheumatol., December 1988, vol. 27(6), pp. 465–468.

Ocular Chrysiasis: D.W. Tierney; J. Am. Optom. Assoc., December 1988, vol. 59(12), pp. 960–962.

**Lead:**

The Biochemical and Clinical Consequences of Lead Poisoning: I.A. al-Saleh; Med. Res. Rev., 1994, vol. 14(4), pp. 415–486.

Childhood Lead Poisoning: H.L. Needleman; Curr. Opin. Neurol., 1994, vol. 7(2), pp. 187–190.

Components of Drinking Water and Risk of Cognitive Impairment in the Elderly: H. Jacqmin, et al.; Am. J. Epidemiol., 1994, vol. 139(1), pp. 48–57.

Environmental Lead and Children's Intelligence: A Systematic Review of the Epidemiological Evidence: S.J. Pocock, et al.; BMJ, 1994, vol. 309(6963), pp. 1189–1197.

Environmental Risk Factors for Osteoporosis: R.A. Goyer, et al.; Environ. Health Perspect., 1994, vol. 102(4), pp. 390–394.

Low-Level Lead Exposure and Cognitive Function in Children: D. Bellinger and K.N. Dietrich; Pediatr. Ann., 1994, vol. 23(11), pp. 600–605.

Pre- and Postnatal Lead Exposure and Behavior Problems in School-Aged Children: D. Bellinger, et al.; Environ. Res., 1994, vol. 66(1), pp. 12–30.

Lead Toxicity: Current Concerns: R.A. Goyer; Environ. Health Perspect., 1993, vol. 100, pp. 177–187.

Perspectives on Lead Toxicity: G. Lockitch; Clin. Biochem., 1993, vol. 26(5), pp. 371–381.

The Relationship Between Cadmium and Lead Burdens and Preterm Labor: U. Fagher, et al.; Int. J. Gynaecol. Obstet., 1993, vol. 40(2), pp. 109–114.

Effects of Low-Level Lead Exposure in Utero: G.P. Wong, et al.; Obstet. Gynecol. Surv., 1992, vol. 47(5), pp. 285–289.

Study of Sperm Characteristics in Persons Occupationally Exposed to Lead: D. Lerda; Am. J. Ind. Med., 1992, vol. 22(4), pp. 567–571.

Lead-Induced Anemia: Dose-Response Relationships and Evidence for a Threshold: J. Schwartz, et al.; Am. J. Pub. Health, February 1990, vol. 80(2), pp. 165–168.

Lead Toxicity: From Overt to Subclinical to Subtle Health Effects: R.A. Goyer; Environ. Health Perspect., June 1990, vol. 86, pp. 177–181.

Occupational Lead Exposure and Pituitary Function: A. Gustafson, et al.; Int. Arch. Occup. Environ. Health, 1989, vol. 61(4), pp. 277–281.

Neurobehavioral Estimation of Children with Life-Long Increased Lead Exposure: A. Benetou-Marantidou, et al.; Arch. Environ. Health, November–December 1988, vol. 43(6), pp. 392–395.

The Persistent Threat of Lead: Medical and Sociological Issues: H.L. Needleman; Curr. Probl. Pediatr., December 1988, vol. 18(12), pp. 697–744.

Thyroid Function As Assessed by Routine Laboratory Tests of Workers with Long-Term Lead Exposure: M. Tuppurainen, et al.; Scand. J. Work Environ. Health, June 1988, vol. 14(3), pp. 175–180.

**Lithium:**

Lithium: The Present and the Future: J. Clin. Psychiatry, 1995, vol. 56(1), pp. 41–48.

Lithium Prophylaxis in Recurrent Affective Illness: Efficacy, Effectiveness and Efficiency: R. Guscott and L. Taylor; Br. J. Psychiatry, 1994, vol. 164(6), pp. 741–746.

Lithium Treatment for People with Learning Disability: Patients' and Carers' Knowledge of Hazards and Attitudes to Treatment: D.J. Clarke and K.J. Pickles; J. Intellect. Disabil. Res., 1994, vol. 38(pt. 2), pp. 187–194.

Review of Clinically Important Drug Interactions with Lithium: N.S. Harvey and S. Merriman; Drug Saf., 1994, vol. 10(6), pp. 455–463.

Association of Maternal Lithium Exposure and Premature Delivery: W.A. Troyer, et al.; J. Perinatol., 1993, vol. 13(2), pp. 123–127.

Maternal Lithium Therapy and Polyhydramnios: M.S. Ang, et al.; Obstet. Gynecol., September 1990, vol. 76(3 Pt. 2), pp. 517–519.

The Use of Lithium in the Medically Ill: K. DasGupta and J.W. Jefferson; Gen. Hosp. Psychiatry, March 1990, vol. 12(2), pp. 83–97.

Lithium-Induced Nephrotic Syndrome: I.K. Wood, et al.; Am. J. Psychiatry, January 1989, vol. 146(1), pp. 84–87.

A Creutzfeldt-Jakob–Like Syndrome due to Lithium Toxicity: S.J. Smith and R.S. Kocen; J. Neurol. Neurosurg. Psychiatry, January 1988, vol. 51(1), pp. 120–123.

Focal Segmental Glomerulosclerosis in Patients Receiving Lithium Carbonate: R.N. Santella, et al.; Am. J. Med., May 1988, vol. 84(5), pp. 951–954.

Lithium-Induced Carpal Tunnel Syndrome: M.P. Deahl; Br. J. Psychiatry, August 1988, vol. 153, pp. 250–251.

Lithium-Induced Downbeat Nystagmus: D.P. Williams, et al.; Arch. Neurol., September 1988, vol. 45(9), pp. 1022–1023.

**Manganese:**

Manganese Intoxication and Chronic Liver Failure: R.A. Hauser, et al; Ann. Neurol., 1994, vol. 36(6), pp. 871–875.

Nervous System Dysfunction Among Workers with Long-Term Exposure to Manganese: D. Mergler, et al.; Environ. Res., 1994, vol. 64(2), pp. 151–180.

Using Psychological Tests for the Early Detection of Neurotoxic Effects of Low Level Manganese Exposure: A. Iregren; Neurotoxicology, 1994, vol. 15(3), pp. 671–677.

Fertility of Male Workers Exposed to Cadmium, Lead, or Manganese: J.P. Gennart, et al.; Am. J. Epidemiol., 1992, vol. 135(11), pp. 1208–1219.

Health Risk Assessment of Long Term Exposure to Chemicals: Application to Cadmium and Manganese: R.R. Lauwerys, et al.; Arch. Toxicol. Suppl., 1992, vol. 15, pp. 97–102.

Manganese As Possible Ecoetiologic Factor in Parkinson's Disease: R.G. Feldman; Ann. N. Y. Acad. Sci., 1992, vol. 648, pp. 266–267.

Preclinical Neurophysiological Signs of Parkinsonism in Occupational Manganese Exposure: A. Wennberg, et al.; Neurotoxicology, 1992, vol. 13(1), pp. 271–274.

Manganese-Induced Parkinsonism: An Outbreak Due to an Unrepaired Ventilation Control System in a Ferromanganese Smelter: J.D. Wang, et al.; Br. J. Ind. Med., December 1989, vol. 46(12), pp. 856–859.

Epidemiological Survey Among Workers Exposed to Manganese: Effects on Lung, Central Nervous System, and Some Biological Indices [published erratum appears in Am. J. Med., 1987, vol. 12(1), pp. 119–120]: H. Roels, et al.; Am. J. Med., 1987, vol. 11(3), pp. 307–327.

The Health Implications of Increased Manganese in the Environment Resulting from the Combustion of Fuel Additives: A Review of the Literature: W.C. Cooper; J. Toxicol. Environ. Health, 1984, vol. 14(1), pp. 23–46.

A Clustering of Prostatic Cancer in an Area with Many Manganese Mines: H. Watanabe, et al.; Tohoku J. Exp. Med., December 1981, vol. 135(4), pp. 441–442.

**Mercury:**

Fractional Mercury Levels in Brazilian Gold Refiners and Miners: S.E. Aks, et al.; J. Toxicol. Clin. Toxicol., 1995, vol. 33(1), pp. 1–10.

Environmental Health: Gold, Mercury and Health: Wkly. Epidemiol. Rec., 1994, vol. 69(37), pp. 275–278.

Inhalational Mercury Poisoning Masquerading As Toxic Shock Syndrome: S.B. Mohan, et al.; Anaesth. Intensive Care, 1994, vol. 22(3), pp. 305–306.

Beryllium, Cadmium, Mercury, and Exposures in the Glass Manufacturing Industry: Working Group Views and Expert Opinions, Lyon, France, February 9–16, 1993: IARC Monogr. Eval. Carcinog. Risks Hum., 1993, vol. 58, pp. 1–415.

Carcinogenicity of Mercury and Mercury Compounds: P. Boffetta, et al.; Scand. J. Work Environ. Health, 1993, vol. 19(1), pp. 1–7.

Effects of Occupational Exposure to Mercury Vapour on the Central Nervous System: S. Langworth, et al.; Br. J. Ind. Med., 1992, vol. 49(8), pp. 545–555.

Elemental Mercury Exposure in Early Pregnancy; J.M. Thorp, Jr., et al.; Obstet. Gynecol., 1992, vol. 79(5 pt 2), pp. 874–876.

Mercury in Dental Amalgam: A Public Health Concern?: R.A. Flanders; J. Public Health Dent., 1992, vol. 52(5), pp. 303–311.

Toxicity of Mercury from Dental Environment and from Amalgam Restorations: Y.K. Fung and M.P. Molvar; J. Toxicol. Clin. Toxicol., 1992, vol. 30(1), pp. 49–61.

Mercury Excretion and Occupational Exposure of Dental Personnel: A. Jokstad; Community Dent. Oral Epidemiol., June 1990, vol. 18(3), pp. 143–148.

Mercury Pigmentation and High Mercury Levels from the Use of a Cosmetic Cream: D.J. Dyall-Smith and J.P. Scurry; Med. J. Aust., October 1, 1990, vol. 153(7), pp. 409–410, 414–415.

Possible Foetotoxic Effects of Mercury Vapour: A Case Report: S. Gelbier and J. Ingram; Public Health, January 1989, vol. 103(1), pp. 35–40.

The Relationship Between Mercury from Dental Amalgam and Mental Health: R.L. Siblerud; Am. J. Psychother., October 1989, vol. 43(4), pp. 575–587.

Were the Hatters of New Jersey "Mad"?: R.P. Wedeen; Am. J. Ind. Med., 1989, vol. 16(2), pp. 225–233.

Cutaneous Manifestations of Acrodynia (Pink Disease): S.M. Dinehart, et al.; Arch. Dermatol., January 1988, vol. 124(1), pp. 107–109.

**Molybdenum:**

Hypersensitivity to Molybdenum As a Possible Trigger of ANA-Negative Systemic Lupus Erythematosus: M. Federmann, et al.; Ann. Rheum. Dis., 1994, vol. 53(6), pp. 403–405.

Lung Cancer Mortality Among a Cohort of Male Chromate Pigment Workers in Japan [published erratum appears in Int. J. Epidemiol., August 1993, vol. 22(4), pp. 757]: K. Kano, et al.; Int. J. Epidemiol., 1993, vol. 22(1), pp. 16–22.

Thiomolybdates in the Treatment of Wilson's Disease [letter, vol. comment]: J.M. Walshe; Arch. Neurol., 1992, vol. 49(2), pp. 132–133.

Trace Elements and Public Health: E.J. Calabrese, et al.; Annu. Rev. Public Health, 1985, vol. 6, pp. 131–146.

**Silver:**

Solubility of Silver Sulfadiazine in Physiological Media and Relevance to Treatment of Thermal Burns with Silver Sulfadiazine Cream: N. Tsipouras, et al; Clin. Chem., 1995, vol. 41(1), pp. 87–91.

Corneal Argyrosis Associated with Silver Soldering: M.W. Scroggs, et al.; Cornea, 1992, vol. 11(3), pp. 264–269.

Silverworker's Finger: An Unusual Occupational Hazard Mimicking a Melanocytic Lesion: P. Sarsfield, et al. Histopathology 1992, vol. 20(1), pp. 73–75.

Connective Tissue Responses to Some Heavy Metals. III. Silver and Dietary Supplements of Ascorbic Acid. Histology and Ultrastructure: G. Ellender and K.N. Ham; Br. J. Experim. Pathol., February 1989, vol. 70(1), pp. 21–39.

Potential Nephrotoxic Effects of Exposure to Silver: K.D. Rosenman, et al.; Br. J. Ind. Med., April 1987, vol. 44(4), pp. 267–272.

**Vanadium:**

Is Vanadium of Human Nutritional Importance Yet?: B.F. Harland and B.A. Harden-Williams; J. Am. Diet. Assoc., 1994, vol. 94(8), pp. 891–894.

Vanadium Salts and the Future Treatment of Diabetes: Y. Shechter and A. Shisheva; Endeavour, 1993, vol. 17(1), pp. 27–31.

Haematological Effects of Vanadium on Living Organisms: H. Zaporowska and W. Wasilewski; Comp. Biochem. Physiol. C, 1992, vol. 102(2), pp. 223–231.

Unusual Occupational Toxins: D.O. Hryhorczuk, et al., Occup. Med., 1992, vol. 7(3), pp. 567–586.

Urinary Vanadium As a Biological Indicator of Exposure to Vanadium: T. Kawai, et al.; Int. Arch. Occup. Environ. Health, 1989, vol. 61(4), pp. 283–287.

Vanadium-Induced Impairment of Haem Synthesis: C. Missenard, et al.; Br. J. Ind. Med., October 1989, vol. 46(10), pp. 744–747.

Vanadium and Manic-Depressive Psychosis: G.J. Naylor; Nutr. Health, 1984, vol. 3(1–2), pp. 79–85.

**Zinc:**

Effect of Pharmacologic Doses of Zinc on the Therapeutic Index of Brain Tumor Chemotherapy with Carmustine: N. Roosen, et al; Cancer Chemother. Pharmacol., 1994, vol. 34(5), pp. 385–392.

Zinc: Health Effects and Research Priorities for the 1990s: C.T. Walsh, et al., Environ. Health Perspect., 1994, vol. 102(suppl. 2), pp. 5–46.

Occupational Asthma Due to Zinc: J.L. Malo, et al.; Eur. Respir. J., 1993, vol. 6(3), pp. 447–450.

Morphologic Findings in Bone Marrow Precursor Cells in Zinc-Induced Copper Deficiency Anemia: A.L. Summerfield, et al.; Am. J. Clin. Pathol., 1992, vol. 97(5), pp. 665–668.

Pulmonary Vascular Lesions in the Adult Respiratory Distress Syndrome Caused by Inhalation of Zinc Chloride Smoke: A Morphometric Study: S. Homma, et al.; Hum. Pathol., 1992, vol. 23(1), pp. 45–50.

A Survey of Chronic Bronchitis Among Brassware Workers: S.K. Rastogi, et al.; Ann. Occup. Hyg., 1992, vol. 36(3), pp. 283–294.

Acute Lung Reaction Due to Zinc Inhalation: J.L. Malo, et al.; Eur. Respir. J., January 1990, vol. 3(1), pp. 111–114.

Cutaneous Reaction to Zinc—A Rare Complication of Insulin Treatment: A Case Report: M. Sandler and H.F. Jordaan; S. Afr. Med. J., April 1, 1989, vol. 75(7), pp. 342–343.

Zinc-Induced Copper Deficiency: H.N. Hoffman, 2d, et al.; Gastroenterology, February 1988, vol. 94(2), pp. 508–512.

# RADIATION SYNDROMES

**Description** The radiation syndromes encompass the various types of tissue injury that result from exposure to ionizing radiation. In general, the potentially harmful effects relate to the total dose and dose rate of radiation received, as well as the specific tissues involved.

**Synonyms**

> Radiation Disease
> Radiation Effects
> Radiation Illness
> Radiation Injuries
> Radiation Reaction
> Radiation Sickness

**Signs and Symptoms** The effects of radiation may be acute, delayed, or chronic, and certain tissues are more sensitive to these effects. In general, tissues with rapid cell turnover, such as lymphoid cells, gonad cells, bone marrow, and enteric mucosa, are the most susceptible to radiation injury. Nerve, bone, muscle, and connective tissues are less radiosensitive.

The overall amount of tissue exposed and the rate of exposure are other important factors in determining the severity of injury. A whole-body dose of 200 **rads** (radiation absorbed dose) is not likely to be fatal, while a whole-body dose of 600 rads may be fatal if the total dose is received over a short period of time. In contrast, a far higher total dose of radiation may be tolerated (as in cancer therapy) if only a small area of tissue is irradiated, and if the dose is given over an extended period of time.

**Whole-body acute irradiation,** such as might occur following an accident at a nuclear power reactor, is associated with 3 distinct syndromes. The **hematopoietic syndrome** may arise following exposure of 200 to 1,000 rads. Symptoms of nausea, vomiting, anorexia, and apathy peak 6 to 12 hours after exposure, and then subside. At 24 to 36 hours postexposure, the victim appears to improve, but atrophy of the lymph nodes, spleen, and bone marrow has begun, with direct cytotoxic effects as well as inhibition of cell regeneration. Pancytopenia follows, with immediate lymphopenia, later neutropenia, and at 3 to 4 weeks postexposure, thrombocytopenia. Death usually occurs within 4 weeks, from superinfection or hemorrhage.

**The gastrointestinal syndrome** typically develops following exposure of 400 rads or more, and results from atrophy of the gastrointestinal mucosa. This syndrome is characterized by nausea, vomiting, and diarrhea, followed by dehydration, diminished plasma volume, and vascular collapse. Death generally occurs within 3 to 10 days.

**The cerebral syndrome** results from very high levels of exposure (3,000 rads or more). Early symptoms include nausea and vomiting, with rapid progression to listlessness, drowsiness, and prostration. Within a few hours, tremors, convulsions, and death ensue.

A further acute syndrome is sometimes seen following therapeutic irradiation for cancer. **Acute radiation sickness** occurs most commonly after abdominal irradiation. Symptoms include nausea, vomiting, headache, malaise, and tachycardia. The etiology is unknown, but the condition is self-limiting within hours or days.

Exposure to **low-level radiation** is associated with delayed effects including amenorrhea, decreased fertility, cataracts, and hematologic abnormalities. Long-term findings include the development of various types of malignancies, as well as a nonspecific shortening of life.

**Local radiation injury** also may lead to various clinical abnormalities. If the bone marrow is exposed to radiation, red and white cell counts may be depressed, and prolonged aplasia may occur. Abdominal radiation may cause diarrhea, ascites, edema, proteinuria, hypertension, and renal failure. Cutaneous radiation injury may result in erythema, telangiectasia, desquamation, and chronic ulceration. Symptoms of thoracic radiation injury include dyspnea and cyanosis; radiation pneumonitis, pericarditis, and myocarditis may also develop. Exposure of the gonads may lead to aspermia or amenorrhea. Ingestion of radium salts has led to the development of osteosarcomas.

The maximum permitted occupational exposure in the United States is currently 5 **rems** (roentgen-equivalent–man) per year. Workers at several nuclear-weapons manufacturing plants, including the Oak Ridge National Laboratory in Tennessee, have been found to have higher-than-normal rates of certain types of cancer, such as leukemia and multiple myeloma. Further investigations are being undertaken to ascertain whether the 5-rem limit should be lowered. Information on maximum permissible dose levels and other important data are available in *Basic Radiation Criteria*, NCRP Report No. 39, published by the National Council on Radiation Protection and Measurements, P.O. Box 30175, Washington, DC 20014.

Diagnosis of chronic or low-level exposure may be difficult, and if suspected, serial hematologic and bone marrow studies and cataract examinations are recommended.

**Etiology** Cellular exposure to radiation causes DNA breakage that may be cytotoxic, mutagenic, or carcinogenic.

Exposure may derive from background ultraviolet radiation; medical use of x-rays and radiotherapy; industrial settings such as the Three Mile Island and Chernobyl nuclear power plants; and military situations such as the explosions over Japan in 1945 and fallout from the Nevada testing site between 1951 and 1958.

There is also current concern about the effects of electromagnetic radiation from household appliances and wiring and from power transmission lines. Conflicting evidence has been seen in epidemiologic studies, and the public health implications are as yet unclear.

**Treatment—Standard** Initial general measures to be taken following acute radiation exposure include removal of all radioactivity through wound irrigation with water and chelating solutions; induction of emesis if radioactive material was ingested; and possible blockage of thyroid uptake with Lugol's solution or saturated solution of potassium iodide. Monitoring includes urine and breath analysis.

Management of the hematopoietic syndrome involves strict isolation and aseptic techniques because of the likelihood of infection and other complications. Treatment measures include platelet transfusions and the administration of antibiotics and fresh blood. Bone-marrow–suppressing agents are usually avoided.

Management of the gastrointestinal syndrome involves replacement of fluid, electrolytes, and plasma as determined by the severity of physical findings. Antiemetics and sedatives are administered as required.

Because the cerebral syndrome is rapidly fatal, treatment is palliative. Routine measures are taken for pain, anxiety, shock, anoxia, and convulsions.

Treatment of the delayed and late effects of chronic low-level radiation exposure requires various approaches, including surgery, whole-blood transfusions, and platelet transfusions.

**Treatment—Investigational** Bone-marrow transplantation has been used as treatment for high-dose whole-body irradiation. This procedure was performed on 13 of the approximately 200 individuals who were exposed to radiation following the accident at the Chernobyl nuclear power station in the Soviet Union. Two patients remained alive 3 years later. Some patients apparently succumbed to graft-versus-host disease, but others died of burns and other direct radiation effects.

Transplantation of fetal hepatocytes into the bone marrow is being investigated as an alternative for bone marrow transplantation, especially in young children whose immune systems have totally failed. Following transplantation, the hepatocytes begin to function like bone marrow cells. There is less likelihood of graft-versus-host disease with this procedure than with bone marrow transplantation, but more research is needed before this approach can be considered safe and effective.

Investigations are also under way to determine the potential hematopoietic benefits of the use of cloned hematopoietic growth factors such as granulocyte or granulocyte-macrophage colony-stimulating factors. Of 8 Brazilian patients with radiation sickness treated with this approach, 4 showed significant improvement. Further research is needed to evaluate safety and effectiveness.

Please contact the agencies listed under Resources, below, for the most current information. Addresses and telephone numbers of these agencies, as well as of individual experts and research centers, may be found in the Master Resources List.

## Resources

**For more information on radiation syndromes:** National Organization for Rare Disorders (NORD); National Association of Radiation Survivors; National Council on Radiation Protection and Measurements; American Cancer Society; Leukemia Society of America; NIH/National Cancer Institute Physician Data Query Phoneline.

## References

The Blood Kinin System of Persons with a History of 1st-Degree Acute Radiation Sickness: V.I. Klimenko, et al.; Vrach. Delo, 1994, vol. 5–6, pp. 81–83.

Hemopoiesis Stimulation by Low-Intensity Laser Radiation in Acute Radiation Sickness Exacerbated by Thermal Trauma: V.M. Ziablitskii, et al.; Radiats. Biol. Radioecol., 1994, vol. 34(2), pp. 210–212.

Determination of Autoantibodies to Antigens of Thymic Epithelial Cells of Clean Up Team Workers and Patients Who Survived Acute Radiation Sickness at Distant Periods After Irradiation: I.M. Beliakov, et al.; Radiobiologiia, 1992, vol. 32(3), pp. 341–348.

Individual Immunological Parameters in Clean-Up Team Members and Patients with Sequelae of Acute Radiation Sickness 5 Years After the Effects of the Chernobyl Accident: A.A. Iarilin, et al.; Radiobiologiia, 1992, vol. 32(6), pp. 771–778.

The Paramagnetic Centers of the Blood in Persons with a History of Acute Radiation Sickness As a Result of the Accident at the Chernobyl Atomic Electric Power Station: V.G. Bebeshko, et al.; Vrach. Delo 1992, vol. (4), pp. 7–10.

Cancer Risk Among Atomic Bomb Survivors: The RERF Life Span Study: Y. Shimizu, et al.; JAMA, August 1, 1990, vol. 264(5), pp. 601–604.

Comparison of Isoeffect Relationships in Radiotherapy: E.O. Voit and P.N. Yi; Bull. Math. Biol., 1990, vol. 52(5), pp. 657–675.

Health Effects of Ionizing Radiation: R.J. Fry and S.A. Fry; Med. Clin. North Am., March 1990, vol. 74(2), pp. 475–488.

Health Effects of Nonionizing Radiation: G.M. Wilkening and C.H. Sutton; Med. Clin. North Am., March 1990, vol. 74(2), pp. 489–507.

Leukemia in Utah and Radioactive Fallout from the Nevada Test Site: A Case-Control Study: W. Stevens, et al.; JAMA, August 1, 1990, vol. 264(5), pp. 585–591.

Microelectronics, Radiation, and Superconductivity: M. Gochfeld; Environ. Health Perspect., June 1990, vol. 86, pp. 285–289.

Bone Marrow Transplantation After the Chernobyl Accident: Alexander Baranov, et al.; N. Engl. J. Med., July 27, 1989, issue 321(4), pp. 205–212.

Evolving Perspectives on the Concept of Dose in Radiobiology and Radiation Protection: A.C. Upton; Health Physics, October 1988, vol. 55(4), pp. 605–614.

Use of Recombinant Granulocyte-Macrophage Colony Stimulating Factor in the Brazil Radiation Accident: A. Butturini, et al.; Lancet 1988, vol. 2, pp. 471–475.

Basic Radiation Protection Criteria: Recommendations of the National Council on Radiation Protection and Measurements: National Council on Radiation Protection and Measurements, 1984.

# 14 | MASTER RESOURCES LIST

In the preceding chapters, each disorder entry contains resources to be consulted for further information or support. These resources range from individual experts to volunteer organizations to research centers. Their addresses and telephone numbers are included in the following Master Resources List.

This list is alphabetized word by word, not letter by letter; for example, The Arc, Arc of Ohio, ARCH.

Prepositions are disregarded among organizations with similar titles. For example, the National Organization *on* Fetal Alcohol Syndrome precedes the National Organization *for* Rare Disorders.

Referrals for the National Institutes of Health are listed alphabetically under NIH.

Disorders that begin with a numeral are listed as if the numeral were a word. For example, 4p- Society is alphabetized as Four p Society.

**Dagfinn Aarskog, M.D.**
Department of Pediatrics
Haukeland Hospital
N-5021 Bergen
Newline, Norway
(For Aarskog syndrome)

**Aarskog Syndrome Support Group**
62 Robin Hill Lane
Levittown, PA 19055-1411
(215) 943-7131
*See also* Dagfinn Aarskog, M.D.
Jerome Gorski, M.D.
Richard A. Lewis, M.D.

**Abiding Hearts**
P.O. Box 5245
Bozeman, MT 59717
(406) 587-7421

**AboutFace**
99 Crowns Lane, 3rd Floor
Toronto, Ontario M5R 3P4
Canada
(800) 225-3223 (U.S.)
(800) 665-3223 (Canada)
(416) 944-3223
*See also* Craniofacial Disorders

**AboutFace USA**
P.O. Box 737
Warrington, PA 18976
(215) 491-0602
(800) 225-3223
*See also* Craniofacial Disorders

**Achondrogenesis**
*See* Robert Campbell, M.D.

**Acidemia, Organic**
*See* British Organic Acidemia Association

**Acoustic Neuroma Association**
P.O. Box 12402
Atlanta, GA 30355
(404) 237-8023

**Acromegaly**
*See* Pituitary Tumor Network Association

**ACTIS**
(AIDS information on privately funded
clinical trials; Spanish-speaking
specialists available)
(800) TRIALS-A
(800) 243-7012 (TDD)
*See also* AIDS

**Addison Disease**
*See* National Adrenal Disease Foundation

**Adrenal Hyperplasia**
*See* Congenital Adrenal Hyperplasia
Support Association, Inc.

**Adrenoleukodystrophy**
*See* Hugo W. Moser, M.D.

**Agenesis of Corpus Callosum Network**
86 North Main Street
Orono, ME 04473
(207) 866-2062

**Agoraphobics in Motion**
605 West Eleven Mile Road
Royal Oak, MI 48067

**AHEPA Cooley's Anemia Foundation**
1909 Q Street, NW
Washington, DC 20009
(202) 232-6300
*See also* Anemia

**Aicardi Syndrome Newsletter, Inc.**
5115 Troy Urbana Road
Casstown, OH 45312-9711
(513) 339-6033
*See also* Richard Allen, M.D.

**AIDS**
*See* ACTIS
AIDS Information Clearinghouse
AIDSLINE
American Autoimmune-Related Diseases
Association
American Foundation for AIDS Research
American Social Health Association
Computerized AIDS Information Network
National AIDS Hotline
National Gay and Lesbian Task Force
National Gay Task Force
National Hemophilia Foundation
National Sexually Transmitted Diseases
Hotline
NIH/National Institute of Allergy and
Infectious Diseases

**AIDS Information Clearinghouse**
(800) 458-5231

**AIDSLINE (National Library of Medicine)**
(800) 638-8480

**Alagille Syndrome (AHD) Alliance**
10630 SW Garden Park Place
Tigard, OR 97223
(503) 639-6217

**Albinism**
*See* National Organization for Albinism and
Hypopigmentation

**Alcaptonuria**
*See* Bert N. La Du, M.D.

**Alcohol Abuse**
*See* Fetal Alcohol Education Program
National Institute on Alcohol Abuse and
Alcoholism
NIH/National Clearinghouse for Alcohol
and Drug Information

**ALD (Adrenoleukodystrophy) Project**
*See* Adrenoleukodystrophy (ALD) Project

**Alexander Graham Bell Association for
the Deaf**
3417 Volta Place NW
Washington, DC 20007-2778
(202) 337-5220
*See also* Hearing Impairment

**Richard Allen, M.D.**
Pediatric Neurology Service 0800/C7123
Outpatient Building
University Hospitals
Ann Arbor, MI 48109-0800
(313) 763-4697
(For Aicardi syndrome)

**Allergy/Asthma**
*See* Allergy Information Association
Allergy Testing
Allergy/Asthma Association Information
Asthma and Allergy Foundation of
America
Environmental Disorders
Latex Allergy Support Service
Mothers of Asthmatics
National Foundation for Asthma
NIH/National Institute of Allergy and
Infectious Diseases

**Allergy Information Association**
25 Poynter Drive, Suite 7
Weston, Ontario MR9 1K8
Canada

**Allergy Testing**
118-21 Queens Boulevard
Forest Hills, NY 11375
(718) 261-3663

**Allergy/Asthma Association Information**
65 Tromley Drive, Suite 10
Etobicoke, Ontario M9B SY7
Canada
(416) 244-9312/244-8585

**Alliance of Genetic Support Groups**
35 Wisconsin Circle, Suite 440
Chevy Chase, MD 20815-7015
(301) 652-5553
(800) 336-GENE
*See also* Chromosomal Abnormalities

**Alopecia Areata International Research,
Inc.**
P.O. Box 1875
Thousand Oaks, CA 91358
(805) 494-4903
*See also* National Alopecia Areata
Foundation

**Bruce S. Alpert, M.D.**
Division of Cardiology
University of Tennessee
848 Adams Avenue
Memphis, TN 38103
(901) 522-3380
(For Marfan syndrome)

**Alpha-1-Antitrypsin Deficiency National
Association**
1829 Portland Avenue
Minneapolis, MN 55404
(612) 871-1747
(800) 425-7421

**Alpha-1-Antitrypsin Deficiency Registry**
David P. Meeker, M.D.
Cleveland Clinic Foundation
Department of Pulmonary Diseases
9500 Euclid Avenue
Cleveland, OH 44195
(216) 444-6505

**Alpha-1 Support Group Newsletter**
819 Bayview Road
Neenah, WI 54956
(414) 727-4576

**Alport Syndrome—Hereditary Nephritis Study**
Department of Physiology, Room #156
University of Utah
410 Chipeta Way
Salt Lake City, UT 84198-1297
(801) 581-5479

**Alstrom Syndrome**
*See* International Alstrom's Syndrome
Newsletter
Jan Marshall, M.D.

**Blanche Alter, M.D.**
Mount Sinai School of Medicine
Fifth Avenue and 100th Street
New York, NY 10029
(For Fanconi anemia)

**Alternative Medicine**
*See* NIH/Office of Alternative Medicine

**Roy D. Altman, M.D.**
University of Miami School of Medicine
Division of Arthritis (VA111)
P.O. Box 016960
Miami, Florida 33101
(305) 547-5735

**Alzheimer Disease**
*See* Alzheimer's Association
Alzheimer's Disease Education and
Referral Center
Denise Juliano, M.S.W.
Linda Nee, M.S.W.
(NIH) National Institute on Aging

**Alzheimer's Association**
919 North Michigan Avenue, Suite 1000
Chicago, IL 60611
(312) 335-8700
(800) 272-3900

**Alzheimer's Disease Education and Referral Center**
P.O. Box 8250
Silver Spring, MD 20907-8250
(301) 495-3311
(800) 438-4380

**Ambiguous Genitalia Support Network**
428 East Elm Street, #4D
Lodi, CA 95240-2310
(209) 369-0414
*See also* International Foundation for
Gender Education
Sexual Disorders

**American Academy of Dermatology**
930 North Meacham Road
P.O. Box 4014
Schaumburg, IL 60168-4014
(708) 330-0230
*See also* Skin Disorders

**American Academy of Environmental Medicine**
P.O. Box 16106
Denver, CO 80216
(303) 622-9755
*See also* Environmental Disorders

**American Amputee Foundation**
P.O. Box 250218
Little Rock, AR 72225
(501) 666-2523
*See also* Amputation

**American Anorexia and Bulimia Association**
293 Central Park West, Suite 1R
New York, NY 10024
(212) 501-8351
*See also* Eating Disorders

**American Association of Kidney Patients**
100 South Ashley Drive, Suite 280
Tampa, FL 33602
(813) 223-7099
(800) 749-2257

**American Association of Orthodontists**
460 North Lindbergh Boulevard
Saint Louis, MO 63141
*See also* Dental Disorders

**American Association of Suicidology**
2459 South Ash
Denver, CO 80222
(303) 692-0985
*See also* National Committee on Youth
Suicide Prevention
Mental Health

**American Association of University Affiliated Programs**
8630 Fenton Street, #410
Silver Spring, MD 20910
(301) 588-8252
(301) 588-3319 (TTY)

**American Autoimmune-Related Diseases Association**
15475 Gratiot Avenue
Detroit, MI 48205
(313) 371-8600
(800) 598-4668
*See also* Immunodeficiency

**American Behçet's Disease Association**
P.O. Box 27494
Tempe, AZ 85285-7494
(602) 320-4001
(800) 723-4238
(602) 821-9606 (TTY)
*See also* J. Desmond O'Duffy

**American Board of Medical Specialties**
(For information on certified physicians)
(800) 776-CERT

**American Brain Tumor Association**
(formerly, Association for Brain Tumor
Research)
2720 River Road, Suite 146
Des Plaines, IL 60018
(708) 827-9910
(800) 886-2282
*See also* Brain Tumors
Cancer

**American Broncho-Esophagological Association (ABEA)**
Vanderbilt University Medical Center
S-6441, Medical Center North
Nashville, TN 37232
(615) 322-7267
*See also* Atresia
Lung Disorders

**American Cancer Society**
1599 Clifton Road NE
Atlanta, GA 30329
(404) 320-3333
(800) 227-2345

**American Chronic Pain Association, Inc.**
P.O. Box 850
Rocklin, CA 95677
(916) 632-0922
*See also* Pain

**American Cleft Palate Cranial Facial Association**
1218 Grandview Avenue
Pittsburgh, PA 15211
(412) 481-1376
(800) 242-5338
*See also* Craniofacial Disorders

**American College of Obstetricians and Gynecologists**
The Resource Center
409 12th Street NW
Washington DC 20024
(202) 863-2518
(202) 638-5577
*See also* Women's Health

**American Council of the Blind, Inc.**
1155 15th Street NW, Suite 720
Washington, DC 20005
(202) 467-5081
(800) 424-8666
*See also* Eye Disorders

**American Council of Blind Parents**
*See* Council of Families with Visual
Impairment

**American Dental Association**
211 East Chicago Avenue
Chicago, IL 60611
(312) 440-2500
*See also* Dental Disorders

**American Diabetes Association**
National Service Center
1660 Duke Street
Alexandria, VA 22314
(703) 549-1500
(800) 342-2383

**American Fertility Society**
1209 Montgomery Highway
Birmingham, AL 35216-2809
(206) 978-5000

**American Foundation for AIDS Research**
733 Third Avenue, 12th Floor
New York, NY 10017-3204
(212) 333-3118

**American Foundation for the Blind**
11 Penn Plaza, Suite 300
New York, NY 10011
(212) 502-7600
(800) 232-5463
(212) 502-7662 (TTY)
Regional Offices:
Atlanta (404) 525-2303
Chicago (312) 269-0095
Dallas (214) 352-7222
San Francisco (415) 392-4845
See also Eye Disorders

**American Foundation for Urologic Disease**
300 West Pratt Street
Baltimore, MD 21201
(800) 242-2383
See also Kidney/Urologic Disorders

**American Hearing Research Foundation**
55 East Washington Street, Suite 2022
Chicago, IL 60602

**American Heart Association**
7272 Greenville Avenue
Dallas, TX 75231-4596
(214) 373-6300
(800) 242-8721
(800) 553-6321 (for the Stroke Connection of the AHA)

**American Humane Association**
P.O. Box 1266
Denver, CO 80201
(303) 792-9900
(For trained hearing dogs)
See also Hearing Impairment

**American Hyperlexia Association**
479 Spring Road
Elmhurst, IL 60126
(708) 530-8551
See also Autism

**American Juvenile Arthritis Organization**
1314 Spring Street NW
Atlanta, GA 30309
(404) 872-7100

**American Kidney Fund**
6110 Executive Boulevard, Suite 1010
Rockville, MD 20852
(301) 881-3052
(800) 638-8299
(800) 492-8361 (in Maryland)
(For treatment and expenses for dialysis patients and transplant recipients/donors)

**American Laryngeal Papilloma Foundation (formerly Christine Lazar)**
2 Hillside Avenue, Suite 5
Rockaway, NJ 07866
(201) 627-1243
See also Recurrent Respiratory Papillomatosis Foundation

**American Leprosy Missions**
1 ALM Way
Greenville, SC 29601
(800) 537-7679
(803) 271-7040
See also National Hansen Disease Center

**American Liver Foundation**
1425 Pompton Avenue
Cedar Grove, NJ 07009-1000
(201) 256-2550
(800) 223-0179

**American Lung Association**
1740 Broadway
New York, NY 10019
(212) 315-8700
(800) 586-4872

**American Lung Association of Connecticut**
45 Ash Street
East Hartford, CT 06108
(203) 289-5401
(800) 992-2263

**American Lupus Society**
260 Maple Street, Suite 123
Ventura, CA 93003
(805) 339-0443
(800) 331-1802
See also Lupus Erythematosus

**American Medical Association**
515 North State Street
Chicago, IL 60610
(312) 464-5000

**American Methadone Treatment Association, Inc.**
253-255 Third Avenue
New York, NY 10010
(212) 566-5555
See also Drug Abuse

**American Paralysis Association**
500 Morris Avenue
Springfield, NJ 07081
(800) 225-0292
(201) 379-2690

**American Paraplegia Society**
75-20 Astoria Boulevard
Jackson Heights, NY 11370-1177
(718) 803-3782
See also Spinal Cord Injuries

**American Porphyria Foundation**
P.O. Box 22712
Houston, TX 77227
(713) 266-9617

**American Printing House for the Blind**
1839 Frankfort Avenue
P.O. Box 6085
Louisville, KY 40206-0085
(502) 895-2405
(800) 223-1839
See also Eye Disorders

**American Pseudo-obstruction and Hirschsprung's Disease Society, Inc.**
P.O. Box 772
Medford, MA 02155-0006
(617) 395-4255
See also Intestinal Pseudo-obstruction

**American Psychiatric Association**
1400 K Street, NW
Washington DC 20005
(202) 682-6000
See also Mental Health

**American Red Cross**
17th and E Streets, NW
Washington, DC 20006
(202) 737-8300

**American Rhinologic Society**
Penn Park Medical Center
2929 Baltimore, Suite 105
Kansas City, MO 64108
See also Nose Disorders

**American Schizophrenia Association**
900 North Federal Highway #330
Boca Raton, FL 33432
See also Mental Health

**American Self-Help Clearinghouse**
Northwest Covenant Healthcare System
25 Pocono Road
Denville, NJ 07834-2995
(201) 625-7101
(201) 625-9053 (TTY)

**American Sickle Cell Anemia Association**
10300 Carnegie Avenue
Cleveland, OH 44106
(216) 229-8600

**American Silicone Implant Survivors (AS-IS), Inc.**
1288 Cork Elm Drive
Kirkwood, MO 63122
(314) 821-0115
See also Breast Implants

**American Sleep Apnea Association**
P.O. Box 66
Belmont, MA 02178
(617) 489-4441
See also Sleep Disorders

**American Sleep Disorders Association**
1610 14th Street NW, Suite 300
Rochester, MN 55901
(507) 287-6006

**American Social Health Association**
P.O. Box 13827
Research Triangle Park, NC 27709
(919) 361-8488
*See also* Sexually Transmitted Disease,
AIDS

**American Society of Adults with
Pseudo-obstruction**
19 Carroll Road
Woburn, MA 01801-6161
(617) 935-9776
*See also* Intestinal Pseudo-obstruction

**American Society of Bariatric Physicians**
5600 South Quebec Street, Suite 109A
Englewood, CO 80111
(303) 779-4833
*See also* Eating Disorders

**American Society for Deaf Children**
P.O. Box 2848
Arden Way, Suite 210
Sacramento, CA 95825-1373
(916) 482-0120
(916) 482-0120 (TTY)
*See also* Hearing Impairment
Children

**American Society of Dermatopathology**
Denver General Hospital 01046
777 Bannock Street
Denver, CO 80204
*See also* Skin Disorders

**American Society of Hypertension**
515 Madison Avenue, 21st Floor
New York, NY 10022
(212) 644-0650
*See also* Heart Disorders
Hypertension

**American Society of Parenteral and
Enteral Nutrition (ASPEN)**
8630 Fenton Street, #412
Silver Spring, MD 20910
(301) 587-6315
*See also* Parent Education Network

**American Society of Plastic and
Reconstructive Surgeons,
International**
444 East Algonquin Road
Arlington Heights, IL 60005
(708) 228-9900
(800) 635-0635 (for physician referrals)
*See also* Institute of Reconstructive Plastic
Surgery

**American Society of Reproductive
Medicine**
1209 Montgomery Highway
Birmingham, AL 35216-2809
(205) 978-5000
*See also* Fertility

**American Speech-Language-Hearing
Association**
10801 Rockville Pike
Rockville, MD 20852
(301) 897-5700
(800) 638-8255
(301) 897-5700 (TTY)
*See also* Hearing Impairment

**American Spinal Injury Association**
250 East Superior Street, Room 619
Chicago, IL 60611
(312) 908-3425
*See also* Spinal Cord Injuries

**American Syringomyelia Alliance
Project, Inc.**
P.O. Box 1586
Longview, TX 75606-1586
(903) 236-7079
(800) 272-7282

**American Tinnitus Association**
P.O. Box 5
Portland, OR 97207
(503) 248-9985
(800) 634-8978
*See also* Ear Disorders
Hearing Impairment

**Stephen S. Amon, M.D.**
California Department of Health Services
Berkeley, CA
(510) 873-6327
(For botulism)

**Amputation**
*See* American Amputee Foundation
National Amputation Foundation
Superkids

**Amyloidosis Network**
602 Bernard Street
Wausau, WI 54401
*See also* Morie A. Gertz, M.D.
Martha Skinner, M.D.

**Amyotrophic Lateral Sclerosis
Association**
21021 Ventura Blvd., Suite 321
Woodland Hills, CA 91364-2206
(818) 340-7500
(800) 782-4747
*See also* Motor Neuron Disease Association

**Amyotrophic Lateral Sclerosis
Association of Greater Philadelphia**
P.O. Box 507
Norristown, PA 19404-0507
(215) 227-3508

**Anemia**
*See* Aplastic Anemia Foundation of America
AHEPA Cooley's Anemia Foundation
Cooley's Anemia Foundation, Inc.
Diamond-Blackfan Anemia Registry
Diamond-Blackfan Anemia Support
Group
Earl J. Goldberg Aplastic Anemia
Foundation
Evans Syndrome Support and Research
Group

Fanconi Anemia Research Fund, Inc.
International Fanconi Registry
(NIH) National Heart, Lung and Blood
Institute Information Center
Sickle Cell

**Anencephaly**
*See* Fighters for Encephaly Support Group

**Angelman Syndrome Foundation, Inc.**
P.O. Box 12437
Gainesville, FL 32604
(904) 332-3303

**Angelman Syndrome Support Group**
Mrs. Sheila Woolven
15 Place Crescent
Waterlooville, NR Portsmouth
Hants, United Kingdom

**Ankylosing Spondylitis Association**
13135 Ventura Boulevard, Suite 300
Studio City, CA 91604-2219
(818) 981-1616
(800) 777-8189

**Anorectal Malformations**
*See* Pull-Thru Network
Alberto Peña, M.D.

**Anorexia and Bulimia Treatment and
Education Center**
621 S. New Ballas Road, Suite 2008-B
Saint Louis, MO 63141
(314) 569-6565
(800) 222-2832
*See also* Eating Disorders

**Anorexia Nervosa and Associated
Disorders, Inc.**
P.O. Box 7
Highland Park, IL 60035
(708) 831-3438
*See also* Eating Disorders

**Anorexia Nervosa and Related Eating
Disorders, Inc.**
P.O. Box 5102
Eugene, OR 97405-0102
(503) 344-1144
*See also* Eating Disorders

**Anxiety Disorders Association of
America**
6000 Executive Boulevard, Suite 513
Rockville, MD 20852
(301) 231-9350
*See also* Eating Disorders

**Any Baby Can, Inc.**
5410 Fredericksburg Road, Suite 104
San Antonio, TX 78229
(210) 377-0222
*See also* Children

**Apert Syndrome Support Group**
8708 Kathy Court
Saint Louis, MO 63126
(314) 965-3356

**Aphasia**
*See* C.A.N.D.L.E.
National Aphasia Association

**Aplastic Anemia Foundation of America**
P.O. Box 22689
Baltimore, MD 21203
(800) 747-2820
*See also* Anemia

**Arachnoiditis Information and Support
Network**
P.O. Box 1166
Ballwin, MO 63021
(314) 394-5741
(201) 239-8870

**Arc, The (a national organization on
mental retardation)**
500 East Border Street, Suite 300
Arlington, TX 76010
(817) 261-6003
(817) 277-0553 (TDD)
(800) 433-5255
*See also* Retarded Infant Services
Mental Health

**Arc of Ohio**
1335 Dublin Road, #205C
Columbus, OH 43215-1000
(800) 589-2726
(614) 487-4720

**ARCH National Resource Center**
800 Eastowne Drive, Suite 105
Chapel Hill, NC 27514
(919) 490-5577
(800) 473-1727

**Arginase Deficiency**
*See* Stephen Cederbaum, M.D.

**Arizona State Ehlers-Danlos Association**
2023 East Adams Street
Tucson, AZ 85719
(602) 327-7956

**Arnold-Chiari Family Network**
67 Spring Street
Weymouth, MA 02188
(617) 337-2368

**Arrhythmia, Sudden Death Due to**
*See* Sudden Arrhythmia Death Syndrome
Foundation
Heart Disorders

**Arteriovenus Malformation (AVM)
Support Group of Nevada, Inc.**
P.O. Box 1261
Fernley, NV 89408
(702) 575-5421

**Arthritis**
*See* American Juvenile Arthritis Organization
Arthritis Foundation
NIH/National Arthritis and
Musculoskeletal and Skin Diseases
Information Clearinghouse
Polychondritis and Rheumatoid Arthritis
Clinic

**Arthritis Foundation**
P.O. Box 7669
Atlanta, GA 30357
(404) 872-7100
(800) 283-7800

**Arthrogryposis**
*See* Arthrogryposis Group
AVENUES
Canadian Arthrogryposis Support Team

**Arthrogryposis Group**
1 The Oaks
Gillingham, Dorset SP8 4SW
United Kingdom

**Asperger Syndrome**
*See* Martha Dencklau, M.D.

**Aspergillosis**
*See* Paul Greenberger, M.D.

**Association Européenne contre les
Leucodystrophes**
7, rue Pasteur, B.P. 267
54005 Nancy CEDEX
France
33-160917500
*See also* Leukodystrophy

**Association for Babies and Children
with Carnitine Deficiency (ABC)**
720 Enterprise Drive
Oak Brook, IL 60521
*See also* Metabolic Disorders

**Association of Birth Defect Children, Inc.**
7910 Woodmont Avenue, Suite 300
Bethesda, MD 20814
(301) 654-6549

**Association for Brain Tumor Research**
*See* American Brain Tumor Association

**Association for the Care of Children's
Health**
7910 Woodmont Avenue, Suite 300
Bethesda, MD 20814
(301) 654-6549
*See also* Children

**Association for Children with Down
Syndrome**
2616 Martin Avenue
Bellmore, NY 11710
(516) 221-4700

**Association for Children with Russell-
Silver Syndrome**
22 Hoyt Street
Madison, NJ 07940-1604
(201) 377-4531
*See also* Children

**Association of Children's Prosthetic and
Orthotic Clinics**
6300 North River Road, Suite 727
Rosemont, IL 60018-4226
(708) 698-1694
*See also* Children
Musculoskeletal Disorders

**Association for Glycogen Storage
Diseases**
P.O. Box 896
Durant, IA 52747
(319) 785-6038
*See also* Metabolic Disorders

**Association for Macular Diseases, Inc.**
210 East 64th Street
New York, NY 10021
(212) 605-3719
*See also* Macular Dystrophy
Eye Disorders

**Association for Male Sexual Dysfunction**
520 East 72nd Street
New York, NY 10021
(212) 794-1616
*See also* Sexual Disorders

**Association for Neurometabolic
Disorders**
5223 Brookfield Lane
Sylvania, OH 43506-1809
(419) 885-1497

**Association for Repetitive Motion
Syndrome**
P.O. Box 514
Santa Rosa, CA 95402-0514
(707) 571-0397
*See also* Ben Carson, M.D.

**Association for Research into Restricted
Growth**
2 Mount Court
81 Central Hill
London SE 19 1 BS
United Kingdom
01-678-2984
*See also* Dwarfism

**Association for Research of Childhood
Cancer**
P.O. Box 251
Buffalo, NY 14225
*See also* Cancer
Children

**Association for Retarded Citizens of the
United States**
*See* The Arc

**Association for Urinary Continence
Control**
785 Park Avenue
New York, NY 10021
(212) 988-8888
*See also* Help for Incontinent People
Kidney/Urologic Disorders

**Association for Voluntary Surgical
Contraception**
122 East 42nd Street
New York, NY 11201
*See also* Fertility

**Asthma and Allergy Foundation of America**
1125 15th Street NW, Suite 502
Washington, DC 20005
(202) 466-7643
(800) 727-8462
*See also* Allergy/Asthma

**Ataxia**
*See* National Ataxia Foundation
Parkinson Disease

**Ataxia Telangiectasia Children's Project**
21645 Cartagena Drive
Boca Raton, FL 33428
(407) 483-2661
(800) 543-5728

**Ataxia Telangiectasia Research Foundation**
344 Copa de Oro Road
Los Angeles, CA 90077
(213) 476-1218

**Atherosclerosis**
*See* International Atherosclerosis Society

**Atresia**
*See* American Broncho-Esophagological Association
Biliary Atresia and Liver Transplant Network, Inc.
TEF/VATER/VACTRL National Support Network

**Atrophy**
*See* Families of Spinal Muscular Atrophy (SMA)

**Attention Deficit Disorders**
*See* Attention Deficit Disorders Association
Children and Adults with Attention Deficit Disorders
National Attention Deficit Disorder Association

**Attention Deficit Disorders Association**
19262 Jamboree Road
Irvine, CA 92715
(800) 487-2282

**Auditory-Verbal International, Inc.**
2121 Eisenhower Avenue, Suite 402
Alexandria, VA 22314
(804) 428-9036

**Arleen Auerbach, M.D.**
International Fanconi Registry
The Rockefeller University
1230 York Avenue
New York, NY 10021
(212) 570-7533
(For Fanconi anemia)

**Autism**
*See* American Hyperlexia Association
Autism Sensory Network
Autism Society of America
Center for the Study of Autism
National Autism Hotline
NIH/National Society for Children and Adults with Autism
Children

**Autism Sensory Network**
7510 Ocean Front Avenue, Suite 650
Bethesda, MD 20814-3015
(301) 657-0881
(800) 328-8476

**Autism Society of America**
7910 Woodmont Avenue, Suite #650
Bethesda, MD 20814-3015
(301) 657-0869
(800) 328-8476

**Autoimmune Diseases**
*See* American Autoimmune-Related Diseases Association

**AVENUES, a National Support Group for Arthrogryposis Multiplex Congenita**
P.O. Box 5192
Sonora, CA 95370-5192
(209) 928-3688

**Awake Network**
Presbyterian University Hospital
Sleep Evaluation Network
Pittsburgh, PA 15213
*See also* Sleep Disorders

**Back Pain**
*See* National Back Pain Association of England

**Balance and Dizziness Disorders**
*See* Ear Disorders

**Sherri Bale, M.D.**
National Institute of Arthritis and Musculoskeletal and Skin Diseases
9000 Rockville Pike
Bethesda, MD 20892
(301) 402-2679.
(For ichthyosis)

**William F. Balistreri, M.D.**
Division of Pediatric Gastroenterology and Nutrition
Children's Hospital Medical Center
Elland and Bethesda Avenues
Cincinnati, OH 45229
(513) 559-4200

**Bardet-Biedl Syndrome**
*See* Laurence-Moon-Bardet-Biedl Syndrome

**Batten Disease Support and Research Association**
2600 Parsons Avenue
Columbus, OH 43207-2972
(614) 445-4161
(800) 448-4570
*See also* Michael J. Bennett, Ph.D.

**Eugene Bauer, M.D.**
Stanford University Medical Center
Department of Dermatology
Edwards Bldg., Room 144
Stanford, CA 94305
(415) 723-2300
(For epidermolysis bullosa)

**Beach Center on Families and Disability**
3111 Haworth Hall
University of Kansas
Lawrence, KS 66045
(913) 864-7600
(913) 864-7600 (TTY)
*See also* Disability Referrals

**Beckwith-Wiedemann Support Network**
3206 Braeburn Circle
Ann Arbor, MI 48108
(313) 973-0263
*See also* Barbara Biesecker

**Behçet Disease**
*See* American Behçet's Disease Association
J. Desmond O'Duffy, M.D

**Benign Essential Blepharospasm Research Foundation, Inc.**
P.O. Box 12468
Beaumont, TX 77726-2468
(409) 832-0788

**Michael J. Bennett, Ph.D.**
Metabolic Disease Center
Baylor University Medical Center
3500 Gaston Avenue
Dallas, TX 75246
(214) 820-4533
(For Batten disease)

**Merrill Benson, M.D.**
Indiana University, Rheumatology A772
1481 West 10th Street
Indianapolis, IN 56201
(317) 635-7401, ext. 2225

**Better Hearing Institute**
P.O. Box 1840
Washington, DC 20013
(703) 642-0580
(800) 327-9355
*See also* Hearing Impairment

**Italo Biaggioni, M.D.**
David Robertson, M.D.
AA 3228 Medical Center North
Vanderbilt University, GCRC
Nashville, TN 37232
(615) 343-6499
(For Shy-Drager syndrome)

**Barbara Biesecker**
NIH/National Center for Human Genome Research
Building 10, Room 10C101
10 Center Drive, MSC 1852
Bethesda, MD 20892
(301) 496-3979
(For Beckwith-Wiedmann syndrome)

**Leslie Biesecker, M.D.**
NIH/National Center for Human Genome Research
Building 49, Room 4A80
Bethesda, MD 20892
(301) 402-2041
(For Pallister-Hall syndrome)

**Big Hearts for Little Hearts**
365 Willis Avenue
Mineola, NY 11501
(516) 741-5522
(For families of children with congenital
heart disease)

**Biocyte Corporation (Cord Blood Stem
Cell Storage Service)**
Holly Pond Plaza
1281 East Main Street
Stamford, CT 06902
(800) 783-6235

**Biliary Atresia and Liver Transplant
Network, Inc.**
Box 190
3835 Richmond Avenue
Staten Island, NY 10312

**Biliary Cirrhosis**
See Primary Biliary Cirrhosis Patient
Support Network

**Edward D. Bird, M.D.**
Brain Tissue Resource Center
Mailman Research Center
McLean Hospital
115 Mill Street
Belmont, MA 02178
(617) 855-2400
See also Brain Tumors

**Birth Defects**
See Association of Birth Defect Children
CHARGE Syndrome Foundation
Kenneth Jones, M.D.
March of Dimes Birth Defects Foundation
National Birth Defects Center
National Birth Defect Registry
Pregnancy Hot Line

**Bladder, Exstrophy**
See National Support Group for Exstrophy
of the Bladder

**Blepharophimosis, Ptosis, and
Epicanthus Inversus Support Group**
SE 820 Meadow Vale Drive
Pullman, WA 99163
(509) 332-6628

**Blind Children's Fund**
2875 Northwind Drive, Suite 211
East Lansing, MI 48823-5040
(517) 333-1725
See also Eye Disorders
Children

**Andrew Blitzer, M.D.**
Department of Clinical Otolaryngology
College of Physicians and Surgeons
Columbia University
New York, NY 10032
(For chronic spasmodic dysphonia)

**Bloom's Syndrome Registry**
Laboratory of Human Genetics
New York Blood Center
310 East 67th Street
New York, NY 10021
(212) 570-3075

**Bone Marrow Transplant (BMT)
Newsletter**
1985 Spruce Avenue
Highland Park, IL 60035
(708) 831-1913

**Bone Marrow Transplants**
See Bone Marrow Transplant (BMT)
Newsletter
Caitlin Raymond International Registry of
Bone Marrow Donor Banks
National Organization for Bone Marrow
Transplants

**Botulism**
See Stephen S. Amon, M.D.

**Brachial Plexus Injury/Erb's Palsy
Support and Information Network**
8347 Valley View Court
Larsen, WI 54947
(441) 836-3843

**Brain and Pituitary Foundation of
America**
281 East Moody Avenue
Fresno, CA 93720-1524
(209) 434-0610

**Brain and Tissue Bank**
University of Maryland
655 Baltimore Street
Baltimore, MD 21201
(800) 841-1539

**Brain and Tissue Bank**
University of Miami School of Medicine
Fox Building, Room 427
1550 NW 10th Avenue
Miami, FL 33136
(800) 59-BRAIN

**Brain Injury Association**
1776 Massachusetts Ave NW, Suite 100
Washington DC 20036-1904
(202) 296-6443
(800) 444-6443 (helpline)

**Brain Research Foundation**
208 South LaSalle Street
Chicago, IL 60604

**Brain Tumor Research Association**
MacLean Hospital
115 Mill Street
Belmont, MA 02178

**Brain Tumor Society**
60 Birmingham Parkway
Boston, MA 02135-1116
(617) 783-0340

**Brain Tumors**
See American Brain Tumor Association
Edward D. Bird, M.D.
Brain and Pituitary Foundation of
America
Brain Research Foundation
Brain and Tissue Bank
Brain Tumor Research Association
Brain Tumor Society
Fred J. Epstein, M.D.
National Brain Tumor Foundation

**Branchio-Oto-Renal Syndrome**
See Tom Fowler

**Breast Cancer Advisory Center**
P.O. Box 224
Kensington, MD 20895
See also National Alliance of Breast Cancer
Organizations
Cancer

**Breast Implants**
See FDA Breast Implant Hotline
Command Trust Network
American Silicone Implant Survivors

**British Organic Acidemia Association**
5 Saxon Road
Ashford, Middlesex TW15 1QL
United Kingdom
See also Urea Cycle Disorders

**British Polio Fellowship**
Bell Close West End Road
Ruislip, Middlesex HA4 6LP
United Kingdom
0895-675-515
See also Polio

**Gary M. Brittenham, M.D.**
Cleveland Metropolitan General Hospital
Cleveland, OH
(For hereditary hemochromatosis)

**Bronchial Diseases**
See Lung Disorders

**Saul Brusilow, M.D.**
301 Children's Medical and Surgical Center
Johns Hopkins Hospital
600 North Wolfe Street
Baltimore, MD 21205
(410) 955-5000
(For urea cycle disorders)

**Rebecca H. Buckley, M.D.**
Michael Hershfield, M.D.
Box 2898
Duke University Hospital
Durham, NC 27710
(919) 684-2922

**Bulimia, Anorexia Self-Help**
6125 Clayton Ave., Suite 215
Saint Louis, MO 63139
See also Eating Disorders

**Bundle Branch Block**
See International Bundle Branch Block
Association

**Burns, Severe**
See International Shriners Headquarters

**Barbara Burton**
347 Manor Road East
Toronto, Ontario M4S 1S6
Canada
(416) 481-9927

**J.C. Bystryn, M.D.**
New York University Hosptial
530 First Avenue
New York, NY
(212) 889-3846
(For malignant melanoma)

**Caitlin Raymond International Registry of Bone Marrow Donor Banks**
University of Massachusetts Medical Center
65 Lake Avenue
Worcester, MA 01655

**C.A.L.M.**
See Children Anguished with Lymphatic Malformations

**Robert Campbell, M.D.**
Santa Rosa Children's Hospital
519 W. Houston Street
San Antonio, Texas
(512) 567-5125
(For expandable rib implantation)

**Canadian Arthrogryposis Support Team**
c/o Medium Chain Acyl-CoA Dehydrognease (MCAD) Family Support Group
2345 Yonge Street, 9th Floor
Toronto, Ontario M4P 2E5
Canada

**Canadian Cystic Fibrosis Foundation**
586 Eglinton Avenue East, Suite 204
Toronto, Ontario M4P 1P2
Canada
See also Cystic Fibrosis Foundation

**Canadian Hemophilia Society**
1450 City Councillors Street, Suite 840
Montreal, Quebec H3A 2E6
Canada
(514) 848-0503

**Canadian Organization for Rare Disorders**
515 Seventh Street South, #100B
Lethbridge, Alberta T1J 2G8
Canada
(403) 329-0665

**Canadian Sickle Cell Society**
1076 Bathurst Street, Suite 305
Toronto, Ontario M5R 3G9
Canada

**Cancer**
See American Brain Tumor Association
American Cancer Society
Association for Research of Childhood Cancer
Breast Cancer Advisory Center
Cancer Survivorship
Candlelighters Childhood Cancer Foundation
CANSURMOUNT
Children's Leukemia Foundation of Michigan
Children's Liver Foundation
Children's PKU Network
Cutaneous Lymphoma Network
Foundation for Childhood Cancer
Hairy Cell Leukemia Foundation
Hereditary Colorectal Cancer Registry
Leukemia Society of America
Li-Fraumeni Syndrome International Registry
Mathews Foundation for Prostate Cancer Research
National Kidney Cancer Association
Nevoid Basal Cell Carcinoma Syndrome Support Network
NIH/National Cancer Institute Physician Data Inquiry
NIH/Office of Cancer Communications
Pituitary Tumor Network Association
Skin Cancer Foundation
Steve Atanas Stavro Familial Gastrointestinal Cancer Registry
Us Too
Brain Tumors
Breast Implants

**Cancer Federation**
P.O. Box 52109
Riverside, CA 92517
(714) 682-7989

**Cancer Survivorship**
Patty Delaney, Cancer Liaison
Dept. of Health and Human Services
Public Health Services
Food and Drug Administration
Rockville, MD 20857
(301) 443-0104

**C.A.N.D.L.E. (Childhood Aphasia, Neurological Disorders, Landau-Kleffner Syndrome, and Epilepsy)**
4414 McCampbell Drive
Montgomery, AL 36106
(334) 271-3947
See also National Aphasia Association
Children
Neurologic Disorders

**Candlelighters Childhood Cancer Foundation**
7910 Woodmont Avenue, Suite 460
Bethesda, MD 20814
(301) 657-8401
(800) 366-2223
See also Cancer
Children

**Robert Canfield, M.D.**
Ethel Siris, M.D.
Thomas Jacobs, M.D.
Columbia Presbyterian Hospital
Department of Medicine
630 W. 168th Street
New York, NY
(212) 694-3526/694-5731
(For Paget disease of bone)

**CANSURMONT (Cancer)**
1599 Clifton Road
Atlanta, GA 30334

**Andrew J. Cant, M.D.**
Newcastle General Hospital
Department of Child Health
Westgate Road
Newcastle-upon-Tyne NE4 6BE
United Kingdom
(091) 273-8811
(091) 272-2641 (fax)
(For severe combined immunodeficiency)

**Cardiac Disorders**
See Heart Disorders

**Cardio-Auditory Syndrome**
See International Long QT Syndrome Registry
Sudden Arrhythmia Death Syndrome Foundation
Heart Disorders

**Cardio-Facial-Cutaneous Syndrome Support Network**
157 Alder Avenue
Egg Harbor Township, NJ 08234
(609) 646-5606

**Caregivers**
See Family Caregiver Alliance
National Family Caregivers Association

**Carnitine Deficiency**
See Association for Babies and Children with Carnitine Deficiency (ABC)

**Carpal Tunnel Syndrome**
See Association for Repetitive Motion Syndrome
Ben Carson, M.D.

**Ben Carson, M.D.**
Children's Center
Johns Hopkins Hospital
Baltimore, MD 21205
(410) 955-7888
(For repetitive motion syndrome; Rasmussen encephalitis)
See also Association for Repetitive Motion Syndrome
Theodore Rasmussen, M.D.

**Suzanne Cassidy, M.D.**
Robert Erickson, M.D.
University of Arizona
Department of Pediatrics
Tuscon, AZ
(For Prader-Willi syndrome)

**Cataplexy**
See Narcolepsy and Cataplexy Foundation of America

**Cataracts**
See Eye Disorders

**Stephen Cederbaum, M.D.**
Department of Psychiatry and Pediatrics
UCLA Medical School
Los Angeles, CA 90024
(310) 825-0402
(For arginase deficiency)

**Celiac Sprue Association/USA**
P.O. Box 31700
Omaha, NE 68131-0700
(402) 558-0600
*See also* Gluten Intolerance Group of North
America
Joseph A. Murray, M.D.

**Center for Accessible Housing**
North Carolina State University
School of Design
Box 8613
Raleigh, NC 27695-8613
(919) 515-3082
*See also* Disability Referrals

**Center for Medical Consumers**
New York, NY
(212) 674-7105
(For reprints of journal articles)

**Center for Medical Genetics**
Blalock 1008
Johns Hopkins Hospital
600 North Wolfe Street
Baltimore, MD 21287-4922
(410) 955-0484

**Center for Rare Diseases and
Disabilities**
Vibeke Manniche, M.D.
Bredgade 25, Sct Annae Passage
Opgang F
1260 Copenhagen K
Denmark
0045 33 91 40 20
*See also* Rare Disease Support Groups

**Center for Research in Sleep Disorders**
1275 East Kemper Road
Cincinnati, OH 45246-3901
(513) 671-3101
(311) 111-6111 (TTY)

**Center for Sickle Cell Disease**
2121 Georgia Avenue NW
Washington, DC 20059
(202) 806-7930

**Center for Stress and Anxiety Disorders**
1535 Western Avenue
Albany, NY 12203
(518) 456-4127
*See also* Eating Disorders

**Center for Substance Abuse Prevention**
National Drug Hotline
Rockwall II
1515 Security Lane
Rockville, MD 20852
(800) 662-HELP
(301) 443-0373 (public education)
*See also* Drug Abuse

**Center for the Study of Autism**
9725 SW Beaverton-Hillsdale Highway,
Suite 230
Beaverton, OR 97005
(610) 643-4121

**Centers for Disease Control**
1600 Clifton Road NE
Atlanta, GA 30333
(404) 639-3534
(404) 332-4555 (recorded message on
vaccines and infectious diseases etc.)
(800) 342-AIDS (AIDS hotline)

**Cerebral Palsy**
*See* United Cerebral Palsy Association

**Arvinda Chakekavarti, M.D.**
Human Genetics Department
University of Pittsburgh
130 Desoto Street
Pittsburgh, PA 15216
(412) 624-3066
(For Hirschsprung disease)

**Sandra Chapman, M.D.**
Callier Center for Communicative Disorders
Dallas Center for Vocal Motor Control
1966 Inwood Road
Dallas, TX 75235

**Charcot-Marie-Tooth Association**
601 Upland Avenue
Upland, PA 19015
(610) 499-7486
(800) 606-2682

**Charcot-Marie-Tooth Disease/Peroneal
Muscular Atrophy Association**
1 Springbank Drive
Saint Catherine's, Ontario L2S 2KI
Canada
(610) 499-7486
(800) 606-2682

**CHARGE Syndrome Foundation**
2004 Parkade Boulevard
Columbia, MO 65202-3121
(314) 442-7604
(800) 442-7604
*See also* Birth Defects
Children

**Chemical Hypersensitivity**
*See* Environmental Disorders

**Chemosensory Clinical Research Center
of Connecticut**
Department of BioStructure
University of Connecticut Health Center
Farmington, CT 06032
(203) 679-2459
*See also* Environmental Disorders

**CHERUB: Association of Families and
Friends of Children with Limb
Disorders**
936 Delaware Avenue
Buffalo, NY 14209
(716) 762-9997
*See also* Superkids, Inc.
Children

**Childhood Disintegrative Network**
56 The Avenue
Nedlands 6009
Western Australia
(61-9) 386-6693
*See also* Children

**Children**
*See* American Society for Deaf Children
Any Baby Can
Association for Children with Down
Syndrome
Association for Children with Russell-
Silver Syndrome
Association for Research of Childhood
Cancer
Association for the Care of Children's
Health
Association of Birth Defect Children
Association of Children's Prosthetic and
Orthotic Clinics (ACPOC)
Ataxia Telangiectasia Children's Project
Blind Children's Fund
C.A.N.D.L.E.
Candlelighters Childhood Cancer
Foundation
CHARGE Syndrome Foundation
CHERUB
Childhood Disintegrative Network
Council of Guilds for Infant Survival
Federation of Families for Children's
Mental Health
For Our Children's Unique Sight (FOCUS)
Foundation Fighting Blindness
Foundation for Childhood Cancer
Help Hospitalized Children's Fund
International Children's Anophthalmia
Network
ITP Society
National Birth Defects Registry
National Birth Defects Center
National Center for Education in Maternal
and Child Health
National Center for Youth with Disabilities
National Information Center for Children
and Youth with Disabilities
National Information Clearinghouse for
Infants with Disabilities and Life-
Threatening Conditions
National Maternal and Child Health
Clearinghouse
NIH/National Institute of Child Health and
Human Development
Research Trust for Metabolic Diseases in
Children
Superkids
Autism
Birth Defects

**Children Afflicted by Toxic Substances**
60 Oser Avenue
Happauge, NY 11788
(516) 273-2287

**Children and Adults with Attention
Deficit Disorders**
499 NW 70th Avenue, Suite 101
Plantation, FL 33317
(305) 587-3700
(800) 233-4050 (for recorded information)
*See also* Attention Deficit Disorders

**Children Anguished with Lymphatic
Malformations**
16 River Bend Road
Montgomery, IL 60538
(708) 906-9028
*See also* National Vascular Malformation
Foundation

**Children's Association for Research on Mucolipidosis IV**
6 Concord Drive
Monsey, NY 10952
(914) 425-0639
*See also* Mucolipidoses/
Mucopolysaccharidoses

**Children's Brain Diseases Foundation for Research**
350 Parnassus, Suite 900
San Francisco, CA 94117
(415) 566-5402

**Children's Craniofacial Association**
9441 LBJ Parkway, Suite 115
Dallas, TX 75243-4522
(214) 994-9831
(800) 535-3643

**Children's Hospice International**
700 Princess Street, LL
Alexandria, VA 22314
(703) 684-0330
(800) 242-4453

**Children's Leukemia Foundation of Michigan**
29777 Telegraph Road, Suite 1651
Southfield, MI 48034
(810) 353-8222
(800) 825-2536
*See also* Cancer

**Children's Liver Foundation**
14245 Ventura Boulevard
Sherman Oaks, CA 91423
(818) 906-3021

**Children's Phenylketonuria (PKU) Network**
P.O. Box 910312
50515 Vista Sorrento Parkway
San Diego, CA 92121-0312
(619) 587-9421
*See also* Phenylketonuria

**Choice in Dying (formerly, Society for the Right to Die)**
200 Varick Street
New York, NY 10014
(212) 366-5540
(800) 989-9455

**Christine Lazar**
*See* American Laryngeal Papilloma
Foundation

**Chromosomal Abnormalities**
*See* Alliance of Genetic Support Groups
Chromosome Deletion Outreach
Chromosome 18 Registry and Research
Society
Contact Group for Trisomy 9p
Cri-du-Chat Society
5p- Society
49XXXXY
4p- Parent Contact Group
Inverted Duplication Exchange and
Advocacy
ML 4 Foundation
Mothers United for Moral Support

National Center for Education in Maternal
and Child Health
National Center on Chromosome
Inversions
National Foundation for Jewish Genetic
Diseases
National Society of Genetic Counselors
National Tay-Sachs and Allied Diseases
Association, Inc.
Parents and Researchers Interested in
Smith-Magenis Syndrome
Spotlight 6
Support Group for 9p-
Support Group for Monosomy 9p
Support Organization for Trisomy
(S.O.F.T.) 18, 13, and Related
Disorders
Support Organization for Trisomy
(S.O.F.T.) Canada, Inc.
Trisomy 9 International Parent Support
Wolf-Hirschhorn Syndrome Support
Group

**Chromosome 4 Ring**
*See* 4p- Parent Contact Group

**Chromosome 5, Trisomy 5p**
*See* 5p- Society

**Chromosome 6 Ring**
*See* Spotlight 6

**Chromosome 9 Ring**
*See* Support Group for 9p-
Support Group for Monosomy 9p

**Chromosome 15 Ring**
*See* Inverted Duplication Exchange and
Advocacy

**Chromosome 17**
*See* Parents and Researchers Interested in
Smith-Magenis Syndrome
Smith-Magenis Syndrome Contact Group

**Chromosome 18 Registry and Research Society**
6302 Fox Head
San Antonio, TX 78247
(210) 657-4968

**Chromosome 49XXXXY**
*See* 49XXXXY

**Chromosome Deletion Outreach**
P.O. Box 280
Driggs, ID 83422
(208) 354-8550

**Chronic Fatigue and Immune Dysfunction Syndrome Society**
P.O. Box 230108
Portland, OR 97223
(503) 684-5261
(800) 442-3437
*See also* Immunodeficiency

**Chronic Granulomatous Disease Association**
2616 Monterey Road
San Marino, CA 91108-1646
(818) 441-4118

**Chronic Granulomatous Disease Registry**
c/o Immune Deficiency Foundation
25 West Chesapeake Avenue, Room 206
Towson, MD 21204
(410) 461-3127

**Chronic Pain Support Group**
P.O. Box 148
Peninsula, OH 44264

**Chronic Spasmodic Dysphonia**
*See* Dysphonia

**George P. Chrousos, M.D.**
National Institutes of Health
Developmental Endocrinology Branch
Building 10, Room 10N262
Bethesda, Maryland 20892

**Harry T. Chugani, M.D.**
UCLA Medical Center
Department of Pediatric Neurology
10833 LeConte
Los Angeles, CA 90024-1752
(215) 825-5946.

**Cirrhosis**
*See* Liver Disorders

**Clearinghouse on Disability Information**
Office of Special Education and
Rehabilitative Services
Department of Education
330 C Street SW
Switzer Building, Room 3132
Washington, DC 20202-2524
(202) 205-8421
*See also* Disability Referrals

**Cleft Palate**
*See* William N. Williams, D.D.S.

**Cleft Palate Foundation**
1218 Grandview Avenue
Pittsburgh, PA 15211
(412) 481-1376
(800) 242-5338 (for parents)
*See also* Craniofacial Disorders

**Clinical Genetics Program**
Children's Hospital
300 Longwood Avenue
Boston, MA 02115
(617) 355-7429

**Clinical Trials funded by the Public Health Service**
*See* CRISP

**Coalition of Heritable Disorders of Connective Tissue**
*See* National Marfan Foundation

**Coalition on Sexuality and Disability, Inc.**
122 East 23rd Street
New York, NY 10010
(212) 242-3900
*See also* Disability Referrals

**Cobalamin Network**
P.O. Box 174
Thetford Center, VT 05075-0174
(802) 785-4029 (after 8:00 P.M. ET)
*See also* Metabolic Disorders

**Cockayne Syndrome**
*See* Share and Care Cockayne Syndrome
Network

**Coffin-Lowry Syndrome Foundation**
P.O. Box 10033
Bainbridge Island, WA 98110
(206) 842-1523

**Command Trust Network**
P.O. Box 17082
Covington, KY 41017
(606) 331-0055
(For information on postsurgical implant
problems)
*See also* Breast Implants

**Communicative Disorders**
*See* National Coalition for Research in
Neurological and Communicative
Disorders

**Computerized AIDS Information Network**
1213 North Highland Avenue
P.O. Box 38777
Hollywood, CA 90038
(213) 464-7400, ext. 450

**Computers for the Mute and Paralyzed**
P.O. Box 1229
Lancaster, Ca 93584
(800) 869-8531

**Cone Dystrophy**
*See* Richard A. Lewis, M.D., M.S.

**Congenital Adrenal Hyperplasia Support**
**Association, Inc.**
801 County Road, #3
Wrenshall, MN 55797
(218) 384-3863

**Congenital Central Hypoventilation**
**Syndrome Family Support Network**
71 Maple Street
Oneonta, NY 13820
(607) 432-8872

**Congenital Heart Anomalies Support,**
**Education, and Resources (CHASER)**
2112 North Wilkins Road
Swanton, OH 43558
(419) 825-5575
*See also* Heart Disorders

**Congenital Nevus Network**
6400 Wurzbach Road, #805
San Antonio, TX 78240-3886
(512) 523-8233
*See also* Giant Congenital Pigmented Nevus
Support Group
Sturge-Weber Foundation

**Contact a Family**
Carol Youngs, Assistant Director
170 Tottenham Court Road
16 Strutton Ground
London W1P0HA
United Kingdom
*See also* Rare Disease Support Groups

**Contact Group for Trisomy 9p**
11 Durgoyne Drive
Bearsden
Glasgow, Scotland
United Kingdom
*See also* Chromosomal Abnormalities

**Contraception**
*See* Fertility
Association for Voluntary Surgical
Contraception

**Cooley's Anemia Foundation, Inc.**
129-09 26th Street, Suite 203
Flushing, NY 11354-1131
(718) 321-2873
(800) 522-7222 (New York State)
*See also* Anemia

**Cord Blood Cell Service**
*See* Biocyte Corporation

**Cornelia de Lange Parent Information**
**Booklet**
Children's Memorial Hospital
8301 Dodge Street
Omaha, NE 68114

**Cornelia de Lange Syndrome Foundation**
60 Dyer Avenue
Collinsville, CT 06022-1273
(203) 693-0159
(800) 223-8355

**Corporation for Menke's Disease**
5720 Buckfield Court
Fort Wayne, IN 46804

**Council of Families with Visual**
**Impairment (formerly, American**
**Council of Blind Parents)**
6212 W. Franklin Street
Richmond, VA 23226
(804) 288-0395
*See also* Eye Disorders

**Council of Guilds for Infant Survival**
P.O. Box 3586
Davenport, IA 52808
(319) 322-4870
*See also* Parent Care
Children

**Council of Regional Networks for**
**Genetics Services**
Jessica G. Davis, M.D.
Cornell University Medical College
1300 York Ave, Genetics Box 53
New York, NY 10102
(212) 746-1496

**Council on Sex Information and**
**Education**
444 Lincoln Blvd., Suite 107
Venice, CA 90291

**Cox Foundation for Mitochondrial**
**Disease**
P.O. Box 156
Hartman, AR 72840-0156
(501) 497-1563

**Craniofacial Abnormalities**
Dept. of Plastic and Maxillofacial Surgery
University of Virginia Medical Center
Box 376
Charlottesville, VA 22908
(804) 924-5801

**Craniofacial Centre Children's Hospital**
300 Longwood Avenue
Boston, MA 02115
(617) 735-6309

**Craniofacial Disorders**
*See* AboutFace
AboutFace USA
American Cleft Palate Cranial Facial
Association
Children's Craniofacial Association
Cleft Palate Foundation
Craniofacial Abnormalities
Craniofacial Centre Children's Hospital
Craniofacial Family Association
Craniofacial Support Group
FACES—National Association for the
Craniofacially Handicapped
Forward Face
Goldenhar Syndrome Research and
Information Fund
Hemifacial Microsomia Family Support
Network
International Center for Skeletal
Dysplasia
Let's Face It
Amy Feldman Lewanda, M.D.
National Craniofacial Foundation
National Foundation for Facial
Reconstruction
National Institute of Dental Research
Orofacial Guild
Prescription Parents
Society for the Rehabilitation of the
Facially Disfigured

**Craniofacial Family Association**
170 Elizabeth Street, Suite 650
Toronto, Ontario M5G 1X8
Canada

**Craniofacial Support Group**
44 Helmsdale Road
Leamington Spa
Warwichshire CV32 7DW
United Kingdom
44 1926 334629

**Cri-du-Chat Society**
Department of Human Genetics
Medical College of Virginia
Box 33, MCV Station
Richmond, VA 23298
(804) 786-9632
*See also* 5p- Society
Chromosomal Abnormalities

**CRISP (Computer Retrieval of
Information on Scientific Projects)**
(301) 435-0650
(For information on biomedical research
funded by the Public Health Service)

**Crohn's and Colitis Foundation of
America, Inc.**
386 Park Avenue South, 17th Floor
New York, NY 10016-8804
(212) 685-3440
(800) 932-2423
*See also* National Foundation of Crohn's
and Colitis

**John T. Curnette, M.D., Ph.D.**
Scripps Research Institute
10666 North Torrey Pines Rd., CAL-1
La Jolla, CA 92037
(619) 554-9784
(For chronic neutropenia)

**Cushing Support and Research
Foundation, Inc.**
65 East India Row, Suite 22B
Boston, MA 02110
(617) 723-3824
*See also* Karen Elkind-Hirsch, Ph.D.
David N. Orth, M.D.
Roy E. Weiss, M.D., Ph.D

**Cutaneous Lymphoma Network**
University Dermatology Consultants
234 Goodman Street, Pavillion A-3
Cincinnati, OH 45269-0523
(513) 558-6955
*See also* Cancer

**Gordon B. Cutler, Jr., M.D.**
National Institutes of Health
9000 Rockville Pike
Building 10, Room 10N260
Bethesda, Maryland 20892
(For Turner syndrome)

**Cyclic Vomiting Syndrome Association**
13180 Caroline Court
Elm Grove, WI 53122
(414) 784-6842
*See also* David Fleisher, M.D.
Neurologic Disorders

**Cystic Fibrosis Foundation**
6931 Arlington Road
Bethesda, MD 20814
(301) 951-4422
(800) 334-4823
*See also* Canadian Cystic Fibrosis
Foundation

**Cystic Fibrosis Research Trust**
Alexandria House
5 Blyth Road
Bromley, Kent BR1 3RS
United Kingdom

**Cystic Hygroma and Lymphangioma
Support Group**
Villa Fontane, Church Road
Worth, Crawley
Sussex RH10 4RT
United Kingdom

**Cystinosis Foundation, Inc.**
1212 Broadway, Suite 830
Oakland, CA 94612
(510) 235-1052
(800) 392-8458
*See also* Jess G. Thoene, M.D.
Jerry A. Schneider, M.D.
William A. Gahl, M.D.

**Cystinuria Support Network**
22814 NE 21st Place
Redmond, WA 98053
(206) 868-2996
*See also* Charles Y.C. Pak, M.D.

**Cytomegalovirus (CMV) Clinic**
Children's Hospital of Saint Paul
345 North Smith Avenue
Saint Paul, MN 55102
*See also* National Congenital CMV Disease
Registry

**DB-Link (National Information
Clearinghouse on Children Who Are
Deaf-Blind)**
354 North Monmouth Avenue
Monmouth, OR 97361
(503) 838-8150
(800) 438-9376
*See also* Hearing Impairment

**Deaf Communications Institute**
P.O. Box 247
Fayville, MA 01745
(617) 872-9496 (Voice and TDD)
*See also* Hearing Impairment

**Deafness Research Foundation**
9 East 38th Street
New York, NY 10016-0003
(212) 684-6556 (Voice and TTY)
(800) 822-1327
*See also* Hearing Impairment

**Martha Dencklau, M.D.**
Johns Hopkins School of Medicine
600 North Wolf Street
Baltimore, MD 21205
(For Asperger syndrome)

**Dental Disorders**
*See* Albert D. Guckes, M.D.
American Association of Orthodontists
American Dental Association
National Foundation of Dentistry for the
Handicapped
NIH/National Institute of Dental Research

**Depression and Related Affective
Disorders Association**
Johns Hopkins Hospital
Meyer 3-181
600 North Wolfe Street
Baltimore, MD 21287-7381
(410) 955-4647
*See also* Mental Health

**Depressives Anonymous: Recovery from
Depression**
329 East 62nd Street
New York, NY 10021
*See also* Mental Health

**Dermatitis Herpetiformis**
*See* Russell P. Hall III, M.D.
Skin Disorders

**Dermatologic Disorders**
*See* Skin Disorders

**Dermatomyositis and Polymyositis
Support Group**
146 Newtown Road
Woolston
Southhampton SO2 9HR
United Kingdom
*See also* Inclusion Body Myositis
Association
National Support Group for Myositis
Skin Disorders

**DES-Action**
Long Island Jewish Hillside Medical Center
New Hyde Park, NY 11040
(516) 775-3450
or
1615 Broadway, Suite 510
Oakland, CA 94612
(510) 465-4011
(For diethysilbestrol, fetal effects)

**DES Cancer Network**
Box 10185
Rochester, NY 14610

**Robert Desnick, M.D.**
Division of Medical Genetics
Mount Sinai Hospital
Annenberg Building, Room 17-76
100th Street and 5th Avenue
New York, NY 10029

**Devereux Foundation**
19 South Waterloo Road, Box 400
Devon, PA 19333-0400
(610) 964-3000
*See also* Mental Health

**Diabetes**
*See* American Diabetes Association
Diabetes Insipidus and Related Disorders
Network
Juvenile Diabetes Foundation
International
NIH/National Diabetes Information
Clearinghouse
Gary L. Robertson
Robert S. Wildin, M.D.

**Diabetes Insipidus and Related
  Disorders Network**
Route 2, Box 198
Creston, IA 50801
(515) 782-7838

**Diamond-Blackfan Anemia Registry**
Adrianna Vlachos, M.D.
Mount Sinai Medical Center
One Gustave Levy Place, Box 1208
New York, NY 10029-6574
(212) 241-6031

**Diamond-Blackfan Anemia Support
  Group**
Ted Gordon-Smith, M.D.
11 Hollyfield Avenue
London N11 3BY
United Kingdom
81-784-2645

**Angelo M. DiGeorge, M.D.**
Temple University School of Medicine
Section of Endocrinology and Metabolism
St. Christopher's Hospital for Children
Erie Avenue at Front Street
Philadelphia, PA 19134
(215) 427-5173

**DiGeorge Syndrome**
See Angelo M. DiGeorge, M.D.
  Frank Greenberg, M.D.
  Information and Support for DiGeorge
    and Shprintzen Syndrome Families
  Craig B. Langman, M.D.

**Digestive Disease**
See Digestive Disease National Coalition
  Joseph Murray, M.D.
  NIH/National Digestive Diseases
    Information Clearinghouse

**Digestive Disease National Coalition**
711 Second Street NE, Suite 200
Washington, DC 20002
(202) 544-7497

**Direct Link for the Disabled**
P.O. Box 1036
Solvang, CA 93464
(805) 688-1603

**Disability Referrals**
See Beach Center on Families and
    Disability
  Center for Accessible Housing
  Clearinghouse on Disability Information
  Coalition on Sexuality and Disability
  Direct Link for the Disabled
  Family Resource Center on Disabilities
  Friends of Disabled Adults
  Higher Education and the Handicapped
    Resource Center
  Learning Disabilities
  Mobility International USA
  National Accessible Apartment
    Clearinghouse
  National Center for Youth with Disabilities
  National Easter Seal Society for Crippled
    Children and Adults
  National Foundation of Dentistry for the
    Handicapped

  National Information Center for Children
    and Youth with Disabilities
  National Library Service for the Blind and
    Physically Handicapped
  National Parent Network on Disabilities
  New York State Institute for Basic
    Research in Developmental Disabilities
  Parent Care
  Rocky Mountain Research and Training
    Institute
  Siblings for Significant Change
  Siblings of Children with Disabilities
  Travelin' Talk
  U.S. Architectural Transportation Barriers
    Compliance Board

**Dissatisfied Parents Together**
128 Branch Road
Vienna, VA 22180
(703) 938-3783
  (For parents of children who have had a
    severe adverse reaction to a vaccine)

**Division of Medical Genetics**
Department of Medicine
University of Calfornia, San Diego
9500 Gilman
La Jolla, CA 92093-0639
(619) 534-4307

**Division of Medical Genetics**
Georgetown University Medical Center
3800 Reservoir Road NW
Washington, DC 20007
(202) 687-8810

**Dizziness and Balance Disorder
  Association**
See Vestibular Disorders Association

**William B. Dobyns, M.D.**
Indiana School of Medicine
Riley Hospital for Children
702 Barnhill Drive
Indianapolis, IN 46202
(For lissencephaly)

**Down Syndrome**
See Association for Children with Down
    Syndrome
  Down Syndrome Association
  National Center for Down's Syndrome
  National Down Syndrome Congress
  National Down Syndrome Society

**Down Syndrome Association**
155 Mitcham Road
Tooting
London SW17 9PG
United Kingdom
081 682-4001

**Drug Abuse**
See Center for Substance Abuse Prevention
  NIH/National Clearinghouse for Alcohol
    and Drug Information
  NIH/National Institute on Drug Abuse

**Thaddeus P. Dryja, M.D.**
Massachusetts Eye and Ear Infirmary
243 Charles Street
Boston, MA 02114
(617) 573-3319
(For retinoblastoma)

**Dubowitz Syndrome Parent Support
  Network**
20 East 46th Street, Room 302
New York, NY 10017
(212) 949-6644

**Dwarfism**
See Association for Research into
    Restricted Growth
  Human Growth Foundation
  Little People of America
  Little People's Research Fund
  Magic Foundation for Children's Growth
  Metatrophic Dysplasia Dwarf Registry
  Parents of Dwarfed Children
  Short Stature Foundation

**Dysautonomia Foundation, Inc.**
20 East 46th Street, Room 302
New York, NY 10017
(212) 949-6644

**Dyslexia**
See Orton Dyslexia Society

**Dysphonia**
See Andrew Blitzer, M.D.
  Sandra Chapman, M.D.
  Christy Ludlow, Ph.D.
  National Spasmodic Dysphonia
    Association
  Our Voice
  Parents of Chronically Ill Children
  Clarence T. Sasaki, M.D.

**Dysplasia, Skeletal**
See International Center for Skeletal
  Dysplasia

**Dystonia Clinical Research Center**
Columbia Presbyterian Hospital
710 West 168th Street
New York, NY 10032

**Dystonia Medical Research Foundation**
1 East Wacker Drive, Suite 2430
Chicago, IL 60601-2001
(312) 755-0198

**Dystrophic Epidermolysis Bullosa
  Research Association**
7 Sandhurst Lodge
Wokingham Road
Crowthrone, Berkshire RG11 7QD
United Kingdom
0344 771961

**Dystrophic Epidermolysis Bullosa
  Research Association of America**
40 Rector Street, 8th Floor
New York, NY 10006
(212) 693-6610

**Ear Anomalies Reconstructed:**
**Atresia/Microtia Support Group**
72 Durand Road
Maplewood, NJ 07040
(201) 761-5438

**Ear Disorders**
*See* American Tinnitus Association
Meniere Crouzon Syndrome Support
Network
Margareta Moller, M.D.
NIH/National Institute on Deafness and
Other Communication Disorders
Vestibular Disorders Association
Hearing Impairment

**E.A.R. Foundation**
2420 Castillo Street
Santa Barbara, CA 93105
(805) 962-7661, ext. 460

**E.A.R. Foundation at Baptist Hospital**
2000 Church Street, Box 111
Nashville, TN 37236
(615) 329-7807
(800) 545-4327 (Voice and TDD)

**Earl J. Goldberg Aplastic Anemia**
**Foundation**
P.O. Box 2231
Glenview, IL 60025
(708) 559-0688

**EASE: Education and Support Exchange**
P.O. Box 1151
Monroeville, PA 15146-1151
(412) 856-9176
*See* Mitochondrial Disease

**Easter Seal Society**
*See* National Easter Seal Society

**Eating Disorders**
*See* American Anorexia and Bulemia
Association
American Society of Bariatric Physicians
Anorexia and Bulemia Treatment and
Education Center
Anorexia Nervosa and Associated
Disorders
Anorexia Nervosa and Related Eating
Disorders
Anxiety Disorders Association of America
Bulimia, Anorexia Self-Help
Center for Stress and Anxiety Disorders
National Anorexic Aid Society
National Association of Anorexia Nervosa
and Associated Disorders
Obesity Foundation

**Ectodermal Dysplasias**
*See* National Foundation for Ectodermal
Dysplasias

**Eczema Association for Science and**
**Education**
1221 South West Yamhill, Suite 303
Portland, OR 97205
(503) 228-4430
*See also* Skin Disorders

**Education and Support Exchange**
*See* EASE

**Ehlers-Danlos National Foundation**
P.O. Box 1212
Southgate, MI 48195
(313) 282-0180

**Ehlers Danlos Support Group**
2 High Garth Road
Richmond, North Yorkshire DC10 4DG
United Kingdom
0423 871651

**Ehlers Danlos Syndrome**
*See* Arizona State Ehlers-Danlos
Association
Ehlers-Danlos National Foundation
Ehlers Danlos Support Group

**David Ehrmann, M.D.**
Department of Medicine
University of Chicago Medical Center
5841 Maryland Avenue, Box 435
(312) 702-965
(For Stein-Leventhal syndrome)

**Elective Mutism Support Group**
99-52 66th Road, 1J
Forest Hills, NY 11375

**John Elefteriades, M.D.**
Cardiothoracic Surgery
Yale University School of Medicine
121 FMB, 333 Cedar Street
New Haven, CT 06520
(203) 785-2705
(For Ondine's curse; sleep apnea)

**Karen Elkind-Hirsch, Ph.D.**
The Methodist Hospital
Department of Medicine-MS b200
6565 Fanin Street
Houston, TX 77030
(713) 793-1088
(For Cushing syndrome)

**Emphysema Anonymous, Inc.**
P.O. Box 3224
Seminole, FL 34642

**Encephalomyelitis**
*See* Myalgic Encephalomyelitis Association

**Encephaly**
*See* Fighters for Encephaly Support Group
Theodore Rasmussen, M.D.

**Endocrine Disorders**
*See* Congenital Adrenal Hyperplasia
Support Association
National Adrenal Diseases Foundation
NIH/Developmental Endocrinology
Branch
NIH/National Institute of Diabetes,
Digestive and Kidney Diseases

**Endometriosis Association**
8585 North 76th Place
Milwaukee, WI 53223
(800) 992-3636
*See* Fertility

**Odile Enjolras, M.D.**
Department of Dermatology
Hospital Tarnier
Paris, France
(For Sturge-Weber syndrome)

**Enteric Feeding**
*See* American Society of Parenteral and
Enteral Nutrition

**Environmental Disorders**
*See* American Academy of Environmental
Medicine
Chemosensory Clinical Research Center
of Connecticut
Hanford Health Information Network
National Association of Radiation
Survivors
National Center for Environmental Health
Strategies
National Council on Radiation Protection
and Measurements
NIH/National Institute of Environmental
Health Sciences
Allergies/Asthma

**Epidermolysis Bullosa**
*See* Eugene Bauer, M.D.
Dystrophic Epidermolysis Bullosa
Research Association of America
Dystrophic Epidermolysis Bullosa
Research Association (U.K.)

**Epidermolytic Hyperkeratosis**
*See* Ervin H. Epstein Jr., M.D.
Robert D. Goldman, M.D.
Leonard Milstone, M.D.

**Epilepsy, Myoclonic Progressive Familial**
*See* Guy A. Rouleau, MD

**Epilepsy Foundation of America**
4351 Garden City Drive
Landover, MD 20785
(301) 459-3700 (Voice and TTY)
(800) 332-1000 (Voice)
(800) 332-2070 (TTY)
*See also* THRESHOLD

**Ervin H. Epstein, Jr., M.D.**
Department of Dermatology
University of California, San Francisco
San Francisco, CA
(415) 647-3992
(For epidermolytic hyperkeratosis)

**Fred J. Epstein, M.D.**
Department of Pediatric Neurosurgery
New York University School of Medicine
550 First Avenue
New York, NY 10016
(212) 263-6419
(For some inoperable brain tumors)

**Erb's Palsy**
*See* Brachial Plexus Injury

**Erythromelalgia and Related Disorders**
**Association of America, Inc.**
P.O. Box 4046
Portland, OR 97208

**Erythromelalgia Syndrome (EMS) Support Group**
c/o Television Workshop
3637 Green Road
Beachwood, OH 44122

**Esophageal Diseases**
*See* Atresia
    American Broncho-Esophagological
    Association

**European Association Against Leukodystrophies**
*See* Association Européenne contre les
    Leucodystrophes

**Evans Syndrome Support and Research Group**
5630 Devon Street
Port Orange, FL 32127
(904) 760-3031
*See also* Anemia

**Exstrophy of the Bladder**
*See* National Support Group for Exstrophy
    of the Bladder
    Kidney/Urologic Disorders

**Extracorporeal Membrane Oxygenation Support Group**
Department of Pediatrics
4th and Indiana Streets
Texas Tech, HSC
Lubbock, TX 79430
(806) 743-2284

**Eye Bank Association of America**
1511 K Street NW, Suite 830
Washington, DC 20005-1401
(301) 628-4280

**Eye Care**
13425 Hidden Meadow Court
Herndon, VA 22071

**Eye Disorders**
*See* American Council of the Blind
    American Foundation for the Blind
    American Printing House for the Blind
    Association for Macular Diseases
    Blind Children's Fund
    Council of Families with Visual
        Impairment
    For Our Children's Unique Sight (FOCUS)
    Foundation Fighting Blindness
    Foundation for Glaucoma Research
    Guiding Eyes for the Blind
    International Children's Anophthalmia
        Network
    International Institute for the Visually
        Impaired
    Richard A. Lewis, M.D.
    Maria A. Musarella, M.D.
    National Association for Parents of the
        Visually Impaired
    National Association for the Visually
        Handicapped
    National Eye Care Project
    National Eye Research Foundation
    National Federation of the Blind
    National Library Service for the Blind and
        Physically Handicapped

National Retinoblastoma Parent Group
National Society to Prevent Blindness
NIH/National Eye Institute
Recording for the Blind
Retinitis Pigmentosa International
Schepens Eye Research Institute
Vision Foundation
Macular Dystrophy

**Fabry Disease**
*See* International Center for Fabry Disease

**FACES—National Association for the Craniofacially Handicapped**
P.O. Box 11082
Chattanooga, TN 37401
(615) 266-1632
(800) 332-2373

**Facial Reconstruction**
*See* National Foundation for Facial
    Reconstruction

**Facioscapulohumeral (FSH) Society**
3 Westwood Road
Lexington, MA 02173
(617) 860-0501
*See also* Muscular Dystrophy, Landouzy-
Dejerine

**Fahr Disease Registry**
Parkinson's Disease and Movement
    Disorders Clinic
Bala V. Manyam, M.D.
Southern Illinois University School of
    Medicine
P.O. Box 19230
Springfield, IL 62794-9230
*See also* Parkinson Disease

**Familial Erythrophagocytic Histiocytosis Support Group**
609 New York Road
Glassboro, NJ 08028
(800) 548-2758

**Familial Erythrophagocytic Lymphohistiocytosis (FEL) Network**
2519 West Twonig
San Antonio, TX 76901
(915) 949-4228

**Familial Polyposis Registry**
Department of Colorectal Surgery
Cleveland Clinic Foundation
9500 Euclid Avenue
Cleveland, OH 44195-5001
(216) 444-6470
*See also* Polyposis

**Families with Maple Syrup Urine Disease**
Route 2, Box 24-19
Flemingsburg, KY 41041
(606) 849-4679
*See also* Kidney/Urologic Disorders

**Families with Moyamoya Support Network**
4900 McGowan Street SE
Cedar Rapids, IA 52403
(319) 364-6847
(800) 261-6692

**Families of Spinal Muscular Atrophy (SMA)**
P.O. Box 196
Libertyville, IL 60048
(708) 367-7620
(800) 886-1762

**Family Caregiver Alliance**
425 Bush Street, Suite 500
San Francisco, CA 94108
(415) 434-3388
(800) 445-8106 (in California)
*See also* National Family Caregivers
    Association

**Family Empowerment Network**
610 Langdon Street, #521
Madison, WI 53703
(608) 262-6590
(800) 462-5254

**Family Resource Center on Disabilities**
20 East Jackson, Room 900
Chicago, IL 60604
(312) 939-3513
(800) 952-4199
(312) 939-3519

**Fanconi Anemia Research Fund, Inc.**
1902 Jefferson Street, Suite 2
Eugene, OR 97405
(503) 687-4658
*See also* Blanche Alter, M.D.
    Arleen Auerbach, M.D.
    International Fanconi Registry
    Johnson M. Liu, M.D.
    Neal S. Young, M.D.

**Food and Drug Administration Breast Implant Hotline**
(800) 532-4440
(For women considering implant surgery)
*See also* Breast Implants

**Federation of Families for Children's Mental Health**
1021 Prince Street
Alexandria, VA 22314-02971
(703) 684-7710

**Fertility**
*See* American Fertility Society
    American Society of Reproductive
        Medicine
    Association for Voluntary Surgical
        Contraception
    Endometriosis Association
    Fertility Research Foundation
    Resolve

**Fertility Research Foundation**
1430 Second Ave.
New York, NY 10021
(212) 744-5000

**Fetal Alcohol Education Program**
7 Kent Street
Brookline, MA 02146
(617) 739-1424
*See also* National Organization on Fetal
    Alcohol Syndrome

**FG Syndrome Support Group**
66 Ford Road
Dagenham, Essex RM10 9JR
United Kingdom
*See also* John M. Opitz, M.D.

**Fibrodysplasia Ossificans Progressiva**
*See* International Fibrodysplasia Ossificans
    Progressiva Association

**Fibromyalgia**
*See* Fibromyalgia Association of Central
    Ohio
    Fibromyalgia Association of Texas
    Fibromyalgia Educational Systems
    Fibromyalgia Network
    National Chronic Fatigue and
        Fibromyalgia Association
    National Fibromyalgia Research
        Association
    Ontario Fibromyalgia Association

**Fibromyalgia Association of Central Ohio**
P.O. 21988
Columbus, OH 43221-0988
(614) 457-4222

**Fibromyalgia Association of Texas**
5650 Forest Lane
Dallas, TX 75230

**Fibromyalgia Educational Systems**
500 Bushaway Road
Wayzata, MN 55391

**Fibromyalgia Network**
P.O. Box 31750
Tucson, AZ 85751-1750
(520) 290-5508
(800) 853-2929

**Fibular Hemimelia**
Superkids Newsletter
60 Clyde Street
Newton, MA 02160

**Fighters for Encephaly Support Group**
332 Brereton Street
Pittsburgh, PA 15219
(412) 687-6437
(412) 331-4365

**Filariasis**
*See* International Filariasis Association

**Finding Our Own Ways**
P.O. Box 1545
Lawrence, KS 66044
*See also* Sexual Disorders

**5p- Society**
11609 Oakmont
Overland Park, KS 66210
(913) 469-8900
*See also* Cri-du-Chat Society
    Chromosomal Abnormalities

**David B. Flannery, M.D.**
Division of Medical Genetics
Department of Pediatrics BG-121
Medical College of Georgia
Augusta, GA 30912
(404) 721-2809
(For Joubert syndrome)

**David Fleisher, M.D.**
Department of Child Health
University of Missouri School of Medicine
Columbia, MO 65212
(314) 882-6993
(For cyclic vomiting)

**Focal Dermal Hypoplasia**
*See* Albert D. Guckes, M.D.
    Dental Disorders

**Food and Drug Administration (FDA)**
Center for Biologics Evaluation and
    Research (CBER)
E-mail: CBER_INFO@A1.CBER.FDA.GOV
(301) 594-1934
(For information on newly approved biotech
    drugs)

**Food and Drug Administration (FDA)**
Office of Consumer Affairs
5600 Fisher Lane, Room 12-A-40
Rockville, MD 20857
(301) 443-4903

**Food and Drug Administration (FDA)**
Office of Orphan Products
5600 Fishers Lane (HF-35; Room 8-73)
Rockville, MD 20857
(301) 443-4903

**For Our Children's Unique Sight (FOCUS)**
1583 Black Eagle Drive, Unit D
San Diego, CA 92126
(619) 271-8488
*See also* Eye Disorders

**49XXXXY**
10001 NE 74th Street
Vancouver, WA 98662-3801
*See also* Chromosomal Abnormalities

**Forward Face**
317 East 34th Street, Suite 901
New York, NY 10016
(212) 684-5860
(800) 422-3223
*See also* Craniofacial Disorders

**Foundation Fighting Blindness**
1401 Mount Royal Avenue
Baltimore, MD 21217-4245
(410) 225-9400/-9404 (TDD)
(800) 683-5555/-5551 (TDD)
*See also* Eye Disorders

**Foundation for Childhood Cancer**
House 52, Road 3/A
Dhanmondi R/A, Dhaka-1209
Bangladesh
India
88-02-865058
*See also* Children

**Foundation for Glaucoma Research**
490 Post Street, Suite 830
San Francisco, CA 94102
(415) 986-3162
*See also* Eye Disorders

**Foundation for Ichthyosis and Related
    Skin Types**
P.O. Box 20921
Raleigh, NC 27619-0921
(919) 782-5728
(800) 545-3286

**Foundation for Nager and Miller
    Syndromes**
333 Country Lane
Glenview, IL 60025-5104
(708) 729-6449
(800) 507-FNMS

**Foundation for Pulmonary Hypertension**
P.O. Box 61540
New Orleans, LA 70161
(504) 533-5888
*See also* Hypertension
    Lung Disorders

**4p- Parent Contact Group**
2048 South 182 Circle
Omaha, NJ 68130
*See also* Wolf-Hirschhorn Syndrome
    Chromosomal Abnormalities

**Tom Fowler**
Boys Town National Research Hospital
Branchio-Oto-Renal Project
555 North 30th Street
Omaha, NE 68131
(800) 835-1468 (voice or TDD)
(For branchio-oto-renal syndrome)

**Fragile X Association of Michigan**
1786 Edinborough Drive
Rochester Hills, MI 48306
(313) 373-3043

**Fragile X Foundation**
P.O. Box 300233
Denver, CO 80220

**Fragile X Syndrome**
*See* Fragile X Association of Michigan
    Fragile X Foundation
    FRAXA Research Foundation
    National Fragile X Foundation
    New York State Institute for Basic
        Research in Developmental Disabilities
    Valerie Simon
    Disability Referrals

**Uta Francke, M.D.**
Howard Hughes Medical Institute
Stanford University School of Medicine
Beckman Center, B205
Stanford, CA 94305
(415) 725-8089
(For Roberts syndrome)

**FRAXA Research Foundation, Inc.**
P.O. Box 935
West Newbury, MA 01985
(508) 462-1990

**Irwin M. Freedberg, M.D.**
New York University Medical Center
Department of Dermatology
550 First Avenue
New York, NY 10016
(212) 340-5245
(For pityriasis rubra pilaris)

**Freeman-Sheldon Gene Mapping Project**
Division of Pediatric Genetics
UREB 413
University of Utah Medical Center
Salt Lake City, UT 84112
(801) 581-8943

**Freeman-Sheldon Parent Support Group**
509 East Northmont Way
Salt Lake City, UT 84103-3324
(801) 364-7060

**Friends of Disabled Adults, Inc.**
4600 Lewis Road
Stone Mountain, GA 30083
(404) 491-9014
See also Disability Referrals

**Friends of the Osteopetrosis Support Trust (FROST)**
37 Reade Road
Holbrook, Ipswich IPG 202
United Kingdom
014 73328083

**Lauren S. Frisch, M.D.**
Reproductive Endocrine Unit
Bartlett Hall Extension, 5th Floor
Massachusetts General Hospital
Fruit Street
Boston, MA 02114
(617) 726-8433, ext. 337

**Frontier's International Vitiligo Foundation**
4 Rozina Court
Owings Mills, MD 21117
(301) 594-0958
See also Skin Disorders

**William A. Gahl, M.D.**
Section of Human Biochemical Genetics
NICHD
Building 10, Room 9S242
Bethesda, MD 20892
(301) 496-9101
(For cystinosis)

**Galactosemia**
See Parents of Galactosemic Children

**Brenda Gallie, M.D.**
Eye Research Institute of Canada
Hospital for Sick Children
399 Bathurst Street
Toronto, Ontario M5T 2F8 Canada
(416) 369-5181
(For retinoblastoma)

**W.R. Gammon, M.D.**
Department of Dermatology
University of North Carolina
137 NC Memorial Hospital
Chapel Hill, NC 27514
(For bullous pemphigoid)

**Ganglioside Sialidase Deficiency**
See ML 4 Foundation
Metabolic Disorders

**Abhimanyu Garg, M.D.,**
University of Texas Southwestern Medical Center
5323 Harry Hines Blvd.
Dallas, TX 75235
(214) 688-2895
(For lipodystrophy)

**Gastrointestinal Cancer, Familial**
See Steve Atanas Stavro Familial Gastrointestinal Cancer Registry

**Gastrointestinal Polyposis and Hereditary Colon Cancer Registry**
Center for Medical Genetics
Johns Hopkins Hospital
600 North Wolfe Street
Baltimore, MD 21287-4922
(410) 955-3875
See also Polyposis

**Gaucher's Disease Foundation**
11140 Rockville Pike, Suite 350
Rockville, MD 20852
(301) 816-1515
(800) 925-8885
See also National Gaucher Foundation
Robert E. Lee, M.D.
Connie Kreps
Ramnik Xavier

**Gay Men's Health Crisis**
129 West 20th Street
New York, NY 10011
(212) 807-6655

**Gazette International Networking Institute**
5100 Oakland Avenue
Saint Louis, MO 63110-1406
(314) 534-0475

**Gender Identification**
See Ambiguous Genitalia Support Network
International Foundation for Gender Education
Sexual Disorders

**Gene Research**
See Genetics Institute
Genome Data Base
National Center for Human Genome Research

**Genetic Diseases**
See Chromosomal Abnormalities

**Genetics Institute, Inc.**
87 Cambridge Park Drive
Cambridge, MA 02140

**Genitalia, Ambiguous**
See Ambiguous Genitalia Support Network

**Genome Data Base and On-Line Mendelian Inheritance in Man**
Lay Gottesman
Applied Research Laboratory
Johns Hopkins University School of Medicine
2024 East Monument Street
Baltimore, MD 21205-2100
(410) 955-7058
(Internet: help@welch.jhu.edu)

**Morie A. Gertz, M.D**
Dept. of Hematology and Internal Medicine
Mayo Clinic
Rochester, MN 55905
(507) 284-2511
(For amyloidosis)

**Giant Congenital Pigmented Nevus Support Group**
12 Twixt Hill Road
Ridgefield, CT 06877
(203) 438-3863
See also Congenital Nevus Network

**Glaucoma**
See Foundation for Glaucoma Research

**Daniel Glaze, M.D.,**
Department of Pediatrics
Rett Syndrome Center
Baylor College of Medicine
Houston, TX 77030
(For Rett syndrome)

**Glutaricaciduria**
See Stephen Goodman, M.D.

**Gluten Intolerance Group of North America**
P.O. Box 23053
Seattle, WA 98102-0353
(206) 325-6980
See also Celiac Sprue Association/USA

**Glycogen Storage Disease**
See Association for Glycogen Storage Diseases

**Rosalie Goldberg**
Robert J. Shprintzen, Ph.D.
Center for Craniofacial Disorders
Albert Einstein College of Medicine
111 East 210th Street
Bronx, NY 10467
(718) 920-4781
(For Shprintzen syndrome)

**Goldenhar Syndrome Research and Information Fund**
8829 Gleneagles Lane
Darien, IL 60561
(708) 910-3939
See also Craniofacial Disorders

**Robert D. Goldman, M.D.**
Department of Cell Biology and Anatomy
Northwestern University Medical School
Chicago, IL
(312) 503-4215
(For epidermolytic hyperkeratosis)

**David Goldstein, M.D.,**
Clinical Neuroscience Branch
(NIH) National Institute of Neurological
    Disorders and Stroke
9000 Rockville Pike
Bethesda, MD 20892
(301) 496-8850
(For Shy-Drager syndrome)

**Stephen Goodman, M.D.**
Department of Pediatrics
Box C233, 4200 East Ninth Avenue
University of Colorado Health Science
    Center
Denver, CO 80262
(For glutaricaciduria)

**Wayne Goodman, M.D.**
Clinical Neuroscience Research Unit
Yale School of Medicine
34 Park Street
New Haven, CT 06508
(203) 298-7334
(For trichotillomania)

**Jerome Gorski, M.D.**
University of Michigan Medical Center
Pediatric Genetics
Room 3570, MSRBII, Box 0688
Ann Arbor, MI 48109-0688
(313) 764-0579
(For Aarskog syndrome)

**Jordan Grafman, Ph.D.**
Cognitive Neuroscience Section
Medical Neurology Branch
NIH/National Institute of Neurological
    Disorders and Stroke
Bldg. 10, Rm. 5C422
Bethesda, MD 20892
(301) 496-0220
(For Pick disease)

**Graft-versus-Host Disease**
See Georgia B. Vogelsang, M.D.

**John M. Graham, Jr., M.D.**
Cedars-Sinai Medical Center
444 South San Vicente Boulevard
Suite 1001
Los Angeles, CA 90048
(310) 855-2211
(For Pallister-Hall syndrome; XYY
    syndrome)

**Granulomatous Disorders**
See Chronic Granulomatous Disease
    Association
    Chronic Granulomatous Disease Registry

**Graves Disease**
See Paul W. Ladenson, M.D.
    National Graves' Disease Foundation

**Frank Greenberg, M.D.**
Baylor College of Medicine
Molecular Genetics
Texas Children's Hospital, Room 0154
6621 Fannin Road
Houston, TX 77030
(713) 798-4951
(For DiGeorge syndrome)

**Paul Greenberger, M.D.**
Northwestern University
Allergy/Immunology Section
303 East Chicago Avenue
Chicago, IL 60611
312-908-8171
(For aspergillosis)

**Group B Strep Association**
P.O. Box 16515
Chapel Hill, NC 27516
(919) 932-5344

**Guardians of Hydrocephalus Research
    Foundation**
2618 Avenue Z
Brooklyn, NY 11235
(718) 743-4473
(800) 458-8655

**Guardianship Services**
See Lifetime Advocacy Plus

**Lisa M. Guay-Woodford, M.D.**
Division of Nephrology
Children's Hospital in Boston
300 Longwood Avenue
Boston, MA 02115
(617) 735-6129
(For polycystic kidney disease)

**Albert D. Guckes, M.D.**
Dental Clinic
National Institute of Dental Research
Bldg. 10, Rm. 6S-255
Bethesda, MD 20892
(301) 496-4371 or 496-2944
(For focal dermal hypoplasia)

**Guiding Eyes for the Blind, Inc.**
611 Granite Springs Road
Yorktown Heights, NY 10598
(914) 245-4024
(For information on guide dogs)
See also Eye Disorders

**Guillain-Barré Syndrome Foundation
    International**
P.O. Box 262
Wynnewood, PA 19096
(610) 667-0131

**Gynecologic Oncology**
See New England Medical Center

**Haemophilia Society**
P.O. Box 9
16 Trinity Street
London SE1 1DE
United Kingdom
01-71-407-1010
See also Hemophilia

**Hairy Cell Leukemia Foundation**
P.O. Box 72
Newtonville, MA 02160
(617) 244-8478
See also Cancer

**Russell P. Hall III, M.D.**
Box 3135
Duke University Medical Center
Durham, NC 27710
(919) 684-3110
(For dermatitis herpetiformis)

**Hallermann-Streiff Support Group**
1367 Beulah Park
Lexington, KY 40597
(606) 273-6928

**Mark Hallet, M.D.**
NIH/National Institute of Neurological
    Disorders and Stroke
9000 Rockville Pike
Bldg. 31, Room 8A06
Bethesda, MD 20892
(301) 496-5751
(For stiff-man syndrome)

**Handicapped**
See Disability Referrals

**Hanford Health Information Network**
1719 Smith Tower
506 Second Avenue
Seattle, WA 98104
(206) 223-7660
(800) 959-7660
(For information on radiation exposure from
    the Hanford site in Washington)
See also Environmental Disorders

**Hansen Disease (Leprosy)**
See American Leprosy Missions
    National Hansen Disease Center

**Hantavirus**
See Navajo Virus

**Frances Harley, M.D.**
Department of Pediatrics
4-120A, C.S.B.
University of Alberta
Edmonton, Alberta TG6 2G3
Canada
(403) 432-6631
(For intestinal pseudo-obstruction)

**Head Injury**
See Brain Injury Association

**Headache**
See National Headache Foundation
    National Migraine Foundation

**Healthy Mothers, Healthy Babies**
409 Twelfth Street SW
Washington, DC 20024
(202) 863-2458

**HEAR NOW**
9745 East Hampden Avenue, Suite 300
Denver, CO 80231
(303) 695-7797
(800) 648-4327
(For free recycled hearing aids)

## Hearing Impairment
See Alexander Graham Bell Association for
    the Deaf
    American Hearing Research Foundation
    American Humane Association (for
    trained hearing dogs)
    American Society for Deaf Children
    American Speech-Language-Hearing
    Association
    American Tinnitus Association
    Better Hearing Institute
    DB-Link
    Deaf Communications Institute
    Deafness Research Foundation
    Hear Now
    International Association of Parents of
    the Deaf
    National Association of the Deaf
    National Information Center on Deafness
    National Crisis Center for the Deaf
    Self-Help for Hard-of-Hearing People
    Ear Disorders

## Heart Disease Research Foundation
50 Court Street
Brooklyn, NY 11201

## Heart Disorders
See American Society of Hypertension
    American Heart Association
    Big Hearts for Little Hearts
    Congenital Heart Anomalies, Support,
    Education, and Resources
    Heart Disease Research Foundation
    International Bundle Branch Block
    Association
    International Long QT Syndrome Registry
    National Stroke Association
    NIH/National Heart, Lung and Blood
    Institute
    Sudden Arrhythmia Death Syndrome
    Foundation

## Hearts and Hands
4115 Thomasville Road
Winston-Salem, NC 27107
(910) 788-1433

## Help for Incontinent People, Inc.
P.O. Box 544
Union, SC 29379
(803) 579-7900
(800) 252-3337
See also Association for Urinary Continence
    Control
    Kidney/Urologic Disorders

## Help Hospitalized Children's Fund
10723 Preston Road #132
Dallas, TX 75230
(214) 696-4351 (fax)

## Helping Hand
12 Arlington Street
Portland, ME 04101

## Helping Hands
109 Chestnut Street
Andover, MA 01810
(617) 475-6888
(617) 475-3388

## Hemifacial Microsomia Family Support
## Network
6 Country Lane Way
Philadelphia, PA 19115
(215) 677-4787
See also Craniofacial Disorders

## Hemimelia
See Fibular Hemimelia

## Hemiplegia, Alternating
See International Foundation for Alternating
    Hemiplegia of Childhood

## Hemochromatosis
See Hemochromatosis Foundation
    Iron Overload Diseases Association
    NIH/National Institute of Diabetes,
    Digestive and Kidney Diseases

## Hemochromatosis Foundation, Inc.
P.O. Box 8569
Albany, NY 12208
(518) 489-0972

## Hemodialysis
See American Association of Kidney
    Patients
    National Association of Patients on
    Hemodialysis and Transplantation

## Hemophilia
See Canadian Hemophilia Society
    Haemophilia Society
    NIH/National Heart, Lung and Blood
    Institute Information Center
    National Hemophilia Foundation
    World Federation of Hemophilia

## Wayne Hening, M.D.
Neurology Service 127
Veterans Administration Medical Center
Lyons, NJ 07939
(For restless legs syndrome)

## Hepatic Disorders
See Liver Disorders

## Hereditary Colorectal Cancer Registry
Johns Hopkins Hospital
550 N. Broadway, #108
Baltimore, MD 21205-2011
(410) 955-3875

## Hereditary Disease Foundation, Inc.
1427 7th Avenue, #2
Santa Monica, CA 90401-9798
(310) 458-4183

## Hereditary Hemorrhagic Telangiectasis
## (HHT) Foundation International, Inc.
P.O. Box 8087
New Haven, CT 06530
(800) 448-6389
(313) 561-2537
See also Martin D. Phillips, M.D.

## Hereditary Hemorrhagic Telangiectasis
## Registry
(Osler-Weber-Rendu Syndrome Registry)
c/o Robert I. White, Jr., M.D.
Yale School of Medicine
Department of Diagnostic Radiology
333 Cedar Street
P.O. Box 3333
New Haven, CT 06510
(203) 785-6938

## Hereditary Nephritis Foundation
P.O. Box 57294
Murray, UT 84157-0294
(801) 262-1465
See also Kidney/Urologic Disorders

## Hermansky-Pudlak Syndrome Network
39 Riveria Court
Malverne, NY 11565-1602
(516) 599-2077
(800) 789-9477

## Hermaphroditism, True
See John Mahoney, M.D.

## Herpes Support Group at Help South Bay
(408) 296-1444
See also Sexually Transmitted Diseases

## Michael Hershfield, M.D.
Duke University Hospital
Box 3049, Room 418
Sands Building, Research Drive
Durham, NC 27710
(919) 684-4184
(For severe combined immunodeficiency;
    PEG-ADA)

## Higher Education and the Handicapped
## Resource Center (HEATH)
One Dupont Circle NW
Washington, DC 20036
(800) 544-3284
See also Disability Referrals

## Hirschsprung Disease
See American Pseudo-obstruction and
    Hirschsprung's Disease Society
    Arvinda Chakekavarti, M.D.

## Histiocytosis Association of America
302 North Broadway
Pitman, NJ 08071
(609) 589-6606
(800) 548-2758

## Histiocytosis-X Association of America
609 New York Road
Glassboro, NJ 08028-2417
(609) 881-4911
(800) 548-2758
See also Diane Komp, M.D.

## Gary S. Hoffman, M.D.
Randi Y. Levitt, M.D.
NIH/National Institute of Allergy and
    Infectious Diseases
9000 Rockville Pike
Bethesda, MD 20892
(301) 496-1124
(For Wegener granulomatosis)

**Holoprosencephaly-Fighters of Defects Support Group**
3032 Brereton Street
Pittsburgh, PA 15219
(412) 687-6437

**Homeopathic Medicine**
See NIH/Office of Alternative Medicine

**Hospice**
See National Hospice Organization
Children's Hospice International
Parent Care

**Human Growth Foundation**
7777 Leesburg Pike, Suite 202 South
Falls Church, VA 22043
(703) 883-1773
(800) 451-6434
See also Dwarfism

**Gary W. Hunninghake, M.D.**
Barbara White, M.D.
Pulmonary Disease Division, C33 GH
Dept. of Internal Medicine
University of Iowa Hospitals and Clinics
Iowa City, IA 52242
(319) 356-4187
(For scleroderma)

**Hunter Syndrome**
See Joseph Muenzer, M.D., Ph.D.

**Huntington Society of Canada**
13 Water Street North, No. 3
PO Box 333
Cambridge, Ontario NIR 5TB
Canada
(519) 622-1002

**Huntington's Disease Society of America**
140 West 22nd Street, 6th Floor
New York, NY 10011
(212) 242-1968
(800) 345-4372

**Hydrocephalus**
See Guardians of Hydrocephalus Research
Foundation
Hydrocephalus Association
Hydrocephalus Parent Support Group
International Federation for
Hydrocephalus and Spina Bifida
National Hydrocephalus Foundation

**Hydrocephalus Association**
870 Market Street, Suite 955
San Francisco, CA 94102-2904
(415) 776-4713

**Hydrocephalus Parent Support Group**
225 Dickerson Street, H-893
San Diego, CA 92103
(619) 695-3139
(619) 726-0507

**Hypercalcemia**
See Infantile Hypercalcaemia Foundation
Ltd.

**Hypertension, Pulmonary**
See American Society of Hypertension

Foundation for Pulmonary Hypertension
John H. Newman, M.D.
United Patients' Association for
Pulmonary Hypertension, Inc.

**Hyperoxaluria**
See Oxalosis and Hyperoxaluria Foundation

**Hyperparathyroidism**
See Paget Foundation

**Hyperplasia, Congenital Hyperplasia**
See Congenital Adrenal Hyperplasia
Support Association
National Adrenal Diseases Foundation

**Hypoglycemia**
See National Hypoglycemia Association

**Hypomyelination**
See Myelin Messenger

**Hypoparathyroidism Newsletter**
c/o James Sander
2835 Salmon
Idaho Falls, ID 83406
(208) 524-3857

**Hypophosphatasia**
See Michael P. Whyte, M.D.

**Hypopigmentation**
See National Organization for Albinism and
Hypopigmentation

**Hypotension, Orthostatic**
See David Robertson, M.D.

**Hysterectomy Education Resources and Service Foundation**
422 Bryn Mawr Avenue
Bala-Cynwyd, PA 19004

**Ichthyosis**
See Foundation for Ichthyosis and Related
Skin Types
Sherri Bale, M.D.

**IgA Nephropathy Support Network**
234 Summit Avenue
Jenkintown, PA 19046
(215) 884-8763
See also Kidney/Urologic Disorders

**Ileitis and Colitis**
See Crohn's and Colitis Foundation of
America, Inc.

**Immune Deficiency Foundation**
25 West Chesapeake Avenue, Suite 206
Towson, MD 21204
(410) 321-6647
(800) 296-4433 (for patients only)

**Immunodeficiency**
See American Autoimmune-Related
Diseases Association
Rebecca H. Buckley, M.D.
Andrew J. Cant, M.D.
Chronic Fatigue and Immune Dysfunction
Syndrome Society
Michael Hershfield, M.D.

Immune Deficiency Foundation
Gareth Morgan, M.D.
National Chronic Fatigue Syndrome and
Fibromyalgia Association

**Imperforate Anus Contact Group**
55 Peverell Road
Bowthorpe, Norwich, Norfolk
United Kingdom
See also Pull-Thru Network

**Impotence Information Center**
(Penis Implants)
(800) 328-3881

**Impotence Support Group**
Sunnybrook Medical Centre
University of Toronto Urology Clinic
2075 Bayview Avenue
Toronto, Ontario M4N 3M5
Canada
(416) 480-4024
(416) 480-4026

**Impotency**
See Impotence Information Center
Impotence Support Group
Impotency Institute of America
The Osbon Foundation

**Impotency Institute of America**
Impotents Anonymous
119 South Ruth Street
Maryville, TN 37801
(615) 983-6064
(800) 669-1603

**Inclusion Body Myositis Association, Inc.**
1420 Huron Court
Harrisonburg, VA 22801
(703) 433-7686
See also National Myositis Association

**Incontinence**
See Association for Urinary Continence
Control
Help for Incontinent People

**Incontinentia Pigmenti Network**
34929 Elm Street
Wayne, MI 48184
(313) 729-7912
See also Richard A. Lewis, M.D.

**Infantile Hypercalcaemia Foundation Ltd.**
37 Mulberry Green
Old Harlow, Essex CM17 OEY
United Kingdom
279-272-14

**Infants with Life-Threatening Illnesses**
See Council of Guilds for Infant Survival
Parent Care

**Infectious Diseases**
See Centers for Disease Control
NIH/National Institute of Allergy and
Infectious Diseases

**Infertility**
*See* Fertility

**Information and Support for DiGeorge and Shprintzen Syndrome Families**
27859 Lassen Street
Castaic, CA 91384-3702
(805) 294-3623

**Inherited Metabolism Disorders Clinic**
Health/Science Center
1056 East 19th Avenue
Denver, CO 80218
(303) 861-6847
*See also* Metabolic Disorders

**Institute of Reconstructive Plastic Surgery**
New York University Medical Center
550 First Avenue
New York, NY 10016
(212) 263-5834
*See also* American Society of Plastic and Reconstructive Surgeons, International

**International Alstrom's Syndrome Newsletter**
1006 Howard Road
Warminster, PA 18974

**International Association of Parents of the Deaf**
814 Thayer Avenue
Silver Spring, MD 20910
(301) 585-5400
*See also* Hearing Impairment

**International Atherosclerosis Society**
6565 Fannin Street
Methodist Hospital
Houston, TX 77030

**International Bundle Branch Block Association**
6631 West 83rd Street
Los Angeles, CA 90045-2899
(213) 670-9132
*See also* Heart Disorders

**International Center for Fabry Disease**
Human Genetics
Mount Sinai Medical Center, Box 1203
Fifth Avenue at 100th Street
New York, NY 10029
(212) 241-6944

**International Center for Skeletal Dysplasia**
Saint Joseph's Hospital
7620 York Road
Towson, MD 21204
(301) 337-1250
(For treatment, not information)
*See also* Craniofacial Disorders

**International Children's Anophthalmia Network (ican)**
Adele Schneider, M.D., or
Jill Stopfer, M.S.
Developmental Medicine and Genetics
Albert Einstein Medical Center
5501 Old York Road Levy 2W
Philadelphia, PA 19141
(215) 456-8722
(800) 580-4226
*See also* Eye Disorders
Children

**International Fanconi Registry**
The Rockefeller University
c/o Arleen Auerbach, Ph.D.
1230 York Avenue
New York, NY 10021
(212) 570-7533
*See also* Fanconi Anemia Research Fund
Anemia

**International Federation for Hydrocephalus and Spina Bifida**
c/o RBU Gata 3
11138 Stockholm
Sweden
Attention: David Bagares

**International Fibrodysplasia Ossificans Progressiva Association**
910 North Jericho Drive
Casselberry, FL 32707
(407) 365-4194

**International Filariasis Association**
Department of Helminthology
London School of Hygiene and Tropical Medicine
Heppel Street
London WC1 E 7HT
United Kingdom

**International Foundation for Alternating Hemiplegia of Childhood**
29 Leonard Road
Melrose, MA 02176-3917
(617) 665-8906

**International Foundation for Gender Education**
P.O. Box 367
Wayland, MA 01778
(617) 894-8340
*See also* Ambiguous Genitalia Support Network

**International Institute for Visually Impaired, 0-7, Inc.**
1975 Rutgers
East Lansing, MI 48823
(517) 322-2666
*See also* Eye Disorders

**International Joseph Diseases Foundation, Inc.**
P.O. Box 2550
Livermore, CA 94551-2550
(510) 371-1287

**International Lesch-Nyhan Disease Association**
11042 Ferndale Street
Philadelphia, PA 19116
(215) 677-4206

**International Long QT Syndrome Registry**
University of Rochester Medical Center
P.O. Box 653
Rochester, NY 14642-8653
(716) 275-5391
*See also* Sudden Arrhythmia Death Syndrome Foundation
Heart Disorders

**International Myeloma Foundation**
2120 Stanley Hills Drive
Los Angeles, CA 90046
(213) 654-3023
(800) 452-2873

**International Opitz Frias Syndrome Association**
116 June Avenue
Nanaimo, BC V9S 4R7
Canada
(604) 754-7088
*See also* Opitz Family Network

**International Peutz-Jeghers Support Group**
Center for Medical Genetics
Johns Hopkins Hospital
Blalock 1008
600 North Wolfe Street
Baltimore, MD 21287-4922
Attention: Anne Krush, M.D.

**International Polio Network**
5100 Oakland Avenue, #206
Saint Louis, MO 63110-1406
(314) 534-0475

**International Progeria Registry**
Human Genetics
Institute for Research
1050 Forest Hill Road
Staten Island, NY 10314
(718) 494-5333

**International Rett Syndrome Association**
9121 Piscataway Road, Suite 2B
Clinton, MD 20735-2561
(301) 856-3334
(800) 818-7388
*See also* Research for Rett Foundation

**International Shriners Headquarters**
2900 Rocky Point Drive
Tampa, FL 33607
(800) 237-5055
(800) 282-9161 (in FL)
(800) 361-7256 (in Canada)
(813) 281-0300
(For severe burns)

**International Tremor Foundation**
833 West Washington Boulevard
Chicago, IL 60607
(312) 733-1893

**Intersex Society of North America**
P.O. Box 31791
San Francisco, CA 94131
(415) 695-0975
See also Sexual Disorders

**Interstitial Cystitis Association of America**
P.O. Box 1553
Madison Square Station
New York, NY 10159
(212) 979-6057
(800) 435-7422
See also Kidney/Urologic Disorders

**Intestinal Multiple Polyposis and Colorectal Cancer (IMPACC)**
P.O. Box 11
Conyngham, PA 18219
(717) 788-3712
(717) 788-1818
See also Polyposis

**Intestinal Pseudo-obstruction**
See American Pseudo-obstruction and Hirschsprung's Disease Society
American Society of Adults with Pseudo-obstruction
Frances Harley, M.D.
Intestinal Pseudoobstruction (IP) Support Network
North American Pediatric Pseudoobstruction Society

**Intestinal Pseudoobstruction (IP) Support Network**
34929 Elm
Wayne, MI 48184
(313) 729-7912

**Intraventricular Hemorrhage (IVH) Parents**
P.O. Box 56-1111
Miami, FL 33256-1111
(305) 232-0381

**Inverted Duplication Exchange and Advocacy**
RD 1, Box 260B
Thomasville, PA 17364-9768
(717) 225-5229
(For chromosome 15 only)
See also Chromosomal Abnormalities

**Iron Overload Diseases Association**
433 Westwind Drive
North Palm Beach, FL 33408
(407) 840-8512
See also Hemochromatosis, Hereditary

**Istituto Di Ricerche Clinciche per le Malattie Rare**
Arrigo Schieppati, M.D.
Erica Daina, M.D.
Villa Camozzi
Via G.B. Camozzi, 3
24020 Ranica
Bergamo, Italy
(035) 516516
(035) 514503 (fax)
(For information on European studies of rare disorders)
See also Rare Disease Support Groups

**ITP Society**
Children's Blood Foundation
333 East 38th Street
New York, NY 10016
(800) 487-7010
See also Children

**Izaac Walton Killam Hospital for Children**
Halifax, Nova Scotia
Canada

**Jervell and Lange-Nielsen Syndrome**
See Sudden Arrhythmia Death Syndrome Foundation
International Long QT Syndrome Registry

**Jewish Genetic Diseases**
See National Foundation for Jewish Genetic Diseases

**Donald R. Johns, M.D.**
Johns Hopkins Hospital
600 North Wolfe Street
Baltimore, MD 21205
(For MELAS syndrome; MERRF syndrome)

**Anne B. Johnson, M.D.**
Department of Pathology, K427
Albert Einstein College of Medicine
1300 Morris Park Avenue
Bronx, NY 10461
(For leukodystrophy research)

**Gilbert N. Jones III**
Susan A. Guckenberger
Southern Illinois University
School of Medicine
Department of Pediatrics
Genetics and Metabolism
P.O. Box 19230
Springfield, IL 62794-9230
(217) 782-8460
(For Wolf-Hirschhorn syndrome)

**Kenneth Jones, M.D.**
Division of Dysmorphology
School of Medicine
University of California
La Jolla, CA
(619) 291-0946

**Joseph Disease**
See International Joseph Diseases Foundation, Inc.
Roger N. Rosenberg, M.D.

**Joubert Syndrome Parents-In-Touch Network**
12348 Summer Meadow Road
Rock, MI 49880
(906) 359-4707
See also David B. Flannery, M.D.

**Denise Juliano, M.S.W.**
Department of Admissions
Neuropsychiatric Research Hospital
2700 Martin Luther King Jr. Avenue SE
Washington, DC 20032
(202) 373-6100
(For Alzheimer disease)

**Juvenile Diabetes Foundation International**
432 Park Avenue South, 16th Floor
New York, NY 10016
(800) 533-2873
(212) 889-7575

**William D. Kaehny, M.D.**
Box C83
University of Colorado Health Science Center
4200 East Ninth Avenue
Denver, CO 80262
(303) 270-7821.
(For polycystic kidney disease)

**Steven Kaler, M.D.**
National Institutes of Health
Building 10, Room 9S-242
9000 Rockville Pike
Bethesda, MD 20892
(301) 496-9101
(For Menkes disease)

**Kearns-Sayre Syndrome**
See Mitochondrial Disorders Foundation of America

**Kernicterus**
See Peter R. Martin, M.D.

**Kidney Cancer**
See National Kidney Cancer Association

**Kidney Foundation**
2 Park Avenue
New York, NY 10016
(212) 899-2210

**Kidney/Urologic Disorders**
See American Association of Kidney Patients
American Foundation for Urologic Disease
American Kidney Fund
Association for Urinary Continence Control
Families with Maple Syrup Urine Disease
Help for Incontinent People
Hereditary Nephritis Foundation
IgA Nephropathy Support Network
Interstitial Cystitis Association of America
Kidney Foundation
National Association of Patients on Hemodialysis and Transplantation
National Exstrophy of the Bladder
National Kidney Cancer Association
National Kidney Foundation
National Kidney of Connecticut
National Support Group for Exstrophy of the Bladder
NIH/National Institute of Diabetes, Digestive and Kidney Diseases
NIH/National Kidney and Urologic Diseases Information Clearinghouse
Simon Foundation
David G. Warnock, M.D.
Polycystic Kidney Disease

**Klinefelter Syndrome**
See Support and Educational Exchange for Klinefelter Syndrome

**Klinefelter Syndrome and Associates**
P.O. Box 119
Roseville, CA 95661-0119

**Klinefelter's Syndrome Association of America**
Route 1, P.O. Box 93
Pine River, WI 54965
(414) 987-5782

**Klinefelter's Syndrome Support Group of Canada**
P.O. Box 5000
Pentanguishene
Ontario LOK 1PO
Canada

**Klippel-Trenaunay Syndrome Support Group**
4610 Wooddale Avenue
Edina, MN 55424-1139
(612) 925-2596

**Diane Komp, M.D.**
Yale University School of Medicine
Department of Pediatrics
P.O. Box 333
New Haven, CT 06510
(203) 785-4640
(For histiocytosis X)

**Korsakoff Syndrome**
See Peter R. Martin, M.D.

**Connie Kreps**
National Institutes of Health
(301) 496-1465
(For Gaucher disease)
See also Ramnik Xavier

**Bert N. La Du, M.D.**
Department of Pharmacology
6322 Medical Sciences, Bldg. 1
University of Michigan School of Medicine
Ann Arbor, MI 48109-0626
(313) 763-6429
(For alcaptonuria and pharmacogenetics)

**Lactic Acidosis Support Group**
P.O. Box 480282
Denver, CO 80248-0282
(303) 287-4953

**Lactic Acidosis Support Trust**
1A Whitley Close
Middlewich, Cheshire CW10 0NQ
United Kingdom
01606-837198

**Paul W. Ladenson, M.D.**
Div. of Endocrinology and Metabolism
Blalock 904
600 North Wolfe Street
Baltimore, MD 21205
(301) 955-3663
(For Graves disease)

**Landau-Kleffner Syndrome**
See C.A.N.D.L.E.
Rush Presbyterian

**Landouzy-Dejerine Muscular Dystrophy**
See Facioscapulohumeral Society

**Craig B. Langman, M.D.**
Samuel S. Gidding, M.D.
Children's Memorial Hospital
Pediatrics/Nephrology, Mail #37
2300 Children's Plaza
Chicago, IL 60614
(312) 880-4000
(For DiGeorge syndrome)

**Laryngeal Papillomatosis**
See American Laryngeal Papilloma
Foundation

**Daniel M. Lasser, M.D.**
Obstetrics and Gynecology
Columbia University
College of Physicians
630 West 168th Street
New York, NY 10032
(212) 305-6784
(For Turcot syndrome; hereditary
medulloblastoma)

**Late Onset Tay-Sachs Foundation**
1303 Paper Mill Road
Erdenheim, PA 19038
(215) 836-9426
(800) 672-2022

**Latex Allergy Support Service**
176 Roosevelt Avenue
Torrington, CT 06790
(203) 482-6869
See also Allergy/Asthma

**Laurence-Moon-Bardet-Biedl Syndrome**
124 Lincoln Drive
Purchase, NY 10577
(914) 251-1163

**Learning Disabilities**
See Learning Disabilities Association of
America
National Center for Learning Disabilities
National Network of Learning-Disabled
Adults
Orton Dyslexia Society
Disability Referrals

**Learning Disabilities Association of America (LDA)**
4156 Library Road
Pittsburgh, PA 15234-1319
(412) 341-1515

**Leber Congenital Amaurosis**
See Richard A. Lewis, M.D.
Maria A. Musarella, M.D.

**Mark Lebwohl, M.D.**
PXE (Pseudoxanthoma Elasticum) Research
Project
Department of Dermatology
Mount Sinai School of Medicine
Fifth Avenue and 100th Street
New York, NY 10029
(212) 876-7199

**David Ledbetter, M.D.**
NIH/Center for Genome Research
9000 Rockville Pike
Bethesda, MD 20892
(For lissencephaly)
See also William B. Dobyns, M.D.

**Robert E. Lee, M.D.,**
University of Pittsburgh Medical School
Department of Pathology
Pittsburgh, Pennsylvania 15261.
(For Gaucher disease)

**Leigh Disease**
See National Leigh's Disease Foundation
Mitochondrial Disorders Foundation of
America

**Marge Lenane**
NIH/National Institute of Mental Health
(301) 496-6081
(For trichotillomania)

**Leprosy**
See American Leprosy Missions
National Hansen Disease Center

**Lesch-Nyhan Disease**
See International Lesch-Nyhan Disease
Association

**Lesch-Nyhan Syndrome Registry**
New York University School of Medicine
Department of Psychiatry
550 First Avenue
New York, NY 10012
(212) 263-6458

**Lethbridge Society for Rare Diseases**
P.O. Box 35
Lethbridge, Alberta T1J 3Y3
Canada
(403) 329-0665
See also Rare Disease Support Groups

**Let's Face It**
P.O. Box 711
Concord, MA 01742
(508) 371-3186
See also Craniofacial Disorders

**Leukemia Society of America**
600 Third Avenue, 4th Floor
New York, NY 10016
(212) 573-8484
(800) 955-4572
See also Cancer

**Leukodystrophy**
See Association Européenne contre les
Leucodystrophes
United Leukodystrophy Foundation
Anne B. Johnson, M.D.

**Amy Feldman Lewanda, M.D.**
Ethylin Wang Jabs, M.D.
CMSC 10
Johns Hopkins Hospital
Baltimore, Maryland 21205
(301) 955-0484
(For craniofacial disorders)

**Richard A. Lewis, M.D., M.S.**
Cullen Eye Institute, NC-206
Baylor College of Medicine
1 Baylor Plaza
Houston, TX 77030
(713) 798-3030
(For inherited retinal disorders, including
Aarskog syndrome, cone dystrophy,
incontinentia pigmenti, Leber congenital
amaurosis)

**Lifetime Advocacy Plus**
(Guardianship services)
424 North 130th Street
Seattle, WA 98133
(206) 367-8055

**Li-Fraumeni Syndrome International
Registry**
Cancer Institute, CE&C
44 Binney Street
Mayer 3A
Boston, MA 02115
(617) 632-3158
(800) 828-6622
See also Cancer

**Limb Disorders**
See CHERUB
Superkids

**Lipid Diseases**
See National Lipid Diseases Foundation

**Lipodystrophy**
See Abhimanyu Garg, M.D.

**Lissencephaly Network**
716 Autumn Ridge Lane
Fort Wayne, IN 46804
(219) 432-4310
See also William B. Dobyns, M.D.
David Ledbetter, M.D.

**Little People of America, Inc.**
P.O. Box 9897
Washington, DC 20016
(301) 589-0730
(800) 243-9273
See also Dwarfism

**Little People's Research Fund, Inc.**
80 Sister Pierre Drive
Towson, MD 21204
(410) 494-0055
(800) 232-5773
See also Dwarfism

**Irene Litvan, M.D.**
NIH/NINDS Experimental Therapeutics
Branch
9000 Rockville Pike
Building 10, Room 5C106
Bethesda, MD 20892
(301) 496-7993
(For progressive supranuclear palsy)

**Johnson M. Liu, M.D.**
NIH/National Heart, Lung and Blood
Institute
Clinical Hematology Branch
9000 Rockville Pike
Building 10, Room 7C103
Bethesda, MD 20892
(301) 496-5093
(For Fanconi anemia)

**Liver Disorders**
See American Liver Foundation
Children's Liver Foundation
Primary Biliary Cirrhosis Patient Support
Network
United Liver Association

**Long QT Syndrome**
See International Long QT Syndrome
Registry

**Lowe's Syndrome Association**
222 Lincoln Street
West Lafayette, IN 47906-2732
(317) 743-3634

**Christy Ludlow, Ph.D.**
(NIH)/National Institute of Deafness and
Other Communication Disorders
Speech Pathology Unit
Building 10, Room 5N226
9000 Rockville Pike
Bethesda, MD 20892
(301) 496-9365
(For spasmodic dysphonia)

**Lung Disorders**
See American Lung Association
American Lung Association of
Connecticut
American Broncho-Esophagological
Association
Foundation for Pulmonary Hypertension
Histiocytosis-X Association
NIH/National Heart, Lung and Blood
Institute

**Lung Line (National Jewish Center)**
(800) 222-LUNG

**Lupus Erythematosus**
See American Lupus Society
Systemic Lupus Erythematosus
Foundation

**Lupus Foundation of America, Inc.**
4 Research Place, Suite 180
Rockville, MD 20850-3226
(301) 670-9292
(800) 558-0121

**Lyme Disease Clinic**
Dana Medical Center, 3rd Floor
789 Howard Avenue
New Haven, CT 06504
(203) 785-7032

**Lyme Disease Clinic**
Marshfield Clinic
1000 North Oak Avenue
Marshfield, WI 54449
(715) 387-5511

**Lyme Disease Foundation, Inc.**
1 Financial Plaza, 18th Floor
Hartford, CT 06103
(203) 525-2000
(800) 886-5963

**Lyme Disease Resource Center**
P.O. Box 9510
Santa Rosa, CA 95405
(707) 575-5133

**Lymphangioma**
See Cystic Hygroma and Lymphangioma
Support Group

**Lymphatic Disorders**
See National Lymphatic and Venous
Diseases Foundation
National Lymphedema Network
NIH/National Heart, Lung and Blood
Institute

**Lymphatic Malformations**
See Children Anguished with Lymphatic
Malformations

**Lymphoproliferative Syndrome**
See James Skare, M.D.

**Macular Degeneration International**
2968 West Ina Road, #106
Tucson, AZ 85741
(520) 797-2525

**Macular Dystrophy**
See Association for Macular Diseases
Stargardt International and Juvenile
Macular Dystrophies
Eye Disorders

**Alice Macynski, R.N.**
NIH/National Institute of Dental Research
9000 Rockville Pike
Building 10, Room 1B-21
Bethesda, Maryland 20892
(301) 496-4371
(For Sjögren syndrome)

**Magic Foundation for Children's Growth**
1327 North Harlem Avenue
Oak Park, IL 60302
(708) 383-0808
(800) 362-4423
See also Dwarfism

**John Mahoney, M.D.**
Dept. of Pediatrics and Psychology
Johns Hopkins University
600 North Wolfe Street
Baltimore, MD 21205
(For true hermaphroditism)

**Make a Wish Foundation of America**
100 West Clarendon #220
Phoenix, AZ 85013
(602) 279-9474
(800) 722-9474

**Male Sexual Dysfunction**
See Association for Male Sexual
Dysfunction
Sexual Disorders

## Malignant Hyperthermia
See Malignant Hyperthermia Association of
the United States
Malignant Hyperthermia Emergencies
Malignant Hyperthermia Clinics
North American Malignant Hyperthermia
Registry

## Malignant Hyperthermia Association of the United States
32 South Main Street
Box 1069
Sherburne, NY 13460-1069
(607) 674-7901
(800) 986-4287

## Malignant Hyperthermia Clinics

Massachusetts General
Department of Anesthesiology
John Ryan, M.D.
Room ACC3
Fruit Street
**Boston**, MA 02114
(617) 726-8800
(For information only)

Thomas E. Nelson, M.D.
University of Texas Health Center
Medical School, Dept. of Anesthesiology
6431 Fannin Street, MSB-5020
**Houston**, TX 77030
(713) 792-5566

Hahnemann Medical School
Department of Anesthesiology
Mail Stop 310
Broad and Vine Streets
**Philadelphia**, PA 19102
(215) 448-7960

Mayo Clinic
Department of Anesthesiology
200 First Street SW
**Rochester**, MN 55905
(507) 285-5601

## Malignant Hyperthermia Emergencies
Medic Alert Foundation International
(209) 634-4917
Ask for INDEX ZERO, Malignant
Hyperthermia Consultant List

## Malignant Melanoma
See J.C. Bystryn, M.D.

## Manic Depressive Association
P.O. Box 753
Northbrook, IL 60062
(312) 446-9009
See also Mental Health

## Maple Syrup Urine Disease
See Families with Maple Syrup Urine
Disease
Kidney/Urologic Disorders

## March of Dimes Birth Defects Foundation
1275 Mamaroneck Avenue
White Plains, NY 10605
(914) 428-7100

## Marfan Syndrome
See Bruce S. Alpert, M.D.
National Marfan Foundation

## Jan Marshall, M.D.
Jackson Laboratory
Bar Harbor, Maine 04609
(207) 288-3371
(For Alstrom syndrome)

## Peter R. Martin, M.D.
Vanderbilt University School of Medicine
A-2205 MCN
Nashville, TN 37232
(614) 322-3527
(For Korsakoff syndrome; kernicterus)

## Mathews Foundation for Prostate Cancer Research
1010 Hurley Way
Sacramento, CA 95825
(916) 567-1400
(800) 422-6237
See also Us Too
Cancer

## Mastocytosis Chronicles
4771 Waynes Trace Road
Hamilton, OH 45011
(513) 726-4605

## Mia McCollin, M.D.
Molecular Neurogenetics Laboratory
Massachusetts General Hospital
Building 149, 13th Street
Charlestown, MA 02129
(617) 726-5725
(For neurofibromatosis)

## McCune-Albright Syndrome
Division of the MAGIC Foundation
c/o Anna Miller
3167 Greensburg Road
North Canton, OH 44720
(216) 896-4455

## Meat Hotline
U.S. Department of Agriculture
(800) 535-4555 (10 A.M.–4 P.M. EST)

## Medic Alert Foundation International
(209) 634-4917

## Medical Genetics
Children's Hospital and Medical Center
Box 5371/4800 Sand Point Way NE
Seattle, WA 98105-0371
(206) 526-2056

## Medium Chain Acyl Dehydrogenase Deficiency
See MCAD Family Support Group

## Medium Chain Acyl-CoA Dehydrogenase (MCAD) Family Support Group
805 Montrose Drive
Greensboro, NC 27410
(910) 547-8682

## Medulloblastoma, Hereditary
See Daniel M. Lasser, M.D.

## MELAS Syndrome
See Donald R. Johns, M.D.
Mitochondrial Disorders Foundation of
America

## Melnick-Needles Syndrome Support Group
4 Kinver Lane
Bexhill-on-Sea
East Sussex TN40 2ST
United Kingdom
01424 217790

## Meniere Crouzon Syndrome Support Network
2375 Valentine Drive #9
Prescott, AZ 96303
See also Margareta Moller, M.D.
Ear Disorders

## Menkes Disease
See Corporation for Menkes Disease
Steven Kaler, M.D.

## Mental Health
See American Association of Suicidology
American Psychiatric Association
American Schizophrenia Society
Depression and Related Affective
Disorders Association
Depressives Anonymous
Devereux Foundation
Federation of Families for Children's
Mental Health
Manic Depressive Association
National Alliance for the Mentally Ill
National Depressive-Manic-Depression
Association
National Institute of Mental Retardation
(Canada)
National Mental Health Association
National Mental Health Consumer
Self-Help Clearinghouse
NIH/National Institute of Mental Health
Obsessive-Compulsive Foundation
The Arc

## MERRF Syndrome
See Donald R. Johns, M.D.
Mitochondrial Disorders Foundation of
America

## Metabolic Disorders
See Association for Babies and Children
with Carnitine Deficiency (ABC)
Association for Glycogen Storage
Diseases
Cobalamin Network
Inherited Metabolism Disorders Clinic
ML 4 Foundation
National Urea Cycle Disorders Foundation
NIH/National Institute for Diabetes,
Digestive and Kidney Disease
Research Trust for Metabolic Diseases in
Children
William Rhead, M.D.

## Metatrophic Dysplasia Dwarf Registry
3393 Geneva Drive
Santa Clara, CA 95051
(408) 244-6354
See also Dwarfism

**Metatrophic Dysplasia Hotline**
3393 Geneva Drive
Santa Clara, CA 95051
(408) 244-6354
*See also* Dwarfism

**Methadone Treatment**
*See* American Methadone Treatment
Association, Inc.

**Michigan State University Human
Genetics**
College of Human Medicine
B240 Life Science Bld.
East Lansing, MI 48824-1317
(517) 353-2030

**Leonard Milstone, M.D.**
Department of Dermatology
Yale University Medical School
New Haven, CT
(203) 937-3833
(For epidermolytic hyperkeratosis)

**Frederick W. Miller, M.D.**
Lisa G. Rider, M.D.
Molecular Immunology Lab, CBER, FDA
National Institutes of Health
Bldg. 29, Rm. 507, HFM-521
8800 Rockville Pike
Bethesda, MD 20892
(301) 496-6913
(For polymyositis/dermatomyositis)

**Miller Syndrome**
*See* Eric A. Wulfsberg, M.D.
Foundation for Nager and Miller
Syndromes

**Mitochondrial Disease**
*See* Cox Foundation for Mitochondrial
Disease
EASE
Mitochondrial Disorders Foundation of
America
Douglas C. Wallace, M.D.

**Mitochondrial Disorders Foundation of
America**
5100-1B Clayton Road, Suite 187
Concord, CA 94521
(510) 798-8798
(800) 838-6332

**ML 4 Foundation (Ganglioside Sialidase
Deficiency)**
6 Concord Drive
Monsey, NY 10952
(914) 425-0639
*See also* Chromosomal Abnormalities

**Mobility International USA**
P.O. Box 10767
Eugene, OR 97440
(503) 343-1284 (Voice and TDD)
*See also* Disability Referrals

**Moebius Syndrome Foundation**
P.O. Box 993
Larchmont, NY 10538
(914) 834-6008

**Moebius Syndrome Support Group**
39521 Rowan Court
Palmdale, CA 93551
(805) 267-2570
(818) 908-9288

**Moebius Syndrome Support Group**
21 Shields Road
Whitley Bay, Tyne and Weir NE25 8UT
United Kingdom

**Molecular Neurogenetics Unit**
Massachusetts General Hospital
East CNY Building 149
13th Street
Charleston, MA 02129
(617) 716-5718

**Margareta Moller, M.D.**
Presbyterian University Hospital
Room 9402, PUH
230 Lothrup Street
Pittsburgh, PA 15213
(412) 624-3376
(For Meniere disease)

**Monosomy**
*See* Chromosomal Abnormalities

**Gareth Morgan, M.D.**
Hospital for Sick Children
Great Ormond Street
London WC1N 3JH
(071) 829-8834
(071) 831-4366 (fax)
(For severe combined immunodeficiency)

**Colleen A. Morris, M.D.**
2040 W. Charleston Blvd., Suite 401
Las Vegas, NV 89102
(702) 385-5411
(For Williams syndrome)

**Hugo W. Moser, M.D.**
Adrenoleukodystrophy (ALD) Project
Kennedy-Krieger Institute
707 North Broadway
Baltimore, MD 21205
(410) 522-5405

**Mothers of Asthmatics**
10875 Main Street, Suite 210
Fairfax, VA 22030
(703) 385-4403
*See also* Allergy/Asthma

**Mothers United for Moral Support
(MUMS)**
National Parent-to-Parent Network
150 Custer Court
Green Bay, WI 54301-1243
(414) 336-5333
*See also* Chromosomal Abnormalities

**Motor Neuron Disease Association**
P.O. 246
Northampton, NN1 2PR
United Kingdom
0604 250505
0604 247726
*See also* Amyotrophic Lateral Sclerosis
Association
Neurologic Disorders

**Mountain States Regional Genetics
Services Network**
c/o Family Planning Center
Attn: Gail Chiarrello
2600 South Broad Street, Suite #1900
Philadelphia, PA 19102-3865
*See also* Genetics

**Moving Forward**
2934 Glenmore Avenue
Kettering, OH 45409
(513) 293-0409
*See also* Neurologic Disorders

**Moyamoya Disease**
*See* Families with Moyamoya Network

**Mucolipidoses/Mucopolysaccharidoses**
*See* Children's Association for Research on
Mucolipidosis Type IV
Mucolipidosis Type IV Foundation
Joseph Muenzer, M.D.
National Lipid Disease Foundation
National Mucopolysaccharidoses/
Mucolipidoses Society
Society of MPS Diseases
Society of Mucopolysaccharide Diseases

**Mucolipidosis Type IV Foundation**
719 East 17th Street
Brooklyn, NY 11230
(718) 434-5067

**Joseph Muenzer, M.D., Ph.D.**
Department of Pediatrics
University of North Carolina
Chapel Hill, NC 27599
(For mucopolysaccharidosis; Hunter
syndrome)

**Multiple Sclerosis**
*See* National Multiple Sclerosis Society

**Joseph A. Murray, M.D.**
Center for Digestive Disease
University of Iowa Hospital and Clinic
200 Hawkins Drive
Iowa City, IA 52242
(319) 356-8246
(For celiac sprue)

**Maria A. Musarella, M.D., F.R.C.S.**
Hospital for Sick Children
Research Institute
555 University Avenue
Toronto, Ontario M5G 1X8
Canada
(416) 598-7506
(For Leber congenital amaurosis and other
inherited retinal disorders )

**Muscular Atrophy**
*See* Families of Spinal Muscular Atrophy

**Muscular Dystrophy**
*See* Muscular Dystrophy Association
Muscular Dystrophy Association of
Canada
Muscular Dystrophy Group of Great
Britain and Northern Ireland
Parent Project for Muscular Dystrophy
Research
Society for Muscular Dystrophy
International

**Muscular Dystrophy Association**
3300 East Sunrise Drive
Tucson, AZ 85718-3208
(602) 529-2000
(800) 572-1717 (Lifeline MDA)

**Muscular Dystrophy Association of Canada**
Shirley Hall
150 Eglinton Avenue East, Suite 400
Toronto, Ontario M4P 1E8
Canada

**Muscular Dystrophy Group of Great Britain and Northern Ireland**
Nattrass House
35 Macaulay Road
London SW4 0QP
United Kingdom
071-720-8055

**Muscular Dystrophy, Landouzy-Dejerine**
See Facioscapulohumeral Society

**Musculoskeletal Disorders**
See Association of Children's Prosthetic and Orthotic Clinics
NIH/National Arthritis and Musculoskeletal and Skin Disorders Information Clearinghouse

**Mutism**
See Elective Mutism Support Group

**Myalgic Encephalomyelitis Association**
Stanhope House
High Street
Essex SS17 0HA
United Kingdom
37-564-2466

**Myasthenia Gravis Foundation**
222 South Riverside Plaza, Suite 1540
Chicago, IL 60606
(312) 258-0522
(800) 541-5454

**Mycosis Fungoides Network**
Department of Dermatology
Pavillion A3
UC Medical Center
Cincinnati, OH 45267-0523
(513) 558-4644

**Myelin Messenger**
Ruth Anderson
HC-29 Box 686
Stable Lane
Prescott, AZ 86301-7435
(520) 776-7556

**Myelitis, Transverse**
See Transverse Myelitis Association

**Myelodysplasia**
See Aplastic Anemia Foundation of America

**Myeloma**
See International Myeloma Foundation

**Myeloproliferative Disease Research Center, Inc.**
950 Park Avenue
New York, NY 10028-0320
(212) 535-8181
(800) 435-7673

**Myoclonus Families United**
1564 East 34th Street
Brooklyn, NY 11234
(718) 252-2133
See also Neurologic Disorders

**Myopathy, Centronuclear and Myotubular**
See X-Linked Myotubular Myopathy Resource Group

**Myositis**
See Inclusion Body Myositis Association
National Myositis Association

**Nager and Miller Syndromes**
See Foundation for Nager and Miller Syndromes
Eric A. Wulfsberg, M.D.

**Sakkubai Naidu, M.D.**
John F. Kennedy Institute for Handicapped Children
707 North Broadway
Baltimore, MD 21205
(For Rett syndrome)

**Narcolepsy**
See Narcolepsy and Sleep Disorders International Newsletter
Narcolepsy and Cataplexy Foundation of America
Narcolepsy Institute
Narcolepsy Network, Inc.
Sleep Disorders

**Narcolepsy and Cataplexy Foundation of America**
445 East 68th Street, Apt. 12L
New York, NY 10021
(212) 570-5506

**Narcolepsy and Sleep Disorders International Newsletter**
P.O. Box 51113
Palo Alto, CA 94303-9559

**Narcolepsy Institute**
Montefiore Medical Center
111 East 210th Street
Bronx, NY 10467
(718) 920-6799

**Narcolepsy Network, Inc.**
P.O. Box 1365
FDR Station
New York, NY 10150
(914) 834-2855

**National Accessible Apartment Clearinghouse**
1111 14th Street NW, 9th Floor
Washington, DC 20005
(800) 421-1221
See also Disability Referrals

**National Adrenal Diseases Foundation**
505 Northern Boulevard
Great Neck, NY 11021
(516) 487-4992
See also Endocrine Disorders

**National AIDS Hotline**
(Centers for Disease Control)
(800) 342-AIDS

**National Alliance of Breast Cancer Organizations**
9 East 37th Street, 10th Floor
New York, NY 10016
(212) 719-0154
See also Breast Cancer Advisory Center

**National Alliance for the Mentally Ill**
200 North Glebe Road, #1015
Arlington, VA 22203-3754
(703) 524-7600
(800) 950-6264

**National Alopecia Areata Foundation**
710 C Street, Suite 11
San Rafael, CA 94901
(415) 456-4644

**National Amputation Foundation, Inc.**
73 Church Street
Malverne, NY 11565
(516) 887-3600
See also Amputation

**National Anorexic Aid Society, Inc.**
1925 East Dublin Granville Road
Columbus, OH 43229
(614) 436-1112
See also Eating Disorders

**National Aphasia Association**
P.O. Box 1887
Murray Hill Station
New York, NY 100156-0611
(800) 922-4622
See also C.A.N.D.L.E.

**National Association of Anorexia Nervosa and Associated Disorders, Inc.**
Box 7
Highland Park, IL 60035
(708) 831-3438
See also Eating Disorders

**National Association of Hospital Hospitality Houses**
4013 West Jackson Street
Muncie, IN 47304
(317) 288-3226
(800) 542-9730

**National Association for Parents of the Visually Impaired**
P.O. Box 317
Watertown, MA 02272-0317
(617) 972-7441
(800) 562-6265
See also Eye Disorders

**National Association of Patients on Hemodialysis and Transplantation**
150 Nassau Street
New York, NY 10038
(212) 619-2720
*See also* American Association of Kidney Patients
Kidney/Urologic Disorders

**National Association of Pseudoxanthoma Elasticum**
1420 Ogden Street
Denver, CO 80218
(303) 832-5055

**National Association of Radiation Survivors**
P.O. Box 278
Live Oak, CA 95953
(800) 798-5102
*See also* National Council on Radiation Protection and Measurements
Environmental Disorders

**National Association for the Craniofacially Handicapped**
*See* FACES

**National Association of the Deaf**
814 Thayer Avenue
Silver Spring, MD 20910
(301) 473-7666
*See also* Hearing Impairment

**National Association for the Visually Handicapped**
22 West 21st Street
New York, NY 10010
(212) 889-3141
*See also* Eye Disorders

**National Ataxia Foundation**
750 Twelve Oaks Center
15500 Wayzata Boulevard
Wayzata, MN 55391
(612) 473-7666
*See also* Parkinson Disease

**National Attention Deficit Disorder Association**
P.O. Box 972
Mentor, OH 44061
(216) 974-4093
(800) 487-2282

**National Autism Hotline**
P.O. Box 507
605 9th Street
Prichard Building
Huntington WV 25710-0507
(304) 525-8014

**National Back Pain Association of England**
31-33 Park Road
Teddington, Middlesex TW11 0AB
United Kingdom
*See also* Pain

**National Birth Defect Registry**
(800) 313-2232

**National Birth Defects Center**
40 Second Avenue, Suite 460
Waltham, MA 02154
(617) 466-9555
*See also* Children

**National Brain Tumor Foundation**
785 Market Street, Suite 1600
San Francisco, CA 94103
(415) 284-0208
(800) 934-3873

**National Center on Chromosome Inversions**
1029 Johnson Street
Des Moines, IA 50315
(515) 287-6798
*See also* Chromosomal Abnormalities

**National Center for Down's Syndrome**
9 Westbourne Road
EDG Baston
Birmingham B-15
United Kingdom
(021) 454-3126

**National Center for Education in Maternal and Child Health**
38th and R Streets NW
Washington, DC 20057
(202) 625-8400
*See also* Chromosomal Abnormalities
Children

**National Center for Environmental Health Strategies**
1100 Rural Avenue
Voorhees, NJ 08043
(609) 429-5358

**National Center of Health Statistics**
Division of Health and Human Services
(301) 436-8500

**National Center for Human Genome Research**
c/o Eleanor Langfelder
(301) 402-0911
*See also* Genome Data Base

**National Center for Learning Disabilities**
381 Park Avenue South #1420
New York, NY 10016
(212) 545-7510

**National Center for Youth with Disabilities**
University of Minnesota, Box 721
420 Delaware Street SE
Minneapolis, MN 55455-0392
(612) 626-2825
(800) 333-6293
*See also* Children
Disability Referrals

**National Chronic Fatigue Syndrome and Fibromyalgia Association**
3521 Broadway, Suite 222
Kansas City, MO 64111
(816) 931-4777
*See also* Immunodeficiency
Fibromyalgia

**National Chronic Pain Outreach Association, Inc.**
7979 Old Georgetown Road, Suite 100
Bethesda, MD 20814
(301) 652-4948

**National Coalition for Research in Neurological and Communicative Disorders**
1250 24th Street NW, Suite 300
Washington DC 20037-1124
(202) 293-5453
*See also* Neurologic Disorders

**National Committee on Youth Suicide Prevention**
825 Washington Street
Norwood, MA 02062
*See also* American Association of Suicidology
Mental Health

**National Congenital CMV Disease Registry**
Clinical Care Center, #1150
6621 Fannin St., MC 3-2371
Houston, TX 77030-2399
(713) 770-4330
*See also* Sturge-Weber Foundation

**National Council on Radiation Protection and Measurements, Inc.**
7910 Woodmont Avenue, Suite 800
Bethesda, MD 20814
(301) 657-2652
*See also* National Association of Radiation Survivors
Environmental Disorders

**National Craniofacial Foundation**
3100 Carlisle Street, Suite 215
Dallas, TX 75204
(800) 535-3643

**National Crisis Center for the Deaf**
University of Virginia Medical Center
Charlottesville, VA 22908
(800) 466-9876 (Voice and TDD)
*See also* Hearing Impairment

**National Depressive-Manic-Depression Association**
(800) 826-3632
*See also* Mental Health

**National Disease Research Interchange**
1880 JFK Boulevard, 6th Floor
Philadelphia, PA 19103
(215) 557-7361
(800) 222-NDRI
(Provides human tissue for biomedical researchers)

**National Down Syndrome Congress**
1605 Chantilly Drive, Suite 250
Atlanta, GA 30324-3269
(800) 232-6372
(404) 633-1555

**National Down Syndrome Society**
666 Broadway, 8th Floor
New York, NY 10012-2317
(212) 460-9330
(800) 221-4602

**National Easter Seal Society, Inc.**
230 West Monroe Street, Suite 1800
Chicago, IL 60606-4802
(312) 726-6200 (voice)
(800) 221-6827
(312) 726-4258 (TDD)
*See also* Disability Referrals

**National Eye Care Project**
P.O. Box 6988
San Francisco, CA 94101
(800) 222-EYES
*See also* Eye Disorders

**National Eye Research Foundation**
910 Skokie Blvd.
Northbrook, IL 60062
*See also* Eye Disorders

**National Family Caregivers Association**
9223 Longbranch Parkway
Silver Spring, MD 20901-3642
(301) 949-3838
*See also* Family Caregiver Alliance

**National Federation of the Blind**
1800 Johnston Street
Baltimore, MD 21230
(410) 659-9314
*See also* Eye Disorders

**National Fibromyalgia Research Association**
P.O. Box 500
Salem, OR 97308

**National Foundation for Asthma**
5301 East Grand Road
Tucson, AZ 85712
*See also* Allergy/Asthma

**National Foundation of Crohn's Colitis, Inc.**
National Headquarters
295 Madison Avenue, Suite #519
New York, NY 10017
(212) 685-3440
*See also* Crohn's and Colitis Foundation of America

**National Foundation of Dentistry for the Handicapped**
1600 Stout Street, Suite 1420
Denver, CO 80202
(303) 573-0264
*See also* Disability Referrals

**National Foundation for Ectodermal Dysplasias**
219 East Main Street
P.O. Box 114
Mascoutah, IL 62258-0114
(618) 566-2020

**National Foundation for Facial Reconstruction**
317 East 34th St., #901
New York, NY 10016
(212) 263-6656
(800) 422-3223
*See also* Craniofacial Disorders

**National Foundation for Jewish Genetic Diseases**
250 Park Avenue, Suite 1000
New York, NY 10017
(212) 371-1030
*See also* Tay-Sachs Disease
Chromosomal Abnormalities

**National Foundation for Vitiligo and Pigment Disorders**
9032 South Woemandy Lane
Centerville, OH 45458
(513) 885-5739
*See also* Skin Disorders

**National Fragile X Foundation**
1441 York St., #303
Denver, CO 80206-2127
(800) 688-8765

**National Gaucher Foundation**
11140 Rockville Pike, Suite 350
Bethesda, MD 20852
(301) 816-1515
(800) 925-8885
*See also* Gaucher's Disease Foundation

**National Gay and Lesbian Task Force**
1734 14th Street NW
Washington, DC 20009
(202) 332-6483
*See also* AIDS

**National Gay Task Force**
80 Fifth Ave, Suite 1601
New York, NY 10011
*See also* AIDS

**National Gay Task Force Crisis Line**
(For information for medical professionals and for patients and their families)
(800) 221-7044 (3 P.M.–9 P.M. ET)

**National Graves' Disease Foundation**
2 Titsy Court
Brevard, NC 28712

**National Hansen Disease Center**
United States Public Health Service Hospital
5445 Point Claire Road
Carville, LA 70721-9607
(504) 642-4740
(800) 642-2477
*See also* American Leprosy Missions

**National Headache Foundation**
5252 North Western Avenue
Chicago, IL 60625
(312) 878-7715
(800) 372-7742
*See also* National Migraine Foundation

**National Health Law Project**
(202) 887-5310
(For legal assistance related to health insurance)

**National Hemophilia Foundation**
110 Greene Street, Suite 303
New York, NY 10012
(212) 219-8180
(800) 424-2634
*See also* Hemophilia
AIDS

**National Hospice Organization**
1901 Fort Myer Drive, Suite 902
Arlington., VA 22209
(703) 243-5900

**National Hydrocephalus Foundation**
22427 S. River Road
Joliet, IL 60436
(815) 467-6548

**National Hypoglycemia Association**
P.O. Box 120
Ridgewood, NJ 07451
(201) 670-1189

**National Incontinentia Pigmenti Foundation**
41 East 57th Street, #601
New York, NY 10022
(212) 207-4636
*See also* Skin Disorders

**National Information Center for Children and Youth with Disabilities (NICHCY)**
P.O. Box 1492
Washington, DC 20009
(202) 884-8200
(800) 695-0285 (Voice and TTY)
*See also* Disability Referrals

**National Information Center on Deafness**
Gallaudet University
800 Florida Avenue NE
Washington, DC 20002-3695
(202) 651-5051 (Voice)
(202) 651-5052 (TDD)
*See also* Hearing Impairment

**National Information Clearinghouse for Infants with Disabilities and Life-Threatening Conditions**
c/o Kathy Mayfield-Smith
University of South Carolina
Center for Developmental Disabilities
Benson Building
Columbia, SC 2908
(800) 922-9234
*See also* Children

**National Information Clearinghouse on Children Who Are Deaf-Blind**
*See* DB-Link

**National Institute of Mental Retardation**
(Canadian Association for the Mentally
 Retarded)
York University
Kinsmen NIMR Building
4700 Keele Street, North York
Toronto, Ontario M3J 1P3
Canada
(416) 661-9611
*See also* Mental Health

**National Institutes of Health**
*See* NIH (National Institutes of Health)

**National Kidney Cancer Association**
1234 Sherman Avenue, Suite 200
Evanston, IL 60202-1375
(708) 332-1051

**National Kidney Foundation**
30 East 33rd Street
New York, NY 10016
(212) 889-2210
(800) 622-9010

**National Kidney Foundation**
 **of Connecticut, Inc.**
920 Farmington Ave.
West Hartford, CT 06107
(203) 232-6054
(800) 441-1280

**National Leigh's Disease Foundation,**
 **Inc.**
608 East Waldron Street
P.O. Box 2222
Corinth, MS 38834-4810
(601) 286-2551
(800) 819-2551

**National Library Service for the Blind**
 **and Physically Handicapped**
Library of Congress
1291 Taylor Street NW
Washington, DC 20542
(202) 707-5100
*See also* Disability Referrals
 Eye Disorders

**National Lipid Diseases Foundation**
1201 Corbin Street
Elizabeth, NJ 07201
(908) 527-8000
*See also* Mucolipidoses/
 Mucopolysaccharidoses

**National Lymphatic and Venous**
 **Diseases Foundation, Inc.**
218 O'Brien Highway
Cambridge, MA 02141
(617) 889-2103
(800) 301-2103
*See also* Lymphatic Disorders

**National Lymphedema Network**
2211 Post Street, Suite 404
San Francisco, CA 94115
(415) 921-2911
(800) 541-3259
*See also* Lymphatic Disorders

**National Marfan Foundation**
382 Main Street
Port Washington, NY 11050
(516) 883-8712
(800) 862-7326
*See also* Coalition for Heritable Disorders of
 Connective Tissue

**National Maternal and Child Health**
 **Clearinghouse**
8201 Greensboro Drive, Suite 600
McLean, VA 22102-3810
(703) 821-8955
*See also* Children

**National Mental Health Association**
1021 Prince Street
Alexandria, VA 22314-2971
(703) 684-7722
(800) 969-6642

**National Mental Health Consumer**
 **Self-Help Clearinghouse**
311 South Juniper Street
Philadelphia, PA 19107
(215) 735-6082
(800) 553-4539

**National Migraine Foundation**
5252 North Western Avenue
Chicago, IL 60625
(800) 843-2256
(800) 523-8858 (in Illinois)
*See also* National Headache Foundation

**National Mucopolysaccharidoses/**
 **Mucolipidoses Society**
17 Kraemer St.
Hicksville, NY 11801
(516) 931-6338
*See also* Mucolipidoses/
 Mucopolysaccharidoses

**National Multiple Sclerosis Society**
1100 New York Avenue NW, Suite 1015
Washington, DC 20005-3934
(202) 408-1500
(800) 344-4867

**National Myositis Association**
7720 B El Camino Road, Suite 367
Rancho LaCosta, CA 92009
(800) 230-0441
*See also* Inclusion Body Myositis
 Association

**National Network of Learning-Disabled**
 **Adults, Inc.**
c/o Bill Butler
P.O. Box 32611
Phoenix, AZ 85064-2611
(602) 941-5112

**National Neurofibromatosis Foundation,**
 **Inc.**
95 Pine Street, 16th Floor
New York, NY 10005
(212) 344-6633
(800) 323-7928

**National Neutropenia Network**
6348 North Milwaukee Avenue
Chicago, IL 60646
(201) 361-9448
(800) 638-8768
*See also* Severe Chronic Neutropenia
 International Registry

**National Niemann-Pick Disease**
 **Foundation, Inc.**
22201 Riverpoint Trail
Carrolltown, VA 23314-3917
(804) 357-6774

**National Organization for Albinism and**
 **Hypopigmentation**
1530 Locust Street, #9
Philadelphia, PA 19102
(215) 545-2322
(800) 473-2310

**National Organization for Bone Marrow**
 **Transplants**
(800) 7A-MATCH

**National Organization on Fetal Alcohol**
 **Syndrome**
1815 H Street NW, Suite 1000
Washington, DC 20006
(202) 785-4585
(800) 666-6327
*See also* Fetal Alcohol Education Program

**National Organization for Rare Disorders**
 **(NORD)**
P.O. Box 8923
New Fairfield, CT 06812-8923
(203) 746-6518
(800) 999-NORD
(203) 746-6481 (fax)
(203) 746-6896 (MAP fax)
(203) 746-6927 (TDD)
*See also* Rare Disease Support Groups

**National Pain Outreach Association**
7979 Old Georgetown Road, Suite 100
Bethesda, MD 20814-2429
(301) 652-4948
*See also* Pain

**National Parent Network on Disabilities**
1600 Prince Street, Suite 115
Alexandria, VA 22314
(703) 684-6763
(703) 684-6763 (TTY)
*See also* Disability Referrals

**National Parkinson's Foundation**
1501 North Ninth Ave NW
Miami, FL 33136
(800) 327-4545
(800) 433-7022 (in Florida)

**National Phenylketonuria (PKU)**
 **Foundation**
6301 Tejas Drive
Pasadena, TX 77503
(713) 487-4802

**National Phenylketonuria (PKU) News**
6869 Woodlawn Avenue NE, Suite 116
Seattle, WA 98115-5469
(206) 525-8140

**National Prune Belly Syndrome Network**
1005 E. Carver Rd.
Tempe, AZ 85284
(602) 730-6364

**National Psoriasis Foundation**
6600 SW 92nd Avenue, Suite 300
Portland, OR 97223-7195
(503) 244-7404
(800) 723-9166
See also Psoriasis Research Association

**National Rehabilitation Information Center**
8455 Colesville Road, Suite 935
Silver Spring, MD 20910
(301) 588-9282
(800) 346-2742
(301) 588-9282 (TDD)

**National Retinoblastoma Parent Group**
110 Allen Road
Bow, NH 03304
(603) 224-4085
See also Eye Disorders

**National Reye's Syndrome Foundation, Inc.**
426 North Lewis Street
P.O. Box 829
Bryan, OH 43506-0829
(419) 636-2679
(800) 233-7393

**National Rosacea Society**
220 South Cook Street, Suite 201
Barrington, IL 60010
(708) 382-8971

**National Scoliosis Foundation, Inc.**
72 Mount Auburn Street
Watertown, MA 02172
(617) 926-0397
See also Scoliosis Association

**National Sexually Transmitted Diseases Hotline**
(800) 227-8922
See also AIDS

**National Sudden Infant Death Syndrome (SIDS) Clearinghouse**
3520 Prospect Street, Suite 1
Washington DC 20057
(202) 625-8410

**National Sjögren's Syndrome Association**
3201 West Evans Drive
Phoenix, AZ 85023-5632
(602) 516-0787
(800) 395-6772

**National Sleep Disorders Foundation**
122 South Robertson Blvd., Suite 201
Los Angeles, CA 90048
(310) 288-0466

**National Sleep Foundation**
1367 Connecticut Ave. NW, Suite 200
Washington, DC 20036
(202) 785-2300

**National Society of Genetic Counselors**
233 Canterbury Drive
Wallingford, PA 19086-6617
(610) 872-7608
See also Chromosomal Abnormalities

**National Society to Prevent Blindness**
500 East Remington Road
Schaumburg, IL 60173
(708) 843-2020
(800) 221-3004 (National Center for Sight)
See also Eye Disorders

**National Spasmodic Dysphonia Association**
P.O. Box 203
Atwood, CA 92601-0203
(714) 961-0945
(800) 714-6732
See also Our Voice

**National Spasmodic Torticollis Association, Inc.**
13545 W. Watertown Plank Road
Box 476
Elm Grove, WI 53122
(414) 797-9912
(800) 487-8385

**National Spinal Cord Injury Association**
545 Concord Avenue, Suite 29
Cambridge, MA 02138-1122
(617) 441-8500
(800) 962-9629 (hotline only)

**National Spinal Cord Injury Hotline**
2201 Argonne Drive
Baltimore, MD 21218
(410) 554-5413
(800) 526-3456

**National Stroke Association**
8480 East Orchard Street #1000
Englewood, CO 80111-5015
(303) 762-9922
(800) 787-6537

**National Stuttering Project**
4601 Irving Street
San Francisco, CA 94122
(415) 556-5324

**National Subacute Sclerosing Panencephalitis Registry**
University of Alabama
School of Medicine
Department of Neurology
2451 Fillingim
Mobile, AL 36615
(205) 471-7834

**National Sudden Infant Death Syndrome (SIDS) Resource Center**
8201 Greenboro Drive, Suite 600
McLean, VA 22102
(703) 821-8955

**National Support Group for Exstrophy of the Bladder**
5075 Medhurst Street
Solon, OH 44139
(216) 248-6851
See also Kidney/Urologic Disorders

**National Support Group for Myositis**
P.O. Box 890
Cooperstown, NY 13326
(607) 547-5446
(800) 230-0441
See also Inclusion Body Myositis
   Association
   Skin Disorders

**National Tay-Sachs and Allied Diseases Association, Inc.**
2001 Beacon Street, Suite 204
Brookline, MA 02146
(617) 277-4463

**National Tuberous Sclerosis Association, Inc.**
8000 Corporate Drive, Suite 120
Landover, MD 20785
(301) 459-9888
(800) 225-6872

**National Ulcer Foundation**
675 Main Street
Melrose, MA 02176

**National Urea Cycle Disorders Foundation**
P.O. Box 32
Sayreville, NJ 08872
(908) 851-2731
(800) 386-8233
See also Metabolic Disorders

**National Vascular Malformation Foundation**
8320 Nightingale Street
Dearborn Heights, MI 48127
(313) 274-1243
See also Children Anguished with
   Lymphatic Malformations

**National Vitiligo Foundation**
P.O. Box 6337
Tyler, TX 75711-6337
(903) 534-2925
See also Skin Disorders

**National Women's Health Network**
514 10th Street, Suite 400
Washington, DC 20004
(202) 628-7814

**National Women's Health Resource Center**
2240 M Street NW, #325
Washington, DC 20037
(202) 293-6045

**Navajo Virus (Hantavirus)**
For information call
(505) 827-2619
(800) 879-3421

**Linda Nee, M.S.W.**
Ronald Polinsky, M.D.
NIH/National Institute of Neurological
   Disorders and Stroke
Medical Neurology Branch
Building 10, Room 5N236
Bethesda, Maryland 20892
(301) 496-8350
(For Alzheimer disease)

**Kenneth H. Nelder, M.D.**
Pseudoxanthoma Elasticum (PXE) Research
    Program
Department of Dermatology
Health Sciences Center
Texas Tech University
Lubbock, TX 79430
(806) 743-2456

**Nephritis**
*See* Hereditary Nephritis Foundation

**Neurofibromatosis**
*See* National Neurofibromatosis
    Foundation, Inc.
    Neurofibromatosis Clinical Facilities
    Neurofibromatosis, Inc.
    Neurofibromatosis (NF)-2 Sharing
        Network
    Mia McCollin, M.D.
    Guy Rouleau, M.D.
    Donald Wright, M.D.

**Neurofibromatosis, Inc.**
8855 Annapolis, Suite #110
Lanham, MD 20706-2924
(301) 577-8984
(800) 942-6825
(410) 461-5213 (TDD)S

**Neurofibromatosis Clinical Facilities**

Massachusetts General Hospital
Department of Neurosurgery
Neurofibromatosis Clinic
Acc 8th Floor, #835
15 Parkman Street
**Boston**, MA 02114
(617) 726-9329
Attention: Mia McCollin, M.D.

Neurofibromatosis Program
University of Chicago
5841 South Maryland Avenue
**Chicago**, IL 60637
(312) 702-6488
Attention: James H. Tonsgard, M.D.

Baylor College of Medicine
Neurofibromatosis Clinic
1 Baylor Plaza
**Houston**, TX 77030
(713) 799-6103
Attention: Vincent Riccardi, M.D.

Cedars-Sinai Birth Defects Center
444 S. San Vincente Blvd., Ste. 1001
**Los Angeles**, CA 90048
(310) 855-2211
Attention: Jana Klein, M.S.

Mount Sinai School of Medicine
Neurofibromatosis Clinic
1 Gustave Levy Place
**New York**, NY 10029
(212) 722-1784
Attention: Allan E. Rubinstein, M.D.

Children's Hospital
Neurofibromatosis Clinic
34th Street and Civic Center Boulevard,
    Room 9028
**Philadelphia**, PA 19104
(215) 590-2920
Attention: Elaine Zackai, M.D.

Children's Hospital
Neurofibromatosis Clinic, Genetics
    Department
111 Michigan Avenue NW, Suite 1950
**Washington**, DC 20010
(202) 884-2187
Attention: Kenneth Rosenbaum, M.D.

Georgetown University Medical Center
Department of Neurosurgery
3800 Reservoir Rd., NW
**Washington**, DC 20007
(202) 687-4972
Attention: Robert L. Martuza, M.D.

---

**Neurofibromatosis (NF)-2 Sharing
    Network**
10074 Cabachon Court
Ellicott City, MD 21241
(410) 461-5213

**Neurogenetics**
*See* Molecular Neurogenetics Unit,
    Massachusetts General Hospital

**Neurologic Disorders**
*See* C.A.N.D.L.E.
    Cyclic Vomiting Syndrome Association
    Motor Neuron Disease Association
    Moving Forward
    Myoclonus Families United
    National Coalition for Research in
        Neurological and Communicative
        Disorders
    Neurological Institute
    NIH/Institute of Neurological Disorders
        and Stroke
    Opsoclonus-Myoclonus Syndrome Parent
        Talk
    Primary Lateral Sclerosis (PLS)
        Newsletter
    Progressive Supranuclear Palsy Research
        Fund
    Restless Legs Syndrome Foundation
    Society for Progressive Supranuclear
        Palsy
    Wallace W. Tourtelotte, M.D.
    Trigeminal Neuralgia Association
    WE MOVE
    Parkinson Disease

**Neurological Institute**
710 West 168th Street
New York, NY 10032
(212) 305-2500

**Neurometabolic Disorders**
*See* Association for Neurometabolic
    Disorders

**Neutropenia**
*See* John T. Curnette, M.D., Ph.D.
    National Neutropenia Network
    Severe Chronic Neutropenia International
        Registry

**Nevoid Basal Cell Carcinoma Syndrome
    (NBCCS) Support Network**
3902 Greencastle Ridge Drive, #204
Burtonsville, MD 20866
(301) 847-1752
(800) 264-8099
(800) 815-4447
*See also* Cancer

**Nevus Network**
1400 South Joyce Street, #1225
Arlington, VA 22202
(703) 920-2349
*See also* Skin Disorders

**Nevus Support Group**
Mrs. R. O'Neill
58 Necton Road
Wheathampstead
Herts AL4 8AU
United Kingdom
*See also* Skin Disorders

**New England Medical Center**
Gynecologic Oncology Group
750 Washington Avenue, Box 232
Boston, MA 02111

**New England Regional Genetics Group**
P.O. Box 670
Mount Desert, ME 04660
(207) 288-2704

**New York Hospital**
Cornell University Medical College
Division of Human Genetics, #HT150
525 East 68th St.
New York, NY 10021
(212) 746-1496

**New York Post-Polio Support Group**
P.O. Box 182
Howard Beach, NY 11414
(718) 835-5536

**New York State Institute for Basic
    Research in Developmental
    Disabilities**
1050 Forest Hill Road
Staten Island, NY 10314
(718) 494-0600
*See also* Sunshine Foundation
    Fragile X Syndrome
    Disability Referrals

**John H. Newman, M.D.**
Vanderbilt University
B1308 Medical Center North
Nashville, TN 37232
(615) 386-6891
(For primary pulmonary hypertension)

**NF-2 Sharing Network**
*See* Neurofibromatosis (NF)-2 Sharing
    Network

**Niemann-Pick Disease Type 3**
*See* National Niemann-Pick Disease
    Foundation

**NIH (National Institutes of Health)**
(301) 496-4000

**NIH/Developmental Endocrinology Branch**
Division of the National Institute of Child Health and Human Development
Bethesda, MD 20892
(301) 496-4686

**NIH/National Arthritis and Musculoskeletal and Skin Diseases**
Information Clearinghouse
One AMS Circle
Bethesda, MD 20892-3675
(301) 495-4484

**NIH/National Cancer Institute**
9000 Rockville Pike
Bethesda, MD 20892
(301) 496-5583

**National Cancer Institute Physician Data Query (PDQ)**
Cancer Information Service
9000 Rockville Pike
Bethesda, MD 20892
(800) 4-CANCER
806-5700 (in Washington, DC, and suburbs)
(800) 638-6070(in Alaska)
(800) 524-1234 (in Oahu, HI); (call collect from neighboring islands)

**NIH/National Center for Human Genome Research**
Ethical, Legal, and Social Issues Branch
Eric Juengst
Room 617, Building 38A
Bethesda, MD 20892
(301) 402-0911

**NIH/National Clearinghouse for Alcohol and Drug Information**
P.O. Box 2345
Rockville, MD 20847-2345
(301) 468-2600
(800) 729-6686
(800) 487-4889

**NIH/National Diabetes Information Clearinghouse**
9000 Rockville Pike
Bethesda, MD 20892
(301) 654-3327

**NIH/National Digestive Diseases Information Clearinghouse**
Two Information Way
Bethesda, MD 20892-3570
(301) 654-3810

**NIH/National Eye Institute**
9000 Rockville Pike
Bethesda, MD 20892
(301) 496-5248

**NIH/National Heart, Lung and Blood Institute**
9000 Rockville Pike
Bethesda, MD 20892-0105
(301) 496-4236

**NIH/National Heart, Lung and Blood Institute Information Center**
P.O. Box 30105
Bethesda, MD 20824-0105
(301) 251-1222

**NIH/National Information Clearinghouse for Infants with Disabilities and Life-Threatening Conditions**
University of South Carolina
Benson Building
Columbia, SC 29208
(800) 922-9234 Ext. 201

**NIH/National Institute on Aging**
9000 Rockville Pike
Bethesda, MD 20892
(301) 496-1752
(800) 222-2225
(800) 438-4380 (for Alzheimer disease)

**NIH/National Institute on Alcohol Abuse and Alcoholism**
5600 Fishers Lane
Rockville, MD 20857
(301) 443-3885

**NIH/National Institute of Allergy and Infectious Diseases**
9000 Rockville Pike
Bethesda, MD 20892
(301) 496-5717

**NIH/National Institute of Arthritis and Musculoskeletal and Skin Diseases**
9000 Rockville Pike
Bethesda, MD 20892
(301) 496-8188

**NIH/National Institute of Child Health and Human Development**
9000 Rockville Pike
Bethesda, MD 20892
(301) 496-5133

**NIH/National Institute of Child Health and Human Development**
Pregnancy and Perinatology Branch
9000 Rockville Pike
Bethesda, MD 20892
(301) 496-5133

**NIH/National Institute on Deafness and Other Communication Disorders**
National Temporal Bone Hearing and Balance Pathology Resource Registry
243 Charles Street
Boston, MA 02114-3096
(617) 573-3711
(800) 822-1327
*See also* Ear Disorders
Hearing Impairment

**NIH/National Institute on Deafness and Other Communication Disorders Information Clearinghouse**
1 Communication Avenue
Bethesda, MD 20892-3456
(800) 241-1044 (voice)
(800) 241-1055 (TDD)
(301) 565-4020

**NIH/National Institute of Dental Research**
9000 Rockville Pike
Bethesda, MD 20892
(301) 496-4261

**NIH/National Institute of Diabetes, Digestive and Kidney Diseases**
9000 Rockville Pike
Bethesda, MD 20892
(301) 496-3583

**NIH/National Institute of Diabetes, Digestive and Kidney Diseases**
Endocrine Diseases Metabolic Diseases Branch
9000 Rockville Pike
Bethesda, MD 20992
(301) 594-7567

**NIH/National Institute on Drug Abuse**
9000 Rockville Pike
Bethesda, MD 20892
(301) 443-6500
(800) 729-6686

**NIH/National Institute of Environmental Health Sciences**
Public Affairs Office
P.O. Box 12233
Research Triangle Park, NC 27709
(919) 541-3345

**NIH/National Institute of Environmental Health Sciences Clearinghouse on Environmental Health Effects (Enviro-Health)**
100 Capitola Drive, Suite 108
Durham, NC 27713
(919-261-9408
(800) 643-4794

**NIH/National Institute of Mental Health**
5600 Fishers Lane
Rockville, MD 20857
(301) 443-4513
(800) 421-4211
(800) 421-4211
(800) 64-PANIC

**NIH/National Institute of Neurological Disorders and Stroke**
9000 Rockville Pike
Bethesda, MD 20892
(301) 496-5751
(800) 352-9424

**NIH/National Institute for Occupational Safety and Health**
(404) 639-3286

**NIH/National Kidney and Urologic Diseases Information Clearinghouse**
9000 Rockville Pike
Bethesda, MD 20892
(301) 468-6345

**NIH/National Oral Health Information
Clearinghouse**
9000 Rockville Pike
Bethesda, MD 20892
(301) 402-7364

**NIH/National Society for Children and
Adults with Autism**
1234 Massachusetts Avenue, Suite 1017
Washington DC 20005
(202) 783-0125

**NIH/Office of Alternative Medicine**
(301) 402-2466

**NIH/Office of Cancer Communications**
Cancer Information Service
9000 Rockville Pike
Bethesda, MD 20892
(800) 422-6237

**NIH/Office of Rare Disease Research**
Steve Groft, M.D.
Federal Building, Room 618
MSC-9120
7550 Wisconsin Avenue
Bethesda, MD 20989-9905
(301) 402-4336
(301) 402-0420 (fax)

**NIH/Office of Recombinant DNA
Activities**
Building 31, Room 4B11
Bethesda, MD 20892

**NIH/Patient Referral Services Unit**
Warren Grant Magnuson Clinical Center
Building #10, Room 2C146
Bethesda, MD 20892
(301) 496-4891

**9p- Chromosome Abnormalities**
*See* Chromosomal Abnormalities

**Noonan Syndrome Support Group**
1278 Pine Avenue
San Jose, CA 95125
(408) 723-5188

**Norrie Disease Association**
Massachusetts General Hospital
E. #6217
149 Thirteenth Street
Charlestown, MA 02129
(617) 726-5718

**North American Malignant Hyperthermia
Registry**
Penn State University
Department of Anesthesia
P.O. Box 850
Hershey, PA 17033-0850
(717) 531-6936

**William L. Nyhan, M.D.**
Professor of Pediatrics
School of Medicine
University of California, San Diego
La Jolla, CA 92093-0609
(619) 534-4150
(For Lesch-Nyhan disease)

**Obesity Foundation**
5600 South Quebec, Suite 160-D
Englewood, CO 80111
(303) 850-0328
*See also* Eating Disorders

**Obsessive-Compulsive Foundation, Inc.**
9 Depot Street
Milford, CT 06460-0070
(203) 878-5669
*See also* Mental Health

**Obstetrics and Gynecology**
*See* American College of Obstetricians and
Gynecologists
Women's Health

**Occupational Hazards and Safety**
*See* NIH/National Institute for Occupational
Safety and Health

**J. Desmond O'Duffy, M.D.**
Division of Rheumatology
Mayo Clinic
200 First Street SW
Rochester, MN 55905
(507) 284-2965
(For Behçet syndrome)

**Olivopontocerebellar Atrophy Support**
Attention: Eva Harris
5243 Beach Blvd.
Jacksonville, FL 32207
(904) 399-8484

**Ollier Disease Support Group**
Bridge House
45 Baring Road
Beaconsfield, Bucks HP9 2 NF
United Kingdom

**Ollier's Disease Self-Help Group**
P.O. Box 52616
Shaw Air Force Base, SC 29152
(803) 775-1757

**Ondine's Curse**
*See* Congenital Central Hypoventilation
Syndrome Family Support Network
John Elefteriades, M.D.
William Tamborlane, Jr., M.D.

**Ontario Fibromyalgia Association**
250 Bloor Street E., Suite 901
Toronto, Ontario M4W 3P2
Canada
(416) 967-1414
(800) 361-1112

**John M. Opitz, M.D.**
Shodar Children's Hospital
P.O. Box 5539
Helena, MT 59604
(406) 444-7500
(For Opitz syndrome; Smith-Lemli-Opitz
syndrome; FG syndrome)

**Opitz Family Network**
P.O. Box 516
Grand Lake, CO 80447
(970) 627-8935
*See also* International Opitz Frias Syndrome

**Opsoclonus-Myoclonus Syndrome
Parent Talk**
724 North Street
Jim Thorpe, PA 18229
(717) 325-3302
*See also* Neurologic Disorders

**Orofacial Guild**
3144 East Jacarda
Orange, CA 92667
*See also* Craniofacial Disorders

**Orphan Drugs**
*See* Food and Drug Administration, Office of
Orphan Drug Products

**David N. Orth, M.D.**
AA-4206 Medical Center North
Vanderbilt University
Nashville, TN 37232
(615) 322-4871
(For Cushing syndrome)

**Orthotics**
*See* Association of Children's Prosthetic
and Orthotic Clinics

**Orton Dyslexia Society**
Chester Bldg., Suite 382
8600 LaSalle Road
Baltimore, MD 21286-2044
(800) 222-3123
(410) 296-0232
*See also* Learning Disabilities

**Osbon Foundation**
(800) 433-4215
(Resource for information on male
impotence)
*See also* Impotence

**Osler-Weber-Rendu Syndrome Registry**
*See* Hereditary Hemorrhagic Telangiectasis
Registry

**Osteogenesis Imperfecta Foundation**
5005 West Laurel Street, Suite 210
Tampa, FL 33607-3836
(813) 282-1161
(800) 981-2663
*See also* Michael P. Whyte, M.D.

**Osteopetrosis**
*See* Friends of the Osteopetrosis Support
Trust

**Ostomy**
*See* United Ostomy Association

**Our Voice (Spasmodic Dysphonia
Newsletter)**
365 West 25th Street, Suite 13E
New York, NY 10001
(212) 929-4299
*See also* National Spasmodic Dysphonia
Association

**Oxalosis and Hyperoxaluria Foundation**
37A Thompson Street
Maynard, MA 01757
(508) 461-0614

**Oxoprolinuria**
See William Rhead, M.D.

**Pachygyria**
See Support Network for Pachygyria,
Agyria, and Lissencephaly

**Pacific Northwest Regional Genetics
Group**
Clinical Services Bldg.
901 East 18th Avenue
Eugene, OR 97403-5254
(503) 346-2610

**Paget Disease of Bone**
See Robert Canfield, M.D.

**Paget Foundation, Inc.**
200 Varick Street, Suite 1004
New York, NY 10014-4810
(212) 229-1582
(800) 237-2438
(For Paget disease of bone and related
disorders)

**Pain**
See American Chronic Pain Association
National Back Pain Association of
England
National Pain Outreach Association

**Charles Y.C. Pak, M.D.**
University of Texas South Western Medical
Center
5323 Harry Hines Boulevard
Dallas, TX 75235
(214) 688-3111
(For cystinuria)

**Pallister-Hall Foundation**
RFD Box 3000
Fairground Road
Bradford, VT 05033
(802) 222-9683
See also Leslie Biesecker, M.D.
John M. Graham, Jr., M.D.

**Pallister-Killian Family Support Group**
3700 Wyndale Court
Fort Worth, TX 76109
(817) 927-8854

**Papillomatosis**
See American Laryngeal Papilloma
Foundation
Recurrent Respiratory Papillomatosis
Foundation

**Paralysis**
See American Paralysis Association
Recurrent Respiratory Papillomatosis
Foundation

**Paraplegia**
See American Paraplegia Society

**Parent Care, Inc.**
9041 Colgate Street
Indianapolis, IN 46268-1210
(317) 872-9913
(For information on improving neonatal
intensive care experiences)
See also Council of Guilds for Infant
Survival
Disability Referrals
Hospice

**Parent Education Network (PEN)**
203 Brookfield Drive
Stratford, WI 54484
(715) 687-4551
(For people on parenteral nutrition or
intravenous feeding)
See also American Society of Parenteral
and Enteral Nutrition

**Parent Project for Muscular Dystrophy
Research**
125 Marymount Court
Middletown, OH 45042
(513) 424-7452
(800) 714-5437

**Parent to Parent**
P.O. Box 704
Cambridge, New Zealand

**Parent to Parent of Georgia**
2900 Woodcock Blvd., Suite 240
Atlanta, GA 30341
(404) 451-5484

**Parenteral and Enteral Nutrition**
See American Society of Parenteral and
Enteral Nutrition
Parent Education Network (PEN)

**Parents and Researchers Interested in
Smith-Magenis Syndrome**
11875 Fawn Ridge Lane
Reston, VA 22094
(703) 709-0568
See also Smith-Magenis Syndrome Contact
Group
Chromosomal Abnormalities

**Parents of Chronically Ill Children**
1527 Maryland Street
Springfield, IL 62702
(217) 522-6810
See also Parent Care
Dysphonia

**Parents of Dwarfed Children**
11524 Colt Terrace
Silver Spring, MD 20902

**Parents of Galactosemic Children, Inc.**
c/o Linda Manis
20981 Solano Way
Boca Raton, FL 33433-1621
(407) 852-0266

**Parkinson Disease**
See Fahr Disease Registry
National Ataxia Foundation
National Parkinson's Foundation
Parkinson's Disease Foundation

Parkinson Disease and Movement
Disorders Clinic
Parkinson's Disease—Movement
Disorders Group
United Parkinson Foundation

**Parkinson Disease and Movement
Disorders Clinic**
Bala V. Manyam, M.D.
Southern Illinois University School of
Medicine
P.O. Box 19230
Springfield, IL 62794-9230
(217) 782-3318

**Parkinson's Disease Foundation**
Columbia Presbyterian Hospital
710 West 168th Street, #336
New York, NY 10032
(212) 923-4700
(800) 457-6676

**Parkinson's Disease—Movement
Disorders Group**
Neurological Institute, Box 57
710 West 168th Street
New York, NY 10032
(212) 305-5779

**Particular Congenital Nevus Network**
6400 Wurzbach Road, 805
San Antonio. TX 78240-3886
(512) 523-8233
See also Skin Disorders

**Pathfinder Family Center**
1600 Second Avenue SW
Minot, ND 56701
(701) 852-9324
(701) 852-9436
(800) 245-5840

**Patient Care Coordinator**
Human Genetics Branch
NIH/National Institute of Child Health and
Human Development
Bethesda, MD 20892
(301) 496-7661.

**Pemphigoid, Bullous**
See W.R. Gammon, M.D.

**Alberto Peña, M.D.**
269-01 76th Avenue
New Hyde Park, NY 10042
(718) 470-3637
(For anorectal malformations)

**PEPCK Deficiency, Mitochondrial and
Cytosolic**
See Mitochondrial Disorders Foundation of
America

**Peutz-Jeghers Syndrome**
See International Peutz-Jeghers Support
Group

**Phenylketonuria (PKU)**
See Children's Phenylketonuria Network
National Phenylketonuria Foundation
National Phenylketonuria News
Phenylketonuria Collaborative Study
Phenylketonuria Parents

**Phenylketonuria (PKU) Collaborative Study**
Children's Hospital of Los Angeles
P.O. Box 54700
Los Angeles, CA 90054
(213) 669-2152

**Phenylketonuria (PKU) Parents**
8 Myrtle Lane
San Anselmo, CA 94960
(415) 457-4632

**Martin D. Phillips, M.D.**
University of Texas
Health Science Center
Houston, TX 77030
(For hereditary hemorrhagic telangiectasia)

**Pick disease**
*See* Jordan Grafman, Ph.D.

**Pilot Parent Exchange**
2818 San Gabriel
Austin, TX 78705
(512) 476-7044

**Pituitary Tumor Network Association**
16350 Ventura Boulevard, Suite 231
Encino, CA 91436
(805) 499-1523
(800) 642-9211
*See also* Cancer

**Pityriasis Rubra Pilaris**
*See* Irwin M. Freedberg, M.D.

**Plastic Surgery**
*See* American Society of Plastic and
    Reconstructive Surgeons, International
    Institute of Reconstructive Plastic
    Surgery

**Polio**
*See* British Polio Fellowship
    International Polio Network
    New York Post-Polio Support Group
    Polio Information Center
    Polio Society
    Post-Polio National, Inc.

**Polio Information Center**
510 Main Street, Suite A446
Roosevelt Island, NY 10044
(212) 223-0353

**Polio Society**
4200 Wisconsin Avenue, Suite 106273
Washington DC 20016
(301) 897-8180

**Paul Poltz**
NIAMS, Bldg. 10, Rm. 9N244
9000 Rockville Pike
Bethesda, MD 20892
(301) 496-1474
*See also* Polymyositis/Dermatomyositis

**Polychondritis and Rheumatoid Arthritis Clinic**
David Trentham, M.D.
Division of Rheumatology
Beth Israel Hospital
330 Brookline Avenue
Boston, MA 02215
(617) 735-2560
*See also* Arthritis Foundation

**Polycystic Kidney Disease**
*See* Lisa M. Guay-Woodford, M.D.
    William D. Kaehny, M.D.

**Polycystic Kidney Research (PKR) Foundation**
4901 Main Street, #320
Kansas City, MO 64112
(816) 931-2600
(800) 753-2873
*See also* Kidney/Urologic Disorders

**Polymyositis**
*See* Frederick W. Miller, M.D.
    National Support Group for Myositis
    Paul Poltz

**Polyposis**
*See* Familial Polyposis Registry
    Gastrointestinal Polyposis and Hereditary
        Colon Cancer Registry
    Intestinal Multiple Polyposis and
        Colorectal Cancer

**Porphyria**
*See* American Porphyria Foundation
    Cecilia Warner, M.D.

**Port Wine Stain**
*See* Congenital Nevus Network
    National Congenital CMV Disease
        Registry
    Sturge-Weber Foundation

**Post-Polio National, Inc.**
(Post-Polio League for Information and
    Outreach, Polio Society)
4200 Wisconsin Ave. NW, Suite 106273
Washington, DC 20016
(301) 897-8180
*See also* Polio

**Prader Willi Association**
223 Main Street
Port Washington, NY 11050
(516) 944-8136
(800) 253-7993

**Prader-Willi Syndrome Association (USA)**
2510 South Brentwood Blvd., Suite 220
Saint Louis, MO 63144-2326
(314) 962-7644
(800) 926-4797

**Prader-Willi Syndrome International Information Forum**
40 Holly Lane
Roslyn Heights, NY 11577
(516) 621-2445
(800) 358-0682

**Pregnancy Hotline**
Jane O'Brien, M.D.
Boston, MA
(617) 291-0946 (fax)
(For those who suspect their child might be
    born with a defect)
*See also* NIH/National Institute of Child
    Health and Human Development
    Pregnancy and Perinatology Branch

**Prescription Parents**
22 Ingersoll Road
Wellesley, MA 02181
(617) 273-2920
(For parents of children with cleft palate)
*See also* Craniofacial Disorders

**Primary Biliary Cirrhosis Patient Support Network**
Box 177
Tamworth, Ontario K0K 3G0
Canada
(613) 379-2534

**Primary Lateral Sclerosis (PLS) Newsletter**
101 Pinta Court
Los Gatos, CA 95032
(408) 356-8227
*See also* Neurologic Disorders

**Progeria**
*See* New York State Institute for Basic
    Research in Developmental Disabilities
    Sunshine Foundation

**Progressive Supranuclear Palsy Research Fund**
Department of Neurology, Room 408
UMDNJ-Robert Wood Johnson Medical
    School
CN19
New Brunswick, NJ 08903
(908) 937-7728
*See also* Society for Progressive
    Supranuclear Palsy
    Irene Litvan, M.D.
    Neurologic Disorders

**Prostate Cancer**
*See* Mathews Foundation for Prostate
    Cancer Research
    Us Too

**Prosthetics**
*See* Association of Children's Prosthetic
    and Orthotic Clinics

**Prune Belly Syndrome**
*See* National Prune Belly Syndrome
    Network

**Pseudohypoparathyroidism (PHP) Self-Help Clearinghouse**
104 Northern Parkway West
Plainview, NY 11803
(516) 681-6308 (noon–6 P.M. ET)

**Pseudomyxoma Peritonei**
*See* Paul H. Sugarbaker, M.D.

**Pseudo-obstruction**
*See* Intestinal Pseudo-obstruction

**Pseudotumor Cerebri Society**
1319 Butternut Street, Suite 3
Syracuse, NY 13208
(315) 464-2553
(800) 926-1230

**Pseudoxanthoma Elasticum (PXE)**
See Mark Lebwohl, M.D.
  National Association for Pseudoxanthoma
  Elasticum
  Kenneth H. Nelder, M.D.

**Psoriasis**
See National Psoriasis Foundation

**Psoriasis Research Association**
107 Vista del Grande
San Carlos, CA 94070
(415) 593-1394
See also National Psoriasis Foundation

**Pull-Thru Network**
62 Edgewood Avenue
Wyckoff, NJ 07481
(201) 981-5977

**Pulmonary Disorders**
See Lung Disorders

**Radiation Disease**
See Environmental Disorders

**Radiation Survivors**
See National Association of Radiation
  Survivors
  National Council on Radiation Protection
  and Measurements

**Rare Disease Support Groups**
See Center for Rare Diseases and
  Disabilities (Denmark)
  Contact a Family (U.K.)
  Istituto di Ricerche Cliniche per le
  Malattie Rare (Italy)
  Lethbridge Society for Rare Diseases
  National Organization for Rare Disorders

**Theodore Rasmussen, M.D.**
Montreal Neurological Hospital
3801 University Street
Montreal H3A 2B4
Canada
(514) 398-6644
(For Rasmussen encephalitis)
See also Ben Carson, M.D.

**Raynaud's Association Trust**
c/o Bladon Crescent
Alsager, Cheshire 5T7 2BG
United Kingdom

**Raynaud's Scleroderma Association**
112 Crewe Road
Alsager, Cheshire ST7 2JA
United Kingdom
027-087-2776

**Reconstruction Surgery for Craniofacial
  or Facial Abnormalities**
See National Foundation for Facial
  Reconstruction

**Recording for the Blind**
545 Fifth Avenue, Suite 1005
New York, NY 10017
(800) 221-4792
See also Eye Disorders

**Recurrent Respiratory Papillomatosis
  Foundation**
50 Wesleyan Drive
Hamilton, NJ 08690
(609) 452-6545
See also American Laryngeal Papilloma
  Foundation

**Reflex Sympathetic Dystrophy Syndrome
  Association (RSDSA)**
116 Haddon Avenue, Suite D
Haddonfield, NJ 08033
(609) 795-8845

**Rehabilitation**
See National Rehabilitation Information
  Center

**Renal Disorders**
See Kidney/Urologic Disorders

**Repetitive Stress Injuries**
See Association for Repetitive Motion
  Syndrome
  Ben Carson, M.D.

**Research for Rett Foundation**
P.O. Box 50347
Mobile, AL 36605
(334) 479-8293
(800) 422-7388
See also International Rett Syndrome
  Association

**Research Trust for Metabolic Diseases
  in Children**
Golden Gate Lodge
Weston Road
Crewe, Cheshire CW1 1XN
United Kingdom
(01270) 250221

**Resolve, Inc.**
Five Water Street
Arlington, MA 02174
(617) 623-0744
See also Fertility

**Restless Legs Syndrome Foundation**
1904 Banbury Road
Raleigh, NC 27608-1120
(919)781-4428
See also Arthur Walters, M.D.
  Wayne Hening, M.D.
  Neurologic Disorders

**Retarded Infant Services**
386 Park Avenue South
New York, NY 10016
(212) 889-5464
See also The Arc

**Retinitis Pigmentosa International**
P.O. Box 900
Woodland Hills, CA 91365
(818) 992-0500
(800) 344-4877
See also Texas Association for Retinitis
  Pigmentosa
  Eye Disorders

**Retinoblastoma**
See National Retinoblastoma Parent Group
  Brenda Gallie, M.D.
  Thaddeus P. Dryja, M.D.

**Rett Syndrome**
See International Rett Syndrome
  Association
  Research for Rett Foundation
  Daniel Glaze, M.D.
  Sakkubai Naidu, M.D.

**Reye Syndrome Society**
Box RS
Benzonia, MI 49616
See also National Reye's Syndrome
  Foundation

**William Rhead, M.D.**
University of Iowa Hospitals and Clinics
Department of Pediatrics
200 Hawkins Drive
Iowa City, IA 52242-1083
(For oxoprolinuria)

**L. Jackson Roberts II, M.D.**
Vanderbilt University Hospital
1161 21st Avenue South
Nashville, TN 37232-2390
(For mastocytosis)

**Roberts Syndrome**
See Uta Francke, M.D.

**David Robertson, M.D.**
Research Database at Vanderbilt University
AA3228 Medical Center North
Vanderbilt University
Nashville, TN 37232-2195
(800) 428-6626
(615) 343-0124
(For orthostatic hypotension)

**Gary L. Robertson**
Northwestern Memorial Hospital
250 East Superior Street
Room 1625
Chicago, IL 60611
(312) 503-0058
(For diabetes insipidus)

**Rocky Mountain Research and Training
  Institute**
6355 Ward Road, Unit 310
Arvada, CO 80004-3823
(303) 420-2942
See also Disability Referrals

**Romano-Ward Syndrome**
See International Long QT Syndrome
  Registry
  Sudden Arrhythmia Death Syndrome
  Foundation

**Rosacea**
*See* National Rosacea Society

**Roger N. Rosenberg, M.D.**
Department of Neurology and Physiology
University of Texas Southwestern Medical
School
5323 Harry Hines Boulevard
Dallas, TX 75235-9036
(214) 688-4800
(For Joseph disease)

**Norman D. Rosenblum, M.D.**
Division of Nephrology
Children's Hospital in Boston
300 Longwood Avenue
Boston, MA 02115
(617) 735-6129
(For polycystic kidney disease)

**Judith Levine Ross, M.D.**
Jefferson Medical College
1025 Walnut Street
Philadelphia, PA 19107-6799
(215) 955-1648
(For Turner syndrome)

**Guy A. Rouleau, M.D.**
Iscia Lopes-Cendes, M.D.
Karen Rye, R.N.
Department of Neurology
Montreal General Hospital
1650 Cedar Ave.
Montreal, Quebec, H3G 1A4
Canada
(514) 937-6011
(For myoclonic progressive familial
epilepsy)
*See also* Neurofibromatosis

**RSH Syndrome**
*See* Smith-Lemli-Opitz/RSH Advocacy and
Exchange
John M. Opitz, M.D.

**Jack H. Rubinstein**
Rubinstein-Taybi Case Documentation
Cincinnati Center for Developmental
Disorders
Pavilion Building
Ell and Bethesda Avenues
Cincinnati, OH 45229-2899
(513) 559-4688

**Rubinstein-Taybi Parent Support Group**
P.O. Box 146
Smith Center, KS 66967-0146
(913) 697-2984

**Rubinstein-Taybi Support Group**
c/o Barbara Baron
46 Windsor Road
Great Harwood
Blackburn, Lancashire BB6 7RR
United Kingdom
0254-889-122

**Rush Presbyterian**
Saint Luke's Medical Center
1753 West Congress Parkway
Chicago, IL 60612
(312) 942-5000
(312) 942-5939

**Russell-Silver Syndrome**
*See* Association for Children with Russell-
Silver Syndrome

**Sarcoidosis Research Institute**
3475 Central Avenue
Memphis, TN 38111-4407
(901) 766-6951

**Clarence T. Sasaki, M.D.**
Yale University School of Medicine
333 Cedar Street
New Haven, CT 06510
(For dysphonia)

**Schepens Eye Research Institute**
20 Staniford Street
Boston, MA 02114-2500
(617) 742-3140
*See also* Eye Disorders

**Jerry A. Schneider, M.D.**
Department of Pediatrics
Basic Science Building
Room 4006/0609F
University of California at San Diego
School of Medicine
La Jolla, CA 92093-0609
(619) 534-6987
(For cystinosis)

**Scleroderma**
*See* Gary W. Hunninghake, M.D.
Scleroderma Federation
Scleroderma Information Exchange
Scleroderma Research Foundation
United Scleroderma Foundation

**Scleroderma Federation, Inc.**
Peabody Office Building
1 Newbury Street
Peabody, MA 01960-3830
(508) 535-6600
(800) 422-1113

**Scleroderma Information Exchange, Inc.**
150 Hines Farm Road
Cranston, RI 02921-1408
(401) 943-3909

**Scleroderma Research Foundation**
2320 Bath Street, Suite 307
Santa Barbara, CA 93105
(805) 563-9133
(800) 441-2873

**Scoliosis Association**
P.O. Box 51353
Raleigh, NC 27609
(919) 846-2639
*See also* National Scoliosis Foundation, Inc.

**Alan Scott, M.D.**
Smith-Kettlewell Eye Research Foundation
2232 Webster Street
San Francisco, CA 94115
(415) 567-0667
(For botulinum toxin)

**Seizure Disorders**
*See* THRESHOLD

**Self-Help for Hard-of-Hearing People,
Inc.**
7910 Woodmont Ave. Suite 1200
Bethesda, MD 20814
(301) 657-2248
(301) 657-2249 (TDD)
*See also* Hearing Impairment

**Severe Chronic Neutropenia
International Registry**
Puget Sound Plaza, #1365
1325 Fourth Avenue
Seattle, WA 98101-2509
(206) 543-9749
(800) 726-4636
*See also* National Neutropenia Network

**Sexual Disorders**
*See* Ambiguous Genitalia Support Network
Association for Male Sexual Dysfunction
Coalition on Sexuality and Disability
Finding Our Own Ways
International Foundation for Gender
Education
Intersex Society of North America

**Sexually Transmitted Diseases**
*See* AIDS
American Social Health Association
Herpes Support Group at Help South Bay

**Share and Care Cockayne Syndrome
Network**
P.O. Box 552
Stanleytown, VA 24168-0552
(703) 629-2369

**Short Stature Foundation**
4521 Campus Drive, #130
Irvine, CA 92715
(714) 258-1833
(800) 243-9273
*See also* Dwarfism

**Shprintzen Syndrome**
*See* Rosalie Goldberg
Velo-Cardio-Facial Syndrome Association

**Shwachman Syndrome Support**
44 Meadowlark Road
Vernon, CT 06066
(203) 870-5454

**Shy-Drager Syndrome Support Group**
1607 Silver Avenue SE
Albuquerque, NM 87106-4443
(505) 243-5118
(800) 737-4999
*See also* David Goldstein, M.D.
Italo Biaggioni, M.D.

**Siblings for Significant Change**
United Charities Building
105 East 22nd Street, Room 710
New York, NY 10010
(212) 420-0776
(800) 841-8251
(Advocacy group for people with disabled
siblings)
*See also* Disability Referrals

**Siblings Information Network**
The A.J. Pappanikou Center
62 Washington Street
Middletown, CT 06457-2844
(203) 344-7500
(203) 344-7590 (TTY)

**Siblings of Children with Disabilities**
c/o Karen A. Swauger
26 Wallace Road
Goffstown, NH 03045
See also Disability Referrals

**Sickle Cell**
See American Sickle Cell Anemia
    Association
  Canadian Sickle Cell Society
  Center for Sickle Cell Disease
  Sickle Cell Association of Ontario
  Sickle Cell Association of Texas Gulf
    Coast
  Sickle Cell Disease Association of
    America
  Triad Sickle Cell Anemia Foundation

**Sickle Cell Association of Ontario**
55 Gateway Blvd.
Don Mills, Ontario M3C 1B4
Canada
(416) 674-6916

**Sickle Cell Association of Texas Gulf
Coast**
2626 South Loop West, Suite 245
Houston, TX 77054
(713) 666-0300

**Sickle Cell Disease Association of
America, Inc.**
200 Corporate Pointe, Suite 495
Culver City, CA 90230-7633
(310) 216-6363
(800) 421-8453

**Paul Sieving, M.D., Ph.D.**
Department of Ophthalmology
University of Michigan Medical Center
Ann Arbor, MI
(For X-linked juvenile retinoschisis)

**Sight Impairment**
See Eye Disorders

**Silicone Breast Implants**
See Breast Implants

**Simon Foundation**
P.O. Box 815
Wilmette, IL 60091
(708) 864-3913
See also Kidney/Urologic Disorders

**Valerie Simon, M.D.**
Michael Reiss, M.D.
Lisa Freund, Ph.D.
Kennedy-Krieger Institute
Behavioral Genetics Unit, Room 103
707 North Broadway Avenue
Baltimore, Maryland 21205
(301) 550-9321
(301) 550-9313 (collect)
(For fragile X syndrome)

**Sjögren Syndrome Foundation**
333 North Broadway
Jericho, NY 11573
(516) 933-6365
See also Alice Macynski, R.N.
    National Sjögren's Syndrome Association

**James Skare, M.D.**
Boston University School of Medicine
Center for Human Genetics
Boston, MA 02118
(617) 638-7086
(For information on X-linked
  lymphoproliferative syndrome studies)

**Skeletal Dysplasia**
See International Center for Skeletal
  Dysplasia

**Skin Cancer Foundation**
245 Fifth Avenue, Suite 2402
New York, NY 10016
(212) 725-5176
(800) 754-6490

**Skin Disease Research Core Centers of
the National Institute of Arthritis and
Musculoskeletal and Skin Diseases**

S. Wright Caughman, M.D.
Department of Dermatology
Emory University School of Medicine
1639 Peirce Drive, Room 5001 WMB
**Atlanta**, GA 30322
(404) 727-5872

Thomas S. Kupper, M.D.
Department of Medicine
Division of Dermatology
Brigham and Women's Hospital
75 Francis Street
**Boston**, MA 02115
(617) 278-0993

Craig A. Elmets, M.D.
Department of Dermatology
University Hospitals of Cleveland
Case Western Reserve University
11100 Euclid Avenue
**Cleveland**, OH 44106
(216) 844-3178

Paul R. Bergstresser, M.D.
Department of Dermatology
University of Texas
Southwest Medical Center
5323 Harry Hines Boulevard
**Dallas**, TX 75235
(214) 648-3493

George P. Stricklin, M.D.
Department of Medicine
Division of Dermatology
Vanderbilt University
1211 21st Avenue South
620 Medical Arts Building
**Nashville**, TN 37212
(615) 936-1135

Robert E. Tigelaar, M.D.
Department of Dermatology
Yale University School of Medicine
333 Cedar Street
**New Haven**, CT 06510
(203) 785-4968

**Skin Disorders**
See American Academy of Dermatology
    American Society of Dermatopathology
    Dermatomyositis and Polymyositis
      Support Group
    Eczema Association for Science and
      Education
    Frontier's International Vitiligo Foundation
    Russell P. Hall III, M.D.
    National Foundation for Vitiligo and
      Pigment Disorders
    National Incontinentia Pigmenti
      Foundation
    National Support Group for Myositis
    Nevus Network
    Nevus Support Group
    Particular Congenital Nevus Network
    Toxic Epidermal Necrolysis Clinical
      Facilities

**Martha Skinner, M.D.**
Alan S. Cohen, M.D
Arthritis Center
Boston University School of Medicine
71 East Concord Street
Boston, MA 02118
(617) 638-4310
(For amyloidosis)

**Gary R. Skuse, Ph.D.**
University of Rochester Medical Center
Division of Genetics
601 Elmwood Avenue, Box 641
Rochester, NY 14642
(716) 275-3463

**Sleep Apnea**
See John Elefteriades, M.D.

**Sleep Disorders**
See American Sleep Apnea Association
    American Sleep Disorders Association
    Awake Network
    Center for Research in Sleep Disorders
    Center for Sleep Disorders
    Narcolepsy and Sleep Disorders
      International Newsletter
    Narcolepsy and Catalexy Foundation of
      America
    Narcolepsy Institute
    Narcolepsy Network
    National Sleep Disorders Foundation
    National Sleep Foundation

**Smell and Taste Research Center**
University of Pennsylvania Hospital
5 Ravdin Building
3400 Spruce Street
Philadelphia, PA 19104
(215) 662-6580

**Smith-Lemli-Opitz/RSH Advocacy and
Exchange**
222 Valley Green Drive
Aston, PA 19014
(610) 494-5287
See also Opitz syndrome

**Smith-Magenis Syndrome Contact Group**
52 Ladeside Close
Newton Mearns, Glasgow
Scotland G77-6TZ
United Kingdom
041-639-9615
*See also* Parents and Researchers
Interested in Smith-Magenis Syndrome

**Social Security Administration Hotline**
(800) 772-1213
(800) 325-0778 (TDD)

**Society of Mucopolysaccharide (MPS) Diseases**
7 Chessfield Park
Buckinghamshire HP6 6RU
United Kingdom

**Society of Mucopolysaccharide (MPS) Diseases, Inc.**
c/o Sheila Lee
204-4912 Ross Street
Red Deer, Alberta T4N 1X7
Canada

**Society for Muscular Dystrophy International**
P.O. Box 479
Bridgewater, Nova Scotia B4V 2X6
Canada
(902) 429-6322

**Society for Progressive Supranuclear Palsy**
J.H. Outpatient Center, #5065
601 North Caroline Street
Baltimore, MD 21287
(410) 955-7357
(800) 457-4777
*See also* Progressive Supranuclear Palsy
Research Fund
Neurologic Disorders

**Society for the Rehabilitation of the Facially Disfigured, Inc.**
550 First Avenue
New York, NY 10016
(212) 340-5400
*See also* National Foundation for Facial
Reconstruction

**Society for the Right to Die**
*See* Choice in Dying

**Juan Sotos, M.D.**
Children's Hospital, C-404
700 Children's Drive
Columbus, OH 43205
(614) 461-2000

**Sotos Syndrome Support Association**
1288 Loughborough Court
Wheaton, IL 60187
(708) 682-8815

**Sotos Syndrome Support Group of Great Britain**
c/o Child Growth Foundation
4 Mayfield Avenue
London W4 1PW
United Kingdom
081-995-0257

**Southeastern Regional Genetics Group**
Emory University
Pediatrics/Medical Genetics
2040 Ridgewood Drive
Atlanta, GA 30322
(404) 727-5844

**Spasmodic Dysphonia**
*See* National Spasmodic Dysphonia
Association
Our Voice

**Spasmodic Torticollis**
*See* National Spasmodic Torticollis
Association

**Spina Bifida Association of America**
4590 MacArthur Boulevard NW
Suite 250
Washington, DC 20007-4226
(202) 944-3285
(800) 621-3141
*See* International Federation for
Hydrocephalus and Spina Bifida

**Spina Bifida Association of Canada**
220 388 Donald Street
Winnipeg, Manitoba R3B 2J4
Canada
(204) 957-1784

**Spinal Cord Injuries**
*See* American Paraplegia Society
American Spinal Injury Association
National Spinal Cord Injury Association
National Spinal Cord Injury Hotline
Spinal Cord Society

**Spinal Cord Society**
Wendell Road
Fergus Falls, MN 56537
(218) 739-5252

**Spinal Muscular Atrophy**
*See* Families of Spinal Muscular Atrophy

**Spondylitis Association of America**
P.O. Box 5872
Sherman Oaks, CA 91413
(818) 981-1616
(800) 777-8189

**Spotlight 6 (Chromosome 6 Disorders)**
2617 Ted Toad Road
Rising Sun, MD 21911
(410) 658-6264
*See also* Chromosomal Disorders

**Stargardt International and Juvenile Macular Dystrophies**
P.O. Box 136
West Chicago, IL 60186
(708) 208-5017
*See also* Macular Dystrophy

**Stein-Leventhal Syndrome**
*See* David Ehrmann, M.D.

**Steve Atanas Stavro Familial Gastrointestinal Cancer Registry**
Mount Sinai, #1157
600 University Ave.
Toronto, Ontario M5G 1X5
Canada
(416) 586-8334
*See also* Cancer

**Stickler Syndrome Support Group**
27 Braycourt Avenue
Walton-on-the-Thames
Surrey KT12 2AZ
United Kingdom
(01932) 229421

**Stiff-Man Syndrome**
*See* Mark Hallet, M.D.

**Streptococcal Infections, Group B**
*See* Group B Strep Association

**Stroke Foundation**
898 Park Avenue
New York, NY 10021
(212) 734-3461
*See also* National Stroke Association
Heart Disorders

**Sturge-Weber Foundation**
P.O. Box 418
Mount Freedom, NJ 07970-0418
(201) 895-4445
(800) 627-5482
*See also* Congenital Nevus Network
Odile Enjolras, M.D.
National CMV Disease Registry

**Stuttering**
*See* National Stuttering Project

**Subacute Sclerosing Panencephalitis**
*See* National Subacute Sclerosing
Panencephalitis Registry

**Substance Abuse**
*See* Center for Substance Abuse Prevention

**Sudden Arrhythmia Death Syndrome Foundation**
P.O. Box 58767
Salt Lake City, UT 84158
(801) 582-1934
(800) 786-7723
*See also* International Long QT Syndrome
Registry
Heart Disorders

**Sudden Infant Death Syndrome**
*See* National Sudden Infant Death Resource
Center
National Sudden Infant Death Syndrome
Clearinghouse
Sudden Infant Death Syndrome (SIDS)
Alliance, Inc.
United Sudden Infant Death Syndrome
Awareness

**Sudden Infant Death Syndrome (SIDS) Alliance, Inc.**
1314 Bedford Avenue, Suite 210
Baltimore, MD 21208
(410) 653-8226
(800) 221-7437

**Paul H. Sugarbaker, M.D.**
The Cancer Institute
Washington Hospital Center
110 Irving Street, NW
Washington, DC 20010-1975
(For pseudomyxoma peritonei)

**Suicide Prevention**
See National Committee on Youth Suicide
     Prevention
     American Association of Suicidology

**Sunshine Foundation**
P.O. Box 255
CR 547N
Loughman, FL 33858
(813) 424-4188
(800) 457-1976
(Provides vacation atmosphere where
     children with progeria are studied)
See also New York State Institute for Basic
     Research in Developmental Disabilities

**Superkids, Inc.**
60 Clyde Street
Newton, MA 02160
(Newsletter for family/friends of children
     with limb abnormalities)
See also Amputation
     CHERUB
     Children

**Support and Educational Exchange for Klinefelter Syndrome**
1417 25th Avenue Drive West
Bradenton, FL 34205-6449
(813) 750-8044

**Support for Families with Children Having Weaver Syndrome**
4357 153rd Ave SE
Bellevue, WA 98006
(206) 747-5382
(416) 948-5401

**Support Group Assistance**
See American Self-Help Clearinghouse

**Support Group for Monosomy 9p**
43304 Kipton Nickle Plate Road
LaGrange, OH 44050
(216) 775-4255
See also Chromosomal Abnormalities

**Support Group for 9p-**
675 North Roundtable Drive
Las Vegas, NV 89110
(702) 453-0788
See also Chromosomal Abnormalities

**Support Network**
c/o Elizabeth E. LaBozetta
1562 Picard Road
Columbus, OH 43227
(614) 235-4032
(For those with serious complications from
     laproscopic gall bladder removal)

**Support Network for Pachygyria, Agyria, Lissencephaly**
2410 South 24th Street #9102
Kansas City, KS 66106
(913) 432-7453

**Support Organization for Trisomy (S.O.F.T.) Canada, Inc.**
760 Brant Street, Suite 420
Burlington, Ontario L7R 4B8
Canada
(800) 668-0696
(416) 632-7755
See also Chromosomal Abnormalities

**Support Organization for Trisomy (S.O.F.T.) 18, 13 and Related Disorders**
2982 South Union Street
Rochester, NY 14624-1926
(716) 594-4621
(800) 716-7638
See also Chromosomal Abnormalities

**Swedish Orphan AB**
Sturplan 15 IV
S-111 45 Stockholm
Sweden

**Syringomyelia**
See American Syringomyelia Alliance
     Project

**Systemic Lupus Erythematosus Foundation, Inc.**
149 Madison Avenue, Suite 608
New York, NY 10016
(212) 685-4118
See also Lupus Erythematosus

**Systemic Lupus Erythematosus Foundation, Inc.**
c/o William L. Nyhan, M.D.
Department of Pediatrics
University of California School of Medicine,
     San Diego
La Jolla, CA 92093-0609
(619) 534-4150
See also Lupus Erythematosus

**William Tamborlane, Jr., M.D.**
Pediatric General Clinical
Research Center
Yale University School of Medicine
333 Cedar Street
New Haven, CT 06510-8064
(203) 432-4771
(For Ondine's curse)

**Tardive Dyskinesia/Tardive Dystonia National Association**
4244 University Way NE
P.O. Box 45732
Seattle, WA 98145-0732
(206) 522-3166

**Tay-Sachs Disease**
See Chromosomal Abnormalities
     Late Onset Tay-Sachs Foundation
     National Tay-Sachs and Allied Diseases
          Association, Inc.
     National Foundation for Jewish Genetic
          Diseases

**Tay-Sachs and Allied Diseases Association**
17 Sydney Road
Barkingside, Ilford
Essex, United Kingdom
01-550-8989

**TEF/VATER/VACTRL National Support Network**
15301 Grey Fox Road
Upper Marlboro, MD 20772
(301) 952-6837
See also Atresia

**Telangiectasia**
See Hereditary Hemorrhagic Telangiectasia

**Temporal Bone Registry**
See NIH/National Institute on Deafness and
     Other Communication Disorders Registry

**Texas Association for Retinitis Pigmentosa**
P.O. Box 8388
Corpus Christi, TX 78412
(512) 852-8515

**Thalidomide Society**
19 Upper Hall Park
Berkhamsted, Herts HP4 2NP
United Kingdom

**Jess G. Thoene, M.D.**
Department of Pediatrics
University of Michigan Medical School
300 NIB, 1182 SE
Ann Arbor, MI 48109-0408
(313) 763-3427
(For cystinosis and other rare disorders)

**THRESHOLD (Intractable Seizure Disorder Support Group and Newsletter)**
26 Stavola Road
Middletown, NJ 07748
(908) 957-0714
See also Epilepsy Foundation of America

**Thrombocytopenia–Absent Radius Syndrome Association (TARSA)**
212 Sherwood Drive
Linwood, NJ 08221
(609) 927-0418 (after 4 P.M. EST)

**Thyroid Foundation of America, Inc.**
R. Sleeper Hl., RSL 350
40 Parkman St.
Boston, MA 02114-2698
(617) 726-8500
(800) 832-8321

**Thyroid Foundation of Canada**
CD/Box 1597
Kingston, Ontario K7L 5C8
Canada
(613) 542-8330

**Tinnitus**
*See* Ear Disorders
Hearing Impairment

**Tissue Samples**
*See* National Disease Research Interchange

**Tourette Syndrome Association, Inc.**
42-40 Bell Blvd.
Bayside, NY 11361
(718) 224-2999
(800) 237-0717

**Tourette Syndrome Association of MD, DC, and VA**
33 University Boulevard East
Silver Spring, MD 20901-2437
(301) 681-4133

**Wallace W. Tourtelotte, M.D.**
National Neurological Research Bank
Neurology Research (W127A)
Veterans Administration
Wadsworth Medical Center
Los Angeles, CA 90073
(213) 824-4307

**Toxic Epidermal Necrolysis Clinical Facilities**

Rockefeller University Hospital
Department of Investigative Dermatology
1230 York Avenue
**New York**, NY 10021
(212) 327-8000

Children's Hospital
Department of Pediatric Dermatology
Dermatology Clinic
34th and Civic Center Boulevard
**Philadelphia**, PA 19104

University of Pennsylvania (diagnosis only)
Dermatology Clinic
34th and Spruce Streets
**Philadelphia**, PA 19104
(215) 662-6535

Washington University School of Medicine
Department of Dermatology
**Saint Louis**, MO 63110
(314) 362-5000

**Toxic Substances**
*See* Environmental Disorders

**Tracheoesophageal Fistula**
*See* TEF/VATER/VACTRL National Support Network

**Transplantation**
*See* National Association of Patients on Hemodialysis and Transplantation

**Transverse Myelitis Association**
3650 Tahoma Place West
Tacoma, WA 98466
(206) 565-8156

**Travelin' Talk**
P.O. Box 3534
Clarksville, TN 37043-3534
(615) 552-6670
(Travel information on access for the disabled)
*See also* Disability Referrals

**Treacher Collins Foundation**
P.O. Box 683
Norwich, VT 05055-0683
(802) 649-3050
(800) 823-2055

**Tremor**
*See* International Tremor Foundation

**Triad Sickle Cell Anemia Foundation**
1102 East Market Street
P.O. Box 20964
Greensboro, NC 27401
(910) 274-1507
(800) 733-8297

**Trichotillomania**
*See* Wayne Goodman, M.D.
Marge Lenane

**Trigeminal Neuralgia Association**
P.O. Box 785
Barnegat Light, NJ 08006-0785
(609) 361-1014
*See also* Neurologic Disorders

**Trisomy 9 International Parent Support**
Children's Hospital, Div. Gen. and Met.
3901 Beaubien Blvd.
Detroit, MI 48201-2196
(313) 745-4513
*See* Chromosomal Abnormalities

**L-Tryptophan Victims Group**
c/o Joanne Hil
(919) 878-5659
*See also* Erythromelalgia Syndrome Support Group
Trisomy and Related Disorders
Chromosomal Abnormalities

**Tuberous Sclerosis**
*See* National Tuberous Sclerosis Association

**Turcot Syndrome and Hereditary Medulloblastoma**
*See* Daniel M. Lasser, M.D.

**Turner Syndrome**
*See* Gordon B. Cutler, Jr., M.D.
Judith Levine Ross, M.D.
Turner Syndrome Support Group of New England
Turner Syndrome Society of Canada
Turner Syndrome Support Group of New England
Turner's Syndrome Society of the U.S.

**Turner Syndrome Society of Canada**
7777 Keel Street, Floor 2
Concord, Ontario L4K 1Y7
Canada
(416) 660-7766

**Turner Syndrome Support Group of New England**
170 Maple Street
Malden, MA 02148
(617) 322-4892

**Turner's Syndrome Society of the U.S.**
811 Twelve Oaks Ct.
15500 Wayzata Blvd.
Wayzata, MN 55391
(612) 475-9944
(800) 365-9944

**Twin to Twin Transfusion Syndrome Foundation, Inc.**
National Office
411 Longbeach Parkway
Bay Village, OH 44140
(216) 899-8887

**Ulcers**
*See* National Ulcer Foundation

**United Cerebral Palsy Association**
1660 L Street NW, Suite 700
Washington, DC 20036
(202) 776-0414
(800) 872-5827
(202) 973-7197 (TTY)

**United Leukodystrophy Foundation**
2304 Highland Drive
Sycamore, IL 60178
(815) 895-3211
(800) 728-5483
*See also* Association Européenne contre les Leucodystrophes

**United Liver Association**
11646 West Pico Boulevard
Los Angeles, CA 90064-2987
(213) 445-4204
(213) 445-4200

**United Ostomy Association**
36 Executive Park, Suite 120
Irvine, CA 92714-6744
(714) 660-8624
(800) 826-0826

**United Parkinson Foundation**
833 West Washington Blvd.
Chicago, IL 60607
(312) 733-1893

**United Patients' Association for Pulmonary Hypertension, Inc.**
P.O. Box 24733
Speedway, IN 46224-0733
(815) 758-4101
(800) 748-7274

**United Scleroderma Foundation, Inc.**
P.O. Box 399
Watsonville, CA 95077-0399
(408) 728-2202
(800) 722-4673

**United Sudden Infant Death Syndrome (SIDS) Awareness, Inc.**
Family and Friends of Sudden Infant Death Syndrome Victims
International Headquarters
3901-3 West Dakin Street
Chicago, IL 60618
(312) 583-3786
*See also* Sudden Infant Death Syndrome

**University of Southern California Medical Center**
2925 Zonal Avenue, Rm. 252
Los Angeles, CA
(213) 226-7616

**Urea Cycle Disorders**
*See* British Organic Acidemia Association
National Urea Cycle Disorders Foundation
Saul Brusilow, M.D.

**Urinary Incontinence**
*See* Association for Urinary Continence Control
H.I.P. (Help for Incontinent People)

**Urologic Disorders**
*See* Kidney/Urologic Disorders

**U.S. Architectural Transportation Barriers Compliance Board**
(800) USA-ABLE
(For information related to the Americans with Disabilities Act)
*See also* Disability Referrals

**Us Too**
300 West Pratt Street, Suite #401
Baltimore MD 21201
(410) 727-2908
(800) 828-7866
(For information on prostate cancer)
*See also* Mathews Foundation for Prostate Cancer Research
Cancer

**Usher Family Support**
4918 42nd Avenue S.
Minneapolis, MN 55417
(612) 724-6982

**Vaccines**
*See* Dissatisfied Parents Together

**VACTRL Association**
*See* TEF/VATER/VACTRL National Support Network

**Vascular Malformation**
*See* National Vascular Malformation Foundation
Arteriovenus Malformation (AVM) Support Group of Nevada

**VATER Association**
*See* TEF/VATER/VACTRL National Support Network

**Velo-Cardio-Facial Syndrome Association**
110-45 Queens Boulevard
Forest Hills, NY 11375-5501
(718) 261-8049
(For DiGeorge syndrome; Shprintzen syndrome)

**Venous Diseases**
*See* National Lymphatic and Venous Diseases Foundation

**Vestibular Disorders Association**
P.O. Box 4467
Portland, OR 97208-4467
(503) 229-7705
(800) 837-8428
*See also* Ear Disorders

**Virginia Commonwealth University Medical College of Virginia Genetics**
Box 980033, MCV
Richmond, VA 23298-0033
(804) 828-9632

**Vision Foundation, Inc.**
818 Mt. Auburn Street
Watertown, MA 02172
(617) 926-4232
(800) 852-3029 (in MA)
*See also* Eye Disorders

**Visual Impairment**
*See* Eye Disorders

**Vitiligo**
*See* Skin Disorders

**VOCAL (Voluntary Organization for Communication and Language)**
336 Brixton Road
London SW9
United Kingdom
071-274-4029

**Georgia B. Vogelsang, M.D.**
Department of Oncology
Johns Hopkins Medical Institutions
Baltimore, MD
(For graft-versus-host disease)

**Von Hippel–Lindau (VHL) Family Alliance**
171 Clinton Road
Brookline, MA 02146-5815
(617) 232-5946
(800) 767-4845

**Von Hippel–Lindau (VHL) Patient and Relative Contact Group**
114 Longfield Road
Littleport, Ely, Cambs CB6 11B
United Kingdom

**Von Hippel–Lindau Syndrome Foundation**
P.O. Box 1516
Tom's River, NJ 08753-1516
(908) 244-7635

**Douglas C. Wallace, M.D.**
Biochemistry Department
Emory University School of Medicine
Atlanta, GA 30322
(For mutational analysis of mitochondrial defects)

**Arthur Walters, M.D.**
Department of Neurology, CN 19
University of Medicine and Dentistry of New Jersey
Robert Wood Johnson Medical School
New Brunswick, NJ 08903-0019
(For restless legs syndrome)

**Cecilia Warner, M.D.**
Div. of Medical and Molecular Genetics
Mount Sinai School of Medicine.
(For acute intermittent porphyria)

**David G. Warnock, M.D.**
Division of Nephrology/NRTC
University of Alabama
647 Tinsley Tower
1900 University Boulevard
Birmingham, AL 35294-0007
(205) 934-3538
(205) 934-1879
(For kidney diseases)

**WE MOVE**
Mount Sinai Medical Center
Gustave L. Levy Place, Box 1052
New York, NY 10029-6574
(212) 241-8567
(800) 437-6682
(For movement disorders)

**Weaver Syndrome**
*See* Support for Families with Children Having Weaver Syndrome

**Wegener's Granulomatosis Support Group, Inc.**
P.O. Box 1518
Platte City, MO 64079-1518
(816) 858-4088
(800) 277-9474
*See also* Gary S. Hoffman, M.D.

**Roy E. Weiss, M.D., Ph.D**
Thyroid Study Unit
University of Chicago
P.O. Box 138
Chicago, IL 60637
(312) 702-6939
(For Cushing syndrome)

**Robert I. White, Jr., M.D.**
Yale University
333 Cedar Street
P.O. Box 3333
New Haven, CT 06510
(203) 785-6938
(For hereditary hemorrhagic telangiectasia)

**Michael P. Whyte, M.D.**
Metabolic Research Unit
Shriners' Hospital for Crippled Children
2001 S. Lindbergh Boulevard
Saint Louis, MO 63131
(314) 432-3600
(For osteogenesis imperfecta;
 hypophosphatasia)

**Robert S. Wildin, M.D.**
Pediatric Genetics, UTMB
301 University Boulevard
Galveston, TX 77555-0359
(409) 772-3466
(For diabetes insipidus)

**William N. Williams, D.D.S.**
College of Dentistry
Box J-424
University of Florida
Gainesville, FL 32610
(904) 392-4370
(For cleft palate)

**Williams Syndrome Association**
P.O. Box 297
Clawson, MI 48017-0297
(810) 541-3630
See also Colleen A. Morris, M.D.

**Wilson's Disease Association**
4 Navaho Drive
Brookfield, CT 06804-3124
(203) 775-4664
(800) 399-0266
Note: Wilson disease is not the same as
 Wilson syndrome.

**Wolf-Hirschhorn Parent Contact Group**
See 4p- Parent Contact Group

**Wolf-Hirschhorn Syndrome Support
 Group**
2B, Harvesters Close
Rainham, Kent ME8 8PA
United Kingdom
(01634) 372218
(01634) 372218 (fax)
See also Gilbert N. Jones III
 Chromosomal Abnormalities

**Women's Health**
See American College of Obstetricians and
 Gynecologists
 National Women's Health Network
 National Women's Health Resource
 Center

**World Federation of Hemophilia**
4616 Saint Catherine's Street West
Montreal, Quebec H3Z 153
Canada
(514) 933-7944

**World Health Organization (WHO)**
525 23rd Street NW
Washington, DC 20037
(202) 861-3200
(202) 861-3305 (library)

**World Life Foundation**
P.O. Box 571
Bedford, TX 76095
(817) 282-1405
(800) 289-5433
(Provides transportation funds for the
 critically ill)

**Donald Wright, M.D.**
Surgical Neurology Branch
NINDS, Building 10A, Room 3E68
Bethesda, MD 20892
(301) 496-2921
(For neurofibromatosis)

**Eric A. Wulfsberg, M.D.**
Karen Supovitz, M.S.
Division of Human Genetics
University of Maryland School of Medicine
Baltimore, MD 20201-1703
(410) 328-3815
(For Miller syndrome)

**Ramnik Xavier**
Massachusetts General Hospital
(617) 726-2066
(For Gaucher disease)

**Xeroderma Pigmentosum Registry**
University of Medicine and Dentistry of
 New Jersey
Department of Pathology, Room C-520
Medical Science Building
185 South Orange Avenue
Newark, NJ 07103-2714
(201) 982-4405

**X-Linked Juvenile Retinoschisis**
See Paul Sieving, M.D.

**X-Linked Myotubular Myopathy
 Resource Group**
2413 Quaker Drive
Texas City, TX 77590
(409) 945-8569

**Neal S. Young, M.D.**
NIH/National Heart, Lung and Blood
 Institute
Clinical Hematology Branch
Building 10, Room 7C103
Bethesda, MD 20892
(301) 496-5093
(For Fanconi anemia)

# 15 | DIRECTORY OF ORPHAN DRUGS APPROVED AND IN DEVELOPMENT

This directory of orphan drugs has been compiled from data supplied by the researchers and manufacturers as of June 1, 1995. Because the Food and Drug Administration makes every effort to expedite approval of orphan drugs, the status may have changed when you consult the listings. For complete information, call the Contact listed in the far right column.

| Condition/Use | Drug Name | Status/Phase | Sponsor/Contact Person |
|---|---|---|---|
| **Acne rosacea** | metronidazole topical gel (Metrogel) | Approved for marketing | Galderma Labs P.O. Box 331329 Ft. Worth, TX 76163 (817) 263-3600 |
| **Adenocarcinoma** *(See also Cancer, Carcinoma)* Colorectal metastatic | fluorouracil (Adrucil) For use in combination with leucovorin | Approved for marketing Exclusive approval | Lederle Laboratories P.O. Box 8299 Philadelphia, PA 19101-2207 G.W. McCarl, M.D. (610) 341-2207 |
| **Acetaminophen overdose** Moderate to severe Intravenous treatment | acetylcysteine (Mucomyst/Mucomyst 10 IV) | | Apothecon P.O. Box 4500 Princeton, NJ 08543 Walter G. Jomp (609) 897-2470 |
| **Adrenal cortical imaging** | iodine-131-68-iodomethyl 19-norcholesterol <NP-59> | Phase III | University of Michigan 1500 E. Medical Center Dr. Ann Arbor, MI 48109-0028 David E. Kuhl, M.D. (313) 936-5388 |
| **AIDS** Adult and pediatric | HIV immune globulin <human>, intravenous | Orphan drug designation granted | North American Biologicals 16500 NW 15 Avenue Miami, FL 33169 Pinya Cohen, Ph.D. (305) 628-7807 |
| | human T-lymphotropic virus Type III gpl 60 antigens | Phase II | MicroGeneSys, Inc. 1000 Research Parkway Meriden, CT 06450 Alex Toles (203) 686-0800 |
| | zidovudine (Retrovir) | Approved for marketing Exclusive approval | Burroughs Wellcome 3030 Cornwallis Rd. Research Triangle Park, NC 27709 Drug Information Service (800) 722-9292 |
| Associated diarrhea | bovine colostrum and special milk collections | Phase I | Donald Hastings, D.V.M. 1030 N. Parkview Drive Bismarck, ND 58501 (701) 223-3036 |
| Pregnant women and their babies | HIV immune globulin <human>, intravenous | Clinical trials | North American Biologicals 16500 NW 15 Avenue Miami, FL 33169 Pinya Cohen, Ph.D. (305) 628-7807 |
| AIDS related non-Hodgkin lymphoma | mitoguazone dihydrochloride | Phase II Pivotal study | ILEX Oncology, Inc. 14960 Omicron Drive San Antonio, TX 78245 Susan Smith (210) 677-8000 |

| Condition/Use | Drug Name | Status/Phase | Sponsor/Contact Person |
|---|---|---|---|
| **AIDS and AIDS-related complex (ARC)**<br>ARC | zidovudine<br>(Retrovir) | Approved for marketing<br>Exclusive approval | Burroughs Wellcome<br>3030 Cornwallis Rd.<br>Research Triangle Park, NC 27709<br>Drug Information Service<br>(800) 722-9292 |
| **Alpha-1-proteinase inhibitor**<br>Replacement therapy in congenital deficiency state (ATT deficiency–related emphysema) | alpha-1-proteinase inhibitor <human><br>(Prolastin) | FDA approval<br>(Orphan drug status) | Bayer<br>400 Morgan Lane<br>West Haven, CT 06516<br>Clinical Information Service<br>(800) 288-8371 |
| **Amenorrhea**<br>Hypothalmic<br>Induction of ovulation | gonadorelin acetate<br>(Lutrepulse) | Approved | Ferring Laboratories<br>400 Rella Blvd.<br>Suffern, NY 10901<br>Isidoro Nudelman, RAC<br>(914) 368-7902 |
| **Amytrophic lateral sclerosis (ALS)** | myotrophin | Phase II/III | Cephalon, Inc.<br>145 Brandywine Pkwy.<br>West Chester, PA 19380<br>Medical Affairs Dept.<br>(610) 344-0200 |
| **Anorexia (loss of appetite)**<br>Stimulation of appetite and prevention of weight loss | dronabinol<br>(Marinol) | Approved for marketing | Unimed Pharmaceuticals, Inc.<br>2150 East Lake Cook Road,<br>  Suite 210<br>Buffalo Grove, IL 60089-1862<br>Robert E. Dudley, Ph.D.<br>(708) 541-2525 |
| **Antithrombin III deficiency**<br>Prevention and treatment | antithrombin III, human<br>(ATnativ) | Approved for marketing | Baxter Healthcare Corp.<br>550 N. Brand Blvd<br>Glendale, CA 91203<br>Mike Herrera<br>(818) 507-5451 |
| **Beta thalassemia** | vx-105 | Phase II | Vertex Pharmaceuticals Inc.<br>40 Allston Street<br>Cambridge, MA 02139-4211<br>Lynne Brum<br>(617) 576-3111 |
| | vx-366 | Phase II | Vertex Pharmaceuticals Inc.<br>40 Allston Street<br>Cambridge, MA 02139-4211<br>Lynne Brum<br>(617) 576-3111 |
| **Blepharospasm** | botulinum toxin-type A<br>(Oculinum) ® | FDA approved | Allergan Pharmaceuticals<br>2525 Dupont Drive<br>Irvine, CA 92715-1599<br>Francine Foerster<br>(714) 752-4500 |

| Condition/Use | Drug Name | Status/Phase | Sponsor/Contact Person |
|---|---|---|---|
| **Blepharospasm** *(continued)*<br>Associated with dystonia<br>in adults | botulinum toxin type A<br>(Botox) | FDA approved | Allergan Pharmaceuticals<br>2525 Dupont Drive<br>Irvine, CA 92715-1599<br>Francine Foerster<br>(714) 752-4500 |
| **Bone marrow<br>transplant**<br>Preparative agent for bone<br>marrow transplant | parenteral busulfan<br>(Busulfanex™) | Pre-NDA | Orphan Medical, Inc.<br>13911 Ridgedale Drive<br>Minnetonka, MN 55303<br>Patti A. Engel<br>(612) 513-6999 |
| Stimulates white blood cell<br>growth in bone marrow<br>transplant patients | sargramostim GMCSF<br>(Leukine) | Approved for marketing | Immunex Corporation<br>51 University Street<br>Seattle, WA 98101<br>Michael Kleinberg<br>(206) 587-0430 |
| **Botulism**<br>Infant | botulism immune<br>globulin | Phase II | California Department<br>Health Services<br>251 Berkeley Way<br>Berkeley, CA 94704<br>Stephen S. Arnon, M.D.<br>(510) 540-2646 |
| **Bronchopulmonary<br>dysplasia**<br>Prevention of, in premature<br>neonates weighing <1500 gm. | superoxide dismatase<br>(OxSODrol) | Phase I | Bio-Technology General<br>70 Wood Avenue, South<br>Iselin, NJ 08830<br>Leah Berkovits<br>(908) 632-8800 |
| **Burns**<br>Severe<br>  Enzymatic debridement | Viananain, comosain<br>(Vianain) | In clinical trials | Genzyme Corporation<br>One Kendall Square<br>Cambridge, MA 02139<br>Scott Furbish, Ph.D.<br>(617) 252-7614 |
| **Cachexia** | atropin<br>(Biotropin) | Phase I completed<br>Not continued at<br>this time | Bio-Technology General<br>70 Wood Avenue, South<br>Iselin, NJ 08830<br>Leah Berkovits<br>(908) 632-8800 |
| Associated with AIDS | (Biotropin) | | Bio-Technology General<br>70 Wood Avenue, South<br>Iselin, NJ 08830<br>Leah Berkovits<br>(908) 632-8800 |
| **Calculi, renal<br>and bladder**<br>Of the apatite or struvite variety | citric acid, glucono-delta-<br>lactone and mag carbonate<br>(Renacidin Irrigation) | Approved for marketing<br>Exclusive approval | United-Guardian, Inc<br>P.O. Box 2500<br>Smithtown, NY 11787<br>Robert Rubinger<br>(516) 273-0900 |

| Condition/Use | Drug Name | Status/Phase | Sponsor/Contact Person |
|---|---|---|---|
| **Cancer**<br>*(See also Adenocarcinoma, Carcinoma)*<br>Cervical | recombinant vaccine human papillomavirus (TA-HPV) | (USA) IND current Phase II trial with NCI commencing 4/95 | Cantab Pharmaceuticals Milton Road Cambridge, CB4, England Dr. J. St. Clair Roberts Tel (44) (0) 1223 423413 Fax (44) (0) 1223 423458 |
| Recurrent invasive or metastatic squamous | dibromodulcitol (Mitolactol) | Phase III completed | Biopharmaceutics, Inc. 990 Station Road Bellport, NY 11713 Dr. Stewart Ehrreich (813) 561-2110 Edward Fine (516) 286-5900 |
| Colorectal, metastatic | 1-leucovorin for use in combination with 5-fluorouracil | Phase III | Lederle Laboratories P.O. Box 8299 Philadelphia, PA 19101-2207 G.W. McCarl, M.D. (610) 341-2207 |
| Lung, nonsmall cell<br>Detection and staging by imaging | technetium Tc 99M anti-nonsmall cell lung cancer murine monoclonal antibody (OncoTrac® Nonsmall Cell Lung Cancer Imaging Kit) | Phase III completed | NeoRx Corporation 410 W. Harrison Seattle, WA 98119 Dee Sweeney (206) 281-7001 |
| Lung, small cell<br>IV therapy | N901-blocked ricin | Phase I/II | ImmunoGen, Inc. 128 Sidney St. Cambridge, MA 02139 Dixie Esseltine, M.D., FRCP (C) (617) 661-9312 |
| Lung, small cell<br>Detection and staging by imaging | technetium Tc 99M anti-small cell lung cancer murine monoclonal antibody (OncoTrac® Small Cell Lung Cancer Imaging Kit) | Orphan status pending PLA pending (Phase: FDA) | NeoRx Corporation 410 W. Harrison Seattle, WA 98119 Dee Sweeney (206) 281-7001 |
| Malignant astrocytoma Grade III/IV (Glioblastoma multiforme) | dibromoducitol (Mitolactol) | Phase III completed | Biopharmaceutics, Inc. 990 Station Road Bellport, NY 11713 Dr. Stewart Ehrreich (813) 561-2110 Edward Fine (516) 286-5900 |
| Ovarian<br>In vivo immunotherapy | MDX-210 MDX-H210 | Phase I/II | Medarex, Inc. 1545 Rt. 22 E, P.O. Box 992 Annandale, NJ 08801 Yashwant M. Deo (908) 713-6010 |
| Pain<br>In cancer patients tolerant to, or unresponsive to intraspinal opiates <epidermal administration> | clonidine hydrochloride | In development | Fujisawa, USA, Inc. 3 Parkway Center, N. Deerfield, IL 60015 D. Buell, M.D. (708) 317-1085 |

| Condition/Use | Drug Name | Status/Phase | Sponsor/Contact Person |
|---|---|---|---|
| **Cancer** *(continued)*<br>Thyroid<br>  Adjunct in diagnosis | human thyroid stimulating<br>hormone <TSH><br>(Thyrogen) | In clinical trials | Genzyme Corporation<br>One Kendall Square<br>Cambridge, MA 02139<br>Scott Furbish, Ph.D.<br>(617) 252-7614 |
| **Carcinoma**<br>*(See also Cancer,<br>Adenocarcinoma)*<br>Bladder, superficial | porfimer sodium<br>(Photofrin®) | Investigational<br>Phase III | QLT Phototherapeutics<br>520 West 6th Avenue<br>Vancouver, British Columbia<br>Canada V5Z 4H5<br>Noel Buskard, M.D.<br>(604) 872-7881 |
| Colorectal | leucovorin<br>leucovorin calcium<br>For use in combination<br>with 5-fluorouracil | Approved for marketing<br>Exclusive approval | Immunex Corporation<br>51 University Street<br>Seattle, WA 98101<br>Michael Kleinberg<br>(206) 587-0430 |
| Esophageal, obstructing<br>and partially obstructing | porfimer sodium<br>(Photofrin®) | NDA submitted | QLT Phototherapeutics<br>520 West 6th Avenue<br>Vancouver, British Columbia<br>Canada V5Z 4H5<br>Noel Buskard, M.D.<br>(604) 872-7881 |
|  | proteo-liposomal<br>Interleukin-2<br>(OncoLipin-2) | Phase I completed<br>Entering phase II | OncoTherapeutics, Inc.<br>1002 Eastpark Boulevard<br>Cranbury, NJ 08512<br>George Emont<br>(609) 655-5300 |
| Renal cell<br>  Metastatic | interleukin-12 | Phase I<br>clinical trials | Hoffmann–La Roche, Inc.<br>340 Kingsland St.<br>Nutley, NJ 07110-1199<br>Darien E. Wilson<br>(201) 562-2232 |
| Metastatic after surgical<br>excision of primary tumor | coumarin<br>(Oncostate Tablets) | Orphan drug designation | Oxford Research, Int'l.<br>1425 Broad Street<br>Clifton, NJ 07013<br>R.J. Doornbos, R.Ph.<br>(201) 777-2800 |
| **Carnitine deficiency**<br>Primary, systemic | l-carnitine<br>(Carnitor) | Approved for marketing<br>Exclusive approval | Sigma Tau Pharmaceuticals<br>200 Orchard Ridge Drive<br>Gaithersburg, MD 20878<br>Ed Helton, VP<br>Regulatory Affairs<br>(301) 948-1041 |
| Secondary | l-carnitine<br>(Carnitor) | Approved for marketing<br>Exclusive approval | Sigma Tau Pharmaceuticals<br>200 Orchard Ridge Drive<br>Gaithersburg, MD 20878<br>Ed Helton, VP<br>Regulatory Affairs<br>(301) 948-1041 |

| Condition/Use | Drug Name | Status/Phase | Sponsor/Contact Person |
|---|---|---|---|
| **Carnitine deficiency** *(continued)* Treatment in patients with end-stage renal disease who require dialysis | l-carnitine (Carnitor) | IND phase III | Sigma Tau Pharmaceuticals 200 Orchard Ridge Drive Gaithersburg, MD 20878 Ed Helton, VP Regulatory Affairs (301) 948-1041 |
| **Central precocious puberty** | leuprolide acetate for depot suspension (Lupron Depot-PED) | Approved for marketing | Tap Pharmaceuticals Inc. 2355 Waukegan Road Deerfield, IL 60015 C.B. Clarke Medical Services (800) 622-2011 |
| | leuprolide acetate (Lupron Injection) | Approved for marketing | Tap Pharmaceuticals Inc. 2355 Waukegan Road Deerfield, IL 60015 C.B. Clarke Medical Services (800) 622-2011 |
| | deslorelin (Somagard) | Phase III clinical studies completed Approved by FDA for sale on cost recovery basis in open phase III protocol for CPP | Roberts Pharmaceuticals 4 Industrial Way, West Eatontown, NJ 07724-2274 Drew Karlan (908) 389-1182 |
| **Cerebral palsy** Treatment of dynamic muscle contracture, pediatric patients | botulinum toxin type a (Botox) | | Allergan Pharmaceuticals 2525 Dupont Drive Irvine, CA 92715-1599 Francine Foerster (714) 752-4500 |
| **Cervical dystonia** | botulimum toxin type A (Botox) | | Allergan Pharmaceuticals 2525 Dupont Drive Irvine, CA 92715-1599 Francine Foerster (714) 752-4500 |
| | botulinum toxin type A (Oculinum) | Approval pending | Allergan Pharmaceuticals 2525 Dupont Drive Irvine, CA 92715 Francine Foerster (714) 752-4500 |
| **Cirrhosis** Primary biliary | ursodeoxycholic acid <ursodiol> (Urso) | Phase II completed Seeking NDA approval | Axcan Pharma, Inc. 597 Laurier Blvd. Mont Saint-Hilaire Quebec J3H 4X8, Canada Dr. Claude Sauriol (514) 467-5138 |
| **Congenital primary ichthyosis** | glyceryl monolaurate (Glylorin™) | Phase III clinical trials planned for late 1995 | Cellegy Pharmaceuticals, Inc. 371 Bel Marin Keys, Suite 210 Novato, CA 94949 Cynthia Selfridge (415) 382-6770 |

| Condition/Use | Drug Name | Status/Phase | Sponsor/Contact Person |
|---|---|---|---|
| **Corneal erosion**<br>Recurrent | dehydrex<br>(DEHYDREX™) | IND III | Holles Labs<br>30 Forest Notch<br>Cohasset, MA 02025<br>Peter Lelecas<br>(617) 383-0741 |
| **Corneal melting syndromes**<br>Of known or presumed immunologic etiopathonenesis, including Mooren's ulcer | cyclosporine 2% ophthalmic ointment | | Allergan Pharmaceuticals<br>2525 Dupont Drive<br>Irvine, CA 92715-1599<br>Francine Foerster<br>(714) 752-4500 |
| **Corneal ulcers**<br>Bacterial | ofloxicin<br>(Ocuflox Ophthalmic Solution) | | Allergan Pharmaceuticals<br>2525 Dupont Drive<br>Irvine, CA 92515-1599<br>Francine Foerster<br>(714) 752-4500 |
| Treatment of nonhealing ulcers or epithelial defects which have been unresponsive to conventional therapy and the underlying cause has been eliminated | fibronectin <human plasma> | Inactive | Melville Biologics<br>155 Duryea Road<br>Melville, NY 11747<br>Dr. Joan C. Pehta<br>(212) 570-3255 |
| **Cryptosporidiosis**<br>In immunocompetent or immunocompromised patients | bovine whey protein concentrate | Phase II<br>clinical trials | Biomune Systems, Inc.<br>540 Arapeen Drive, Suite 202<br>Salt Lake City, UT 84108<br>Frank A. Eldredge, Ph.D.<br>(801) 582-2345 |
| **Cushing syndrome**<br>For use in differentiating pituitary and ectopic production of ACTH in patients with ACTH-dependent Cushing syndrome | ovine corticorelin trifulate releasing hormone<br>(Acthrel) | FDA approval | Ferring Labs, Inc.<br>400 Rella Blvd.<br>Suffern, NY 10901<br>Isidoro Nudelman, RAC<br>(914) 368-7902 |
| **Cutaneous fistulas**<br>Adjunct to nonoperative management in the stomach, duodeneum, small intestine (jejunum and ileum) or pancreas | somatostatin<br>(Zecnil) | Phase III | Ferring Labs, Inc.<br>400 Rella Blvd.<br>Suffern, NY 10901<br>Isidoro Nudelman, RAC<br>(914) 368-7902 |
| **Cystic fibrosis** | gelsolin | Preclinical | Biogen, Inc.<br>14 Cambridge Center<br>Cambridge, MA 02124<br>Kathryn Bloom<br>(617) 679-2000 |
| | cystic fibrosis gene therapy | Preclinical | Genzyme Corporation<br>One Kendall Square<br>Cambridge, MA 02139<br>Scott Furbish, Ph.D.<br>(617) 252-7614 |

| Condition/Use | Drug Name | Status/Phase | Sponsor/Contact Person |
|---|---|---|---|
| **Cystic fibrosis** *(continued)* | amiloride <aerosolized> | Phase III clinical trials | Glaxo, Inc. 5 Moore Drive Research Triangle Park, NC 27709 Drug Information Service (800) 334-0089 |
| | tobramycin solution for inhalation | Phase III | PathoGenesis Corporation 201 Elliott Ave., W. Seattle, WA 98119 Bruce Montgomery, M.D. (206) 467-8100 |
| | synthetic pulmonary surfactant | Phase II | Burroughs Wellcome Co. 3030 Cornwallis Rd. Research Triangle Park, NC 27709 Drug Information Service (800) 722-9292 |
| Transmembrane conductance regulator | cystic fibrosis transmembrane conductance regulator protein replacement therapy | Preclinical | Genzyme Corporation One Kendall Square Cambridge, MA 02139 Scott Furbish, Ph.D. (617) 252-7614 |
| Treatment and prevention pulmonary infections due to *Pseudomonas aeruginosa* in patients with CF | mucoid exopolysaccharide pseudomonas hyperimmune globulin | Phase II | Univax Corporation 12280 Wilkins Avenue Rockville, MD 20852 Scott Harkonen, M.D. (301) 770-3099 |
| **Cystine nephrolithiasis** Prevention in patients with homozygous cystinuria | tiopronin (Thiola) | Approved for marketing Exclusive approval | Mission Pharmacal Company 2391 N.E. Loop 410, Suite 109 San Antonio, TX 78217 Dan K. Crawford (800) 531-3333 (800) 292-7364 (In Texas) |
| **Cystinosis, nephropathic** | phosphocysteamine | Phase III Clinical trials completed | Medea Research Laboratories 200 Wilson Street Pt. Jefferson Station, NY 11776 Dorothy Mangano (516) 331-7718 |
| | cysteamine <2-amino-ethanethiol> | IND II/III Completed | Jess G. Thoene, M.D. University of Michigan Medical School 300 NIB, 1182 SE Ann Arbor, MI 48109-0408 (313) 763-3427 |
| | <cysteamine bitartrate> (Cystagon™) | Approved for marketing | Chronimed 13911 Ridgedale Drive Minnetonka, MN 55305 Mark Peterson, R.Ph. (800) 444-5951 |
| **Cystitis** Interstitial | sodium pentosan polysulphate (Elmiron) | Phase III—Clinical trials complete NDA submitted | Baker-Norton Pharmaceuticals 8800 N.W. 36th Street Miami, FL 33078 Fred Sherman, M.D. (800) 347-4774 |

| Condition/Use | Drug Name | Status/Phase | Sponsor/Contact Person |
|---|---|---|---|
| **Cytomegalovirus**<br>Primary | cytomegalovirus immune glubulin <human> | Approved for marketing | MedImmune, Inc.<br>35 West Watkins Mill Road<br>Gaithersburg, MD 20878<br>David Wright<br>(301) 417-0770 |
| **Dermatitis Herpetiformis** | sulfapyridine | Phase III<br>(Available for compassionate use) | Jacobus Pharmaceutical Co.<br>37 Cleveland Lane<br>Princeton, NJ 08540<br>Neil J. Lewis, Ph.D.<br>(609) 921-7447 |
| | dapsone | Approved | Jacobus Pharmaceutical Co.<br>37 Cleveland Lane<br>Princeton, NJ 08540<br>Neil J. Lewis, Ph.D.<br>(609) 921-7447 |
| **Digitalis intoxication**<br>Potentially life-threatening in patients who are refractory to management by conventional therapy | digoxin immune fab <ovine><br>(Digibind) | Approved for marketing<br>Exclusive approval | Burroughs-Wellcome<br>3030 Cornwallis Rd.<br>Research Triangle Park, NC 27709<br>Drug Information Service<br>(800) 722-9292 |
| **Disseminated *M. avium* complex** | aminosidine | Phase I<br>completing preclinical | Thomas P. Kanyok, Pharm.D.<br>University of Illinois<br>833 South Wood Street<br>Room 164, M/C 886<br>Chicago, IL 60612<br>(312) 996-8369 |
| **Duchenne muscular dystrophy (DMD)** | mazindol<br>(Sanorex) | Investigational | Platon J. Collipp, M.D.<br>176 Memorial Drive<br>Jesup, GA 31545<br>(912) 427-9378 |
| **Epilepsy**<br>Drug-resistant generalized tonic-clonic (GTC) | antiepilepsirine<br>(llepcimide) | Pending approval | Children's Hospital<br>700 Children's Drive<br>Columbus, OH 43205<br>Phil Walson<br>(614) 472-6477 |
| **Esophageal varices** | terlipressin<br>(Glypressin) | Phase III | Ferring Labs., Inc<br>400 Rella Blvd.<br>Suffern, NY 10901<br>Isidoro Nudelman, RAC<br>(914) 368-7902 |
| Bleeding | somatostatin | Phase II | UCB Pharma, Inc.<br>Smyrna, GA |
| **Erythropoictic protoporphyria** | L-cysteine-HCL | Phase III<br>Study in progress | Tyson and Associates<br>12832 Chadron Avenue<br>Hawthorne, CA 90250<br>Don Tyson, President<br>(310) 625-1080 |

| Condition/Use | Drug Name | Status/Phase | Sponsor/Contact Person |
|---|---|---|---|
| **Familial amyotrophic lateral sclerosis (FALS)** <br> Associated with a mutation of the gene for Cu, Zn superoxide dismutase | orgotein for injection <bovine Cu, Zn superoxide dismutase> | Preclinical development | OXIS International, Inc. <br> 6040 N. Cutter Circle, Suite 317 <br> Portland, OR 92717-3935 <br> Lynda M. Taylor <br> (800) 547-3686 <br> (503) 283-3911 |
| **Familial hypercholesterolemia** <br> Homozygous | sodium dichloroacetate <DCA> | Phase II limited studies completed | Peter Stacpoole, Ph.D., M.D. <br> University of Florida <br> P.O. Box 100226 <br> Gainesville, FL 32610-0277 <br> (904) 392-2321 |
| **Familial spastic paraparesis** | L-threonine | Phase II clinical trials | Interneuron Pharmaceuticals <br> One Ledgemont Center <br> 99 Hayden Ave., Suite 340 <br> Lexington, MA 02173 <br> Bobby W. Sandage, Jr., Ph.D. <br> (617) 861-8444 |
| **Farbry disease** | ceramide trihexosidase/ alpha-galactosidase A | Preclinical | Genzyme <br> One Kendall Square <br> Cambridge, MA 02139 <br> Scott Furbish, Ph.D. <br> (617) 252-7614 |
| **Gallbladder disease** <br> Dissolution of cholesterol gallstones retained in the common bile duct | monoctanoin (Moctanin) | Approved for marketing Exclusive approval | Ethitek <br> 7701 N. Austin Avenue <br> Skokie, IL 60077 <br> Dennis Emig <br> (708) 675-6616 |
| **Gaucher disease** <br> Replacement therapy—Type I | glucocerebrosidase-beta glucosidase <placenta derived> (Ceredase) alglucenase inject. | Approved for marketing | Genzyme <br> One Kendall Square <br> Cambridge, MA 02139 <br> Scott Furbish, Ph.D. <br> (617) 252-7614 |
| Replacement therapy Types I, II and III | glucerase (Cerezyme) | Approved for Type I | Genzyme <br> One Kendall Square <br> Cambridge, MA 02139 <br> Scott Furbish, Ph.D. <br> (617) 252-7614 |
| Replacement therapy, patients deficient in glucocerebrosidase | peg-glucocerebrosidase | Phase I clinical trials | Enzon, Inc. <br> 20 Kingsbridge Road <br> Piscataway, NJ 08854 <br> Anna T. Viau, Ph.D. |
| **Glaucoma** <br> Control of scarring associated with failure of glaucoma surgery | mitomycin-C (MitoSert) | Phase III clinical studies | IOP Inc. <br> 3100 Airway Avenue <br> Costa Mesa, CA 92626 <br> Jason Malecka <br> (714) 549-1185 |

| Condition/Use | Drug Name | Status/Phase | Sponsor/Contact Person |
|---|---|---|---|
| **Glioblastoma multiforme** | crisnatol mesylate | Phase III trial | ILEX Oncology, Inc.<br>14960 Omicron Drive<br>San Antonio, TX 78245<br>Susan Smith<br>(210) 677-8000 |
| **Glioma**<br>Recurrent malignant<br>For localized placement<br>in the brain | biodegradable polymer<br>implant containing<br>carmustine<br>(Gliadel) | Phase III completed<br>NDA filing and a<br>treatment IND application<br>planned 4th qtr. 1995 | Guilford Pharmaceuticals<br>6611 Tributary Street<br>Baltimore, MD 21224<br>Earl W. Henry, M.D.<br>(410) 631-6302 |
| **Grafts**<br>Prevention of graft loss<br>of meshed autografts<br>on excised burn wounds | Mafenide acetate solution<br>(Sulfamylon solution) | Orphan-approved | Dow Hickam Pharmaceuticals<br>10410 Corporate Drive<br>Sugar Land, TX 77478<br>Barbara Thomas Smith<br>(713) 240-7411 |
| **Graft-versus-host disease**<br>**(GVHD)**<br>Prevention of acute graft-<br>versus-host disease following<br>bone marrow transplantation | dacliximab<br>(Zenapax™) | Phase III | Hoffmann–La Roche, Inc.<br>340 Kingsland Street<br>Nutley, NJ 07110-1199<br>Darien Wilson<br>(201) 562-2232 |
| **Graft rejection**<br>Following penetrating<br>keratoplasty | cyclosporine 2% ophthalmic<br>ointment | | Allergan Pharmaceuticals<br>2525 Dupont Drive<br>Irvine, CA 92715-1599<br>Francine Foerster<br>(714) 752-4500 |
| Prevention of acute rejection<br>of human organ transplants | anti-CD45 monoclonal anti-<br>bodies | | Baxter Healthcare Corp.<br>1620 Waukegan Road<br>McGaw Park, Il 60085<br>Marsha Wolfson, M.D.<br>(708) 473-6343 |
| **Growth and puberty**<br>Constitutional delay | sublingual testosterone<br>(Androtest-SL ) | Phase II | Bio-Technology General<br>70 Wood Avenue, South<br>Iselin, NJ 08830<br>Leah Berkovits<br>(908) 632-8800 |
| | oxandrolone<br>(Oxandrin) | Phase III completed<br>(Placebo-controlled<br>and open-labeled)<br>Treatment IND | Bio-Technology General<br>70 Wood Avenue, South<br>Iselin, NJ 08830<br>Leah Berkovits<br>(908) 632-8800 |
| **Growth hormone**<br>**deficiency** | somatorelin | Phase III | ICN Pharmaceuticals, Inc.<br>3300 Hyland Avenue<br>Costa Mesa, CA 92626<br>Humberto Fernandez, M.D.<br>(714) 545-0100 |
| **Homocystinuria** | betaine anhydrous powder<br>(Cystadane™) | Pre-NDA | Orphan Medical, Inc.<br>13911 Ridgedale Drive<br>Minnetonka, MN 55305<br>Patti A. Engel<br>(612) 513-6999 |

| Condition/Use | Drug Name | Status/Phase | Sponsor/Contact Person |
|---|---|---|---|
| **Hemophilia A**<br>Prophylaxis and treatment of bleeding episodes/surgery | recombinate antihemophilic factor VIII (Kogenate) | FDA approval (Orphan drug status) | Bayer<br>400 Morgan Lane<br>West Haven, CT 06516<br>Clinical Information Service<br>(800) 288-8371 |
| Mild von Willebrand disease | desmopressin acetate, nasal spray 1.5 mg/ml concentration (Stimate) | Approved 3/7/94 | Armour Pharmaceutical Co.<br>500 Arcola Road, Box 1200<br>Collegeville, PA 19426-0107<br>Arlene Santhouse, R.Ph.<br>(610) 454-2872 |
| **Hemophilia B** | rhFactor IX | Phase I/II clinical testing | Genetics Institute, Inc.<br>87 Cambridge Park Drive<br>Cambridge, MA 02140<br>Dennis Harp<br>(617) 498-8498 |
| | Factor IX <human> (Mononine) | Approved 8/20/92 | Armour Pharmaceutical Co.<br>500 Arcola Road<br>Box 1200<br>Collegeville, PA 19426-0107<br>Arlene Santhouse, R.Ph.<br>(610) 454-2872 |
| **Hemmorrhagic fever**<br>Renal failure syndrome | ribavirin | Inactive | ICN Pharmaceuticals, Inc.<br>3300 Hyland Avenue<br>Costa Mesa, CA 92626<br>Humberto Fernandez, M.D.<br>(714) 545-0100 |
| **Hepatitis**<br>Alcoholic | oxandrolone (Hepandrin) | Phase III | Bio-Technology General<br>70 Wood Avenue, South<br>Iselin, NJ 08830<br>Leah Berkovits<br>(909) 632-8800 |
| **Hepatitis B** | interferon beta recombinant <human> IFN-B-la | Phase II | Biogen, Inc.<br>14 Cambridge Center<br>Cambridge, MA 02142<br>Kathryn Bloom<br>(617) 679-2000 |
| Liver transplant patients | Hepatitis B immune globulin <human>, intravenous (HBIG, Intravenous) | Orphan drug designation | North American Biologicals<br>16500 NW 15 Ave.<br>Miami, FL 33169<br>Pinya Cohen, Ph.D.<br>(305) 628-7807 |
| **Hepatitis C** | interferon beta recombinant <human> IFN-B-la | Phase II | Biogen, Inc.<br>14 Cambridge Center<br>Cambridge, MA 02142<br>Kathryn Bloom<br>(617) 679-2000 |

| Condition/Use | Drug Name | Status/Phase | Sponsor/Contact Person |
|---|---|---|---|
| **Hepatitis C** *(continued)*<br>In liver transplant patients | Hepatitis C immune globulin , intravenous | FDA application pending | North American Biologicals<br>16500 N.W. 15 Avenue<br>Miami, FL 33169<br>Pinya Cohen, Ph.D.<br>(305) 628-7807 |
| **Herpes simplex encephalitis**<br>In individuals afflicted with AIDS | PR-225 (redox-acyclovir) | Preclinical | Pharmos Corporation<br>2 Innovation Drive<br>Alachua, FL 32615<br>Emil Pop, Ph.D.<br>(904) 462-1210 |
| **HIV**<br>Infection | vx-478<br>protease inhibitor | Phase I | Burroughs Wellcome Co.<br>3030 Cornwallis Road<br>Research Triangle Park, NC 27709<br>Drug Information Service<br>(800) 722-9292 |
| | 935U | Phase I/II | Burroughs Wellcome Co.<br>3030 Cornwallis Road<br>Research Triangle Park, NC 27709<br>Drug Information Service<br>(800) 722-9292 |
| | 524U | Phase I | Burroughs Wellcome Co.<br>3030 Cornwallis Road<br>Research Triangle Park, NC 27709<br>Drug Information Service<br>(800) 722-9292 |
| | 1592U | Phase I | Burroughs Wellcome Co.<br>3030 Cornwallis Road<br>Research Triangle Park, NC 27709<br>Drug Information Service<br>(800) 722-9292 |
| | 589C | Phase II | Burroughs Wellcome Co.<br>3030 Cornwallis Road<br>Research Triangle Park, NC 27709<br>Drug Information Service<br>(800) 722-9292 |
| Combination therapy with AZT as well as monotherapy | zalcitabine<br>(HIVID®) | Approved | Hoffmann–La Roche, Inc.<br>340 Kingsland St.<br>Nutley, NJ 07110-1199<br>Gail Levinson<br>(201) 562-2218 |
| Maternal transmission | zidovudine<br>(Retrovir) | Approved | Burroughs Wellcome<br>3030 Cornwallis Road<br>Research Triangle Park, NC 27709<br>Drug Information Service<br>(800) 722-9292 |
| Wasting syndrome | oxandrolone<br>(Oxandrin) | Phase II | Bio-Technology General<br>70 Wood Avenue, South<br>Iselin, NJ 08830<br>Leah Berkovits<br>(908) 632-8800 |

| Condition/Use | Drug Name | Status/Phase | Sponsor/Contact Person |
|---|---|---|---|
| **Hyaline membrane disease (HMD)** (Also known as Infant respiratory distress syndrome <IRDS>) Prevention of HMD, in infants born at 32 weeks gestation or less | synthetic pulmonary surfactant (Exosurf) | Approved for marketing | Burroughs Wellcome 3030 Cornwallis Rd. Research Triangle Park, NC 27709 Drug Information Service (800) 722-9292 |
| Prevention and treatment in premature newborns | berectant intratracheal suspension <modified bovine lung surfactant extract> (Survanta) | Approved Currently marketed | Ross Laboratories 625 Cleveland Ave. Columbus, OH 43216 Elizabeth M. Zola, Pharm.D. (614) 624-7677 |
| Treatment of established HMD at all gestational ages | synthetic pulmonary surfactant (Exosurf) | Approved | Burroughs Wellcome 3030 Cornwallis Rd. Research Triangle Park, NC 27709 Drug Information Service (800) 722-9292 |
| **Hyperammonemia** Urea cycle enzymopathies | 10% sodium benzoate and 10% sodium phenylacetate (Ucephan) | Oral form approved for marketing | McGaw, Inc. 2525 McGaw Ave. Irvine, CA 92714 Order Services (800) 624-2963 |
| **Hyperbilirubimenia** In newborn infants unresponsive to phototherapy | flumecinol (Zixoryn) | Phase II | Farmacon 90 Grove Street, Suite 109 Ridgefield, CT 06877 Dr. Laszlo L. Darko (203) 438-7331 |
| **Hypercalcemia** Of a malignancy | etidronate disodium (Didronel) | Approved for marketing | MGI Pharma, Inc. 9900 Bren Road, Suite 300E Minneapolis, MN 55343 Rajesh Shrotriya, M.D. (612) 935-7335 |
| **Hypercalciuria, absorptive** Control and prevention of type I with calcium nephrolithiasis | cellulose sodium phosphate (Calcibind) | Approved for marketing Exclusive approval | Mission Pharmacal Company 2391 N.E. Loop 410, Suite 109 San Antonio, TX 78217 Dan K. Crawford (800) 531-3333 (800) 292-7364 (In Texas) |
| **Hyperekplexia** (Startle disease) | clonazepam (Klonopin) | Phase III | Hoffmann–La Roche, Inc. 340 Kingsland Street Nutley, NJ 07110-1199 Alfred Wasilewski (201) 562-2231 |

| Condition/Use | Drug Name | Status/Phase | Sponsor/Contact Person |
|---|---|---|---|
| **Hyperphosphatemia**<br>In end-stage renal disease (ESRD) | calcium acetate (PhosLo) | Approved for marketing<br>On market | Braintree Laboratories<br>60 Columbian St., PO Box 850929<br>Braintree, MA 02185<br>Peter Kenney<br>(617) 843-2202 |
| **Hyphema** | aminocaproic acid topical (Caprogel™) | Clinicals | Orphan Medical, Inc.<br>13911 Ridgedale Drive<br>Minnetonka, MN 55303<br>Patti A. Engel<br>(612) 513-6999 |
| **Hypocalcemia**<br>Diagnostic agent for use in patients with clinical and laboratory evidence of hypocalcemia due to hypoparathyroidism or pseudohypoparathyroidism | teriparatide (Parathar®) | Approved for marketing | Rhone-Poulenc Rorer<br>500 Arcola Road<br>P.O. Box 1200<br>Collegeville, PA 19426-0107<br>Dr. Arthur Stokes<br>(610) 454-8295 |
| **Hypocitraturia**<br>Prevention and control of calcium renal stones | potassium citrate (Urocit-K) | Approved for marketing<br>Exclusive approval | Mission Pharmacal Company<br>2391 N.E. Loop 410, Suite 109<br>San Antonio, TX 78217<br>Dan K. Crawford<br>(800) 531-3333<br>(800) 292-7364 (In Texas) |
| **Hypotension**<br>Idiopathic orthostatic | midodrine HCL (Pro-Amatine) | NDA filed April 1988<br>Under review | Roberts Pharmaceuticals<br>4 Industrial Way, West<br>Eatontown, NJ 07724-2224<br>Drew Karlan<br>(908) 389-1182 |
| **Immune thrombocytopenic purpura (IYP)** | $Rh_0$<D> immune globulin (WinRho SD) | PLA review | Univax Corporation<br>12280 Wilkins Avenue<br>Rockville, MD 20852<br>Scott Harkonan, M.D.<br>(301) 770-3099 |
| **Kaposi sarcoma**<br>AIDS-related | interferon alfa-2-A <recombinant> (Roferon®-A) | Approved for marketing | Hoffmann—La Roche, Inc.<br>340 Kingsland St.<br>Nutley, NJ 07110-1199<br>Alfred Wasilewski<br>(201) 562-2231 |
| HIV associated, advanced | liposomal duanorubicin in citrate buffer (DuanoXome) | Phase II–III trials completed<br>Submitted to FDA | Vestar, Inc.<br>650 Cliffside Drive<br>San Dimas, CA 91773<br>Geoffrey Mukwaya, M.D.<br>(909) 394-4066 |
| **Kidney stones**<br>Control and prevention of infection stones (struvite) | acetohydroximic acid (Lithostat) | Approved for marketing<br>Exclusive approval | Mission Pharmacal Company<br>2391 N.E. Loop 410, Suite 109<br>San Antonio, TX 78217<br>Dan K. Crawford<br>(800) 531-3333<br>(800) 292-7364 (In Texas) |

| Condition/Use | Drug Name | Status/Phase | Sponsor/Contact Person |
|---|---|---|---|
| **Lactic acidosis**<br>Congenital | sodium dichloroacetate <DCA> | Phase III<br>trials under way | Peter Stacpoole, Ph.D., M.D<br>University of Florida<br>P.O. Box 100226<br>Gainesville, FL 32610-0277<br>(904) 392-2321 |
| **Lambert-Eaton myasthenic syndrome** | dynamine | Phase II | Mayo Clinic Foundation<br>200 S. W. 1st Ave.<br>Rochester, MN 55905<br>Kathleen McEvoy, M.D., Ph.D.<br>(507) 284-4234 |
| | 3.4-diaminopyridine | Phase II | Jacobus Pharmaceutical Co.<br>37 Cleveland Lane<br>Princeton, NJ 08540<br>Neil J. Lewis, Ph.D.<br>(609) 921-7447 |
| **Lennox-Gastaut syndrome** | felbamate | Approved for marketing | Wallace Laboratories<br>P.O. Box 1001<br>Cranbury, NJ 08512<br>A. Rosenberg, M.D.<br>(609) 951-2002 |
| **Leukemia**<br>Acute, adult | amsacrine<br>(Amsidyl) | Investigational | Warner-Lambert<br>2800 Plymouth Road<br>Ann Arbor, MI 48106-1047<br>William R. Grove, M.S.<br>(800) 521-0999 |
| Acute myelogenous | decitabine <5-aza-2'-deoxycytidine, DCA> | IND filed<br>Phase II studies ongoing | Pharmachemie, USA, Inc.<br>P.O. Box 145<br>Oradell, NJ 07649<br>J. David Hayden, Pres.<br>(201) 265-1942 |
| Acute lymphocytic (ALL)<br>Diluent for intrathecally administered agents | elliott's B solution<br>(Elliott's B™) | Pre-NDA | Orphan Medical, Inc.<br>13911 Ridgedale Drive<br>Minnetonka, MN 55305<br>Patti A. Engel<br>(612) 513-6999 |
| | pegaspargase<br>(PEG-I-asparaginase)<br>(Oncaspar) | Approved Feb. 94 | Enzon, Inc.<br>20 Kingsbridge Road<br>Piscataway, NJ 08854<br>Anna T. Viau, Ph.D.<br>(908) 980-4677 |
| Acute T-cell leukemia and related T-cell | Anti-CD6-blocked ricin | Phase I | ImmunoGen, Inc.<br>128 Sidney Street<br>Cambridge, MA 02139<br>Dixie Esseltine, M.D., FRCP (C)<br>(617) 661-9312 |
| Non-T-cell, Acute lymphocytic (ALL)<br>Ex vivo purging of leukemic cells from bone marrow, subsequent to reinfusion adult and pediatric patients. | Anti-B4-blocked ricin | Phase I/II | ImmunoGen, Inc.<br>128 Sidney Street<br>Cambridge, MA 02139<br>Dixie Esseltine, M.D., FRCP (C)<br>(617) 661-9312 |

| Condition/Use | Drug Name | Status/Phase | Sponsor/Contact Person |
|---|---|---|---|
| **Leukemia** (continued)<br>Pediatric (ALL) | idarubicin | Investigational | Pharmacia, Inc.<br>P.O. Box 16529<br>Columbus, OH 43216-6529<br>M. Gerber<br>(614) 764-8155 |
| Acute myeloid (AML)<br>Acute nonlymphocytic (ANLL)<br>In adults | idarubicin<br>(Idamycin) | Approved | Pharmacia, Inc.<br>P.O. Box 16529<br>Columbus, OH 43216-6529<br>D. McDaniel<br>(614) 764-4004 |
| Acute myelocytic<br>Ex vivo purging of leukemic<br>cells from the bone marrow<br>of acute patients | Anti-MY9-blocked ricin | Phase I/II | ImmunoGen, Inc.<br>128 Sidney Street<br>Cambridge, MA 02139<br>Dixie Esseltine, M.D., FRCP (C)<br>(617) 661-9312 |
| Acute Myeloid<br>Adjunctive treatment | mdx-11<br>(PM-81) | Phase II | Medarex, Inc.<br>1545 Rt. 22 E, P.O. Box 992<br>Annandale, NJ 08801<br>Yashwant M. Deo<br>(908) 713-6010 |
| Acute promyelocytic | all-trans retinoic acid<br>tretinoin<br>(Vesanoid®) | NDA pending<br>FDA Advisory Committee<br>recommended approval | Hoffmann–La Roche, Inc.<br>340 Kingsland St.<br>Nutley, NJ 07110-1199<br>Alfred Wasilewski<br>(201) 562-2231 |
| | fludarabine monophosphate<br>(Fludara) | Approved | Berlex Laboratories<br>P.O. Box 4099<br>Richmond, CA 94804-0099<br>Howard Robin<br>(510) 262-5054 |
| Chronic myelogenous | interferon alfa-2A<br><recombinant><br>(Referon-A®) | NDA pending<br>FDA Advisory Committee<br>recommended approval | Hoffmann–La Roche, Inc.<br>340 Kingsland Street<br>Nutley, NJ 07110-1199<br>Alfred Wasilewski<br>(201) 562-2231 |
| Hairy cell | pentostatin | Approved for marketing | Warner-Lambert<br>2800 Plymouth Rd.<br>Ann Arbor, MI 48105<br>Mark Meyer, Pharm.D., M.S.<br>(800) 521-8999 |
| Myelocytic, acute & chronic,<br>AML & CML<br>I.V. therapy to treat AML<br>patients and CML patients<br>in blast crisis | Anti-MY9-blocked ricin | Phase I/II | ImmunoGen, Inc.<br>128 Sidney Street<br>Cambridge, MA 02139<br>Dixie Esseltine, M.D., FRCP (C)<br>(617) 661-9312 |
| **Liver disease**<br>Treatment/prevention of<br>TPN-associated | choline chloride | Phase II trials | Alan L. Buchman, M.D., M.S.P.H.<br>6550 Fannin, Suite 1122<br>Houston, TX 77030<br>(713) 790-2171 |

| Condition/Use | Drug Name | Status/Phase | Sponsor/Contact Person |
|---|---|---|---|
| **Lymphoma**<br>B-cell<br>  I.V. therapy of non-Hodgkins<br>  lymphoma (NHL) | Anti-B4-blocked ricin | Phase III | ImmunoGen, Inc.<br>128 Sidney St.<br>Cambridge, MA 02139<br>Dixie Esseltine, M.D., FRCP (C)<br>(617) 661-9312 |
| B-cell<br>  I.V. therapy of non-Hodgkins<br>  lymphoma (NHL)<br>    HIV associated NHL | Anti-B4-blocked ricin | Phase II | ImmunoGen, Inc.<br>128 Sidney Street<br>Cambridge, MA 02139<br>Dixie Esseltine, M.D., FRCP (C)<br>(617) 661-9312 |
| I.V. therapy of B-cell<br>non-Hodgkins lymphoma (NHL) | Anti-B4-DC1 | Phase I<br>(IND application submitted,<br>Orphan drug application<br>anticipated in near future) | ImmunoGen, Inc.<br>148 Sidney St.<br>Cambridge, MA 02139<br>Dixie Esseltine, M.D., FRCP (C)<br>(617) 661-9312 |
| Non-Hodgkin | fludarabine monophosphate<br>(Fludara) | Phase II | Berlex Laboratories<br>P.O. Box 4099<br>Richmond, CA 94804-0099<br>Howard Robin<br>(510) 262-5054 |
| T-cell | 2-amino-1,5-dihydr0-7-<br><C-pryidinylmethyl><br>-4H-pyrrolo [3,2-d]<br>pyrimindin-4-one<br>(peldesine) | Orphan drug status<br>Clinical studies | Biocryst Pharmaceuticals, Inc.<br>2190 Parkway Lake Drive<br>Birmingham, AL 35244<br>William J. Cook, M.D., Ph.D<br>(205) 444-4600 |
| Cutaneous T-cell lymphoma<br>Acute T-cell leukemia-<br>lymphoma and related T-cell<br>malignancies | Anti-CD6-blocked ricin | Phase I | ImmunoGen, Inc.<br>128 Sidney Street<br>Cambridge, MA 02139<br>Dixie Esseltine, M.D., FRCP (C)<br>(617) 661-9312 |
| **Malaria** | atovaquone<br>(Mepron) | Phase III | Burroughs Wellcome Co.<br>3030 Cornwallis Rd.<br>Research Triangle Park, NC 27709<br>Drug Information Service<br>(800) 722-9292 |
| Associated lactic acidosis | sodium dichloroacetate<br><DCA> | Phase II<br>trials completed | Peter Stacpoole, Ph.D., M.D.<br>University of Florida<br>P.O. Box 100226<br>Gainesville, FL 32610-0277<br>(904) 392-2321 |
| Treatment and prophylaxis<br>and plasmodium | mefloquine HCL<br>(Larium®) | Approved for marketing | Hoffmann–La Roche, Inc.<br>340 Kingsland St.<br>Nutley, NJ 07110-1199<br>Diane Donlon<br>(201) 562-2203 |
| **Mastocytosis** | cromolyn sodium<br>(Gastrocrom) | Approved for marketing<br>Available | Fisons Corporation<br>P.O. Box 1766<br>Rochester, NY 14603<br>Elizabeth Likly<br>(716) 274-5955 |

| Condition/Use | Drug Name | Status/Phase | Sponsor/Contact Person |
|---|---|---|---|
| **Melanoma**<br>Metastatic<br> Detecting by imaging | melanoma murine monoclonal antibody (OncoTrac® Melanoma Imaging Kit) | Phase III completed<br>Orphan status granted | NeoRx Corp.<br>410 W. Harrison<br>Seattle, WA 98119<br>Dee Sweeney<br>(206) 281-7001 |
| Stage II–IV | melanoma theraccine <therapeutic vaccine> (Melacine) | Phase III | Ribi ImmunoChem Research<br>553 Old Corvallis Road<br>Hamilton, MT 59840-3131<br>Kenneth B. Von Eschen, Ph.D.<br>(406) 363-6214 |
| Stage III–IV | melanoma theraccine <therapeutic vaccine> (Melacine) | Phase III<br>controlled study<br>completed<br>No PLA planned | Ribi ImmunoChem Research<br>553 Old Corvallis Road<br>Hamilton, MT 59840-3131<br>Kenneth B. Von Eschen, Ph.D.<br>(406) 363-6214 |
| Stage III–IV | melanoma theraccine (Melacine) + interferon-alpha 2b | Phase III<br>controlled study<br>Study protocol/IND<br>allowed by FDA 5/95<br>Patient enrollment<br>to begin in 1995 | Ribi ImmunoChem Research<br>553 Old Corvallis Road<br>Hamilton, MT 59840-3131<br>Kenneth B. Von Eschen, Ph.D.<br>(406) 363-6214 |
| **Meningitis**<br>Neoplastic | depofoam encapsulated (DepoCyt) | Phase III<br>Clinical trials | DepoTech Corporation<br>11025 Torrey Pines Road,<br>  Suite 100<br>La Jolla, CA 92037<br>Craig Wichner<br>(619) 625-2424 |
| **Multiple sclerosis** | interferon beta, recombinant human (Betaseron) | Approved | Berlex Laboratories<br>P.O. Box 4099<br>Richmond, CA 94804-0099<br>Howard Robin<br>(510) 262-5054 |
| | interferon beta, recombinant <human> INF-B-la (Avonex™) | Phase III complete<br>Regulatory filings<br>planned first half 1995<br>for U.S. and Europe | Biogen, Inc.<br>14 Cambridge Center<br>Cambridge, MA 02142<br>Kathryn Bloom<br>(617) 679-2000 |
| | copolymer 1 <cop 1> | Phase III<br>NDA in preparation | Lemmon Company<br>1510 Delp Drive<br>Kulpsville, PA 19443<br>Dr. Stanley Scheindlin<br>(800) 523-6542 |
| | 4-aminopyridine/ fampridine | Phase II/III | Elan Pharmaceutical<br>1300 Gould Drive<br>Gainesville, GA 30504<br>Dr. David Tierney<br>(404) 534-8239 |

| Condition/Use | Drug Name | Status/Phase | Sponsor/Contact Person |
|---|---|---|---|
| **Mycobacterium avium (MAC) complex**<br>Prevention of MAC in patients with AIDS and with CD4 counts less than 200/MM$^3$ | rifabutin (Mycobutin) | Approved | Pharmacia, Inc.<br>P.O. Box 16529<br>Columbus, OH 43216-6529<br>Dr. Beverley Wynne<br>(614) 764-8159 |
| Treatment of MAC in patients with AIDS | rifabutin (Mycobutin) | Investigational | Pharmacia, Inc.<br>P.O. Box 16529<br>Columbus, OH 43216-6529<br>Dr. Beverley Wynne<br>(614) 764-8159 |
| **Myelodyplastic syndromes**<br>Treatment | RII retinamide | Orphan drug status granted in 1993<br>Filing IND 1995 | Sparta Pharmaceuticals<br>P.O. Box 13288<br>Research Triangle Park, NC 27709<br>Dr. William McCulloch<br>(919) 361-3461 |
| **Myoclonus** | piracetam | Phase II | UCB Pharma, Inc.<br>Smyrna, Ga |
| Postanoxic | I-5 Hydroxytryptophan <I-5HTP> | Compassionate use under a protocol | Circa Pharmaceutical, Inc<br>33 Ralph Avenue<br>Copiague, NY 11726<br>Monica A. Paccione<br>(516) 842-8383 |
| **Narcolepsy**<br>Treatment symptoms associated with narcolepsy | gamma hydroxybutyrate | Research | Orphan Medical, Inc.<br>13911 Ridgedale Drive<br>Minnetonka, MN 55303<br>Patti A. Engel<br>(612) 513-6999 |
| Excessive sleepiness | modafinil | Phase III | Cephalon, Inc.<br>145 Brandywine Parkway<br>West Chester, PA 19380<br>Medical Affairs Dept.<br>(610) 344-0200 |
| **Neuralgia**<br>Trigeminal | L-baclofen | Phase II clinical trials | Dr. Michael J. Soso<br>Neurology Department<br>University of Pittsburgh<br>322 Scaife Hall<br>Pittsburgh, PA 15261<br>(412) 648-2022 |
| **Neurosyphilis**<br>AIDS-associated | PR-239 (redox penicillin) | Preclinical | Pharmos Corporation<br>2 Innovation Drive<br>Alachua, FL 32615<br>Emil Pop, Ph.D.<br>(904) 462-1210 |
| **Opiate addiction** | buprenorphine hydrochloride | NDA pending | Reckitt & Colman Pharm.<br>1901 Huguenot Road<br>Richmond, VA 23235<br>Charles O'Keeffe<br>(804) 379-1090 |

| Condition/Use | Drug Name | Status/Phase | Sponsor/Contact Person |
|---|---|---|---|
| **Opiate addiction** (continued) | buprenorphine in combination with naloxone | NDA pending | Reckitt & Colman Pharm. 1901 Huguenot Road Richmond, VA 23235 Charles O'Keeffe (804) 379-1090 |
| **Panencephalitis (SSPE)** Subacute sclerosing | inosine pranobex inosine dimepranol acedoben (Isoprinosine) | Orphan drug designation 1988 NDA & IND withdrawn 1992, with option to re-open Reopening NDA under evaluation | Newport Synthesis, Ltd. 1582 Deere Avenue Irvine, CA 92714-4811 Mrs. Jean Dreyer (714) 222-9902 |
| **Parkinson disease** Adjuvant to levodopa and carbidopa treatment of idio-pathic Parkinson disease (paralysis agitans) , post-encephalitic parkinsonism, and symptomatic parkinsonism | selegiline HCL (Eldepryl) | Approved for marketing | Somerset Pharmaceuticals 777 South Harbour Island Blvd., Suite 880 Tampa, FL 33602 Dana G. Barnett (800) 892-8889 |
| **Penicillin hypersensitivity** | benzylpenicilloyl polylysine/MDM (Pre-Pen/MDM) | Phase III | Schwarz Pharma P.O. Box 2038 Milwaukee, WI 53201 Mary Anne Krupski (800) 472-9309 |
| **Peripheral arterial occlusive disease** Severe | alprostadil (Vasoprost for Injection) | Phase III | Schwarz Pharma P.O. Box 2038 Milwaukee, WI 53201 Mary Anne Krupski (800) 472-9309 |
| **Pheochromocytoma/ neuroblastoma** Diagnostic adjunct | I-131 MIBG (Iobenguane Sulfate I-131 Injection) | Orphan Drug NDA filed Approved 3/25/94 | CIS-US, Inc. 10 DeAngelo Drive Bedford, MA 01730 Mary E. Donovan (617) 275-7120 |
| **Pituitary gland** Diagnostic measure of capacity of pituitary gland to release growth hormone | NG-29 (Somatrel) | Phase III | Ferring Labs, Inc. 400 Rella Blvd. Suffern, NY 10901 Isidoro Nudelman, RAC (914) 368-7902 |
| **Pneumocystis carinii pneumonia (PCP)** | (Mepron) | Approved for marketing | Burroughs Wellcome 3030 Cornwallis Rd. Research Triangle Park, NC 27709 Drug Information Service (800) 722-9292 |
| Prevention | dapsone | Pre NDA | Jacobus Pharmaceutical Co. 37 Cleveland Lane Princeton, NJ 08540 Neil J. Lewis, Ph.D. (609) 921-7447 |

| Condition/Use | Drug Name | Status/Phase | Sponsor/Contact Person |
|---|---|---|---|
| **Pneumocystis carinii pneumonia (PCP)** (continued) <br> Treatment | dapsone in conjunction with trimethoprim | Pre-NDA | Jacobus Pharmaceuticals Co. <br> 37 Cleveland Lane <br> Princeton, NJ 08540 <br> Neil J. Lewis, Ph.D. <br> (609) 921-7447 |
| Prevention, in patients at high risk | pentamidine isethionate <inhalation> (Pneumopent) | Pending approval <br> NDA | Fisons Corporation <br> P.O. Box 1766 <br> Rochester, NY 14603 <br> Elizabeth Likly <br> (716) 274-5955 |
| **Poisoning** <br> Antidote <br>   Ethylene glycol and methanol poisoning | 4-MP (Antizol™) | Pre-NDA | Orphan Medical, Inc. <br> 13911 Ridgedale Drive <br> Minnetonka, MN 55303 <br> Patti A. Engel <br> (612) 513-6999 |
| **Polycythemia vera** | anagrelide (Agrelin) | Phase III | Roberts Pharmaceuticals <br> 4 Industrial Way, West <br> Eatontown, NJ 07724-2274 <br> Drew Karlan <br> (908) 389-1182 |
| **Porphyria** <br> Acute, intermittent (AIP) <br> Amelioration of recurrent attacks temporarily related to the menstrual cycle in susceptible women and similar symptoms which occur in other patients with AIP, porphyria variegata, and hereditary coproporphyria | hemin (Panhematin) | Approved for marketing <br> Exclusive approval | Abbott Laboratories <br> Pharmaceutical Products Div. <br> North Chicago, IL 60064 <br> Tom Gesell, Pharm.D. <br> (708) 938-0618 |
| Acute, intermittent, hereditary coproporphyria, variegate porphyria | heme arginate (Normosang) | Investigational <br> Orphan drug designation | Karl E. Anderson, M.D. <br> University of Texas <br> Medical Branch at Galveston <br> 700 Harborside Drive <br> Galveston, TX 77555-1109 <br> (409) 772-4661 |
| Acute | heme plus zinc-mesoporphyrin (HEMEX) | IND under review | Herbert L. Bonkovsky, M.D. <br> University of Massachusetts <br>   Medical Center <br> 55 Lake Avenue, North <br> Worcester, MA 01655 <br> (508) 856-3068 |
| **Primary pulmonary hypertension (PPH)** | epoprostenol (Flolan) | NDA filed <br> FDA Advisory Committee recommended approval | Burroughs Wellcome <br> 3030 Cornwallis Rd. <br> Research Triangle Park, NC 27709 <br> Drug Information Service <br> (800) 722-9292 |
| Chronic PPH with no detectable secondary cause | epoprostenol, prostacyclin (Flolan) | Approved | Burroughs Wellcome <br> 3030 Cornwallis Rd. <br> Research Triangle Park, NC 27709 <br> Drug Information Service <br> (800) 722-9292 |

| Condition/Use | Drug Name | Status/Phase | Sponsor/Contact Person |
|---|---|---|---|
| **Protein malnutrition**<br>In peritoneal dialysis patients | Peritoneal dialysis solution with 1.1% amino acids (Nutrineal) | Phase III | Baxter Healthcare Corp.<br>Renal Division<br>1620 Waukegan Road<br>McGaw Park, IL 60085<br>Marsha Wolfson, M.D.<br>(708) 473-6343 |
| **Pseudomembranous enterocolitis**<br>Caused by toxins A and B elaborated by *clostridium difficile* | bacitracin (Altracin) | Clinical studies completed Preparing for submission to FDA | A.L. Laboratories, Inc.<br>1 Executive Drive<br>P.O. Box 1299<br>Fort Lee, NJ 07024<br>Dr. Bernard Brown<br>(201) 947-7774 |
| **Pulmonary hypertension**<br>In newborns (persistent) | nitric oxide | Investigational | Ohmeda Pharmaceutical Products Division<br>110 Allen Rd., P.O. Box 804<br>Liberty Corner, NJ 07938-0804<br>Bob Outwater<br>Sr. Dir., Reg. Affairs<br>(908) 604-7704 |
| **Radiation proctitis**<br>Treatment | short chain fatty acid enema Colomed™ | Clinicals | Orphan Medical, Inc.<br>13911 Ridgedale Drive<br>Minnetonka, MN 55303<br>Patti A. Engel<br>(612) 513-6999 |
| **Renal failure**<br>Acute | anaritide acetate (Auriculin®) | Phase III | Scios Nova Inc.<br>2450 Bayshore Parkway<br>Mountain View, CA 94043<br>Kira Bacon<br>(415) 966-1550 |
| **Renal transplant**<br>Improvement early renal allograft function | anaritide acetate (Auriculin®) | Phase II | Scios Nova Inc.<br>2450 Bayshore Parkway<br>Mountain View, CA 94043<br>Kira Bacon<br>(415) 966-1550 |
| Prevention of acute renal allograft rejection | dacliximab (Zenapax™ | Phase III | Hoffmann–La Roche, Inc.<br>340 Kingsland Street<br>Nutley, NJ 07110-1199<br>Diane Donlon<br>(201) 562-2203 |
| **Respiratory distress syndrome**<br>Adult | L-2-oxothiazolidine-4-carboxylic (Procysteine) | | Free Radical Sciences<br>245 First Street<br>Cambridge, MA 02142<br>Michael Sullivan<br>(617) 374-1224 |

| Condition/Use | Drug Name | Status/Phase | Sponsor/Contact Person |
|---|---|---|---|
| **Respiratory Distress Syndrome** (continued) | | | |
| Infant | pulmonary surfactant replacement | Preclinical | Scios Nova, Inc. 2450 Bayshore Parkway Mountain View, CA 94043 Kira Bacon (415) 966-1550 |
| Infant Associated with prematurity Prevention | protirelin | Phase III | UCB Pharma, Inc. Smyrna, GA |
| **Respiratory failure** Treatment and prevention, due to pulmonary surfactant deficiency | surface active extract of saline lavage of bovine lungs (Infasurf) | NDA submitted | Ony, Inc. 1576 Sweet Home Rd. Amherst, NY 14228 Edmund Egan, M.D. (716) 636-9096 |
| Caused by Meconium Aspiration Syndrome, persistent pulmonary hypertension, or pneumonia and sepsis in full-term newborn infants | berectant intratracheal suspension <modified bovine lung surfactant extract> (Survanta) | Phase III | Ross Laboratories 625 Cleveland Ave. Columbus, OH 43216 Elizabeth M. Zola (614) 624-7677 |
| **Retinitis pigmentosa** | (VisionAid) | Investigational Orphan drug and IND submitted | Platon J. Collipp, M.D. 176 Memorial Drive Jesup, GA 31545 (912) 427-9378 |
| **Sarcoma** Osteogenic | methotrexate sodium (Methotrexate) | Approved for marketing | Lederle Laboratories P.O. Box 8299 Philadelphia, PA 19101-2207 G.W. McCarl, M.D. (610) 341-2207 |
| | leucovorin leucovorin calcium For use with methotrexate | Approved for marketing Exclusive approval | Immunex Corporation 51 University Street Seattle, WA 98101 Michael Kleinberg (206) 587-0430 |
| | 1-leucovorin for use in combination with methotrexate | NDA submitted | Lederle Laboratories P.O. Box 8299 Philadelphia, PA 19101-2207 G.W. McCarl, M.D. (610) 341-2207 |
| **Severe combined immunodeficiency disease (SCID)** ADA-deficiency related | pegademase bovine (ADAGEN Injection) | Approved 1990 | Enzon, Inc. 20 Kingsbridge Road Piscataway, NJ 08854 Anna T. Viau, Ph.D. (908) 980-4677 |
| **Sickle cell disease** | vx-105 | Phase II | Vertex Pharmaceuticals Inc. 40 Allston Street Cambridge, MA 02139-4211 Lynne Brum (617) 576-3111 |

| Condition/Use | Drug Name | Status/Phase | Sponsor/Contact Person |
|---|---|---|---|
| **Sickle cell disease** (continued) | vx-366 | Phase II | Vertex Pharmaceuticals Inc.<br>40 Allston Street<br>Cambridge, MA 02139-4211<br>Lynne Brum<br>(617) 576-3111 |
| | sodium phenylbutyrate | IND/2 | George Dover, M.D.<br>Johns Hopkins Medical Inst.<br>720 Rutland Avenue<br>Ross 1125<br>Baltimore, MD 21287-2539<br>(410) 955-3886 |
| Crisis | poloxamer 188<br>(Rheothrx Copolymer) | Phase II | Burroughs Wellcome Co.<br>3030 Cornwallis Rd.<br>Research Triangle Park, NC 27709<br>Drug Information Service<br>(800) 722-9292 |
| | polymeric oxygen<br><ozone/oxygen> | (Approved in Cuba only)<br>Seeking research groups<br>in U.S. | Capmed, USA<br>P.O. Box 14<br>Byrn Mawr, PA 19010<br>James A. Caplan<br>(215) 472-9740 |
| Prophylactic treatment of<br>sickle cell disease to reduce<br>the incidence of crisis | polymeric oxygen<br><ozone/oxygen> | (Approved in Cuba only)<br>Seeking research groups<br>in U.S. | Capmed, USA<br>P.O. Box 14<br>Byrn Mawr, PA 19010<br>James A. Caplan<br>(215) 472-9740 |
| Ulcers | polymeric oxygen<br><ozone/oxygen> | (Approved in Cuba only)<br>Seeking research groups<br>in U.S. | Capmed, USA<br>P.O. Box 14<br>Byrn Mawr, PA 19010<br>James A. Caplan<br>(215) 472-9740 |
| | polymeric oxygen<br><ozone/oxygen> | (Approved in Cuba only)<br>Seeking research groups<br>in U.S. | Capmed, USA<br>P.O. Box 14<br>Byrn Mawr, PA 19010<br>James A. Caplan<br>(215) 472-9740 |
| **Sjogren Syndrome**<br>Xerostomia and kerato-<br>conjunctivitis sicca | pilocarpine hydrochloride<br>(Salagen Tablets) | Phase III | MGI Pharma, Inc.<br>9900 Bren Road, East, Suite 300E<br>Minneapolis, MN 55343<br>Rajesh Shrotriya, M.D.<br>(612) 935-7335 |
| **Spasticity**<br>Cerebral origin | baclofen <intrathecal><br>(Lioresal® Intrathecal)<br>baclofen injection | Treatment IND | Medtronic Neurological Division<br>800 53rd Ave., N.E.<br>Minneapolis, MN 55421<br>Gail Davison<br>(800) 328-0810 |
| Severe, chronic<br>Of spinal cord origin | baclofen <intrathecal><br>(Lioresal®Intrathecal)<br>baclofen injection | Commercially available | Medtronic Neurological Division<br>800 53rd Ave., N.E.<br>Minneapolis, MN 55421<br>Rita Hirsch<br>(800) 328-0810 |

| Condition/Use | Drug Name | Status/Phase | Sponsor/Contact Person |
|---|---|---|---|
| **Status epilepticus**<br>Grand mal type, emergency rescue treatment | PR-122<br>(redox-phenytoin) | Preclinical | Pharmos Corporation<br>2 Innovation Drive<br>Alachua, FL 32615<br>Emil Pop, Ph.D.<br>(904) 462-1210 |
| | PR-320<br>(Molecusol carbamazepine) | Preclinical | Pharmos Corporation<br>2 Innovation Drive<br>Alachua, FL 32615<br>Emil Pop, Ph.D.<br>(904) 462-1210 |
| **Strabismus**<br>Adult | Botulinum<br>(Oculinum) | Approved by FDA | Allergan Pharmaceuticals<br>2525 Dupont Drive<br>Irvine, CA 92715-1599<br>Francine Foerster<br>(714) 752-4500 |
| **Streptococcal infection**<br>Treatment of neonates with disseminated Group B infection | group B streptococcus immune globulin | Phase I | Univax Corporation<br>12280 Wilkins Avenue<br>Rockville, MD 20852<br>Scott Harkonen, M.D.<br>(301) 770-3099 |
| **Systemic lupus erythematosus (SLE)** | GL701<br>(DHEA, dehydroepiandrosterone) | Phase III<br>clinical trials | Genelabs Technologies<br>505 Penobscot Drive<br>Redwood City, CA 94063<br>Kenneth J. Gorelick, M.D.<br>(415) 369-9500 |
| | Monoclonal antibody 3E10 | Phase I<br>clinical studies | MedClone<br>17500 Red Hill Avenue, Suite 100<br>Irvine, CA 92714<br>Martin L. Lee, Ph.D.<br>(818) 985-8920<br>Karen K. Yamamoto, Ph.D.<br>(714) 798-5932 |
| **Thalassemia** | sodium phenylbutyrate | IND/2 | George Dover, M.D.<br>Johns Hopkins Medical Inst.<br>720 Rutland Avenue<br>Ross 1125<br>Baltimore, MD 21287-2539<br>(410) 955-3886 |
| **Toxoplasmosis**<br>Prevention | depsone<br>in conjunction with<br>pyrimethamine | Pre NDA | Jacobus Pharmaceutical Co.<br>37 Cleveland Lane<br>Princeton, NJ 08540<br>Neil J. Lewis, Ph.D.<br>(609) 921-7447 |
| **Thrombocythemia**<br>Essential | anagrelide<br>(Agrelin) | Phase III<br>Approved for sale on cost recovery basis | Roberts Pharmaceuticals<br>4 Industrial Way, West<br>Eatontown, NY 07724-2274<br>Drew Karlan<br>(908) 389-1182 |

| Condition/Use | Drug Name | Status/Phase | Sponsor/Contact Person |
|---|---|---|---|
| **Thrombocytosis**<br>In chronic myelogenous leukemia | anagrelide<br>(Agrelin) | Phase III | Roberts Pharmaceuticals<br>4 Industrial Way, West<br>Eatontown, NJ 07724-2274<br>Drew Karlan<br>(908) 389-1182 |
| **Thrombosis**<br>Prevention and treatment in patients with hereditary AT-III deficiency<br>  In connection with surgical or obstetrical procedures or thromboembolus | antithrombin III human<br>(ATnativ) | Approved for marketing<br>Exclusive approval | Baxter Healthcare Corp.<br>550 N. Brand Blvd<br>Glendale, CA 91203<br>Mike Herrera<br>(818) 328-5451 |
| Replacement therapy in congenital deficiency state (AT deficiency related thrombosis) | antithrombin III<br>(THROMBATE III) | FDA approval | Bayer<br>400 Morgan Lane<br>West Haven, CT 06516<br>Clinical Information Service<br>(800) 288-8371 |
| **Toxoplasma gondii encephalitis**<br>In patients with or without AIDS<br>In combination with pyrimethamine | sulfadiazine | Approved for marketing | Eon Labs Manufacturing Co.<br>227-15 N. Conduit Avenue<br>Laurelton, NY 11413<br>Martha Constantino<br>(718) 276-8600 |
| **Toxoplasmosis**<br>Prevention in immunocompromised patients | dapsone<br>CD4<100 | Pre-NDA | Jacobus Pharmaceutical Co.<br>37 Cleveland Lane<br>Princeton, NJ 08540<br>Neil J. Lewis, Ph.D.<br>(609) 921-7447 |
| **Trapanosoma Brucei**<br>Gambiense sleeping sickness | eflornithineHCL <dfmo><br>(Ornidyl) | Approved for marketing | Marion Merrell Dow Inc.<br>9300 Ward Parkway<br>Kansas City, MO 64114<br>Product Communications<br>(800) 362-7466 |
| **Tuberculosis** | aminosidine | Pending FDA approval<br>begin phase III end 1995 | Thomas P. Kanyok, Pharm.D.<br>University of Illinois<br>833 South Wood Street<br>Room 164, M/C 886<br>Chicago, IL 60612<br>(312) 996-8639 |
| Short course | rifampin, isoniazid pyrazinamide<br>(Rifater V) | Approved for marketing | Marion Merrell Dow Inc.<br>9300 Ward Parkway<br>Kansas City, MO 64114<br>Product Communications<br>(800) 362-7466 |
| When use of oral form of drug is not feasible | rifampin<br>(Rifadin I.V.) | Approved for marketing | Marion Merrell Dow Inc.<br>9300 Ward Parkway<br>Kansas City, MO 64114<br>Product Communications<br>(800) 362-7466 |

| Condition/Use | Drug Name | Status/Phase | Sponsor/Contact Person |
|---|---|---|---|
| **Tuberculosis** (continued)<br>Drug resistant | aminosalicylic acid<br>(PASER Granules) | Approved | Jacobus Pharmaceutical Co.<br>37 Cleveland Ave.<br>Princeton, NJ 08540<br>Neil J. Lewis, Ph.D.<br>(609) 921-7447 |
| **Tumors**<br>Brain and central<br>nervous system | protco-liposomal<br>Interleukin-2<br>(OncoLipin-2) | Phase I completed<br>Entering phase II | OncoTherapeutics, Inc.<br>1002 Eastpark Boulevard<br>Cranbury, NJ 08512<br>George Emont<br>(609) 655-5300 |
| **Turner syndrome** | ethinyl estradiol, USP<br>(Estrafem) | Phase III | Bio-Technology General<br>70 Wood Avenue, South<br>Iselin, NJ 08830<br>Leah Berkovits<br>(908) 632-8800 |
| | oxandrolone<br>(Oxandrin) | Phase III<br>(Placebo-controlled<br>and treatment IND) | Bio-Technology General<br>70 Wood Avenue, South<br>Iselin, NJ 08830<br>Leah Berkovits<br>(908) 632-8800 |
| **Ulcerative colitis**<br>Treatment of active phase,<br>with involvement restricted<br>to left side of colon | short chain fatty acid<br>solution | Investigational | Richard Breuer, M.D.<br>2500 Ridge Avenue<br>Evanston, IL 60201<br>(708) 869-5636 |
| **Urea cycle disorders**<br>Deficiencies of carbamyl<br>phosphate synthetase, ornithine<br>transcarbamylase and<br>argininosuccinate synthetase | sodium phenylbutyrate (oral) | NDA submitted | Saul W. Brusilow, M.D.<br>Johns Hopkins Medical Inst.<br>600 North Wolfe St.<br>Park 336<br>Baltimore, MD 21287<br>(410) 955-0885 |
| Deficiencies of carbamyl<br>phosphate synthetase, ornithine<br>transcarbamylase and<br>argininosuccinate synthetase | sodium benzoate/sodium<br>phenylacetate combination<br>in intravenous dosage form | IND/3 | Saul W. Brusilow, M.D.<br>Johns Hopkins Medical Inst.<br>600 North Wolfe St.<br>Park 336<br>Baltimore, MD 21287<br>(410) 955-0885 |
| **Uremic osteodystrophy** | dihydroxycholecalciferol | Phase III | Lemmon Company<br>1510 Delp Drive<br>Kulpsville, PA 19443<br>Dr. Stanley Scheindlin<br>(800) 523-6542 |
| **Uric acid nephrolithiasis**<br>Prevention and control | potassium citrate<br>(Urocit-K) | Approved for marketing<br>Exclusive approval | Mission Pharmacal Company<br>2391 N.E. Loop 410, Suite 109<br>San Antonio, TX 78217<br>Dan K. Crawford<br>(800) 531-3333<br>(800) 292-7364 (In Texas) |

| Condition/Use | Drug Name | Status/Phase | Sponsor/Contact Person |
|---|---|---|---|
| **Urolithiasis** <br> Avoidance of complication of calcium stone formation | potassium citrate (Urocit-K) | Approved for marketing | Mission Pharmacal Company <br> 2391 N.E. Loop 410, Suite 109 <br> San Antonio, TX 78217 <br> Dan K. Crawford <br> (800) 531-3333 <br> (800) 292-7364 (In Texas) |
| Treatment and prevention of life-threatening urolithiasis | sotalol HCL (Betapace) | Approved | Berlex Laboratories <br> 300 Fairfield Road <br> Wayne, NJ 07470-4100 <br> H. Joseph Reiser <br> (201) 305-5073 |
| | cromolyn sodium 4% ophthalmic solution (Opticrom 4% Ophthalmic Sol.) | Approved for marketing <br> Currently unavailable | Fisons Corporation <br> P.O. Box 1766 <br> Rochester, NY 14603 <br> Elizabeth Likly <br> (716) 274-5955 |
| **Vernal conjunctivitis** | lodoxamide tromethamine ophthalmic solution (Alomide®) | Approved for marketing | Alcon Laboratories, Inc. <br> 6201 South Freeway <br> Fort Worth, TX 76134-2099 <br> Stuart Raetzman <br> (817) 568-6102 |
| **Vernal keratitis** | lodoxamide tromethamine ophthalmic solution (Alomide®) | Approved for marketing | Alcon Laboratories, Inc. <br> 6201 South Freeway <br> Fort Worth, TX 76134-2099 <br> Stuart Raetzman <br> (817) 568-6102 |
| **Vernal keratoconjunctivitis** | lodoxamide tromethamine ophthalmic solution (Alomide®) | Approved for marketing | Alcon Laboratories, Inc. <br> 6201 South Freeway <br> Fort Worth, TX 76134-2099 <br> Stuart Raetzman <br> (817) 568-6102 |
| | cromolyn sodium (Gastrocrom) | Currently unavailable | Fisons Corporation <br> P.O. Box 1766 <br> Rochester, NY 14603 <br> Sue Scott <br> (716) 274-5974 |
| **Visceral leishmaniasis (kala-azar)** | aminosidine | Phase III | Thomas P. Kanyok, Pharm.D. <br> University of Illinois <br> 833 South Wood Street <br> Room 164, M/C 886 <br> Chicago, IL 60612 <br> (312) 996-8639 |
| **von Willebrand disease** | antihemophilic factor, human pasteurized (Humate-P) | Orphan status pending FDA approval | Armour Pharmaceutical Co. <br> 500 Arciola Road <br> P.O. Box 1200 <br> Collegeville, PA 19426-0107 <br> Arlene Santhouse, R.Ph. <br> (610) 454-2872 |
| **Vulvar dystrophies** <br> Lichen sclerosus atrophicus in particular | 2% testosterone propionate ointment (Vulvan) | IND submission process. FDA approval to begin clinical trials | Star Pharmaceuticals, Inc. <br> 1990 N.W. 44th Street <br> Pompano Beach, FL 33064 <br> Scott L. Davidson, Pres. <br> (305) 971-7718 |

| Condition/Use | Drug Name | Status/Phase | Sponsor/Contact Person |
|---|---|---|---|
| **West's syndrome**<br>Infantile spasms | CCD 1042 | Phase II | CoCensys<br>213 Technology Drive<br>Irvine, CA 92718<br>Donald W. Ashbrook, Ph.D.<br>(714) 753-6132 |
| **Wilson disease**<br>Initial therapy | ammonium tetrathiomolybdate | IND | George J. Brewer, M.D.<br>University of Michigan Medical<br>  School<br>4708 Medical Science Building II<br>Ann Arbor, MI 48109-0618<br>(313) 764-5499 |
|  | zinc acetate | Phase III<br>NDA submitted<br>Now under review | Lemmon Company<br>Kulpsville, PA 19443<br>Dr. Stanley Scheindlin<br>(800) 523-6542 |
| In patients intolerant of penicillamine | trientine HCL<br>(Syprine) | Approved for marketing<br>Exclusive Approval | Merck Sharp & Dohme<br>Merck National Service Cntr.<br>West Point, PA 19486<br>Medical Services<br>(800) 672-6372 |
| **Xeroderma pigmentosum**<br>Prevention of cutaneous<br>neoplasms and other skin<br>abnormalities | endonuclease V, liposome<br>encapsulated<br>[T4N5] | Phase II completed<br>Phase III starting | Applied Genetics, Inc.<br>205 Buffalo Ave.<br>Freeport, NY 11520<br>Jonathan Klein<br>(516) 868-9026 |
| **Xerostomia**<br>Radiation induced in<br>head and neck cancer patients | pilocarpine hydrochloride<br>(Salagen Tablets) | Approved | MGI Pharma, Inc.<br>9900 Bren Road, East, Suite 300E<br>Minneapolis, MN 55343<br>Rajesh Shrotriya, M.D.<br>(612) 935-7335 |

# INDEX OF SYMPTOMS AND KEY WORDS

*Note:* **Boldface** pages locate main articles.

Black measles. *See* Rocky Mountain spotted fever (RMSF)
Blackouts, sleep apnea and, 265
Bladder
  cancer of, 698
  exstrophy of, 693–94
  impaired control of
    cerebral palsy and, 285
    Devic disease and, 297
    spina bifida occulta and, 376
  missing, sirenomelia sequence and, 137
  paralysis of, syringomyelia and, 380
Bladder and bowel dysfunction
  late syphilis and, 584
  multiple sclerosis (MS) and, 332
  Shy-Drager syndrome and, 374
Blastomycosis, **530–31**
Bleeding. *See also* Hemorrhage
  into abdomen, wandering spleen and, 685
  congenital afibrinogenemia and, 444
  into epidermis and mucous membranes, aplastic anemia and, 448
  essential thrombocythemia and, 505
  excessive
    from cuts and injuries, Bernard-Soulier syndrome and, 460
    on injury, Chédiak-Higashi syndrome and, 463
    from mouth during dental work, May-Hegglin anomaly and, 489
  gastrointestinal
    congenital hepatic fibrosis and, 677
    gold poisoning and, 831
    idiopathic thrombocytopenic purpura (ITP) and, 498
    polyarteritis nodosa (PAN) and, 773
    retroperitoneal fibrosis and, 780
    von Willebrand disease and, 507
    Wiskott-Aldrich syndrome and, 599
    Zellweger syndrome and, 248
  genitourinary, idiopathic thrombocytopenic purpura (ITP) and, 498
  internal
    slow, factor XIII deficiency and, 466
    uncontrolled, without apparent cause, hemophilia and, 475
  in nose, prolonged, von Willebrand disease and, 507
  Peutz-Jeghers syndrome and, 681
  rectal
    familial polyposis and, 672
    Gardner syndrome and, 673
  subcutaneous, thrombasthenia and, 504
  from umbilical cord, factor XIII deficiency and, 466
  vaginal, idiopathic thrombocytopenic purpura (ITP) and, 498
Bleeding diathesis, 441
  TORCH syndrome and, 586
Bleeding tendency, 437–41
  Ehlers-Danlos syndromes (EDS) and, 758
  hereditary fructose intolerance and, 193
  Shwachman syndrome and, 501
  thrombasthenia and, 505
Blennorrheal idiopathic arthritis. *See* Reiter syndrome
Blepharitis, Hay-Wells syndrome and, 633
Blepharophimosis
  blepharophimosis, ptosis, epicanthus inversus and, 793
  cerebro-oculo-facio-skeletal (COFS) syndrome and, 287
  Dubowitz syndrome and, 58
  fronto-facio-nasal dysplasia and, 76
Blepharophimosis, ptosis, epicanthus inversus syndrome (BPES), **793**
Blepharospasm. *See* Benign essential blepharospasm (BEB)
Blepharospasm oromandibular dystonic syndrome. *See* Meige syndrome
Blessig cysts, 813
Blindness. *See also* Color blindness; Night blindness (nyctalopia); Vision
  Alpers disease and, 260
  Alstrom syndrome and, 716
  Behçet syndrome and, 755
  congenital toxoplasmosis and, 589
  cortical
    MELAS syndrome and, 213
    Sturge-Weber syndrome and, 143
    subacute sclerosing panencephalitis (SSPE) and, 582
  day, cone dystrophy and, 797
  Erdheim-Chester disease and, 190
  Hermansky-Pudlak syndrome and, 477
  infantile metachromatic leukodystrophy and, 324
  Krabbe leukodystrophy and, 323
  late syphilis and, 584
  Maroteaux-Lamy syndrome and, 211
  Norrie disease and, 809
  olivopontocerebellar atrophy III and, 357
  papillitis and, 809
  Reiter syndrome and, 779
  Sandhoff disease and, 238
  temporary
    conversion disorder and, 292
    Takayasu arteritis and episodes of, 753

Weill-Marchsani syndrome and, 159
Blind spots, multiple sclerosis (MS) and, 332
Blinking
  excessive, Tourette syndrome and, 386
  frequent or forceful, benign essential blepharospasm (BEB) and, 279
  inability to control, corticobasal degeneration and, 292
Blistering
  from acantholysis, pemphigus and, 652
  blisters with central hair follicle, Grover disease and, 631
  following minor trauma to hands and feet, epidermolysis bullosa (EB) and, 621–22
  itching and burning, dermatitis herpetiformis (DH) and, 617
  large, easily broken, toxic epidermal necrolysis (TEN) and, 658
  of mucous membranes, benign mucosal pemphigoid and, 650
  subepidermal, bullous pemphigoid and, 651
  of sun-exposed skin
    porphyria cutanea tarda and, 232
    variegate porphyria and, 234
  Wells syndrome and, 661
Bloating, wandering spleen and, 686
Bloch-Siemens-Sulzberger syndrome. *See* Incontinentia pigmenti
Bloch-Sulzberger syndrome. *See* Incontinentia pigmenti
Blood clots
  antiphospholipid syndrome and, 524
  neuroleptic malignant syndrome and, 353
  renal cell carcinoma and, 461
Blood clotting mechanisms, disruption of
  amyloid arthropathy and, 749
  Hageman factor deficiency and, 471
  malignant hyperthermia and, 97
Blood coagulation, decreased, celiac sprue and, 670
Blood counts, abnormal, histiocytosis X and, 478
Blood pressure. *See also* Hypertension; Hypotension
  dramatic drop in, meningococcemia and, 564
  high, Desmin storage myopathy and, 345
  imperceptible, Takayasu arteritis and, 753
  unstable, familial dysautonomia and, 304
Bloody and purulent discharge, Wegener granulomatosis and, 508
Bloom syndrome, **21–22**. *See also* Dubowitz syndrome
Blue diaper syndrome, **183**
Blue disease. *See* Rocky Mountain spotted fever (RMSF)
Blue fever. *See* Rocky Mountain spotted fever (RMSF)
Blue rubber bleb nevus, **22**. *See also* Cavernous hemangioma; Hemangioma-thrombocytopenia syndrome; Maffucci syndrome
Blurred vision. *See under* Vision
Bobble-head doll syndrome, 267
Body development
  asymmetrical, chromosome 14, trisomy mosaic and, 41
  unbalanced, cutis marmorata telangiectatica congenita and, 615
Body weight. *See* Birth weight; Weight
Boerhaave syndrome, 679
Bone(s)
  alterations in structure, Fairbank disease and, 65
  brittle and easily broken, Cushing syndrome and. *See also* Bone fractures
  deformed, in arms, legs and elbows, acrodysostosis and, 10
  density
    increased, osteopetrosis and, 115
    mild-to-moderate increased, trichodentoosseous syndrome and, 148
  dislocations and abnormalities of, Larsen syndrome and, 94
  excessive development of, epidermal nevus syndrome and, 621
  long. *See* Long bones
  malformations, Schinzel type acrocallosal syndrome and, 9
  softening, thinning, or deteriorating
    Gaucher disease and, 194
    hypophosphatemic rickets and, 705
    mastocytosis and, 488
  wormian. *See* Wormian bones
Bone decalcification, phenylketonuria and, 225
Bone fractures
  easy, osteogenesis imperfecta and, 114
  from extreme twisting and contracting of muscles, stiff-man syndrome and, 378
  frequent, osteopetrosis and, 115
  Gorham disease and, 763
  hereditary sensory neuropathy type II and, 356
  hypophosphatemic rickets and, 705
  Maffucci syndrome and, 96
  Menkes disease and, 214
  Ollier disease and, 770
  McCune-Albright syndrome and, 736
  proneness to, McCune-Albright syndrome and, 736
  vitamin D-deficiency rickets and, 740
Bone lesions
  blastomycosis and, 530
  polyostotic fibrous dysplasia and, 71
Bone loss, Gorham disease and, 763

Bone marrow
  atrophy of, hematopoietic syndrome and, 836
  cystine crystals in, cystinosis and, 188
  damage, histiocytosis X and, 478
  decreased density in, osteopetrosis and, 115
  depression, gold poisoning and, 831
  formation of foam cells in, Niemann-Pick disease and, 222
  transient suppression, typhoid fever and, 592
Bone pain
  chronic myelogenous leukemia and, 481
  cystic fibrosis and, 406
  Engelmann disease and, 63
  and joint, fibrous dysplasia and, 71
  late congenital syphilis and, 585
  multiple myeloma and, 490
  Paget disease of bone and, 772
  severe, Oroya fever and, 529
Bone tumor-epidermoid cyst-polyposis. See Gardner syndrome
Bonnet-Dechaume-Blanc syndrome. See Wyburn-Mason syndrome
Bonnevie-Ulrich syndrome. See Turner syndrome
Bony spinal canal, erosion of, syringomyelia and, 380
Borborygmi, glucose-galactose malabsorption and, 676
Borjeson-Forssman-Lehmann syndrome. See Borjeson syndrome
Borjeson syndrome, 22–23. See also Frölich syndrome
Bossing, frontal. See Frontal bossing
Botulism, 531–32
Bouba. See Yaws
Bourneville Pringle syndrome. See Tuberous sclerosis (TS)
Bovine smallpox. See Cowpox
Bowel
  cancer, familial polyposis and, 672
  dysmotility, mixed connective tissue disease and, 769
  rotated improperly, Ivemark syndrome and, 86
Bowel control
  difficulty in gaining, cerebral palsy and, 285
  loss of
    Devic disease and, 297
    Kugelberg-Welander syndrome and, 320
Bowen-Conradi Hutterite syndrome. See Bowen Hutterite syndrome
Bowen-Conradi syndrome. See Bowen Hutterite syndrome
Bowen disease, 612–13. See also Bowenoid papulosis; Paget disease
  of the breast; Squamous cell carcinoma, cutaneous
Bowen Hutterite syndrome, 23–24
Bowenoid papulosis, 613
Bowlegs
  hypophosphatemic rickets and, 705
  vitamin D-deficiency rickets and, 740
Brachial neuritis. See Parsonnage-Turner syndrome
Brachial plexus, injury to upper, Erb palsy and, 302
Brachial plexus neuritis. See Parsonnage-Turner syndrome
Brachiocephalic ischemia. See Arteritis, Takayasu
Brachmann-de Lange syndrome. See Cornelia de Lange syndrome
Brachycephaly, Saethre-Chotzen syndrome and, 132
Brachydactyly
  oral-facial-digital syndrome and, 113
  Saethre-Chotzen syndrome and, 132
  with webbing, Carpenter syndrome and, 27
Bradbury-Eggleston syndrome (idiopathic orthostatic hypotension),
    374–75
Bradycardia
  Chagas disease and, 536
  Dandy-Walker syndrome and, 295
  fever and, Dengue fever and, 542
  Gilbert syndrome and, 675
  Guillain-Barré syndrome and, 307
  infantile apnea and, 265
Bradykinesia
  corticobasal degeneration and, 292
  progressive supranuclear palsy (PSP) and, 368
  vitamin E deficiency and, 245
Bradypnea, Dandy-Walker syndrome and, 295
Brain
  abnormally small, EEC syndrome and, 62
  absence of brain tissue, anencephaly and, 13
  arteriovenous malformations of, 614
  larger than normal, cutis marmorata telangiectatica congenita and,
    615
  lipomata on frontal lobe of, fronto-facio-nasal dysplasia and, 76
  missing areas or unusual development of, Fryns syndrome and, 77
  nevi in, blue rubber bleb nevus and, 22
  uneven atrophy of, Pick disease and, 365
Brain abscesses
  nocardiosis and, 566
  predisposition to, atrial septal defects and, 401
Brain damage
  osteopetrosis and, 115
  propionic acidemia and, 176
Brain demyelination
  Balo disease and, 277
  childhood ALD and, 177

neonatal ALD and, 177, 178
Brain hernia, Roberts syndrome and, 128
Brain stem, compression of, achondroplasia and, 8
Brain tumor. See Astrocytoma, benign
Branched chain ketonuria. See Maple syrup urine disease
Brancher deficiency. See Andersen disease
Branchial fistula, branchio-oto-renal syndrome and, 24
Branchio-oculo-facial syndrome, 24. See also Branchio-oto-renal
    syndrome
Branchio-oto-renal syndrome, 24–25. See also Fraser syndrome;
    Renal agenesis, bilateral
Brandt syndrome. See Acrodermatitis enteropathica (AE)
Brandywine type dentinogenesis imperfecta. See Dentinogenesis
    imperfecta, type III
Brazilian achondrogenesis. See Achondrogenesis
Brazilian trypansomiasis. See Chagas disease
Breakbone fever. See Dengue fever
Breast(s)
  absent or abnormally developed
    with normal nipple development in women, Tay syndrome and,
      657
    Poland syndrome and, 124
  atrophy, Sheehan syndrome and, 742
  early development in females
    Kabuki makeup syndrome and, 89
    precocious puberty and, 738
  enlarged, in men, and secreting milk, Forbes-Albright syndrome
    and, 726
  failure to develop, Bardet-Biedl syndrome and, 19
  late development in, McCune-Albright syndrome and, 736
  Paget disease of, 494–95
  reduction in size of, Achard-Thiers syndrome and, 710
Breath
  fishy odor, trimethylaminuria and, 243
  shortness of
    AAT deficiency and, 397
    eosinophilic gastroenteritis (EG) and, 675
    hantavirus pulmonary syndrome and, 554
    lymphangiomyomatosis and, 484
    thrombotic thrombocytopenic purpura (TTP) and, 500
  urine-like odor, Alport syndrome and, 692
Breathing
  difficulties
    acquired autoimmune hemolytic anemia and, 451
    during activity or feeding, ventricular septal defects and, 427
    bronchopulmonary dysplasia and, 403
    congenital lobar emphysema and, 411
    exertion-produced, warm-antibody hemolytic anemia and, 454
    Farber disease and, 192
    Guillain-Barré syndrome and, 307
    histiocytosis X and, 478
    megaloblastic anemia and, 455
    in newborn, Miller syndrome and, 105
    Opitz syndrome and, 112
    sideroblastic anemia and, 456
    due to spasms of tongue, throat, and respiratory tract, Meige
      syndrome and, 328
  inability, except when sitting upright, mitral valve prolapse
    syndrome (MVPS) and, 418
  irregular, formaldehyde poisoning and, 829
  labored, hemolytic-uremic syndrome (HUS) and, 695
  noisy
    Hurler syndrome and, 202
    Maroteaux-Lamy syndrome and, 211
  periods of deep, abnormal (in infants), Joubert syndrome and, 315
  rapid
    pheochromocytoma and, 495
    and shallow, ventricular septal defects and, 427
    and shallow, with moderate exercise, fibrosing alveolitis and, 399
  temporary cessation of, infantile apnea and, 265
Breda's disease. See Yaws
Breech birth
  bilateral renal agenesis and, 703
  Smith-Lemli-Opitz syndrome and, 137
Brissaud II. See Tourette syndrome
Brittle bone disease. See Osteogenesis imperfecta (OI)
Broad beta disease, 402–3
Broad thumb-hallux syndrome. See Rubinstein-Taybi syndrome
Brocq-Duhring disease. See Dermatitis herpetiformis (DH)
Bronchial hyperreactivity, cobalt poisoning and, 831
Bronchiectasis, 90
  central, allergic bronchopulmonary aspergillosis and, 526
  Kartagener syndrome and, 89, 90
  paroxysmal coughing and, pertussis and, 568
  yellow nail syndrome and, 429
Bronchiolar constriction, anaphylaxis and, 523
Bronchitis. See also Alpha-1-antitrypsin (AAT) deficiency; Pertussis
  frequent, precipitating heart failure, cor triatriatum and, 405
  vanadium poisoning and, 831
  yellow nail syndrome and, 429

pointed, leprechaunism and, 95
prominent, Coffin-Lowry syndrome and, 46
protruding, Binder-type maxillonasal dysplasia and, 102
receding
  bilateral renal agenesis and, 703
  chromosome 11q- syndrome and, 37
  chromosome 11q- syndrome and, 37
  Hutchinson-Gilford syndrome and, 84
  Tay syndrome and, 657
  Treacher Collins syndrome and, 147
small
  chromosome 9 ring and, 33
  cri du chat syndrome and, 51
Chiropractic, xvi, xix
Chloracne, 607
Choanal atresia or stenosis
  Antley-Bixler syndrome and, 15
  CHARGE association and, 30
  Marshall-Smith syndrome and, 100
Choking
  ataxia telangiectasia and, 275
  esophageal atresia and tracheoesophageal fistula and, 64
  Friedreich ataxia and, 272
  furious rabies syndrome and, 573
  Marie ataxia and, 273
  Rubinstein-Taybi syndrome and, 129
Cholangitis, primary sclerosing, 551
Cholelithiasis
  hereditary spherocytic hemolytic anemia and, 453
  thalassemia major and, 502
Cholera, **538–39**
Cholestasis, 663. *See also* Vitamin E deficiency
  gold poisoning and, 831
  neonatal hepatitis and, 556
  with peripheral pulmonary stenosis. *See* Alagille syndrome
Cholestasis-lymphedema syndrome, 667
Cholesterol
  elevated level of, broad beta disease and, 402
  high levels, at birth, congenital syphilis and, 585
  increased amounts in large thoracic and abdominal organs, Niemann-Pick disease and, 222
  low plasma
    acanthocytosis and, 443
    Tangier disease and, 241
Chondrodysplasia, Murk-Jansen type. *See* Metaphyseal chondrodysplasia, Jansen type
Chondrodysplasia punctata, 2, 61
  Binder-type maxillonasal dysplasia and, 102
Chondrodysplasia punctata. *See* Conradi-Hünermann syndrome
Chondrodysplasia (rhizomelic type), 48
Chondrodystrophia calcificans congenita. *See* Conradi-Hünermann syndrome
Chondrodystrophic myotonia. *See* Schwartz-Jampel syndrome
Chondrodystrophy. *See also* Achondroplasia
  with clubfeet. *See* Diastrophic dysplasia
  epiphyseal. *See* Dysplasia epiphysealis hemimelica
  hyperplastic. *See* Metatrophic dysplasia I
  hypochondroplasia, 85
Chondroectodermal dysplasia, 18
Chondrogenesis imperfecta. *See* Achondrogenesis
Chondropathia tuberosa. *See* Tietze syndrome
Chondrosarcoma
  Maffucci syndrome and, 96
  Ollier disease and, 770
Chorea. *See also* Myoclonus
  antiphospholipid syndrome and, 524
  Kufs disease and, 319
  olivopontocerebellar atrophy I and, 357
  rheumatic fever and, 575
  tardive dyskinesia and, 380
  of trunk and limbs, neuroacanthocytosis and, 352
Chorea minor. *See* Sydenham chorea
Choreic movements, chronic, glutaricaciduria I and, 196
Choreiform movements, Huntington disease and, 310
Choreoacanthocytosis. *See* Neuroacanthocytosis
Choreoathetosis
  bilateral, kernicterus and, 317
  Hallervorden-Spatz disease and, 308
Choriocapillaris, subretinal neovascular membrane growing from, serpiginous choroiditis and, 795
Chorioretinal anomalies. *See* Aicardi syndrome
Chorioretinitis
  Behçet syndrome and, 755
  congenital toxoplasmosis and, 586, 589
  TORCH syndrome and, 586
Choroid, angiomas in, Sturge-Weber syndrome and, 143
Choroidal sclerosis. *See* Choroideremia
Choroideremia, 789, **794–95**. *See also* Alstrom syndrome
Choroiditis, serpiginous, **795–96**, 801
Chotzen syndrome. *See* Saethre-Chotzen syndrome

Christmas disease. *See* Factor IX deficiency; Hemophilia
Christmas tree syndrome. *See* Jejunal atresia
Christ-Siemens-Touraine syndrome, 633
Chromaffin cell tumor. *See* Pheochromocytoma
Chromium poisoning, 831
13q- Chromosomal syndrome. *See* Chromosome 13q- syndrome
Chromosomal triplication. *See* Trisomy
Chromosome 3, deletion of distal 3p. *See* Chromosome 3, monosomy 3p2
Chromosome 3, monosomy 3p2, **31**
Chromosome 4, trisomy 4p. *See* Trisomy 4p
Chromosome 4q-syndrome, **37**
Chromosome 4 ring, **31–32**
Chromosome 5p- syndrome. *See* Cri du chat syndrome
Chromosome 5 trisomy 5p, **40–41**
Chromosome 6 ring, **32–33**
Chromosome 9 ring, **33**
Chromosome 11q- syndrome, **37–38**. *See also* Chromosome 4q-syndrome; Triploid syndrome
Chromosome 13q- mosaicism, 38
Chromosome 13q- syndrome, **38–39**. *See also* Holoprosencephaly
Chromosome 13 ring, 38
Chromosome 14, trisomy mosaic, **41–42**
Chromosome 14 ring, **33–34**
Chromosome 15 ring, **34**
Chromosome 17, interstitial deletion 17p-. *See* Smith-Magenis syndrome
Chromosome 18, Monosomy 18q. *See* Chromosome 18q- syndrome
Chromosome 18, Trisomy 18, 23
Chromosome 18 long arm deletion syndrome. *See* Chromosome 18q- syndrome
Chromosome 18p- syndrome, **39**. *See also* Holoprosencephaly; 13q-syndrome; Triploid syndrome
Chromosome 18q- syndrome, **39–40**
Chromosome 18 ring, **35**
Chromosome 21 ring, **35–36**
Chromosome 22, trisomy mosaic, **42–43**
Chromosome 22 ring, **36–37**
Chromosome number 4 short arm deletion syndrome. *See* Wolf-Hirschhorn syndrome (WHS)
Chromosome triploidy syndrome. *See* Triploid syndrome
Chronic adhesive arachnoiditis. *See* Arachnoiditis
Chronic adrenocortical insufficiency. *See* Addison disease
Chronic asthenia. *See* Neurasthenia
Chronic dysphagocytosis. *See* Granulomatous disease, chronic (CGD)
Chronic EBV infection, 547
Chronic encephalitis and epilepsy. *See* Encephalitis, Rasmussen
Chronic familial icterus. *See* Anemia, hemolytic, hereditary spherocytic
Chronic granulocytic leukemia. *See* Leukemia, chronic myelogenous
Chronic granulomatous disease, 789. *See also* Neutropenia, chronic
Chronic hematogenous TB, 591
Chronic hiccups, **288**
Chronic idiopathic jaundice. *See* Dubin-Johnson syndrome
Chronic idiopathic polyneuritis, 307
Chronic inflammatory demyelinating polyneuropathy (CIDP), **289**. *See also* Multiple sclerosis (MS)
Chronic localized encephalitis. *See* Encephalitis, Rasmussen
Chronic lymphatic leukemia, 454
Chronic lymphocytic leukemia, 491
Chronic lymphocytic thyroiditis. *See* Hashimoto disease
Chronic meningococcemia, 564
Chronic multiple tics. *See* Tourette syndrome
Chronic myelocytic leukemia. *See* Leukemia, chronic myelogenous
Chronic myeloid leukemia. *See* Leukemia, chronic myelogenous
Chronic progressive chorea. *See* Huntington disease
Chronic renal failure, 694
Chronic sinobronchial disease and dextrocardia. *See* Kartagener syndrome
Chronic spasmodic dysphonia (CSD), **289–90**
Chronic stuttering, 290
Chronic tics, 387
Chronic vomiting in childhood. *See* Cyclic vomiting syndrome
Churg-Strauss syndrome, **404–5**. *See also* Aspergillosis; Granulomatous disease, chronic (CGD); Lymphomatoid granulomatosis; Polyarteritis nodosa (PAN); Vasculitis
Chylangioma. *See* Lymphangioma, cavernous
Chylomicrons
  failure to form, following meal, acanthocytosis and, 443
  massive accumulation in blood plasma, hyperchylomicronemia and, 203
Chylous effusions, Waldmann disease and, 685
Chylous pleural effusion, Gorham disease and, 763
Chyluria due to longstanding lymphatic obstruction, filariasis and, 550
Cicatricial pemphigoid. *See* Pemphigoid, benign mucosal
Ciguatera fish poisoning, 822, **827–28**
Ciliary dysentery. *See* Balantidiasis
Ciliary dyskinesia. *See* Polynesian bronchiectasis
Ciliary vessel vasculitis, Wegener granulomatosis and, 508
Circulatory collapse

persistent truncus arteriosus and, 426
Pierre Robin syndrome and, 123
renal cell carcinoma and, 461
rheumatic fever and, 575
with right-sided valvular cardiac disease, carcinoid syndrome and, 719
Whipple disease and, 598
Conical cornea. See Keratoconus
Conjugated hyperbilirubinemia. See Dubin-Johnson syndrome
Conjunctiva
  angiomas in, Sturge-Weber syndrome and, 143
  cobblestone-like changes in upper palpebral, vernal keratoconjunctivitis and, 803
  cystine crystals in, cystinosis and, 188
  inflammation of
    and redness, benign mucosal pemphigoid and, 650
    vernal keratoconjunctivitis and, 803
  redness of, ligneous conjunctivitis and, 798
  scarring, benign mucosal pemphigoid and, 650
  shiny, pearly spots of triangular-shaped tissue (Bitôt spots) on, keratomalacia and, 805
  xerosis of, keratomalacia and, 805
Conjunctival edema, Graves disease and, 727
Conjunctival hemorrhage, leptospirosis and, 560
Conjunctivitis, ligneous, **798–99**
Conjunctivitis (pink eye), 798, 803
  acne rosacea and, 607
  acrodermatitis enteropathica (AE) and, 608
  bilateral, Kawasaki syndrome and, 764
  leprosy and, 559
  painful, with purulent discharge, Stevens-Johnson syndrome and, 581
  Reiter syndrome and, 779
  Wegener granulomatosis and, 508
Connective tissue disorder, Marden-Walker type. See Marden-Walker syndrome
Conn syndrome, **720–21**
Conradi disease. See Conradi-Hünermann syndrome
Conradi-Hünermann syndrome, **48–49**, 61. See also Dysplasia epiphysealis hemimelica; Fairbank disease; Ichthyosis; Keratitis-ichthyosis-deafness (KID) syndrome; Maxillonasal dysplasia, Binder-type
Consciousness
  alterations of, Weil syndrome and, 597
  disturbance of, moyamoya disease and, 331
  unexpected partial or total recurring loss of, Romano-Ward syndrome and, 424
Constipation
  acute intermittent porphyria and, 229
  ALA-D porphyria and, 230
  blue diaper syndrome and, 183
  botulism and, 531
  Chagas disease and, 536
  chronic, Rubinstein-Taybi syndrome and, 129
  congenital generalized fibromatosis and, 70
  FG syndrome and, 69
  Floating-Harbor syndrome and, 72
  Gardner syndrome and, 673
  hereditary coproporphyria porphyria and, 233
  Hirschsprung disease and, 678
  in infancy, Williams syndrome and, 162
  intermittent diarrhea and, pernicious anemia and, 456
  intestinal pseudoobstruction and, 678
  oculo-gastrointestinal muscular dystrophy and, 339
  pheochromocytoma and, 495
  resistant to treatment, duodenal atresia or stenosis and, 58
  wandering spleen and, 686
Constitutional aplastic anemia. See Anemia, Fanconi
Constitutional eczema. See Dermatitis, atopic
Constitutional erythroid hypoplasia. See Anemia, Diamond-Blackfan
Constitutional liver dysfunction. See Gilbert syndrome
Constitutional thrombopathy. See von Willebrand disease
Constrictive median neuropathy. See Carpal tunnel syndrome (CTS)
Constructional apraxia, 266
Contact dermatitis, 523, 548, 661. See also Anaphylaxis; Dermatitis, atopic; Urticaria, cholinergic; Urticaria, cold
  chromium poisoning and, 831
Contact lens wear, intolerance to, vernal conjunctivitis and, 803
Continuous muscle fiber activity syndrome. See Isaacs syndrome
Contortions of muscles, involuntary, torsion dystonia and, 385
Contractural arachnodactyly, congenital. See Beals syndrome
Contractures
  Duchenne muscular dystrophy and, 335
  of feet at birth, Wieacker syndrome and, 393
  multiple with arachnodactyly. See Beals syndrome
  Pallister-Killian syndrome and, 118
Conversion disorder, **291–92**
Convulsions. See also Epilepsy
  alcohol withdrawal in infants and, 67
  congenital syphilis and, 585

contralateral, malignant astrocytoma and, 271
Dandy-Walker syndrome and, 295
dehydration with, in infants, diabetes insipidus (DI) and, 725
glioblastomas in frontal lobe and, 468
hydrocephalus and, 312
infantile metachromatic leukodystrophy and, 324
kernicterus and, 317
Kufs disease and, 320
Menkes disease and, 214
radiation exposure and, cerebral radiation syndrome and, 837
vitamin D-deficiency rickets and, 740
Whipple disease and, 598
Convulsive seizures, cerebral palsy and, 285
Cooley anemia. See Thalassemia major
Coordination
  difficulty with
    Creutzfeldt-Jakob disease and, 293
    of extremities, Joseph disease and, 314
    eye-hand, agenesis of the corpus callosum (ACC) and, 257
    glioblastomas in temporal lobe and, 468
    in late teens or early 20s, Kufs disease and, 319
    Shy-Drager syndrome and, 374
    tetrahydrobiopterin deficiencies and, 242
    of upper extremities, parenchymatous cortical degeneration of the cerebellum and, 361
  impaired muscle
    ataxia telangiectasia and, 274
    congenital hypomyelination neuropathy and, 354
  loss or lack of
    Asperger syndrome and, 270
    ataxic cerebral palsy and, 286
    Seitelberger disease and, 374
    Wilson disease and, 247
Copper, excess stored, Wilson disease and, 247
Copper depletion, molybdenum poisoning and, 831
Copper poisoning, 831
Coprolalia, 386
Coprolalia-generalized tic disorder. See Tourette syndrome
Coproporphyrin, excess, in urine and stool, hereditary coproporphyria porphyria and, 234
Cor biloculare (complete atrioventricular septal defect). See Atrioventricular septal defect
Cori disease. See Glycogen storage disease III (GSD III)
Cornea
  angiomas in, Sturge-Weber syndrome and, 143
  arcus lipidus corneae, broad beta disease and, 402
  clouding of. See also Corneal opacities
    achondrogenesis and, 7
    Bowen Hutterite syndrome and, 23
    De Barsey syndrome and, 757
    focal dermal hypoplasia and, 627
    Hurler syndrome and, 202
    Hutchinson-Gilford syndrome and, 84
    Miller-Dieker syndrome and, 325
    Morquio disease and, 216
    mucolipidosis IV and, 218
    phocomelia syndrome and, 122
    Roberts syndrome and, 128
    X-linked ichthyosis and, 642
    Zellweger syndrome and, 248
  cone-shaped, keratoconus and, 804
  cystine crystals in, cystinosis and, 188
  diminished, Ehlers-Danlos syndromes (EDS) and, 759
  Kayser-Fleischer ring (rusty-brown deposit), Wilson disease and, 247
  opaque ring around outer edge of, Rieger syndrome and, 127
  small, Hallermann-Streiff syndrome and, 82
  tumors of, xeroderma pigmentosum and, 662
  xerosis of, keratomalacia and, 805
Corneal anesthesia, inadvertent injury and blindness due to, leprosy and, 559
Corneal clouding-cutis laxa-mental retardation. See De Barsey syndrome
Corneal deposits, Tangier disease and, 241
Corneal edema
  Cogan-Reese syndrome and, 802
  essential iris atrophy and, 803
Corneal flatness, Marfan syndrome and, 98
Corneal inflammation
  insensitivity of eye to pain from foreign objects and, familial dysautonomia and, 304
  KID syndrome and, 644
Corneal lesions, berylliosis and, 826
Corneal opacities
  at about 8 years of age, Sly syndrome and, 240
  Fryns syndrome and, 77
  a-mannosidosis and, 210
  Maroteaux-Lamy syndrome and, 211
  mucolipidosis II and, 217
  mucolipidosis III and, 218

conductive
 Klippel-Feil syndrome and, 91
 Treacher Collins syndrome and, 147
congenital rubella and, 578
congenital sensorineural, Waardenburg syndrome and, 158
craniometaphyseal dysplasia and, 49
Goldenhar syndrome and, 78
KID syndrome and, 644
LEOPARD syndrome and, 646
Maroteaux-Lamy syndrome and, 211
multiple sulfatase deficiency and, 220
neurosensory, Tay syndrome and, 657
Norrie disease and, 809
osteopetrosis and, 115
partial, Cockayne syndrome and, 45
profound, Sanfilippo syndrome and, 239
sensorineural, FG syndrome and, 69
Stickler syndrome and, 142
thrombopathic thrombocytopenia and, 460
Deafness, congenital, and functional heart disease. *See* Jervell and
 Lange-Nielsen syndrome
Deafness, sensorineural, with imperforate anus and hypoplastic
 thumbs. *See* Townes-Brocks syndrome
Deafness-myopia-cataract-saddle nose, Marshall type. *See* Marshall
 syndrome
De Barsey syndrome, **757–58**. *See also* Cutis laxa
Debre syndrome. *See* Cat-scratch disease
Decerebrate dementia. *See* Subacute sclerosing panencephalitis
 (SSPE)
Decompression sickness, 771
Deefferented state. *See* Locked-in syndrome
Deep vein thrombosis, essential thrombocythemia and, 505
Defecation, loss of physiologic urge for, Hirschsprung disease and,
 678
Degenerative chorea. *See* Huntington disease
Degenerative lumbar spinal stenosis. *See* Spinal stenosis
DeGeorge anomaly, 438
Degos disease, **408–9**
 antiphospholipid syndrome and, 524
Dehydration
 celiac sprue and, 670
 childhood ALD and, 177
 congenital adrenal hyperplasia (CAH) and, 713
 from diarrhea
 Addison disease and, 712
 carcinoid syndrome and, 719
 gastrointestinal radiation syndrome and, 836
 gastroschisis and, 77
 hemolytic-uremic syndrome (HUS) and, 695
 21—hydroxylase deficiency and, 714
 with hypernatremia in infants, diabetes insipidus (DI) and, 725
 meningococcal meningitis and, 562
 mercury poisoning and, 831
 methylmalonic acidemia and, 175
 microvillus inclusion disease and, 680
 peeling of large sheets of skin, toxic epidermal necrolysis
 (TEN) and, 658
 polycystic kidney diseases (PKD) and, 702
 propionic acidemia and, 176
 from vomiting, Addison disease and, 712
Dejerine-Landouzy muscular dystrophy. *See* Muscular dystrophy,
 Landouzy-Dejerine
Dejerine-Roussy syndrome. *See* Thalamic syndrome
Dejerine-Sottas disease, **296**. *See also* Charcot-Marie-Tooth disease;
 Chronic inflammatory demyelinating polyneuropathy (CIDP);
 Multiple sclerosis (MS); Roussy-Lévy syndrome
 congenital hypomyelination neuropathy and, 354
Delayed hypersensitivity. *See* Dermatitis, contact
Delayed speech and language development, 340
Deletion on long arm of chromosome 11. *See* Chromosome 11q-
 syndrome
Deletion on the short arm of 11p13, 38
Delinquency due to frustration with classroom performance, dyslexia
 and, 299
Delirium
 arsenic poisoning and, 830
 Rocky Mountain spotted fever (RMSF) and, 576
 typhoid fever and, 592
Delleman-Oorthuys syndrome. *See* Oculo-cerebro-cutaneous
 syndrome
Delleman syndrome. *See* Oculo-cerebro-cutaneous syndrome
Delta hepatitis. *See* Hepatitis D
Delta storage pool disease. *See* Hermansky-Pudlak syndrome
Dementia
 AIDS-related dementia complex, 516, 517
 in children, childhood ALD and, 177
 corticobasal degeneration and, 292
 Fahr disease and, 303
 Hallervorden-Spatz disease and, 308
 Hartnup disease and, 199

Huntington disease and, 310
Klüver-Bucy syndrome and, 318
late syphilis and, 584
lipodystrophy and, 735
metachromatic leukodystrophy and, 324
olivopontocerebellar atrophy and, 357
progressive
 MELAS syndrome and, 213
 MERRF syndrome and, 215
 subacute sclerosing panencephalitis (SSPE) and, 582
progressive myoclonic epilepsy and, 343
progressive supranuclear palsy (PSP) and, 368
Seitelberger disease and, 374
senile, Binswanger disease and, 281
severe
 Pick disease and, 365
 Rett syndrome and, 371
Sjögren syndrome (SjS) and, 783
subacute cerebellar degeneration and, 285
DeMorgan or ruby spots. *See* Hemorrhagic telangiectasia, hereditary
De Morsier syndrome. *See* Septo-optic dysplasia
Demyelinating polyneuropathy. *See* Conversion disorder
Demyelination, Rosenberg-Chutorian syndrome and, 372
Dengue fever, **542–43**
Dengue hemorrhagic fever, 542
Dengue shock syndrome, 542
Dental caries
 chromosome 18p- syndrome and, 39
 Cockayne syndrome and, 45
 high occurrence of, chromosome 18p- syndrome and, 39
 hypophosphatemic rickets and, 705
 Sjögren syndrome (SjS) and, 783
Dental defects, osteopetrosis and, 115
Dental development, retarded, Coffin-Siris syndrome and, 47
Dentin dysplasia, coronal, **53**. *See also* Dentin dysplasia, radicular;
 Dentinogenesis imperfecta, type III
Dentin dysplasia, radicular, **54**. *See also* Dentin dysplasia, coronal;
 Dentinogenesis imperfecta, type III
Dentin dysplasia, type I. *See* Dentin dysplasia, radicular
Dentin dysplasia, type II. *See* Dentin dysplasia, coronal
Dentinogenesis, osteogenesis imperfecta and, 114
Dentinogenesis imperfecta, Shields type II. *See* Dentinogenesis
 imperfecta, type I
Dentinogenesis imperfecta, Shields type III. *See* Dentinogenesis
 imperfecta, type III
Dentinogenesis imperfecta, type I, 54
Dentinogenesis imperfecta, type III, **54–55**. *See also* Dentin
 dysplasia, coronal
Dentition. *See* Teeth
Dento-oculo-osseous dysplasia. *See* Oculo-dento-digital dysplasia
Denys-Drash syndrome, **723–24**. *See also* WAGR syndrome
Depakene, fetal effects from. *See* Fetal valproate syndrome
Depakote, fetal effects from. *See* Fetal valproate syndrome
Depakote sprinkle, fetal effects from. *See* Fetal valproate syndrome
Depersonalization disorder, **296–97**
Depersonalization neurosis. *See* Depersonalization disorder
Depressed cellular immunity, 433
Depression
 acute intermittent porphyria and, 229
 in adolescence, familial dysautonomia and, 304
 Binswanger disease and, 281
 congenital adrenal hyperplasia (CAH) and, 713
 Dercum disease and, 724
 hepatorenal syndrome and, 695
 hyperactivity combined with, anorexia nervosa and, 263
 idiopathic edema and, 480
 interstitial cystitis and, 697
 Kawasaki syndrome and, 765
 lead poisoning and, 831
 myalgic encephalomyelitis and, 547
 neurasthenia and, 352
 Parkinson disease and, 362
 polymyalgia rheumatica and, 774
 rabies and, 572
 systemic lupus erythematosus (SLE) and, 784
 Wolfram syndrome and, 164
Dercum disease, **724**
Dermatan sulfate, elevated urinary, multiple sulfatase deficiency and,
 220
Dermatitis
 atopic, 523. *See also* Anaphylaxis; Contact dermatitis
 ichthyosis vulgaris and, 641
 after blood transfusion or bone marrow transplant, graft-versus-
 host disease and, 552
 chronic granulomatous disease and, 470
 contact. *See* Contact dermatitis
 erythematous over extensor surfaces of joints,
 polymyositis/dermatomyositis and, 775
 gold poisoning and, 831

in arms and legs, meningococcemia and, 564
  Buerger disease and, 756
  fingertip, Raynaud disease and phenomenon and, 777
Gardener-Diamond syndrome, 499
Gardner syndrome, 663, **673**. *See also* Cronkhite-Canada disease;
  Familial polyposis; Fibromatosis, congenital generalized;
  Peutz-Jeghers syndrome
Gas, excessive foul, cystic fibrosis and, 406
Gasser syndrome. *See* Hemolytic-uremic syndrome (HUS)
Gastric atony, amyloidosis and, 749
Gastric carcinoma, 467, 674
Gastric lymphoma, non-Hodgkin type, **467–68**. *See also* Gastritis,
  giant hypertrophic
Gastric neurasthenia, 352
Gastric varices, AAT deficiency and, 397
Gastrinoma. *See* Zollinger-Ellison syndrome
Gastritis, giant hypertrophic, **674**. *See also* Waldmann disease
Gastrocnemius, short, trismus pseudocamptodactyly syndrome and,
  150
Gastroenteritis
  chromium poisoning and, 831
  eosinophilic (EG), 663, **674–75**
  lithium poisoning and, 831
  silver poisoning and, 831
Gastroesophageal laceration-hemorrhage syndrome. *See* Mallory-
  Weiss syndrome
Gastrointestinal bleeding
  gold poisoning and, 831
  polyarteritis nodosa (PAN) and, 773
  prolonged, von Willebrand disease and, 507
Gastrointestinal disturbances
  arsenic poisoning and, 830
  cobalt poisoning and, 831
  cold-antibody hemolytic anemia and, 452
  copper poisoning and, 831
  mercury poisoning and, 831
  zinc poisoning and, 831
Gastrointestinal polyposis with ectodermal changes. *See* Cronkhite-
  Canada disease
Gastrointestinal radiation syndrome, 836
Gastrointestinal tract
  diverticula of, cutis laxa and, 615
  nevi in, blue rubber bleb nevus and, 22
Gastroschisis, **77–78**
Gaucher disease, **194–95**, 320. *See also* Banti syndrome; Fabry
  disease; Gorham disease; Hajdu-Cheney syndrome; Niemann-
  Pick disease; Osteonecrosis; Refsum syndrome; Sandhoff
  disease
Gaucher-Schlagenhaufer. *See* Gaucher disease
Gaze
  downward, hydrocephalus and, 312
  loss of upward, kernicterus and, 317
  loss of vertical, progressive supranuclear palsy (PSP) and, 368
Gaze palsy, corticobasal degeneration and, 292
Gee-Herter disease. *See* Celiac sprue
Gee-Thaysen disease. *See* Celiac sprue
Gélineau syndrome. *See* Narcolepsy
Gel phenomenon, ankylosing spondylitis and, 750
Genee-Wiedemann syndrome. *See* Miller syndrome
Generalized anaphylaxis. *See* Anaphylaxis
Generalized anxiety disorder, 359
Generalized congenital osteosclerosis. *See* Osteopetrosis
Generalized glycogenosis. *See* Pompe disease
Generalized or systemic chondromalacia. *See* Relapsing
  polychondritis
Genetic counseling, 2–3
Genital hypertrophy, lipodystrophy and, 734, 735
Genitalia
  abnormal
    chromosome 9 ring and, 33
    trisomy 13 syndrome and, 153
  ambiguous
    morphologically ambiguous external, true hermaphroditism and,
      731
    Reifenstein syndrome and, 739
    WAGR syndrome and, 816
  atrophy, Sheehan syndrome and, 742
  displacement of external, caudal regression syndrome and, 29
  edema on, hereditary angioedema and, 457
  female
    abnormalities of external, 21—Hydroxylase deficiency and, 714
    masculinization of external, congenital adrenal hyperplasia
      (CAH) and, 713
    underdeveloped, Tay syndrome and, 657
  hypoplastic external, 133
  itchy, patchy, crusty areas on, extramammary Paget disease and,
    495
  male
    failure to masculinize, congenital lipoid hyperplasia and, 714
    immature into adulthood, cutis laxa and, 615

males born with female or ambiguous external
  17-20—Desmolase deficiency and, 714
  17—Hydroxylase deficiency and, 714
  3—hydroxysteroid dehydrogenase deficiency and, 714
  sex-reversal, Smith-Lemli-Opitz syndrome and, 137
Genital lesions, reddish brown or violet, sometimes velvety, Bowenoid
  papulosis and, 613
Genitourinary defects, Wilms tumor and, 509
Genitourinary TB, 591
Genuine hyperhidrosis. *See* Hyperhidrosis
Genu valgum
  cleidocranial dysplasia and, 43
  Dyggve-Melchior-Clausen syndrome and, 59
  Ellis-van Creveld syndrome and, 62
  Goodman syndrome and, 79
  Jackson-Weiss syndrome and, 87
  Morquio disease and, 216
  Summitt syndrome and, 144
Genu varum
  chromosome 18q- syndrome and, 40
  Dyggve-Melchior-Clausen syndrome and, 59
  Schmid-type metaphyseal chondrodysplasia and, 104
Geographic choroiditis. *See* Choroiditis, serpiginous
Geographic helicoid serpiginous choroidopathy. *See* Choroiditis,
  serpiginous
Geographic tongue, 632
Gerhardt disease. *See* Erythromelalgia
German measles. *See* Rubella
Gerstmann syndrome, **306–7**
Gianotti-Crosti syndrome, **629–30**. *See also* Mucha-Habermann
  disease
Giant benign lymphoma. *See* Castleman disease
Giant-cell arteritis, 745, 746, 752–53
Giant cell cirrhosis of newborn. *See* Hepatitis, neonatal
Giant cell disease. *See* Hepatitis, neonatal
Giant-cell glioblastoma. *See* Astrocytoma, malignant; Glioblastoma
  multiforme
Giant cell hepatitis. *See* Hepatitis, neonatal
Giant cyst of the retina. *See* Senile retinoschisis
Giant tongue. *See* Macroglossia
*Giardia lamblia* infection, primary agammaglobulinemias and, 444
Giardiasis, **551–52**
Gibbus, mucolipidosis II and, 217
Gibraltar fever. *See* Brucellosis
Gigantism, 711
  Beckwith-Wiedemann syndrome and, 20
  McCune-Albright syndrome and, 736
Gilbert-Dreyfus syndrome. *See* Reifenstein syndrome
Gilbert-Lereboullet syndrome. *See* Gilbert syndrome
Gilbert syndrome, 663, **675–76**. *See also* Cholestasis
Gilchrist disease. *See* Blastomycosis
Gilford syndrome. *See* Hutchinson-Gilford syndrome
Gilles de la Tourette syndrome. *See* Tourette syndrome
Gingival hyperplasia, mucolipidosis II and, 217
Gingival swelling, histiocytosis X and, 478
Gingivitis, Sjögren syndrome (SjS) and, 783
Glanzmann disease. *See* Thrombasthenia
Glanzmann-Naegeli syndrome. *See* Thrombasthenia
Glaucoma
  Alstrom syndrome and, 716
  aniridia (AN) and, 792
  Coats disease and, 797
  cutis marmorata telangiectatica congenita and, 615
  dominant juvenile-onset open-angle, 792
  essential iris atrophy and, 803
  Hallermann-Streiff syndrome and, 82
  Lowe syndrome and, 209
  Marshall syndrome and, 100
  myopia with associated, Ehlers-Danlos syndromes (EDS) and, 759
  neovascular, Eales disease and, 800
  peripheral uveitis (pars planitis) and, 810
  Reiter syndrome and, 779
  retinoblastoma and, 812
  Rieger syndrome and, 127
  SHORT syndrome and, 134
  Sturge-Weber syndrome and, 143
  Vogt-Koyanagi-Harada syndrome and, 595
  Weill-Marchsani syndrome and, 159
Glaucoma simplex, Stickler syndrome and, 142
Glioblastoma multiforme, **468–69**. *See also* Astrocytoma, malignant
Glioma, Maffucci syndrome and, 96
Globoid leukodystrophy. *See* Leukodystrophy, Krabbe
Glomerular cystic disease, 702
Glomerular failure, cystinosis and, 188
Glomerulonephritis, 692
  erythema nodosum leprosum and, 559
  Goodpasture syndrome and, 413
  systemic lupus erythematosus (SLE) and, 784
  Wegener granulomatosis and, 508
Glossitis, 632

Weill-Marchesani syndrome and, 159
Palato-oto-digital syndrome. *See* Oto-palatal-digital syndrome
Paleness. *See* Pallor
Palilalia, Tourette syndrome and, 386
Pallidopyramidal syndrome. *See* Parkinson disease
Pallister-Hall syndrome, **117–18**
Pallister-Killian syndrome, **118–19**
Pallister mosaic aneuploidy. *See* Pallister-Killian syndrome
Pallister mosaic syndrome. *See* Pallister-Killian syndrome
Pallister-W syndrome, **119**
Pallor. *See also* Anemia
    Aase-Smith syndrome and, 6
    atrial flutter and, 428
    bone pain and, multiple myeloma and, 490
    dramatic stark white, of fingers and toes, Raynaud disease and
        phenomenon and, 777
    endocardial fibroelastosis (EFE) and, 412
    Goodpasture syndrome and, 413
    medullary cystic disease and, 700
    megaloblastic anemia and, 455
    myelofibrosis-osteosclerosis (MOS) and, 492
    paroxysmal nocturnal hemoglobinuria (PNH) and, 474
    pheochromocytoma and, 495
    pure red cell aplasia and, 497
    thalassemia minor and, 503
    thrombotic thrombocytopenic purpura (TTP) and, 500
    urine-like breath odor in association with, Alport syndrome and,
        692
    warm-antibody hemolytic anemia and, 454
    Wilms tumor and, 509, 816
Palmar fascia, nodules and bands in, Dupuytren contracture and, 758
Palmoplantar keratoderma, Hay-Wells syndrome and, 633
Palms of hands
    deep creases in, trisomy 8 and, 151
    erythematous, Kawasaki syndrome and, 764
    hyperkeratosis of, arsenic poisoning and, 830
    keratoderma on, lamellar recessive ichthyosis and, 640
    pebbly, KID syndrome and, 644
    pronounced markings, ichthyosis vulgaris and, 641
    scaling on, pityriasis rubra pilaris (PRP) and, 653
    symmetrical red scaling, peeling plaques on, erythrokeratolysis
        hiemalis and, 626
    thick and hard skin on, ichthyosis hystrix, Curth-Macklin type and,
        639
    xanthomas on, broad beta disease and, 402
Palpebral (eyelid) slant, antimongoloid, Noonan syndrome and, 110
Palpebral fissure
    almond-shaped, Prader-Willi syndrome and, 125
    Brown syndrome and, 794
    downward slanting
        Cardio-facio-cutaneous syndrome and, 27
        Coffin-Lowry syndrome and, 46
        mild, Cohen syndrome and, 47
        Miller syndrome and, 105
        Opitz syndrome and, 112
        oto-palato-digital syndrome and, 116
        and short, FG syndrome and, 69
        Weaver syndrome and, 159
    enlarged, remaining open even during sleep, Bell's palsy and, 278
    short, fetal alcohol syndrome and, 67
    slanted
        slightly, Goodman syndrome and, 79
        trisomy 13 syndrome and, 152
Palpitations
    acquired autoimmune hemolytic anemia and, 451
    megaloblastic anemia and, 455
    mitral valve prolapse syndrome (MVPS) and, 418
    neurasthenia and, 352
    panic-anxiety syndrome and, 359
    pheochromocytoma and, 495
    thalassemia major and, 502
    warm-antibody hemolytic anemia and, 454
Palsy. *See* Cerebral palsy
Pancreatic adenocarcinomas, Maffucci syndrome and, 96
Pancreatic cholera, 538, 719
Pancreatic cysts, asphyxiating thoracic dystrophy and, 18
Pancreatic fibrosis. *See* Cystic fibrosis (CF)
Pancreatic insufficiency, Schmidt syndrome and, 741
Pancreatic ulcerogenic tumor syndrome. *See* Zollinger-Ellison
        syndrome
Pancreatitis. *See also* Alpha-1-antitrypsin (AAT) deficiency
    cystic fibrosis and, 406
    hyperchylomicronemia and, 203
Pancytopenia
    dyskeratosis congenita and, 619
    hematopoietic syndrome and, 836
    osteopetrosis and, 115
Panhypopituitarism, 267
Panic, sleep paralysis and, 349

Panic-anxiety syndrome, **358–59**. *See also* Depersonalization
        disorder; Neurasthenia
Panic disorder. *See* Panic-anxiety syndrome
Panmural fibrosis. *See* Interstitial cystitis
Panmyelopathy. *See* Anemia, aplastic
Panmyelophthisis. *See* Anemia, aplastic
Papilledema
    cryptococcosis and, 540
    Dandy-Walker syndrome and, 295
    diencephalic syndrome and, 298
    moyamoya disease and, 331
    with progressive visual loss, pseudotumor cerebri and, 368
Papillitis, **809–10**. *See also* Leber hereditary optic neuropathy
Papillotonic pseudotabes. *See* Adie syndrome
Papule(s)
    follicular, itchy, sharply pointed, horn-like, and brownish-red to
        rosy yellow, pityriasis rubra pilaris (PRP) and, 653
    with gray-brown scales or crusts, Darier disease and, 616
    itching and burning, dermatitis herpetiformis (DH) and, 617
    large flat, duration 20 to 25 days, Gianotti-Crosti syndrome and,
        629
    leprosy and, 558
    painless, nonitchy, cat-scratch disease and, 534
    pink or brown crusty, Bowen disease and, 612
    reddish-brown, pruritic, urticaria pigmentosa and, 659
    soft, brownish-red, lupus miliaris disseminatus faciei and, 559
    waxy-looking, amyloidosis and, 749
    Wegener granulomatosis and, 508
Paracoccidioidal granuloma. *See* Paracoccidiodomycosis (PCM)
Paracoccidioidomycosis (PCM), **567–68**. *See also* Tuberculosis (TB)
Paradoxical embolism, atrial septal defects and, 401
Paradoxical myotonia, paramyotonia congenita and, 360
Paralysis
    abdominal muscle, myelitis and, 342
    of all voluntary muscles, locked-in syndrome and, 326
    arachnoiditis and, 268
    Baló disease and, 277
    benign astrocytoma and, 270
    of bladder, syringomyelia and, 380
    Canavan leukodystrophy and, 322
    chronic inflammatory demyelinating polyneuropathy (CIDP) and,
        289
    conversion disorder and, 292
    cranial nerve, myalgic encephalomyelitis (ME) and, 547
    of extremities and muscles of respiratory system, ALA-D porphyria
        and, 230
    of eye, centronuclear myopathy and, 344
    facial
        Bell's palsy and, 278
        peripheral, Melkersson-Rosenthal syndrome and, 329
    ipsilateral to wound, Brown-Séquard syndrome and, 282
    of legs
        caudal regression syndrome and, 29
        spina bifida and, 376
        spinal stenosis and, 377
    leprosy and, 558
    malignant astrocytoma and, 270
    multiple exostoses and, 64
    multiple sclerosis (MS) and, 332
    muscular, ciguatera fish poisoning and, 827
    paramyotonia congenita and, 360
    partial, Alpers disease and, 260
    phosphoglycerate kinase deficiency and, 227
    of respiratory muscles, pseudocholinesterase deficiency and, 235
    of shoulder and upper extremity, Erb palsy and, 302
    simian B virus infection and, 580
    sleep, 349
    spastic, of all limbs, Nezelof syndrome and, 494
    transient, Conn syndrome and, 721
    vocal cord, syringobulbia and, 379
Paralysis agitans. *See* Parkinson disease
Paralysis periodica paramyotonica. *See* Paramyotonia congenita
Paralytic ileus, 679
Paralytic rabies syndrome, 573
Paramyotonia congenita, **359–60**
Paranasal swelling, marked symmetrical, Goundou and, 600
Paraneoplastic cerebellar degeneration, 284
Parangi. *See* Yaws
Paranoia, acute intermittent porphyria and, 229
Paraparesis of lower limbs, Devic disease and, 297
Parapemphigus. *See* Pemphigoid, bullous
Paraplegia
    arachnoid cysts and, 267
    hereditary spastic, **360–61**. *See also* Isaacs syndrome
    Krabbe leukodystrophy and, 323
Paraproteinemia, Waldenstrom macroglobulinemia and, 596
Parasitemia, filariasis and, 550
Paratyphoid fever, 592
Parenchymatous cortical degeneration of the cerebellum, **361**. *See*
        *also* Joseph disease

Pigmented autosomal recessive hypomaturation type amelogenesis imperfecta, 11
Pineal gland, neoplasia of, retinoblastoma and, 812
Pink eye. See Conjunctivitis
Pink tetralogy of Fallot (acyanotic tetralogy of fallot). See Tetralogy of Fallot
Pinna
    cystlike swellings on, diastrophic dysplasia and, 55
    malformed, Treacher Collins syndrome and, 147
Pins and needles in fingers, Raynaud disease and phenomenon and, 777
Pinta, 569–70. See also Bejel; Syphilis, acquired; Syphilis, congenital; Yaws
Pipecolic acid, increased plasma, neonatal ALD and, 178
Pitted autosomal dominant hypoplastic type amelogenesis imperfecta, 11
Pituitary dwarfism II. See Growth hormone insensitivity syndrome (GHIS)
Pituitary fossa, apparently empty, empty sella syndrome and, 300
Pituitary gland
    absent
        holoprosencephaly and, 309
        partial or complete, caudal regression syndrome and, 29
    enlarged, Nelson syndrome and, 737
    hyperfunction, McCune-Albright syndrome and, 736
Pituitary tumor after adrenalectomy. See Nelson syndrome
Pityriasis lichenoides et varioliformis acuta. See Mucha-Habermann disease
Pityriasis rosea, 648
Pityriasis rubra pilaris (PRP), 653–54
Placenta, unusually large, triploid syndrome and, 149
Placental infarcts, aplasia cutis congenita and, 611
Plagiocephaly. See Craniosynostosis, primary
Plantar extensors, abnormal reflexes of, adrenoleukodystrophy and, 177
Plantar fasciitis, Reiter syndrome and, 779
Plaques
    discoid, mixed connective tissue disease (MCTD) and, 769
    of dry papules in axillary, pubic, and nipple area, Fox-Fordyce disease and, 629
    of eruptive xanthomas, hyperchylomicronemia and, 203
    erythematous, silvery-gray, sharply demarcated, psoriatic arthritis and, 776
    erythematous scaling, with shifting configuration, erythrokeratodermia variabilis and, 625
    firm, hard, oval-shaped, with ivory centers and encircled by violet ring, scleroderma and, 781
    hyperkeratotic
        distributed symmetrically, erythrokeratodermia symmetrica progressiva and, 624
        often foul-smelling, Darier disease and, 616
    keratotic, erythrokeratodermia variabilis and, 625
    large, dry, scaly, rough, and red, pityriasis rubra pilaris (PRP) and, 653
    large ecchymotic, Cronkhite-Canada disease and, 670
    leprosy and, 558
    in retina, multiple yellow-white, acute posterior multifocal placoid pigment epitheliopathy and, 801
    symmetrical red scaling, peeling, erythrokeratolysis hiemalis and, 626
    yellow or white, pseudoxanthoma elasticum (PXE) and, 654
Plasma cell leukemia, 490
Plasma cell myeloma. See Multiple myeloma
Plasma porphyrin fluorescence, variegate porphyria and, 234
Plasma thromboplastin component deficiency. See Factor IX deficiency
Plasma transglutaminase deficiency. See Factor XIII deficiency
Plasma volume, diminished, radiation exposure and, 836
Platelets
    abnormal appearance and failure to aggregate normally, thrombasthenia and, 504
    circulating, structural and functional abnormalities in, Wiskott-Aldrich syndrome and, 599
    disorders of function, 437, 440
    giant, oddly shaped, May-Hegglin anomaly and, 489
    lower than normal concentration
        Bernard-Soulier syndrome and, 460
        Chédiak-Higashi syndrome and, 463
    storage pool-deficient, Hermansky-Pudlak syndrome and, 477
Platelet-vessel interaction, disorders due to abnormalities of, 440
Play
    imaginative, absent or repetitious, Asperger syndrome and, 270
    strong, ritualistic, repetitive component, autism and, 276
Pleocytosis in cerebrospinal fluid, leptospirosis and, 560
Pleural effusion, hereditary lymphedema and, 485
Pleural TB, 591
Pleurisy, systemic lupus erythematosus (SLE) and, 784
Pleuritic pain, familial Mediterranean fever (FMF) and, 760
Pleuritis, acanthocheilonemiasis and, 516
PLEVA. See Mucha-Habermann disease

Pneumocystis carinii infections, acquired immune deficiency syndrome (AIDS) and, 516, 517
Pneumonia. See also a-1-antitrypsin (AAT) deficiency; Pulmonary alveolar proteinosis; Typhoid
    achalasia and, 666
    Aspergillus, 526
    cerebro-costo-mandibular syndrome and, 29
    chronic, blastomycosis and, 530
    chronic granulomatous disease and, 470
    chronic neutropenia and, 566
    congenital syphilis and, 585
    desquamative interstitial, 399
    eosinophilic, 555
    frequent, precipitating heart failure, cor triatriatum and, 405
    interstitial, 411, 555
    lower lobe, tuberculosis (TB) and, 590
    nocardiosis and, 566
    Pneumocystis carinii
        acquired immune deficiency syndrome (AIDS) and, 516, 517
        Nezelof syndrome and, 493
        severe combined immunodeficiency (SCID) and, 578
    psittacosis and, 571
    Q fever and, 572
    recurrent, Bowen Hutterite syndrome and, 23
    Stevens-Johnson syndrome and, 581
    susceptibility to, multiple myeloma and, 490
Pneumonitis, 437
    esophageal atresia and tracheoesophageal fistula and, 64
    gold poisoning and, 831
    Q fever and, 572
    systemic lupus erythematosus (SLE) and, 784
    toxoplasmosis in immunosuppressed patient and, 589
Pneumorenal syndrome. See Goodpasture syndrome
Pneumothorax
    bilateral renal agenesis and, 703
    cystic fibrosis and, 406
    Marfan syndrome and, 98
POEMS syndrome, 570
Poland syndrome, 124
Polio, late effects. See Post-polio syndrome
Poliodystrophia cerebri progressiva. See Alpers disease
Poliomyelitis virus, infection by. See also Post-polio syndrome
    primary agammaglobulinemias and, 444
Polio sequelae. See Post-polio syndrome
Pollitt syndrome, 657
Polyarteritis nodosa, 753–54
Polyarteritis nodosa (PAN), 745, 753–54, 773. See also Antiphospholipid syndrome; Buerger disease; Churg-Strauss syndrome; Granulomatous disease, chronic (CGD); Systemic lupus erythematosus (SLE); Vasculitis
Polyarthralgia
    asymmetric, Churg-Strauss syndrome and, 404
    erythema nodosum leprosum and, 559
Polyarthritis
    Behçet syndrome and, 755
    rheumatic fever and, 574
    streptococcal, 574
Polyarthritis enterica. See Reiter syndrome
Polycystic bilateral ovarian syndrome. See Stein-Leventhal syndrome
Polycystic kidney diseases (PKD), 689, 702–3. See also Carcinoma, renal cell; Hepatorenal syndrome; Loken-Senior syndrome; Medullary cystic disease
    congenital hepatic fibrosis and, 677
Polycystic liver disease, 682
Polycythemia
    atrial septal defects and, 401
    hereditary hemorrhagic telangiectasia and, 476
    tetralogy of Fallot and, 425
    ventricular septal defects and, 427
Polycythemia vera, 433, 496–97. See also Leukemia, chronic myelogenous; Osteonecrosis
Polydactyly
    asphyxiating thoracic dystrophy and, 18
    Bardet-Biedl syndrome and, 19
    Ellis-van Creveld syndrome and, 62
    with flexed fingers, trisomy 13 syndrome and, 152–53
    focal dermal hypoplasia and, 627
    hereditary spherocytic hemolytic anemia and, 453
    Klippel-Trenaunay syndrome and, 92
    Meckel syndrome and, 102, 103
    Moebius syndrome and, 106
    postaxial
        Goodman syndrome and, 79
        unilateral, Simpson-Golabi-Behmel syndrome and, 136
    Schinzel type acrocallosal syndrome and, 9
    VACTERL association and, 156
Polydipsia
    Achard-Thiers syndrome and, 710
    acromegaly and, 711
    Bartter syndrome and, 718

Rachitic rosary, vitamin D-deficiency rickets and, 740
Radial aplasia-amegakaryocytic thrombocytopenia syndrome. *See* Thrombocytopenia-absent radius (TAR) syndrome
Radial aplasia-thrombocytopenia syndrome. *See* Thrombocytopenia-absent radius (TAR) syndrome
Radial limb dysplasia, VACTERL association and, 156
Radiation effects. *See* Radiation syndromes
Radiation pneumonitis, thoracic radiation injury and, 837
Radiation syndromes, 822, **836–38**
Radicular dentin dysplasia. *See* Dentin dysplasia, radicular
Radiohumeral synostosis, Antley-Bixler syndrome and, 15
Radioulnar synostosis, Apert syndrome and, 16
Radius, radii
    absent or underdeveloped
        Baller-Gerold syndrome and, 18
        thrombocytopenia-absent radius syndrome and, 145
    aplasia of, Fanconi anemia and, 450
    curvature of lower, dyschondrosteosis and, 60
    dislocation of head of, oto-palato-digital syndrome and, 116
    hypoplastic
        Aase-Smith syndrome and, 6
        Seckel syndrome and, 133
    partial dislocation of, dyschondrosteosis and, 60
    short, bowed and flared, Melnick-Needles syndrome and, 103
    synostosis of, LADD syndrome and, 93
Rage, episodes of, tuberous sclerosis (TS) and, 389
Rales
    cystic fibrosis and, 406
    extrinsic allergic alveolitis and, 398
    fine, moist, endocardial fibroelastosis (EFE) and, 412
    at high altitude, acute mountain sickness and, 825
    hypoplastic left heart syndrome and, 415
    toxocariasis and, 588
Ramsay Hunt syndrome, 343. *See also* Bell's palsy
Range of motion, limitation of, osteonecrosis and, 771
Raphe nucleus encephalopathy. *See* Encephalomyelitis, myalgic (ME)
Rapp-Hodgkins syndrome, 62, 633
Rash, skin
    acquired immune deficiency syndrome (AIDS) and, 516
    angioimmunoblastic with dysproteinemia lymphadenopathy (AILD) and, 483
    beginning on wrists and ankles and spreading centrally, Rocky Mountain spotted fever (RMSF) and, 576
    bejel and, 529
    cat-scratch disease and, 534
    chikungunya and, 537
    Churg-Strauss syndrome and, 404
    congenital syphilis and, 585
    congenital toxoplasmosis and, 589
    eczematoid, phenylketonuria and, 225
    erythema marginatum, lasting only for hours, rheumatic fever and, 575
    erythematous, multiple carboxylase deficiency and, 220
    erythematous butterfly, across bridge of nose and cheeks, systemic lupus erythematosus (SLE) and, 784
    erythematous vesicular, berylliosis and, 826
    itchy and burning, with papules, pustules, and vesicles, Mucha-Habermann disease and, 648
    Kawasaki syndrome and, 764
    leptospirosis and, 560
    maculopapular, on trunk and spreading peripherally, Dengue fever and, 542
    malar, mixed connective tissue disease (MCTD) and, 769
    meningococcal meningitis and, 562
    meningococcemia and, 564
    Netherton syndrome and, 648
    numerous vesicles on exposed skin, cowpox and, 539
    purpuric, Wegener granulomatosis and, 508
    red
        and diffusely thickened, KID syndrome and, 644
        recurrent, Mucha-Habermann disease and, 648
        and scaly, after exposure to sunlight, Hartnup disease and, 199
        spreading over entire body, meningococcemia and, 564
    rose spots, typhoid fever and, 592
    scaly or greasy, histiocytosis X and, 478
    Sjögren syndrome (SjS) and, 783
    small, reddish or purplish, and psoriatic (pintids), pinta and, 569
    small nodular lesions, usually on face and extremities, verruga peruana and, 529
    "sunburn," with desquamation on palms and soles, toxic shock syndrome (TSS) and, 586
    after vaccination, generalized vaccinia and, 539
    vesicular, hand-foot-mouth syndrome and, 553–54
Rasmussen encephalitis, 546–47
Raynaud disease and phenomenon, 747, **777–78**. *See also* Cryoglobulinemia, essential mixed; Fabry disease; Hemorrhagic telangiectasia, hereditary; Mixed connective tissue disease (MCTD); Perniosis; Urticaria, cold
    in fingers, polymyositis/dermatomyositis and, 774
    mixed connective tissue disease (MCTD) and, 769

scleroderma and, 781
    systemic lupus erythematosus (SLE) and, 784
    Takayasu arteritis and, 753
    Waldenstrom macroglobulinemia and, 596
Reactive arthritis, Reiter syndrome, 778–79
Reading ability
    dyslexia and confusion of letters, 298
    inability to read, simultanagnosia and, 258
REAR syndrome, 156
Recessive dystrophic epidermolysis bullosa, 622
Recklinghausen disease (NF 1). *See* Neurofibromatosis (NF)
Rectal bleeding
    chronic, familial polyposis and, 672
    Gardner syndrome and, 673
Rectal mucosa, cystine crystals in, cystinosis and, 188
Rectal prolapse, cystic fibrosis and, 406
Rectum
    absence of
        bilateral renal agenesis and, 703
        sirenomelia sequence and, 137
    bleeding in, Klippel-Trenaunay syndrome and, 92
    fistulas involving, VACTERL association and, 156
    itchy, patchy, crusty areas on, extramammary Paget disease and, 495
    open into vagina, imperforate anus and, 85
    underdeveloped, achondrogenesis and, 7
    yellow-orange, Tangier disease and, 241
Rectus muscles, separation of, trisomy 18 syndrome and, 154
Recurrent aphthous stomatitis. *See* Sutton disease II
Recurrent polyserositis. *See* Familial Mediterranean fever (FMF)
Red cell casts, Wegener granulomatosis and, 508
Reed-Sternberg cells in lymph nodes, Hodgkin disease and, 479
Reflexes
    abnormal
        Dandy-Walker syndrome and, 295
        hydrocephalus and, 312
        Marie ataxia and, 274
    absence of
        Dejerine-Sottas disease and, 296
        Seitelberger disease and, 374
        syringomyelia and, 380
    changes, medulloblastoma and, 328
    cough, poor, ataxia telangiectasia and, 275
    extensor plantar, Creutzfeldt-Jakob disease and, 293
    hyperactive, pernicious anemia and, 456
    in legs, decreased or absent, hereditary sensory neuropathy type I and, 355
    slowed, Kugelberg-Welander syndrome and, 320
    stretch, loss of, acanthocytosis and, 443
Reflexes, deep tendon
    absence of
        Becker muscular dystrophy and, 334
        Charcot-Marie-Tooth disease and, 287
        Devic disease and, 297
        Guillain-Barré syndrome and, 307
        nemaline myopathy and, 350
        peripheral neuropathy and, 365
    hyperactive, amyotrophic lateral sclerosis (ALS) and, 262
    increased deep
        Gaucher disease and, 194
        phenylketonuria and, 226
Reflexes, tendon
    absent or reduced
        Andersen disease and, 179
        chronic inflammatory demyelinating polyneuropathy and, 289
        familial dysautonomia and, 304
        Fukuyama type muscular dystrophy and, 337
        giant axonal neuropathy and, 354
        hereditary sensory neuropathy type II and, 356
        neuroacanthocytosis and, 352
        Werdnig-Hoffmann disease and, 391
    Fukuyama type muscular dystrophy and, 337
    hyperactive, myalgic encephalomyelitis (ME) and, 547
    increased, hereditary spastic paraplegia and, 360
Reflex neurovascular dystrophy. *See* Reflex sympathetic dystrophy syndrome (RSDS)
Reflex sympathetic dystrophy syndrome (RSDS), **369–70**. *See also* Thalamic syndrome
Refractory anemia. *See* Anemia, aplastic
Refrigeration palsy. *See* Bell's palsy
Refsum syndrome, **238**, 251. *See also* Adrenoleukodystrophy (ALD); Alexander disease; Charcot-Marie-Tooth disease; Erythrokeratodermia variabilis; Keratitis-ichthyosis-deafness (KID) syndrome; Niemann-Pick disease; Pelizaeus-Merzbacher brain sclerosis; Rosenberg-Chutorian syndrome; Roussy-Lévy syndrome; Zellweger syndrome
Regurgitation
    Chagas disease and, 536
    esophageal atresia and tracheoesophageal fistula and, 64
    nighttime, achalasia and, 666

toxocariasis and, 588
Whipple disease, 513, **598–99**. *See also* Celiac sprue
Whistling face syndrome. *See* Freeman-Sheldon syndrome
Whistling face-windmill vane hand syndrome. *See* Freeman-Sheldon
    syndrome
White blood cells
    elevated levels of
        incontinentia pigmenti and, 643
        Reiter syndrome and, 779
    lower levels of, methylmalonic acidemia and, 175
White-Darier disease. *See* Darier disease
White spot disease. *See* Lichen sclerosus et atrophicus (LSA); Vitiligo
Whitlow, hereditary sensory neuropathy type II and, 356
Whitnall-Norman syndrome. *See* Norrie disease
Whole-body acute irradiation, 836
Whooping cough. *See* Pertussis
Widow's peak
    Aarskog syndrome and, 6
    Opitz syndrome and, 112
Wieacker syndrome, **393**
Wildervanck syndrome, **161–62**. *See also* Duane syndrome; Klippel-
    Feil syndrome
Willebrand-Juergens disease. *See* von Willebrand disease
Williams-Beuren syndrome. *See* Williams syndrome
Williams syndrome, 2, **162–63**. *See also* Leprechaunism
Willi-Prader syndrome. *See* Prader-Willi syndrome
Wilms tumor, **509–10**. *See also* Chromosome 11q- syndrome;
    Deletion on the short arm of 11p13; Denys-Drash syndrome
    aniridia (AN) and, 792
    Beckwith-Wiedemann syndrome and, 20
    WAGR syndrome and, 816
Wilms tumor-aniridia-gonadoblastoma-mental retardation syndrome.
    *See* WAGR syndrome
Wilms tumor association, 1
Wilms tumor-pseudohermaphroditism-nephropathy. *See* Denys-
    Drash syndrome
Wilms tumor-pseuodohermaphroditism-glomerulopathy. *See* Denys-
    Drash syndrome
Wilson disease, **247–48**, 251. *See also* Benign essential
    blepharospasm (BEB); Conversion disorder; Cystinosis;
    Epilepsy, myoclonic progressive familial; Fanconi syndrome;
    Heavy metal poisoning; Huntington disease; Menkes disease;
    Neuroacanthocytosis; Rickets, hypophosphatemic; Sydenham
    chorea
Winchester-Grossman syndrome. *See* Winchester syndrome
Winchester syndrome, **163**
Winking, see-saw, oral-facial-digital syndrome and, 113
Wiskott-Aldrich syndrome, 435, 436, 438, **599–600**. *See also*
    Agammaglobulinemias, primary; DiGeorge syndrome; Job
    syndrome; May-Hegglin anomaly; Nezelof syndrome;
    Thrombasthenia
Withdrawal, fetal alcohol syndrome and, 67
Withdrawal from barbiturates and substance intoxications, 359
Witkop tooth-nail syndrome. *See* Tooth and nail syndrome
Wolff-Parkinson-White (WPW) syndrome, 395, **428–29**
Wolf-Hirschhorn syndrome (WHS), **164**. *See also* Chromosome 4q-
    syndrome; Chromosome 13q- syndrome
Wolfram syndrome, **164–65**. *See also* Rosenberg-Chutorian
    syndrome
Wolf syndrome. *See* Wolf-Hirschhorn syndrome (WHS)
Woody Guthrie disease. *See* Huntington disease
Wormian bones
    Hajdu-Cheney syndrome and, 764
    Menkes disease and, 214

Wound botulism, 531–32
Wrist
    bowed, dyschondrosteosis and, 60
    compromised range of motion, Kienboeck disease and, 766
    deformities in, Ollier disease and, 770
    enlarged and possibly hyperextensible, Morquio disease and, 216
    fusion of bones in, Townes-Brocks syndrome and, 146
    tetany spasms of, vitamin D-deficiency rickets and, 740
Wrist-biting, Smith-Magenis syndrome and, 138
Wrist drop, Landouzy-Dejerine muscular dystrophy and, 337
Wuchereriasis. *See* Filariasis

Xanthogranulomatosis, generalized. *See* Erdheim-Chester disease
Xanthomas
    broad beta disease and, 402
    primary biliary cirrhosis and, 683
    raised, whitish-yellow nodules containing milky fluid, on red base,
        hyperchylomicronemia and, 203
    von Gierke disease and, 246
Xanthoma tuberosum. *See* Broad beta disease
Xeroderma pigmentosum, **662**
Xerophthalmia. *See* Keratomalacia
Xerostomia
    amyloidosis and, 749
    Sjögren syndrome and, 783
Xerotic keratitis. *See* Keratomalacia
X-linked adult-onset spinobulbar muscular atrophy. *See* Kennedy
    disease
X-linked adult spinal muscular atrophy. *See* Kennedy disease
X-linked agammaglobulinemia, 433, 436, 444
X-linked centronuclear myopathy, 344
X-linked copper deficiency. *See* Menkes disease
X-linked hypophosphatemia. *See* Rickets, hypophosphatemic
X-linked juvenile retinoschisis (RS), **818–19**. *See also* Senile
    retinoschisis
X-linked lymphoproliferative (XLP) syndrome, 436, **510–11**
X-linked mental retardation and macroorchidism. *See* Fragile X
    syndrome
X-linked spondyloepiphyseal dysplasia. *See* Spondyloepiphyseal
    dysplasia tarda
X-linked vitamin D-resistant rickets. *See* Rickets, hypophosphatemic
XYY syndrome, **165–66**
    Sotos syndrome and, 139

Yaws, **600–601**. *See also* Bejel; Pinta; Syphilis, acquired; Syphilis,
    congenital
Yelling in startle reaction, jumping Frenchmen of Maine and, 316
Yellow fundus reflex, Coats disease and, 797
Yellow nail syndrome, **429–30**
Yknodysostosis, 43
Young female arteritis. *See* Arteritis, Takayasu

Zanier-Roubicek syndrome, 633
Zellweger syndrome, **248**. *See also* Adrenoleukodystrophy (ALD);
    Alagille syndrome; Hepatitis, neonatal
Ziehen-Oppenheim disease. *See* Torsion dystonia
Zinc deficiency, congenital. *See* Acrodermatitis enteropathica (AE)
Zinc poisoning, 831
Zinsser-Cole-Engman syndrome. *See* Dyskeratosis congenita
Zollinger-Ellison syndrome, **744**. *See also* Carcinoid syndrome;
    Gastric lymphoma, non-Hodgkin type

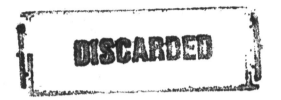